Targeted Therapy in
Translational Cancer Research

# TRANSLATIONAL ONCOLOGY

SERIES EDITORS

## ROBERT C. BAST, MD

Vice President for Translational Research
The University of Texas MD Anderson Cancer Center
Houston, TX, USA

## MAURIE MARKMAN, MD

Senior Vice President for Clinical Affairs
Cancer Treatment Centers of America

Clinical Professor of Medicine
Drexel University College of Medicine
Philadelphia, PA, USA

## ERNEST HAWK, MD, MPH

Vice President, Division of OVP, Cancer Prevention and Population Sciences
The University of Texas MD Anderson Cancer Center
Houston, TX, USA

# Targeted Therapy in Translational Cancer Research

EDITED BY

## Apostolia-Maria Tsimberidou, MD, PhD

Department of Investigational Cancer Therapeutics
The University of Texas MD Anderson Cancer Center
Houston, TX, USA

## Razelle Kurzrock, MD

Center for Personalized Cancer Therapy
UC San Diego Moores Cancer Center
La Jolla, CA, USA

## Kenneth C. Anderson, MD, PhD

LeBow Institute for Myeloma Therapeutics and Jerome Lipper Myeloma Center
Department of Medical Oncology, Dana-Farber Cancer Institute
Harvard Medical School
Boston, MA, USA

WILEY Blackwell

Published by John Wiley & Sons, Inc., Hoboken, New Jersey
Published simultaneously in Canada

For general information on our other products and services or for technical support, please contact our Customer Care Department within the United States at (800) 762-2974, outside the United States at (317) 572-3993 or fax (317) 572-4002.

Wiley also publishes its books in a variety of electronic formats. Some content that appears in print may not be available in electronic formats. For more information about Wiley products, visit our web site at www.wiley.com.

*Library of Congress Cataloging-in-Publication Data:*

Targeted therapy in translational cancer research / edited by Apostolia-Maria Tsimberidou, Razelle Kurzrock, Kenneth C. Anderson.
        p. ; cm. – (Translational oncology)
    Includes bibliographical references and index.
    ISBN 978-1-118-46857-9 (cloth)
    I. Tsimberidou, Apostolia-Maria, editor.    II. Kurzrock, Razelle, editor.    III. Anderson, Kenneth C., editor.    IV. Series: Translational oncology (Series)
    [DNLM: 1. Molecular Targeted Therapy.    2. Neoplasms–drug therapy.    3. Immunotherapy.    4. Individualized Medicine.    5. Translational Medical Research.    QZ 267]
    RC271.I45
    616.99′4061–dc23
                                                                                                2015015320

Printed in Singapore by Markono Print Media Pte Ltd

10  9  8  7  6  5  4  3  2  1

# Contents

# List of Contributors

**James Abbruzzese,** MD
Division of Medical Oncology
Duke Cancer Institute
Durham, NC, USA

**Maen Abdelrahim,** MD, PhD
Department of Internal Medicine
Baylor College of Medicine
Houston, TX, USA

**Abass Alavi,** MD, MD(Hon.), PhD(Hon.), DSc(Hon.)
Department of Radiology
Hospital of the University of Pennsylvania
Philadelphia, PA, USA

**Kenneth C. Anderson,** MD, PhD
LeBow Institute for Myeloma Therapeutics and Jerome Lipper Myeloma
Center
Department of Medical Oncology, Dana-Farber Cancer Institute
Harvard Medical School
Boston, MA, USA

**Michael Andreeff,** MD, PhD
Section of Molecular Hematology and Therapy
Department of Leukemia
The University of Texas MD Anderson Cancer Center
Houston, TX, USA

**Analia Azaro,** MD
Early Clinical Drug Development Group
Vall d'Hebron Institute of Oncology
Universitat Autonoma de Barcelona
Barcelona, Spain

**Susana Banerjee,** MBBS, MA, MRCP, PhD
The Royal Marsden Hospital
London, UK

**Robert C. Bast,** MD
The University of Texas MD Anderson Cancer Center
Houston, TX, USA

**Susanne H. C. Baumeister,** MD
Department of Pediatric Oncology
Dana-Farber Cancer Institute
Boston, MA

Division of Hematology-Oncology
Boston Children's Hospital
Harvard Medical School
Boston, MA

**Giada Bianchi,** MD
LeBow Institute for Myeloma Therapeutics and Jerome Lipper Myeloma
Center
Department of Medical Oncology, Dana-Farber Cancer Institute
Harvard Medical School
Boston, MA, USA

**Patrick Boland,** MD
Department of Medicine
Temple University School of Medicine
Philadelphia, PA, USA

**Jessica L. Bowser,** PhD
Department of Pathology
The University of Texas MD Anderson Cancer Center
Houston, TX, USA

**Russell R. Broaddus,** MD, PhD
Department of Pathology
The University of Texas MD Anderson Cancer Center
Houston, TX, USA

**Harold J. Burstein,** MD, PhD
Dana-Farber Cancer Institute
Brigham and Women's Hospital
Harvard Medical School
Boston, MA, USA

**Lewis C. Cantley,** PhD
Meyer Cancer Center at Weill Cornell Medical College
New York, NY, USA

**Robert L. Coleman,** MD
Department of Gynecologic Oncology and Reproductive Medicine
Center for RNA Interference and Non-Coding RNA
The University of Texas MD Anderson Cancer Center
Houston, TX, USA

**Anthony P. Conley,** MD
Department of Sarcoma Medical Oncology
The University of Texas MD Anderson Cancer Center
Houston, TX, USA

**Jorge Cortes,** MD
Department of Leukemia
The University of Texas MD Anderson Cancer Center
Houston, TX, USA

**M. Angelica Cortez,** PhD
Department of Experimental Radiation Oncology
The University of Texas MD Anderson Cancer Center
Houston, TX, USA

**Carlo M. Croce, MD**
Department of Molecular Virology, Immunology and Medical Genetics
Comprehensive Cancer Center
Ohio State University
Columbus, OH, USA

**Jasmine Quynh Dao, MD**
Children's Cancer Hospital
The University of Texas MD Anderson Cancer Center
Houston, TX, USA

**John F. de Groot, MD**
Department of Neuro-Oncology
The University of Texas MD Anderson Cancer Center
Houston, TX, USA

**Yves A. DeClerck, MD**
Division of Hematology-Oncology
Department of Pediatrics and Department of Biochemistry and Molecular
Biology
The Saban Research Institute of Children's Hospital Los Angeles
Los Angeles, CA, USA

Department of Medicine
Committee on Clinical Pharmacology and Pharmacogenomics
The University of Chicago
Chicago, IL, USA

**Gianpiero Di Leva, PhD**
Department of Molecular Virology, Immunology and Medical Genetics
Comprehensive Cancer Center
Ohio State University
Columbus, OH, USA

**Glenn Dranoff, MD, PhD**
Department of Medicine, Harvard Medical School
Human Gene Transfer Laboratory Core, Dana-Farber Cancer Institute
Boston, MA, USA

**Hua Fang, PhD**
Division of Hematology-Oncology
The Saban Research Institute of Children's Hospital Los Angeles
Los Angeles, CA, USA

Department of Medicine
Committee on Clinical Pharmacology and Pharmacogenomics
The University of Chicago
Chicago, IL, USA

**Omotayo Fasan, MRCP**
Department of Medicine
Temple University School of Medicine
Philadelphia, PA, USA

Department of Hematologic Oncology and Blood Disorders
Levine Cancer Institute
Charlotte, NC, USA

**Keith T. Flaherty, MD**
Massachusetts General Hospital Cancer Center
Boston, MA, USA

**David Fogelman, MD**
Department of Gastrointestinal Medical Oncology
The University of Texas MD Anderson Cancer Center
Houston, TX, USA

**Matthew D. Galsky, MD**
Division of Hematology and Medical Oncology
The Tisch Cancer Institute
Mount Sinai School of Medicine
New York, NY, USA

**Guillermo García-Manero, MD**
Department of Leukemia
The University of Texas MD Anderson Cancer Center
Houston, TX, USA

**Benjamin A. Gartrell, MD**
Department of Medical Oncology
Montefiore Medical Center
The Albert Einstein College of Medicine
Bronx, NY, USA

**Gabriel Ghiaur, MD, PhD**
The Sidney Kimmel Comprehensive Cancer Center
The Johns Hopkins University School of Medicine
Baltimore, MD, USA

**Michael C. Haffner, MD**
The Sidney Kimmel Comprehensive Cancer Center and Brady Urological
Institute
The Johns Hopkins University School of Medicine
Baltimore, MD, USA

**Roy S. Herbst, MD, PhD**
Department of Medicine
Division of Medical Oncology
Yale Comprehensive Cancer Center
New Haven, CT, USA

**Ashley M. Holder, MD**
The University of Texas MD Anderson Cancer Center
Houston, TX, USA

**David Hong, MD**
Department of Investigational Cancer Therapeutics
The University of Texas MD Anderson Cancer Center
Houston, TX, USA

**Jean-Pierre J. Issa, MD**
Fels Institute for Cancer Research and Molecular Biology
Temple University School of Medicine
Philadelphia, USA

**Elias Jabbour, MD**
Department of Leukemia
The University of Texas MD Anderson Cancer Center
Houston, TX, USA

**Nitin Jain, MD**
Department of Leukemia
The University of Texas MD Anderson Cancer Center
Houston, TX, USA

**Preetesh Jain, MD, DM, PhD**
Department of Leukemia
The University of Texas MD Anderson Cancer Center
Houston, TX, USA

**Filip Janku,** MD, PhD
Department of Investigational Cancer Therapeutics (Phase I Clinical Trials Program)
Division of Cancer Medicine
The University of Texas MD Anderson Cancer Center
Houston, TX, USA

**Milind Javle,** MD
Department of Gastrointestinal Medical Oncology
The University of Texas MD Anderson Cancer Center
Houston, TX, USA

**Richard J. Jones,** MD
The Sidney Kimmel Comprehensive Cancer Center
The Johns Hopkins University School of Medicine
Baltimore, MD, USA

**Stan Kaye,** MD
The Royal Marsden hospital and The Institute of Cancer Research
London, UK

**Samuel J. Klempner,** MD
Division of Hematology/Oncology
University of California Irvine Health
Orange, CA, USA

**Birgit Knoechel,** MD, PhD
Boston Children's Hospital
Dana-Farber Cancer Institute
Harvard Medical School
Boston, MA, USA

**Kensuke Kojima,** MD, PhD
Section of Molecular Hematology and Therapy
Department of Leukemia
The University of Texas MD Anderson Cancer Center
Houston, TX, USA

**Scott Kopetz,** MD, PhD, FACP
Department of Gastrointestinal Medical Oncology
The University of Texas MD Anderson Cancer Center
Houston, TX, USA

**Patricia Kropf,** MD
Department of Medicine
Temple University School of Medicine
Philadelphia, PA, USA

**Razelle Kurzrock,** MD
Center for Personalized Cancer Therapy
UC San Diego Moores Cancer Center
La Jolla, CA, USA

**Jens G. Lohr,** MD, PhD
Dana-Farber Cancer Institute
Boston, MA, USA

Harvard Medical School
Boston, MA, USA

**David Menter,** PhD
Department of Gastrointestinal Medical Oncology
The University of Texas MD Anderson Cancer Center
Houston, TX, USA

**Funda Meric-Bernstam,** MD
Department of Investigational Cancer Therapeutics
Institute for Personalized Cancer Therapy
Department of Surgical Oncology
The University of Texas MD Anderson Cancer Center
Houston, TX, USA

**Larissa A. Meyer,** MD, MPH
Department of Gynecologic Oncology and Reproductive Medicine
The University of Texas MD Anderson Cancer Center
Houston, TX, USA

**Marcus M. Monroe,** MD
Department of Otolaryngology
University of Utah School of Medicine
Salt Lake City, UT

**Guillermo Montalbán-Bravo,** MD
Department of Hematology
Hospital Universitario La Paz
Madrid, Spain

**Daniel Morgensztern,** MD
Department of Medicine
Division of Medical Oncology
Washington University School of Medicine
St. Louis, MO, USA

**Javier Munoz,** MD, FACP
Division of Hematology/Oncology
Banner MD Anderson Cancer Center
Gilbert, AZ, USA

**Andrea P. Myers,** MD, PhD
Novartis Pharmaceuticals
Cambridge, MA, USA

**Jeffrey N. Myers,** MD, PhD
Department of Head and Neck Surgery
The University of Texas MD Anderson Cancer Center
Houston, TX, USA

**William G. Nelson,** MD, PhD
The Sidney Kimmel Comprehensive Cancer Center and Brady Urological Institute
The Johns Hopkins University School of Medicine
Baltimore, MD, USA

**Barbara J. O'Brien,** MD
Department of Neuro-Oncology
The University of Texas MD Anderson Cancer Center
Houston, TX, USA

**Susan O'Brien,** MD
Department of Leukemia
The University of Texas MD Anderson Cancer Center
Houston, TX, USA

**William K. Oh,** MD
Division of Hematology and Medical Oncology
The Tisch Cancer Institute
Mount Sinai School of Medicine
New York, NY, USA

**Shreyaskumar Patel,** MD
Department of Sarcoma Medical Oncology
The University of Texas MD Anderson Cancer Center
Houston, TX, USA

**Saeed Rafii,** MD, PhD, MRCP
Institute of Cancer Sciences
The University of Manchester and The Christie Hospital
Manchester, UK

**Farhad Ravandi-Kashani,** MD
Department of Leukemia
The University of Texas MD Anderson Cancer Center
Houston, TX, USA

**Vinod Ravi,** MD
Department of Sarcoma Medical Oncology
The University of Texas MD Anderson Cancer Center
Houston, TX, USA

**Jordi Rodon,** MD
Early Clinical Drug Development Group
Vall d'Hebron Institute of Oncology
Universitat Autonoma de Barcelona
Barcelona, Spain

**Rabih Said,** MD, MPH
Department of Investigational Cancer Therapeutics
The University of Texas MD Anderson Cancer Center
Department of Internal Medicine
The University of Texas Health Science Center
Houston, TX, USA

**Allison C. Sharrow,** PhD
Department of Pathology
Johns Hopkins University School of Medicine
Baltimore, MD, USA

Department of Cancer Immunotherapeutics and Tumor Immunology
Beckman Research Institute
City of Hope Comprehensive Cancer Center
Duarte, CA, USA

**Alexander C. Small,** MD
Division of Hematology and Medical Oncology
The Tisch Cancer Institute
Mount Sinai School of Medicine
New York, NY, USA

**Sonali M. Smith,** MD
Department of Medicine
The University of Chicago
Chicago, IL, USA

**Anil K. Sood,** MD
Department of Gynecologic Oncology and Reproductive Medicine
Center for RNA Interference and Non-Coding RNA
Department of Cancer Biology
The University of Texas MD Anderson Cancer Center
Houston, TX, USA

**Richard M. Stone,** MD
Department of Medical Oncology
Dana-Farber Cancer Institute
Boston, MA, USA

**Chad Tang,** MD
Department of Radiation Oncology
The University of Texas MD Anderson Cancer Center
Houston, TX, USA

**Morgan Taylor,** MD
Department of Gynecologic Oncology and Reproductive Medicine
The University of Texas MD Anderson Cancer Center
Houston, TX, USA

**Drew A. Torigian,** MD, MA, FSAR
Department of Radiology
Hospital of the University of Pennsylvania
Philadelphia, PA, USA

**Davis Torrejon,** MD
Early Clinical Drug Development Group
Vall d'Hebron Institute of Oncology
Universitat Autonoma de Barcelona
Barcelona, Spain

**Apostolia-Maria Tsimberidou,** MD, PhD
Department of Investigational Cancer Therapeutics
The University of Texas MD Anderson Cancer Center
Houston, TX, USA

**Thanh-Trang Vo,** PhD
Department of Molecular Biology and Biochemistry
University of California Irvine
Irvine, CA, USA

**Julie M. Vose,** MD, MBA
Division of Hematology/Oncology
University of Nebraska Medical Center
Omaha, NE, USA

**Saiama N. Waqar,** MBBS, MSCI
Department of Medicine
Division of Medical Oncology
Washington University School of Medicine
St. Louis, MO, USA

**Shiao-Pei Weathers,** MD
Department of Neuro-Oncology
The University of Texas MD Anderson Cancer Center
Houston, TX, USA

**James W. Welsh,** MD
Department of Radiation Oncology
The University of Texas MD Anderson Cancer Center
Houston, TX, USA

**Shannon N. Westin,** MD, MPH
Department of Gynecologic Oncology and Reproductive Medicine
The University of Texas MD Anderson Cancer Center
Houston, TX, USA

**Ofir Wolach,** MD
Adult Leukemia Program
Department of Medical Oncology
Dana-Farber Cancer Institute
Boston, MA, USA

**Scott E. Woodman,** MD, PhD
Departments of Melanoma Medical Oncology and Systems Biology
The University of Texas MD Anderson Cancer Center
Houston, TX, USA

**Srinivasan Yegnasubramanian,** MD, PhD
The Sidney Kimmel Comprehensive Cancer Center and Brady Urological
Institute
The Johns Hopkins University School of Medicine
Baltimore, MD, USA

**Jian Q. (Michael) Yu,** MD, FRCPC
Department of Diagnostic Imaging
Fox Chase Cancer Center
Philadelphia, PA, USA

**W. K. Alfred Yung,** MD
Department of Neuro-Oncology
The University of Texas MD Anderson Cancer Center
Houston, TX, USA

**Patrick A. Zweidler-McKay,** MD, PhD
Children's Cancer Hospital
The University of Texas MD Anderson Cancer Center
Houston, TX, USA

# Series Foreword

While our knowledge of cancer at a cellular and molecular level has increased exponentially over the last decades, progress in the clinic has been more gradual, largely depending upon empirical trials using combinations of individually active anti-cancer drugs to treat the average patient. The challenge for the immediate future is to accelerate the pace of progress in clinical cancer care by enhancing the bidirectional interaction between laboratory and clinic. Our new understanding of human cancer biology and the heterogeneity of cancers at a molecular level must be used to identify novel targets for therapy, prevention, and detection focused on each individual. Barriers must be removed to facilitate the flow of targeted agents and fresh approaches from the laboratory to the clinic, while returning relevant human specimens, images, and data from the clinic to the laboratory for further analysis.

*An Introduction to Translational Cancer Research* provides a brief overview of current understanding of human cancer biology that is driving interests in targeted therapy and personalized management. Further development of molecular diagnostics should facilitate earlier detection, more precise prognostication, and prediction of response across the spectrum of cancer development. Targeted therapy has already had a dramatic impact on several forms of cancer and strategies are being developed to identify small groups of patients who would benefit from novel targeted drugs in combination with each other or with more conventional surgery, radiotherapy, or chemotherapy. Development of personalized interventions—whether preventive or therapeutic in nature—will require multidisciplinary teams of investigators and the infrastructure to match patient samples and agents in real time.

To accelerate translational cancer research, greater alignment will be required between academic institutions, the National Cancer Institute, the Food and Drug Administration, foundations, pharma, and community oncologists. Ultimately, new approaches to prevention, detection, and therapy must be sustainable. In the long run, translational research and personalized management can reduce the cost of cancer care, which has escalated in recent years. More accurate and specific identification of at-risk members and risk stratification will be helpful to minimize the risks of over-diagnosis and over-treatment, while maximizing the benefits of screening, early detection, and preventive intervention. Patients who would benefit most can be identified and funds saved by avoiding treatment in those whose cancers would not respond. Participation and education of community oncologists will be required, as will modification of practice patterns. For progress in the clinic to occur at an optimal pace, leaders of translational teams must envision a clear path to bring new concepts and new agents from the laboratory to the clinic, to complete pharmaceutical or biological development, to obtain regulatory approval and to bring new strategies for detection, prevention, and treatment to patients in the community.

In a series of additional volumes regarding *translational cancer research*, several topics are explored in greater depth, including *gene therapy by viral and non-viral vectors, biomarkers, immunotherapy*, and this volume concerning *targeted therapy*. The purpose of these books has been not only to describe different strategies for controlling particular forms of cancer but also to identify some of the barriers to translation using different reagents or different strategies around common therapeutic or diagnostic modalities. Potential barriers are many and include the need for a deeper understanding of science, methods to overcome the challenge of tumor heterogeneity, the development of targeted therapies, the availability of patients with an appropriate phenotype and genotype within a research center with the investigators, research teams and infrastructure required for clinical/translational research and the design of novel trials, adequate financial support, a viable connection to diagnostic and pharmaceutical development, and a strategy for regulatory approval as well as for dissemination in the community.

*Targeted Therapy in Translational Cancer Research* considers many of these areas. Principles are beginning to emerge for identifying therapeutic targets. A critical issue is how best to combine therapies against different targets within the same cancer if we are to develop effective personalized care. Tumor initiating cells must be eliminated as well as their progeny. Not only the cancer cells but tumor vessels and microenvironment can be targeted. While a separate volume will consider *immunotherapy*, a chapter on principles of immunotherapeutic targeting has been included, because of the rapid progress in this area. A better understanding of epigenetic and miRNA regulation has suggested new approaches to targeted therapy. The current status of targeted therapy for individual hematologic neoplasms and solid cancers has been reviewed extensively. As several major molecular targets and signaling pathways—TP53, PARP, Met, Kit, PI3K, and Ras/MAP—are important to cancers at multiple sites, chapters have also been devoted to strategies for their inhibition. Overall, this volume includes substantial perspective regarding the translational potential of targeted therapy that should provide useful information for investigators and clinicians.

*Robert C. Bast*
*Maurie Markman*
*Ernest Hawk*

# Foreword

As a busy clinical oncologist/hematologist striving to be current in preparing to see a new patient, or as a clinical investigator trying to determine what might be the best new approach for the patient with advanced refractory cancer, this volume titled *Targeted Therapy in Translational Cancer Research* can be of enormous help. In addition, for the young or experienced bench scientist this offering gives both a basic background and an important grounding in the current field of clinical targeted therapies.

The above comments should come as no surprise given the deep experience of the editors and the contributors to this volume.

In a review of the parts of this volume there is excellent coverage of (a) the principles of targeted therapies; (b) specific targeted therapies in the hematologic and solid malignancies; and (c) coverage of targeted therapies for specific molecular aberrations. As one drills down into the well-written individual chapters there is excellent coverage of the current state of the art plus meaningful coverage of how the field is evolving.

It is gratifying to see chapters on functional imaging, the issue of combining targeted therapies, targeted immunotherapies, the microenvironment, microRNAs, and tackling tough targets such as Ras and TP53.

The chapter on specific organ types of cancer are both practical for us to catch up on the best treatments and yet comprehensive enough to see how the treatments are evolving.

All in all, this is a wonderful volume to aid all of us in a practical and deeper understanding of targeted therapies. Congratulations to the contributors and editors of this special volume.

*Daniel D. Von Hoff, MD, FACP*

# Preface: Bench to Bedside and Back

In the last decade, emergent technologies have enhanced our understanding of genomic, transcriptional, proteomic, epigenetic, and immune mechanisms in carcinogenesis. This improved understanding has enabled the development of targeted cancer therapies and transformed conventional treatment paradigms; it has provided the framework for the discovery of new targets, for validation of novel agents, for combination therapies predicated upon scientific rationale, and for clinical trials that have already markedly improved the prognosis and outcome of patients with cancer. Excitingly, the implication of immunomodulatory targets in carcinogenesis has led to the development of new promising drugs based on the central principle that breaking tolerance using immune checkpoint blockers can achieve durable responses. Moreover, although distinct pathways are initially analyzed independently, interdependent and compensatory mechanisms have derived innovative combinations of targeted, immunomodulating, antiangiogenic, and/or chemotherapeutic agents, which have additive or synergistic cytotoxicity and can overcome resistance to conventional therapies. Continued progress will require improved genomic classification of the various tumor types, delineation of the mechanisms of resistance to treatment and disease progression, and improved understanding of metastasis, ultimately allowing for provision of therapies designed to target tumor heterogeneity early in the disease course.

This edition of *Targeted Therapy in Translational Cancer Research* for the Translational Oncology series provides a comprehensive overview of recent developments in our understanding of tumor biology, elucidates the roles of targets and pathways involved in carcinogenesis, and describes current state-of-the-art anticancer therapy, as well as the most promising areas of translational research and targeted therapy. Basic principles of targeted therapy, including immunotherapy and the roles of cancer stem cells, the microenvironment, angiogenesis, epigenetics, microRNAs, and functional imaging in precision medicine, are highlighted. Major advances in the therapeutic management of hematologic malignancies and solid tumors using conventional therapy, targeted therapy, immunotherapy, or novel treatment modalities are summarized. Importantly, advances in technology and bioinformatic analyses of complex data have already allowed for improved characterization of tumor biology, function, and dynamic tumoral changes over time, thereby allowing for improved cancer diagnosis, prognosis, and therapy.

We are on the threshold of translating discoveries in cancer biology into unprecedented durable responses and improved clinical outcomes in the majority of patients with cancer. In this unique time in history, the discovery of novel therapeutic approaches targeting the molecular basis of cancer will allow for implementation of precision medicine, with the promise of potentially curative, well-tolerated therapies. *Targeted Therapy in Translational Cancer Research* was written to increase the awareness and access of basic and clinical researchers, caregivers, and patients alike to cutting-edge "bench to bedside and back" breakthroughs, which have transformed the diagnosis, prognosis, and treatment of cancer.

*Apostolia-Maria Tsimberidou*
*Kenneth C. Anderson*

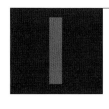

# PART I

# Principles of Targeted Therapies

# CHAPTER 1

# Toward Personalized Therapy for Cancer

*Ashley M. Holder[1] and Funda Meric-Bernstam[2,3,4]*

[1] The University of Texas MD Anderson Cancer Center, Houston, TX, USA
[2] Department of Investigational Cancer Therapeutics, Houston, TX, USA
[3] Institute for Personalized Cancer Therapy, Houston, TX, USA
[4] Department of Surgical Oncology, The University of Texas MD Anderson Cancer Center, Houston, TX, USA

## Introduction

Personalized cancer care is grounded in the principle that the patient's genotype and molecular characterization of a tumor and its microenvironment can identify the most effective cancer management for each patient while reducing toxicity. By tailoring therapy to a specific tumor, the approach of personalized cancer therapy is expected to save critical treatment time and healthcare costs by avoiding the selection of less beneficial therapies. Thus, the objective of personalized cancer therapy is to harvest information about the tumor—its DNA, RNA, proteins, and metabolism—within the context of the tumor microenvironment and the patient's genotype to inform treatment decisions. However, much work remains to be done before this concept can be translated from the research environment to the clinical setting.

Several complementary components are necessary to achieve personalized medicine throughout the continuum of cancer care (Figure 1.1). The first phase of personalized cancer care includes risk assessment, in order to identify patients at higher cancer risk, appropriately modifying screening strategies and frequency, and offering preventive strategies. Once a cancer diagnosis is made, the care of the patient enters the second phase of personalized care—molecular characterization of the tumor to assess patient prognosis. Accordingly, patients at a high risk of recurrence can receive more intensive therapy, while patients at low risk may receive less toxic systemic therapy or may avoid additional therapy altogether.

The third phase in personalized care involves in-depth molecular characterization of the tumor to identify potential therapeutic targets and to test for established and putative predictive markers, that is, markers predictive of response to specific therapies. Markers predictive of adverse events can be used to select regimens with the least toxicity. Early response to therapy may be monitored with pharmacodynamic markers of response.

Furthermore, as efficacy of treatment for recurrent disease improves, a growing role for biomarkers is likely to develop in monitoring early recurrence and providing a personalized program for survivorship. Although currently standardized follow-up schedules based on cancer histology and stage exist for most cancer types, more precise determination of expected prognosis (i.e., likelihood of recurrence) based on molecular subtype would personalize cancer follow-up, including the frequency of follow-up visits and the need for specialist follow-up. As many cancer treatments have long-term unintended effects, personalized survivorship programs can offer more intensive screening for patients at higher risk of developing these side effects.

## Personalized Targeted Therapy

### Principles of Molecular Therapeutics

Even in therapy-sensitive cancers such as breast cancer, only a subgroup of cancer patients achieve a pathologic complete response with currently available standard chemotherapy, underscoring the need to develop novel targeted therapies.[1,2] Therefore, an important component of personalized therapy is the delivery of individualized "targeted" therapy, directed toward molecular aberrations in specific tumors. The principle of molecular therapy is to target molecular differences between cancer cells and normal cells. To implement molecular therapeutics, targets must first be identified using genomic and proteomic techniques. Notably, numerous differences exist between cancer cells and normal cells; differentiating between cancer "drivers" that play a key role in cancer progression and survival and "passengers" that are present but not critical for cancer maintenance is a challenging but surmountable component, critical to the success of targeted therapies. Extensive preclinical studies are needed for functional characterization of the effect of specific gene alterations on cancer initiation and progression and cancer cell survival. The ideal target is usually differentially expressed or activated in cancer cells conferring cell growth and survival advantage. Thus, target inhibition induces cancer cell cytostasis or, more preferably, cancer cell death.

### Predictors of Response for Patient Selection

In addition to the need for compelling therapeutic targets, drugs that inhibit the identified targets, ideally through selective inhibition, are necessary to minimize off-target toxicity. Biomarkers to detect the presence of the target within the tumor are employed to select patients who will benefit from the targeted therapy. Often, the presence of the target is pursued as a potential predictive marker; however, expression of the target itself may not be sufficient to

*Targeted Therapy in Translational Cancer Research*, First Edition. Edited by Apostolia-Maria Tsimberidou, Razelle Kurzrock and Kenneth C. Anderson.
© 2016 John Wiley & Sons, Inc. Published 2016 by John Wiley & Sons, Inc.

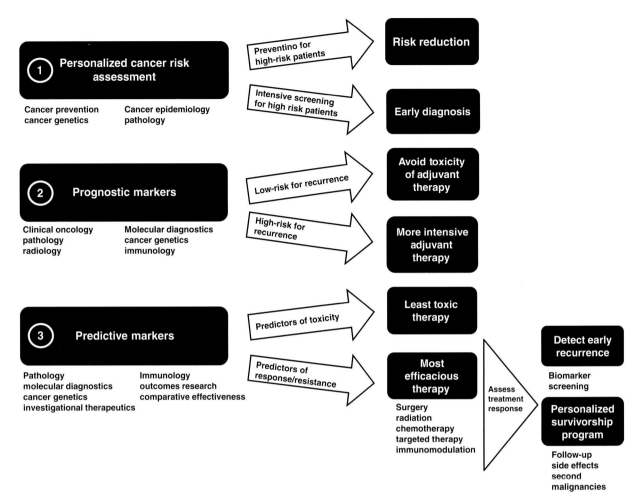

**Figure 1.1** The cancer care continuum for personalized medicine.

confer sensitivity to a therapy. For example, in colorectal cancer EGFR expression assessed by immunohistochemistry (IHC) is not considered to be a reproducible marker of sensitivity to cetuximab.[3] In contrast, patients with colorectal cancers bearing mutated *K-ras* have reproducibly been shown not to benefit from cetuximab, whereas patients with tumors bearing wild-type *K-ras* do benefit.[4–6] As this example demonstrates, predictive markers of response, sensitivity, and resistance must be carefully developed. Even still, most clinically approved targeted therapies have low rates of objective tumor response in single agent therapy. Furthermore, predictive markers of response and clinical benefit remain elusive. Thus, it is important that extensive preclinical modeling to identify markers of response and resistance be performed early in drug development. For targeted therapies with strong rationale for predictive markers, trials can be conducted in patients selected for or enriched for certain markers.

### Pharmacodynamic Markers of Response

Early in drug development, pharmacodynamic markers of biological effect must be discovered to determine whether the putative target is inhibited by the novel therapeutic agent and to measure the extent of target inhibition and downstream signaling inhibition. Biological inhibition of the target can be assessed in surrogate tissue samples, such as skin biopsies, hair follicles, peripheral blood mononuclear cells, or platelets. However, ultimately there is value added in determining the effect of the drug on tumor cells by obtaining pre-treatment and on-treatment biopsies.

Another important goal for molecular therapeutics is the development of early biomarkers of response. The traditional approach to assessing response in clinical trials has been to treat patients for two to three cycles and then evaluate treatment response with repeat imaging. However, with the implementation of targeted therapies, the discovery of pharmacodynamic markers of response that can assess response earlier would spare patients from unnecessary toxicity, save the healthcare system the cost of administering ineffective therapy, and facilitate the transfer to alternate therapeutic regimens without further disease progression. Through assessment of biomarkers pre-treatment and on-treatment with repeat biopsies, pharmacodynamic markers of response within the tumor can be examined after only one cycle of therapy or even earlier; likewise, the biopsy assessment would permit correlation with radiographic response or clinical benefit on standard response assessment. In addition, an on-treatment biopsy can provide further information about adaptive responses to the current treatment. This insight can assist in planning future studies of rational combinatorial therapy. An area yet to be explored is the use of individual adaptive responses to personalize combination therapies chosen.

Although obtaining pre- and on-treatment biopsies to assess pharmacodynamic markers of response is theoretically appealing, this process presents several challenges. One barrier to early assessment of treatment response is that measurement of target inhibition itself may be difficult. Pathway activation is often determined through assessment of phosphorylation of downstream mediators, and phospho-specific residues are known to be relatively unstable.[7,8] The acquisition of a biopsy may also change the readout of the pathway and cell proliferation. Cold ischemia time and intratumoral heterogeneity of the specimen can alter the measurable targets within the sample. There are no widely accepted approaches for quantitative assessment of downstream signaling; though IHC, reverse-phase protein array (RPPA), enzyme-linked immunosorbent assay (ELISA), and bead-based multiplex proteomics are all currently utilized, they have limitations. To minimize variability in assessment of treatment response, researchers and clinicians must collaborate to optimize and standardize specimen collection and assay selection for each desired target within a tissue type.

Another valid concern is the significant cost added to clinical trials by pre- and on-treatment biopsies. Further, these biopsies introduce additional problems, such as biopsy quality and potential increased morbidity. Despite the increasing number of early trials incorporating biopsies for pharmacodynamic assessment, only a small fraction of phase I trials that included biomarkers made use of the biomarker results for dose selection.[9] Some have proposed that if the drug does not show preliminary evidence of antitumor efficacy in an early trial, the biopsies will be uninformative. However, even if antitumor efficacy is not observed, pharmacodynamic assessment may serve other important roles, such as determining whether there was lack of or insufficient target inhibition. These results could uncover the need to modify treatment dose or schedule. Furthermore, if there were inhibition of target but with inadequate treatment response, the information gathered from the biopsy could suggest that the target may not be the primary driver in that tumor type or that there may be alternate resistance mechanisms within the tumor.

### Early Successes in Personalized Therapy

Despite the challenges to biomarker selection, targeted therapy development, and treatment response assessment, the field of personalized cancer therapy has generated early successes incorporating biomarkers and targeted therapies to transform cancer treatment.

## Prognostic Stratification and Prediction of Chemotherapy Benefit in Hormone Receptor-Positive Breast Cancer

Several RNA-based prognosticators have recently been developed. Two of these commercially available multi-marker assays for breast cancer prognostication are notable as they are widely utilized. In two independent analyses of phase III clinical trials, one in node-negative and one in node-positive breast cancer with tamoxifen-alone control arms, the Oncotype Dx (Genomic Health) RT-PCR-based 21-gene recurrence score was shown to identify a group of patients with low recurrence scores, who do not appear to benefit from chemotherapy and a second group, with high scores, who do benefit from chemotherapy. The role of chemotherapy in breast cancer patients with hormone receptor-positive, node-negative, intermediate recurrence score tumors and hormone receptor-positive, node-positive, low and intermediate recurrence score tumors is being assessed prospectively in the TAILORx and RxPONDER studies, respectively. In a non-randomized clinical setting, the Mammoprint 70-gene signature was shown to be prognostic in node negative and 1–3 node positive patients and to predict chemotherapy benefit in the high-risk group.[10–12] The Mammoprint is being prospective validated in the large adjuvant MINDACT (Microarray In Node-negative Disease May Avoid ChemoTherapy) clinical trial. For both Oncotype and Mammoprint assays, the discordance rates between the assay prediction and clinical-pathologic risk categories are approximately 30%. Clinical utility studies demonstrate that assay use results in a change in treatment decision in 25–30% of cases, most commonly from chemo-endocrine therapy to endocrine therapy alone.[13] The widespread use of these tools in clinical practice suggests that clinicians not only are seeking prognostic tools to assist in counseling patients and treatment planning but also are willing to modify their clinical practice to incorporate new technological adjuncts.

## HER2-Targeted Therapy in Breast Cancer

Twenty percent of breast cancers display HER2 amplification, which is associated with a poorer prognosis compared to those without HER2 overexpression.[14,15] However, treatment of these breast cancers in the adjuvant setting with trastuzumab, a monoclonal antibody targeting the extracellular domain of the protein encoded for by HER2, has been shown to improve survival in both early stage and metastatic breast cancers with HER2 amplification.[16–19] This initial success was rapidly followed by development of additional anti-HER2 therapies such as lapatinib, pertuzumab, and T-DM1. Even still, many HER2-positive tumors do not respond to HER2-targeted therapy, suggesting that additional biomarkers are needed to predict intrinsic resistance and the emergence of acquired resistance.

## BRAF Inhibitors in BRAF Mutant Melanoma

B-Raf is a member of the Raf kinase family of serine–threonine kinases that activates the MAP/ERK signaling pathway. Mutations in BRAF have been detected in 40–60% of melanomas.[20,21] Less than a decade after the development of the RAF inhibitor vemurafenib, a phase III randomized trial confirmed that the BRAF V600E mutation was a response-specific predictive biomarker for treatment of melanoma with vemurafenib. Patients with therapy-naïve metastatic melanoma harboring the BRAF V600E mutation had significantly longer progression free and overall survival when treated with vemurafenib compared to standard chemotherapy.[22] The rapid clinical development of B-Raf inhibitors exemplifies how molecular identification of a driver aberration can be rapidly translated into a clinically effective therapy. However, in spite of the impressive response rates (48% for vemurafenib compared with 5% for dacarbazine), responses were short-lived, demonstrating the need for combinatorial therapy with other drugs or immunotherapy to obtain durable responses.

## Strategies for Comprehensive Molecular Characterization

With the advent of high-throughput technologies, interest in the utilization of multimarker technologies to assist in tumor molecular classification and selection of optimal personalized therapy has intensified. A brief summary of strategies commonly utilized for comprehensive molecular characterization is provided below and in Table 1.1.

**Table 1.1** Strategies for comprehensive molecular characterization.

| Technology | Detection target | Tissue requirement | Advantages | Disadvantages |
|---|---|---|---|---|
| **DNA** | | | | |
| Hot spot mutation testing | Single nucleotide variations | Blood, fresh/frozen tissue or FFPE | Minimal DNA required<br>Cost effective<br>High throughput | Limited to hot spot mutations assayed |
| Targeted gene sequencing | Mutations in candidate genes | Fresh/frozen tissue or FFPE | Complete sequencing of open reading frames | Larger amount of tissue required<br>Must differentiate germline SNPs from somatic mutations<br>Limited gene panel |
| Whole exome and genome sequencing | Mutations | Fresh or high-quality frozen tissue | Valuable target discovery<br>Comprehensive | FFPE not optimized<br>Predicting functional impact of mutation<br>Expensive |
| DNA methylation screening | Methylation | Blood, fresh or high-quality frozen tissue | High throughput | High-quality frozen material required |
| **RNA** | | | | |
| Quantitative PCR | Relative gene expression | Blood, fresh or high-quality frozen tissue | Monitor treatment effect on pathway expression | Quantitates relative to housekeeping gene |
| Microarray-based gene expression profiling | Relative mRNA or miRNA expression | Blood, fresh or high-quality frozen tissue | Monitor treatment effect on pathway expression<br>High throughput<br>Cost effective | Reproducibility of results due to sample preparation and type of platform |
| RNA sequencing | Absolute RNA abundance, splicing variants, mutations, fusions | Fresh/frozen tissue | Monitor treatment effect on pathways<br>High throughput<br>Base pair resolution | "Reads" are proxies for mRNA abundance<br>Reproducibility monitoring<br>Need to reconstruct short "reads" |
| Ribosome footprinting | Quantitate expression | Fresh/frozen tissue | Information on protein abundance regulation | Does not quantitate proteins but only translation efficiency |
| **Protein** | | | | |
| Stable isotopic labeling with amino acids in cell culture (SILAC) | Relative protein concentration | Fresh/frozen tissue or FFPE | High throughput<br>High accuracy and sensitivity | Isotopic labeling may not be feasible |
| High-resolution tandem mass spectrometry | Absolute protein quantification | Blood, fresh/frozen tissue or FFPE | Cost effective | Dependent on calibration or reference standards |
| RPPA | Relative protein expression and activation | Blood, fresh/frozen tissue or FFPE | Cost effective<br>High throughput | Proteins must have high-quality antibodies available |
| Immunohistochemistry | Relative protein expression and activation | Fresh/frozen tissue or FFPE | Tissue morphology<br>Intratumoral location | Proteins must have high-quality antibodies available<br>Low throughput<br>Larger amount of sample required |
| Metabolomics | Metabolite expression and pathway activation | Blood, urine, or fresh/frozen tissue | High throughput | Sample harvest conditions can alter results |

## Genomic Profiling

Much of the effort in biomarker discovery for personalized cancer therapy has been directed at genomic markers, in part because of targeted therapies entering the market with DNA-based predictive markers, such as *BRAF* V600E as a predictor of response to BRAF inhibitors, and also because of the recent advances allowing multiplex genomic testing to be performed in a rapid, reproducible, and relatively cost-effective manner.

Recently, several high-throughput genotyping methods have moved into the Clinical Laboratory Improvement Amendments (CLIA) environment including the MassARRAY System (Sequenom), SNaPshot technology (Applied Biosystems), and ion semiconductor sequencing (Ion Torrent Technology). Multiplex hot spot mutation testing, also referred to as high-throughput SNP genotyping, has many advantages: requiring minimal DNA, accommodating formalin-fixed paraffin-embedded (FFPE) tissue, processing multiple samples simultaneously, detecting mutations present in a small proportion (5%) of cells, and being relatively cost-effective. However, this technique is limited to evaluating only the hot spot mutations being assayed. Hot spot genotyping does not have the capability to provide full coverage of all tumor suppressor genes, to detect new mutations in known cancer-related genes, or to discover novel cancer-related genes.

In addition to high-throughput SNP genotyping, targeted sequencing has recently become available in the CLIA environment. Target enrichment allows for selective capture of genomic regions of interest (usually exomes) and subsequent sequencing of cancer-relevant genes, including actionable targets, and common mutations. This technique has several benefits: complete sequencing of genes, including tumor suppressor genes; directing analytical resources to the most relevant genes in a select panel (e.g., 200–400); and accommodating FFPE tissue. The drawbacks of targeted exome sequencing are the larger amounts of tissue required, the need to differentiate germline SNPs from somatic mutations, and the limitations of novel gene discovery resulting from the limited gene panel. Sequencing alone will also not capture other critical alterations such as epigenetic changes.

As the cost for whole exome sequencing (WES) and whole genome sequencing (WGS) has decreased, the utility of these approaches in personalized cancer therapy is now being explored. The advantage of these techniques is the comprehensive genomic analysis of the tumor, yielding mutational, gene copy number, and rearrangement data. This complete examination can detect changes resulting in oncogene activation or tumor suppressor gene inactivation, perhaps uncovering alterations in the exome or genome that are essential for the maintenance of the malignant phenotype. In addition, the genomic data harvested from WES and WGS can aid in the development of novel targeted therapies, and assist in the selection of currently available treatments likely to be most effective. However, the minimum quantity of DNA required is significantly greater than other genomic techniques, and WES/WGS analysis of FFPE samples is only being optimized now. Even still, WES and WGS are prone to high rates of false positive and false negative calls, especially in samples with low tumor cellularity, necessitating validation with additional technologies. Possible solutions to these concerns are creating a standardized algorithm for calling single nucleotide variants (SNVs) and stringent standards to assess the reliability of calls in the CLIA environment. Despite the development of tools to assist in calling SNVs, hurdles to incorporating WES and WGS in personalized cancer therapy involve predicting the functional impact of every mutation and prioritizing each

mutation as a driver or passenger. In addition, the large amount of data generated from WES/WGS creates considerable challenges to the capacity and security of information storage, as well as to the timely turnaround of bioinformatic analysis.

Next-generation targeted sequencing and WES/WGS approaches also have the advantage of providing information on DNA copy number. Other high-throughput technologies being pursued to assess copy number alterations include comparative genomic hybridization, single nucleotide polymorphism arrays, digital karyotyping, and molecular inversion probes.[23, 24]

## Epigenetic Profiling

Genomic technologies can detect genetic alterations that yield response-predictive biomarkers; however, the frequency of mutations in some cancers is quite low. An alternative to mutational analysis is epigenetic or DNA methylation screening. Epigenetic profiling of immortalized cancer cell lines can uncover associations between methylated genes and therapeutic sensitivity. Inactivation of DNA mismatch repair genes can be assessed using epigenetic tools that can then provide prognostic stratification for clinical application, such as CpG island methylator phenotype (CIMP) in colorectal cancer.[25] In addition, methylation screening can detect activation of oncogenic signaling through the silencing of pathway signaling regulators. To detect mechanisms of resistance, methylation screening of a tumor pre- and post-treatment can identify epigenetic changes following chemotherapy that may alter the antitumor efficacy of other agents, such as the use of the methylating agent temozolomide based on the methylation status of the MGMT promoter in glioblastoma.[26, 27]

## Transcriptional Profiling

To produce an individualized signature of a patient's tumor, gene expression profiling utilizes mRNA, microRNA, and non-coding RNA. This unique transcriptome can then be used for classification of unique molecular subtypes, prognostic assessment, and to predict therapeutic responsiveness of tumors. In addition, transcriptional profiling of cancers before and after neoadjuvant systemic therapy can provide crucial information about the effect of treatment on the regulation of pathways and biological processes, potentially revealing new targets for therapy.[28]

Other technologies such as exon junction arrays and genome tiling arrays use probes to the expected splice sites for each gene, thus allowing detection of splicing isoforms. As interest in massive parallel sequencing of RNA (RNA-seq) has intensified, RNA-based technologies are continuing to evolve rapidly. Compared with traditional transcriptional profiling with microarray technology, RNA-seq has the ability to detect other abnormalities in the cancer transcriptome in addition to changes in RNA expression, including alternative splicing, novel transcripts, and gene fusion.[29] Furthermore, RT-PCR-based multiplex assays, such as Oncotype Dx, that assess expression of selected RNA panels are likely to have sustained utility.

## Proteomic Profiling

IHC is a well-validated tool to assess therapeutic biomarkers, such as the estrogen receptor in breast cancer. However, IHC has limitations as a low-throughput technology requiring larger amounts of sample and considerable clinical manpower and expense to process and interpret each biomarker of interest. An advantage of IHC is its visualization of the protein of interest within the tumor, providing information about intratumoral location and tissue morphology.

The development of a multiplex method for IHC could transport this worthwhile and validated tool into the realm of personalized oncology.

Other assays, such as ELISA, and new-generation assays, such as bead-based multiplexed proteomic assays, can allow for assessment of a panel of proteins but still present challenges regarding not only linear range and challenges in absolute quantitation but also scalability to a large sample set. Mass-spectrometry-based proteomics remains a powerful discovery tool. RPPA is a protein array designed that allows the measurement of protein expression levels in a large number of biological samples simultaneously in a quantitative manner. Briefly, lysates from cell lines, tissue lysates, or biological fluids can be spotted onto reverse-phase protein microarrays and probed with a panel of high-quality, monospecific antibodies. RPPA is a relatively cost-effective, high-throughput method to identify cancer subtypes, resistance biomarkers, and functional pathways. One drawback of RPPA is that it is limited to proteins for which high-quality antibodies are available. Given that most biomarkers and drug targets are proteins, proteomics has an advantage over transcriptional profiling for monitoring therapeutic response, discovering novel targets, and exposing mechanisms of pathway resistance in a personalized manner. The proteomic signature can also guide treatment selection by stratifying tumors into molecular categories and allowing the clinical team to incorporate the most efficacious therapy into the treatment plan. Further, RPPA is mainly utilized through comparison of a sample with other samples in a set. Approaches to normalize expression of a sample compared to controls are needed to transition this approach from a discovery tool to a point-of-care assay. Large-scale validation of proteomic signatures as well as proteomic platforms must be achieved before proteomic profiles can enter wide-spread clinical use.

## Metabolomics

Metabolomics utilizes mass spectrometry, nuclear magnetic resonance, and gas and liquid chromatography to reveal small molecule metabolites and metabolic pathway alterations essential for the maintenance of the malignant phenotype. Metabolic screening can also aid in the early detection of cancers, especially those for which screening is difficult, by assessing biomarkers not only in tumor tissues but also in patients' body fluids. Alterations in mitochondrial metabolism, a characteristic of invasive cancer, can differentiate malignancy from normal tissues. *In vivo* metabolic screening for staging and monitoring cancer is achieved through PET imaging technology that capitalizes on the increased metabolic activity of malignant cells to expose residual disease and metastases. Alterations in imaging may also occur with different tumor subtypes. For example, mutations in the isocitrate dehydrogenase (IDH) genes are frequently found in gliomas. This results in the production of an oncometabolite, 2-hydroxyglutarate (2-HG), which can be detected noninvasively in gliomas with IDH mutations using magnetic resonance spectroscopy.[30]

## Integrated Multi-analyte Analysis

With increasing access to high-throughput technologies and the ability to perform assays on smaller amount of tissues, the frontier of multi-analyte analysis is expanding to incorporate DNA, RNA, and protein data, to perform integrated analysis for better molecular classification of tumors, and to identify the most suitable actionable targets. Although such a systems biology approach may indeed be the future of personalized medicine, integrated analysis of high-throughput sequencing is still in the pilot stages.[31,32]

Greater emphasis on big data, and sharing of clinically annotated high-throughput data, is likely to improve predictive algorithms.

## A Personalized Approach to Investigational Therapy Selection

Increasingly, genomic characterization directs patients to specific clinical trials targeting the aberrant gene product or downstream signaling pathway. Routine comprehensive testing of patients with advanced disease could facilitate faster delivery of effective therapies to patients, while enriching for patients with matched aberrations in targeted therapy trials and accelerating accrual in those trials. Comprehensive testing is of the greatest value to patients who are interested in participating in clinical trials, are potentially eligible for therapeutic trials, and are able to access a menu of actively accruing targeted therapy trials. Unfortunately, most patients have limited access to pathway-matched investigational targeted therapies due to lack of relevant trials or lack of availability in early clinical trials.

Standardized molecular testing in the CLIA environment can facilitate a variety of phase II clinical trial designs (Figure 1.2). In one commonly used approach, a biomarker can be used for patient selection for treatment with an agent targeting that alteration or the downstream pathway activated by that alteration (Figure 1.2a), or for randomization between standard of care or the targeted therapy (Figure 1.2b). Alternately, the biomarker can be used for prospective stratification, but all patients may be treated in a single arm study with the targeted therapy (Figure 1.2c) or randomized to targeted therapy or standard therapy (Figure 1.2d). In umbrella trials, patients are allocated to one of several treatments based on their biomarker profile (Figure 1.2e). In adaptive trials, patients are initially randomly allocated but subsequently allocated by biomarkers linked to therapeutic approaches discovered in the initial part of the treatment (Figure 1.2f) (e.g., ISPY 2, BATTLE trials 20).[33–38] One common strategy is to match patients to trials based on a chosen molecular aberration, such as enrolling patients with *PIK3CA*-mutant breast cancer in trials that have the presence of a *PIK3CA* mutation as an eligibility criterion (Figure 1.2a). However, biomarker assessment can also enrich trials without biomarker eligibility criteria through the enrollment of patients with pathway aberrations, for example, matching patients with *PIK3CA* mutations in trials with agents targeting the PI3K pathway. Ultimately, this technique may enhance the clinical benefit achieved for enrolled patients, as supported by a study in which matching treatment delivered to patient tumor genotype improved response rate even in early clinical trials.[39] However, it should be noted that the response and clinical benefit rates observed in this study may not be representative of the general population due to small sample size and lack of randomization.

There is also increasing interest in treating individual patients through off-label use of drugs targeting an aberration approved for another indication or compassionate use of agents in clinical trials that do not "fit" the patient characteristics. Cancer centers need to determine ways to facilitate treatment of these patients on "N-of-1" studies (Figure 1.2g).[40–42] "N-of-1" trials use clinicopathologic molecular characteristics to select an individualized therapy plan. The most significant challenge is in quantifying benefit of an "N-of-1" effort; the test is of the process and not the individual biomarker/drug pairing. Clinical benefit has been suggested in "N-of-1" settings by measuring time-to-progression on the trial drug compared to time-to-progression on the most recent treatment.[43,44]

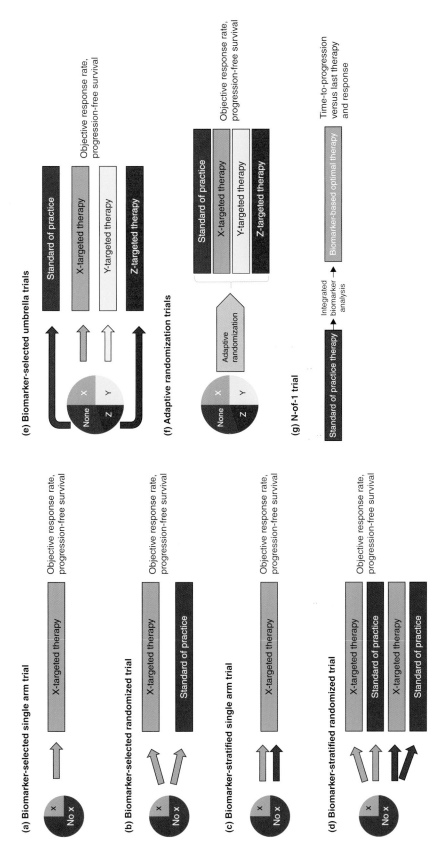

**Figure 1.2** Biomarker-driven clinical trials. (a, b) Biomarker-selected single arm trials may deliver targeted therapy to patients selected for a specific genomic alteration or other biomarker or may randomize patients with a biomarker to investigational therapy or standard of care therapy. (c, d) Patients may be stratified based on the biomarker status, and patients with or without the biomarker may receive the investigational therapy or they may be randomized between standard of care therapy and the investigational arm. (e) In umbrella trials, multiple biomarkers may be simultaneously assessed, and patients allocated to treatment based on biomarker status. (f) In adaptive trials, initially patients can be randomly allocated between treatment arms, but subsequently the allocation is adaptive, based on disease control or other short-term endpoints in each biomarker subtype for each therapy. (g) In N-of-1 trials, patients are given a therapeutic regimen assessed to match their genomic/molecular profile most closely.

Collaborations with industry are needed to access novel investigational drugs that may be of benefit in these trials. Biomarker-selected trials for rare alterations are especially challenging. Collaboration across institutions is necessary to enroll across a variety of institutions, usually leveraging local testing for enrollment. The efficiency of such trials is increased with the increasing utilization of "basket trials," trials that test the efficacy of agents either in a histology-independent manner, or by accruing a variety of tumor types, with planned analysis in disease-specific cohorts.

With increasing multiplex testing, patients are frequently found to have more than one actionable alteration. Novel strategies are needed to rapidly test novel combination therapies, either targeting more than one alteration at a time, or targeting one actionable gene and additional survival pathway shown to be associated with intrinsic or acquired resistance.

The design of clinical trials inherently poses significant challenges not only to biomarker discovery but also to validating the benefit of targeted therapies. Phase I trials often contain heavily pretreated patients, adding additional complexity to the challenges of tumor heterogeneity and molecular evolution. Phase II trials can have small sample sizes with inadequate power for biomarker validation. In addition, to validate a biomarker, patients with and without the biomarker must be treated with a drug; however, this methodology also raises ethical concerns about treating patients in non-marker matched trials if strong rationale exists for the biomarker's predictive benefit. However, if genomic markers were used at the onset during the development of a drug and therapies were proven effective, studies in populations with and without markers still would have been of importance to determine the predictive value of a marker. Another challenge is that even in phase III trials of targeted therapies may yield few objective responders as many novel treatments are cytostatic but not cytotoxic. One commonly utilized strategy for discovery in phase I, II, and III trials is to select patients for additional analysis through an unusual responder protocol; this method focuses efforts on patients who fail to respond as predicted or who achieve notably better results on a treatment regimen.

## Challenges to Personalized Cancer Therapy

Although personalized therapy holds much promise, biomarker-based treatment is utilized in only a few cancer types at this time. Furthermore, no data has demonstrated that comprehensive molecular profiling provides added value for the patient or decreases healthcare costs. Before personalized therapy can be implemented, several challenges must be overcome; these obstacles are discussed below.

### Tumor Heterogeneity

From variation among the proportion of cancer cells having specific mutations to variation among the types of mutations, tumors have considerable heterogeneity. Presently available multiplex technologies can detect mutations that exist in as few as 5% of a tumor's cells; in-depth sequencing may be able to detect even rarer tumors. It is currently not known whether a minimum proportion of tumor cells must contain a somatic mutation to observe an effect on tumor biology, response to targeted therapies, or resistance to alternate pathway inhibitors. The relative tumor cellularity also influences the "percentage mutant" through the relative proportion of normal DNA in the total DNA analyzed. In select cases with low tumor cellularity, microdissection of tumor cells may be necessary prior to

genomic screening, resulting in markedly increased cost. Addressing this issue is critical to determining the genomic sequencing coverage-depth necessary to make clinical decisions.

### Molecular Evolution

Biomarker assessment of archival tissue, typically the primary tumor specimen, often serves as the basis for patient treatment decisions. However, tumors evolve as the disease progresses, acquiring additional mutations that provide a growth or survival advantage and selecting for a population of subclones. In a study of pancreatic cancer metastases and matched primary tumors, sequencing revealed that the clonal populations that resulted in distant metastases were also represented in the primary tumor; however, these clones had genetically evolved from the parental non-metastatic clone.[45] Furthermore, it is not yet known whether "founder mutations" that exist in parental clones or "progressor mutations" that arise following clonal evolution are better therapeutic targets. It is also unclear if the concordance of biomarkers between primary and recurrent tumors differ by cancer tissue of origin. In breast cancer, discordance in the standard of care markers—estrogen receptor, progesterone receptor, and human epidermal growth factor receptor-2 (HER2)—between the primary tumor and metastases has been observed and is associated with poorer outcomes.[46] Similarly, there is discordance in immunohistochemical markers of phosphatidylinositol 3-kinase (PI3K) pathway activation, as well as in PIK3CA mutation status between primary and recurrent breast cancers.[47,48] Interestingly, the discordance observed is not only attributable to metastases acquiring additional aberrations but also from loss of aberrations that had been detected in the primary tumor. In contrast to PIK3CA mutation status in breast cancer, a high concordance in K-Ras status between primary tumors and matched liver metastases has been reported[49] To inform the selection of samples for biomarker assessment, additional studies are needed to establish the concordance of key biomarkers among different cancer tissues of origin and different metastatic sites.

Cancer cells adapt and acquire resistance through several mechanisms upon prolonged treatment with targeted therapy. One method is through loss of the target, as observed in a study of breast cancer patients treated with neoadjuvant trastuzumab-based chemotherapy; on post-treatment biopsy, a third of the samples from patients who did not have a complete pathologic response now displayed loss of the HER2 amplification that had been present in their pretreatment biopsies.[50] Another means by which cancers develop resistance is the acquisition of additional genomic aberrations. In lung cancer, a second mutation in *EGFR* (T790M) and MET amplification have been described as two mechanisms of drug resistance to the EGFR inhibitors erlotinib and gefitinib.[51-53] Subpopulations of cells with MET amplification were identified even prior to drug exposure, suggesting that drug treatment effectively selects for these subpopulations.[54] To reveal mechanisms of acquired drug resistance, sequential tumor biopsies and systematic genetic and histological analyses were performed in 37 patients with drug-resistant non-small cell lung cancers (NSCLC) harboring *EGFR* mutations.[55] Across sequential biopsies, every tumor retained the activating *EGFR* mutations; some developed known mechanisms of resistance, including the *EGFR* T790M mutation and MET amplifications. Others displayed novel genetic changes, including EGFR amplification, *PIK3CA* mutations, and markers of epithelial-to-mesenchymal transition. Some tumors transformed into small cell lung cancers (SCLC) that were sensitive to standard SCLC treatments. Serial biopsies in three patients revealed that genetic aberrations were lost after cessation of EGFR inhibitor treatment, yet these cancers then became sensitive to a second round of EGFR inhibitor treatment.

These studies emphasize the importance of re-characterizing tumors at the time of relapse to identify mechanisms of resistance and to design more efficacious combinatorial therapies. Assessing cancers throughout the disease course introduces additional challenges: the cost associated with image-guided biopsies, concerns about biopsy quality, the morbidity of biopsies, and the understanding that all distant sites of metastasis may not develop identical mechanisms of resistance. To evaluate the molecular evolution of a patient's cancer in a safer and more cost-effective manner, less invasive approaches—including biomarker analysis of circulating tumor cells or circulating free DNA and functional imaging—must be optimized for clinical application.

## Strategies for Biomarker Analysis

The traditional approach to biomarker analysis is the point-of-care assessment of relevant biomarkers prior to treatment with a specific therapy, such as *BRAF* mutational screening to select treatments for metastatic melanoma. There are now increasing numbers of phase I and II trials accruing patients with specific somatic mutations, thereby necessitating pretreatment testing. Although the approach limits the quantity of biomarkers assessed, this strategy introduces delays in treatment initiation for patients. Even in highly efficient molecular diagnostic labs, the retrieval of archival tissue blocks often requires many days to weeks, especially if the samples are in an extramural location. After several weeks of waiting, many patients learn their tumors lack the necessary biomarker for trial eligibility and thus will have experienced an unnecessary treatment delay. This delay can be even more sizeable for biomarkers requiring WES or WGS, as the testing and analysis takes several weeks, well beyond a clinically acceptable window for biomarker turnaround time for treatment planning.

One strategy to prevent these delays in biomarker analysis is comprehensive multi-marker testing performed at the time of presentation, allowing for earlier determination of treatment options. However, this approach relies on the examination of archival blocks and thus may not encompass changes due to molecular evolution. Alternatively, point-of-care biopsies can be obtained, eliminating the time lost in the retrieval of archival tissue and potentially accounting for molecular evolution. This approach introduces additional costs and morbidity to obtain the biopsy and does not eliminate the delays in biomarker assessment.

## Biopsy and Tumor Specimen Quality

Biopsy quality is another challenge to implementation of personalized oncology. Even with dedicated radiologists and pathologists, one study of lung cancer patients found that 16.7% of research biopsies are inadequate for biomarker assessment.[56] This percentage may be even higher in other tumor types, in patients who have received several previous treatment regimens, and in the application to technologies requiring large DNA quantities and high tumor cellularity. Furthermore, as more patients receive effective neoadjuvant therapy, even surgical excisions may provide samples with minimal tumor cellularity. Surgical samples also deteriorate with prolonged specimen storage, resulting in lower-quality data even from robust DNA-based assays. These quality and quantity concerns underscore the need to develop biomarker analysis of minimally invasive samples, including circulating tumor cells, circulating free DNA and bone marrow micrometastases.

## Biomedical Informatics and Decision Support

An additional challenge to personalized cancer therapy is the bioinformatics and medical informatics capacity and medical decision support that must be leveraged to provide reliable results in a timely fashion and to supply the clinical team with accessible tools for designing treatment strategies. The rapidly growing field of bioinformatics must evolve with technology to develop standardized algorithms for calling SNVs, predicting functional impact of mutations, and prioritizing mutations to differentiate drivers from passengers. Institutions must also build a medical informatics infrastructure to facilitate therapy selection and monitoring. Systems need to be built to analyze and inform the expected outcome for a patient treated with standard regimens based on their molecular profile. These teams must also monitor patient toxicity and the response to treatment of the primary tumor and any metastases, while analyzing that data in the context of the patient's biomarker status. Medical decision support must provide clinicians with user-friendly software to identify and prioritize actionable targets revealed in biomarker assessment, while incorporating patient health information, prior treatment response, and relevant data from published literature. The personnel and technological needs to design and support these valuable clinical tools add substantial cost.

## Resource Allocation

The implementation of personalized cancer medicine is a costly endeavor. In light of the current economic decline, policymakers and insurance providers are scrutinizing healthcare spending and rising costs. Although better validated and thus more reliable, CLIA testing for biomarker assessment is expensive. To contain costs and maintain accuracy, CLIA laboratories that perform large volumes of high-throughput testing, analysis, and validation must be designated as testing centers for the comprehensive tumor assessment that is critical to personalized cancer therapy. Academic cancer centers with governmental and philanthropic funding to support and advance biomarker testing must assume a leadership role in the personalized cancer therapy movement. These centers must maintain current grants and seek out additional funding sources to maintain ongoing research into targeted therapies and the clinical trials essential for their evaluation. Lastly, buy-in from insurance providers is crucial to the success of personalized cancer therapy, as partial or complete failure to reimburse for comprehensive testing and cancer treatment—including biomarker analysis, routine pre-, on-, and post-treatment biopsies, and novel targeted therapies—will hinder advancement of the field and restrict the personalization of treatment to the affluent minority.

## Collaboration and Regulation

To execute cancer treatment in a personalized manner, academia and industry must collaborate on biomarker discovery and validation to develop novel targeted therapies and expedite their evaluation in clinical trials. Likewise, clinicians and researchers must connect in order to translate laboratory breakthroughs into predictive biomarkers, innovative treatment design. Increased studies on biomarkers of toxicity can also lead to reduction of patient toxicity. Furthermore, knowledge-sharing and collaborative training of clinical and research personnel will improve communication and effectiveness in the multidisciplinary team approach to cancer treatment. Clinical research committees and institutional review boards must recruit, maintain, and develop members with expertise in biomarkers, genomics, and proteomics, to ensure the safety of patients while also not introducing delays to the approval of research protocols and clinical trials.

## Summary

Personalized cancer therapy stems from the premise that comprehensive molecular characterization of the patient's tumor will result in the most effective treatment design for each patient while minimizing individual toxicity. Utilizing current and developing assays, each tumor can be assessed for preventative, prognostic, and predictive biomarkers, while also uncovering novel actionable targets. Early successes, such as *BRAF* mutational screening of melanomas to select for treatment with BRAF inhibitors, have provided encouragement to a field facing significant challenges. Tumor heterogeneity and molecular evolution add considerable complexity to biomarker assessment and treatment design, while funding, personnel, and regulatory issues are a cause for concern at the institutional level. Although much must be accomplished before this model enters widespread use in the clinic, we must not be discouraged. Personalized cancer therapy long-term will not only be in the best interest of our patients but also financially advantageous. Our goal must be to treat each and every patient with the most effective treatment, the first time, to attain prolonged responses and ultimately to achieve cures.

## References

1　Cristofanilli M, Gonzalez-Angulo A, Sneige N, et al. Invasive lobular carcinoma classic type: response to primary chemotherapy and survival outcomes. *J Clin Oncol.* 2005;23(1):41–48.

2　Caudle AS, Gonzalez-Angulo AM, Hunt KK, et al. Predictors of tumor progression during neoadjuvant chemotherapy in breast cancer. *J Clin Oncol.* 2010;28(11):1821–1828.

3　Deschoolmeester V, Baay M, Specenier P, Lardon F, Vermorken JB. A review of the most promising biomarkers in colorectal cancer: one step closer to targeted therapy. *Oncologist.* 2010;15(7):699–731.

4　Karapetis CS, Khambata-Ford S, Jonker DJ, et al. K-ras mutations and benefit from cetuximab in advanced colorectal cancer. *N Engl J Med.* 2008;359(17):1757–1765.

5　Lievre A, Bachet JB, Le Corre D, et al. KRAS mutation status is predictive of response to cetuximab therapy in colorectal cancer. *Cancer Res.* 2006;66(8):3992–3995.

6　Linardou H, Dahabreh IJ, Kanaloupiti D, et al. Assessment of somatic k-RAS mutations as a mechanism associated with resistance to EGFR-targeted agents: a systematic review and meta-analysis of studies in advanced non-small-cell lung cancer and metastatic colorectal cancer. *Lancet Oncol.* 2008;9(10):962–972.

7　Pinhel IF, Macneill FA, Hills MJ, et al. Extreme loss of immunoreactive p-Akt and p-Erk1/2 during routine fixation of primary breast cancer. *Breast Cancer Res.* 2010;12(5):R76.

8　Baker AF, Dragovich T, Ihle NT, Williams R, Fenoglio-Preiser C, Powis G. Stability of phosphoprotein as a biological marker of tumor signaling. *Clin Cancer Res.* 2005;11(12):4338–4340.

9　Goulart BH, Clark JW, Pien HH, Roberts TG, Finkelstein SN, Chabner BA. Trends in the use and role of biomarkers in phase I oncology trials. *Clin Cancer Res.* 2007;13(22 Pt 1):6719–6726.

10　van 't Veer LJ, Dai H, van de Vijver MJ, et al. Gene expression profiling predicts clinical outcome of breast cancer. *Nature.* 2002;415(6871):530–536.

11　Mook S, Schmidt MK, Viale G, et al. The 70-gene prognosis-signature predicts disease outcome in breast cancer patients with 1–3 positive lymph nodes in an independent validation study. *Breast Cancer Res Treat.* 2009;116(2):295–302.

12　Knauer M, Straver M, Rutgers E, et al. The 70-gene MammaPrint signature is predictive for chemotherapy benefit in early breast cancer. *Breast* 2009; 18(suppl. 1):S36–S37.

13　Albain KS, Paik S, van't Veer L. Prediction of adjuvant chemotherapy benefit in endocrine responsive, early breast cancer using multigene assays. *Breast.* 2009;18:S141–S145.

14　Slamon DJ, Clark GM, Wong SG, Levin WJ, Ullrich A, McGuire WL. Human breast cancer: correlation of relapse and survival with amplification of the HER-2/neu oncogene. *Science.* 1987;235(4785):177–182.

15　Seshadri R, Firgaira FA, Horsfall DJ, McCaul K, Setlur V, Kitchen P. Clinical significance of HER-2/neu oncogene amplification in primary breast cancer. *J Clin Oncol.* 1993;11(10):1936–1942.

16　Dawood S, Broglio K, Buzdar AU, Hortobagyi GN, Giordano SH. Prognosis of women with metastatic breast cancer by HER2 status and trastuzumab treatment: an institutional-based review. *J Clin Oncol.* 2010;28(1):92–98.

17　Romond EH, Perez EA, Bryant J, et al. Trastuzumab plus adjuvant chemotherapy for operable HER2-positive breast cancer. *N Engl J Med.* 2005;353(16):1673–1684.

18　Piccart-Gebhart MJ, Procter M, Leyland-Jones B, et al. Trastuzumab after adjuvant chemotherapy in HER2-positive breast cancer. *N Engl J Med.* 2005;353(16):1659–1672.

19　Joensuu H, Kellokumpu-Lehtinen PL, Bono P, et al. Adjuvant docetaxel or vinorelbine with or without trastuzumab for breast cancer. *N Engl J Med.* 2006;354(8):809–820.

20　Shinozaki M, Fujimoto A, Morton DL, Hoon DS. Incidence of BRAF oncogene mutation and clinical relevance for primary cutaneous melanomas. *Clin Cancer Res.* 2004;10(5):1753–1757.

21　Kumar R, Angelini S, Czene K, et al. BRAF mutations in metastatic melanoma: a possible association with clinical outcome. *Clin Cancer Res.* 2003;9(9):3362–3368.

22　Chapman PB, Hauschild A, Robert C, et al. Improved survival with vemurafenib in melanoma with BRAF V600E mutation. *N Engl J Med.* 2011;364(26):2507–2516.

23　Leary RJ, Cummins J, Wang TL, Velculescu VE. Digital karyotyping. *Nat Protoc.* 2007;2(8):1973–1986.

24　Thompson PA, Brewster AM, Kim-Anh D, et al. Selective genomic copy number imbalances and probability of recurrence in early-stage breast cancer. *PloS One.* 2011;6(8):e23543.

25　Hinoue T, Weisenberger DJ, Lange CP, et al. Genome-scale analysis of aberrant DNA methylation in colorectal cancer. *Genome Res.* 2012;22(2):271–282.

26　Bobola MS, Tseng SH, Blank A, Berger MS, Silber JR. Role of O6-methylguanine-DNA methyltransferase in resistance of human brain tumor cell lines to the clinically relevant methylating agents temozolomide and streptozotocin. *Clin Cancer Res.* 1996;2(4):735–41.

27　Hegi ME, Diserens AC, Godard S, et al. Clinical trial substantiates the predictive value of O-6-methylguanine-DNA methyltransferase promoter methylation in glioblastoma patients treated with temozolomide. *Clin Cancer Res.* 2004;10(6):1871–1874.

28　Gonzalez-Angulo AM, Iwamoto T, Liu S, et al. Gene expression, molecular class changes, and pathway analysis after neoadjuvant systemic therapy for breast cancer. *Clin Cancer Res.* 2012;18(4):1109–1119.

29　Wu Y, Wang X, Wu F, et al. Transcriptome profiling of the cancer, adjacent non-tumor and distant normal tissues from a colorectal cancer patient by deep sequencing. *PloS One.* 2012;7(8):e41001.

30　Andronesi OC, Kim GS, Gerstner E, et al. Detection of 2-hydroxyglutarate in IDH-mutated glioma patients by in vivo spectral-editing and 2D correlation magnetic resonance spectroscopy. *Sci Transl Med*. 2012;4(116):116ra4.

31 Gonzalez-Angulo AM, Hennessy BT, Mills GB. Future of personalized medicine in oncology: a systems biology approach. *J Clin Oncol*. 2010;28(16):2777–2783.

32 Roychowdhury S, Iyer MK, Robinson DR, et al. Personalized oncology through integrative high-throughput sequencing: a pilot study. *Sci Transl Med*. 2011;3(111):111ra21.

33 Rubin EH, Anderson KM, Gause CK. The BATTLE trial: a bold step toward improving the efficiency of biomarker-based drug development. *Cancer Discov*. 2011;1(1):17–20.

34 Sequist LV, Muzikansky A, Engelman JA. A new BATTLE in the evolving war on cancer. *Cancer Discov*. 2011;1(1):14–16.

35 Esserman LJ, Berry DA, Demichele A, et al. pathologic complete response predicts recurrence-free survival more effectively by cancer subset: results from the I-SPY 1 TRIAL–CALGB 150007/150012, ACRIN 6657. *J Clin Oncol*. 2012;30(26):3242–3249.

36 Esserman LJ, Berry DA, Cheang MC, et al. Chemotherapy response and recurrence-free survival in neoadjuvant breast cancer depends on biomarker profiles: results from the I-SPY 1 TRIAL (CALGB 150007/150012; ACRIN 6657). *Breast Cancer Res Treat*. 2012;132(3): 1049–1062.

37 Lin C, Buxton MB, Moore D, et al. Locally advanced breast cancers are more likely to present as Interval Cancers: results from the I-SPY 1 TRIAL (CALGB 150007/150012, ACRIN 6657, InterSPORE Trial). *Breast Cancer Res Treat*. 2012;132(3):871–879.

38 Barker AD, Sigman CC, Kelloff GJ, Hylton NM, Berry DA, Esserman LJ. I-SPY 2: an adaptive breast cancer trial design in the setting of neoadjuvant chemotherapy. *Clin Pharmacol Ther*. 2009;86(1):97–100.

39 Janku F, Tsimberidou AM, Garrido-Laguna I, et al. PIK3CA mutations in patients with advanced cancers treated with PI3K/AKT/mTOR axis inhibitors. *Mol Cancer Ther*. 2011;10(3):558–565.

40 Von Hoff DD, Stephenson JJ Jr., Rosen P, et al. Pilot study using molecular profiling of patients' tumors to find potential targets and select treatments for their refractory cancers. *J Clin Oncol*. 2010;28(33):4877–4883.

41 Nakagawa M, Morimoto M, Takechi H, et al. The new primary chemotherapy with S-1 and docetaxel for advanced breast cancer: a first report of N-1 trial. *J Clin Oncol*. 2012;30(suppl.): Abstract e11560.

42 Guyatt G, Sackett D, Taylor DW, Chong J, Roberts R, Pugsley S. Determining optimal therapy–randomized trials in individual patients. *N Engl J Med*. 1986;314(14):889–892.

43 Lillie EO, Patay B, Diamant J, Issell B, Topol EJ, Schork NJ. The n-of-1 clinical trial: the ultimate strategy for individualizing medicine? *Per Med*. 2011;8(2):161–173.

44 Zucker DR, Ruthazer R, Schmid CH. Individual (N-of-1) trials can be combined to give population comparative treatment effect estimates: methodologic considerations. *J Clin Epidemiol*. 2010;63(12):1312–1323.

45 Yachida S, Jones S, Bozic I, et al. Distant metastasis occurs late during the genetic evolution of pancreatic cancer. *Nature*. 2010;467(7319):1114–1117.

46 Liedtke C, Broglio K, Moulder S, et al. Prognostic impact of discordance between triple-receptor measurements in primary and recurrent breast cancer. *Ann Oncol*. 2009;20(12):1953–1958.

47 Akcakanat A, Sahin A, Shaye AN, Velasco MA, Meric-Bernstam F. Comparison of Akt/mTOR signaling in primary breast tumors and matched distant metastases. *Cancer*. 2008;112(11):2352–2358.

48 Gonzalez-Angulo AM, Ferrer-Lozano J, Stemke-Hale K, et al. PI3K pathway mutations and PTEN levels in primary and metastatic breast cancer. *Mol Cancer Ther*. 2011;10(6):1093–1101.

49 Knijn N, Mekenkamp LJ, Klomp M, et al. KRAS mutation analysis: a comparison between primary tumours and matched liver metastases in 305 colorectal cancer patients. *Br J Cancer*. 2011;104(6):1020–1026.

50 Mittendorf EA, Wu Y, Scaltriti M, et al. Loss of HER2 amplification following trastuzumab-based neoadjuvant systemic therapy and survival outcomes. *Clin Cancer Res*. 2009;15(23):7381–7388.

51 Pao W, Miller VA, Politi KA, et al. Acquired resistance of lung adenocarcinomas to gefitinib or erlotinib is associated with a second mutation in the EGFR kinase domain. *PLoS Med*. 2005;2(3):e73.

52 Engelman JA, Zejnullahu K, Mitsudomi T, et al. MET amplification leads to gefitinib resistance in lung cancer by activating ERBB3 signaling. *Science*. 2007;316(5827):1039–1043.

53 Bean J, Brennan C, Shih JY, et al. MET amplification occurs with or without T790M mutations in EGFR mutant lung tumors with acquired resistance to gefitinib or erlotinib. *Proc Natl Acad Sci USA*. 2007;104(52):20932–20937.

54 Turke AB, Zejnullahu K, Wu YL, et al. Preexistence and clonal selection of MET amplification in EGFR mutant NSCLC. *Cancer Cell*. 2010;17(1):77–88.

55 Sequist LV, Waltman BA, Dias-Santagata D, et al. Genotypic and histological evolution of lung cancers acquiring resistance to EGFR inhibitors. *Sci Transl Med*. 2011;3(75):75ra26.

56 Kim ES, Herbst RS, Wistuba II, et al. The BATTLE trial: personalizing therapy for lung cancer. *Cancer Discov*. 2011;1(1):44–53.

## CHAPTER 2

# Combining Targeted Therapies

*Jordi Rodon[1], Analia Azaro[1], Davis Torrejon[1], and Razelle Kurzrock[2]*

[1]Early Clinical Drug Development Group, Vall d'Hebron Institute of Oncology, Universitat Autonoma de Barcelona, Barcelona, Spain
[2]Center for Personalized Cancer Therapy, UC San Diego Moores Cancer Center, La Jolla, CA, USA

## Rationale for Drug Combination of Targeted Agents

Combining therapies has been successful in many areas of medicine such as hypertension, hypercholesterolemia, tuberculosis, AIDS, and cancer. Hodgkin's disease, colon cancer, prostate cancer, and breast cancer[1-3] are good examples of therapeutic success in response to combining chemotherapeutic agents, hormone therapies, and/or biological agents.

The approval of targeted therapies, such as imatinib for the treatment of chronic myeloid leukemia and trastuzumab for epidermal growth factor receptor 2 (HER2)-positive breast cancer, heralded the era of personalized cancer treatment.[4,5]

Despite advances in defining the molecular pathways that produce cancer growth and invasion, progress in developing therapies that effectively target those pathways has been hampered by their inherent complexity. Many cancer cells have redundant signaling pathways that act as backup or bypass pathways, thereby fostering adaptation to drug inhibition of the primary driving pathway and consequent drug resistance. Early on, it became apparent that single agent application of these therapies, while sometimes resulting in remarkable antitumor effects, was often not enough to eradicate disease, and clinical responses have generally been transitory. In addition, some of these treatments have had limited efficacy, and only a few of them have attained regulatory approval. Success there has primarily been observed in subpopulations of patients with a given disease[6-8] such as erlotinib for mutated non-small cell lung cancer.[9]

Some of the reasons for the lack of activity of single agent, targeted therapies include:

- Resistance mechanisms due to a mutation or genetic event affecting the target of the drug itself, so that the kinase is still able to drive the growth of the tumor despite the continued presence of the drug, such as secondary mutations that may abrogate the salutary effects of targeted agents. For example, KIT mutations that are associated with decreased drug binding may attenuate the beneficial effects of imatinib in gastrointestinal stromal tumors[9]; a similar mechanism occurs in BRAF mutant melanoma and medulloblastoma treated with a BRAF inhibitor or an SMO inhibitor, respectively.[10,11]

- Other aberrations activate downstream proteins, bypassing the inhibited kinase. These bypasses activate downstream signaling pathways so that the tumor no longer needs the target to grow, such as phosphatidylinositol-3-kinase (PI3K), which circumvents the effects of the targeted agent.[12] In a similar way, pharmacological inhibition of downstream molecules such as PI3K or BRAF may activate upstream molecules through compensatory pathways (HER2, EGFR, PDGFR or IGF1R).[13-17]

- Redundant aberrant signaling pathways are activated by genetic perturbations at different levels.[18]

It seems rational, then, to design drug combinations for cancer treatment that will target various loci in underlying aberrant signal transduction pathways to enhance the antiproliferative effect of treatment. Here we review strategies adopted to examine combinatorial therapy, which include the goal of hitting more than one target by specifically inhibiting signal transduction cascades and suppressing specific mechanisms of action. Two complex considerations are: which agents to combine, given the heterogeneity of tumors and their various underlying perturbations including secondary mutations and feedback loops, and how to translate findings from the bench to the bedside or directly from the bedside.

## Deciding Between "Dirty" Drugs or a Cocktail of "Clean" Drugs

Several strategies evolved out of the empirical and rational drug development process with the goal of hitting more than one target.

One approach has been using highly selective drugs ("clean" drugs) designed to specifically inhibit signal transduction cascades. This group includes monoclonal antibodies, antisense oligonucleotides, any gene therapy strategy, and a minority of tyrosine kinase inhibitors such as erlotinib and lapatinib (which are mainly selective for the tyrosine kinase domains of epidermal growth factor receptor 1 (EGFR) and HER2).

At the other extreme are the drugs that were rationally developed to inhibit a specific mechanism of action, irrespective of the selective consequences of this inhibition, rather than having a unique molecular effect. These include histone deacetylase inhibitors (HDAC), proteasome inhibitors, heat shock protein inhibitors, demethylating agents, and others. Because these agents target multiple client

*Targeted Therapy in Translational Cancer Research*, First Edition. Edited by Apostolia-Maria Tsimberidou, Razelle Kurzrock and Kenneth C. Anderson.
© 2016 John Wiley & Sons, Inc. Published 2016 by John Wiley & Sons, Inc.

proteins, their intercellular effects are highly unpredictable in the absence of being able to comprehensively identify specific cellular targets.[19-21] Current technology cannot address the entire proteome vis-à-vis these agents, yet because these drugs affect many cancer gene products, they have been validated as anticancer treatments.

Somewhere between these two extremes are two more strategies. One, the use of multitargeted kinase inhibitors (tyrosine and serine/threonine kinase inhibitors), was developed from either empirical, high-throughput screening of large compound libraries against one target, or selective profiling against several or a full panel of protein kinases. Each compound may have a unique inhibition profile against many kinases and, in fact, these drugs have been called "promiscuous." Drugs such as sorafenib were discovered using this approach.

On the other hand, combinatorial chemistry and chemoinformatics (computational chemistry) have allowed drugs to be engineered with rationally designed selectivity for specific kinases by composing the drug with different pharmacophores, groups important for specific ligand binding. An example is the efforts of Shokat and colleagues, with the goal of inhibiting PI3K and the mammalian target of rapamycin (mTOR) by designing a drug that fills the "chemical space" between those two kinases.[22] In an analogous approach, a drug with two specific binding domains has been developed by producing bispecific antibodies and DARPins (designed ankyrin repeat proteins).[23-26]

Although using multitargeted agents may seem to be a more pragmatic approach, a scientifically appealing approach is to utilize cocktails composed of "clean" drugs. This strategy has several theoretical advantages over single-agent multitargeted therapy:
- It can maximize cell kill while minimizing host toxicities by using agents with non-overlapping dose-limiting toxicities.
- It can increase the range of activity against tumor cells with endogenous resistance to specific types of therapy.
- Finally, it may prevent or slow the development of newly resistant tumor cells.[27]

In summary, the approach of combining highly specific agents can be more precisely targeted when, at least to a degree, the specific entity being inhibited is known, thus abrogating off-target effects such as toxicities. However, clinical experience so far suggests that the effects of multitargeted "dirty" drugs are as good or better than those of highly specific agents. For example, Cabozantinib, a MET inhibitor as well as a vascular endothelial growth factor receptor (VEGFR) inhibitor, has proven to be very active,[28], whereas anti-MET antibodies such as onartuzumab[28, 29] have a more discrete antitumor activity in monotherapy.[29]

## Principles and Strategies for Combining Agents Targeting Signaling Pathways

While combinations of targeted therapies have a commonality with combinations of chemotherapeutic agents, targeted therapies often do not have a direct dose–response–toxicity correlation. Therefore, in the case of targeted agents, established maximum tolerated doses may not be able to be used in combination. Thus, the recommended dose of a given targeted therapy to be used in combination may be below the maximum tolerated dose and guided instead by target inhibition, i.e., a biologically effective dose.[30]

Many of the basic principles for combinations of chemotherapy, antibiotics, and antiretrovirals apply when planning combinations of molecular targeted anticancer agents. Still, many nuances should be mentioned. Table 2.1 provides a comparison of the principles underlying the use of combined cytotoxic agents versus combining targeted agents.

**Table 2.1** Comparing principles underlying the use of combined cytotoxic agents versus combining targeted agents.

| Principles underlying the use of cytotoxic agents in combination | Application to target agents in combination |
| --- | --- |
| Drugs known to be active as single agents should be selected for use in combinations; preferentially drugs that induce complete remission should be included | It applies but, although single agent activity is needed for approval, this could be rare for some MTAs. Targeted agents in combination may induce remissions due to synergistic effects (synthetic lethality) but not as single agents. |
| Drugs with different dose-limiting toxicities should be combined | It applies. Still, off-target sequelae may limit some combinations while side effects due to on-target effects (mechanism-based toxicities) could be medically managed to maintain the therapeutic effect. |
| Full or nearly full therapeutic doses should be utilized for each drug in the combination | It applies, but with many exceptions. Biologically effective doses should be considered if the combination at maximum tolerated doses is not achievable. Pharmacodynamic synergism may allow decreasing the dose of MTA in some combinations while maintaining efficacy. |
| Drugs should be given at consistent intervals, and the treatment-free period should be as short as possible to allow for recovery for the most sensitive normal tissues | It generally applies to the MTA. The PK/PD relationship should drive the dosing schedule. Treatment-free periods may depend on the mechanisms of action of the drugs and their tolerabilities/toxicities. |
| Drugs with different mechanisms of action and with additive or synergistic cytotoxic effects on the tumor should be combined | It generally applies to the MTA. Some drugs with similar mechanism of action could be combined for enhancement of the pathway inhibition (i.e., trastuzumab and lapatinib). |
| Drugs with different patterns of resistance should be used to minimize cross-resistance | It applies to the MTA. Combinations of MTAs are needed since tumors develop many different abnormalities that activate many signaling pathways. Oncogene addiction is a rare phenomenon (i.e., imatinib and CML). |

*Source*: Adapted from Takimoto 2007, Reference 31 with permission from Elsevier.
MTA: molecularly targeted agent; PK: pharmacokinetic; PD: pharmacodynamic.

The strategies for combining targeted therapies are diverse and could be summarized as follows[32]:

- Targeting diverse signaling pathways to produce an additive effect through synergism, which may be achieved by inhibition at the receptor level (EGFR and VEGFR, estrogen receptor (ER) and HER2); or, alternatively, effecting dual inhibition of parallel signaling pathways (i.e., inhibition of mitogen-activated protein kinase (MAPK) and PI3K).[17,33–35] By combined inhibition of separate, critical, pathways, one could avoid resistance mechanisms that result from the activation of an alternative pathway that circumvents inhibition of a primary signaling receptor after it has occurred. For example, amplification of C-MET circumvents the antitumor effects of EGFR inhibition with erlotinib in EGFR-mutant lung cancer cells.[17,33–35] Something similar happens in some cases of resistance to VEGF inhibitors, when blocking DLL4-Notch signaling enhances the efficacy of VEGF inhibitors.[36] In other cases, there would be biological cooperation when employing different mechanisms of action (i.e., temsirolimus and bevacizumab for renal cell cancer) or targeting different cell populations (i.e., combining EGFR inhibitors with HER2 inhibitors for EGFR-positive and HER2-positive cells).

- Superinhibition. Inhibiting a single target such as a receptor using two different strategies, such as combining a monoclonal antibody against the extracellular domain with small molecule inhibition of the tyrosine kinase domain (cetuximab/erlotinib, trastuzumab/lapatinib)[37] or using two monoclonal antibodies against different epitopes (trastuzumab/pertuzumab.[38,39] Although this strategy evolved from observing incomplete signal transduction interruption with a single agent, the use of an antibody and a small molecule may have unexpected extra benefits,[40] especially since recent data suggest that some receptor kinases, such as EGFR, also signal through non-kinase pathways.[41] Also, mutations conferring drug resistance may produce conformational changes that result in reduced sensitivity to a given molecular targeted agent's inhibitory effect. In this case, combination therapy directed against the same target but with different drugs may inhibit multiple alternate conformational forms of the target. An example of success using this approach was combining imatinib and dasatinib, either given together or in sequence, as the primary treatment of chronic myelogenous leukemia.[42] A similar effect has been observed in treating *C-KIT*-mutated gastrointestinal stromal tumor (GIST).[43]

- Inhibiting sequential steps in a single pathway, which includes both upstream and downstream signals. The goal of this strategy is to interrupt signaling at its origin (the receptor), as well as disrupting the intermediate relays that amplify it (e.g., combining EGFR and mTOR inhibition.[44–46] This is the case with PI3K, which mediates the signaling of cell surface receptors such as HER2, EGFR, C-MET, or the insulin-like growth factor receptor. Blocking both the receptor and the downstream PI3K pathway may produce supra-additive effects.[47–49] This approach also has the benefit of overcoming known mechanisms of resistance (K-Ras mutations and sensitivity to EGFR inhibition[6]; phosphatase and tensin homolog (PTEN) loss and PI3K mutations and resistance to HER2-targeted therapies.[50] Additionally, two discrete cell populations may be targeted this way, i.e., HER2+ cells vs. p95HER2 cells, EGFR+ cells vs. EGFRvIII cells.[51–53]

- Combining a targeted agent and a modulator of the target. Some examples are the combined use of trastuzumab, crizotinib or imatinib, and an HSP90 inhibitor. HSP90 serves a chaperone function, protecting key intracellular proteins against degradation and inducing the folding of mutant proteins. In oncogene-addicted tumors (to HER2, ALK or C-Kit respectively), preclinical experiments have shown that inhibition of HSP90 blocks client proteins, with a subsequent rapid turnover and a synergistic effect with specific inhibitors.[27,36,54]

- Inhibiting different functional pathways (e.g., survival and angiogenesis) described as the "hallmarks of cancer" (acquired capabilities necessary for tumor growth and progression). Progress in molecular biology has elucidated the key mechanisms of tumorigenesis. At the same time, the biotechnology industry has developed inhibitors for a variety of these functions that contribute to the survival of most tumor cells. Therefore, co-targeting multiple core hallmark capabilities with drug combinations (i.e., an inhibitor of invasion/metastasis such as a cMET inhibitor, with an inhibitor of angiogenesis such as a VEFGR inhibitor) may result in more effective and durable therapies for human cancer.

- Empiric combinations or a "let the data talk" approach. This strategy is based on the fact that a clear understanding of how various molecular pathways interact is frequently lacking, and that combinations of effective drugs can be found by an empirical, high throughout analysis of compound libraries. An example is the use of a synthetic lethality paradigm, wherein cells are treated with an initial drug and an siRNA library is used to define potential targets for synergistic combinations.[55] Alternatively, one can limit the plethora of possible empirical combinations by mathematical modeling, such as directed discovery algorithms[56,57] where second generation combinations are built upon the results of a first set of agents tested, and so on.

- Cytotoxic enhancement or normal tissue protection. One agent modulates the repair of the damage performed by the second agent (Pi3K inhibitor and PARP inhibitor).[58] Or, additionally, one agent may reduce early/late side effects without compromising tumor control, that is, BRAF inhibitors and the reduction in skin tumors seen when combined with MEK inhibitors.[59]

## Combining Targeted and Immune Therapies

Generally, when combining targeted agents that inhibit signaling pathways, the rationale is based on biological cooperation whereby related pathways are inhibited, including intracellular signaling and feedback loops. In some other instances, combining targeted agents seeks the biological cooperation of unrelated mechanisms that the cancer cells need for survival. But there is also a case for "spatial cooperation," combining agents that target different cell populations such as immune cells and cancer cells or the stroma and cancer cells. During the last decades, significant advancement in cancer immune therapy has made combining immune therapy with anticancer targeted therapies possible.

The strategies that can be exploited include[60]:

- Additive effect of apoptosis induced after inhibition of the target in an oncogene-addicted tumor (BRAF and BRAF inhibitors) and cell-mediated cytotoxicity when T-cells are activated (CTL4 and ipilitumumab.[61,62]

- Targeted therapies such as trastuzumab can induce rapid tumor regression, with a consequent decrease in tumor-associated immunosuppression. This may allow a favorable window-of-opportunity for immunotherapy to achieve more potent cytotoxicity. This may also occur if targeted therapies only potentiate tumor cell senescence, facilitating tumor clearance by T cells.[47]

- The cell kill mediated by some drugs may release large amounts of cell debris containing antigens that can contribute to the activation of dendritic cells and the immune response.[63]
- Immunotherapy might consolidate the tumor responses that are achieved with targeted therapy into durable ones and reduce the risk of the emergence of potentially drug-resistant tumor cell clones.
- Some targeted agents may have indirect but beneficial effects on the immune system that can be exploited by combining them with agents that give intrinsic immunity an extra boost.[64] For example, bevacizumab seems to increase dendritic cell maturation, shifting differentiation toward mature dendritic cells instead of myeloid-derived suppressor cells, and increases priming of T cells, which could be exploited by combining bevacizumab with a specific antibody for cytotoxic T lymphocyte-associated antigen 4 (CTLA4). A similar response has been observed with cetuximab combined with vaccines.[65–69]
- Combining two agents that act on the immune system.[70] One agent may be a vaccine, and the other a coadjuvant agent that stimulates the immune system (granulocyte macrophage colony-stimulating factor (GMC-SF)).[71] Another example is to combine a vaccine with an enhancer of cell-mediated cytotoxicity (anti-PD-1 antibody).[72]
- These effects indicate that the timing, dose, and sequence of administration of the targeted therapy agent combined with immunotherapy need to be carefully investigated.[62]

## Preliminary Data: Building the Hypothesis and Rationale for the Trial

One key question that needs to be elucidated is when do we have enough information to provide an appropriate rationale for instituting a phase I trial?

Various lines of evidence can address that question:

1 **Literature based or rationale based on basic scientific theory.** Combinations are based on the different pathways that are relevant to cancer and the way they interact, as viewed by basic science, i.e., HER2 activation upregulates VEGF, so the combined inhibition of HER2 and VEGF is likely to be effective.[73] The main difficulty with this approach is that responses to genetic alterations and pharmacological inhibition of a pertinent protein product can diverge considerably,[74] so observations based on *in vitro* target downregulation cannot always be translated to pharmacological modulation without formal preclinical experimentation.

2 **Empirical approach.** A plus B act synergistically in a panel of diverse cell lines (chemosensitivity assays as in a combination high throughput screening platform –cHTSTM– or "COMBO-Plate"[75]) or synergism observed after screening a library composed of many combinations of compounds. The main difficulty with this approach is that the mechanism of action of targeted therapies may require testing in an animal model, rather than in isolated cell cultures, if the microenvironment or immunity is affected, and even in these cases, correlation between *in vivo* testing and the clinic is not that clear.

3 **Observation-based approach.** This approach is based on preclinical *in vitro* and *in vivo* tests of candidate drugs in different tumor models (cell lines, xenografts, orthotopic tumors, primary cultures, and animal models). The sequence of thought is: when we treat with A preclinically, we observe upregulation of X. B is an inhibitor of X. Preclinically A+B work synergistically. A

clinical trial of A+B is therefore justified (i.e., EGFR and IGFR inhibitors).[55] This is the most extensive approach, but currently, because most cell lines are well profiled, there is a great risk of biasing the results by selecting "adequate" models that "prove" the hypothesis, i.e., asking the answer.

4 **Highly sophisticated approach.** The rationale for this strategy is based on transgenic mice harboring specific mutations or engineered models with conditional expression or suppression of target genes. The main problem for drug development is that this kind of model, which is ideal for describing mechanisms of action, is vastly divergent from "real" tumors. There is thus a disjuncture between the bench and the bedside.

5 **Pragmatic approach.** This approach is based on clinical experience more than on results from preclinical assays. The progression of thought underlying this strategy is: A is active in a specific disease (at least in some cases). B is also active in the same disease (at least in some cases). A and B are well tolerated and do not appear to have overlapping toxicities, so A+B should be more efficient together than as single agents (or at least in more cases) and a trial is warranted (i.e., sorafenib plus temsirolimus in renal cell carcinoma).[76] The main difficulty with this approach is the risk of missing potentially beneficial activity in diseases for which A or B was not active as single agents. However, a significant advantage to this approach is that it is possible to impact the clinical setting in a short period of time.

## The Value of Preclinical *In Vivo* Models

Most of the sources of evidence used to build rationales underlying drug combinations are tested *in vivo* for the efficacy of the suggested combination. Other goals of *in vivo* testing include pharmacokinetic modeling (peak concentration, $C_{max}$; area under the concentration $\times$ time of elimination curve) and correlation with antitumor effect (pharmacokinetic/pharmacodynamics (PK/PD) modeling).

However, such *in vivo* models have many limitations when evaluating targeted agents,[77] that are especially relevant to drug combinations:

- Animal models that are used are immune tolerant (immunosuppressed) to allow the growth of the tumor. Because of this, the contribution of the immune system to targeted agents (trastuzumab) and the efficacy of vaccines or immune modulators and combinations cannot be studied (agents such as thalidomide, lenalidomide, aminolevulinic acid, and levamisole).[78] This is also important for safety evaluation. All protein formulations contain at least low levels of aggregates, which could modulate immune reactions in non-compromised subjects.[79]
- There may be important differences between the human and animal response derived from the lack of genetic diversity of the animals.
- The presence or structure of the target may vary between humans and animals. For example, mice and humans differ in the composition of the peptide and in the response of antigen-presenting cells to VEGF, and the immune effects of VEGF may be different when translating preclinical results into early clinical testing. Different analogous drugs should be used in each species, as was done with M Ab A.4.6.1 or bevacizumab.[16,80–82]
- Occasionally, resistance mechanisms or feedback loops cannot be modeled in animals, but only *in silico* or *in vitro*. Also, stroma–tumor interaction in humans and in xenografts cannot be compared.

In such cases, a pragmatic approach, with limited preclinical data but a strong rationale and perhaps single agent activity in the clinical setting of each drug, could be sufficient for testing a combination, thereby avoiding unnecessary and uninformative *in vivo* testing.

## First Step, Regulatory Issues to Consider Before a Hands-On Approach

Before clinical testing, a drug must be evaluated preclinically, and information about its pharmacology (pharmacokinetics and metabolism, pharmacodynamics, and toxicology in at least two different species) and efficacy must be appraised by the US Food and Drug Administration (FDA), a procedure that is, interestingly, not necessary for many drug combinations, or the European Medicine Agency (EMA).

Most regulatory documents used for guidance in the FDA process involve preclinical testing of a single agent, and the requirements for data needed to determine the initial doses to be tested in clinical trials can vary among regulatory bodies. Data should include the conduct of nonclinical safety studies of variable duration to assess the toxicity profile of the new chemical entity, reproduction toxicities (ICH S5 (R2) CPMP/ICH/386/95), and genotoxicitiy (ICH S2B R1 EMA CHMP/ICH126642/2008) studies. Sometimes, carcinogenic (ICH S1 CPMP/ICH/140/95) potential, immunotoxicity (ICH S8 CHMP/167235/2004), phototoxicity, juvenile animal toxicity, and abuse liability (ICH M3 R2 Note 6) assessments are also required. For anticancer pharmaceuticals, which need a more expeditious development procedure, ICH S9 facilitates and accelerates development by being more flexible in design and timing requirements for nonclinical studies (ICH S9 CHMP/ICH/646107/2008).

To streamline the nonclinical toxicity studies required to support clinical investigations, and to find a common ground across regulatory agencies, these requirements were revised in ICH guideline M3 and its two revisions of 1997 (R1) and 2008 (R2). But it quickly became clear that developing drug combinations in cancer needed special attention, especially when each drug had first been explored individually. The FDA's "Combination Rule" 21 CFR 300.50 refers to fixed combinations and required isolating the contribution of each agent to treatment effect through factorial designs (A vs. B vs. A+B). However, some phase II trials were initiated with full doses of each compound, without a run-in to assess the safety of the combination. This approach seems most feasible when the drugs have non-overlapping or few toxicities and is often safe and successful. Nonetheless, at times, unexpected serious toxicities have been encountered, e.g., several cases of microangiopathic hemolytic anemia in patients with solid tumors receiving bevacizumab and sunitinib were reported recently, and the FDA has shut down clinical trials testing this combination.

To address this particular setting, key players in drug development were consulted, including the FDA, representatives from pharmaceutical companies, well-known investigators and patient advocates. Following the conclusions from those meetings, the FDA issued a draft of the "Guidance for Industry Codevelopment of Two or More Unmarketed Investigational Drugs for Use in Combination" that has been sent for comments. This document reflects the different scenarios of drug combinations and defines different degrees of preclinical studies required to initiate clinical trials of a drug combination.

In order to coordinate regulatory policies, European and US agencies have exchanged information to conduct collaborative inspections through the Pilot EMA-FDA GCP initiative (EMA-FDA Pilot GCP initiative. 18 July 2011 EXT/INS/GCP/56289/2011).

The ultimate arbiter today for assessing the need for preclinical studies for combination treatment seems to be the reigning culture among different academic centers and Institutional Review Boards (IRB) that govern decisions about whether there is a sufficient rationale for and presumptive safety that warrants testing a combination. It appears clear that for many drugs, the clinical experience with each compound provides sufficient data to safely combine the drugs in the clinic, and to be a powerful predictor of efficacious rational drug combinations. Further, combining two or more drugs, each of which has activity in a specific type of cancer, often significantly improves response rates. Whether it does so because cumulative subsets of disease are impacted or because individuals with cancer have multiple aberrations, or both, remains unclear and may vary from tumor to tumor.

## Clinical Scenarios and Clinical Trial Design

Potential combinations of anticancer agents include varied permutations of experimental agents and/or standards of care (e.g., chemotherapy, targeted agents, and immunomodulators). Before clinical trials of combination therapies can be initiated, rational preclinical models should guide clinical trial design and will illuminate issues such as dosing regimens (administering two drugs concomitantly or sequentially), drug interactions affecting pharmacokinetics, and interactive toxic effects. The characteristics of the individual compounds and the patient population of interest should also influence the trial design.

### Clinical Scenarios

Phase I trials of targeted agent drug combinations are best served by utilizing new approaches that can improve efficiency and increase our understanding of how best to test agents in combination. Since it is clear that the characteristics of targeted therapies are very diverse, and consequently drug combinations are also multitudinous, no one-size-fits-all approach can be used in designing phase I trial.[83-85]

Conceptually, these different scenarios can be broken down into three classes of drug combinations that define specific drug development plans:

- **Scenario 1.** The combination of A + B demonstrates potential antitumor activity, but neither drug is active (or they are minimally active) as single agents. This is the case, for example, for combinations directed toward synthetic lethality (i.e., a PARP inhibitor plus a PI3K inhibitor (Kimbung, Biskup, et al.)). There are three important variables: the administration regimen (A with B, A before B, or B before A), the ratio of drug A to drug B, and dose of each drug in the combination. The development plan for the combination requires a phase I trial using a factorial design (since monotherapy makes no sense, one could do a short run-in with drug A, and then add B, so all patients receive the combination) followed by a phase II design with a fixed ratio and dose and concomitant administration (A+B) compared with the standard of care (SOC).
- **Scenario 2 (uni-enhancement).** Drug A is active, but potentially modulated by the administration of Drug B, which by itself is inactive. The minimally active agent's role frequently is to prevent resistance or inhibit redundant pathway activation (i.e., erlotinib plus a MET inhibitor, or letrozol plus a CDK 4/6).[33] Each drug should have been evaluated separately in a prior phase I trial. Then, the combination requires a phase I exploration where the dose of A is fixed and the dose of B is modulated, and vice versa,

to explore the influence of the inactive drug on the safety, efficacy, and pharmacodynamics of the active compound. Next, a randomized phase II design (A vs. AB vs. SOC) will further evaluate the combination.[86]

- **Scenario 3 (co-enhancement).** Both drugs are active independently, but the combination is expected to be more effective than either agent alone (i.e., trastuzumab or letrozole plus a PI3K inhibitor, a PI3K plus a MEK inhibitor).[87] A formal phase I trial of each drug is necessary prior to studying the combination. The phase I trial of the combination will be designed around a testable hypothesis such as: A and B can be given at full dose; A modulates the pharmacokinetics of B; A modulates the pharmacodynamics of B; or A increases the toxicity of B. If there is a possible pharmacodynamic interaction (e.g., one may increase the toxicity of the other), consider designing the trial so that patients receive one drug alone in the first treatment cycle, followed by the combination in subsequent cycles. The phase II trial should evaluate the effect of each drug and the combination (A vs. B vs. A+B vs. SOC).

A phase I trial might not be necessary under certain circumstances. Preclinical data may suggest that a pharmacokinetic interaction is unlikely, as indicated by *in vitro* studies and knowledge of the metabolism and transport mechanics of both drugs. In addition, a drug combination may progress directly into a phase II study if *in vivo* animal studies demonstrated that both drugs can be safely given together at the full doses without increased toxicity compared to monotherapy. If there is no formal phase I trial, the safety of the full dose of the combination should be tested as an initial cohort in the phase II study.

## Pharmacology and Drug–Drug Interactions

When selecting the most appropriate drugs for clinically testing a combination, it is important to consider the pharmacology of each drug, routes of delivery, and potential drug–drug interactions.

The interaction between two given drugs could be due to pharmacodynamic or pharmacokinetic interaction (via inhibition or induction of metabolic enzymes or transporters). The latter occurs when one drug influences the absorption, distribution, metabolism, and/or excretion of another. Today, it is common practice and FDA mandatory[88] to preclinically test potential drug interactions of novel combinations. Several *in vitro* methods assess drug interaction issues pertaining to transportation and enzyme inhibition and/or induction. The major paradigm shift in the field has been associated with the use of modern human tissue preparations such as human liver slices, freshly isolated human liver cells, primary culture of human hepatocytes, sub-cellular fractions such as microsomes, cytosol and S9 fractions, recombinant human enzymes (CYP and UGT), transgenic cell lines, and cell-based reporter assays (reviewed in References 89–91).

Still, the prediction of *in vivo* drug interactions from *in vitro* metabolic data remains highly controversial, since *in vitro* data do not necessarily translate directly into relative extents of inhibition *in vivo*. The assays referred to above, therefore, are more likely to be useful in halting further development of potentially problematic drug combinations if alternative ones are available.

Information regarding interaction of drugs with biologics, and with monoclonal antibodies in particular, is scarce, and a formal assessment of these types of relationships is inherently complicated. Drug–drug interactions are more frequent when combining two small molecules, than when a small molecule is combined with an antibody.[92,93] The explanation for this is that two small molecules

are more likely to share the same metabolic mechanisms (hepatic metabolism, renal excretion, and biliary excretion).

However, certain interactions between cytokines and small molecules and between therapeutic proteins and small molecules have been described,[94–96] and drug–drug interaction studies should be considered on a case-by-case basis.

## Obtaining Access to Clinical Trial Drugs

The importance of collaborations in developing combination therapies is key because of the inability of a single investigator or drug company to have the resources necessary to effectively and expediently confront the complex mechanisms by which cancer cells become resistant to treatment. Obtaining the desired drug(s) for the trial can be problematic due to the limited options surrounding approved targeted therapies. For one, in order for a drug to be approved in the first place, significant activity has to be demonstrated. This requires time, and also it may be difficult to prove the activity of single agents. For combining investigational agents, the Cancer Therapy Evaluation Program (CTEP) of the National Institutes of Health (NCI) has experimental access to some of these drugs and it has championed clinical trials combining targeted therapies.[97] Table 2.2 summarizes different sources of targeted therapies to be used in combination studies, especially those still in development.

## Clinical Trial Design for Exploring Drug Combinations

Trial design is another important consideration. The design of the clinical trial may be key for proof of concept ("hitting the target") or may eliminate, early in development, combinations that will eventually fail.

Since the realization that molecularly targeted therapies likely behave differently from classical cytotoxic chemotherapeutic agents, many proposals have advocated changing how early clinical trials are conducted, including their endpoints, when targeted therapies are being tested.[103] Some of these proposals have been incorporated into the design of phase I and phase II trials and have been successful. Still, the way that we perform combination trials has rarely changed, and few guidelines or proposals of novel designs for testing combinations have been discussed. In our organization, some of these proposals, with variations, are being considered for clinical trials (Figure 2.1).

- **Multiple permissible maximum tolerated doses.**[104] The model is a two-dimensional escalation matrix with many potential dose levels that can be explored sequentially, but with several cohorts potentially enrolling at the same time (Figure 2.1a). This design seems appropriate in clinical scenario 3 depicted above. In some cases, one could dose escalate both drugs at the same time (see diagonal orientation in Figure 2.1b), especially if no overlapping toxicities are expected. A more prudent variant is to increase the dose of each drug, one at a time like a staircase (Figure 2.1c). In any case, if there are toxicities that prevent further dose escalation in diagonal, alternative cohorts can be opened to explore high doses of drug A and low doses of drug B, or alternately, low doses of drug A and high doses of drug B, or intermediate doses of both drugs (Figure 2.1d). This dose escalation scheme allows the definition of several MTDs. A 3D model could be developed combining three drugs (i.e., bevacizumab/sorafenib/temsirolimus) with rules based on mechanism-related toxicities required to stop escalation in one of the directions (Figure 2.1f).

**Table 2.2** Potential sources of targeted drugs.

| Sources of targeted agents to combine | PRO/CON | Examples |
|---|---|---|
| Combining several approved drugs (sorafenib, lapatinib, decitabine, and others) | PRO: Available to any institution that would like to sponsor the trial<br>Academic freedom to explore combinations that may be interesting in indications that may not be profitable<br>CON: Extremely expensive trial if agents are not provided by pharmaceutical companies<br>Approval of a molecular targeted therapy requires single agent activity and much time<br>Possible combinations are very limited while there are many more biologically reasonable combinations | Bevacizumab plus temsirolimus<br>Erlotinib plus trastuzumab<br>Cetuximab, bevacizumab, and erlotinib[98] |
| Combining with drugs provided by National Institutes of Health (NCI) through the Cancer Therapy Evaluation Program (CTEP) | PRO: Combinations of an investigational MTA with other agents in settings that may not be in the development plan of companies are possible. Combinations of several investigational agents may be possible. NCI mentoring.<br>CON: Competitive<br>Although an agreement with the NCI and a pharmaceutical company is in place, the pharmaceutical company still has to approve the trial<br>Time-consuming and slow approval. NCI has a priority list of indications and combinations.<br>NCI-CTEP has limited agreements with pharmaceutical companies, and most of the available drugs may not be new drugs or the best-in-class | 17-Allyaminoglendanamycin (17 AAG) HSP-90 inhibitor and imatinib (commercially available)<br>Vorinostat and 5-Azacytidine (commercially available) |
| Combining with drugs approved for other indications (rapamycin, statins, PARP inhibitors, verapamil, COX2 inhibitors) | PRO: Drugs are available and cheap<br>CON: Drugs may not be the best ones for the inhibition of a specific target<br>Drugs approved for other indications that may have anticancer effects are limited | Erlotinib and celecoxib[99] |
| Combining drugs from the same sponsor | PRO: Pharmaceutical companies may be highly motivated. Quick design and organization of the trial. No economic or regulatory issues.<br>CON: Drug companies vary in the size of their pipeline. Drugs may be in different development phases. Available MTA may not be the best in-class. | Antiangiogenic agents such as AMG 386 (peptibody that inhibits angiopoietin 1 and 2) and AMG 706 (multi-kinase inhibitor targeting vascular endothelial growth factor (VEGF), platelet-derived growth factor (PDGF) and c-kit receptors) |
| Combining drugs from two related companies (in co-development or merging) | PRO: Pharmaceutical companies may be highly motivated. Quick design and organization of the trial.<br>CON: Royalty and patent issues may slow or limit the approval of the proposal. Available MTA may not be the best in-class. | MK0646 (IGF1R inhibitor from Merck) and deforolimus (AP23573 developed by Ariad and acquired by Merck) |
| Combining MTAs from different companies by designing an investigator-initiated co-development plan | PRO: All possible combinations could be explored.<br>CON: Time consuming. Regulatory, copyright, patent and royalty issues may be very difficult to overcome. Development plans from different companies may differ or even compete, in their drug development plans. | RAD001 and erlotinib[100]<br>RAD001 and trastuzumab |
| Combining with drugs that have been shelved (orphan or abandoned drugs such as farnesyltransferase inhibitors) | PRO: Drugs may be inexpensive and easy to obtain if development plans have been abandoned<br>CON: Drug supply may be an issue if production is not maintained | Tipifarnib and fulvestrant[101]<br>Tipifarnib and imatinib[102] |

MTA: molecular targeted therapy.

- The classical design is based on the most active drug being used as a backbone, with the other drug added in a sequential dose escalation scheme. Not all potential dose levels are explored since there is a pre-established prioritization of the most active drug (in Figure 2.1e, the most active drug would be drug B). This design fits better with the requirements of clinical scenario 2.

- Synergy finder. Here the treatment leads in with drug A and after assessment, drug B is added (Figure 2.1g). This design fits better with the requirements of clinical scenarios 1 and 2. Assessments at different time points (biomarker, efficacy, toxicity) are used to determine molecular synergy. If several drug candidates are to be evaluated, an arm for each combination can be developed and patients are allocated by adaptive randomization based on such assessments, for example, EGFR inhibitor plus dasatinib vs. EGFR inhibitor plus MET inhibitor with the endpoint being overcoming resistance to EGFR inhibitors.[105] A similar objective could be achieved with a phase 0 trial combining targeted therapies for biomarker testing. The doses of both drugs in the combination must be well known, and there must be no expectation of interaction among drugs, and the biomarker must already be validated.[106,107]

- Drug-resistance evaluation. In this clinical trial design, patients are treated with drug A. At disease progression, drug B can be added (Figure 2.1h). If several mechanisms of resistance are

evaluated, different combinations could be explored (A+B, A+C, A+D). This design can be used in clinical scenarios 2 and 3.
- Multiple agents compared in a single study also designated "complete phase I." Here, an array of different combinations, schedules, or timings are being assessed (Figure 2.1i). In this trial design, one drug could remain the same in each arm with the second drug being variable. In looking for comparisons of efficacy, an adaptive randomization scheme could explore multiple combinations or schedules in a rational way (Figure 2.1j).
- Histology-independent clinical trial. Patients are selected on the basis of the presence of a molecular marker, regardless of the anatomic origin of their tumor. This approach is based on

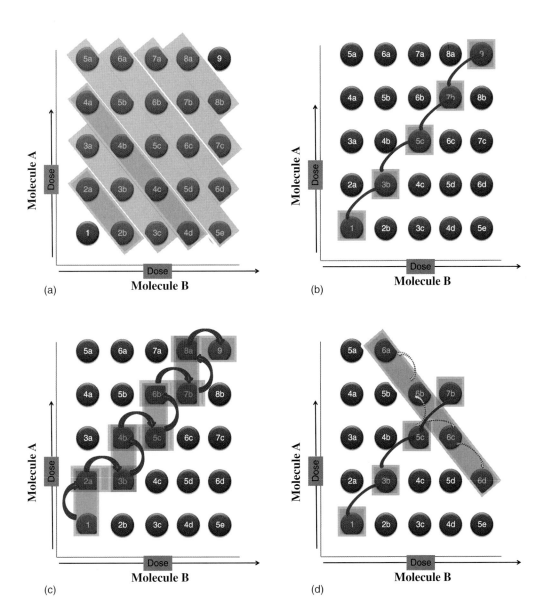

**Figure 2.1** Proposal of novel trial designs exploring combinations of targeted therapies. Combining two drugs depicts a 2D matrix of possible dose levels (a). In some cases, dose escalation can proceed without exploring all those potential dose levels; dose escalation can proceed in a diagonal orientation (b), by increasing the dose of each drug, one at a time like a staircase (c) or by starting at full doses of one drug and escalating the dose of the other (e). In case side effects are seen, dose escalation can diverge and several alternative cohorts can be opened (d), allowing exploration of multiple MTDs. In the case of combining 3 drugs, the matrix of dose levels is in 3D (f). In looking for synergy, one could begin with one drug, and after an assessment, the other one is added (g). When exploring the role of one drug for overcoming drug-resistance of the principal one, patients could be treated with the principal one and at disease progression, the second drug is added (h). Multiple combinations or schedules can be compared in a single study with or without an adaptive randomization methodology (i and j).

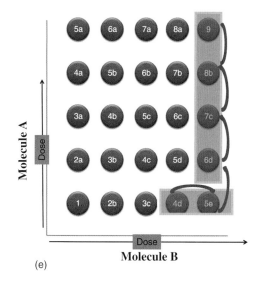

(e)

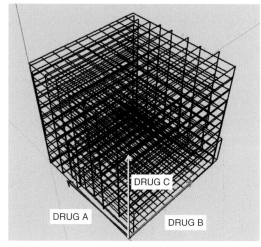

(f)

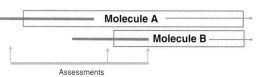

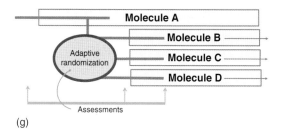

(g)

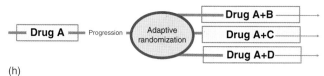

(h)

**Complete phase I study:**
**Multiple combinations compared in a single study**

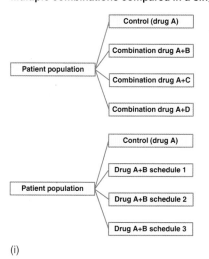

(i)

**Multiple combinations compared with adaptive randomization**

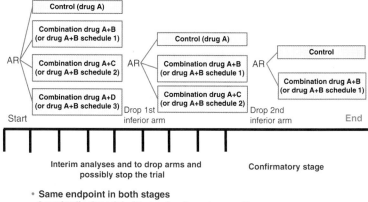

- Same endpoint in both stages
- Longitudinal model of tumor burden, etc. over time

AR: Adaptive randomization

(j)

Figure 2.1 (*Continued*)

the concept that tumors with a similar genetic background (and oncogene addiction) may respond similarly, and specific targeted therapies may be active in specific genetic backgrounds, i.e., mutation or amplifications in PI3K-alpha (mutations are frequent in breast and bowel cancers, while amplifications are present in more than 50% of ovarian, cervix, and lung cancers).[108–110] This approach is applicable to the study of single targeted agents, as well as combination regimens.

Early clinical trials are becoming an arena for hypothesis testing, and ideas such as mechanism(s) of action and proof of concept, optimal biologic dose, and the incorporation of pharmacodynamic endpoints will need to be incorporated into their designs. Whether these concepts change how we test drug combinations has yet to be shown.

## Conclusions

The ultimate design for demonstrating the efficacy of a drug or drug combination is the randomized controlled trial (RCT), which has important limitations. One can answer only a very limited number of questions per trial, such as the appropriate use of drugs or comparing various (but not many) drug regimens. Currently, in clinical trials the regimens to be compared are pre-set and patients are assigned to different arms randomly, regardless of their genetic drivers. "Personalized medicine," on the other hand, refers to tailoring medical treatment to the individual characteristics of each patient or tumor.[111] It is necessary to develop and validate markers for identifying patients who will benefit from particular interventions or to tailor therapeutic regimens to individual underlying variations in mutations and aberrations.[112,113] Parallel to molecular diagnosis is the requirement for the design of clinical trials to be flexible enough to study matching patient tumor molecular profiles with appropriate drug combinations that are targeted to specific patient subpopulations.[114,115]

Recent and continuing developments in high-throughput and multiplexed assay platforms, as well as in disciplines such as bioinformatics and biostatistics, will shape the future of clinical trials. Applying novel techniques in a comprehensive approach, based upon the interrelations among targets and the mechanisms of action underlying cancer (Systems Biology),[57,116,117] may lead to comprehensive diagnostic tools (Systems Pathology).[118] The era of molecular diagnosis is here, since whole genome sequencing in real time is a near reality.[119]

But even if we are able to define the molecular context of a tumor, we lack the ability to test the combination of more than two targeted drugs in a rational way. Even given numerous lines of evidence pointing to the need for combining agents directed at several (more than three) targets in order to get a meaningful antitumor effect,[120,121] how best to clinically test the inhibition of multiple targets remains largely empirical. Designing and testing combinations of multiple drugs (cocktails of monoclonal antibodies [MoAbs], or RNA therapeutics, and others) will require innovation in regulatory and clinical trial design in the future.

## References

1 Bosset JF, Collette L, Calais G, et al. Chemotherapy with preoperative radiotherapy in rectal cancer. *N Engl J Med*. 2006;355(11):1114–1123.

2 Hurwitz H, Fehrenbacher L, Novotny W, et al. Bevacizumab plus irinotecan, fluorouracil, and leucovorin for metastatic colorectal cancer. *N Engl J Med*. 2004;350(23):2335–2342.

3 Klijn JG, Beex LV, Mauriac L, et al. Combined treatment with buserelin and tamoxifen in premenopausal metastatic breast cancer: a randomized study. *J Natl Cancer Inst*. 2000;92(11):903–911.

4 O'Brien SG, Guilhot F, Larson RA, et al. Imatinib compared with interferon and low-dose cytarabine for newly diagnosed chronic-phase chronic myeloid leukemia. *N Engl J Med*. 2003;348(11):994–1004.

5 Slamon DJ, Leyland-Jones B, Shak S, et al. Use of chemotherapy plus a monoclonal antibody against HER2 for metastatic breast cancer that overexpresses HER2. *N Engl J Med*. 2001;344(11):783–792.

6 Amado RG, Wolf M, Peeters M, et al. Wild-type KRAS is required for panitumumab efficacy in patients with metastatic colorectal cancer. *J Clin Oncol*. 2008;26(10):1626–1634.

7 Di Nicolantonio F, Martini M, Molinari F, et al. Wild-type BRAF is required for response to panitumumab or cetuximab in metastatic colorectal cancer. *J Clin Oncol*. 2008;26(35):5705–5712.

8 Seidman AD, Berry D, Cirrincione C, et al. Randomized phase III trial of weekly compared with every-3-weeks paclitaxel for metastatic breast cancer, with trastuzumab for all HER-2 overexpressors and random assignment to trastuzumab or not in HER-2 nonoverexpressors: final results of Cancer and Leukemia Group B protocol 9840. *J Clin Oncol*. 2008;26(10):1642–1649.

9 Heinrich MC, Owzar K, Corless CL, et al. Correlation of kinase genotype and clinical outcome in the North American Intergroup Phase III Trial of imatinib mesylate for treatment of advanced gastrointestinal stromal tumor: CALGB 150105 Study by Cancer and Leukemia Group B and Southwest Oncology Group. *J Clin Oncol*. 2008;26(33):5360–5367.

10 Poulikakos PI, Persaud Y, Janakiraman M, et al. RAF inhibitor resistance is mediated by dimerization of aberrantly spliced BRAF(V600E). *Nature*. 2011;480(7377):387–390.

11 Yauch RL, Dijkgraaf GJ, Alicke B, et al. Smoothened mutation confers resistance to a Hedgehog pathway inhibitor in medulloblastoma. *Science*. 2009;326(5952):572–574.

12 Eichhorn PJ, Gili M, Scaltriti M, et al. Phosphatidylinositol 3-kinase hyperactivation results in lapatinib resistance that is reversed by the mTOR/phosphatidylinositol 3-kinase inhibitor NVP-BEZ235. *Cancer Res*. 2008;68(22):9221–9230.

13 Nazarian R, Shi H, Wang Q, et al. Melanomas acquire resistance to B-RAF(V600E) inhibition by RTK or N-RAS upregulation. *Nature*. 2010;468(7326):973–977.

14 Prahallad A, Sun C, Huang S, et al. Unresponsiveness of colon cancer to BRAF(V600E) inhibition through feedback activation of EGFR. *Nature*. 2012;483(7387):100–103.

15 Serra V, Scaltriti M, Prudkin L, et al. PI3K inhibition results in enhanced HER signaling and acquired ERK dependency in HER2-overexpressing breast cancer. *Oncogene*. 2011;30(22):2547–2557.

16 Block MS, Nevala WK, Leontovich AA, Markovic SN. Differential response of human and mouse dendritic cells to VEGF determines interspecies discrepancies in tumor-mediated TH1/TH2 polarity shift. *Clin Cancer Res*. 2011;17(7):1776–1783.

17 Villanueva J, Vultur A, Lee JT, et al. Acquired resistance to BRAF inhibitors mediated by a RAF kinase switch in melanoma can be overcome by cotargeting MEK and IGF-1R/PI3K. *Cancer Cell*. 2010;18(6):683–695.

18 Stommel JM, Kimmelman AC, Ying H, et al. Coactivation of receptor tyrosine kinases affects the response of tumor cells to targeted therapies. *Science*. 2007;318(5848):287–290.

19 Adams J. The proteasome: a suitable antineoplastic target. *Nat Rev Cancer*. 2004;4(5):349–360.

20 Goetz MP, Toft DO, Ames MM, Erlichman C. The Hsp90 chaperone complex as a novel target for cancer therapy. *Ann Oncol.* 2003;14(8):1169–1176.

21 Mork CN, Faller DV, Spanjaard RA. A mechanistic approach to anticancer therapy: targeting the cell cycle with histone deacetylase inhibitors. *Curr Pharm Des.* 2005;11(9):1091–1104.

22 Apsel B, Blair JA, Gonzalez B, et al. Targeted polypharmacology: discovery of dual inhibitors of tyrosine and phosphoinositide kinases. *Nat Chem Biol.* 2008;4(11):691–699.

23 Kiewe P, Hasmuller S, Kahlert S, et al. Phase I trial of the trifunctional anti-HER2 x anti-CD3 antibody ertumaxomab in metastatic breast cancer. *Clin Cancer Res.* 2006;12(10):3085–3091.

24 Lu D, Zhang H, Koo H, et al. A fully human recombinant IgG-like bispecific antibody to both the epidermal growth factor receptor and the insulin-like growth factor receptor for enhanced antitumor activity. *J Biol Chem.* 2005;280(20):19665–19672.

25 Boersma YL, Pluckthun A. DARPins and other repeat protein scaffolds: advances in engineering and applications. *Curr Opin Biotechnol.* 2011;22(6):849–857.

26 Stumpp MT, Binz HK, Amstutz P. DARPins: a new generation of protein therapeutics. *Drug Discov Today.* 2008;13(15–16):695–701.

27 Bauer S, Yu LK, Demetri GD, Fletcher JA. Heat shock protein 90 inhibition in imatinib-resistant gastrointestinal stromal tumor. *Cancer Res.* 2006;66(18):9153–9161.

28 Kurzrock R, Sherman SI, Ball DW, et al. Activity of XL184 (Cabozantinib), an oral tyrosine kinase inhibitor, in patients with medullary thyroid cancer. *J Clin Oncol.* 2011;29(19):2660–2666.

29 Catenacci DV, Henderson L, Xiao SY, et al. Durable complete response of metastatic gastric cancer with anti-Met therapy followed by resistance at recurrence. *Cancer Discov.* 2011;1(7):573–579.

30 Parulekar WR, Eisenhauer EA. Phase I trial design for solid tumor studies of targeted, non-cytotoxic agents: theory and practice. *J Natl Cancer Inst.* 2004;96(13):990–997.

31 Takimoto C. Principles of oncologic pharmacotherapy. In: Pazdur R, Coia LR, Hoskins WJ, Wagman LD, eds. *Cancer Management: A Multidisciplinary Approach,* 10th Ed. Darien, CT: CMP Medica; 2007.

32 Kwak EL, Clark JW, Chabner B. Targeted agents: the rules of combination. *Clin Cancer Res.* 2007;13(18 Pt 1):5232–5237.

33 Engelman JA, Zejnullahu K, Mitsudomi T, et al. MET amplification leads to gefitinib resistance in lung cancer by activating ERBB3 signaling. *Science.* 2007;316(5827):1039–1043.

34 Wee S, Jagani Z, Xiang KX, et al. PI3K pathway activation mediates resistance to MEK inhibitors in KRAS mutant cancers. *Cancer Res.* 2009;69(10):4286–4293.

35 Yu K, Toral-Barza L, Shi C, Zhang WG, Zask A. Response and determinants of cancer cell susceptibility to PI3K inhibitors: combined targeting of PI3K and Mek1 as an effective anticancer strategy. *Cancer Biol Ther.* 2008;7(2):307–315.

36 Modi S, Stopeck AT, Gordon MS, et al. Combination of trastuzumab and tanespimycin (17-AAG, KOS-953) is safe and active in trastuzumab-refractory HER-2 overexpressing breast cancer: a phase I dose-escalation study. *J Clin Oncol.* 2007;25(34):5410–5417.

37 Huang S, Armstrong EA, Benavente S, Chinnaiyan P, Harari PM. Dual-agent molecular targeting of the epidermal growth factor receptor (EGFR): combining anti-EGFR antibody with tyrosine kinase inhibitor. *Cancer Res.* 2004;64(15):5355–5362.

38 Baselga J, Bradbury I, Eidtmann H, et al. Lapatinib with trastuzumab for HER2-positive early breast cancer (NeoALTTO): a randomised, open-label, multicentre, phase 3 trial. *Lancet.* 2012;379(9816):633–640.

39 Nahta R, Hung MC, Esteva FJ. The HER-2-targeting antibodies trastuzumab and pertuzumab synergistically inhibit the survival of breast cancer cells. *Cancer Res.* 2004;64(7):2343–2346.

40 Scaltriti M, Verma C, Guzman M, et al. Lapatinib, a HER2 tyrosine kinase inhibitor, induces stabilization and accumulation of HER2 and potentiates trastuzumab-dependent cell cytotoxicity. *Oncogene.* 2009;28(6):803–814.

41 Weihua Z, Tsan R, Huang WC, et al. Survival of cancer cells is maintained by EGFR independent of its kinase activity. *Cancer Cell.* 2008;13(5):385–393.

42 Guilhot F, Apperley J, Kim DW, et al. Dasatinib induces significant hematologic and cytogenetic responses in patients with imatinib-resistant or -intolerant chronic myeloid leukemia in accelerated phase. *Blood.* 2007;109(10):4143–4150.

43 Demetri GD, van Oosterom AT, Garrett CR, et al. Efficacy and safety of sunitinib in patients with advanced gastrointestinal stromal tumour after failure of imatinib: a randomised controlled trial. *Lancet.* 2006;368(9544):1329–1338.

44 Bianco R, Garofalo S, Rosa R, et al. Inhibition of mTOR pathway by everolimus cooperates with EGFR inhibitors in human tumours sensitive and resistant to anti-EGFR drugs. *Br J Cancer.* 2008;98(5):923–930.

45 Buck E, Eyzaguirre A, Brown E, et al. Rapamycin synergizes with the epidermal growth factor receptor inhibitor erlotinib in non-small-cell lung, pancreatic, colon, and breast tumors. *Mol Cancer Ther.* 2006;5(11):2676–2684.

46 Ramalingam S, Forster J, Naret C, et al. Dual inhibition of the epidermal growth factor receptor with cetuximab, an IgG1 monoclonal antibody, and gefitinib, a tyrosine kinase inhibitor, in patients with refractory non-small cell lung cancer (NSCLC): a phase I study. *J Thorac Oncol.* 2008;3(3):258–264.

47 Disis ML, Wallace DR, Gooley TA, et al. Concurrent trastuzumab and HER2/neu-specific vaccination in patients with metastatic breast cancer. *J Clin Oncol.* 2009;27(28):4685–4692.

48 Ma PC, Schaefer E, Christensen JG, Salgia R. A selective small molecule c-MET Inhibitor, PHA665752, cooperates with rapamycin. *Clin Cancer Res.* 2005;11(6):2312–2319.

49 O'Reilly KE, Rojo F, She QB, et al. mTOR inhibition induces upstream receptor tyrosine kinase signaling and activates Akt. *Cancer Res.* 2006;66(3):1500–1508.

50 Berns K, Horlings HM, Hennessy BT, et al. A functional genetic approach identifies the PI3K pathway as a major determinant of trastuzumab resistance in breast cancer. *Cancer Cell.* 2007;12(4):395–402.

51 Ji H, Zhao X, Yuza Y, et al. Epidermal growth factor receptor variant III mutations in lung tumorigenesis and sensitivity to tyrosine kinase inhibitors. *Proc Natl Acad Sci U S A.* 2006;103(20):7817–7822.

52 Mellinghoff IK, Wang MY, Vivanco I, et al. Molecular determinants of the response of glioblastomas to EGFR kinase inhibitors. *N Engl J Med.* 2005;353(19):2012–2024.

53 Scaltriti M, Rojo F, Ocana A, et al. Expression of p95HER2, a truncated form of the HER2 receptor, and response to anti-HER2 therapies in breast cancer. *J Natl Cancer Inst.* 2007;99(8):628–638.

54 Modi S, Stopeck A, Linden H, et al. HSP90 inhibition is effective in breast cancer: a phase II trial of tanespimycin (17-AAG) plus trastuzumab in patients with HER2-positive metastatic breast cancer progressing on trastuzumab. *Clin Cancer Res.* 2011;17(15):5132–5139.

55 Iglehart JD, Silver DP. Synthetic lethality—a new direction in cancer-drug development. *N Engl J Med.* 2009;361(2):189–191.

56 Miller JZR, Barrett B. Directed discovery of novel drug cocktails. Santa Fe Institute Working Paper 05-07-031; 2005.

57 Nelander S, Wang W, Nilsson B, et al. Models from experiments: combinatorial drug perturbations of cancer cells. *Mol Syst Biol.* 2008;4:216.

58 Kimbung S, Biskup E, Johansson I, et al. Co-targeting of the PI3K pathway improves the response of BRCA1 deficient breast cancer cells to PARP1 inhibition. *Cancer Lett.* 2012;319(2):232–241.

59 Flaherty KT, Infante JR, Daud A, et al. Combined BRAF and MEK inhibition in melanoma with BRAF V600 mutations. *N Engl J Med.* 2012;367(18):1694–1703.

60 Vanneman M, Dranoff G. Combining immunotherapy and targeted therapies in cancer treatment. *Nat Rev Cancer.* 2012;12(4):237–251.

61 Boni A, Cogdill AP, Dang P, et al. Selective BRAFV600E inhibition enhances T-cell recognition of melanoma without affecting lymphocyte function. *Cancer Res.* 2010;70(13):5213–5219.

62 Ribas A, Hodi FS, Callahan M, Konto C, Wolchok J. Hepatotoxicity with combination of vemurafenib and ipilimumab. *N Engl J Med.* 2013;368(14):1365–1366.

63 Chakraborty M, Abrams SI, Coleman CN, Camphausen K, Schlom J, Hodge JW. External beam radiation of tumors alters phenotype of tumor cells to render them susceptible to vaccine-mediated T-cell killing. *Cancer Res.* 2004;64(12):4328–4337.

64 Pedersen AE, Buus S, Claesson MH. Treatment of transplanted CT26 tumour with dendritic cell vaccine in combination with blockade of vascular endothelial growth factor receptor 2 and CTLA-4. *Cancer Lett.* 2006;235(2):229–238.

65 Araki K, Turner AP, Shaffer VO, et al. mTOR regulates memory CD8 T-cell differentiation. *Nature.* 2009;460(7251):108–112.

66 Correale P, Botta C, Cusi MG, et al. Cetuximab +/− chemotherapy enhances dendritic cell-mediated phagocytosis of colon cancer cells and ignites a highly efficient colon cancer antigen-specific cytotoxic T-cell response in vitro. *Int J Cancer.* 2012;130(7):1577–1589.

67 Hsu YF, Ajona D, Corrales L, et al. Complement activation mediates cetuximab inhibition of non-small cell lung cancer tumor growth in vivo. *Mol Cancer.* 2010;9:139.

68 Yao S, Zhu Y, Chen L. Advances in targeting cell surface signalling molecules for immune modulation. *Nat Rev Drug Discov.* 2013;12(2):130–146.

69 McNeel DG, Smith HA, Eickhoff JC, et al. Phase I trial of tremelimumab in combination with short-term androgen deprivation in patients with PSA-recurrent prostate cancer. *Cancer Immunol Immunother.* 2012;61(7):1137–1147.

70 Wolchok JD, Kluger H, Callahan MK, et al. Nivolumab plus ipilimumab in advanced melanoma. *N Engl J Med.* 2013;369(2):122–133.

71 Jaffee EM, Hruban RH, Biedrzycki B, et al. Novel allogeneic granulocyte-macrophage colony-stimulating factor-secreting tumor vaccine for pancreatic cancer: a phase I trial of safety and immune activation. *J Clin Oncol.* 2001;19(1):145–156.

72 Flies DB, Sandler BJ, Sznol M, Chen L. Blockade of the B7-H1/PD-1 pathway for cancer immunotherapy. *Yale J Biol Med.* 2011;84(4):409–421.

73 Wen XF, Yang G, Mao W, et al. HER2 signaling modulates the equilibrium between pro- and antiangiogenic factors via distinct pathways: implications for HER2-targeted antibody therapy. *Oncogene.* 2006;25(52):6986–6996.

74 Weiss WA, Taylor SS, Shokat KM. Recognizing and exploiting differences between RNAi and small-molecule inhibitors. *Nat Chem Biol.* 2007;3(12):739–744.

75 Lehar J, Krueger AS, Avery W, et al. Synergistic drug combinations tend to improve therapeutically relevant selectivity. *Nat Biotechnol.* 2009;27(7):659–666.

76 Molina AM, Feldman DR, Voss MH, et al. Phase 1 trial of everolimus plus sunitinib in patients with metastatic renal cell carcinoma. *Cancer.* 2012;118(7):1868–1876.

77 Becher OJ, Holland EC. Genetically engineered models have advantages over xenografts for preclinical studies. *Cancer Res.* 2006;66(7):3355–3358, discussion 8–9.

78 Holbeck SL, Collins JM, Doroshow JH. Analysis of Food and Drug Administration-approved anticancer agents in the NCI60 panel of human tumor cell lines. *Mol Cancer Ther.* 2010;9(5):1451–1460.

79 Brinks V, Jiskoot W, Schellekens H. Immunogenicity of therapeutic proteins: the use of animal models. *Pharm Res.* 2011;28(10):2379–2385.

80 Ferrara N, Hillan KJ, Gerber HP, Novotny W. Discovery and development of bevacizumab, an anti-VEGF antibody for treating cancer. *Nat Rev Drug Discov.* 2004;3(5):391–400.

81 Gerber HP, Kowalski J, Sherman D, Eberhard DA, Ferrara N. Complete inhibition of rhabdomyosarcoma xenograft growth and neovascularization requires blockade of both tumor and host vascular endothelial growth factor. *Cancer Res.* 2000;60(22):6253–6258.

82 Presta LG, Chen H, O'Connor SJ, et al. Humanization of an anti-vascular endothelial growth factor monoclonal antibody for the therapy of solid tumors and other disorders. *Cancer Res.* 1997;57(20):4593–4599.

83 Clark A, Ellis M, Erlichman C, Lutzker S, Zwiebel J. Development of rational drug combinations with investigational targeted agents. *Oncologist.* 2010;15(5):496–499.

84 Hamberg P, Ratain MJ, Lesaffre E, Verweij J. Dose-escalation models for combination phase I trials in oncology. *Eur J Cancer.* 2010;46(16):2870–2878.

85 Humphrey RW, Brockway-Lunardi LM, Bonk DT, et al. Opportunities and challenges in the development of experimental drug combinations for cancer. *J Natl Cancer Inst.* 2011;103(16):1222–1226.

86 Seymour L, Ivy SP, Sargent D, et al. The design of phase II clinical trials testing cancer therapeutics: consensus recommendations from the clinical trial design task force of the national cancer institute investigational drug steering committee. *Clin Cancer Res.* 2010;16(6):1764–1769.

87 Shimizu T, Tolcher AW, Papadopoulos KP, et al. The clinical effect of the dual-targeting strategy involving PI3K/AKT/mTOR and RAS/MEK/ERK pathways in patients with advanced cancer. *Clin Cancer Res.* 2012;18(8):2316–2325.

88 Zhang L, Zhang YD, Zhao P, Huang SM. Predicting drug-drug interactions: an FDA perspective. *Aaps J.* 2009;11(2):300–306.

89 Aszalos A. Drug–drug interactions affected by the transporter protein, P-glycoprotein (ABCB1, MDR1) I. Preclinical aspects. *Drug Discov Today.* 2007;12(19–20):833–837.

90 Gomez-Lechon MJ, Donato MT, Castell JV, Jover R. Human hepatocytes in primary culture: the choice to investigate drug metabolism in man. *Curr Drug Metab.* 2004;5(5):443–462.

91 Hariparsad N, Sane RS, Strom SC, Desai PB. In vitro methods in human drug biotransformation research: implications for cancer chemotherapy. *Toxicol In Vitro.* 2006;20(2):135–153.

92 Dirks NL, Meibohm B. Population pharmacokinetics of therapeutic monoclonal antibodies. *Clin Pharmacokinet.* 2010;49(10):633–659.

93 Herbst RS, Johnson DH, Mininberg E, et al. Phase I/II trial evaluating the anti-vascular endothelial growth factor monoclonal antibody bevacizumab in combination with the HER-1/epidermal growth factor receptor tyrosine kinase inhibitor erlotinib for patients with recurrent non-small-cell lung cancer. *J Clin Oncol.* 2005;23(11):2544–2555.

94 Huang SM, Zhao H, Lee JI, et al. Therapeutic protein–drug interactions and implications for drug development. *Clin Pharmacol Ther.* 2010;87(4):497–503.

95 Lee JI, Zhang L, Men AY, Kenna LA, Huang SM. CYP-mediated therapeutic protein–drug interactions: clinical findings, proposed mechanisms and regulatory implications. *Clin Pharmacokinet.* 2010;49(5):295–310.

96  Schmitt C, Kuhn B, Zhang X, Kivitz AJ, Grange S. Disease—drug–drug interaction involving tocilizumab and simvastatin in patients with rheumatoid arthritis. *Clin Pharmacol Ther*. 2011;89(5):735–740.

97  Goldman B. For investigational targeted drugs, combination trials pose challenges. *J Natl Cancer Inst*. 2003;95(23):1744–1746.

98  Lin CC, Calvo E, Papadopoulos KP, et al. Phase I study of cetuximab, erlotinib, and bevacizumab in patients with advanced solid tumors. *Cancer Chemother Pharmacol*. 2009;63(6):1065–1071.

99  Reckamp KL, Krysan K, Morrow JD, et al. A phase I trial to determine the optimal biological dose of celecoxib when combined with erlotinib in advanced non-small cell lung cancer. *Clin Cancer Res*. 2006;12(11 Pt 1):3381–3388.

100  Johnson BE, Jackman D, Janne PA. Rationale for a phase I trial of erlotinib and the mammalian target of rapamycin inhibitor everolimus (RAD001) for patients with relapsed non small cell lung cancer. *Clin Cancer Res*. 2007;13(15 Pt 2):s4628–s4631.

101  Li T, Christos PJ, Sparano JA, et al. Phase II trial of the farnesyltransferase inhibitor tipifarnib plus fulvestrant in hormone receptor-positive metastatic breast cancer: New York Cancer Consortium Trial P6205. *Ann Oncol*. 2009;20(4):642–647.

102  Cortes J, Quintas-Cardama A, Garcia-Manero G, et al. Phase 1 study of tipifarnib in combination with imatinib for patients with chronic myelogenous leukemia in chronic phase after imatinib failure. *Cancer*. 2007;110(9):2000–2006.

103  El-Maraghi RH, Eisenhauer EA. Review of phase II trial designs used in studies of molecular targeted agents: outcomes and predictors of success in phase III. *J Clin Oncol*. 2008;26(8):1346–1354.

104  Braun TM, Alonzo TA. Beyond the 3+3 method: expanded algorithms for dose- escalation in phase I oncology trials of two agents. *Clin Trials*. 2011;8(3):247–259.

105  Xu L, Kikuchi E, Xu C, et al. Combined EGFR/MET or EGFR/HSP90 inhibition is effective in the treatment of lung cancers codriven by mutant EGFR containing T790M and MET. *Cancer Res*. 2012;72(13):3302–3311.

106  Doroshow JH, Parchment RE. Oncologic phase 0 trials incorporating clinical pharmacodynamics: from concept to patient. *Clin Cancer Res*. 2008;14(12):3658–3663.

107  Kummar S, Kinders R, Rubinstein L, et al. Compressing drug development timelines in oncology using phase "0" trials. *Nat Rev Cancer*. 2007;7(2):131–139.

108  Bertelsen BI, Steine SJ, Sandvei R, Molven A, Laerum OD. Molecular analysis of the PI3K-AKT pathway in uterine cervical neoplasia: frequent PIK3CA amplification and AKT phosphorylation. *Int J Cancer*. 2006;118(8):1877–1883.

109  Levine DA, Bogomolniy F, Yee CJ, et al. Frequent mutation of the PIK3CA gene in ovarian and breast cancers. *Clin Cancer Res*. 2005;11(8):2875–2878.

110  Samuels Y, Wang Z, Bardelli A, et al. High frequency of mutations of the PIK3CA gene in human cancers. *Science*. 2004;304(5670):554.

111  Woodcock J. The prospects for "personalized medicine" in drug development and drug therapy. *Clin Pharmacol Ther*. 2007;81(2):164–169.

112  Frank R, Hargreaves R. Clinical biomarkers in drug discovery and development. *Nat Rev Drug Discov*. 2003;2(7):566–580.

113  Peck RW. Driving earlier clinical attrition: if you want to find the needle, burn down the haystack. Considerations for biomarker development. *Drug Discov Today*. 2007;12(7–8):289–294.

114  Tsimberidou AM, Iskander NG, Hong DS, et al. Personalized medicine in a phase I clinical trials program: the MD Anderson Cancer Center initiative. *Clin Cancer Res*. 2012;18(22):6373–6383.

115  Von Hoff DD, Stephenson JJ Jr., Rosen P, et al. Pilot study using molecular profiling of patients' tumors to find potential targets and select treatments for their refractory cancers. *J Clin Oncol*. 2010;28(33):4877–4883.

116  van der Greef J, Hankemeier T, McBurney RN. Metabolomics-based systems biology and personalized medicine: moving towards n = 1 clinical trials? *Pharmacogenomics*. 2006;7(7):1087–1094.

117  Verhaak RG, Hoadley KA, Purdom E, et al. Integrated genomic analysis identifies clinically relevant subtypes of glioblastoma characterized by abnormalities in PDGFRA, IDH1, EGFR, and NF1. *Cancer Cell*. 2010;17(1):98–110.

118  Saidi O, Cordon-Cardo C, Costa J. Technology insight: will systems pathology replace the pathologist? *Nat Clin Pract Urol*. 2007;4(1):39–45.

119  Sundquist A, Ronaghi M, Tang H, Pevzner P, Batzoglou S. Whole-genome sequencing and assembly with high-throughput, short-read technologies. *PLoS ONE*. 2007;2(5):e484.

120  Takahashi K, Tanabe K, Ohnuki M, et al. Induction of pluripotent stem cells from adult human fibroblasts by defined factors. *Cell*. 2007;131(5):861–872.

121  Yu J, Vodyanik MA, Smuga-Otto K, et al. Induced pluripotent stem cell lines derived from human somatic cells. *Science*. 2007;318(5858):1917–1920.

## CHAPTER 3

# Principles of Targeted Immunotherapy

*Susanne H.C. Baumeister[1,2] and Glenn Dranoff[3,4]*

[1]Department of Pediatric Oncology, Dana-Farber Cancer Institute, Boston, MA
[2]Division of Hematology-Oncology, Boston Children's Hospital, Harvard Medical School, Boston, MA
[3]Department of Medicine, Harvard Medical School, Boston, MA, USA
[4]Human Gene Transfer Laboratory Core, Dana-Farber Cancer Institute, Boston, MA, USA

## Introduction

While the immune system's evolution to fight pathogens is universally recognized, the natural propensity for antitumor immunity had been a subject of debate for many years. However, there is now a wealth of compelling evidence that the immune system has an important role in controlling cancer, both from studies in mice[1,2] and humans.[3] Apart from numerous reports on tumor rejection by T cells in animal models, the presence of T cells inside tumors can significantly correlate with overall survival, as shown for patients with non-Hodgkin lymphoma (NHL)[4] and colon cancer.[5] It is also well established that tumors have evolved to develop an immunosuppressive microenvironment. In this process, called immunoediting,[6] cancer cells develop immune escape mechanisms that predominantly interfere with antigen presentation, T-cell activation, and differentiation, gradually leading to a loss of control by T cells.[7] Compelling evidence of tumor immunosurveillance in humans is provided by paraneoplastic diseases, which are neurological disorders manifesting as an autoimmune consequence of an antitumor response, reports of rare spontaneous tumor regressions in melanoma and renal cell carcinoma,[8] particularly following infection,[9] and the higher incidence of melanoma in patients on chronic pharmacological immunosuppression following organ transplantation.[10] It is also clear from an expanding body of preclinical and clinical experiences that the immune system can be manipulated in increasingly sophisticated ways to prevent, control, or aid in the control of established cancers.

The pursuit of successfully targeted immunotherapy relies on careful consideration of the appropriate target antigen and the quality of pre-existing immunological memory. Tumor-associated antigens (TAAs) that are unique to the tumor and not expressed on healthy tissues often require priming of the immune system, but are advantageous since an induced immune response toward the tumor is unlikely to have autoimmune side effects. Antigens that are over-expressed on tumor cells, but also present on some healthy tissues, might have led to depletion of high-avidity clones through negative selection and have polarized existing memory T cells (Tm) toward tolerance. Effective immunotherapy in this scenario requires breaking of tolerance and possibly induction of undesired autoimmunity. While clinical application of immunotherapy as a standard of care

was limited to the use of monoclonal antibodies (mAb), cytokines, and bone marrow transplantation for decades, cancer immunotherapy is now entering an exciting new era, with FDA approval of the first cancer vaccine (Sipuleucel -T) in castration-resistant metastatic prostate cancer (mCRPC) and anti-CTLA-4 mAb for the treatment of melanoma (Table 3.1).

## Principles of Immunotherapy

### Hematopoietic stem cell transplantation

Allogeneic hematopoietic stem cell transplantation (HSCT) is a well-established curative treatment for many hematologic malignancies. In conventional HSCT, patients receive myeloablative preparative chemotherapy regimens with or without total body irradiation to eliminate residual tumor cells and suppress host immunity in order to prevent rejection of donor hematopoietic stem cells. While the conditioning regimen is important, immune reconstitution and immune recognition of residual tumor cells by donor cells in a process termed graft-versus-leukemia (GVL) is critical for eradication of tumor cells and long-term cure. This was shown poignantly by PCR-based evaluation of bcr/abl transcripts in 92 chronic myeloid leukemia (CML) patients, where 80% of patients still had detectable bcr/abl transcripts within 6 months after transplant. Six to twelve months after transplant, 88% of patients receiving a T-cell depleted transplant remained PCR positive compared to 30% who received unmodified marrow.[11] Contrary to the patient's own immune cells, donor cells are not tolerant to tumor cells and may recognize tumor cells through expression of TAAs as well as minor histocompatibility antigens (mHA). While recipient and donor are generally matched for the major-histocompatibility (MHC) loci on chromosome 6, immune recognition of mHAs encoded by genetic polymorphisms throughout the human genome may occur.[12] Clinically, GVL was initially evidenced by reports that recipients of syngeneic stem cells were more likely to relapse than HLA-matched allogeneic recipients, who developed graft-versus-host-disease (GVHD).[13] Since then a large body of clinical literature established that patients experiencing GVHD were less likely to relapse, that leukemia remissions could occur in association with worsening GVHD[14] as well as after stopping immunosuppressive

*Targeted Therapy in Translational Cancer Research*, First Edition. Edited by Apostolia-Maria Tsimberidou, Razelle Kurzrock and Kenneth C. Anderson.
© 2016 John Wiley & Sons, Inc. Published 2016 by John Wiley & Sons, Inc.

**Table 3.1** Overview of currently approved immunotherapies for cancer.

| Approved cancer immunotherapies | Indication |
| --- | --- |
| **Therapeutic vaccines** | |
| Sipuleucel -T | Prostate cancer |
| **Prophylactic vaccines** | |
| Hepatitis B vaccine | Hepatocellular carcinoma |
| Human papillomavirus vaccine | Cervical cancer |
| **Cellular therapies** | |
| Allogeneic hematopoietic stem cell transplant | Hematologic malignancies |
| Donor lymphocyte infusion | Hematologic malignancies |
| **Monoclonal antibodies** | |
| Rituximab | NHL,CLL |
| Trastuzumab | Breast cancer |
| Gemtuzumab | AML |
| Alemtuzumab | CLL |
| 90Y-ibritumomab tiuxetan | NHL |
| 131I-tositumomab | NHL |
| Cetuximab | Colorectal cancer |
| Bevacizumab | Colorectal cancer, lung cancer |
| Panitumumab | Colorectal cancer |
| Ofatumumab | CLL |
| Ipilimumab | Melanoma |
| Brentuximabvedotin | Hodgkin lymphoma, anaplastic large cell lymphoma |
| **Cytokines** | |
| Interferon-α | Melanoma, renal cell carcinoma |
| Interleukin-2 | Melanoma, renal cell carcinoma |
| TNF-α | Melanoma, soft tissue sarcoma |

NHL, non-Hodgkin lymphoma; CLL, chronic lymphoblastic leukemia; AML, acute myeloid leukemia.

medications for prevention of GVHD,[15] and that T-cell depletion of grafts is associated with higher relapse rates.[16] Based on these findings, Kolb et al. first showed that donor lymphocyte infusions without additional chemotherapy or radiation could induce disease remissions in patients with relapsed CML after allogeneic HSCT.[17] Moreover, non-myeloablative reduced intensity conditioning regimens are now used increasingly, particularly for medically fragile patients. They are designed to facilitate engraftment of donor stem cells, but rely on elimination of the recipient's normal stem cells and tumor cells through the donor's immune cells.

Unfortunately, the most efficient GVL responses often arise in the setting of GVHD. Efforts have focused on defining the immunological mechanisms contributing to GVL in order to allow targeted exploitation of the beneficial GVL effect while preventing the significant morbidity and mortality related to GVHD. Distinction between the nature and tissue-specific expression of antigens targeted by GVL versus GVHD is crucial. As shown in a recent phase I trial, adoptive transfer of T cells specific for minor H antigens is feasible, but restricted expression of the mHA on tumor or hematopoietic cells is crucial for a favorable toxicity profile.[18,19] Genomic approaches are likely to identify previously unknown mHAs that could be targeted.[20] Another area of interest concerns the role of alloreactive NK cells, which mediate a GVL effect in myeloid leukemias but curiously do not cause GVHD. NK cells express inhibitory Killer Immunoglobulin-like receptors (KIR) that prevent NK-cell mediated attack against autologous MHC-class I+ cells. NK-cell alloreactivity ensues when inhibitory KIRs fail to encounter the HLA-I allele they are specific for. This is being explored in the haploidentical HSCT setting, where HLA-I mismatch occurs and KIR mismatching is possible. While the initial clinical success reported by Ruggeri et al.[21] was not consistently reproduced by other groups,[22] this may be in part due to different definitions of KIR-mismatch utilized in the studies. As our understanding of ideal NK-cell receptor typing becomes more sophisticated, NK-cell mediated GVL is conceptually of great interest. Multiple ongoing clinical trials explore alloreactive NK cells either in the setting of haploidentical HSCT (NCT00145626) or allogeneic NK cell infusion after autologous HSCT for lymphoma (NCT00330166) or neuroblastoma (NCT00698009).

## Vaccines

Vaccination for the prevention of infectious diseases has been one of medicine's great successes and indeed vaccines providing protection against oncogenic viruses effectively protect against certain cancers as well. The Centers for Disease Control and Prevention (CDC) estimates that approximately 26,000 new cervical cancers each year are attributable to human papillomavirus (HPV).[23] Thus the implementation of a quadrivalent HPV vaccine since 2007[24,25] has tremendous public health implications, and is now recommended for female and male adolescents.[26] Another well-established example is Hepatitis B virus vaccination in the prevention of hepatocellular carcinoma.[27] Analogous to the difficulty of controlling chronic viral infections by way of a vaccine, the generation of therapeutic cancer vaccines is much more challenging, given that such vaccine must overcome pre-established tumor tolerance. However, the discovery that patients can harbor CD8+ and CD4+ T cells specific for antigens expressed in their tumors[28] gave rise to the idea that a therapeutic cancer vaccine could amplify this pre-existing reaction and possibly induce new immune responses.

Vaccination strategies involving dendritic cells (DCs) have been developed owing to the crucial role DCs play in the orchestration of an adaptive immune response. Under steady state conditions, immature DCs take up antigen. The immune response induced by a DC depends on the subtype of DC, the signals it receives via pattern recognition receptors, and the presence of appropriate maturation signals. They can induce a variety of immune responses, including CD8+ T-cell responses, CD4+ Th1-, Th2-, Th17-, follicular helper T-cell-, or regulatory T-cell (Treg) responses. Antigen presentation by immature DCs in the absence of maturation signals leads to immune tolerance. It is crucial to consider the complexity of DC biology in the context of DC vaccine design.[29] Delivery of the tumor-antigen to DCs and provision of maturation signals can be provided *ex vivo* or *in vivo*. Due to low frequencies of DCs in the peripheral blood, *ex vivo* approaches generate DCs from monocytes under culture conditions with different cytokine combinations (most commonly GM-CSF and IL-4, which induces inflammatory DCs[30]) and then culture them with the desired antigen. Such combinations have been clinically tested for more than a decade,[31] concluding that they are safe and can induce expansion of circulating tumor-specific CD4+ and CD8+ T cells, with objective and potentially long-lasting responses in some patients.[32,33] Most notably, Sipuleucel-T, a vaccine based on enriched blood APCs that are briefly cultured with a fusion protein of prostatic acid phosphatase and GM-CSF, resulted in prolonged median survival of metastatic prostate cancer patients in phase III trials,[34] and is the first tumor vaccine to receive FDA approval. Another approach targets DCs *in vivo*. This can be achieved by fusing the selected antigen to an antibody directed against a DC surface receptor and has been shown to elicit potent antigen-specific CD4+ and CD8+ T-cell responses.[35] The choice of DC receptor that is targeted determines in part the elicited immune response, as distinct DC subsets elicit and polarize different immune responses.[36] The engagement of some DC receptors by such targeting antibodies also provides activation signals, which are important to avoid the induction of T-cell anergy. In fact, it is now accepted that the adjuvant component of vaccines (even non-DC based vaccines) primarily acts by triggering DC maturation.

Largely due to poor understanding of the mechanisms of immunization and the role of DCs, many early trials unsuccessfully treated patients with short-peptide-based vaccines in the absence of effective adjuvants.[37] Due to their pharmacokinetic properties, short peptides may be rapidly cleared and in the absence of an adjuvant that can effectively trigger DC-maturation, may promote tolerance rather than immunity. However, the administration of a short-peptide derived from the melanocyte differentiation antigen gp100 in conjunction with IL-2 was recently reported to augment tumor responses and prolong progression-free survival compared to IL-2 alone in advanced melanoma.[38] Another promising approach involves the use of longer peptides (~20-mer), which require further processing by DCs, but have the potential to prime against a greater variety of antigens and capture CD8+ and CD4+ lymphocyte responses compared to those peptides (10–12-mers) which fit the MHC-class I antigen-binding groove unedited. A long-peptide vaccine against HPV-16 oncoproteins administered in incomplete Freund's adjuvant to patients with vulvar intraepithelial neoplasia proved to have good efficacy, including complete responses, in a phase II trial.[39] These favorable results may reflect the selection of viral gene products for immunization, which might be more readily recognized as foreign by the host. In contrast, a long-peptide vaccine derived from p53, a tumor suppressor mutated in many cancers, delivered in the emulsion-adjuvant Montanide induced no tumor regressions in advanced ovarian cancer patients, underscoring the pre-existing tolerance to self and the need to optimize these formulations further.[40]

Given that they harbor a wider profile of epitopes, full-length protein vaccines are being pursued. While a diverse set of targets has been explored, many belong to a class referred to as cancer testes antigens. These antigens are expressed by a large variety of tumor cells, as well as in the immune-privileged environment of the testes or placenta, but not on healthy tissues. Two cancer testes antigens, MAGE-A3 and NY-ESO-1, have been explored in clinical trials.[41,42] Phase I and II trials have been conducted with adjuvant-mixed, recombinant MAGE-A3 protein or peptide vaccines in melanoma and NSCLC, demonstrating potent antitumor B and T cell responses, tumor-specific cell persistence for years after vaccination, and encouraging clinical effects.[43,44] MAGRIT, a large, randomized phase III trial including >2500 patients, is currently underway. This trial uses a recombinant fusion protein encoding MAGE-A3 in HLA-A2-positive NSCLC patients, together with an ASO2B adjuvant consisting of a saponin/lipid-A emulsion combined with TLR4 and TLR9 agonists.[45]

Whole-cell vaccines have the advantage of containing the broadest range of tumor-antigens (including mutated proteins), and a meta-analysis of 173 immunotherapy trials in a variety of solid tumors revealed that patients vaccinated with whole tumor-antigen

had low, but significantly higher objective response rates than patients in trials which used molecularly defined tumor antigens.[46] Whole tumor cells engineered to secrete GM-CSF and irradiated prior to injection (GVAX) reached furthest in clinical development. Several phase I clinical trials of GVAX were performed in patients with metastatic melanoma, NSCLC, renal cell carcinoma, prostate cancer, ovarian carcinoma, multiple myeloma, and myeloid leukemias.[47] In the initial studies, autologous tumor cells were engineered to secrete GM-CSF via retroviral or adenoviral gene transfer. Other approaches include stable transfection of allogeneic tumor cell lines with GM-CSF encoding plasmids, or admixture of autologous tumor cells with a standardized GM-CSF secreting K562 bystander cell line. These early stage trials were not powered to assess clinical endpoints, but consistently demonstrated biological activity with immune cell infiltration at the sites of vaccination, and dense infiltrates of intra-tumoral CD4+ and CD8+ lymphocytes and plasma cells that effectuated extensive tumor necrosis. Although some patients had promising results to GVAX in preceding trials, a phase III trial in prostate cancer using allogeneic tumor cell lines as the immunogen did not demonstrate clinical efficacy,[48] indicating that this strategy may be most effective when autologous tumor cells are used, or perhaps when combined with other immune-modulating therapies. Sequential immunotherapy, with administration of anti-CTLA4-mAb to patients immunized with GVAX 1–4 months prior, evoked objective responses of metastatic melanoma with minimal toxicities. Tumor necrosis was highly associated with a favorable CD8+/FoxP3+ ratio in tumor infiltrating T cells, suggesting the underlying therapeutic mechanism of sequential therapy to be the induction of cytotoxic T cells coupled with a loss of immune suppression.[49] Concomitant use of allogeneic GVAX and ipilimumab in a recent phase I trial for mCRPC was safe and triggered immune activation and a decline in prostate-specific antigen in select patients.[50] Furthermore, administration of GVAX early after allogeneic bone marrow transplantation was shown to be safe and immunogenic. Intriguingly, some long-term responders demonstrated a significant decrease in soluble NKG2D levels and normalization of NKG2D expression on cytotoxic lymphocytes, suggestive of a potentiated GVL effect.[51]

Attention has also been drawn to idiotype vaccines. The clonal immunoglobulin idiotype, displayed on the surface of most malignant B cells, is a patient- and tumor-specific antigen that can be used for therapeutic vaccination. One phase III trial using an idiotype vaccine conjugated with KLH and administered with GM-CSF (BiovaxID) indicated prolonged progression-free survival; however, several other trials have not corroborated these results, which might be related to differences in vaccine manufacture or patient selection.[52]

Another vaccination strategy employs viral vectors encoding tumor antigens, with the idea that strong immune responses against the viral vaccine components enhance the reactivity against the tumor antigen. One such phase II trial, PROSTVAC, involved initial inoculation of recombinant vaccinia virus encoding PSA along with co-stimulatory and adhesion molecules intended to render infected cells into surrogate antigen-presenting cells. Subsequently, a similarly configured fowlpox vector was administered in a prime-boost strategy. For additional immune stimulation, GM-CSF was administered with the vectors. This trial demonstrated an overall survival (OS) benefit of 25.1 months in the treatment versus 16.6 in the control group receiving empty vector plus saline.[53] On the basis of these encouraging results, a phase III trial has been launched.

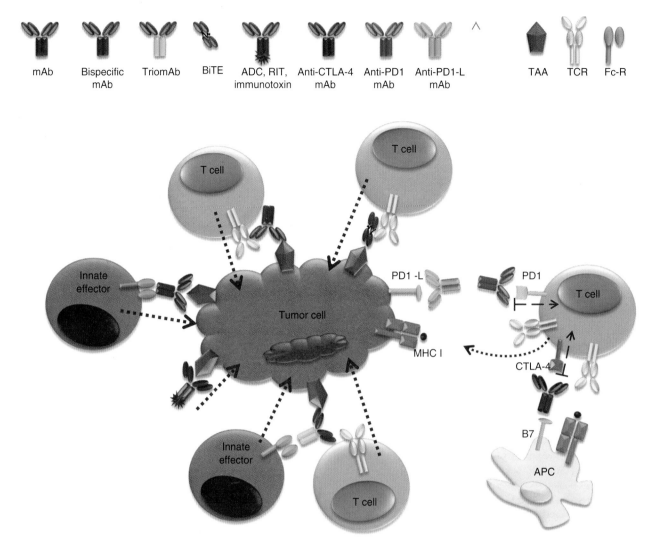

**Figure 3.1** Antibody-based immunotherapy. Various iterations of monoclonal antibodies (mAbs) have been developed for the treatment of cancer. Unconjugated mAbs bind to their target and engage NK cells, macrophages, dendritic cells as well as soluble complement components via the Fc-component of the mAb. These resulting effector functions include ADCC (antibody-dependent cellular cytotoxicity), CMC (complement-mediated cytotoxicity—not depicted), and ADCP (antibody-dependent phagocytosis—not depicted). Bispecific mAbs and BiTEs are engineered to bind to the TAA (tumor-associated antigen) and engage CD3 on CTLs (cytotoxic lymphocytes), thereby activating CTLs against tumor cells, independent of their TCR (T-cell receptor) specificity. TriomAbs additionally recruit NK cells and macrophages via their Fc-receptor. Immunoconjugates such as ADC (antibody-drug conjugates), RIT (radioimmunotherapies), immunotoxins, or ADEPT (antibody-dependent enzyme prodrug therapies) deliver cytotoxic agents directly to the target cell. Antagonistic mAbs to CTLA-4, PD1 or PD1-L block ligand–receptor interactions that otherwise deliver inhibitory signals to the T cell and allow targeted cellular cytotoxicity to ensue.

## Antibody-Based Immunotherapy

First conceptualized by Paul Ehrlich over a century ago, the specific recognition of antigens expressed by pathogens or tumor cells by an antibody holds great promise for immunotherapy that is affordable, feasible and effective. While the majority of antibody-based therapy relies on antibody-mediated recognition of surface antigens preferentially expressed by tumor cells, others interfere with tumor cell growth by disrupting negative regulatory and survival pathways as well as ligand–receptor mediated cell growth. Another crucial mechanism in this therapeutic modality is the recruitment of innate effectors toward tumor cells via the Fc domain of the antibody, which can trigger antibody-dependent cellular cytotoxicity (ADCC), complement-mediated cytotoxicity (CMC) and antibody-dependent phagocytosis (ADCP). Via the ADCP pathway, antibodies entice antigen-presenting cells such as DCs or macrophages to take up, process and present on MHCs a variety of tumor contents (not only the antibody-targeted antigen) and induce a CD4+ and CD8+ T-cell response.[54] This allows induction of humoral and cellular immunological memory and is termed the "vaccinal effect", since therapeutic antibodies promote not only direct tumor cell death, but also vaccine-like antitumor effects. Clinically, this has been shown to be relevant in solid tumors and lymphomas.[55] However, conventional antibodies do not trigger T-cell immunity directly. A promising approach to recruit and activate T cells directly at the site of the tumor cell is the development of bispecific antibodies (bsAb). Variations of bsAbs will be described below; however the underlying concept is that some of these bsAbs are specific not only to the tumor antigen, but also CD3, thereby activating T cells (Figure 3.1).

## Antibody Therapy Targeted Toward Tumor-Associated Antigens

**Unconjugated antibodies.** Rituximab, a genetically engineered chimeric mouse anti-human CD20 monoclonal Ab (mAb), was the first mAb to be approved in the treatment of cancer and is now a well-established component of therapeutic regimens for CD20+ NHL (diffuse large B-cell lymphoma and follicular lymphoma) and chronic lymphocytic leukemia in the United States and Europe.[56] The murine Fab domain of rituximab binds CD20 on tumor cells with high affinity while the humanized Fc domain crosslinks with Fc receptors on tumor cells and Fc receptors on monocytes, NK cells, and granulocytes. The mechanism of cytotoxicity mediated by rituximab is postulated to be via ADCC and CMC, although rituximab has also been shown to induce apoptosis, including sensitizing-resistant lymphoma cells to chemotherapy- and Fas ligand-induced apoptosis, which appears to be Fc-independent.[57] This synergism led to the use of combined chemotherapy regimens in clinical practice. It has also been suggested that rituximab may have a vaccinal effect, leading to T-cell priming and anti-lymphoma immunity beyond the immediate cytotoxic effect of rituximab. Another effective unconjugated mAb is used in the treatment of high-risk neuroblastoma, where the administration of an antibody directed against the tumor-associated disialoganglioside GD2 in conjunction with IL-2, GM-CSF and isoretinoin after intensive multimodal therapy has been shown to improve event-free survival (EFS) and OS compared to isoretinoin alone.[58]

**Bispecific antibodies.** The concept of using bispecific antibodies to engage cytotoxic T cells for cancer cell lysis was first shown by Staerz et al.[59] These constructs have become more sophisticated, but follow the principle of dual specificity for CD3+ as well as the surface target antigen of interest. BiTE antibodies have been constructed to more than 10 different target antigens including CD19, EpCAM, HER2/neu, EGFR, CEA, CD33, EphA2, and MCSP. Key hallmarks distinguishing them from other bispecific constructs are high potency at picomolar range, target cell-dependent activation of T cells and support of serial lysis at low E:T ratios. Conventional EGFR-blocking antibodies such as cetuximab are known to mediate an ADCC effect via FcR, but likely act predominantly by blocking EGFR, based on analyses showing that patients with downstream mutations in KRAS and BRAF genes do not have an overall survival advantage.[60] EGFR-BiTE Abs, however, can activate a T cell via CD3 when engaging a tumor cell and have been shown to lyse even KRAS-mutated colorectal cancer cell lines.[61] The epithelial adhesion molecule EpCAM is frequently expressed on human adeno- and some squamous cell carcinomas, but also on cancer stem cells.[62,63] MT110[64] and an EpCAM BiTE are being tested in a phase I trial for lung, gastrointestinal, breast, ovarian, and prostate cancers (NCT00635596). Blinatumomab, a CD19 BiTE, has shown encouraging phase II results eliminating minimal residual disease in patients with pre-B-ALL[65] and in advanced NHL.[66]

Further variations of bsAbs, so-called TriomAbs, are specific for the surface antigen of interest and engage T cells via CD3, but additionally recruit NK cells and macrophages via Fc-Receptor. Catumaxomab, a TriomAb against EpCAM has been shown to effectively kill tumor cells *in vivo* and *in vitro* and to produce protective immunity,[67] likely through memory T cells. Following its success in a phase II/III clinical trial, it was approved in Europe in 2009 for the treatment of malignant ascites in a variety of EpCAM+ abdominal tumors. Other TriomAbs are in phase I/II clinical trials, such as a CD20-TriomAb in the therapy of B-cell lymphoma in conjunction with DLI after allogeneic HSCT (NCT01138579)

and ertumaxomab a TriomAb against HER2/neu, in advanced breast cancer and other HER2/neu positive advanced solid tumors (NCT01569412). An anti-GD2 TriomAb has so far been tested in animal models of neuroblastoma.[68]

Several techniques of creating optimized bispecific mAbs are emerging: Systematic analysis of binding affinities toward a second antigen after random mutation of the light-chain complementarity-determining regions (CDRs) for a parent antibody[69] created bsAbs with two identical Fab regions targeting VEGFA and HER2 or EGFR and HER3, with improved binding affinities compared to the parent antibody. The CovX-Body technology fuses two peptide pharmacophores together and links this complex to a universal scaffold antibody with a known Fc function. This allows for rapid, reproducible and specific creation of bispecific antibodies. CVX-241, a CovX-Body targeting the angiogenesis ligands VEGFA and Ang2, demonstrated significantly inhibited tumor growth when combined with the chemotherapeutic agent irinotecan in breast and skin carcinoma xenograft models,[70] and was evaluated in a phase I clinical trial (NCT01004822). An alternative approach is based on linking the variable regions from two different antibodies. One such antibody, MM-111, targeting HER2 and HER3 is currently in a phase I trial (NCT00911898).

**Toxin-labeled antibodies.** Given the possibility of delivering cytotoxic agents directly to the tumor cell site via mAbs that target TAAs, various immunoconjugates were developed. In this iteration, mAbs were linked to radionuclides (radioimmunotherapies or RITs), drugs (antibody-drug conjugates or ADCs), toxins (immunotoxins) and enzymes (antibody-directed enzyme prodrug therapy, or ADEPT) to boost the cytotoxic mAb effects on target cells. The three currently FDA-approved immunoconjugates are all for hematologic malignancies: Two RITs targeting CD20 have been FDA-approved: $Y^{90}$-ibritumomab tiuxetan, an RIT, first approved in 2002, is currently approved for the use in follicular NHL or relapsed or refractory low-grade NHL. $^{131}I$-tositumomab was FDA-approved in 2003 and is now indicated in the treatment of CD20+ relapsed or refractory follicular or transformed NHL.[71,72]

The most clinically advanced immunotoxin, BL22, is bound to a modified Pseudomonas exotoxin and directed against CD22. It has shown significant promise in phase II trials for the treatment of hairy cell leukemia.[73] A very promising recent immunoconjugate, brentuximab vedotin, carries the antimitotic drug monomethyl auristatin E and targets CD30. It has shown remarkable efficacy in patients with relapsed or refractory Hodgkin lymphomas (HL) or anaplastic large-cell lymphomas (ALCL)[74] and was shown to be safe and effective in patients after autologous HSCT. This led to brentuximab's accelerated FDA approval for the treatment of HL and ALCL.[74,75] Its efficacy in other CD30+ malignancies is currently being tested in phase II trials (NCT01461538 and NCT01421667). Furthermore, multiple clinical trials are testing its safety and efficacy in conjunction with combination chemotherapy as a front-line agent (NCT01060904). It may also have therapeutic benefit in patients with GVHD[76] (NCT01596218).

## Modulation of Regulatory Pathways

Under physiologic conditions, the balance between co-stimulatory and inhibitory signals (so-called immune checkpoints) is critical to allow for an efficient T-cell activation while modulating the duration and amplitude of the T-cell response and protecting against autoimmunity.[77] These checkpoints include upregulation of inhibitory receptors such as CTLA-4 and PD-1 by T cells. However, dysregulation can occur in the process of immunoediting, such that inhibitory ligands and receptors are often overexpressed on tumor cells or non-transformed cells in the tumor microenvironment.[78] Since many of these immune checkpoints are mediated by ligand–receptor interactions, their inhibitory functions may be blockable with mAbs. In contrast to TAA-specific mAbs described above, these mAbs do not target the tumor, but rather lymphocyte receptors and their ligands, thereby unleashing their potential antitumor activity.

CTLA-4 was the first inhibitory receptor to be clinically targeted. CTLA-4 is upregulated on activated T cells, where it dampens T-cell activation upon engagement with the B7 receptors on dendritic cells through various mechanisms. Although expressed by CD8+ T-lymphocytes, its major physiological impact is on downregulation of CD4+helper T-cell activity and upregulation of the activity of Tregs, which express CTLA-4 constitutively, given that it is a target gene of the forkhead transcription factor FoxP3.[79] Although the exact mechanism by which CTLA-4 enhances Treg function is not known, numerous studies have shown that the ratio of effector T cells to Tregs in the tumor microenvironment plays a crucial role in the control of tumors and correlates with outcome.[80, 81]

Pioneered by Allison and colleagues, effective tumor regressions were achieved in preclinical models using single agent anti-CTLA-4 mAb for immunogenic tumors.[82] Poorly immunogenic tumors did not respond to anti-CTLA-4 mAb alone, but significant regression was achieved when given with GVAX.[83] Based on these results, two fully humanized anti-CTLA-4 mAbs, ipilimumab and tremelimumab, entered phase I clinical trials in 2000, and demonstrated ~10% objective response rates in patients with refractory metastatic melanoma receiving either GVAX[84] or gp100 peptide vaccines.[85] While the first phase III trial with tremelimumab plus dacarbazine compared to dacarbazine alone did not show benefit at the dose used,[86] a later trial comparing ipilimumab plus dacarbazine versus dacarbazine plus placebo showed improved outcomes with ipilimumab.[87] In the first phase III trial with ipilimumab, either alone or in combination with a gp100 peptide vaccine, "ippy" was the first drug to demonstrate a survival benefit in patients with melanoma in a randomized trial.[88] Importantly, up to 30% of patients may experience severe immune-related side effects, which modestly correlate with response, the most common being colitis. Careful clinical management using steroids and TNF-blockade has improved overall morbidity and mortality, although some adverse effects such as hypophysitis, may be long-lasting or irreversible, though readily managed with hormonal replacement therapy. In 2011, ipilimumab was approved by FDA as a second- or first-line agent for the treatment of advanced melanoma. Several phase II trials of ipilimumab in prostate cancer, either alone (NCT01498978), in combination with GM-CSF (NCT01530984), or with androgen-ablation (NCT01377389, NCT00170157) are ongoing. Other clinical trials are evaluating ipilimumab in conjunction with the BRAF-inhibitor vemurafenib (NCT01400451) or the anti-VEGF mAb bevacizumab for melanoma (NCT00790010), as well as the combination of ipilimumab with chemotherapy for NSCLC and other solid tumors (NCT01331525, NCT01473940).

Another important immune checkpoint is PD-1. PD-1 is expressed on activated T cells, as well as activated B cells and NK cells. Upon binding its ligands PDL1 or PDL2, kinases involved in T-cell activation are inhibited. However, analogously to CTLA-4, PD1 is also expressed on Tregs, where it enhances proliferation upon PD1-engagement by ligand.[89] Whereas CTLA-4 regulates the immune response at the time of T-cell activation in the lymphoid organs, PD1 primarily limits the activity of T cells in peripheral tissues. Numerous reports have demonstrated that PD1 ligands are commonly upregulated on the tumor cell surface in a variety of human malignancies where they mediate immune resistance[78, 90] as well as on myeloid cells in the tumor microenvironment.[91] Conversely, tumor infiltrating lymphocytes have increased expression of PD1, though this partly represents the presence of Tregs in the tumor microenvironment. Several studies in mouse models demonstrated enhancement of antitumor immunity through blockade of PD1 or its ligands. They also suggested a favorable safety profile opposite CTLA-4 given a comparatively mild phenotype of PD1, PDL1, and PDL2 knockout mice. There is now a growing experience with anti-PD1mAbs clinically. The first phase I trial using a fully human anti-PD1 mAb yielded very promising results in patients with a variety of solid tumors, including one complete response.[92] The latest data from a phase I trial evaluating an anti-PD1 mAb in patients with advanced melanoma, NSCLC, prostate cancer, renal-cell, or colorectal cancer, demonstrated an objective response rate of 36% in patients with PDL1+ tumors, with quite durable responses and a safety profile comparable to ipilimumab.[93] Concurrently, a multicenter phase I trial with anti-PD1-Ligand mAb reported an objective response rate of 6–17% depending on the underlying malignancy (without consideration of PDL1-expression).[94] Several phase I and II trials are currently ongoing, which investigate PD1-blockade for various malignancies either alone (NCT01354431), with ipilimumab (NCT01024231), with gp100-, MART-1- or NY-ESO-1- peptide vaccines (NCT01176461) or in conjunction with chemotherapeutic agents (NCT01176461). Several other immune checkpoint molecules are emerging as candidates for therapeutic blockade such as LAG3, 2B4, BTLA, TIM3, A2aR and KIR. Another therapeutic target undergoing evaluation in early trials is the stimulation of co-stimulatory pathways, such as 41BB (CD137) or ICOS.[95]

## T-Cell Based Immunotherapy

The ability of lymphocytes to eradicate tumor cells was first demonstrated in metastatic melanoma, for which the T-cell cytokine interleukin IL-2, now an FDA-approved therapy, can mediate measurable responses in 15% of patients.[96–98] Furthermore, tumor infiltrating lymphocytes (TIL) can be isolated, expanded and adoptively transferred back into the patient.[99] Non-myeloablative chemotherapy and 12 Gy total body irradiation prior to TIL-infusion resulted in clinical response rates of 72% with 40% complete responses in selected patients.[100] However, TILs cannot be obtained in all patients. Based on this limitation, Morgan et al. developed an approach by which genes encoding the alpha and beta chains for a TCR recognizing the TAA MART-1 were cloned from a TIL clone of a patient with metastatic melanoma who demonstrated near complete regression after adoptive transfer of TILs.[101] T cells of several HLA-matched patients with metastatic melanoma were then transduced to express the anti-MART-1 TCR utilizing retroviral gene transfer. Select patients with sustained high levels of circulating engineered T cells had objective regression of metastatic melanoma lesions.[102]

A different and more widely used approach, which is not restricted to HLA-type, involves the gene transfer of chimeric antigen-receptor T cells (CARs). This method, pioneered by Eshhar and colleagues,[103–105] links a tumor-specific antibody or other extracellular domain recognizing the desired TAA to an intracellular signaling domain capable of activating the T cell upon ligation of the extracellular domain.[106–108] Once T cells are transduced to express the CAR, they acquire specificity for the TAA (Figure 3.2). CARs recognize tumor antigens in a HLA-independent manner, which has several advantages: First, it obviates the need for

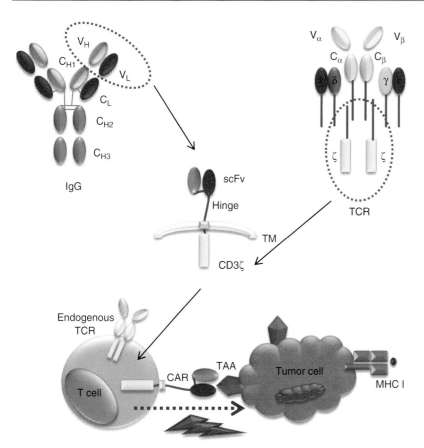

**Figure 3.2** Chimeric antigen-receptor (CARs) T cells. T cells can be transduced to express chimeric antigen-receptors (CARs) that endow them with specificity to a particular TAA. Although many iterations have been developed, the CAR commonly consists of a sFcv (single-chain variable fragment) derived from an mAb against a TAA which is linked to an ITAM (immunoreceptor tyrosine-based activation motif) such as the CD3ζ-chain. Frequently, additional intracellular co-stimulatory domains are included (not depicted here). CAR+ T-cells can recognize TAAs independent of their MHC-presentation and become activated upon binding to the TAA.

HLA-matching and allows universal use of the respective CAR-construct for the transduction of patient T cells and large-scale production of CARs for clinical use. Secondly, the ability of CARs to recognize TAAs independent of their presentation on MHC molecules allows CAR+ T-cells to attack tumor cells in the immunosuppressive tumor microenvironment, where MHC-downregulation is a major evasion mechanism. While CAR+ T-cells are typically manufactured individually from a patient's autologous T cells, a more recent approach focused on the creation of "universal" allogeneic T cells modified to eliminate their endogenous TCR, (which might otherwise mediate GVHD in the allogeneic setting), while maintaining CAR-specificity to the TAA.[109] If complete elimination of TCR can be reached, it might allow cost-effective off-the-shelf therapy with universal allogeneic T cells.

Several generations of CARs have been developed. First generation CARs typically comprise an extracellular single-chain variable fragment (scFv) of a monoclonal antibody and an intracellular immunoreceptor tyrosine-based activation motif (ITAM) consisting of the CD3ζ-chain or rarely FcεRIγ. While such CARs deliver "signal 1" resulting in T-cell activation, target cell lysis, modest IL-2 secretion, and *in vivo* antitumor function, they lack "signal 2", the absence of which leads to T-cell anergy under physiological conditions. Second generation CARs therefore include an intracellular co-stimulatory signaling domain such as CD28, ICOS or a TNFR family member (4–1BB or OX40) to mimic physiologic T-cell activation and enhance T-cell proliferation, IL-2 synthesis and expression of the anti-apoptotic protein Bcl-xL. The choice of co-stimulatory molecule may play a crucial role and more is not necessarily better. Compared to CD28 domains, 4–1BB signaling domains show a reduced propensity to trigger IL-2 and TNF-α,[110] but this may

be associated with sustained clinical activity and reduced risk of cytokine storm. Furthermore, decreased IL-2 levels may be beneficial, given that substantial doses of IL-2 can elicit Treg-mediated suppression of CAR+ T-cells.[111]

CARs have been developed against a variety of targets for use across a wide range of tumors. CD19, a B-cell marker expressed on most B-cell malignancies, yet not on hematopoietic stem cells, is a frequently targeted epitope, whose "on target/off tumor" toxicity is limited to B-cell aplasia. Several phase I/II clinical trials have evaluated the safety and efficacy of CD19 CAR+ T-cells in patients with CLL, acute lymphoblastic leukemia (ALL) and NHL. While they differ in their use of single-chain variable fragments, CD28[112] versus 4–1BB[113] co-stimulatory domains, the addition of IL-2,[114] preparatory conditioning regimens and ultimately efficacy, all report complete and partial remissions at least in some patients. Kalos et al. reported on three patients with advanced CLL treated with chemotherapy followed by split infusion of a CD19–41BB-zetaCAR.[115] Two of the treated patients achieved a complete and one patient a partial remission.[113] The use of CD19 CAR+ T-cells is further being explored in the post-HSCT setting (NCT01475058).

Some of the early proof-of-principle clinical trials included CARs directed against Carboxy-anhydrase-IX (CAIX) for the treatment of renal cell carcinoma,[116] folate-receptor for metastatic ovarian cancer,[117] CD20 for Non-Hodgkin and mantle cell lymphomas[118] and CD171 for neuroblastoma.[119] These phase I trials demonstrated minimal or manageable toxicities, modest efficacy and generally poor persistence of T cells. One adverse event was reported for a patient with metastatic colon cancer, who received a large dose of HER2/CD28/41BB-zeta-CAR+ T-cells, which also recognized low level HER2 expression in healthy lung tissue and led to pulmonary toxicity and subsequent cytokine storm.[120] With cautious dose escalation regimens, CAR+ T-cell therapy has since been explored on clinical trials without significant toxicities. The integration of an inducible suicide gene (HSV-tk or inducible caspase 9), as has been explored for the treatment and prevention of GVHD,[121, 122] has been suggested, but not implemented in clinical CAR trials thus far. Other examples of CARs that are being evaluated on clinical trials include HER2 for sarcomas (NCT00902044), glioblastomas (NCT01109095), advanced osteosarcoma (NCT00902044) and CD30 for the treatment of HL and NHLs (NCT01316146).

Given the variable persistence of CAR+ T-cells, some groups have explored the concept of transducing EBV+ or CMV+ T-cells from patients, conferring improved persistence and avoiding theoretical off-target toxicity. This approach has shown encouraging results in a clinical anti-GD2-CAR+ trial treating patients with neuroblastoma, who received both EBV+ GD2-CAR+ T-cells and polyclonal, activated GD2-CAR+ T-cells,[123] although CAR+ T-cell persistence was concordant with percentage of CD4+ T-cells and central memory T cells, rather than virus-specific T cells.[124] This further underlines the potential of optimizing current CAR technology not only by systematically comparing co-stimulatory domains, but also by carefully considering and selecting the ideal T-lymphocyte subset/phenotype.[125, 126] Furthermore, several interesting CAR constructs have been explored in preclinical models: Examples include a CAR containing the NKG2D-receptor, which targets the natural ligands of NKG2D, which are overexpressed on a multitude of tumors,[127] a polypeptide against VEGFR-2,[128] IL-12 secreting CAR+ T-cells[129] and an anti-FITC CAR, which could be utilized as a "universal" CAR construct recognizing a variety of TAAs, marked by FITC-conjugated therapeutic molecules specific for the TAA of interest.[108]

### Emerging New Targets

There is increasing evidence that immunosuppressive enzymes, such as indoleamine 2,3-dioxygenase (IDO) and Arginase are expressed by many tumor cells as well as infiltrating myeloid suppressor cells.[130, 131] These enzymes locally deplete amino acids essential for anabolic T-lymphocyte function or produce ligands for cytosolic receptors that can alter lymphocyte function. Inhibition of these enzymes in an effort to enhance intratumoral inflammation by molecular analogues through competitive inhibition of suicide substrates is a promising approach.[132, 133] Another interesting area is the manipulation and normalization of tumor vasculature in combination with immunotherapy. VEGF blockade has shown to increase T cell homing to tumors[134] and can enhance the efficacy of immunotherapy in mouse models.[135] Lastly, inflammatory pathways such as STAT3 and NF-κB signaling, cytokines such as IL-6, IL-17, IL-23 and TNF-α have shown to be important in tumor promotion.[136] Targeted inhibition of these circuits may not only antagonize tumor progression, but also enhance the efficacy of immunotherapy.

### Immune Response Criteria

A topic of cancer immunotherapy that should not be underestimated is how to accurately assess clinical efficacy. There is a clear need to develop validated biomarkers that can be used to monitor the development of an immune response following therapy, and identify those that best correlate with and predict clinical efficacy.[137] Traditionally, the response evaluation criteria in solid tumors (RECIST) or modified WHO criteria have been used to assess tumor regression. While this is an appropriate measure of chemotherapy-induced responses, these criteria do not adequately measure clinical efficacy of immunotherapy. In fact, in the early phase of treatment, lesions might increase in size, due to infiltration by immune cells and the inflammatory reaction they induce. False-negative interpretation as progression could shut down the most promising immunotherapy regimens. A randomized phase III trial with CTLA-4 blockade in stage IV melanoma, which showed a twofold improved overall survival for recipients of anti-CTLA-4mAb, most clearly illustrated that lesions might initially increase in size and that immunotherapy responses develop more slowly than chemotherapy responses, reflecting the gradual build-up of a lasting immune response.[88] To this end, collaborative efforts to standardize laboratory protocols for biomarkers and to implement new immune-related response criteria (irRC) are underway.[138, 139]

## Conclusion

Critical advances in understanding the complex interactions between the regulatory and antitumor components of the immune system in the tumor microenvironment and beyond are ongoing and will continue to contribute greatly to the design of optimized targeted cancer immunotherapy. A multitude of strategies to improve the immune system's control of cancer are underway, both with experimental and increasingly with approved clinical therapies. While at first sight, the overall median survival advantage may not always be overwhelming when using immunotherapy alone, it is crucial to keep in mind that these are results from phase I–III studies, which are performed in patients with progressive disease who have failed all established therapies and are the results of mono immunotherapy. Success in cancer therapy in general has only been achieved by employing multi-agent or multimodality treatments, such as combination of different chemotherapy agents or a combination of radiotherapy and chemotherapy, and this is likely to be the case with cancer immunotherapy as well. Several studies suggest that the immune system has the ability to increase the efficacy of existing therapeutic modalities in cancer, and the prospect of a synergistic effect of immunotherapy is highly encouraging. While small molecule kinase-inhibitors can effectuate impressive tumor responses, these drugs are frequently limited by the emergence of drug resistance. The full effect of immunotherapy is not immediate, but once developed can offer a sustained response that is unparalleled by other therapeutic modalities. The combination of targeted molecular therapy with targeted immunotherapy may thus prove to be particularly efficacious and well tolerated.[140]

## References

1 Shankaran V, Ikeda H, Bruce AT, et al. IFNgamma and lymphocytes prevent primary tumour development and shape tumour immunogenicity. *Nature*. 2001;410(6832):1107–1111.

2 Dunn GP, Bruce AT, Ikeda H, Old LJ, Schreiber RD. Cancer immunoediting: from immunosurveillance to tumor escape. *Nat Immunol*. 2002;3(11):991–998.

3 Finn OJ. Cancer immunology. *N Engl J Med*. 2008;358(25):2704–2715.

4 Wahlin BE, Sander B, Christensson B, Kimby E. CD8+ T-cell content in diagnostic lymph nodes measured by flow cytometry is a predictor of survival in follicular lymphoma. *Clin Cancer Res*. 2007;13(2 Pt 1):388–397.

5  Galon J, Costes A, Sanchez-Cabo F, et al. Type, density, and location of immune cells within human colorectal tumors predict clinical outcome. *Science*. 2006;313(5795):1960–1964.

6  Schreiber RD, Old LJ, Smyth MJ. Cancer immunoediting: integrating immunity's roles in cancer suppression and promotion. *Science*. 2011;331(6024):1565–1570.

7  Rabinovich GA, Gabrilovich D, Sotomayor EM. Immunosuppressive strategies that are mediated by tumor cells. *Annu Rev Immunol*. 2007;25:267–296.

8  Kalialis LV, Drzewiecki KT, Klyver H. Spontaneous regression of metastases from melanoma: review of the literature. *Melanoma Res*. 2009;19(5):275–282.

9  Nauts HC. Bacteria and cancer–antagonisms and benefits. *Cancer Surv*. 1989;8(4):713–723.

10  McCann J, Can skin cancers be minimized or prevented in organ transplant patients? *J Natl Cancer Inst*. 1999;91(11):911–913.

11  Pichert G, Roy DC, Gonin R, et al. Distinct patterns of minimal residual disease associated with graft-versus-host disease after allogeneic bone marrow transplantation for chronic myelogenous leukemia. *J Clin Oncol*. 1995;13(7):1704–1713.

12  Mullally A, Ritz J. Beyond HLA: the significance of genomic variation for allogeneic hematopoietic stem cell transplantation. *Blood*. 2007;109(4):1355–1362.

13  Weiden PL, Flournoy N, Thomas ED, et al. Antileukemic effect of graft-versus-host disease in human recipients of allogeneic-marrow grafts. *N Engl J Med*. 1979;300(19):1068–1073.

14  Tricot G, Vesole DH, Jagannath S, Hilton J, Munshi N, Barlogie B. Graft-versus-myeloma effect: proof of principle. *Blood*. 1996;87(3):1196–1198.

15  Libura J, Hoffmann T, Passweg J, et al. Graft-versus-myeloma after withdrawal of immunosuppression following allogeneic peripheral stem cell transplantation. *Bone Marrow Transplant*. 1999;24(8):925–927.

16  Goldman JM, Gale RP, Horowitz MM, et al. Bone marrow transplantation for chronic myelogenous leukemia in chronic phase. Increased risk for relapse associated with T-cell depletion. *Ann Intern Med*. 1988;108(6):806–814.

17  Kolb HJ, Mittermüller J, Clemm C, et al. Donor leukocyte transfusions for treatment of recurrent chronic myelogenous leukemia in marrow transplant patients. *Blood*. 1990;76(12):2462–2465.

18  Bleakley M, Riddell SR. Exploiting T cells specific for human minor histocompatibility antigens for therapy of leukemia. *Immunol Cell Biol*. 2011;89(3):396–407.

19  Warren EH, Fujii N, Akatsuka Y, et al. Therapy of relapsed leukemia after allogeneic hematopoietic cell transplantation with T cells specific for minor histocompatibility antigens. *Blood*. 2010;115(19):3869–3878.

20  Chapman M, Warren EH 3rd, Wu CJ. Applications of next-generation sequencing to blood and marrow transplantation. *Biol Blood Marrow Transplant*. 2012;18(1 suppl):S151–S160.

21  Ruggeri L, Capanni M, Urbani E, et al. Effectiveness of donor natural killer cell alloreactivity in mismatched hematopoietic transplants. *Science*. 2002;295(5562):2097–2100.

22  Leung W. Use of NK cell activity in cure by transplant. *Br J Haematol*. 2011;155(1):14–29.

23  Centers for Disease Control and Prevention (CDC). Human papillomavirus-associated cancers – United States, 2004–2008. *MMWR Morb Mortal Wkly Rep*. 2012;61:258–261.

24  Lowy DR, Schiller JT. Prophylactic human papillomavirus vaccines. *J Clin Invest*. 2006;116(5):1167–1173.

25  Garland SM, Hernandez-Avila M, Wheeler CM, et al. Quadrivalent vaccine against human papillomavirus to prevent anogenital diseases. *N Engl J Med*. 2007;356(19):1928–1943.

26  Committee on Infectious Diseases. HPV vaccine recommendations. *Pediatrics*. 2012;129(3):602–605.

27  McMahon BJ, Bulkow LR, Singleton RJ, et al. Elimination of hepatocellular carcinoma and acute hepatitis B in children 25 years after a hepatitis B newborn and catch-up immunization program. *Hepatology*. 2011;54(3):801–807.

28  Boon T, Coulie PG, Van den Eynde BJ, van der Bruggen P. Human T cell responses against melanoma. *Annu Rev Immunol*. 2006;24:175–208.

29  Palucka K, Banchereau J. Cancer immunotherapy via dendritic cells. *Nat Rev Cancer*. 2012;12(4):265–277.

30  Romani N, Gruner S, Brang D, et al. Proliferating dendritic cell progenitors in human blood. *J Exp Med*. 1994;180(1):83–93.

31  Ueno H, Schmitt N, Klechevsky E, et al. Harnessing human dendritic cell subsets for medicine. *Immunol Rev*. 2010;234(1):199–212.

32  Palucka K, Ueno H, Roberts L, Fay J, Banchereau J. Dendritic cells: are they clinically relevant? *Cancer J*. 2010;16(4):318–324.

33  Draube A, Klein-González N, Mattheus S, et al. Dendritic cell based tumor vaccination in prostate and renal cell cancer: a systematic review and meta-analysis. *PLoS One*. 2011;6(4):e18801.

34  Kantoff PW, Higano CS, Shore ND, et al. Sipuleucel-T immunotherapy for castration-resistant prostate cancer. *N Engl J Med*. 2010;363(5):411–422.

35  Bonifaz LC, Bonnyay DP, Charalambous A, et al. In vivo targeting of antigens to maturing dendritic cells via the DEC-205 receptor improves T cell vaccination. *J Exp Med*. 2004;199(6):815–824.

36  Dudziak D, Kamphorst AO, Heidkamp GF, et al. Differential antigen processing by dendritic cell subsets in vivo. *Science*. 2007;315(5808):107–111.

37  Rosenberg SA, Yang JC, Restifo NP. Cancer immunotherapy: moving beyond current vaccines. *Nat Med*. 2004;10(9):909–915.

38  Schwartzentruber DJ, Lawson DH, Richards JM, et al. gp100 peptide vaccine and interleukin-2 in patients with advanced melanoma. *N Engl J Med*. 2011;364(22):2119–2127.

39  Kenter GG, Welters MJ, Valentijn AR, et al. Vaccination against HPV-16 oncoproteins for vulvar intraepithelial neoplasia. *N Engl J Med*. 2009;361(19):1838–1847.

40  Leffers N, Lambeck AJ, Gooden MJ, et al. Immunization with a P53 synthetic long peptide vaccine induces P53-specific immune responses in ovarian cancer patients, a phase II trial. *Int J Cancer*. 2009;125(9):2104–2113.

41  Gnjatic S, Nishikawa H, Jungbluth AA, et al. NY-ESO-1: review of an immunogenic tumor antigen. *Adv Cancer Res*. 2006;95:1–30.

42  Valmori D, Souleimanian NE, Tosello V, et al. Vaccination with NY-ESO-1 protein and CpG in Montanide induces integrated antibody/Th1 responses and CD8 T cells through cross-priming. *Proc Natl Acad Sci U S A*. 2007;104(21):8947–8952.

43  Atanackovic D, Altorki NK, Cao Y, et al. Booster vaccination of cancer patients with MAGE-A3 protein reveals long-term immunological memory or tolerance depending on priming. *Proc Natl Acad Sci U S A*. 2008;105(5):1650–1655.

44  Brichard VG, Lejeune D. GSK's antigen-specific cancer immunotherapy programme: pilot results leading to phase III clinical development. *Vaccine*. 2007;25(suppl 2):B61–B71.

45  Tyagi P, Mirakhur B. MAGRIT: the largest-ever phase III lung cancer trial aims to establish a novel tumor-specific approach to therapy. *Clin Lung Cancer*. 2009;10(5):371–374.

46  Neller MA, Lopez JA, Schmidt CW. Antigens for cancer immunotherapy. *Semin Immunol*. 2008;20(5):286–295.

47 Jinushi M, Hodi FS, Dranoff G. Enhancing the clinical activity of granulocyte-macrophage colony-stimulating factor-secreting tumor cell vaccines. *Immunol Rev.* 2008;222:287–298.

48 Copier J, Dalgleish A. Whole-cell vaccines: a failure or a success waiting to happen? *Curr Opin Mol Ther.* 2010;12(1):14–20.

49 Hodi FS, Butler M, Oble DA, et al. Immunologic and clinical effects of antibody blockade of cytotoxic T lymphocyte-associated antigen 4 in previously vaccinated cancer patients. *Proc Natl Acad Sci U S A.* 2008;105(8):3005–3010.

50 van den Eertwegh AJ, Versluis J, van den Berg HP, et al. Combined immunotherapy with granulocyte-macrophage colony-stimulating factor-transduced allogeneic prostate cancer cells and ipilimumab in patients with metastatic castration-resistant prostate cancer: a phase 1 dose-escalation trial. *Lancet Oncol.* 2012;13(5):509–517.

51 Ho VT, Vanneman M, Kim H, et al. Biologic activity of irradiated, autologous, GM-CSF-secreting leukemia cell vaccines early after allogeneic stem cell transplantation. *Proc Natl Acad Sci U S A.* 2009;106(37):15825–15830.

52 Bendandi M. Idiotype vaccines for lymphoma: proof-of-principles and clinical trial failures. *Nat Rev Cancer.* 2009;9(9):675–681.

53 Kantoff PW, Schuetz TJ, Blumenstein BA, et al. Overall survival analysis of a phase II randomized controlled trial of a Poxviral-based PSA-targeted immunotherapy in metastatic castration-resistant prostate cancer. *J Clin Oncol.* 2010;28(7):1099–1105.

54 Dhodapkar KM, Krasovsky J, Williamson B, Dhodapkar MV. Antitumor monoclonal antibodies enhance cross-presentation of cellular antigens and the generation of myeloma-specific killer T cells by dendritic cells. *J Exp Med.* 2002;195(1):125–133.

55 Hilchey SP, Hyrien O, Mosmann TR, et al. Rituximab immunotherapy results in the induction of a lymphoma idiotype-specific T-cell response in patients with follicular lymphoma: support for a "vaccinal effect" of rituximab. *Blood.* 2009;113(16):3809–3812.

56 Keating GM. Rituximab: a review of its use in chronic lymphocytic leukaemia, low-grade or follicular lymphoma and diffuse large B-cell lymphoma. *Drugs.* 2010;70(11):1445–1476.

57 Vega MI, Huerta-Yepez S, Martinez-Paniagua M, et al. Rituximab-mediated cell signaling and chemo/immuno-sensitization of drug-resistant B-NHL is independent of its Fc functions. *Clin Cancer Res.* 2009;15(21):6582–6594.

58 Yu AL, Gilman AL, Ozkaynak MF, et al. Anti-GD2 antibody with GM-CSF, interleukin-2, and isotretinoin for neuroblastoma. *N Engl J Med.* 2010;363(14):1324–1334.

59 Staerz UD, Kanagawa O, Bevan MJ. Hybrid antibodies can target sites for attack by T cells. *Nature.* 1985;314(6012):628–631.

60 Karapetis CS, Khambata-Ford S, Jonker DJ, et al. K-ras mutations and benefit from cetuximab in advanced colorectal cancer. *N Engl J Med.* 2008;359(17):1757–1765.

61 Lutterbuese R. Raum T, Kischel R, et al. T cell-engaging BiTE antibodies specific for EGFR potently eliminate KRAS- and BRAF-mutated colorectal cancer cells. *Proc Natl Acad Sci U S A.* 2010;107(28):12605–12610.

62 Maetzel D, Denzel S, Mack B, et al. Nuclear signalling by tumour-associated antigen EpCAM. *Nat Cell Biol.* 2009;11(2):162–171.

63 Cioffi M, Dorado J, Baeuerle PA, Heeschen C. EpCAM/CD3-Bispecific T-cell engaging antibody MT110 eliminates primary human pancreatic cancer stem cells. *Clin Cancer Res.* 2012;18(2):465–474.

64 Brischwein K, Schlereth B, Guller B, et al. MT110: a novel bispecific single-chain antibody construct with high efficacy in eradicating established tumors. *Mol Immunol.* 2006;43(8):1129–1143.

65 Topp MS, Kufer P, Gökbuget N, et al. Targeted therapy with the T-cell-engaging antibody blinatumomab of chemotherapy-refractory minimal residual disease in B-lineage acute lymphoblastic leukemia patients results in high response rate and prolonged leukemia-free survival. *J Clin Oncol.* 2011;29(18):2493–2498.

66 Bargou R, Leo E, Zugmaier G, et al. Tumor regression in cancer patients by very low doses of a T cell-engaging antibody. *Science.* 2008;321(5891):974–977.

67 Ruf P, Lindhofer H. Induction of a long-lasting antitumor immunity by a trifunctional bispecific antibody. *Blood.* 2001;98(8):2526–2534.

68 Manzke O, Russello O, Leenen C, Diehl V, Bohlen H, Berthold F. Immunotherapeutic strategies in neuroblastoma: antitumoral activity of deglycosylated Ricin A conjugated anti-GD2 antibodies and anti-CD3xanti-GD2 bispecific antibodies. *Med Pediatr Oncol.* 2001;36(1):185–189.

69 Schaefer G, Haber L, Crocker LM, et al. A two-in-one antibody against HER3 and EGFR has superior inhibitory activity compared with monospecific antibodies. *Cancer Cell.* 2011;20(4):472–486.

70 Doppalapudi VR, Huang J, Liu D, et al. Chemical generation of bispecific antibodies. *Proc Natl Acad Sci U S A.* 2010;107(52):22611–22616.

71 Kaminski MS, Estes J, Zasadny KR, et al. Radioimmunotherapy with iodine (131)I tositumomab for relapsed or refractory B-cell non-Hodgkin lymphoma: updated results and long-term follow-up of the University of Michigan experience. *Blood.* 2000;96(4):1259–1266.

72 Kaminski MS, Tuck M, Estes J, et al. 131I-tositumomab therapy as initial treatment for follicular lymphoma. *N Engl J Med.* 2005;352(5):441–449.

73 Kreitman RJ, Stetler-Stevenson M, Margulies I, et al. Phase II trial of recombinant immunotoxin RFB4(dsFv)-PE38 (BL22) in patients with hairy cell leukemia. *J Clin Oncol.* 2009;27(18):2983–2990.

74 Younes A, Bartlett NL, Leonard JP, et al. Brentuximab vedotin (SGN-35) for relapsed CD30-positive lymphomas. *N Engl J Med.* 2010;363(19):1812–1821.

75 Younes A, Yasothan U, Kirkpatrick P. Brentuximab vedotin. *Nat Rev Drug Discov.* 2012;11(1):19–20.

76 Chen YB, McDonough S, Hasserjian R, et al. Expression of CD30 in patients with acute graft-vs.-host disease. *Blood.* 2012;120(3):691–696.

77 Pardoll DM. The blockade of immune checkpoints in cancer immunotherapy. *Nat Rev Cancer.* 2012;12(4):252–264.

78 Zou W, Chen L. Inhibitory B7-family molecules in the tumour microenvironment. *Nat Rev Immunol.* 2008;8(6):467–477.

79 Wing K, Onishi Y, Prieto-Martin P, et al. CTLA-4 control over Foxp3+ regulatory T cell function. *Science.* 2008;322(5899):271–275.

80 Curiel TJ, Coukos G, Zou L, et al. Specific recruitment of regulatory T cells in ovarian carcinoma fosters immune privilege and predicts reduced survival. *Nat Med.* 2004;10(9):942–949.

81 Koyama K, Kagamu H, Miura S, et al. Reciprocal CD4 +T-cell balance of effector CD62Llow CD4+ and CD62LhighCD25+ CD4+ regulatory T cells in small cell lung cancer reflects disease stage. *Clin Cancer Res.* 2008;14(21):6770–6779.

82 Leach DR, Krummel MF, Allison JP. Enhancement of antitumor immunity by CTLA-4 blockade. *Science.* 1996;271(5256):1734–1736.

83 van Elsas A, Hurwitz AA, Allison JP. Combination immunotherapy of B16 melanoma using anti-cytotoxic T lymphocyte-associated antigen 4 (CTLA-4) and granulocyte/macrophage colony-stimulating factor (GM-CSF)-producing vaccines induces rejection of subcutaneous and metastatic tumors accompanied by autoimmune depigmentation. *J Exp Med.* 1999;190(3):355–366.

84 Hodi FS, Mihm MC, Soiffer RJ, et al. Biologic activity of cytotoxic T lymphocyte-associated antigen 4 antibody blockade in previously vaccinated metastatic melanoma and ovarian carcinoma patients. *Proc Natl Acad Sci U S A.* 2003;100(8):4712–4717.

85  Phan GQ, Yang JC, Sherry RM, et al. Cancer regression and autoimmunity induced by cytotoxic T lymphocyte-associated antigen 4 blockade in patients with metastatic melanoma. *Proc Natl Acad Sci U S A*. 2003;100(14):8372–8377.

86  Ribas A. Clinical development of the anti-CTLA-4 antibody tremelimumab. *Semin Oncol*. 2010;37(5):450–454.

87  Robert C. Thomas L, Bondarenko I, et al. Ipilimumab plus dacarbazine for previously untreated metastatic melanoma. *N Engl J Med*. 2011;364(26):2517–2526.

88  Hodi FS, O'Day SJ, McDermott DF, et al. Improved survival with ipilimumab in patients with metastatic melanoma. *N Engl J Med*. 2010;363(8):711–723.

89  Francisco LM, Salinas VH, Brown KE, et al. PD-L1 regulates the development, maintenance, and function of induced regulatory T cells. *J Exp Med*. 2009;206(13):3015–3029.

90  Dong H, Strome SE, Salomao DR, et al. Tumor-associated B7-H1 promotes T-cell apoptosis: a potential mechanism of immune evasion. *Nat Med*. 2002;8(8):793–800.

91  Kuang DM, Zhao Q, Peng C, et al. Activated monocytes in peritumoral stroma of hepatocellular carcinoma foster immune privilege and disease progression through PD-L1. *J Exp Med*. 2009;206(6):1327–1337.

92  Brahmer JR, Drake CG, Wollner I, et al. Phase I study of single-agent anti-programmed death-1 (MDX-1106) in refractory solid tumors: safety, clinical activity, pharmacodynamics, and immunologic correlates. *J Clin Oncol*. 2010;28(19):3167–3175.

93  Topalian SL, Hodi FS, Brahmer JR, et al. Safety, activity, and immune correlates of anti-PD-1 antibody in cancer. *N Engl J Med*. 2012;366(26):2443–2454.

94  Brahmer JR, Tykodi SS, Chow LQ, et al. Safety and Activity of Anti-PD-L1 antibody in patients with advanced cancer. *N Engl J Med*. 2012;366(26):2455–2465.

95  Liakou CI, Kamat A, Tang DN, et al. CTLA-4 blockade increases IFNgamma-producing CD4+ICOShi cells to shift the ratio of effector to regulatory T cells in cancer patients. *Proc Natl Acad Sci U S A*. 2008;105(39):14987–14992.

96  Rosenberg SA, Yang JC, White DE, Steinberg SM. Durability of complete responses in patients with metastatic cancer treated with high-dose interleukin-2: identification of the antigens mediating response. *Ann Surg*. 1998;228(3):307–319.

97  Atkins MB, Kunkel L, Sznol M, Rosenberg SA. High-dose recombinant interleukin-2 therapy in patients with metastatic melanoma: long-term survival update. *Cancer J Sci Am*. 2000;6(suppl 1):S11–S14.

98  Atkins MB, Lotze MT, Dutcher JP, et al. High-dose recombinant interleukin 2 therapy for patients with metastatic melanoma: analysis of 270 patients treated between 1985 and 1993. *J Clin Oncol*. 1999;17(7):2105–2116.

99  Dudley ME, Wunderlich JR, Shelton TE, Even J, Rosenberg SA. Generation of tumor-infiltrating lymphocyte cultures for use in adoptive transfer therapy for melanoma patients. *J Immunother*. 2003;26(4):332–342.

100  Rosenberg SA, Yang JC, Sherry RM, et al. Durable complete responses in heavily pretreated patients with metastatic melanoma using T-cell transfer immunotherapy. *Clin Cancer Res*. 2011;17(13):4550–4557.

101  Dudley ME, Wunderlich JR, Robbins PF, et al. Cancer regression and autoimmunity in patients after clonal repopulation with antitumor lymphocytes. *Science*. 2002;298(5594):850–854.

102  Morgan RA, Dudley ME, Wunderlich JR, et al. Cancer regression in patients after transfer of genetically engineered lymphocytes. *Science*. 2006;314(5796):126–129.

103  Gross G, Eshhar Z. Endowing T cells with antibody specificity using chimeric T cell receptors. *Faseb J*.1992;6(15):3370–3378.

104  Gross G, Gorochov G, Waks T, Eshhar Z. Generation of effector T cells expressing chimeric T cell receptor with antibody type-specificity. *Transplant Proc*. 1989;21(1 Pt 1):127–130.

105  Gross G, Waks T, Eshhar Z. Expression of immunoglobulin-T-cell receptor chimeric molecules as functional receptors with antibody-type specificity. *Proc Natl Acad Sci U S A*. 1989;86(24):10024–10028.

106  Jena B, Dotti G, Cooper LJ. Redirecting T-cell specificity by introducing a tumor-specific chimeric antigen receptor. *Blood*. 2010;116(7):1035–1044.

107  Gilham DE, Debets R, Pule M, Hawkins RE, Abken H. CAR-T cells and solid tumors: tuning T cells to challenge an inveterate foe. *Trends Mol Med*. 2012;18(7):377–384.

108  Curran KJ, Pegram HJ, Brentjens RJ. Chimeric antigen receptors for T cell immunotherapy: current understanding and future direction. *J Gene Med*. 2012;14(6):405–415.

109  Torikai H, Reik A, Liu PQ, et al. A foundation for "universal" T-cell based immunotherapy: T-cells engineered to express a CD19-specific chimeric-antigen-receptor and eliminate expression of endogenous TCR. *Blood*. 2012;119(24):5697–5705.

110  Milone MC, Fish JD, Carpenito C, et al. Chimeric receptors containing CD137 signal transduction domains mediate enhanced survival of T cells and increased antileukemic efficacy in vivo. *Mol Ther*. 2009;17(8):1453–1464.

111  Lee JC, Hayman E, Pegram HJ, et al. In vivo inhibition of human CD19-targeted effector T cells by natural T regulatory cells in a xenotransplant murine model of B cell malignancy. *Cancer Res*. 2011;71(8):2871–2881.

112  Brentjens RJ, Rivière I, Park JH, et al. Safety and persistence of adoptively transferred autologous CD19-targeted T cells in patients with relapsed or chemotherapy refractory B-cell leukemias. *Blood*. 2011;118(18):4817–4828.

113  Kalos M, Levine BL, Porter DL, et al. T cells with chimeric antigen receptors have potent antitumor effects and can establish memory in patients with advanced leukemia. *Sci Transl Med*. 2011;3(95):95ra73.

114  Kochenderfer JN, Dudley ME, Feldman SA, et al. B-cell depletion and remissions of malignancy along with cytokine-associated toxicity in a clinical trial of anti-CD19 chimeric-antigen-receptor-transduced T cells. *Blood*. 2012;119(12):2709–2720.

115  Porter DL, Kalos M, Zheng Z, Levine B, June C. Chimeric antigen receptor therapy for B-cell malignancies. *J Cancer*. 2011;2:331–332.

116  Lamers CH, Sleijfer S, Vulto AG, et al. Treatment of metastatic renal cell carcinoma with autologous T-lymphocytes genetically retargeted against carbonic anhydrase IX: first clinical experience. *J Clin Oncol*. 2006;24(13):e20–e22.

117  Kershaw MH, Westwood JA, Parker LL, et al. A phase I study on adoptive immunotherapy using gene-modified T cells for ovarian cancer. *Clin Cancer Res*. 2006;12(20 Pt 1):6106–6115.

118  Till BG, Jensen MC, Wang J, et al. Adoptive immunotherapy for indolent non-Hodgkin lymphoma and mantle cell lymphoma using genetically modified autologous CD20-specific T cells. *Blood*. 2008;112(6):2261–2271.

119  Park JR, Digiusto DL, Slovak M, et al. Adoptive transfer of chimeric antigen receptor re-directed cytolytic T lymphocyte clones in patients with neuroblastoma. *Mol Ther*. 2007;15(4):825–833.

120  Morgan RA, Yang JC, Kitano M, Dudley ME, Laurencot CM, Rosenberg SA. Case report of a serious adverse event following the administration of T cells transduced with a chimeric antigen receptor recognizing ERBB2. *Mol Ther*. 2010;18(4):843–851.

121  Bonini C, Ferrari G, Verzeletti S, et al. HSV-TK gene transfer into donor lymphocytes for control of allogeneic graft-versus-leukemia. *Science*. 1997;276(5319):1719–1724.

122 Tey SK, Dotti G, Rooney CM, Heslop HE, Brenner MK. Inducible caspase 9 suicide gene to improve the safety of allodepleted T cells after haploidentical stem cell transplantation. *Biol Blood Marrow Transplant*. 2007;13(8):913–924.

123 Pule MA, Savoldo B, Myers GD, et al. Virus-specific T cells engineered to coexpress tumor-specific receptors: persistence and antitumor activity in individuals with neuroblastoma. *Nat Med*. 2008;14(11):1264–1270.

124 Louis CU, Savoldo B, Dotti G, et al. Antitumor activity and long-term fate of chimeric antigen receptor-positive T cells in patients with neuroblastoma. *Blood*. 2011;118(23):6050–6056.

125 Turtle CJ, Riddell SR. Genetically retargeting CD8+ lymphocyte subsets for cancer immunotherapy. *Curr Opin Immunol*. 2011;23(2):299–305.

126 Terakura S, Yamamoto TN, Gardner RA, Turtle CJ, Jensen MC, Riddell SR. Generation of CD19-chimeric antigen receptor modified CD8+ T cells derived from virus-specific central memory T cells. *Blood*. 2012;119(1):72–82.

127 Zhang T, Lemoi BA, Sentman CL. Chimeric NK-receptor-bearing T cells mediate antitumor immunotherapy. *Blood*. 2005;106(5):1544–1551.

128 Niederman TM, Ghogawala Z, Carter BS, Tompkins HS, Russell MM, Mulligan RC. Antitumor activity of cytotoxic T lymphocytes engineered to target vascular endothelial growth factor receptors. *Proc Natl Acad Sci U S A*. 2002;99(10):7009–7014.

129 Pegram HJ, Lee JC, Hayman EG, et al. Tumor-targeted T cells modified to secrete IL-12 eradicate systemic tumors without need for prior conditioning. *Blood*. 2012;119(18):4133–4141.

130 Mellor AL, Keskin DB, Johnson T, Chandler P, Munn DH. Cells expressing indoleamine 2,3-dioxygenase inhibit T cell responses. *J Immunol*. 2002;168(8):3771–3776.

131 Rodriguez PC, Ochoa AC. Arginine regulation by myeloid derived suppressor cells and tolerance in cancer: mechanisms and therapeutic perspectives. *Immunol Rev*. 2008;222:180–191.

132 Qian F, Villella J, Wallace PK, et al. Efficacy of levo-1-methyl tryptophan and dextro-1-methyl tryptophan in reversing indoleamine-2,3-dioxygenase-mediated arrest of T-cell proliferation in human epithelial ovarian cancer. *Cancer Res*. 2009;69(13):5498–5504.

133 Reisser D, Onier-Cherix N, Jeannin JF. Arginase activity is inhibited by L-NAME, both in vitro and in vivo. *J Enzyme Inhib Med Chem*. 2002;17(4):267–270.

134 Manning EA, Ullman JG, Leatherman JM, et al. A vascular endothelial growth factor receptor-2 inhibitor enhances antitumor immunity through an immune-based mechanism. *Clin Cancer Res*. 2007;13(13):3951–3959.

135 Shrimali RK, Yu Z, Theoret MR, Chinnasamy D, Restifo NP, Rosenberg SA. Antiangiogenic agents can increase lymphocyte infiltration into tumor and enhance the effectiveness of adoptive immunotherapy of cancer. *Cancer Res*. 2010;70(15):6171–6180.

136 Wang L, Yi T, Kortylewski M, Pardoll DM, Zeng D, Yu H. IL-17 can promote tumor growth through an IL-6-Stat3 signaling pathway. *J Exp Med*. 2009;206(7):1457–1464.

137 Fox BA, Schendel DJ, Butterfield LH, et al. Defining the critical hurdles in cancer immunotherapy. *J Transl Med*. 2011;9(1):214.

138 Wolchok JD, Hoos A, O'Day S, et al. Guidelines for the evaluation of immune therapy activity in solid tumors: immune-related response criteria. *Clin Cancer Res*. 2009;15(23):7412–7420.

139 Hoos A, Eggermont AM, Janetzki S, et al. Improved endpoints for cancer immunotherapy trials. *J Natl Cancer Inst*. 2010;102(18):1388–1397.

140 Vanneman M, Dranoff G. Combining immunotherapy and targeted therapies in cancer treatment. *Nat Rev Cancer*. 2012;12(4):237–251.

# CHAPTER 4

# Cancer Stem Cell Principles

*Allison C. Sharrow[1,2], Gabriel Ghiaur[3], and Richard J. Jones[3]*

[1]Department of Pathology, Johns Hopkins University School of Medicine, Baltimore, MD, USA

[2]Department of Cancer Immunotherapeutics and Tumor Immunology, Beckman Research Institute, City of Hope Comprehensive Cancer Center, Duarte, CA, USA

[3]The Sidney Kimmel Comprehensive Cancer Center, The Johns Hopkins University School of Medicine, Baltimore, MD, USA

## Background

Therapeutic advances over the past three decades now allow most cancer patients to achieve major clinical responses. Although clinical responses can clearly decrease side effects and improve quality of life, most patients with advanced cancer still eventually relapse and die of their disease. The cancer stem cell concept may explain why dramatic responses often fail to translate into cures. This hypothesis proposes that a malignancy maintains a similar hierarchical structure to the normal tissue of origin, such that the bulk of the tumor primarily represents the differentiated progeny of rarer cancer stem cells with self-renewal capacity. Initial responses in cancer would represent therapeutic effectiveness against the differentiated cancer cells making up the bulk of the tumor. Rare, biologically distinct cancer stem cells that are relatively resistant to these therapies could persist and cause relapse (Figure 4.1). This pattern of activity is analogous to mowing a dandelion; although the visible portion of the weed will be eliminated, the unseen root remains and will eventually lead to regrowth. If the cancer stem cells could be effectively targeted, durable remissions (i.e., cures) could possibly be obtained, but perhaps only after significant delays that could obscure effectiveness. Such a treatment effect mimics attacking just the root of the dandelion. Although this has no immediately discernible effect on the weed, over time, the weed should eventually wither and die if its root has been eliminated. Although cells meeting the definition for cancer stem cells have now been described in most malignancies, there remains healthy skepticism about their true biological significance.

## Historical Perspective

Carl Nordling first proposed the multi-step model of carcinogenesis in 1953.[1] In this model of carcinogenesis, further refined by Ashley,[2] Knudson[3] and Nowell,[4] inherited and/or environmentally induced mutations lead to the development of pre-malignant cells. Such cells further accumulate genetic mutations until one reaches a critical state that confers a growth and/or survival advantage

over its normal counterparts and gives rise to a fully malignant tumor. As postulated by Ashley, cancer-initiating cells must survive long enough to accumulate the three to seven genetic mutations necessary to generate cancer.[2] Moreover, these cells must already possess proliferative capacity or develop it anew as a consequence of genetic mutation(s). The inherent longevity and extensive proliferative capacity of tissue stem cells make them ideal candidate cancer-initiating cells. In contrast, most terminally differentiated cells are short-lived with only a limited number of divisions remaining in their differentiation program, thus making it unlikely that they would be able to produce tumors. Differentiated cells could only acquire the multiple genetic mutations required for malignant tumor growth if these mutations occurred simultaneously or in rapid succession, such as in the generation of induced pluripotent stem cells.

Observations during the early 1950s on the DNA content of cells led several groups to hypothesize that only a fraction of the cells in tumors were capable of normal and regular mitosis; these groups used the term tumor stem cells, suggesting that these cells were responsible for malignant growth by producing both new tumor stem cells as well as the rest of the population.[5,6] Additional evidence that only a small subset of cancer cells were responsible for cancer growth came from clinical studies in the early 1960s. Assays on leukemia patients injected with tritiated thymidine demonstrated that cell division appeared to take place only in the bone marrow, with the leukemia cells that were released into the blood unable to undergo further divisions.[7] In 1985, Sabbath et al. showed that clonogenic leukemia cells were usually less differentiated than the bulk leukemia cells, with some exhibiting cell surface markers similar to normal hematopoietic stem cells.[8]

Since the cancer-initiating cell in this model possesses self-renewal capacity and at least some differentiation potential—two of the defining features of normal stem cells—this cell naturally came to be called a cancer stem cell. Alternatively, it is also conceptually possible that the low clonogenicity of cancer is the result of all cells within a cancer retaining the capacity to proliferate, but only at a low rate (stochastic growth, Figure 4.1). Which of these two scenarios accounts for the low clonogenicity of most cancers has been debated for years, as the necessary methodology for addressing the question has been lacking until recently.

Funding: NIH grants P01CA15396, P01CA70790, DOD grant W81XWH-09-1-0129

## Cancer stem cell model

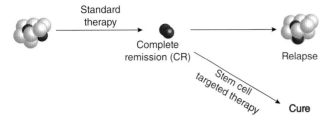

## Stochastic model

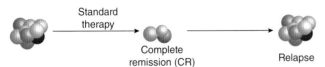

**Figure 4.1** Cancer stem cell concept versus stochastic model of tumor growth. The cancer stem cell concept proposes that most cancers are broadly organized in a similar hierarchical structure to their tissue of origin: relatively rare populations of stem-like cells, termed cancer stem cells (depicted in red), give rise to more prevalent differentiated cells. It further hypothesizes that current treatment methods eliminate the differentiated cells, but leave behind the drug-resistant cancer stem cells that eventually regenerate the tumor and lead to relapse; accordingly, cure requires treatments that target the drug-resistant cancer stem cells. Conversely, the stochastic model suggests that some cancer cells will escape therapy as a result of chemotherapy response following first order kinetics, and any remaining cancer cell can regenerate the tumor. Under this model, it would not be necessary to specifically target a subset of cells, but rather better targeting of the total population is needed.

## Cancer Stem Cells in Hematologic Malignancies

### Chronic Myeloid Leukemia

Given that hematopoiesis is the best characterized somatic stem cell system, it is not surprising that cancer stem cells have been best characterized in hematologic malignancies. There is now universal agreement that the cancer-initiating event in chronic myeloid leukemia occurs in an early hematopoietic cell, if not the hematopoietic stem cell itself. Evidence supporting the cancer stem cell concept in chronic myeloid leukemia dates back to the 1960s. Fialkow et al. demonstrated that erythrocytes and granulocytes in chronic myeloid leukemia share a common cancer stem cell.[9] The stem cell origin of chronic myeloid leukemia was confirmed in the 1990s when several groups, using characteristics known to define normal hematopoietic stem cells, identified and isolated chronic myeloid leukemia cells capable of expansion in culture.[10] Moreover, chronic myeloid leukemia stem cells not only phenotypically resembled normal hematopoietic stem cells, but their gene expression patterns also closely resembled those of normal hematopoietic stem cells.[11] The classic phenotype of hematopoietic stem cells, also expressed by CML stem cells, is the expression of CD34 and aldehyde dehydrogenase 1 ($ALDH^{high}$) with lack of expression of lineage-specific markers such as CD38. CD34 is expressed on the surface of normal hematopoietic stem cells and may help these cells attach to the bone marrow supportive components. CD38 is absent from the surface of normal hematopoietic stem cells and is expressed when these cells transition into progenitor cells. The aldehyde dehydrogenase

family of enzymes is responsible for oxidation of intracellular aldehydes. The aldehyde dehydrogenase 1 (ALDH1) family, also called retinaldehyde dehydrogenases, plays an important role in the conversion of vitamin A into retinoic acid, which is a required co-factor for the growth of stem cells.

### Acute Myeloid Leukemia

Acute myeloid leukemia was the first cancer in which malignant cells with the ability to recapitulate the disease in an immunocompromised mouse were identified.[12] The growth of human cells after xenotransplantation into immunocompromised mice is a widely accepted model for the study of stem cells, which are better able to grow, or engraft, after transplantation than their terminally differentiated progeny. Studying the cells that are produced after xenotransplantation also reveals the differentiation capacity of the transplanted cells. Most early studies on acute myeloid leukemia stem cells found that they, like chronic myeloid leukemia stem cells, exhibited a hematopoietic stem cell phenotype ($CD34^+CD38^-ALDH^{high}$). However, the exact surface phenotype of acute myeloid leukemia stem cells continues to be a subject of debate, perhaps because of the heterogeneity of the disease. Acute myeloid leukemia cells with the ability to proliferate in immunocompromised mice have been found in both $CD38^-$ and $CD38^+$ populations, as well as in $CD34^-$ populations.[13] The current uncertainty about the phenotype of the acute myeloid leukemia stem cells has led many investigators to advocate for a functional definition of these cells: those leukemic cells capable of engrafting immunodeficient mice.[13–15] Yet, this current "gold standard" for the identification of acute myeloid leukemia stem cells has proven to be somewhat problematic. Many acute myeloid leukemia samples will not engraft in immunodeficient mice, and the assay is cumbersome and often non-quantitative.[16,17] In addition, the clinical implications of this assay are unclear.[17]

### Multiple Myeloma

In 1968, Bergsagel and Valeriote used the term tumor stem cells to describe the small fraction of mouse multiple myeloma cells that were capable of clonogenic growth.[18] Subsequent studies by Hamburger and Salmon confirmed these findings with clinical myeloma specimens, revealing a cloning efficiency ranging from approximately 1:1000 to 1:100,000 cells.[19] Insufficient tools existed at the time to distinguish whether this low clonogenic potential was the result of proliferative capacity exclusively restricted to a small subset of cancer cells or was stochastic, that is, every cell had growth capacity but only at a low, random rate. Recent work suggested that the bulk plasma cells in myeloma are the terminally differentiated progeny of myeloma stem cells that have a similar phenotype to memory B cells and express high levels of ALDH1.[20,21] Moreover, the putative myeloma stem cells and the plasma cells that comprise the bulk of the tumor exhibited disparate drug sensitivities. The putative myeloma stem cells were also resistant to most clinically active agents (e.g., dexamethasone, lenalidomide, bortezomib), perhaps in part by co-opting normal stem cells' intrinsic defense mechanisms such as quiescence, efflux pumps, and detoxifying enzymes.[20,21] In addition, the stem cell niche may also protect cancer stem cells as it does normal stem cells.

### Lymphomas

The hallmark of classic Hodgkin's lymphoma, Hodgkin and Reed–Sternberg (HRS) cells, are derived from B cells but are unlike any normal cells of that lineage, and their limited proliferative potential belies the clinical aggressiveness of the disease. More than 20 years ago, Newcom et al. identified subclones of mononuclear B cells that appeared to be responsible for the production of the HRS cells in a Hodgkin's lymphoma cell line.[22] These findings were recently confirmed in several other Hodgkin's lymphoma cell lines.[23] Moreover, ALDH1-expressing memory B cells that exhibited identical clonal immunoglobulin gene rearrangements as the patients' HRS cells could be isolated from the peripheral blood of most newly diagnosed Hodgkin's lymphoma patients.[23] Thus, as in multiple myeloma, the cancer-initiating cells in Hodgkin's lymphoma appear to be memory B cells. There is also evidence for cancer stem cells in mantle cell lymphoma. B cells with high ALDH1 activity were identified in human mantle cell lymphoma cell lines, as well as in patients with newly diagnosed disease.[24] These cells were found to be relatively quiescent and resistant to many classic chemotherapeutic agents used to treat this condition.[24]

## Cancer Stem Cells in Solid Tumors

Identification and characterization of cancer stem cells from hematologic malignancies was founded on decades of experience in human hematopoiesis, including well-understood purification methodology and both *in vivo* and *in vitro* functional assays. Limited understanding of the cellular markers and biology associated with normal differentiation of solid organs has hampered the study of cancer stem cells in solid tumors, if they indeed exist. Because of this, research into cancer stem cells in solid tumors lagged substantially behind that for hematologic malignancies and was initially based on findings in liquid malignancies

### Breast Cancer

The first evidence of cancer stem cells in a solid tumor came from studies of breast cancer in 2003.[25] Breast cancer cells with a $CD44^+CD24^{-/low}Lineage^-$ phenotype were able to form tumors in immunocompromised mice with lower cell numbers than their bulk counterparts; these cells also reproduced the phenotypic diversity of the original tumor.[25] CD44 is a receptor for hyaluronic acid and plays an important role in cell–cell interactions, cell adhesion, migration, and metastasis, properties likely exhibited by putative cancer stem cells. CD24 is widely expressed and often upregulated in cancer, but its function is only well defined in B cells. Further work provided additional characterization of these putative breast cancer stem cells. They lacked expression of cytokeratin 14, cytokeratin 18, CD10, and epithelial specific antigen (EPCAM), which are markers of differentiated breast cancer cells.[26] Like putative hematologic malignancy cancer stem cells, these cells also displayed gene expression patterns consistent with normal stem cells including oct-4 (a transcription factor important for stem cell self-renewal), telomerase activity, the anti-apoptotic protein survivin, and lack of expression of connexin 43 (a protein important for forming gap junctions).[26] Based on markers of cancer stem cells in hematopoietic malignancies, the population was further refined as $CD133^{+\,27}$ and $ALDH^{high}$.[27,28] CD133 binds cholesterol and appears to suppress differentiation, making it a commonly used marker for the identification of cancer stem cells.

### Brain Tumors

The description of a population of cells with cancer stem cell properties in breast cancer was followed quickly by the discovery of a putative cancer stem cell population in brain cancer. $CD133^+$ brain cancer cells, but not $CD133^-$ cells, were found to generate tumors

after xenotransplantation into mice.[29] More recently, putative brain cancer stem cells were shown to also express ALDH1[30,31] and other stem cell markers, such as sox2 (suppresses neuronal differentiation), Musashi (may maintain neuronal stem cells in an undifferentiated state), and nestin (required for survival of neuronal progenitor cells).[32] Similar to hematologic cancer stem cells, putative glioblastoma stem cells were found to be relatively more resistant to radiotherapy than the differentiated cells that make up the bulk of the tumor mass.[32]

### Ovarian Cancer

Ovarian carcinoma is one of the most responsive solid tumors, but as with many hematologic malignancy patients, few women are cured despite the majority achieving initial complete remissions.[33] The first evidence for a cancer stem cell population in ovarian cancer was published in 2005 when cells from patient samples that grew under non-adherent culture conditions were found to express cytokeratin 18, vimentin, c-met, epidermal growth factor receptor, CD44, and Slug.[34] Cytokeratin 18 and vimentin are intermediate filaments with different expression patterns. Cytokeratin 18 is commonly expressed in epithelial cells, while vimentin is primarily found in mesenchymal cells. C-met regulates proliferation and survival. Epidermal growth factor receptor is widely expressed in epithelial tissues including normal and cancerous ovarian cells. Slug plays a role in the development of epithelial cancers. Since then, several groups have proposed a variety of markers for the identification of ovarian cancer stem cells, including Hoechst side population,[35,36] CD133,[37,38] CD44,[36,39,40] c-kit (important for stem cell maintenance),[39] CD24,[41] and ALDH1.[36,42] Hoechst side population marks cells with increased expression of ATP-binding cassette (ABC) membrane transport pumps, a common feature of stem cells.

### Prostate Cancer

$CD44^+$integrin $\alpha_2\beta_1{}^{high}CD133^+$ putative prostate cancer stem cells exhibiting self-renewal and high proliferative potential were described in 2005.[43] Integrins are involved in cellular adhesion, and the different isoforms vary in their tissue distribution and function. The $\alpha_2\beta_1$ type binds laminin, collagen, fibronectin, and E-cadherin. Further experiments showed that $CD44^+$ cells were more tumorigenic and lead to more metastases than $CD44^-$ cells.[44] Putative prostate cancer stem cells also expressed the stem cell genes β-catenin, smoothened, Oct-3/4,[44] and NF-κB.[45] β-catenin regulates the growth and adhesion of epithelial cells, and mutations are associated with several types of cancer. Smoothened is an indirect receptor for the developmentally conserved Hedgehog ligands; hedgehog signaling is important for directionality in the developing embryo, and plays a role in regulating adult tissue homeostasis. The NF-κB pathway is nearly universally expressed and has a wide array of functions, including regulating differentiation, cell growth, tumorigenesis, and apoptosis. When NF-κB signaling was blocked, the putative prostate cancer stem cells, but not normal stem cells, underwent apoptosis *in vitro*, suggesting a possible treatment approach.[45]

### Gastrointestinal Malignancies

Over the past 5 years, most gastrointestinal tumors have been shown to harbor rare cancer cells with stem-like properties. A population of cells expressing CD133 has been reported in colon cancer.[46,47] These cells were more tumorigenic than the predominant $CD133^-$ cells,[46,47] lacked expression of the gastrointestinal differentiation marker cytokeratin 20, and had the ability to differentiate into cytokeratin 20-expressing $CD133^-$ cells.[47] Putative colon cancer stem cells have also been shown to express ALDH1.[48] Cells with increased tumorigenicity were identified in gastric cancer cell lines on the basis of Hoechst side population,[49] CD44,[50,51] CD24,[51] and ALDH1 expression.[52] To date, there are only limited cancer stem cell studies in gastric cancer clinical specimens.

CD44[+]CD24[+]EPCAM[+] pancreatic cancer cells were found to better form tumors in immunocompromised mice than CD44[−], CD24[−], or EPCAM[−] cells.[53] These putative pancreatic cancer stem cells had self-renewal capacity, regenerated the phenotypic diversity of the tumor, and had upregulation of the Hedgehog signaling pathway.[53] Another group found that CD133[+] pancreatic cancer cells were also highly tumorigenic in a xenograft mouse model and regenerated the phenotypic diversity of the original tumor.[54] These putative pancreatic cancer stem cells also lacked expression of the differentiation marker cytokeratin (CK5, 6, 8, 17 and 19) and expressed CXCR4, which is an important receptor for the cell migration signal SDF-1.[54] The same CD133[+] putative stem cell population was also more resistant to chemotherapy.[54] ALDH1 has been shown to further enrich for pancreatic cancer stem cell activity.[55] CD44[+]CD24[+]ALDH[high] cells were more tumorigenic than cells expressing just one of the markers.[55]

CD90[+] and CD44[+] liver cancer cells were found to be tumorigenic in immunocompromised mice.[56] There was some overlap between these populations, but it is unclear if CD90[+]CD44[+] cells were more tumorigenic than either marker alone. They also found overlap with CD90[+] and other potential cancer stem cell antigens, including CD133, EPCAM, CXCR4, CD24, and KDR.[56] KDR is a vascular endothelial growth factor receptor that regulates endothelial cell proliferation, survival, and migration. Putative liver cancer stem cells isolated from the blood of patients were able to form tumors in immunocompromised mice, suggesting that circulating liver cancer stem cells may be responsible for metastasis.[56]

### Other Cancers

Putative cancer stem cells have also been identified in most other malignancies, including lung cancer,[57–61] melanoma,[62] head and neck cancer,[63] bladder cancer,[64] and sarcomas.[65–69] These putative cancer stem cells have generally been identified using the same markers used to identify cancer stem cells in hematologic and other solid organ malignancies described above, including ALDH1, CD44, CD24, CD133, and Hoechst side population. However, similar to acute myeloid leukemia, there is no consensus on the phenotype of cancer stem cells from most cancers, if they exist. It is possible that each of these markers identifies different stages of cellular differentiation that can all have the ability to generate tumors. Another possibility is that each of these markers defines separate, but overlapping, populations. Nevertheless, the putative cancer stem cells from most malignancies have been shown to have many stem-like features, including high clonogenic capacity *in vitro* and *in vivo*, expression of putative stem cell pathways, the ability to regenerate the phenotypic diversity of the tumor, and relative drug resistance.

### Controversy and Clinical Relevance

Despite conceptual support and laboratory evidence for the existence of stem-like cells in most malignancies, many investigators have proposed that cancer stem cells may be nothing more than laboratory curiosities, primarily reflecting the limitations of current models for assessing tumorigenic potential.[70] This controversy is highlighted by a study that compared the growth of primary melanoma cells in mice with different levels of immunocompetence. NOD/SCID mice lack T and B cells, while NOD/SCID-IL2Rγ[−/−] (NSG) mice additionally lack natural killer cells. Although only about 1 in 100,000 unselected melanoma cells produced tumors in NOD/SCID mice, as few as 1 in 4 melanoma cells were tumorigenic when transplanted into NSG mice.[71] However, despite being considered the gold standard assay for cancer stem cells by many in the field, there is no reason to assume that growth in immunocompromised mice is in fact a relevant assay for cancer stem cell function.

Perhaps the strongest reason for skepticism regarding the cancer stem cell concept has been the limited evidence that such cells have clinical relevance. Importantly, until recently, there has been no definitive data showing that cancer stem cells from any malignancy are in fact responsible for disease progression or relapse. Relapse could result from a tumor's stochastic first-order kinetic response to drugs or the development of a therapeutic resistance mechanism by any cell within a malignancy (Figure 4.1). The inability to directly observe early events in carcinogenesis makes definitively determining the cell of origin for cancer problematic. Regardless of where in the differentiation hierarchy of a tissue the initiating event occurred or whether the cells are tumorigenic in immunocompromised mice, the most clinically important cancer cells are those that survive therapy and lead to relapse. Even if every cell in a cancer possessed tumorigenic potential, the presence of a discrete subset resistant to treatment—perhaps as a result of stem cell properties—would have undeniable clinical significance.

Possibly the first evidence suggesting biological and clinical relevance for cancer stem cells was data showing that lung,[58] pancreatic,[55] and ovarian cancer[42,72] clinical specimens expressing the stem cell marker ALDH1 were associated with poor prognoses. Metastatic pancreatic cancer also has been shown to exhibit higher expression of ALDH1 than the primary tumor, suggesting that the cancer stem cells may be responsible for metastases.[55] Evidence further implicating cancer stem cells as the metastasis-initiating cells comes from observations in several cancers that these cells circulate in the blood.[20,23,73,74] In addition, human pancreatic cancer xenografts in mice are enriched for CD133[+] cancer stem cells following treatment of the mice with chemotherapy.[54] However, these data are primarily correlations, and not direct evidence for the role of cancer stem cells in treatment resistance and relapse.

If cancer stem cells are indeed more resistant to therapy than the bulk tumor cells, then minimal residual disease after treatment should be enriched for these cells. Furthermore, the presence of cancer stem cells after therapy should predict recurrence. Indeed, residual breast cancer cell populations persisting after treatment are enriched for phenotypic cancer stem cells.[75,76] Similarly, patients with myelodysplastic syndrome continue to harbor a population of phenotypically distinct cancer stem cells after clinically effective treatment.[77] Based on their persistence, these cells appeared to be resistant to chemotherapy treatment and thus may have accounted for disease relapse.

Only recently, however, has the detection of phenotypic cancer stem cells been found to correlate with relapse. Minimal residual disease detected during complete remission in acute myeloid leukemia patients was enriched for phenotypic cancer stem cells.[78] Moreover, the presence of these cells after therapy highly correlated with subsequent clinical relapse.[78] Also, the persistence of detectable circulating cancer stem cells after treatment in patients with Hodgkin's lymphoma was associated with a greater chance of relapse.[79] Although confirmation in larger numbers of patients is required, these reports provide evidence of clinical relevance for cancer stem cells. If confirmed, screening for cancer stem cells after treatment should provide an early window into prognosis and help personalize treatment. At present, the only available therapy that targets stem cells is allogeneic blood or marrow transplantation (BMT), but its inherent toxicity and limited spectrum of activity (i.e., little activity against solid tumors) limit its applicability. The ability to predict relapse by detecting persistent cancer stem cells would allow clinicians to better determine which patients with hematopoietic malignancies would benefit from allogeneic BMT.[78,79]

## Targeting Cancer Stem Cells

The search for novel anticancer therapies has generally focused on targets that are specific for, or overexpressed in, selected cancers. However, attacking cancer-specific targets has met with variable success, and many of the most effective anticancer therapies show limited or even no tumor selectivity. Targeting a cancer-specific pathway could have limited effectiveness for several reasons. It is likely that many cancers have already acquired multiple oncogenic mutations capable of driving tumor growth. In such cases, targeting only one pathway will likely be ineffective. Furthermore, even when the initiating oncogenic event is targeted, inherent stem cell properties may make the target inaccessible or irrelevant in cancer stem cells. For example, the quiescence of stem cells may make them resistant to drugs targeting dividing cells. The high expression of cell membrane efflux pumps such as MDR1 and ABCG2 by stem cells also limits drug availability to cellular targets. Moreover, stem cells have survival mechanisms that do not depend on the targeted oncogene.

However, properties shared with normal stem cells may not only be responsible for cancer stem cell resistance to many anticancer agents, but they could also serve as the targets for novel therapies active across many malignancies. Prospective targets shared with normal stem cells may have particularly strong anticancer potential since their conserved expression suggests a critical function retained by the cancer stem cell. Emerging data suggest that cancer stem cells across a wide spectrum of malignancies exhibit shared stem-cell-related biological characteristics, such as Hedgehog signaling[80] and telomerase expression.[81] While the bulk cells of various tumors have distinct biology and thus require distinct treatments, the therapies targeting cancer stem cells of different malignancies may prove to be more universally applicable. Using such treatments either in combination with debulking therapy or as subsequent maintenance therapy may improve cure rates. Successfully targeting cancer stem cells could not only improve patient outcomes, but also provide the ultimate evidence for the cancer stem cell concept.

In fact, preliminary data suggest that inhibition of stem cell pathways, even when they are not mutated or overexpressed, may produce potent antitumor activity across a range of malignancies, possibly because of the key roles these pathways play in stem cell maintenance and growth. Hedgehog signaling appears key to the growth and survival of several malignancies including glioblastoma, breast cancer, pancreatic cancer, multiple myeloma, and chronic myeloid leukemia.[80] Moreover, Hedgehog pathway blockade, while having little or no effect on the differentiated cells, markedly inhibits myeloma stem cell growth *in vitro* and leads to their terminal differentiation.[82] Based on these results, clinical trials targeting cancer stem cells with Hedgehog inhibitors are underway. Telomerase is expressed in a variety of cancers, and inhibition of telomerase has been reported to have activity against a variety of putative cancer stem cells *in vitro*.[83–86] Trials targeting telomerase in cancer stem cells are also underway. Another approach potentially applicable to cancer stem cells is to augment their differentiation. Such induction of terminal differentiation appears to eliminate cancer stem cells *in vitro,* and clinical trials attempting to induce terminal differentiation of cancer stem cells clinically are also underway.[87]

The potential for toxicity is an obvious concern for targets shared with normal stem cells. However, there are several potential differences between normal stem cells and cancer stem cells that may provide a therapeutic ratio for shared targets. Normal stem cells have normal cell cycle checkpoints that are likely to protect them from cellular damage or crisis. The stage of differentiation at which cancers arise may also provide selectivity for approaches targeting cancer stem cells. Although many cancers may arise from normal cells with stem cell properties, these cells may not be the most primitive tissue stem cells. For example, if a therapy equally eliminated both myeloma stem cells and their normal counterparts, memory B cells, the existence of more primitive normal hematopoietic stem cells should replenish the normal B-cell pool.

A difference in the interplay between telomere length and telomerase is another example how a stem cell pathway may provide a therapeutic ratio between cancer stem cells and their normal counterparts. Normal stem cells require telomerase to prevent telomere shortening and replicative senescence. However, even in the absence of telomerase, normal stem cells can maintain replicative capacity for some period of time because of their relatively long telomeres. Accordingly, mice lacking functional telomerase showed very limited abnormalities until the fourth generation.[88] In addition, the major cause of death in dyskeratosis congenita, a congenital disease that results from loss of function mutations in telomerase components, is bone marrow failure, but this usually does not manifest until the second to fourth decade of life.[89] In contrast, uninterrupted telomerase activity may be absolutely required for the maintenance and growth of most malignancies in order to stabilize the short telomeres that appear to characterize cancer stem cells.[90] In fact, crossing telomerase knockout mice with mice genetically predisposed to cancer significantly lowered the development of cancers in these mice.[91,92] Thus, the differences in telomere length between normal (long) and cancer (short) stem cells could render telomerase inhibition selectively toxic to cancer.

The rarity of many cancer stem cells (often <1% of the total tumor cells) has both limited their study and potentially masked cancer stem cell responses to treatment. Any therapeutic impact on the rare cancer stem cells may be imperceptible, hidden by the bulk cancer cells. Current detection methods are insufficient to resolve differences in the size of this minute cancer stem cell population with treatment. Hence, therapies which are effective against only the differentiated cells, but inactive against cancer stem cells, may appear overly promising, while highly active agents against cancer stem cells may appear falsely ineffective if they have little impact on the differentiated cancer bulk. Accordingly, new clinical methodologies are necessary to successfully assess the effects of potential cancer stem cell therapies. Evaluating the efficacy of treatments against cancer stem cells should be possible by testing these treatments after eliminating the bulk tumor cells. In cancers that often show an initial remission followed by relapse, potential therapies could be administered during remission to determine if they increase the duration of remission. For some cancers, such as hematopoietic malignancies, the fate of cancer stem cells could also be assessed using the same detection methods developed for laboratory research.

## Conclusions

Initial responses to cancer treatment represent therapeutic effectiveness against the cancer cells making up the bulk of the tumor. However, emerging data suggest that initially effective therapy may have little activity against the biologically distinct cancer stem cells, which may be responsible for relapse. Nevertheless, there remains a healthy skepticism regarding the cancer stem cell hypothesis. This uncertainty has been based on discrepant phenotypic findings, conflicting results from the current gold standard xenograft transplant assay, and limited evidence for clinical significance. However, new data showing that putative cancer stem cells are enriched in minimal residual disease and may therefore be responsible for relapse provides strong support for the cancer stem cell concept.

Traditional response criteria measure tumor bulk and may not reflect changes in populations of rare cancer stem cells. Therapy selectively directed at cancer stem cells will not immediately eliminate the differentiated tumor cells and will be prematurely abandoned if usual response criteria are used. Thus, novel clinical methodology for studying cancer stem cell-targeted therapy is needed. In order to also eliminate the bulk cells, cancer stem cell targeted therapy will need to be administered in combination with debulking therapy or during remission as maintenance therapy.

## References

1. Nordling CO. A new theory on cancer-inducing mechanism. *Br J Cancer*. 1953;7(1):68–72.
2. Ashley DJ. The two "hit" and multiple "hit" theories of carcinogenesis. *Br J Cancer*. 1969;23(2):313–328.
3. Knudson AG Jr. Mutation and cancer: statistical study of retinoblastoma. *Proc Natl Acad Sci U S A*. 1971;68(4):820–823.
4. Nowell PC. The clonal evolution of tumor cell populations. *Science*. 1976;194(4260):23–28.
5. Richards BM. Deoxyribose nucleic acid values in tumour cells with reference to the stem-cell theory of tumour growth. *Nature*. 1955;175(4449):259–261.
6. Makino S. The role of tumor stem-cells in regrowth of the tumor following drastic applications. *Acta Unio Int Contra Cancrum*. 1959;15(suppl. 1):196–198.
7. Killmann SA, Cronkite EP, Robertson JS, Fliedner TM, Bond VP. Estimation of phases of the life cycle in leukemic cells from labeling in human beings in vivo with tritiated thymidine. *Lab Invest*. 1963;12(7):671–684.
8. Sabbath KD, Ball ED, Larcom P, Davis RB, Griffin JD. Heterogeneity of clonogenic cells in acute myeloblastic leukemia. *J Clin Invest*. 1985;75(2):746–753.
9. Fialkow PJ, Gartler SM, Yoshida A. Clonal origin of chronic myelocytic leukemia in man. *Proc Natl Acad Sci U S A*. 1967;58(4):1468–1471.
10. Bedi A, Zehnbauer BA, Collector MI, et al. BCR-ABL gene rearrangement and expression of primitive hematopoietic progenitors in chronic myeloid leukemia. *Blood*. 1993;81(11):2898–2902.
11. Gerber JM, Qin L, Kowalski J, et al. Characterization of chronic myeloid leukemia stem cells. *Am J Hematol*. 2011;86(1):31–37.
12. Lapidot T, Sirard C, Vormoor J, et al. A cell initiating human acute myeloid leukaemia after transplantation into SCID mice. *Nature*. 1994;367(6464):645–648.
13. Sarry JE, Murphy K, Perry R, et al. Human acute myelogenous leukemia stem cells are rare and heterogeneous when assayed in NOD/SCID/IL2Rgammac-deficient mice. *J Clin Invest*. 2011;121(1):384–395.
14. Taussig DC, Miraki-Moud F, Anjos-Afonso F, et al. Anti-CD38 antibody-mediated clearance of human repopulating cells masks the heterogeneity of leukemia-initiating cells. *Blood*. 2008;112(3):568–575.
15. Taussig DC, Vargaftig J, Miraki-Moud F, et al. Leukemia-initiating cells from some acute myeloid leukemia patients with mutated nucleophosmin reside in the CD34àí fraction. *Blood*. 2010;115(10):1976–1984.
16. Pearce DJ, Taussig D, Zibara K, et al. AML engraftment in the NOD/SCID assay reflects the outcome of AML: implications for our understanding of the heterogeneity of AML. *Blood*. 2006;107(3):1166–1173.
17. Rombouts WJ, Martens AC, Ploemacher RE. Identification of variables determining the engraftment potential of human acute myeloid leukemia in the immunodeficient NOD/SCID human chimera model. *Leukemia*. 2000;14(5):889–897.
18. Bergsagel DE, Valeriote FA. Growth characteristics of a mouse plasma cell tumor. *Cancer Res*. 1968;28(11):2187–2196.
19. Hamburger AW, Salmon SE. Primary bioassay of human tumor stem cells. *Science*. 1977;197(4302):461–463.
20. Matsui W, Huff CA, Wang Q, et al. Characterization of clonogenic multiple myeloma cells. *Blood*. 2004;103(6):2332–2336.
21. Matsui W, Wang Q, Barber JP, et al. Clonogenic multiple myeloma progenitors, stem cell properties, and drug resistance. *Cancer Res*. 2008;68(1):190–197.
22. Newcom SR, Kadin ME, Phillips C. L-428 Reed-Sternberg cells and mononuclear Hodgkin's cells arise from a single cloned mononuclear cell. *Int J Cell Cloning*. 1988;6(6):417–431.
23. Jones RJ, Gocke CD, Kasamon YL, et al. Circulating clonotypic B cells in classic Hodgkin lymphoma. *Blood*. 2009;113(23):5920–5926.
24. Brennan SK., Meade B, Wang Q, Merchant AA, Kowalski J, Matsui W. Mantle cell lymphoma activation enhances bortezomib sensitivity. *Blood*. 2010;116(20):4185–4191.
25. Al-Hajj M, Wicha MS, Benito-Hernandez A, Morrison SJ, Clarke MF. Prospective identification of tumorigenic breast cancer cells. *Proc Natl Acad Sci U S A*. 2003;100(7):3983–3988.
26. Ponti D, Costa A, Zaffaroni N, et al. Isolation and in vitro propagation of tumorigenic breast cancer cells with stem/progenitor cell properties. *Cancer Res*. 2005;65(13):5506–5511.
27. Croker AK, Goodale D, Chu J, et al. High aldehyde dehydrogenase and expression of cancer stem cell markers selects for breast cancer cells with enhanced malignant and metastatic ability. *J Cell Mol Med*. 2009;13(8B):2236–2252.
28. Ginestier C, Hur MH, Charafe-Jauffret E, et al. ALDH1 is a marker of normal and malignant human mammary stem cells and a predictor of poor clinical outcome. *Cell Stem Cell*. 2007;1:555–567.
29. Singh SK, Hawkins C, Clarke ID, et al. Identification of human brain tumour initiating cells. *Nature*. 2004;432:396–401.
30. Rasper M, Schäfer A, Piontek G, et al. Aldehyde dehydrogenase 1 positive glioblastoma cells show brain tumor stem cell capacity. *Neuro Oncol*. 2010;12(10):1024–1033.
31. Choi SA, Lee JY, Phi JH, et al. Identification of brain tumour initiating cells using the stem cell marker aldehyde dehydrogenase. *Eur J Cancer*. 2014;50(1):137–149.
32. Bao S, Wu Q, McLendon RE, et al. Glioma stem cells promote radioresistance by preferential activation of the DNA damage response. *Nature*. 2006;444(7120):756–760.
33. Armstrong DK, Bundy B, Wenzel L, et al. Intraperitoneal cisplatin and paclitaxel in ovarian cancer. *N Engl J Med*. 2006;354(1):34–43.

34 Bapat SA, Mali AM, Koppikar CB, Kurrey NK, et al. Stem and progenitor-like cells contribute to the aggressive behavior of human epithelial ovarian cancer. *Cancer Res.* 2005;65(8):3025–3029.

35 Szotek PP, Pieretti-Vanmarcke R, Masiakos PT, et al. Ovarian cancer side population defines cells with stem cell-like characteristics and Mullerian Inhibiting Substance responsiveness. *Proc Natl Acad Sci U S A.* 2006;103(30):11154–11159.

36 Yasuda K, Torigoe T, Morita R, et al. Ovarian cancer stem cells are enriched in side population and aldehyde dehydrogenase bright overlapping population. *PLoS ONE.* 2013;8(8):e68187.

37 Baba T, Convery PA, Matsumura N, et al. Epigenetic regulation of CD133 and tumorigenicity of CD133 +ovarian cancer cells. *Oncogene.* 2009;28(2):209–218.

38 Ferrandina G, Bonanno G, Pierelli L, et al. Expression of CD133–1 and CD133–2 in ovarian cancer. *Int J Gynecol Cancer.* 2008;18(3):506–514.

39 Zhang S, Balch C, Chan MW, et al. Identification and characterization of ovarian cancer-initiating cells from primary human tumors. *Cancer Res.* 2008;68(11):4311–4320.

40 Alvero AB, Chen R, Fu HH, et al. Molecular phenotyping of human ovarian cancer stem cells unravels the mechanisms for repair and chemoresistance. *Cell Cycle.* 2009;8(1):158–166.

41 Gao MQ, Choi YP, Kang S, Youn JH, Cho NH. CD24 +cells from hierarchically organized ovarian cancer are enriched in cancer stem cells. *Oncogene.* 2010;29:2672–2680.

42 Landen CN Jr, Goodman B, Katre AA, et al. Targeting aldehyde dehydrogenase cancer stem cells in ovarian cancer. *Mol Cancer Ther.* 2010;9(12):3186–3199.

43 Collins AT, Berry PA, Hyde C, Stower MJ, Maitland NJ. Prospective identification of tumorigenic prostate cancer stem cells. *Cancer Res.* 2005;65(23):10946–10951.

44 Patrawala LCalhoun T, Schneider-Broussard R, et al. Highly purified CD44+ prostate cancer cells from xenograft human tumors are enriched in tumorigenic and metastatic progenitor cells. *Oncogene.* 2006;25(12):1696–1708.

45 Birnie R, Bryce SD, Roome C, et al. Gene expression profiling of human prostate cancer stem cells reveals a pro-inflammatory phenotype and the importance of extracellular matrix interactions. *Genome Biol.* 2008;9(5):R83.

46 O'Brien CA, Pollett A, Gallinger S, Dick JE. A human colon cancer cell capable of initiating tumour growth in immunodeficient mice. *Nature.* 2007;445:106–110.

47 Ricci-Vitiani L, Lombardi DG, Pilozzi E, et al. Identification and expansion of human colon-cancer-initiating cells. *Nature.* 2007;445(7123):111–115.

48 Huang EH, Hynes MJ, Zhang T, et al. Aldehyde dehydrogenase 1 is a marker for normal and malignant human colonic stem cells (SC) and tracks SC overpopulation during colon tumorigenesis. *Cancer Res.* 2009;69(8):3382–3389.

49 Fukuda K, Saikawa Y, Ohashi M, et al. Tumor initiating potential of side population cells in human gastric cancer. *Int J Oncol.* 2009;34(5):1201–1207.

50 Takaishi S, Okumura T, Tu S, et al. Identification of gastric cancer stem cells using the cell surface marker CD44. *Stem Cells.* 2009;27(5):1006–1020.

51 Zhang C, Li C, He F, Cai Y, Yang H. Identification of CD44+CD24+ gastric cancer stem cells. *J Cancer Res Clin Oncol.* 2011;137(11):1679–1686.

52 Zhi QM, Chen XH, Ji J, et al. Salinomycin can effectively kill ALDHhigh stem-like cells on gastric cancer. *Biomed Pharmacother.* 2011;65(7):509–515.

53 Li C, Heidt DG, Dalerba P, et al. Identification of pancreatic cancer stem cells. *Cancer Res.* 2007;67(3):1030–1037.

54 Hermann PC, Huber SL, Herrler T, et al. Distinct populations of cancer stem cells determine tumor growth and metastatic activity in human pancreatic cancer. *Cell.* 2007;1(3):313–323.

55 Rasheed ZA, Yang J, Wang Q, et al. Prognostic significance of tumorigenic cells with mesenchymal features in pancreatic adenocarcinoma. *J Nat Cancer Inst.* 2010;102(5):340–351.

56 Yang ZF, Ho DW, Ng MN, et al. Significance of CD90+ cancer stem cells in human liver cancer. *Cancer Cell.* 2008;13(2):153–166.

57 Eramo A, Lotti F, Sette G, et al. Identification and expansion of the tumorigenic lung cancer stem cell population. *Cell Death Differ.* 2007;15(3):504–514.

58 Jiang F, Qiu Q, Khanna A, et al. Aldehyde dehydrogenase 1 is a tumor stem cell-associated marker in lung cancer. *Mol Cancer Res.* 2009;7(3):330–338.

59 Liu J, Xiao Z, Wong SK, et al. Lung cancer tumorigenicity and drug resistance are maintained through ALDH hi CD44 hi tumor initiating cells. *Oncotarget.* 2013;4:1698–1711.

60 Cortes-Dericks L, Froment L, Boesch R, Schmid RA, Karoubi G. Cisplatin-resistant cells in malignant pleural mesothelioma cell lines show ALDHhighCD44+ phenotype and sphere-forming capacity. *BMC Cancer.* 2014;14(1):304.

61 Shao C, Sullivan JP, Girard L, et al. Essential role of aldehyde dehydrogenase 1A3 (ALDH1A3) for the maintenance of non-small cell lung cancer stem cells is associated with the STAT3 pathway. *Clin Cancer Res.* 2014;20(15):4154–4166.

62 Schatton T, Murphy GF, Frank NY, et al. Identification of cells initiating human melanomas. *Nature.* 2008;451:345–349.

63 Prince, ME, Sivanandan R, Kaczorowski A, et al. Identification of a subpopulation of cells with cancer stem cell properties in head and neck squamous cell carcinoma. *Proc Natl Acad Sci U S A.* 2007;104(3):973–978.

64 Chan KS, Espinosa I, Chao M, et al. Identification, molecular characterization, clinical prognosis, and therapeutic targeting of human bladder tumor-initiating cells. *Proc Natl Acad Sci U S A.* 2009;106(33):14016–14021.

65 Suvà ML, Riggi N, Stehle JC, et al. Identification of cancer stem cells in Ewing's sarcoma. *Cancer Res.* 2009;69(5):1776–1781.

66 Yang M, Yan M, Zhang R, Li J, Luo Z. Side population cells isolated from human osteosarcoma are enriched with tumor-initiating cells. *Cancer Sci.* 2011;102(10):1774–1781.

67 Tirino V, Desiderio V, Paino F, et al. Human primary bone sarcomas contain CD133+ cancer stem cells displaying high tumorigenicity in vivo. *FASEB J.* 2011;25(6):2022–2030.

68 Awad O, Yustein JT, Shah P, et al. High ALDH activity identifies chemotherapy-resistant ewing's sarcoma stem cells that retain sensitivity to EWS-FLI1 inhibition. *PLoS ONE.* 2010;5(11):e13943.

69 Honoki K, Fujii H, Kubo A, et al. Possible involvement of stem-like populations with elevated ALDH1 in sarcomas for chemotherapeutic drug resistance. *Oncol Rep.* 2010;24(2):501–505.

70 Kelly PN, Dakic A, Adams JM, Nutt SL, Strasser A. Tumor growth need not be driven by rare cancer stem cells. *Science.* 2007;317(5836):337.

71 Quintana E, Shackleton M, Sabel MS, Fullen DR, Johnson TM, Morrison SJ. Efficient tumour formation by single human melanoma cells. *Nature.* 2008;456(7222):593–598.

72 Liu S, Liu C, Min X, et al. Prognostic value of cancer stem cell marker aldehyde dehydrogenase in ovarian cancer: a Meta-Analysis. *PLoS ONE.* 2013;8(11):e81050.

73 Petzer AL, Eaves CJ, Lansdorp PM, Ponchio L, Barnett MJ, Eaves AC. Characterization of primitive subpopulations of normal and leukemic

cells present in the blood of patients with newly diagnosed as well as established chronic myeloid leukemia. *Blood*. 1996;88(6):2162–2171.

74 Riethdorf S, Pantel K. Disseminated tumor cells in bone marrow and circulating tumor cells in blood of breast cancer patients: current state of detection and characterization. *Pathobiology*. 2008;75(2):140–148.

75 Creighton CJ, Li X, Landis M, et al. Residual breast cancers after conventional therapy display mesenchymal as well as tumor-initiating features. *Proc Natl Acad Sci U S A*. 2009;106(33):13820–13825.

76 Tanei T, Morimoto K, Shimazu K, et al. Association of breast cancer stem cells identified by aldehyde dehydrogenase 1 expression with resistance to sequential paclitaxel and epirubicin-based chemotherapy for breast cancers. *Clin Cancer Res*. 2009;15(12):4234–4241.

77 Tehranchi R, Woll PS, Anderson K, et al. Persistent malignant stem cells in del(5q) myelodysplasia in remission. *N Engl J Med*. 2010;363(11):1025–1037.

78 Gerber JM, Smith BD, Ngwang B, et al. A clinically relevant population of leukemic CD34+CD38- cells in acute myeloid leukemia. *Blood*. 2012;119(15):3571–3577.

79 Kasamon YL, Jacene HA, Gocke CD, et al. Phase 2 study of rituximab-ABVD in classical Hodgkin lymphoma. *Blood*. 2012;119(18):4129–4132.

80 Merchant AA, Matsui W. Targeting Hedgehog–a cancer stem cell pathway. *Clin Cancer Res*. 2010;16(12):3130–3140.

81 Harley CB. Telomerase and cancer therapeutics. *Nat Rev Cancer*. 2008;8(3):167–179.

82 Peacock CD, Wang Q, Gessel GS, et al. Hedgehog signaling maintains a tumor stem cell compartment in multiple myeloma. *Proc Natl Acad Sci U S A*. 2007;104(10):4048–4053.

83 Brennan SK, Wang Q, Tressler R, et al. Telomerase inhibition targets clonogenic multiple myeloma cells through telomere length-dependent and independent mechanisms. *PLoS ONE*. 2010;5(9):e12487.

84 Castelo-Branco P, Zhang C, Lipman T, et al. Neural tumor-initiating cells have distinct telomere maintenance and can be safely targeted for telomerase inhibition. *Clin Cancer Res*. 2011;17(1):111–121.

85 Joseph I, Tressler R, Bassett E, et al. The telomerase inhibitor imetelstat depletes cancer stem cells in breast and pancreatic cancer cell lines. *Cancer Res*. 2010;70(22):9494–9504.

86 Serrano D, Bleau AM, Fernandez-Garcia I, et al. Inhibition of telomerase activity preferentially targets aldehyde dehydrogenase-positive cancer stem-like cells in lung cancer. *Mol Cancer*. 2011;10(96):96.

87 Schenk T, Chen WC, Göllner S, et al. Inhibition of the LSD1 (KDM1A) demethylase reactivates the all trans retinoic acid differentiation pathway in acute myeloid leukemia. *Nat Med*. 2012;18(4):605–611.

88 Hao LY, Armanios M, Strong MA, et al. Short telomeres, even in the presence of telomerase, limit tissue renewal capacity. *Cell*. 2005;123(6):1121–1131.

89 Knight S, Vulliamy T, Copplestone A, Gluckman E, Mason P, Dokal I. Dyskeratosis Congenita (DC) Registry: identification of new features of DC. *Br J Haematol*. 1998;103(4):990–996.

90 Ju Z, Rudolph KL. Telomeres and telomerase in cancer stem cells. *Eur J Cancer*. 2006;42(9):1197–1203.

91 Greenberg RA, Chin L, Femino A, et al. Short dysfunctional telomeres impair tumorigenesis in the INK4adelta2/3 cancer-prone mouse. *Cell*. 1999;97(4):515–525.

92 Rudolph KL, Millard M, Bosenberg MW, DePinho RA. Telomere dysfunction and evolution of intestinal carcinoma in mice and humans. *Nat Genet*. 2001;28(2):155–159.

# CHAPTER 5

# The Tumor Microenvironment as a Target for Therapeutic Intervention

*Hua Fang[1,2] and Yves A. DeClerck[1,2,3]*

[1]Division of Hematology-Oncology, The Saban Research Institute of Children's Hospital Los Angeles, Los Angeles, CA, USA

[2]Department of Medicine and Committee on Clinical Pharmacology and Pharmacogenomics, University of Chicago, Chicago, IL, USA

[3]Department of Pediatrics and Department of Biochemistry and Molecular Biology, The Saban Research Institute of Children's Hospital Los Angeles, Los Angeles, CA, USA

## Introduction

### The Tumor Microenvironment: Toward a Nonreductionist View of Cancer Biology

Over the last several decades we have witnessed dramatic progress in our understanding of the roles that genes play in cancer initiation and progression. The Human Genome project completed at the turn of the century combined with The Cancer Genome Atlas project to be soon completed are providing a comprehensive map of all genetic and epigenetic alterations that are the causes and/or consequences of malignant transformation. At the same time, we are harvesting some of the fruits of our efforts to obtain a fundamental and molecular understanding of cancer, in the form of new therapeutic agents that specifically target the product of genetic alterations responsible for driving cancer progression. Such therapies are rapidly revolutionizing the way we care for cancer patients by allowing a personalized approach to cancer diagnosis and treatment. There remain, however, multiple and important challenges. Among some of the most significant ones are the tremendous heterogeneity that exists within a single tumor and the ability of tumor cells to become resistant to therapies through mutations or activation of alternate pathways. Another important hurdle is the need to fully appreciate and understand that tumors are not just composed of malignant and genetically affected cells but contain a variety of nonmalignant cells and are embedded in an extracellular matrix (ECM) of a highly complex nature. These known as the tumor microenvironment (TME) are not innocent bystanders.

In the early 1970s, some seminal observations made by various laboratories had already pointed to the fact that cancer is not only a disease of the genes. In 1971, J. Folkman and his laboratory opened an entirely new field of investigation as they proposed the concept of angiogenesis, a highly integrated ecosystem between tumor cells and capillary endothelial cells (EC) where tumor cells stimulate the growth of EC and vice-versa.[1] Also fundamental were the observations made in the 1980s by I. J. Fidler and colleagues, who reported that the primary environment (orthotopic implantation) of tumor cells was essential for their ability to grow and metastasize,[2] and

by L.A. Liotta and colleagues, who identified basement membrane-degrading proteases produced by metastatic tumor cells.[3] Demonstrating that inhibition of β-1 integrin in a three-dimensional culture model of breast cancer cells led to a striking morphological and functional reversion of malignant breast cancer cells to a normal phenotype, M. Bissell and colleagues in 1997 suggested that the phenotype of the TME could even be dominant over the cellular genotype of a cancer cell.[4] The work of these laboratories and many others, too numerous to mention here, led to the recognition at the beginning of the 21st century that our view of cancer biology may have been too reductionist.[5] We were also reminded of the importance of some seminal observations made in the 19th century by Virchow, who first recognized the potential role of macrophages and inflammation in cancer,[5] and by Paget, who suspected the critical selective role that the environment of an organ (soil) plays in supporting the development of a metastatic tumor (seed)[6] (Figure 5.1). As a result, over the last decade there has been a resurgent interest in the study of the interactions between tumor cells and the TME, which has led to a molecular understanding of their roles in cancer initiation and progression.[7,8] Such understanding now allows the identification of agents that either interfere with the interactions between tumor cells and their microenvironment or inhibit signaling pathways specifically activated upon contact between tumor cells and the TME. In this chapter, after a brief review of the major components of the TME and of the mechanisms of interactions between tumor cells and the microenvironment, we summarize existing and emerging therapeutic strategies that target the TME and provide examples of agents currently used clinically or in pre-clinical and clinical development. Targeted immunotherapy against cancer, which is not covered in this chapter, is the subject of a separate chapter.

## Components of the TME

The microenvironment of tumors is highly complex as it is made up of a large variety of nonmalignant cells, including vascular and lymphatic EC, pericytes, fibroblasts and myofibroblasts, and

---

*Targeted Therapy in Translational Cancer Research*, First Edition. Edited by Apostolia-Maria Tsimberidou, Razelle Kurzrock and Kenneth C. Anderson.
© 2016 John Wiley & Sons, Inc. Published 2016 by John Wiley & Sons, Inc.

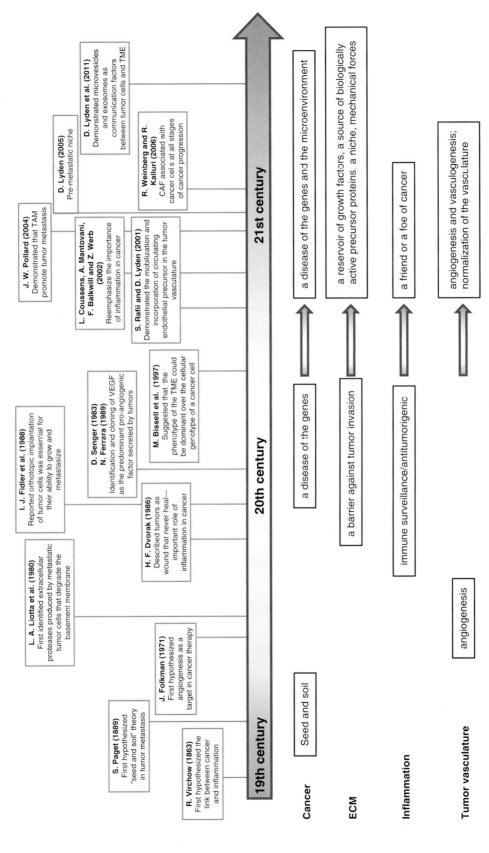

**Figure 5.1** Evolution of the concept of the tumor microenvironment in cancer biology: some milestone discoveries.

adaptive and innate immune cells. Depending on the location of the primary or the metastatic tumor, more specialized cells like osteoblasts and osteoclasts (bone), astrocytes and glial cells (brain), kupfer cells (liver), and adipocytes (bone marrow, omentum) actively contribute. The presence of the ECM adds another level of complexity to the TME, not only because of its highly diverse composition and structure but also because it acts as a reservoir for growth factors, cytokines and chemokines, and exerts dynamic mechanical forces on tumor cells. Here, we have selected for discussion some unique features of these components on the basis of their therapeutic relevance.

## The Tumor Vasculature

Tumor angiogenesis is an intricate process which is tightly regulated by pro- and antiangiogenic factors produced by both malignant cells and nonmalignant cells through autocrine and paracrine signaling pathways. The onset of angiogenesis, known as "angiogenic switch," is induced when the pro-angiogenic factors are favored.[9] Vascular endothelial growth factor (VEGF/VEGF-A) is the predominant pro-angiogenic factor involved in EC activation,[10] but many other growth factors are also pro-angiogenic, such as fibroblast growth factor (FGF), platelet-derived growth factor (PDGF), and epidermal growth factor (EGF).[9] Conversely, a number of endogenous inhibitors of angiogenesis (e.g., thrombospondin, angiostatin, endostatin) can also be detected in the circulation and act as intrinsic barriers of angiogenesis by incipient neoplasias.[11–13] Different from the normal vasculature characterized by an organized formation of mature EC covered with pericytes, the tumor vasculature is typically abnormal with a deficit in pericytes and perivascular cells, and an increased permeability, resulting in a leaky vascular system.[14] The formation of a tumor vasculature was initially considered to be solely dependent on the ability of neighboring mature EC to invade a small tumor mass, a process called angiogenesis.[1] It is now well recognized that bone marrow-derived endothelial progenitor cells also contribute to the tumor vasculature through a process known as vasculogenesis.[15]

## Immune Inflammatory Cells and Tumor-Associated Macrophages

The association between cancer and inflammation has been known for a long time, but our understanding of its role has only recently improved significantly.[16,17] The presence of innate and adaptive immune cells in tumors was initially considered to be the sign of an effective attack of the immune system against cancer. It is now recognized that immune cells can also promote cancer initiation, progression, and metastasis.[18] Our understanding of this dual role of immune cells in cancer progression is centered on the concept of polarization of the immune system toward either $T_H1$-type (generally antitumor) or $T_H2$-type (generally pro-tumor). While initially described for CD4+ T-cells, it is now well accepted that $T_H1$- and $T_H2$-type factors regulate the phenotype and bioactivity of essentially all immune cell subtypes. For example, macrophages can be directed toward a behavior that is antitumorigenic (so-called M1) or pro-tumorigenic (so-called M2).[19] The polarization of the immune system is characterized by metabolic changes and the production of specific cytokines by immune cells. $T_H1$-type-driven immune cells express high levels of inducible nitric oxide synthase (iNOS), which converts arginine into citrullin and nitric oxide (NO), and secrete inflammatory cytokines such as TNF-$\alpha$, interleukin (IL)-23 and IL-12. M1 macrophages express specific

cell surface markers like CD11c, and their polarity is influenced by granulocyte-macrophage colony stimulating factor (GM-CSF/CSF-2). $T_H$-2-driven immune cells express high levels of Arginase-1 that catalyze arginine hydrolysis and secrete high levels of specific cytokines such as IL-10 and IL-6. M2 macrophages typically express the cell surface markers CD163 and CD 206, and the polarity is promoted by macrophage colony stimulating factor (M-CSF/CSF-1).[20] Tumor-associated macrophages (TAM)—which are polarized toward M2—have emerged as being among the most important players in inflammation and cancer. Their contribution to cancer metastasis and drug resistance is now well recognized.[21]

## Mesenchymal-Derived Cells

Fibroblasts are the most abundant cell type in connective tissues. Activated fibroblasts (sometimes referred to as myofibroblasts) are often found in association with cancer cells and are known as carcinoma-associated fibroblasts (CAF). CAF are the most prominent cell type within the stroma of many cancers, most notably breast, prostate, and pancreatic carcinomas.[22] They are a source of specific proteins like fibroblast activation protein α (FAPα, a dipeptidyl peptidase) and fibroblast-specific protein-1 (FSP1 or S100A4). These cells either represent local resident cells or are recruited from distant organs, in particular the bone marrow, or are generated from normal or transformed epithelial cells via epithelial-mesenchymal transition (EMT). Fibroblast activation is induced by various growth factors (e.g., transforming growth factor-β or TGF-β, EGF, PDGF, FGF2) that are released by injured epithelial cells and infiltrating macrophages. CAF can also be directly activated by cell–cell communication.[22] CAF communicate among themselves as well as with cancer cells and immune cells directly through cell contact and indirectly through paracrine/exocrine signals, proteases, and by their ability to modulate the ECM. Their role in cancer is not entirely understood but they have been shown to promote tumor growth, angiogenesis, and metastasis.[22] They also can contribute to the formation of a rigid ECM and suppress antitumor immunity.[23]

## The ECM

Tumor cells and stromal cells are embedded in a large diversity of ECM proteins that provide a three-dimensional structure supporting malignant and normal cells. The ECM is much more than a barrier against tumor cell invasion, which was the focus of investigation in the 1980s. The ECM is a rich reservoir of growth factors and controls their bioavailability. Upon degradation of the ECM by extracellular proteases like serine proteases of the plasmin-plasminogen activator family or the matrix metalloproteinases (MMPs), growth factors are released as soluble proteins and can interact with a larger number of cells.[24] The degradation of the ECM by these proteases also results in the release of soluble biologically active proteolytic fragments that inhibit angiogenesis.[13] The ECM is also used by tumor cells as a point of attachment to allow them to survive and migrate. Adhesion of tumor cells to ECM proteins, like vitronectin and fibronectin that are abundant in the pre-metastatic niche, plays a critical role in invasion and metastasis. The ECM also exerts mechanical forces on the stroma and on tumor cells which affect gene expression and cell behavior. The presence of a stiff ECM is typically a sign of a more aggressive form of cancer.[25] Lysyl oxidase (LOX), which promotes the cross-linking of collagens, is frequently elevated in tumors. Such a stiff matrix with highly cross-linked collagen molecules stimulates tumor progression through enhanced integrin signaling.[26]

The ECM thus has a dual role in tumor progression. It can be anti-tumorigenic by forming a barrier against tumor invasion and metastasis and by sequestering growth factors. It can be pro-tumorigenic by providing a stiff environment that promotes growth and survival of malignant cells. Similarly, degradation of the ECM can facilitate tumor progression and metastasis but also has antitumorigenic and antiangiogenic effects.

## The Hypoxic Nature of the TME

Most of the attention has focused on intra-tumoral hypoxia and its role in angiogenesis. However, hypoxia has important functions other than stimulating the production of VEGF and promoting the proliferation of EC. Tumor cells adapt to the hypoxic environment to survive, using mechanisms that promote genomic instability, deregulated DNA repair system and expression of proto-oncogenes[27] which stimulates tumor invasiveness and metastasis, and induce tumor resistance to radiotherapy and chemotherapy.[28,29] Furthermore, hypoxia through the expression of hypoxia-inducible factor-1(HIF-1)$\alpha$ and -2$\alpha$ regulates the polarization of macrophages into a $T_H1$ type phenotype (M1) or a $T_H2$ type phenotype (M2).[30]

## Complex Communication Between Tumor Cells and Their Microenvironment

The understanding of mechanisms by which tumor cells communicate with their microenvironment has been the subject of extensive investigation over the last decade, with the anticipation that such investigation will identify targets for therapeutic intervention. Both adhesion-dependent and adhesion-independent mechanisms contribute. Adhesion-dependent mechanisms typically involve heterotypic adhesion between tumor cells and stromal cells or the ECM via cell adhesion molecules (CAM) such as integrins. For example, as they switch toward a radial growth phase and invade the dermis, melanoma cells increase their expression of the vitronectin-binding $\alpha_v\beta_3$ and $\alpha_v\beta_5$ integrins abundantly present around blood vessels[31] which provides a mechanism promoting intravasation. Similarly, the expression of the $\beta_1$ integrin by myeloma cells allows them to establish contact with bone marrow stromal cells, which upregulates the production of IL-6 by stromal cells and in turn activates osteoclasts promoting the proliferation and survival of myeloma cells through signal transduction and transcriptional activator (STAT) 3.[32]

Adhesion-independent mechanisms of communication between tumor cells and stromal cells or the ECM also play an important role. Many of these interactions occur through the production by tumor cells of soluble factors that stimulate stromal cells, and vice versa. Some of these factors, which are considered for targeted therapeutic intervention, are described here. Stromal-derived factor-1 (SDF-1), also known as chemokine (C-X-C motif) ligand-12 (CXCL-12), is secreted by many stromal cells, in particular osteoblasts in the bone marrow environment. Many tumor cells express the receptor for SDF-1/CXCL-12 (CXCR-4) and are thus attracted to the bone marrow niche by the same mechanism that retains hematopoietic stem cells (HSC) in the bone marrow. Metastatic circulating tumor cells compete with HSC for occupancy in the osteoblastic niche.[33] Another critical soluble factor in the TME is CSF-1 (MCSF), which is secreted by tumor cells and attracts CSF-1 receptor-expressing monocytes/macrophages into the tumor, promoting their M2 polarization. The expression of CSF-1 by tumor cells is stimulated by IL-4 made by lymphocytes, thus providing a communication network among lymphocytes, macrophages, and

tumor cells.[21] Our laboratory has shown that the production of prostaglandin-E2 and galectin-3 binding protein by neuroblastoma cells are two mechanisms that upregulate the expression and secretion of IL-6 by bone marrow mesenchymal cells. IL-6 then stimulates osteoclasts and promotes neuroblastoma cell survival and proliferation.[34,35]

In addition to secreted soluble chemokines/cytokines and growth factors, there has been recent evidence that the shedding of microvesicles and exosomes by tumor cells and stromal cells provides an important mechanism of communication between tumor cells and their microenvironment.[36] For example, it has been recently shown in a mouse model that exosomes from highly metastatic melanomas increased the metastatic behavior of primary tumors by educating bone marrow progenitors through activation of the receptor tyrosine kinase MET.[37] The recent observation that exosomes not only contain proteins but also nucleic acids including DNA and micro-RNA opens a new field of investigation on the communication between tumor cells and stromal cells in the TME.

## Therapeutic Targeting of the TME

The strategies that are developed to target the TME are numerous. For didactic purposes, we have grouped them into the following four categories (Table 5.1)[38]: (1) strategies that target the tumor vasculature, (2) strategies that target cancer-associated inflammation, (3) strategies that target the communication between tumor cells and the TME, and (4) strategies that target the tumor hypoxic microenvironment.

## Targeting the Tumor Vasculature

So far, angiogenesis-targeted strategies are mainly focusing on inhibiting EC activation by interfering with angiogenic factors. This approach has produced a rapidly expanding group of antiangiogenic agents that are at various stages of clinical investigation or are already in clinical application.

### VEGF Signaling Pathway and Anti-VEGF Agents

The VEGF family comprises five VEGF glycoproteins (VEGF-A, B, C, D, and E) and placental growth factors 1 and 2.[10] VEGF-A or VEGF is abundantly produced by tumor cells, CAF, TAM, and other inflammatory cells due to hypoxia, acidic pH, hypoglycemia, and several inducing cytokines and growth factors (e.g., IL-6, PDGF, FGF, insulin-like growth facor-1 or IGF-1).[39] As a potent pro-angiogenic growth factor, VEGF binds to two homologous receptors on vascular EC, VEGF receptor-1 (VEGFR-1, Flt-1) and VEGF receptor-2 (VEGFR-2/KDR). Binding of VEGF to VEGFR-1 and -2 results in receptor dimerization and ligand-dependent receptor tyrosine kinase phosphorylation, thereby activating intracellular signaling pathways involved in EC survival, proliferation, migration, sprouting, and tube formation.[40] A third receptor, VEGF receptor-3 (Flt-4), has been shown to involve VEGF-C and VEGF-D-mediated lymphangiogenesis.[39]

Considering the important functions of VEGF signaling in tumor angiogenesis, growth, invasion and metastasis, several VEGF- and VEGFR- antagonists have been developed. The most advanced agent is bevacizumab (Avastin), a recombinant humanized VEGF-neutralizing antibody, which has been approved by the Food and Drug Administration (FDA) for the treatment of several metastatic cancers including colorectal, renal, nonsmall cell lung cancer, and glioblastoma, in general in combination with cytotoxic therapies.

**Table 5.1** Agents targeting the tumor microenvironment. Fang and Declerck 2013 [38]. Reproduced by permission of American Association for Cancer Research (AACR).

| Category | Pathway | Target | Agent | Mechanism of action | Indication | Clinical status |
|---|---|---|---|---|---|---|
| **Tumor vasculature** | VEGF signaling | VEGF | Bevacizumab (Avastin) | Humanized monoclonal Ab against VEGF | Metastatic colorectal cancer, metastatic renal cell carcinoma, nonsmall cell lung cancer, glioblastoma | FDA approved |
| | | VEGFR | Ramucirumab (Cyramza) | VEGFR-2 neutralizing Ab | Advanced or metastatic gastric cancer or gastro-oesophageal junction adenocarcinoma with disease progression on or after fluoropyrimidine- or platinum-containing chemotherapy | FDA approved |
| | | VEGFR | Sunitinib (Sutent) | TKI of VEGFR1-3, PDGFR, c-Kit | Advanced renal cell carcinoma, pancreatic neuroendocrine tumors, gastrointestinal stromal tumors | FDA approved |
| | | VEGFR | Sorafenib (Nexavar) | TKI of VEGFR2, PDGFRβ, Raf | Advanced renal cell carcinoma, unresectable hepatocellular carcinoma | FDA approved |
| | | VEGFR | Pazopanib (Votrient) | TKI of VEGFR1-3, PDGFR, c-Kit | Advanced renal cell carcinoma, soft tissue sarcoma | FDA approved |
| | FGF signaling | FGFR | BMS-582664 (Brivanib) | FGFR and VEGFR | Hepatocellular carcinoma, colorectal cancer | Phase II/III |
| | PDGF signaling | PDGF | SU6668 | PDGFR, VEGFR, and FGFR | Not specific | Phase I |
| | EGFR signaling | EGFR | Cetuximab (Erbitux) | Monoclonal Ab against EGFR | Metastatic colorectal cancer, head and neck squamous carcinoma | FDA approved |
| | | EGFR | Panitumumab | Monoclonal Ab against EGFR | Metastatic colorectal cancer | FDA approved |
| | | EGFR | Erlotinib | TKI of EGFR | Nonsmall cell lung cancer and pancreatic cancer | FDA approved |
| | | EGFR | Gefitinib | TKI of EGFR | Nonsmall cell lung cancer | FDA approved |
| **Inflammation** | IL-6/JAK/STAT3 signaling | IL-6 | CNTO-328 (Siltuximab) | Monoclonal neutralizing Ab against IL-6 | Prostate cancer, multiple myeloma, metastatic renal cell carcinoma, ovarian cancer | Phase I/II |
| | | IL-6R | Tocilizumab | An IL-6R blocking antibody | N/A | Preclinical |
| | | JAK1/2 | AZD1480 | Small molecule inhibitor of Jak1/2 | Solid tumors | Phase I |
| | | JAK1/2 | Ruxolitinib (INCB018424) | Small molecule inhibitor of Jak1/2 | Advanced breast cancer, advanced hematologic malignancies, metastatic pancreatic adenocarcinoma | Phase II |
| | | STAT3 | STAT3 decoy | STAT3 DNA competitor | Head and neck cancer | Phase 0 |

*(continued)*

**Table 5.1** (Continued)

| Category | Pathway | Target | Agent | Mechanism of action | Indication | Clinical status |
|---|---|---|---|---|---|---|
| | NF-κB signaling | IKK | PS-1145 | Small molecule inhibitor of IKK kinases | B-cell lymphoma cells, prostate cancer | Preclinical |
| | | 26S proteasome | Bortezomib (Velcade) | Inhibitor of 26S proteasome disrupting IκB degradation | Multiple myeloma, mantle cell lymphoma | FDA approved |
| | | NF-κB | Curcumin | Phytochemical extract from turmeric that suppress NF-κB activation and NF-κB-dependent gene expression | Colon cancer, pancreatic cancer, breast cancer, multiple myeloma, prostate cancer | Phase I/II |
| | | NF-κB | Arsenic | NF-κB inhibitor | Acute promyelocytic leukemia | Phase I/II |
| | TNF-α signaling | TNF-α | Etanercept (Enbrel) | Recombinant inhibitory TNF-α receptors | Recurrent ovarian cancer, metastatic breast cancer, chronic lymphocytic leukemia | Phase I/II |
| | | TNF-α | Infliximab (cA2, Remicade) | Neutralizing Ab against TNF-α | Renal cell carcinoma | Phase II |
| | COX2 signaling | COX2 | Celecoxib | COX2 inhibitor | Nonsmall cell lung cancer, nasopharyngeal carcinoma, hormone sensitive prostate cancer | Phase II/III |
| | TGFβ signaling | TGFβ | AP12009 (trabedersen) | Antisense phosphorothioate oligodeoxynucleotide for TGFβ2 | Anaplastic astrocytoma, glioblastoma | Phase II/III |
| | | TGFβ | Soluble TGFβ receptor II/III | TGFβ ligand traps | Metastatic pancreatic cancer model, colon cancer model | Preclinical |
| | | TGFβ | Soluble TGFβ receptor II fusion protein | TGFβ ligand traps | Pancreatic cancer and melanoma model | Preclinical |
| | | TGFβR | LY2109761 | Small molecule inhibitor for TGFβ-receptor kinase | Metastatic pancreatic and colorectal cancer model | Preclinical |
| | | TGFβR | SB-431542 | Small molecule inhibitor for TGFβ-receptor kinase | N/A | Preclinical |
| | | Interaction between TGFβ ligands and receptors | 2G7 | Neutralizing Ab minimizing the interaction between ligands and receptors | Breast cancer model | Preclinical |
| | | Interaction between TGFβ ligands and receptors | 1D11 | Neutralizing Ab minimizing the interaction between ligands and receptors | Breast cancer model | Preclinical |

| | Target | Agent | Mechanism | Cancer/Model | Stage |
|---|---|---|---|---|---|
| Macrophage recruitment | CCL2 | CNTO888 (carlumab) | Neutralizing antibody to human CCL2 | Castration-resistant prostate cancer | Phase I/II |
| | CCL2 | Bindarit | A small molecule inhibitor of CCL2 | Prostate and breast cancer model | Preclinical |
| | CSF-1 | Mouse CSF-1 antisense oligonucleotides, CSF-1 or CSF-1 receptor small interfering RNAs | CSF-1 antibodies and antisense oligonucleotides | Breast cancer model | Preclinical |
| | CSF-1 receptor | Ki20227 | TKI of CSF-1 receptor | Bone metastasis mouse model | Preclinical |
| | CSF-1 receptor | JNJ-28312141 | TKI of CSF-1 receptor | Lung adenocarcinoma, breast cancer, acute myeloid leukemia models | Preclinical |
| **Interactions between tumor cells and their microenvironment** Integrin signaling | $\alpha_v\beta_3$ and $\alpha_v\beta_5$ | Cilengitide | RGD peptide as an inhibitor of $\alpha_v\beta_3$ and $\alpha_v\beta_5$ integrins | Glioblastoma, prostate cancer, metastatic melanoma, refractory high-grade glioma in children, advanced nonsmall cell lung cancer | Phase II/III |
| | $\alpha_v\beta_3$ | Etaracizumab (Medi-522) | Monoclonal Ab against $\alpha_v\beta_3$ integrin | Prostate cancer, colorectal cancer, melanoma | Phase I/II |
| | $\alpha_v$ | Intetumumab (CNTO 95) | Monoclonal Ab against $\alpha_v$ integrin | Prostate cancer, melanoma | Phase I/II |
| RANK/RANKL signaling | RANKL | Denosumab | Monoclonal Ab against RANKL | Bone metastases from solid tumors, patients at high risk of fracture with nonmetastatic prostate cancer on androgen-deprivation therapy or adjuvant aromatase inhibitor therapy for breast cancer | FDA approved |
| PTHrP signaling | PTHrP | CAL | Monoclonal Ab against PTHrP | Bone metastatic breast cancer | Phase I/II |
| **Hypoxia** Hypoxic environment | Hypoxia | Tirapazamine (TPZ) | Bioreductive prodrug of an aromatic N-oxide generating a DNA-reactive free radical | Cervix cancer, advanced head and neck squamous carcinoma | Phase III |
| | Hypoxia | TH-302 | Bioreductive prodrug of a 2-nitroimidazole-based nitrogen mustard | Multiple myeloma, advanced renal cell carcinoma, soft tissue sarcoma, pancreatic adenocarcinoma, nonsmall cell lung cancer | Phase I/II/III |

*(continued)*

**Table 5.1** (*Continued*)

| Category | Pathway | Target | Agent | Mechanism of action | Indication | Clinical status |
|---|---|---|---|---|---|---|
| | | Hypoxia | PR-104 | Bioreductive prodrug of a 3,5-dinitrobenzamide nitrogen mustard | Leukemia, solid tumors | Phase I/II |
| | | Hypoxia | AQ4N | Bioreductive prodrug of an aliphatic N-oxide generating a DNA intercalator | Glioblastoma, non-Hodgkin's lymphoma; leukemia | Phase I/II |
| | HIF-1α signaling | HIF-1α | EZN-2968 | HIF-1α antisense mRNA | Advanced solid tumors, lymphoma | Phase I |
| | | HIF-1α | PX-478 | Small molecule inhibitor of HIF-1α | Advanced solid tumors, lymphoma | Phase I |
| | UPR signaling | 26S proteasome | Bortezomib (Velcade) | Inhibitor of 26S proteasome that cause ER stress | Multiple myeloma, mantle cell lymphoma | FDA approved |
| | | 26S proteasome | Nelfinavir | Inhibitor of 26S proteasome that causes ER stress, impairs HIF-1α and VEGF expression | Colorectal cancer | Phase I/II |
| | | HSP90 | IPI-504 (Retaspimycin) | Small molecule inhibitor of HSP90 that is in part responsible for protein folding | Castration-resistant prostate cancer, gastrointestinal stromal tumors, breast cancer, lung cancer | Phase I/II |
| | | HSP90 | 17-AAG (Tanespimycin) | Small molecule inhibitor of HSP90 that is in part responsible for protein folding | Metastatic breast cancer | Phase II/III |

VEGF, vascular endothelial growth factor; Ab, antibody; VEGFR, vascular endothelial growth factor receptor; FDA, Food and Drug Administration; HER2, human epidermal growth factor receptor 2; FGF, fibroblast growth factor; FGFR, fibroblast growth factor receptor; PDGF, platelet-derived growth factor; EGFR, epidermal growth factor receptor; TKI, tyrosine kinase inhibitor; IL-6, interleukin-6; IL-6R, interleukin-6 receptor; JAK, Janus kinase; STAT3, signal transducer and activator of transcription 3; NF-κB, nuclear factor-kappaB; IKK, inhibitor of kappaB kinase complex; TNFα, tumor necrosis factor α; COX2, prostaglandin–endoperoxide synthase 2; TGFβ, transforming growth factor β; TGFβR, transforming growth factor β receptor; CCL-2, chemokine (C–C motif) ligand 2; CSF-1, colony stimulating factor-1; RGD, arginine–glycine–aspartic acid; RANK, receptor activator of nuclear factor kappaB ligand; RANKL, receptor activator of nuclear factor kappaB ligand; PTHrP, parathyroid hormone–related protein; HIF-1α, hypoxia-inducible factor-1α; UPR, unfolded protein response; ER, endoplasmic reticulum; HSP, heat shock protein; N/A, not available.

Alternatively, VEGF signaling may also be inhibited by small molecule receptor tyrosine kinase inhibitors (e.g., sunitinib/Sutent, sorafenib/Nexavar, and pazopanib/Votrient) or by receptor-specific antibodies (e.g., Ramucirumab, an antibody against VEGFR-2). Sunitinib, sorafenib, and pazopanib have already been approved by the FDA, in most cases for advanced renal cell carcinoma. Ramucirumab (Cyramza) was also recently approved by the FDA for use as monotherapy in the treatment of advanced or metastatic gastric cancer or gastro-oesophageal junction adenocarcinoma in patients who experience disease progression on or after fluoropyrimidine- or platinum-containing chemotherapy.[41, 42] In another phase III trial in stage IV nonsmall cell lung cancer (NSCLC) patients, Ramucirumab plus docetaxel versus placebo plus docetaxel improved patients' overall survival as second-line treatment.[43]

## Beyond VEGF Signaling

In cancer, multiple redundant signaling pathways are involved in angiogenesis, and suppressing one pathway may promote another, which accounts for the relatively limited efficacy of some inhibitors and for acquired resistance to anti-VEGF therapies in the clinical setting. Highlighting the need to develop more effective antiangiogenic agents is the recent decision of the FDA to withdraw Avastin from approval for breast cancer because of a lack of benefit that outweighed its serious and potentially life-threatening side effects in patients with breast cancer.

**FGF signaling pathway.** FGF are a family of growth factors that interact with high-affinity tyrosine kinase FGF receptors (FGFR), involved in the regulation of multiple fundamental pathways and cellular behaviors.[44] The prototype FGF family member, FGF2, is a potent mitogen of different cell types including vascular EC and fibroblasts, that acts synergistically with VEGF to increase tumor blood vessel growth and maturation.[45] Emerging evidence suggests that the upregulation of FGF provides a mechanism of resistance to anti-VEGF therapy.[46] Most FGF/FGFR-targeting agents are still in an early stage of development[45] and the most advanced agent is BMS-582664 (brivanib), an oral dual inhibitor of VEGFR and FGFR tyrosine kinases, which is currently being tested in multiple phase II/III clinical trials. In a phase II open-label study in patients with advanced hepatocellular carcinoma (HCC) who had failed prior antiangiogenic treatment with sorafenib, brivanib has shown promising antitumor activity with a manageable safety profile.[47] However, in a recent multinational, randomized, double-blind, phase III trial that compared brivanib with sorafenib as first-line treatment for HCC, the primary end point of overall survival noninferiority for brivanib versus sorafenib was not met.[48] Both agents had similar antitumor activity, based on secondary efficacy end points. Brivanib had an acceptable safety profile, but was less well-tolerated than sorafenib.

**PDGF signaling pathway.** PDGF and its receptors PDGFR have been detected in various human cancers, and PDGFR is upregulated in the tumor vasculature, particularly in pericytes during tumor progression. In addition to promoting cell migration, survival, and proliferation, PDGF signaling also regulates angiogenesis by inducing VEGF expression and by recruiting pericytes to mature blood vessels.[49] SU6668, a small molecule kinase inhibitor for PDGFR, VEGFR, and FGFR, has currently completed phase I clinical trials in patients with advanced solid tumors but the data have shown relatively low plasma levels that may limit its usage as single agent.[50]

**EGFR signaling pathway.** EGF receptor (EGFR) is a member of HER growth factor receptor family, a group of homologous recep-tor tyrosine kinases known to modulate normal cell growth and differentiation.[51] In solid tumors, VEGF and EGFR pathways are linked, thus promoting angiogenesis,[52] and resistance to EGFR targeting therapy is accompanied by an increase in VEGF levels.[53] Both tumor cells and tumor-associated EC express EGFR, and aberrant EGFR expression correlates with poor prognosis. Inhibition of EGFR therefore has a dual function, inhibiting tumor cells and also EC. The EGFR signaling pathway modulates angiogenesis by upregulating VEGF or other key pro-angiogenic factors (e.g., FGF).[54] Several EGFR-neutralizing antibodies (e.g., cetuximab, panitumumab) and small inhibitors (e.g., erlotinib, gefitinib) have been approved by the FDA and have been incorporated into the standard care for different types of cancers.

## Targeting Cancer-Associated Inflammation

Among the key endogenous factors involved in cancer-related inflammation are transcriptional factors such as nuclear factor-κB (NF-κB) and STAT3, inflammatory cytokines/chemokines and growth factors such as IL-1β, IL-6, tumor necrosis factor-α (TNF-α), TGF-β, as well as COX2.[16, 17] In addition to targeting cancer-related inflammatory factors and the signaling pathways they activate, interfering with the recruitment and/or polarization of TAM is another strategy explored. The overall goal of these approaches is to convert a tumor-promoting microenvironment into a tumor-inhibiting one.

### IL-6/JAK/STAT3 Signaling Pathway

STAT3 signaling pathway has been the focus of much attention over the last several years as it plays a central role in cancer-associated inflammation.[55] STAT3 is typically phosphorylated and activated by Janus kinases (JAK). Upon activation, phosphorylated STAT3 dimerizes and translocates into the nucleus where it transcriptionally activates a large group of genes that promote survival, proliferation, angiogenesis, and also inflammation.[56] In many instances, STAT3 activation in the TME is induced by IL-6, a potent, pleiotropic inflammatory cytokine[57] that belongs to a larger family of cytokines signaling through a common signaling receptor, gp130, expressed on many cell types. IL-6 also binds to the membrane-bound IL-6 receptor (gp 80 or IL-6R) or a soluble form of the IL-6R receptor (sIL-6R), which upon dimerization with gp130 activates the associated JAK.[58] Activation of STAT3 in tumor cells transcriptionally upregulates a large number of genes encoding for cytokines, chemokines, and growth factors that activate STAT3 in tumor-associated immune cells. This STAT3 "feed-forward loop" is established through a crosstalk between tumor cells and tumor-associated immune cells.[59] Our laboratory, for instance, has shown that the activation of STAT3 in neuroblastoma cells is mediated by IL-6 and sIL-6R, produced by bone marrow stromal cells[34] and TAM.[60]

Given the importance of aberrant IL-6/JAK/STAT3 signaling in cancers, each molecular player in this signaling pathway may serve as a potential target for cancer therapy. Strategies to inhibit such pathways have therefore focused on (1) blocking IL-6/IL-6R interaction by large molecules (mAb), (2) blocking JAK phosphorylation of STAT3 by small molecule inhibitors of JAK kinase activity, and (3) inhibiting STAT3 DNA binding activity. An IL-6 neutralizing antibody (siltuximab/CNTO-328) is being tested in a number of phase I/II clinical trials. When given in combination with mitoxantrone/prednisone in patients with metastatic castration-resistant prostate cancer, siltuximab was found to be of no additional benefit,[61] however, it has been shown to stabilize disease and induce partial responses in patients with platinum-resistant ovarian cancer[62] and metastatic renal cell carcinoma.[63] A humanized anti-IL-6R blocking antibody (tocilizumab) has been recently approved for the treatment of rheumatoid arthritis[64] and will likely be tested in cancers. Ruxolitinib (INCB018424), a JAK2 specific inhibitor, which was shown to significantly decrease circulating pro-inflammatory cytokines in a phase III clinical trial in patients with myelofibrosis,[65] is currently being tested in multiple phase II clinical trials for several cancer types, including advanced hematologic malignancies, advanced breast cancers, and metastatic pancreatic adenocarcinoma. In two phase II studies in patients with relapsed/refractory leukemias[66] and polycythemia vera,[67] respectively, Ruxolitinib was well tolerated and showed rapid and durable antitumor activity. Another JAK1/2 inhibitor AZD1480[68] is being tested in phase I clinical trials for solid tumors. A STAT3 transcription factor decoy, which directly binds to STAT3 with high affinity and suppresses the binding of STAT3 to DNA, has recently been developed. A phase 0 (biological effect) clinical trial of this STAT3 decoy directly injected into the tumors of patients with head and neck cancer prior to surgical resection showed that it binds with high affinity to STAT3 protein, reduces cellular viability, and suppresses STAT3 target gene expression in cancer cells.[69] Further clinical investigations are warranted.

## NF-κB Signaling Pathway

NF-κB is a generic term for a family of transcriptional factors that also play pivotal roles in both inflammation-induced tumorigenesis and antitumor immunity.[70,71] The NF-κB signaling pathway is highly interconnected with the STAT3 signaling pathway. Both pathways are often simultaneously activated in tumor cells and in tumor-associated myeloid cells, inducing the expression of a highly overlapping repertoire of proliferative, antiapoptotic, angiogenic, pro-inflammatory, and metastatic genes.[55] However, STAT3 opposes the activation of antitumor immunity programs activated by NF-κB when both are active in the same cells.[55] NF-kB in cancer can either enhance or inhibit inflammation depending on the cancer type and the mechanism of carcinogenesis involved.[72] NF-κB plays a role in bone metastasis where it is activated in osteoclasts upon stimulation of the receptor activator of nuclear factor kappa-B (RANK) by its ligand RANKL produced by tumor cells and by osteoblasts.[73] Under physiological conditions, NF-κB is present in the cytosol in an inactive state through interaction with the inhibitor of κB (IκB) family of proteins. Activation of most forms of NF-κB depends on phosphorylation-induced ubiquitination of IκB proteins, which is modulated by the IκB kinase (IKK) complex.[74] Once poly-ubiquitinated, IκB proteins undergo rapid degradation through the 26S proteasome.

To date, most efforts in targeting NF-κB signaling have concentrated on the development of specific inhibitors for IKKβ subunit.[75] For example, PS-1145, a small molecule inhibitor of IKKβ, was found to be selectively toxic for subtypes of diffuse large B-cell lymphoma cells that are associated with NF-κB.[76] The alternative approaches include (1) targeting proteasomes to disrupt the degradation of IκBs, by agents like bortezomib (Velcade) used in multiple myeloma[77] and (2) directly targeting NF-κB-dependent gene expression with agents like curcumin and arsenic. But it is now clear that IKKβ has many NF-κB independent functions and its inhibition could result in undesired effects.[74]

## TNF-α Signaling Pathway

TNF-α is another important mediator of cancer-related inflammation and its function is dose-dependent. In animal models, high doses of TNF-α have a significant anticancer effect through stimulation of T-cell-mediated immunity and the destruction of blood vessels.[78] Conversely, physiologic and lower levels of TNF-α may enhance tumor growth and metastasis by inducing the production of pro-inflammatory cytokines/chemokines (e.g., IL-6), pro-angiogenic factors (e.g., VEGF, FGF), and proteases (e.g., MMP).[78,79]

At least two TNF-α antagonists have been tested in patients with advanced cancers. The first antagonist is etanercept (Enbrel), a recombinant humanized soluble p75 TNF-α trapping receptor that binds to TNF-α tested in several phase I/II clinical trials. Etanercept in combination with rituximab (a mAb against B cells) is well tolerated and has produced durable remissions in chronic lymphocytic leukemia patients.[80] Similarly, etanercept as single agent has resulted in disease stabilization and some partial responses in patients with recurrent ovarian cancer[81] and has shown safety and biological activity in metastatic breast cancer.[82] The second TNF-α antagonist, infliximab (cA2, Remicade), is a chimeric human–mouse monoclonal antibody. In several phase II clinical trials for renal cell carcinoma, infliximab produced stable disease or partial responses as single agent[83] but did not provide additional therapeutic benefits when combined with sorafenib.[84]

## COX2 Signaling Pathway

COX2, an inducible enzyme responsible for the synthesis of prostanoids (prostaglandins, prostacyclin and thromboxane) from the precursor arachidonic acid, plays a major role in inflammation. COX2 overexpression is observed in both cancer and stroma cells during tumor progression, which is partially induced by anticancer therapies. Elevated levels of COX2 in tumors are associated with increased angiogenesis, tumor invasion, and promotion of tumor cell resistance to apoptosis.[85,86]

Celecoxib, a COX2 inhibitor, has shown efficacy in preventing colon cancer in patients with inflammatory bowel diseases, but was not adopted clinically due to its unacceptable cardiac toxicity.[87] The therapeutic administration of celecoxib has been tested in a number of phase II/III clinical trials for multiple cancers and has shown mixed clinical results. Whereas it has improved the efficacy of conventional therapy in locally advanced undifferentiated nasopharyngeal carcinoma patients,[88] it had no effect in hormone-sensitive prostate cancer[89] or advanced nonsmall cell lung cancer.[90]

## TGF-β Signaling Pathway

TGF-β-mediated signaling has a dual role in the regulation of cancer: it is tumor suppressive in pre-malignant cells, whereas it has a pro-tumorigenic activity during the later stages of carcinoma progression.[91] Autocrine TGF-β signaling can cause EMT in cancer cells, which increases cell invasion and metastasis. Paracrine TGF-β signaling can promote angiogenesis and also contribute to an immunosuppressive environment by suppressing T-lymphocytes and natural killer cells.[92] TGF-β signaling is particularly important in tumor bone metastasis due to its sequestration in the bone. During osteoclastic bone resorption, TGF-β is released from the bone matrix and accelerates the formation of osteolytic bone metastasis.

Several strategies to inhibit TGF-β activity have been developed, in particular[93]: (1) blocking the production of TGF-β with antisense molecules (e.g., AP12009/trabedersen), (2) blocking the activity of

TGF-β with neutralizing antibodies (e.g., 2G7, 1D11), (3) blocking the interaction between TGF-β and its receptors with soluble forms of TGF-β receptors (e.g., soluble TGF-βRII/TGF-βRIII, TGF-βRII:Fc fusion proteins), and (4) blocking TGF-β-mediated receptor signaling by small molecule tyrosine kinase inhibitors of TGF-βRII and TGF-βRIII (e.g., LY2109761, SB-431542). Among agents inhibiting TGF-β, AP12009 (trabedersen), an 18-oligomer antisense phosphorothioate oligodeoxynucleotide that prevents the production of TGF-β2 is at the most advanced stage of development. In a phase II clinical trial for patients with brain tumors, the addition of AP12009 to conventional chemotherapy resulted in a significant increase in 14-month tumor control rate in anaplastic astrocytoma patients and in an increase in 2 and 3 year survival in a subgroup of glioblastoma patients.[94]

## Beyond Inflammatory Signaling Pathways—Inhibiting TAM

Another recently proposed approach to target cancer-associated inflammation has been to inhibit the recruitment of TAM by targeting monocyte chemo-attractants.[20] One such strategy has been to target the chemokine CCL2, also known as monocyte chemotactic protein-1 (MCP-1), or the growth factor CSF-1. CCL2 and CSF-1 promote M2-like polarization of macrophages, a characteristic of TAM.

A neutralizing monoclonal antibody to human CCL2, CNTO888 (carlumab), was tested in two phase I trials, showing good tolerance with evidence of transient-free CCL2 suppression and antitumor activity.[95, 96] Similarly, in another phase II trial in patients with metastatic castration-resistant prostate cancer (CRPC),[97] carlumab was well tolerated and suppression of free CCL2 serum concentrations was briefly observed. However, carlumab as a single agent did not block the CCL2/CCR2 axis or show antitumor activity in metastatic CRPC. Bindarit, a small molecule inhibitor of CCL2, has also shown anticancer activity in preclinical models of prostate and breast cancer, with a significant decrease in the infiltration of TAM and myeloid-derived suppressor cells in tumors.[98] Similarly, anti-CSF-1 antibodies and antisense oligonucleotides suppress macrophage infiltration and xenograft mammary tumor growth in mice.[99, 100] Tyrosine kinase inhibitors of CSF-1 receptor (also known as c-fms) have also been developed. Ki20227 has been shown to suppress osteolysis in a bone metastasis mouse model[101] and JNJ-28312141 to inhibit angiogenesis and bone metastasis in preclinical models of solid tumors and acute myeloid leukemia.[102]

## Targeting Communications Between Tumor Cells and TME

### Communication Between Tumor Cells and ECM

Integrins are clustered at the cell surface in complexes known as focal adhesions and play a significant role in tumor-associated signaling events involving cell growth, anchorage-dependent differentiation, adhesion, motility, apoptosis, and angiogenesis.[103, 104] Tumor cells also express integrins, which potentiate tumor metastasis by facilitating migration and invasion. Integrin inhibition can thus affect both tumor cells and EC. So far most of the efforts have been at targeting integrin of the αv family.

Cilengitide (EMD 121974), a cyclic RGD pentapeptide, is the first potent integrin inhibitor for both $\alpha_v\beta_3$ and $\alpha_v\beta_5$ that has reached clinical trials.[105] Multiple phase II trials were conducted in different types of cancer, including recurrent glioblastoma,[106] refractory or relapsed high-grade gliomas in children,[107] advanced nonsmall

cell lung cancer,[108] metastatic melanoma,[109] and castration-resistant prostate cancer.[110] Overall, cilengitide monotherapy was found to be well tolerated but exhibited little antitumor activity, warranting additional studies that integrate cilengitide into combinatorial regimens. Etaracizumab (MEDI-522), a monoclonal antibody against the human $\alpha_v\beta_3$ integrin, and intetumumab (CNTO 95), a monoclonal antibody against the human $\alpha_v$ integrin, are also under investigation for multiple phase I/II clinical trials. Intetumumab has shown a favorable safety profile and a trend toward improved overall survival in a phase II clinical trial of advanced melanoma patients.[111] In contrast, in another phase II trial of advanced melanoma patients, etaracizumab (MEDI-522) did not provide any therapeutic benefit.[112]

## Communication Between Tumor Cells and the Bone Microenvironment

The bone is the most common metastatic site for many different types of cancer, especially breast and prostate cancer and myelomas.[113] The mechanisms involved in bone metastasis have been well characterized.[114] Tumor cells secrete parathyroid hormone-related peptide (PTHrP), which promotes the expression of RANKL at the surface of osteoblasts. RANKL then binds to its receptor RANK on osteoclast precursors and promotes their differentiation into active osteoclasts, leading to excessive bone loss. RANKL is inhibited by a natural inhibitor, osteoprotegerin (OPG). At the same time, tumor growth in the bone is accelerated by the release of growth factors (e.g., FGF, PDGF, TGF-β) from the bone matrix. Thus, both RANK/RANKL and PTHrP have been considered as therapeutic targets.

A humanized monoclonal antibody targeting PTHrP, CAL, has completed a phase I/II study for breast cancer patients with bone metastasis. However, no results have been reported. Denosumab, a fully humanized monoclonal antibody that specifically targets RANKL, is the first RANKL inhibitor to be approved by the FDA. In 2010, denosumab was first approved by the FDA for use in postmenopausal women with risk of osteoporosis and later for the prevention of skeletal-related events[105] in patients with bone metastases from solid tumors. In 2011, the FDA granted approval for denosumab as a treatment to increase bone mass in patients who are at high risk of fracture from receiving androgen deprivation therapy for nonmetastatic prostate cancer or adjuvant aromatase inhibitor therapy for breast cancer.

## Targeting Hypoxia in the TME

Hypoxia represents a compelling therapeutic target in the TME, and two strategies—bioreductive prodrugs and molecularly targeted agents—have been explored so far.[115]

### Profiting from Hypoxia with Bioreductive Prodrugs

The first strategy for targeting hypoxia consists of the use of bioreductive prodrugs such as Tirapazamine (TPZ), TH-302, PR-104, or AQ4N, which are activated by enzymatic reduction (bioreduction) into toxic products in hypoxic tissues.[115] Among those bioreductive prodrugs, TPZ is the most investigated. In the presence of hypoxia, TPZ is metabolized by an intracellular reductase to form highly reactive radical species capable of inducing DNA single- and double-strand breaks and other chromosomal aberrations that result in cell death. Despite promising results from preclinical studies and early-phase clinical trials, several phase III trials have however failed to demonstrate any benefit of adding TPZ to chemotherapy or radiation therapy on the survival of patients with nonsmall cell lung cancer, head and neck cancer, or cervical carcinoma limited to pelvis.[116,117] Other bioreductive prodrugs—TH-302, PR-104, AQ4N—are currently being investigated in a number of phase I/II clinical trials. No efficacy results have been released at this point.

### Targeting HIF-1α Signaling

HIF-1α is a transcription factor that is activated in response to intratumoral hypoxia and plays a pivotal role in adaptation of tumor cells to hypoxia.[118] Multiple agents developed as HIF inhibitors are currently being evaluated in clinical trials. Among the most important ones are EZN-2968, a HIF-1α antisense mRNA, and PX-478, a small molecule inhibitor of HIF derived from melphalan by oxidation of the nitrogen mustard moiety.[119] In a pilot clinical trial of EZN-2968 in patients with refractory solid tumors, preliminary proof of concept for modulation of HIF-1α mRNA and protein expression and target genes in tumor biopsies following the administration of EZN-2968 was demonstrated.[120]

### Targeting Unfolded Protein Response Signaling

Severe hypoxia leads to increased levels of unfolded proteins in the endoplasmic reticulum (ER), leading to the induction of unfolded protein response (UPR). UPR suppresses protein synthesis, stimulates protein degradation in the ER, and activates apoptosis or autophagy to resolve ER stress.[121] One therapeutic strategy to target UPR signaling seeks to exacerbate ER stress in order to overwhelm the UPR on the assumption that it is near capacity in hypoxic cells.[121] Agents having such action include inhibitors of 26S proteasome (such as bortezomib, nelfinavir) and inhibitors of HSP90 (such as IPI-504, 17-AAG). Bortezomib has been approved by the FDA for multiple myeloma and mantle cell lymphoma, and nelfinavir is still under investigation in phase I trials. A phase II trial of IPI-504 (retaspimycin) used as a single agent was shown to have a minimal effect on tumor burden and an unacceptable toxicity in patients with castration-resistant prostate cancer.[122] In another multicenter phase II trial in patients with HER2-positive metastatic breast cancer, IPI-504 plus trastuzumab were well tolerated but only showed modest clinical activity without meeting criteria for trial expansion.[123] In contrast, 17-AAG (tanespimycin) has shown significant additional benefit when combined with trastuzumab in patients with HER2-positive metastatic breast cancer in another phase II trial,[124] clearly warranting further clinical investigation.

## Lessons Learned and Conclusions

### What Have We Learned So Far?

With more than a decade of experience using drugs that more specifically target the TME, it is appropriate to ask the question of "what we have learned?" as we continue to move forward. Among the many lessons learned, we want to highlight three in particular in this chapter.

### Lesson 1: Targeting the TME Can Be Toxic

As clinical studies using agents targeting the TME were initiated, it was somewhat assumed that these agents would be much less toxic than the cytotoxic agents used in chemotherapy. It is now clear that this is not the case as many initially promising studies on agents targeting the TME had to be discontinued because of unacceptable and often unanticipated toxicity. The reasons are multiple and complex.

The first and most obvious reason is that many agents targeting the TME alter the homeostatic balance in normal organs and tissues, as was well illustrated in the case of small molecule inhibitors of MMPs. Cell and ECM proteins in tissues are not static but are subject to a constant and dynamic turnover that requires a delicate balance between growth and death, synthesis and degradation, and activation and inhibition of specific proteolytic processes or pathways. By disturbing the balance between MMP activation and inhibition, inhibitors of MMPs were found to increase collagen deposition in tissues and to cause musculoskeletal pain and inflammation that although reversible, necessitated stopping their use in one third of the patients.[125] Similarly, the use of Avastin in clinical trials has been associated with significant toxicities, in particular hypertension, proteinuria, thromboembolism, and congestive heart failure, caused in part by a decrease in NO production associated with vasoconstriction and a lack of vascular integrity causing proteinuria, hemorrhage, and thrombosis. As previously discussed, these side effects have resulted in the FDA's decision to remove Avastin from previous approval in breast cancer.[126] However, this is not always the case. One would have anticipated that inhibition of the proteasome by drugs like Bortezomib would be associated with major toxicities, considering the central role the proteasome complex is playing in the degradation of ubiquinated proteins. Somewhat surprisingly this drug, which has been tested in more than 200 clinical trials, is relatively well tolerated and has controllable toxicity, primarily neuropathy and thrombocytopenia.[127]

A second reason is that agents targeting the TME often target cells or pathways that are not always the enemy of cancer cells. This is again well illustrated in the case of MMP inhibitors, which were found to inhibit not only MMPs used by tumor cells for invasion but also MMPs involved in the production of antiangiogenic peptides by cleavage of precursor proteins.[125] Similarly, targeting NF-κB or TGF-β can have significant side effects as these pathways, depending on the state of tumor progression, can either promote or inhibit tumor growth. As agents targeting inflammation trail behind antiangiogenic therapies in clinical development, it will be important to remember the lessons learned from the testing of MMP and angiogenesis inhibitors and to consider the role of these agents within the dynamic context of an immune system that can be pro- as well as antitumorigenic.

### Lesson 2: Targeting the TME Does Not Prevent Resistance

Because agents targeting the TME are affecting nonmalignant cells, it was initially assumed that—in contrast to their malignant counterparts—they would not be subjected to genomic instability, and that the acquisition of resistance would not be a significant problem. This, however, has not been the case as we have seen with Avastin. Based on a systems biology approach, it could in fact be predicted that the redundancy of angiogenic signals might limit the efficacy of antiangiogenic monotherapies.[128] In support of this idea, it has been recently shown that tumors become refractory or even evade the inhibition of a single pro-angiogenic pathway like VEGF by upregulating compensatory angiogenic factors or other pathways that are favorable to tumor cells.[129,130] Another important consideration is that drugs that target the TME often do not only target pathways activated in nonmalignant cells but also in malignant cells which are prone to develop either drug resistance or to activate bypass mechanisms.

### Lesson 3: Targeting the TME Requires Knowing the Optimal Biological Dose

Somewhat unfortunately, agents targeting the TME have been tested in clinical trials often at their maximal tolerated dose (MTD), which has been the strategy for chemotherapy trials where it is often assumed that more is better. However, this may not be the case when targeting the TME. One of the objectives in targeting the TME is in fact to re-establish a disrupted homeostasis in a "malignant organ" rather than to flip the balance in an entirely opposite direction by "over-hitting" the target at MTD. The complex relationship between the ECM and tumor cells illustrates well this latter point.

Determining the optimal biological dose (OBD) of TME-targeting agents may thus be more important than finding their MTD. This requires: (1) that the drug hits the target, (2) that the target is altered by the drug, (3) that the tumor is altered by hitting the target, and (4) that giving a higher dose fails to improve outcomes further.[131] It will therefore be critical to develop "companion" biomarkers that can serve as indicators of the effect of agents targeting the TME. Sensitive functional imaging techniques and molecular markers such as cytokines and chemokines profiles and immunometrics and immunoscore[132] are likely to play an important role in our evaluation of clinical trials targeting the TME.

### Final Remarks

It has now been 10 years since the FDA's approval of Avastin as the first drug specifically targeting the TME in cancer. Since this milestone, we have witnessed a dramatic increase in the pre-clinical development and clinical testing of agents that target the TME. Several of them are already part of the standard treatment in patients with specific cancers, while others are still at the early stages of clinical testing. So far, strategies targeting the tumor vasculature appear to be the most successful, as demonstrated by the large number of agents approved by the FDA. Strategies inhibiting the pro-tumorigenic inflammatory response of the TME are rapidly being developed with agents either targeting TAM and their recruitment or pro-tumorigenic inflammatory pathways activated in tumor cells and stromal cells. Inhibition of tumor cell–stroma interactions is another strategy where new agents are also rapidly emerging.

As more agents targeting the TME are proposed for clinical trials, it is important to remember that there are several questions in regard to their activity and place in our therapeutic arsenal against cancer that remain to be answered. One, for example, is whether these agents are most effective when used alone or in combination with chemotherapy, radiation therapy, or other molecularly targeted therapy. Recent data suggest that the TME is an important contributor to therapeutic resistance.[133] Thus combining agents targeting the TME with chemotherapeutic agents to prevent the emergence of minimal residual disease from drug-resistant tumor cells may be critical. If those TME-targeting agents are used in combination with myeloablative agents, it will be important to determine whether some agents such as those inhibiting the recruitment of bone marrow-derived cells should be specifically used between courses of intensive and myelosuppressive therapy to prevent the release of precursor cells into the blood circulation.[134] Another question is whether some agents would be more effective at early stages on cancer progression and others at later stages (i.e., TGF-β inhibitors), considering the dynamic changes in the pro- or anti-tumorigenic functions of the TME during cancer progression. As discussed above, the question of the development of resistance to agents targeting the TME remains an important consideration.

As we are rapidly entering the era of precision cancer treatment and are using a genomic and biomarker-integrated approach to determine the best front line therapies for cancer patients, it will be equally important to develop reliable biomarkers that indicate the type of TME present in a specific tumor. For example, precise molecular or cellular information on the nature of immune cells present in a specific tumor and on their polarization could be as critical as the identification of the driver(s) mutation(s) that should be targeted. The development of such TME biomarkers and molecular signatures that reflect the TME should be an exciting and valuable research direction in the TME over the next several years.

### Acknowledgment

This manuscript was in part supported by grant U54 CA163117 to Y.A.D from the National Institutes of Health/National Cancer Institute. HF is supported by a training grant (T32GM007019) from the National Institutes of Health, Clinical Therapeutics.

### References

1 Folkman J. Tumor angiogenesis: therapeutic implications. *N Engl J Med*. 1971;285:1182–1186. doi:10.1056/NEJM197111182852108.

2 Morikawa K, Walker SM, Nakajima M, Pathak S, Jessup JM, Fidler IJ. Influence of organ environment on the growth, selection, and metastasis of human colon carcinoma cells in nude mice. *Cancer Res*. 1988;48:6863–6871.

3 Liotta LA, Tryggvason K, Garbisa S, Hart I, Foltz CM, Shafie S. Metastatic potential correlates with enzymatic degradation of basement membrane collagen. *Nature*. 1980;284:67–68.

4 Weaver VM, Petersen OW, Wang F, et al. Reversion of the malignant phenotype of human breast cells in three-dimensional culture and in vivo by integrin blocking antibodies. *J Cell Biol*. 1997;137:231–245.

5 Balkwill F, Mantovani A. Inflammation and cancer: back to Virchow? *Lancet*. 2001;357:539–545. doi:S0140-6736(00)04046-0 [pii].

6 Fidler IJ, Poste G. The "seed and soil" hypothesis revisited. *Lancet Oncol*. 2008;9:808. doi:S1470-2045(08)70201-8 [pii].

7 Hanahan D, Weinberg RA. Hallmarks of cancer: the next generation. *Cell*. 2011;144:646–674. doi:S0092-8674(11)00127-9 [pii].

8 Hanahan D, Coussens LM. Accessories to the crime: functions of cells recruited to the tumor microenvironment. *Cancer Cell*. 2012;21:309–322. doi:S1535-6108(12)00082-7 [pii].

9 Bergers G, Benjamin LE. Tumorigenesis and the angiogenic switch. *Nat Rev Cancer*. 2003;3:401–410. doi:10.1038/nrc1093. nrc1093 [pii].

10 Ferrara N, Davis-Smyth T. The biology of vascular endothelial growth factor. *Endocr Rev*. 1997;18:4–25.

11 Ribatti D. Endogenous inhibitors of angiogenesis: a historical review. *Leuk Res*. 2009;33:638–644. doi:S0145-2126(08)00507-9 [pii].

12 Folkman J. Angiogenesis. *Annu Rev Med*. 2006;57:1–18. doi:10.1146/annurev.med.57.121304.131306.

13 Nyberg P, Xie L, Kalluri R. Endogenous inhibitors of angiogenesis. *Cancer Res*. 2005;65:3967–3979. doi:65/10/3967 [pii].

14 Jain RK. Normalization of tumor vasculature: an emerging concept in antiangiogenic therapy. *Science*. 2005;307:58–62. doi:307/5706/58 [pii].

15 Rafii S, Lyden D, Benezra R, Hattori K, Heissig B. Vascular and haematopoietic stem cells: novel targets for anti-angiogenesis therapy? *Nat Rev Cancer*. 2002;2:826–835. doi:10.1038/nrc925. nrc925 [pii].

16 Grivennikov SI, Greten FR, Karin M. Immunity, inflammation, and cancer. *Cell*. 2010;140:883–899. doi:S0092-8674(10)00060-7 [pii].

17 Mantovani A, Allavena P, Sica A, Balkwill F. Cancer-related inflammation. *Nature*. 2008;454:436–444. doi:nature07205 [pii].

18 de Visser KE, Eichten A, Coussens LM. Paradoxical roles of the immune system during cancer development. *Nat Rev Cancer*. 2006;6:24–37. doi:nrc1782 [pii].

19 Biswas SK, Mantovani A. Macrophage plasticity and interaction with lymphocyte subsets: cancer as a paradigm. *Nat Immunol*. 2010;11:889–896. doi:ni.1937 [pii].

20 Sica A, Mantovani A. Macrophage plasticity and polarization: in vivo veritas. *J Clin Invest*. 2012;122:787–795. doi:10.1172/JCI59643. 59643 [pii].

21 Qian BZ, Pollard JW. Macrophage diversity enhances tumor progression and metastasis. *Cell*. 2010;141:39–51. doi:S0092-8674(10)00287-4 [pii].

22 Kalluri R, Zeisberg M. Fibroblasts in cancer. *Nat Rev Cancer*. 2006; 6:392–401.

23 Kraman M, Bambrough PJ, Arnold JN, et al. Suppression of antitumor immunity by stromal cells expressing fibroblast activation protein-alpha. *Science*. 2010;330:827–830. doi:330/6005/827 [pii].

24 Ferrara N. Binding to the extracellular matrix and proteolytic processing: two key mechanisms regulating vascular endothelial growth factor action. *Mol Biol Cell*. 2010;21:687–690. doi:21/5/687 [pii].

25 Lo CM, Wang HB, Dembo M, Wang YL. Cell movement is guided by the rigidity of the substrate. *Biophys J*. 2000;79:144–152. doi:S0006-3495(00)76279-5 [pii].

26 Levental KR, Yu H, Kass L, et al. Matrix crosslinking forces tumor progression by enhancing integrin signaling. *Cell*. 2009;139:891–906. doi:S0092-8674(09)01353-1 [pii].

27 Bristow RG, Hill RP. Hypoxia and metabolism. Hypoxia, DNA repair and genetic instability. *Nat Rev Cancer*. 2008;8:180–192. doi:nrc2344 [pii].

28 Vaupel P, Kelleher DK, Hockel M. Oxygen status of malignant tumors: pathogenesis of hypoxia and significance for tumor therapy. *Semin Oncol*. 2001;28:29–35.

29 Overgaard J. Hypoxic radiosensitization: adored and ignored. *J Clin Oncol*. 2007;25:4066–4074. doi:25/26/4066 [pii].

30 Keith B, Johnson RS, Simon MC. HIF1alpha and HIF2alpha: sibling rivalry in hypoxic tumour growth and progression. *Nat Rev Cancer*. 2012;12:9–22. doi:10.1038/nrc3183. nrc3183 [pii].

31 Varner JA, Cheresh DA. Integrins and cancer. *Curr Opin Cell Biol*. 1996;8:724–730. doi:S0955-0674(96)80115-3 [pii].

32 Shain KH, Yarde DN, Meads MB, et al. Beta1 integrin adhesion enhances IL-6-mediated STAT3 signaling in myeloma cells: implications for microenvironment influence on tumor survival and proliferation. *Cancer Res*. 2009;69:1009–1015. doi:0008-5472.CAN-08-2419 [pii].

33 Shiozawa Y, Pedersen EA, Havens AM, et al. Human prostate cancer metastases target the hematopoietic stem cell niche to establish footholds in mouse bone marrow. *J Clin Invest*. 2011;121:1298–1312. doi:10.1172/JCI43414. 43414 [pii].

34 Ara T, Song L, Shimada H, et al. Interleukin-6 in the bone marrow microenvironment promotes the growth and survival of neuroblastoma cells. *Cancer Res*. 2009;69:329–337. doi:69/1/329 [pii].

35 Silverman AM, Nakata R, Shimada H, Sposto R, DeClerck YA. A galectin-3-dependent pathway upregulates interleukin-6 in the microenvironment of human neuroblastoma. *Cancer Res*. 2012;72:2228–2238. doi:0008-5472.CAN-11-2165 [pii].

36 Peinado H, Lavotshkin S, Lyden D. The secreted factors responsible for pre-metastatic niche formation: old sayings and new thoughts. *Semin Cancer Biol*. 2011;21:139–146. doi:S1044-579X(11)00003-4 [pii].

37 Peinado H, Alečković M, Lavotshkin S, et al. Melanoma exosomes educate bone marrow progenitor cells toward a pro-metastatic phenotype through MET. *Nat Med*. doi:10.1038/nm.2753. nm.2753 [pii].

38 Fang H, Declerck YA. Targeting the tumor microenvironment: from understanding pathways to effective clinical trials. *Cancer Res*. 2013;73:4965–4977. doi:10.1158/0008-5472.CAN-13-0661. 0008-5472.CAN-13-0661 [pii].

39 Ferrara N. Vascular endothelial growth factor as a target for anticancer therapy. *Oncologist*. 2004;9(suppl 1):2–10.

40 Ferrara N, Gerber HP, LeCouter J. The biology of VEGF and its receptors. *Nat Med*. 2003;9:669–676. doi:10.1038/nm0603-669. nm0603-669 [pii].

41 Poole RM, Vaidya A. Ramucirumab: first global approval. *Drugs*. 2014;74:1047–1058. doi:10.1007/s40265-014-0244-2.

42 Fuchs CS, Tomasek J, Yong CJ, et al. Ramucirumab monotherapy for previously treated advanced gastric or gastro-oesophageal junction adenocarcinoma (REGARD): an international, randomised, multicentre, placebo-controlled, phase 3 trial. *Lancet*. 2014;383:31–39. doi:10.1016/S0140-6736(13)61719-5.

43 Garon EB, Ciuleanu TE, Arrieta O, et al. Ramucirumab plus docetaxel versus placebo plus docetaxel for second-line treatment of stage IV non-small-cell lung cancer after disease progression on platinum-based therapy (REVEL): a multicentre, double-blind, randomised phase 3 trial. *Lancet*. 2014;384(9944):665–673. doi:10.1016/S0140-6736(14)60845-X.

44 Itoh N, Ornitz DM. Evolution of the Fgf and Fgfr gene families. *Trends Genet*. 2004;20:563–569. doi:S0168-9525(04)00241-0 [pii].

45 Lieu C, Heymach J, Overman M, Tran H, Kopetz, S, Beyond VEGF: inhibition of the fibroblast growth factor pathway and antiangiogenesis. *Clin Cancer Res*. 2011;17:6130–6139. doi:1078-0432.CCR-11-0659 [pii].

46 Batchelor TT, Sorensen AG, di Tomaso E, et al. AZD2171, a pan-VEGF receptor tyrosine kinase inhibitor, normalizes tumor vasculature and alleviates edema in glioblastoma patients. *Cancer Cell*. 2007;11:83–95. doi:S1535-6108(06)00370-9 [pii].

47 Finn RS, Kang YK, Mulcahy M, et al. Phase II, open-label study of brivanib as second-line therapy in patients with advanced hepatocellular carcinoma. *Clin Cancer Res*. 2012;18:2090–2098. doi:1078-0432.CCR-11-1991 [pii].

48 Johnson PJ, Qin S, Park JW, et al. Brivanib versus sorafenib as first-line therapy in patients with unresectable, advanced hepatocellular carcinoma: results from the randomized phase III BRISK-FL study. *J Clin Oncol*. 2013;31:3517–3524. doi:10.1200/JCO.2012.48.4410.

49 Andrae J, Gallini R, Betsholtz C. Role of platelet-derived growth factors in physiology and medicine. *Genes Dev*. 2008;22:1276–1312. doi:22/10/1276 [pii].

50 Xiong HQ, Herbst R, Faria SC, et al. A phase I surrogate endpoint study of SU6668 in patients with solid tumors. *Invest New Drugs*. 2004;22:459–466. doi:10.1023/B:DRUG.0000036688.96453.8d. 5273870 [pii].

51 Carpenter G. Receptors for epidermal growth factor and other polypeptide mitogens. *Annu Rev Biochem*. 1987;56:881–914. doi:10.1146/annurev.bi.56.070187.004313.

52 Ellis LM. Epidermal growth factor receptor in tumor angiogenesis. *Hematol Oncol Clin North Am*. 2004;18:1007–1021, viii. doi:S0889-8588(04)00050-4 [pii].

53 Larsen AK, Ouaret DEI, Ouadrani K, Petitprez A, Targeting EGFR and VEGF(R) pathway cross-talk in tumor survival and angiogenesis. *Pharmacol Ther*. 2011;131:80–90. doi:S0163-7258(11)00078-7 [pii].

54 Wheeler DL, Dunn EF, Harari PM. Understanding resistance to EGFR inhibitors-impact on future treatment strategies. *Nat Rev Clin Oncol.* 2010;7:493–507. doi:nrclinonc.2010.97 [pii].

55 Yu H, Pardoll D, Jove R. STATs in cancer inflammation and immunity: a leading role for STAT3. *Nat Rev Cancer.* 2009;9:798–809. doi:nrc2734 [pii].

56 Mertens C, Darnell JE Jr, SnapShot: JAK-STAT signaling. *Cell.* 2007;131:612. doi:S0092-8674(07)01353-0 [pii].

57 Bromberg J, Wang TC. Inflammation and cancer: IL-6 and STAT3 complete the link. *Cancer Cell.* 2009;15:79–80. doi:S1535-6108(09)00006-3 [pii].

58 Sansone P, Bromberg J. Targeting the interleukin-6/Jak/stat pathway in human malignancies. *J Clin Oncol.* 2012;30:1005–1014. doi:JCO.2010. 31.8907 [pii].

59 Yu H, Kortylewski M, Pardoll D. Crosstalk between cancer and immune cells: role of STAT3 in the tumour microenvironment. *Nat Rev Immunol.* 1995;7:41–51. doi:nri1995 [pii].

60 Song L, Asgharzadeh S, Salo J, et al. Valpha24-invariant NKT cells mediate antitumor activity via killing of tumor-associated macrophages. *J Clin Invest.* 2009;119:1524–1536. doi:37869 [pii].

61 Fizazi K, De Bono JS, Flechon A, et al. Randomised phase II study of siltuximab (CNTO 328), an anti-IL-6 monoclonal antibody, in combination with mitoxantrone/prednisone versus mitoxantrone/prednisone alone in metastatic castration-resistant prostate cancer. *Eur J Cancer.* 2012;48:85–93. doi:S0959-8049(11)00821-5 [pii].

62 Coward J, Kulbe H, Chakravarty P, et al. Interleukin-6 as a therapeutic target in human ovarian cancer. *Clin Cancer Res.* 2011;17:6083–6096. doi:1078-0432.CCR-11-0945 [pii].

63 Rossi JF, Négrier S, James ND, et al. A phase I/II study of siltuximab (CNTO 328), an anti-interleukin-6 monoclonal antibody, in metastatic renal cell cancer. *Br J Cancer.* 2010;103:1154–1162. doi:6605872 [pii]. 10.1038/sj.bjc.6605872.

64 Nakashima Y, Kondo M, Harada H, et al. Clinical evaluation of tocilizumab for patients with active rheumatoid arthritis refractory to anti-TNF biologics: tocilizumab in combination with methotrexate. *Mod Rheumatol.* 2010;20:343–352. doi:10.1007/s10165-010-0290-x.

65 Verstovsek S. Therapeutic potential of JAK2 inhibitors. *Hematology Am Soc Hematol Educ Program.* 2009;636–642. doi:2009/1/636 [pii].

66 Eghtedar A, Verstovsek S, Estrov Z, et al. Phase 2 study of the JAK kinase inhibitor ruxolitinib in patients with refractory leukemias, including postmyeloproliferative neoplasm acute myeloid leukemia. *Blood.* 2012;119:4614–4618. doi:10.1182/blood-2011-12-400051.

67 Verstovsek S, Passamonti F, Rambaldi A, et al. A phase 2 study of ruxolitinib, an oral JAK1 and JAK2 Inhibitor, in patients with advanced polycythemia vera who are refractory or intolerant to hydroxyurea. *Cancer.* 2014;120:513–520. doi:10.1002/cncr.28441.

68 Xin H, Herrmann A, Reckamp K, et al. Antiangiogenic and antimetastatic activity of JAK inhibitor AZD1480. *Cancer Res.* 2011;71: 6601–6610. doi:0008-5472.CAN-11-1217 [pii].

69 Sen M, Thomas SM, Kim S, et al. First-in-human trial of a STAT3 decoy oligonucleotide abrogates target gene expression in head and neck tumors: implications for cancer therapy. *Cancer Discov.* doi:2159-8290.CD-12-0191 [pii].

70 Karin M, Greten FR. NF-kappaB: linking inflammation and immunity to cancer development and progression. *Nat Rev Immunol.* 2005;5:749–759. doi:nri1703 [pii].

71 Pikarsky E, Porat RM, Stein I, et al. NF-kappaB functions as a tumour promoter in inflammation-associated cancer. *Nature.* 2004;431:461–466. doi:10.1038/nature02924. nature02924 [pii].

72 Ben-Neriah Y, Karin M. Inflammation meets cancer, with NF-kappaB as the matchmaker. *Nat Immunol.* 2011;12:715–723. doi:10.1038/ni.2060. ni.2060 [pii].

73 Kingsley LA, Fournier PG, Chirgwin JM, Guise TA. Molecular biology of bone metastasis. *Mol Cancer Ther.* 2007;6:2609–2617. doi:6/10/2609 [pii].

74 Perkins ND. The diverse and complex roles of NF-kappaB subunits in cancer. *Nat Rev Cancer.* 2012;12:121–132. doi:10.1038/nrc3204. nrc3204 [pii].

75 Karin M, Yamamoto Y, Wang QM. The IKK NF-kappa B system: a treasure trove for drug development. *Nat Rev Drug Discov.* 2004;3:17–26. doi:10.1038/nrd1279. nrd1279 [pii].

76 Lam LT, Davis RE, Pierce J, et al. Small molecule inhibitors of IkappaB kinase are selectively toxic for subgroups of diffuse large B-cell lymphoma defined by gene expression profiling. *Clin Cancer Res.* 2005;11:28–40. doi:11/1/28 [pii].

77 Cavo M. Proteasome inhibitor bortezomib for the treatment of multiple myeloma. *Leukemia.* 2006;20:1341–1352. doi:2404278 [pii].

78 Balkwill F. TNF-alpha in promotion and progression of cancer. *Cancer Metastasis Rev.* 2006;25:409–416. doi:10.1007/s10555-006-9005-3.

79 Locksley RM, Killeen N, Lenardo MJ. The TNF and TNF receptor superfamilies: integrating mammalian biology. *Cell.* 2001;104:487–501. doi:S0092-8674(01)00237-9 [pii].

80 Woyach JA, Lin TS, Lucas MS, et al. A phase I/II study of rituximab and etanercept in patients with chronic lymphocytic leukemia and small lymphocytic lymphoma. *Leukemia.* 2009;23:912–918. doi:leu2008385 [pii].

81 Madhusudan S, Muthuramalingam SR, Braybrooke JP, et al. Study of etanercept, a tumor necrosis factor-alpha inhibitor, in recurrent ovarian cancer. *J Clin Oncol.* 2005;23:5950–5959. doi:23/25/5950 [pii].

82 Madhusudan S, Foster M, Muthuramalingam SR, et al. A phase II study of etanercept (Enbrel), a tumor necrosis factor alpha inhibitor in patients with metastatic breast cancer. *Clin Cancer Res.* 2004;10:6528–6534. doi:10/19/6528 [pii].

83 Harrison ML, Obermueller E, Maisey NR, et al. Tumor necrosis factor alpha as a new target for renal cell carcinoma: two sequential phase II trials of infliximab at standard and high dose. *J Clin Oncol.* 2007;25:4542–4549. doi:25/29/4542 [pii].

84 Larkin JM, Ferguson TR, Pickering LM, et al. A phase I/II trial of sorafenib and infliximab in advanced renal cell carcinoma. *Br J Cancer.* 2010;103:1149–1153. doi:6605889 [pii].

85 Tsujii M, Kawano S, Tsuji S, Sawaoka H, Hori M, DuBois RN. Cyclooxygenase regulates angiogenesis induced by colon cancer cells. *Cell.* 1998;93:705–716. doi:S0092-8674(00)81433-6 [pii].

86 Fosslien E. Biochemistry of cyclooxygenase (COX)-2 inhibitors and molecular pathology of COX-2 in neoplasia. *Crit Rev Clin Lab Sci.* 2000;37:431–502. doi:10.1080/10408360091174286.

87 Dubois RN. New, long-term insights from the adenoma prevention with celecoxib trial on a promising but troubled class of drugs. *Cancer Prev Res (Phila).* 2009;2:285–287. doi:1940-6207.CAPR-09-0038 [pii].

88 Mohammadianpanah M, Razmjou-Ghalaei S, Shafizad A, et al. Efficacy and safety of concurrent chemoradiation with weekly cisplatin +/- low-dose celecoxib in locally advanced undifferentiated nasopharyngeal carcinoma: a phase II-III clinical trial. *J Cancer Res Ther.* 2011;7:442–447. doi:10.4103/0973-1482.92013.

89 James ND, Sydes MR, Mason MD, et al. Celecoxib plus hormone therapy versus hormone therapy alone for hormone-sensitive prostate cancer: first results from the STAMPEDE multiarm, multistage, randomised controlled trial. *Lancet Oncol.* 2012;13:549–558. doi:S1470-2045(12)70088-8 [pii].

90 Groen HJ, Sietsma H, Vincent A, et al. Randomized, placebo-controlled phase III study of docetaxel plus carboplatin with celecoxib and cyclooxygenase-2 expression as a biomarker for patients with advanced non-small-cell lung cancer: the NVALT-4 study. *J Clin Oncol.* 2011;29:4320–4326. doi:JCO.2011.35.5214 [pii].

91 Massague J. TGFbeta in cancer. *Cell.* 2008;134:215–230. doi:S0092-8674(08)00878-7 [pii].

92 Bierie B, Moses HL. Tumour microenvironment: TGFbeta: the molecular Jekyll and Hyde of cancer. *Nat Rev Cancer.* 2006;6:506–520. doi:nrc1926 [pii].

93 Achyut BR, Yang L. Transforming growth factor-beta in the gastrointestinal and hepatic tumor microenvironment. *Gastroenterology.* 2011;141:1167–1178. doi:S0016-5085(11)01083-3 [pii].

94 Bogdahn U, Hau P, Stockhammer G, et al. Targeted therapy for high-grade glioma with the TGF-beta2 inhibitor trabedersen: results of a randomized and controlled phase IIb study. *Neuro Oncol.* 2011;13:132–142. doi:noq142 [pii].

95 Brana I, Calles A, LoRusso PM, et al. Carlumab, an anti-C-C chemokine ligand 2 monoclonal antibody, in combination with four chemotherapy regimens for the treatment of patients with solid tumors: an open-label, multicenter phase 1b study. *Target Oncol.* doi:10.1007/s11523-014-0320-2.

96 Sandhu SK, Papadopoulos K, Fong PC, et al. A first-in-human, first-in-class, phase I study of carlumab (CNTO 888), a human monoclonal antibody against CC-chemokine ligand 2 in patients with solid tumors. *Cancer Chemother Pharmacol.* 2013;71:1041–1050. doi:10.1007/s00280-013-2099-8.

97 Pienta KJ, Machiels JP, Schrijvers D, et al. Phase 2 study of carlumab (CNTO 888), a human monoclonal antibody against CC-chemokine ligand 2 (CCL2), in metastatic castration-resistant prostate cancer. *Invest New Drugs.* 2013;31:760–768. doi:10.1007/s10637-012-9869-8.

98 Zollo M, Di Dato V, Spano D, et al. Targeting monocyte chemotactic protein-1 synthesis with bindarit induces tumor regression in prostate and breast cancer animal models. *Clin Exp Metastasis.* 2012;29:585–601. doi:10.1007/s10585-012-9473-5.

99 Aharinejad S, Abraham D, Paulus P, et al. Colony-stimulating factor-1 antisense treatment suppresses growth of human tumor xenografts in mice. *Cancer Res.* 2002;62:5317–5324.

100 Aharinejad S, Paulus P, Sioud M, et al. Colony-stimulating factor-1 blockade by antisense oligonucleotides and small interfering RNAs suppresses growth of human mammary tumor xenografts in mice. *Cancer Res.* 2004;64:5378–5384. doi:10.1158/0008-5472.CAN-04-0961. 64/15/5378 [pii].

101 Ohno H, Kubo K, Murooka H, et al. A c-fms tyrosine kinase inhibitor, Ki20227, suppresses osteoclast differentiation and osteolytic bone destruction in a bone metastasis model. *Mol Cancer Ther.* 2006;5:2634–2643. doi:5/11/2634 [pii].

102 Manthey CL, Johnson DL, Illig CR, et al. JNJ-28312141, a novel orally active colony-stimulating factor-1 receptor/FMS-related receptor tyrosine kinase-3 receptor tyrosine kinase inhibitor with potential utility in solid tumors, bone metastases, and acute myeloid leukemia. *Mol Cancer Ther.* 2009;8:3151–3161. doi:1535-7163.MCT-09-0255 [pii].

103 Hynes RO. Integrins: bidirectional, allosteric signaling machines. *Cell.* 2002;110:673–687. doi:S0092867402009716 [pii].

104 Brooks PC, Clark RA, Cheresh DA. Requirement of vascular integrin alpha v beta 3 for angiogenesis. *Science.* 1994;264:569–571.

105 Dechantsreiter MA, Planker E, Mathä B, et al. N-Methylated cyclic RGD peptides as highly active and selective alpha(V)beta(3) integrin antagonists. *J Med Chem.* 1999;42:3033–3040. doi:10.1021/jm970832g. jm970832g [pii].

106 Reardon DA, Fink KL, Mikkelsen T, et al. Randomized phase II study of cilengitide, an integrin-targeting arginine-glycine-aspartic acid peptide, in recurrent glioblastoma multiforme. *J Clin Oncol.* 2008;26:5610–5617. doi:JCO.2008.16.7510 [pii].

107 MacDonald TJ, Vezina G, Stewart CF, et al. Phase II study of cilengitide in the treatment of refractory or relapsed high-grade gliomas in children: a report from the Children's Oncology Group. *Neuro Oncol.* 2013;15:1438–1444. doi:10.1093/neuonc/not058.

108 Manegold C, Vansteenkiste J, Cardenal F, et al. Randomized phase II study of three doses of the integrin inhibitor cilengitide versus docetaxel as second-line treatment for patients with advanced non-small-cell lung cancer. *Invest New Drugs.* 2013;31:175–182. doi:10.1007/s10637-012-9842-6.

109 Kim KB, Prieto V, Joseph RW, et al. A randomized phase II study of cilengitide (EMD 121974) in patients with metastatic melanoma. *Melanoma Res.* 2012;22:294–301. doi:10.1097/CMR.0b013e32835312e4.

110 Alva A, Slovin S, Daignault S, et al. Phase II study of cilengitide (EMD 121974, NSC 707544) in patients with non-metastatic castration resistant prostate cancer, NCI-6735. A study by the DOD/PCF prostate cancer clinical trials consortium. *Invest New Drugs.* 2012;30:749–757. doi:10.1007/s10637-010-9573-5.

111 O'Day S, Pavlick A, Loquai C, et al. A randomised, phase II study of intetumumab, an anti-alphav-integrin mAb, alone and with dacarbazine in stage IV melanoma. *Br J Cancer.* 2011;105:346–352. doi:10.1038/bjc.2011.183. bjc2011183 [pii].

112 Hersey P, Sosman J, O'Day S, et al. A randomized phase 2 study of etaracizumab, a monoclonal antibody against integrin alpha(v)beta(3), + or − dacarbazine in patients with stage IV metastatic melanoma. *Cancer.* 2010;116:1526–1534. doi:10.1002/cncr.24821.

113 Coleman RE. Clinical features of metastatic bone disease and risk of skeletal morbidity. *Clin Cancer Res.* 2006;12:6243s–6249s. doi:12/20/6243s [pii].

114 Onishi T, Hayashi N, Theriault RL, Hortobagyi GN, Ueno NT. Future directions of bone-targeted therapy for metastatic breast cancer. *Nat Rev Clin Oncol.* 2010;7:641–651. doi:nrclinonc.2010.134 [pii].

115 Wilson WR, Hay MP. Targeting hypoxia in cancer therapy. *Nat Rev Cancer.* 2011;11:393–410. doi:nrc3064 [pii].

116 Reddy SB, Williamson SK. Tirapazamine: a novel agent targeting hypoxic tumor cells. *Expert Opin Invest Drugs.* 2009;18:77–87. doi:10.1517/13543780802567250.

117 DiSilvestro PA, Ali S, Craighead PS, et al. Phase III randomized trial of weekly cisplatin and irradiation versus cisplatin and tirapazamine and irradiation in stages IB2, IIA, IIB, IIIB, and IVA cervical carcinoma limited to the pelvis: a Gynecologic Oncology Group study. *J Clin Oncol.* 2014;32:458–464. doi:10.1200/JCO.2013.51.4265.

118 Semenza GL. Targeting HIF-1 for cancer therapy. *Nat Rev Cancer.* 2003;3:721–732. doi:10.1038/nrc1187. nrc1187 [pii].

119 Xia Y, Choi HK, Lee K. Recent advances in hypoxia-inducible factor (HIF)-1 inhibitors. *Eur J Med Chem.* 2012;49:24–40. doi:S0223-5234(12)00048-7 [pii].

120 Jeong W, Rapisarda A, Park SR, et al. Pilot trial of EZN-2968, an antisense oligonucleotide inhibitor of hypoxia-inducible factor-1 alpha (HIF-1alpha), in patients with refractory solid tumors. *Cancer Chemother Pharmacol.* 2014;73:343–348. doi:10.1007/s00280-013-2362-z.

121 Wouters BG, Koritzinsky M. Hypoxia signalling through mTOR and the unfolded protein response in cancer. *Nat Rev Cancer.* 2008;8:851–864. doi:nrc2501 [pii].

122 Oh WK, Galsky MD, Stadler WM, et al. Multicenter phase II trial of the heat shock protein 90 inhibitor, retaspimycin hydrochloride

(IPI-504), in patients with castration-resistant prostate cancer. *Urology.* 2011;78:626–630. doi:S0090-4295(11)00471-7 [pii].

123 Modi S, et al. A multicenter trial evaluating retaspimycin HCL (IPI-504) plus trastuzumab in patients with advanced or metastatic HER2-positive breast cancer. *Breast Cancer Res Treat.* 2013;139(1):107–113. doi:10.1007/s10549-013-2510-5.

124 Modi S, Stopeck A, Linden H, et al. HSP90 inhibition is effective in breast cancer: a phase II trial of tanespimycin (17-AAG) plus trastuzumab in patients with HER2-positive metastatic breast cancer progressing on trastuzumab. *Clin Cancer Res.* 2011;17:5132–5139. doi:1078-0432.CCR-11-0072 [pii].

125 Coussens LM, Fingleton B, Matrisian LM. Matrix metalloproteinase inhibitors and cancer: trials and tribulations. *Science.* 2002;295:2387–2392. doi:10.1126/science.1067100. 295/5564/2387 [pii].

126 Dienstmann R, Ades F, Saini KS, Metzger-Filho O. Benefit-risk assessment of bevacizumab in the treatment of breast cancer. *Drug Saf.* 2012;35:15–25. doi:10.2165/11595910-000000000-00000.

127 Cvek B. Proteasome inhibitors. *Prog Mol Biol Transl Sci.* 2012; 109:161–226. doi:10.1016/B978-0-12-397863-9.00005-5. B978-0-12-397863-9.00005-5 [pii].

128 Abdollahi A, Folkman J. Evading tumor evasion: current concepts and perspectives of anti-angiogenic cancer therapy. *Drug Resist Updat.* 2010;13:16–28. doi:10.1016/j.drup.2009.12.001. S1368-7646(09)00077-6 [pii].

129 Bergers G, Hanahan D. Modes of resistance to anti-angiogenic therapy. *Nat Rev Cancer.* 2008;8:592–603. doi:10.1038/nrc2442. nrc2442 [pii].

130 Lu KV, Chang JP, Parachoniak CA, et al. VEGF inhibits tumor cell invasion and mesenchymal transition through a MET/VEGFR2 complex. *Cancer Cell.* 2012;22:21–35. doi:10.1016/j.ccr.2012.05.037. S1535-6108(12)00252-8 [pii].

131 Marshall JL. Maximum-tolerated dose, optimum biologic dose, or optimum clinical value: dosing determination of cancer therapies. *J Clin Oncol.* 2012;30:2815–2816. doi:10.1200/JCO.2012.43.4233. JCO.2012.43.4233 [pii].

132 Coussens LM, Zitvogel L, Palucka AK. Neutralizing tumor-promoting chronic inflammation: a magic bullet? *Science.* 2013;339:286–291. doi:10.1126/science.1232227. 339/6117/286 [pii].

133 Meads MB, Gatenby RA, Dalton WS. Environment-mediated drug resistance: a major contributor to minimal residual disease. *Nat Rev Cancer.* 2009;9:665–674. doi:10.1038/nrc2714. nrc2714 [pii].

134 Ferrara N, Kerbel RS. Angiogenesis as a therapeutic target. *Nature.* 2005;438:967–974. doi:nature04483 [pii].

## CHAPTER 6

# The Role of Angiogenesis in Cancer

*Morgan Taylor[1], Robert L. Coleman[1,2], and Anil K. Sood[1,2,3]*

[1] Department of Gynecologic Oncology and Reproductive Medicine, The University of Texas MD Anderson Cancer Center, Houston, TX, USA

[2] Center for RNA Interference and Non-Coding RNA, The University of Texas MD Anderson Cancer Center, Houston, TX, USA

[3] Department of Cancer Biology, The University of Texas MD Anderson Cancer Center, Houston, TX, USA

In the 1960s, Judah Folkman first discovered that a tumor could not grow beyond the perfusion of its vasculature.[1] Although hypervascularity of tumors was well described, the idea that tumor expansion required the parallel expansion of its vasculature was a new idea that Folkman hypothesized, along with the logical next step: tumors themselves release factors to induce growth of surrounding blood vessels.[2] Experimental evidence for his hypotheses would steadily accumulate, leading to the acceptance of angiogenesis as a hallmark of malignancy.[3]

As the numerous factors and their respective roles in tumor angiogenesis have been elucidated, molecular targeting of this essential process has been undertaken as well. Nine different therapies against the dominant pathway (i.e., vascular endothelial growth factor (VEGF) ligands and their receptors) have been approved by the Food and Drug Administration (FDA) for their antineoplastic efficacy.[4] Despite these advances, the full potential of antiangiogenic therapies has yet to be reached.[5] The search for better therapies continues, as do efforts to overcome resistance and discover predictive biomarkers. Both basic scientists and practicing clinicians have important roles in solving these issues; this chapter will provide an understanding of tumor angiogenesis and antiangiogenic therapy from its molecular beginnings to clinical applications.

## How Vessels Are Formed

It is important to differentiate the production of *de novo* blood vessels from angioblasts, called *vasculogenesis*, from the sprouting of new vessels from existing vasculature, called *angiogenesis*.[6,7] Angiogenesis, following an initial proangiogenic stimulus, involves endothelial cells (ECs) breaking free from the blood vessel, migrating to an adjacent habitat, forming tubes through proliferation, and finally becoming enwrapped by pericytes during the maturation process. In tumor angiogenesis, this sprouting is encouraged by tumor signals, and tumor stem cells may even differentiate into tumor endothelium, thereby contributing to the neovascular milieu. Before the signal to sprout occurs, cells are held in a quiescent state by autocrine signaling and, especially, pericytes.[8,9] Pericytes provide factors that promote survival but inhibit proliferation. VEGF is likely one of these factors, produced locally by pericytes in response to platelet-derived growth factor (PDGF)-BB, providing ECs with a local source of survival signals.

For many solid tumors, the initial events on the path to neovascularization likely involve vascular "co-option," whereby metastatic cancer cells grow along preexisting vessels.[6,10] Subsequently, the host vasculature becomes de-stabilized, resulting in central necrosis. Under hypoxic strain, tumor cells provide the stimulus for angiogenesis through VEGF, angiopoietin (ANG)-2, or fibroblast growth factors (FGFs). VEGF signaling causes the basement membranes of ECs to degrade. This, along with ANG-2 stimulation of pericytes, promotes pericyte separation. ECs can now invade the neighboring extracellular matrix (ECM) to create a migration column. VEGF stimulation also increases expression of delta-like ligand 4 (DLL4) in ECs, which inhibits neighboring tip selection through Notch. Whichever cell manages the greatest inhibitory signaling will push the others to the stalk and claim the tip position. Stalk cells then proliferate to lengthen the stalk and establish the lumen. Union with an opposing vessel branch is mediated via myeloid bridge cells, allowing blood flow to become established. Pericytes are recruited by PDGF-BB, ANG-1, and other signaling molecules to cover the new vessel and provide stability.

Alternative mechanisms of neovascularization are also important to mention, as they represent avenues for resistance and future therapeutic targets.[6,10] Vascular mimicry is a process whereby tumor cells can mimic the expression of vascular cells and form their own tubes that allow blood flow to facilitate tumor growth. Evidence of this process has been observed in several cancers, including melanoma, ovarian cancer, and glioblastoma multiforme (GBM).[11–15] Researchers have further shown that an overall majority of tumor ECs were derived originally from tumors and that selective targeting of these cells retarded the growth of xenografts.[16]

## Angiogenesis Pathways

### VEGF Family

In 1986, Dvorak and colleagues discovered a 35–45-kD polypeptide with a role in vascular permeability.[17] Later studies produced its sequence and final name, VEGF, and began attributing to VEGF various functions within both normal and tumor-driven angiogenesis.[10,18] The initial form was named VEGF-A; more proteins were added to a family that now comprises VEGF A-E and includes two placental growth factors (PGF-1, -2). Secondary to alternative splicing, VEGF-A itself has four isoforms denoted by the number of

*Targeted Therapy in Translational Cancer Research*, First Edition. Edited by Apostolia-Maria Tsimberidou, Razelle Kurzrock and Kenneth C. Anderson.
© 2016 John Wiley & Sons, Inc. Published 2016 by John Wiley & Sons, Inc.

amino acids: 121, 165, 189, and 206. VEGF-165 is the major isoform expressed in both normal and tumor cells and is crucial to tumor angiogenesis.[10]

VEGF-A is expressed in a diverse panel of cells, from macrophages to osteoblasts. Its expression and secretion by tumor cells occurs in response to conditions often present in solid tumors—hypoxia, low pH, and cellular stress.[10] Vascular ECs predominantly express two VEGF receptors: fms-like tyrosine kinase and kinase insert domain-containing receptor, also respectively known as VEGF receptor 1 and 2 (VEGFR-1, -2). These receptors share seven extracellular immunoglobulin-like domains, one transmembrane segment, and an intracellular tyrosine kinase sequence with an interjected kinase-insert domain. After VEGF binding and receptor dimerization, the tyrosine kinase is phosphorylated. VEGFR-1 is vital for developmental and physiologic angiogenesis, but VEGFR-2 appears to be the main mediator of VEGF-A's effect on tumor angiogenesis.

Activation of the VEGF receptors promotes signaling pathways that lead to increased vessel permeability, EC proliferation and migration, and stabilization of newly formed blood vessels. More distantly, secreted VEGF can summon endothelial progenitor cells from the bone marrow to participate in new vessel formation. The ability of VEGF to increase vascular permeability allows plasma proteins capable of contributing to tumor progression to leak into the ECM, a role that is clinically recognizable by the presence of malignant pleural effusion or ascites. Proteins such as matrix metalloproteinases can then break down the ECM to create space for further cell proliferation or for other extravasating proteins, such as fibrinogen, which can then act as a medium for new vessel growth. VEGF also influences ECs to migrate to these areas and proliferate. The latter effect is secondary to activating the protein kinase C-Raf-Mek-Erk pathway. Despite the subsequent development of poorly formed vessels by these ECs, VEGF ensures their survival by phosphoinositide 3-kinase (PI3K)/AKT pathway stimulation.

## FGF Family

Armelin first showed in 1973 that pituitary gland extracts stimulated 3T3 cells and suggested the organ as a "source of fibroblast growth factor [FGF] *in vivo*".[19] The protein was purified in 1974 by Gospodarowicz.[20] Researchers have since identified a family of FGF ligands, 18 in all, that have similar structure and size (the largest is 34 kDa). However, FGF-1 and particularly FGF-2 were found most important for angiogenesis, initially in the context of perfusing healing wounds.[21,22]

The ECM holds most of the FGFs, which are secreted glycoproteins. Ligands are thought to be mobilized by tumors through either enzymatic liberation of matrix FGF or tumor cell expression/secretion. FGF Receptor 1-IIIc and 2-IIIc can both be highly expressed in ECs, and, when activated by FGFs, they lead to dimerization, activation of an intracellular kinase, and phosphorylation of its own tyrosine residues. Further downstream events lead to MAPK and PKC activation. The end result is proliferation and migration of these cells along with concurrent ECM breakdown.

## PDGF Family

In 1974, a factor from platelets was discovered that could stimulate fibroblasts and smooth muscle cells after activation by thrombin.[23] This factor became known as PDGF and consisted of two distinct polypeptide chains, denoted A and B. Homodimeric versions were eventually discovered, as well as other related polypeptides, PDGF-C and -D. PDGF-AB is the only heterodimer, however,

and its infrequency *in vivo* suggests the dominance of the homodimeric forms (hereafter denoted PDGF-A, -B, -C, and -D). The functions of PDGF-B in tumor angiogenesis have been particularly well-studied, though it is not the only form that contributes to this process.[8,9]

The ECs of newly sprouted vessels secrete PDGF-B as a chemoattractant for nearby pericytes, as well as a promoter for vascular smooth muscle cell proliferation. These pericytes, recruited either locally or from perivascular progenitors, play a substantial role in stabilizing vessels in the microvasculature either by constructing the surrounding ECM or by providing factors related to endothelial differentiation. Pericytes responding to this signal express the tyrosine kinase receptor PDGFR-β, which dimerizes upon ligand binding with another beta receptor and can activate multiple signaling cascades, including Ras-mitogen-activated protein kinase (MAPK), PI3K, and phospholipase C-gamma. The importance of PDGF-B and its receptor in pericyte coverage can be seen in knockout models, where pericyte deficiency leads to vessel dysfunction, subsequent microhemorrhage and edema, and resultant postnatal lethality.[9] Although the degree of pericyte coverage varies among different malignancies, tumor vessels with fewer pericytes tend to be more sensitive to anti-VEGF therapy; this treatment prunes unprotected blood vessels, leaving an increased percentage of pericyte-covered vessels behind. This observation crafted the rationale for adding PDGF-B/PDGFR-β inhibitors to anti-VEGF therapy.

## ANG-TIE

In 1992, Partenen and co-workers first reported a novel human tyrosine kinase receptor expressed in ECs and their precursors, which they named TIE ("tyrosine kinase with Ig and EGF homology domains").[24,25] The next year, Sato and colleagues subcategorized this class of receptors into two members, TIE-1 and -2. The main ligands to TIE-2 are ANG-1, which functions as an agonist, and ANG-2, which normally functions as an ANG-1 antagonist. However, ANG-2 can function as a partial agonist under certain conditions such as lack of ANG-1 expression or when ANG-2 is present in high concentration. A TIE-1 ligand has not yet been found. This class of receptors and ligands regulates the end of angiogenesis when vessels mature and influences continued vessel quiescence during adulthood.

Malignant cells initially grow along available normal vasculature in a process known as vessel co-option. Subsequent activation of associated ECs leads to apoptosis in these cells and vessel regression via ANG-2 signaling. The resultant hypoxia in tumors leads to VEGF upregulation and tumor-derived angiogenesis. The effect of ligand overexpression is typically antitumorigenic for ANG-1 via its stimulation of pericytes. Given ANG-1's role in vessel maturation, it is not surprising that the changes to blood vessels after anti-VEGF therapy (increased pericyte coverage) are orchestrated by ANG-1. ANG-2 expression, on the other hand, appears very important in early tumorigenesis. Its role as an antagonist to ANG-1's stimulation of pericyte recruitment causes pericyte dropout, and this decreased coverage causes increased permeability to factors, such as cytokines or myeloid cells, that later act as building blocks for VEGF-induced angiogenesis.

## Notch

In 1914, John S. Dexter first noted a heritable abnormality in the wings of *Drosophila* where notches were present at the tips, and Thomas Hunt Morgan would identify the first allele of the "Notch" gene a few years later.[26,27] It codes for a single-pass transmembrane receptor that is characterized by 36 epidermal growth factor-like repeats and a few cysteine-rich Notch/lineage defective (LIN)-12 repeats extracellularly, with its intracellular domain consisting of six ankyrin repeats, a glutamine-rich domain, and a PEST sequence. Ligands for this receptor are also single-pass transmembrane proteins, named DLL4 and Jagged-1; after surface expression, they are thought to interact with the Notch receptor on neighboring cells. The Notch family of ligands and receptors is a conserved pathway necessary for normal development of the embryo, tissue homeostasis, and stem-cell regulation after adulthood.[28, 29] Within these roles, it participates in several elements of EC activity during angiogenesis.

VEGFR-2 activation during angiogenesis leads to increased levels of DLL4 in what will become the tip cell, or the cell within the preexisting vessel that migrates as its neighboring stalk cells divide behind it to form an associated stalk. This DLL4 will bind and activate the Notch receptor in the adjacent stalk cells, which causes VEGFR-2 endocytosis and a decline in stalk-cell sensitivity to VEGF. Jagged-1 also antagonizes any reciprocal Notch activation by the stalk cells. These actions further establish the tip cell's role. Inhibiting this process through blocking or silencing DLL4/Notch leads to a greater number of vessels, but these vessels are largely nonfunctional, resulting in reduced tumor growth.

### Integrins

Several reviews have summarized the relationship between integrins and cancer, specifically angiogenesis.[30] Integrins, as a class, are structurally similar receptors for polypeptides in the ECM and immunoglobulin superfamily. These receptors are heterodimers of various glycoproteins divided into two subgroups, alpha and beta, of which there are 18 and 8 members, respectively. Some receptors recognize single, others multiple, ligands, and these ligands can be cell-surface associated. These include proteins such as collagen, laminin, fibronectin, fibrinogen, vitronectin, and cell-adhesion molecules.

The $\alpha v \beta 3$ integrin, in particular, has received considerable attention in the study of tumor angiogenesis and exemplifies functions of its class within angiogenesis. Whereas normal vasculature does not express this receptor, human tumor endothelium does. This upregulation is thought to occur in response to growth factors associated with angiogenesis, such as basic FGF, tumor necrosis factor-alpha, and interleukin (IL)-8. Studies suggest it contributes to cell survival and migration of ECs recruited for the creation of new tumor vessels, as promoting ligation leads to survival through MAPK, focal adhesion kinase, and SRC signaling, whereas inhibiting integrin ligation pathways leads to cell death via caspase 8. Ligand binding results in receptor cluster formation. These receptors have no enzymatic abilities themselves, but their clustering promotes the assembly and activation of associated kinases and adaptor proteins into focal adhesion complexes.

## Therapies Targeting the VEGF Pathway

A search for open studies at the National Institutes of Health clinical trials registry produced around 50 distinct antiangiogenic drugs that are currently being investigated in approximately 250 overlapping categories of cancer and other neoplasms.[31, 32] Many of these therapies target combinations of various ligands and receptors within the VEGF pathway, much like currently approved treatments. A significant number of VEGF pathway inhibitors are in the midst of phase III evaluation (Table 6.1). A detailed discussion of all potential therapies targeting this pathway, or even all those in

**Table 6.1** VEGF pathway inhibitors with ongoing phase III trials.

| Type | Drug | Target | Cancers |
|---|---|---|---|
| Heparanase inhibitor | Muparfostat | Endo-beta-D-glucuronidase heparanase, FGF-1/2, VEGF | HCC |
| Monoclonal antibody | Bevacizumab | VEGF | Breast cancer, gastrointestinal carcinoid cancer, GBM, NSCLC, ovarian cancer |
| | Ramucirumab | VEGFR-2 | Breast cancer, CRC, gastric cancer, HCC, NSCLC, ovarian cancer |
| Peptibody | Trebananib | ANG-1/2 | Ovarian cancer |
| Tyrosine kinase inhibitor | Cabozantinib | AXL, c-Kit, FLT-3, MET, RET, TIE-2, TrkB, VEGFR-1/2/3 | Prostate cancer, MTC |
| | Dovitinib | c-Kit, CSF1R, FGFR-1/2/3, FLT-3, PDGFR-β, TrkA, VEGFR-1/2/3 | RCC |
| | Lenvatinib | VEGFR-2/3 | HCC, thyroid carcinoma |
| | Masitinib | c-Kit, FAK, FGFR-3, PDGFR-α/β | GIST, MM, pancreatic cancer |
| | Nintedanib | FGFR-1/2/3, FLT-3, Lck, Lyn, PDGFR-α/β, Src, VEGFR-1/2/3 | NSCLC, ovarian cancer |
| | Pazopanib | c-Kit, PDGFR-α/β, VEGFR-1/2/3 | Ovarian cancer, RCC |
| | Sorafenib | PDGFR-β, RAF, VEGFR-2 | Breast cancer, HCC, RCC, thyroid cancer |
| | Sunitinib | c-Kit, FLT-3, PDGFR-β, VEGFR-2 | RCC |
| | Tivozanib | VEGFR-1/2/3 | RCC |

Cancer abbreviations: CRC, colorectal cancer; GBM, glioblastoma multiforme; GIST, gastrointestinal stromal tumor; HCC, hepatocellular carcinoma; MM, multiple myeloma; MTC, medullary thyroid cancer; NSCLC, non-small cell lung cancer; RCC, renal cell cancer; STS, soft tissue sarcoma.

Target abbreviations: ANG, angiopoietin; CSF1R, colony-stimulating factor 1 receptor; FAK, focal adhesion kinase; FLT-3, Fms-like tyrosine kinase 3; FGF, fibroblast growth factor; FGFR, fibroblast growth factor receptor; Lck, lymphocyte-specific protein tyrosine kinase; MET, hepatocyte growth factor receptor; PDGFR, platelet-derived growth factor receptor, TIE-2; TrkA, neurotrophic tyrosine kinase receptor type 1; TrkB, neurotrophic tyrosine kinase receptor type 2; VEGF, vascular endothelial growth factor; VEGFR, vascular endothelial growth factor receptor.

**Table 6.2** Approved VEGF pathway inhibitors in cancer.

| Drug | Indication | Improvement in RR (%) | Improvement in median PFS (mos) | Improvement in median OS (mos) |
|---|---|---|---|---|
| Bevacizumab | Metastatic CRC | 10.0 | 4.4 | 4.7 |
| | Metastatic CRC (2nd line) | 14.1 | 2.6 | 2.1 |
| | Metastatic CRC (progressive) | NS | 1.7 | 1.4 |
| | NSCLC | 20.0 | 1.7 | 2.0 |
| | GBM (2nd line) | | Phase II data only | |
| | Metastatic RCC | 18.0 | 4.8 | NS |
| Sunitinib | GIST (2nd line) | 7.0 | 4.5 | NS |
| | Metastatic RCC | 35.0 | 6.0 | 4.6 |
| | pNET | 9.3 | 4.8 | NR |
| Sorafenib | Metastatic RCC (2nd line) | 8.0 | 2.7 | NS |
| | Unresectable HCC | 1.0 | NS | 2.8 |
| Pazopanib | Metastatic RCC | 27.0 | 5.0 | NS |
| | Metastatic STS (2nd line) | 4.0 | 3.0 | 1.9 |
| Vandetanib | Metastatic MTC | 32.0 | 11.2[a] | NR |
| Axitinib | Metastatic RCC (2nd line) | 10.0 | 2.0 | NS |
| Aflibercept | Metastatic CRC (2nd line) | 8.7 | 2.2 | 1.4 |
| Regorafenib | Metastatic CRC (3rd line) | 0.6 | 0.3 | 1.4 |
| | GIST (3rd line) | 3.0 | 3.9 | NS |
| Cabozantinib | Metastatic MTC | 28.0 | 7.2 | PR |

Cancer and statistical abbreviations: CRC, colorectal cancer; GBM, glioblastoma multiforme; GIST, gastrointestinal stromal tumor; MTC, medullary thyroid cancer; NR, not reported; NS, nonsignificant; NSCLC, non-small cell lung cancer; OS, overall survival; PFS, progression-free survival; pNET, pancreatic neuroendocrine tumor; PR, pending report; RCC, renal cell cancer; RR, response rate; STS, soft tissue sarcoma.

[a]Predicted by Weibull Model.

advanced-phase trials, will not be attempted here. As well, agents known or hypothesized to affect angiogenesis indirectly, for example, thalidomide will not be covered in this chapter. Instead, we will focus on the nine approved drugs targeting the VEGF pathway and their current indications.[4,31,32]

The United States FDA has now approved the anti-VEGF monoclonal antibody bevacizumab (2004) for metastatic colorectal cancer (CRC); metastatic nonsquamous, non-small cell lung cancer; progressive GBM; and metastatic renal cell carcinoma (RCC) (Table 6.2). The majority of the remaining approvals have been tyrosine kinase inhibitors (TKIs) that have multiple targets. Sorafenib (2005) inhibits Raf, VEGFR-2, and PDGFR-β kinases and is used to treat advanced RCC and unresectable hepatocellular carcinoma (HCC). Sunitinib (2006) targets several enzymes including VEGFR-2, PDGFR-β, c-kit, and FLT3; current approved indications include imatinib-resistant gastrointestinal stromal tumors, metastatic RCC, and metastatic progressive neuroendocrine tumors. Pazopanib (2009) is approved for treatment of advanced RCC and soft tissue sarcomas as a pan-VEGFR inhibitor with added effects on PDGFR-α/β and c-kit. Metastatic medullary thyroid cancer gained two TKI therapies, vandetanib and cabozantinib (2011 and 2012), both of which target VEGFR among other kinases. Axitinib was approved in early 2012 for advanced RCC, and its inhibitory effects closely resemble those of pazopanib. Regorafenib, also released in 2012, targets VEGFR-2/TIE-2 and has been used to treat metastatic CRC and advanced gastrointestinal stromal tumors. Besides bevacizumab, the only other non-TKI antiangiogenic therapy to gain approval has been ziv-aflibercept (2012) or VEGF Trap, a protein containing fused extracellular domains of VEGFR-1 and -2 to allow VEGF-A/B inhibition. It can be used for metastatic CRC that is oxaliplatin resistant.

Beyond new therapeutics, increased antiangiogenic effect is being sought with traditional cytotoxics by giving lower doses at more frequent intervals, termed metronomic or semimetronomic dosing.[33,34] The primary targets of this approach are the proliferating endothelial cells providing the substance of new tumor vasculature.[35–37]

In 2009, the Japanese Gynecologic Oncology Group (JGOG) found that a semi-metronomic regimen of weekly low-dose paclitaxel and carboplatin in advanced ovarian cancer patients showed improved survival over the standard regimen, given every 3 weeks.[38] Additional trials with this approach in combination with intraperitoneal platinum are underway.[39] Additionally, a German trial recently offered 10-year survival data that supported more frequent dosing in node-positive breast cancer.[40] Further studies are ongoing to explore the utility of metronomic regimens in cancer therapy.[31,32]

## Toxicities

Reported toxicities of anti-VEGF therapy include hypertension, proteinuria, arterial thromboembolic events, cardiomyopathy, hemorrhage, wound complications, gastrointestinal perforation or fistula formation, and reversible posterior leukoencephalopathy syndrome. A well-written and relatively comprehensive review of these exists,[41] so we have chosen to focus on the most-studied adverse effect of anti-VEGF therapies, hypertension. Hypertension is both a prevalent preexisting morbidity in cancer patients (38%) and one of the more common high-grade (combined grade III and IV) adverse effects of VEGF antagonism.[42,43] A 2010 meta-analysis of high-grade hypertension resulting from bevacizumab found an overall incidence of 7.9%, ranging from 1.8% to 22.0%.[43] Studies of sunitinib and sorafenib have found comparable results.[44, 45]

Both dose and tumor type affect risk. When the dose of bevacizumab is increased from 2.5 to 5.0 mg/kg/week, the relative risk for all-grade hypertension more than doubles.[42] However, the relative risk of high-grade hypertension increases more modestly (RR: 4.78 vs. RR: 5.39). Across tumor types, patients with RCR, pancreatic cancer, and CRC were particularly at risk for high-grade hypertension. How hypertension develops from VEGF antagonism is not completely understood. It is thought that a downstream decrease in nitric-oxide synthase activity and nitric oxide production results in vasoconstriction and renal retention of sodium. A decrease in the number of functional arterioles and capillaries leading to vascular stiffness and capillary rarefaction after therapy may also play a role.[46, 47] The Investigational Drug Steering Committee of the National Cancer Institute convened a panel in 2010 that provided recommendations for managing the blood pressure in patients receiving these agents.[42] Their recommendations include (1) recognizing and treating preexisting hypertension prior to using antiangiogenic therapy; (2) actively monitoring blood pressure during therapy, especially in the first several weeks; and (3) continuing medical optimization of blood pressure during therapy, with discontinuation or dose reduction of anti-VEGF therapy if blood pressure goals are not met despite intervention.

As can be expected, the other major toxicities are also of a mostly vascular nature,[47] and we will very briefly touch on some of these. Disruption of VEGF-mediated glomerular endothelial integrity can lead to proteinuria, though this is rare with the multikinase inhibitors and infrequently is severe enough to require intervention. Although cardiac toxicity leading to congestive heart failure or electrophysiological perturbations has not been well characterized for all antiangiogenic drugs, New York Heart Association functional class III–IV congestive heart failure has been reported in up to 8% of patients taking sunitinib.[47] Given this finding and the potential consequences, oncologists should be wary if confronted with symptoms of heart failure, even if progressive disease may seem to be the most likely cause.

Though guidelines are lacking, a small increase in arterial or venous thromboembolic events has been seen in trials of some antiangiogenic drugs, and clinicians should monitor patients with risk factors or those who suffer from such events. There can be a tendency for increased bleeding events with these therapies, although serious episodes have been infrequent. Many physicians recommend discontinuing these agents the month before and after surgery, as well as using them with caution in patients with bleeding diatheses, whether acquired or iatrogenic. The recommendation regarding delay around the time of major surgery also results from a significantly higher rate of wound healing complications (three- to fourfold higher) when VEGF targeting was initiated with chemotherapy within the first 28 post-operative days.[48] Finally, the non-TKI agents have been associated with bowel perforation, especially in patients with ovarian cancer and in patients receiving any additional antiangiogenic drugs (e.g., erlotinib).[47] It has also been demonstrated in frontline ovarian cancer trials with chemotherapy and bevacizumab to be substantially higher in patients with intrinsic inflammatory bowel disease, diverticular disease, and colitis.[49] There has also been concern in patients with known involvement of the bowel wall by tumor.[47] Mechanistically, these associations are rational given these agents' known interference with normal wound healing. Clinicians should prudently select patients and be vigilant for suggestive symptomatology.

## Resistance to Antiangiogenic Therapy

Despite showing the ability to contribute to patient survival even in aggressive malignancies, antiangiogenic therapy has generally delayed tumor progression only temporarily.[50, 51] Because the details of many hypothesized resistance mechanisms are incomplete, these mechanisms are difficult to categorize by adaptations arising from the cancer cell itself (tumor dependent) versus the tumor microenvironment (tumor independent).

Resistance to antiangiogenesis drugs can be considered as intrinsic or evasive.[50] Although a particular mechanism may span both categories, these terms essentially denote preexisting *versus* adaptive resistance, respectively. The intrinsic mode of resistance is characterized by the "absence of a discernible (even transitory) beneficial effect of an angiogenesis inhibitor, even when the subject's tumour(s) is serially analysed".[50] This does not indicate stasis but, in fact, continued growth through antiangiogenic treatment. Evidence suggests that this resistance arises from (1) preexisting expression of several proangiogenic molecules such as FGFs, ephrins, or ANG; (2) already present inflammatory cells protecting vessels; (3) hypovascular tumors arising from a natively hypoxic environment; and (4) tumors with early invasive qualities that co-opt existing vasculature instead of growing new vessels. We will refer readers to their article for a more detailed discussion, and instead focus on the various hypothesized mechanisms for resistance, be they preexisting or acquired.

### Redundant Proangiogenic Signaling

Studies suggest that targeting specific angiogenic factors can be circumvented by selecting cell populations that simply express uninhibited members of the proangiogenic family. In pancreatic models, the initial arrest in vessel formation and tumor growth with VEGF inhibition succumbs to eventual acceleration of both activities after 10–14 days.[52] The concomitant upregulation of FGF-1, FGF-2, Ephrin-A1 (Eph-A1), Eph-A2, and ANG-1 is thought to explain this behavior, especially given the attenuation of rebound tumor growth by FGF Trap.

Clinical studies of GBM patients have analogously shown that elevated circulating FGF2 levels are associated with disease relapse following treatment with VEGFR inhibitors.[53] Because mice without tumors showed increased tissue expression of several angiogenic factors after treatment with sunitinib, these elevations cannot yet be definitely implicated in renewed tumor angiogenesis and growth in humans.[54] From the vantage of intrinsic resistance, however, the transition seen in breast cancer progression, where predominant VEGF expression gives way to more diverse signaling (including FGF2 expression) and nonresponsive tumors, supports this mechanism.[55]

### Recruiting Progenitor Cells from the Bone Marrow

The resultant hypoxia after anti-VEGF treatment can bring not only other proangiogenic molecules but also new cells that affect the microenvironment.[50] Bone marrow-derived cells (BMDCs) are the progenitors of ECs, pericytes, and monocytes. Influx of these three types of cells can lead to revascularization as they contribute to new vessels, protect the vasculature, and provide supportive paracrine signaling, respectively. By first studying ischemia in normal tissue then in malignancies prone to hypoxia, researchers have implicated the hypoxia-inducible factor (HIF)1-alpha pathway in BMDC recruitment, finding that absence of this signaling impairs both

BMDC numbers and subsequent growth. Further evidence for this mechanism, as mentioned above, comes from investigating intrinsic resistance. Characterizing tumors unaffected by anti-VEGF treatment showed a preexisting infiltrate of CD11b+Gr1+ myeloid cells, which express various proangiogenic molecules.[56] Inhibiting this infiltrate restores sensitivity to anti-VEGF therapy, providing a possible new avenue for targeted therapy seeking to abrogate developing or preexisting tumor resistance.

## Normalization of Tumor Vasculature

It is thought that anti-VEGF treatment may lead to vascular normalization in tumors. Larger vessels become smaller, tortuous vessels straighter, and theoretically the resulting blood flow becomes less stagnant. As well, remaining vessels exhibit greater stability through greater numbers of associated pericytes. Whether this change in response to anti-VEGF therapy would be beneficial for the tumor or for the patient remains unclear.[50,51]

Evidence suggests that inhibiting VEGF signaling (a survival signal) to ECs causes these cells to attempt pericyte recruitment. These pericytes then provide the degree of paracrine VEGF signaling necessary to promote continued survival. The end result is that vessels that successfully recruit pericytes are maintained, and the rest are pruned by therapy. The logical thought that added inhibition of pericyte recruitment would then cause more tumor vessel destruction and further therapeutic effect, however, has some caveats. Although inhibiting tumor angiogenesis and growth become more pronounced with combination therapy, so does metastasis. This and other evidence suggest pericytes also have a role in decreasing tumor intravasation.

Of note, a potential route of targeting these preexisting tumor vessels has emerged in the form of a class of drugs called vascular disrupting agents (VDAs).[57] These drugs, which are either flavonoid or tubulin-binding compounds, disrupt the morphology of tumor endothelial cells and lead to vascular collapse and tumor necrosis. Although these agents have not shown great promise as monotherapy, vessel repopulation after treatment necessitates angiogenesis, providing a rationale for combination with antiangiogenic therapies. Mouse models have confirmed the potential efficacy of this approach and a combination of VDA (fosbretabulin) with bevacizumab is currently being evaluated for recurrent ovarian cancer in clinical trials.[31,32]

## Invasion Without Angiogenesis

This mechanism was first described in a mouse model of GBM treated with VEGF inhibitors or with genetic disruption of several angiogenic molecules including VEGF, HIF1-alpha, and MMP9.[58-60] Although growth was slowed, a more invasive phenotype was promoted, with new, more invasive lesions forming in neighboring areas. The cells, unable to spread through neovascularization, instead traveled along existing vessels in multiple directions. A similar phenotype has been noted clinically in certain GBM patients after anti-VEGF treatment with the development of multiple invasive foci.[61] Several possible mechanisms have been suggested, but this phenomenon is still under study.

The GBM example is not an isolated incident; the possibility that antiangiogenic inhibitors lead to more aggressive malignancies through evasive actions by the tumor is an important topic.[5] Further research will be needed to investigate the potential implications, including the relative importance of metastatic potential in preclinical testing, and how therapeutic resistance should be best integrated into mouse models of malignancy.

## Biomarkers

Within the context of targeted therapy, biomarkers are primarily biologic indicators that can prognosticate tumor behavior, predict tumor response, gauge the pharmacodynamics of drugs, detect the development of resistance, or point toward toxicity.[62] These indicators could allow us to individualize therapy, to quickly optimize dosing regimens, to halt ineffective treatment, and to preempt adverse effects. Despite the many candidates, unfortunately none have been validated for antiangiogenic therapy.

### Hypertension

Hypertension is a long-recognized adverse effect of therapy directed, at least in part, against VEGF. Proposed mechanisms include decreased nitric oxide production, decreased capillary density, and renovascular mechanisms. Researchers have suggested that high blood pressure signifies greater antitumor effects, giving the measurement predictive value. A recent, large retrospective analysis looked at hypertension as a biomarker in three trials, totaling over 500 patients, where sunitinib was used to treat metastatic RCC.[63] Elevated blood pressure was significantly associated with greater progression-free survival and overall survival, although hypertension was neither necessary nor sufficient for clinical benefit. Prospective studies are needed to validate these findings.

### Circulating Proteins or Cells

Researchers have also studied factors that can be measured in the circulation. The most intuitive and most widely studied molecule is VEGF itself.[62] Pretreatment levels in the plasma have shown some correlations with progression-free survival, but the directionality has varied by drug type for reasons that remain unknown. Studies of these baseline values have not found a correlation with the ability to predict treatment efficacy. Circulating levels of related molecules, such as other VEGF family members and VEGFRs, have been considered but require further study. Outside of VEGF-related proteins, studies have found evidence that the extent of increase in IL-6 levels after treatment with bevacizumab in rectal and ovarian cancer (or after treatment with sunitinib in advanced HCC) is associated with worse outcomes. Researchers have also examined whether antiangiogenic drugs may change the levels of circulating ECs or their progenitors, which could then be used as a marker.[64] However, the relatively low amounts of these cells in the blood and the advanced technologies needed for their characterization have limited widespread use.

### Gene Polymorphisms

Although circulating VEGF is currently not a promising marker, its genotype may prove to be. The VEGF-2578AA genotype, in particular, has been associated with superior overall survival in a combined bevacizumab plus chemotherapy arm in metastatic breast cancer.[65] In another study, a polymorphism in the gene for IL-8 that leads to increased expression of the protein appeared to be a molecular predictor of response, though further studies are needed.[66]

### Imaging Biomarkers

Imaging-based measurements of various vascular parameters have been used in clinical trials to evaluate earlier changes in pharmacodynamics after antiangiogenic therapy. Whether these changes could be the basis for a predictive biomarker is still being investigated, but this represents the most exciting area of biomarker development for these therapies.

The majority of these parameters originate from computed tomography and dynamic contrast-enhanced magnetic resonance imaging performed in clinical studies of RCC, HCC, and high-grade glioma.[62] Essentially, dynamic changes in contrast concentration within the tumor vasculature are used to describe aspects of blood flow (K-trans) and blood/plasma volume within the tumor. Current models of anti-VEGF mechanisms are consistent with changes in these parameters, with pruning of abnormal vasculature leading to decreased blood flow, blood volume, and tumoral edema.

Despite some heterogeneity between studies with regard to methodology, a general trend emerges. Pretreatment K-trans and biomarkers for acute change (size, K-trans) appear to have prognostic significance in metastatic RCC, high-grade glioma, and recurrent or persistent ovarian cancer.[64] Their predictive capability (e.g., CT perfusion scanning) is now entering into clinical development[31,32] [GOG 0262]) but will need validation in well-designed, large prospective trials, and across different agents and tumor types.

## Concluding Remarks

Definite gains have been made following the translation of Folkman's initial hypothesis into new therapeutic modalities, and the advances in antiangiogenic therapy will positively affect many patients. However, the benefits to cancer patients in terms of survival have been modest.[67] For the majority of patients taking these drugs, the potential payoff comes in months, not years. A deeper understanding of drug actions and tumor responses is required to optimize current therapies with regard to pharmacodynamics and patient selection. As well, understanding the basis of nonresponse and adaptive resistance in tumors will aid in developing new therapies that target resistance mechanisms. Nevertheless, antiangiogenesis therapies hold potential to further improve the outcome of cancer patients, and their use will likely continue to expand.

## References

1 Folkman MJ, Long DM, Becker FF. Growth and metastasis of tumor in organ culture. *Cancer.* 1963;16:453–467.

2 Folkman J. Tumor angiogenesis: therapeutic implications. *N Engl J Med.* 1971;285:1182–1186.

3 Hanahan D, Weinberg RA. Hallmarks of cancer: the next generation. *Cell.* 2011;144(5):646–674.

4 http://www.fda.gov/default.html. Accessed March 23, 2013.

5 Ebos JM, Kerbel RS. Antiangiogenic therapy: impact on invasion, disease progression, and metastasis. *Nat Rev Clin Oncol.* 2011;8(4):210–221.

6 Weis SM, Cheresh DA. Tumor angiogenesis: molecular pathways and therapeutic targets. *Nat Med.* 2011;17(11):1359–1370.

7 Carmeliet P. Angiogenesis in health and disease. *Nat Med.* 2003;9(6):653–660.

8 Carmeliet P, Jain RK. Molecular mechanisms and clinical applications of angiogenesis. *Nature.* 2011;473(7347):298–307.

9 Matsuo K, Lu C, Shazad MMK, et al. Role of pericytes in resistance to antiangiogenic therapy. In: Bagley R, ed. *The Tumor Microenvironment.* New York, NY: Springer; 2010:311–324.

10 Frumovitz M, Sood AK. Vascular endothelial growth factor (VEGF) pathway as a therapeutic target in gynecologic malignancies. *Gynecol Oncol.* 2007;104(3):768–778.

11 Shen R, Ye Y, Chen L, Yan Q, Barsky SH, Gao J. Precancerous stem cells can serve as tumor vasculogenic progenitors. *PLoS ONE.* 2008;3(2):e1652.

12 Bussolati B, Grange C, Sapino A, Camussi G. Endothelial cell differentiation of human breast tumour stem/progenitor cells. *J Cell Mol Med.* 2009;13:309–319.

13 Bussolati B, Bruno S, Grange C, Ferrando U, Camussi G. Identification of a tumor-initiating stem cell population in human renal carcinomas. *FASEB J.* 2008;22:3696–3705.

14 Alvero AB, Fu HH, Holmberg J, et al. Stem-like ovarian cancer cells can serve as tumor vascular progenitors. *Stem Cells.* 2009;27:2405–2413.

15 Wang R, Chadalavada K, Wilshire J, et al. Glioblastoma stem-like cells give rise to tumour endothelium. *Nature.* 2010;468:829–833.

16 Ricci-Vitiani L, Pallini R, Biffoni M, et al. Tumour vascularization via endothelial differentiation of glioblastoma stem-like cells. *Nature.* 2010;468:824–828.

17 Senger DR, Galli SJ, Dvorak AM, Perruzzi CA, Harvey VS, Dvorak HF. Tumor cells secrete a vascular permeability factor that promotes accumulation of ascites fluid. *Science.* 1983;219(4587):983–985.

18 Leung DW, Cachianes G, Kuang WJ, Goeddel DV, Ferrara N. Vascular endothelial growth factor is a secreted angiogenic mitogen. *Science.* 1989;246(4935):1306–1309.

19 Armelin HA. Pituitary extracts and steroid hormones in the control of 3T3 cell growth (mouse fibroblasts/growth factor). *Proc Natl Acad Sci U S A.* 1973;70(9):2702–2706.

20 Gospodarowicz D. Localisation of a fibroblast growth factor and its effect along and with hydrocortisone on 3T3 cell growth. *Nature.* 1974;249(5453):123–127.

21 Werner S, Grose R. Regulation of wound healing by growth factors and cytokines. *Physiol Rev.* 2003;83:835–870.

22 Turner N, Grose R. Fibroblast growth factor signalling: From development to cancer. *Nat Rev Cancer.* 2010;10(2):116–129.

23 Andrae J, Gallini R, Betsholtz C. Role of platelet-derived growth factors in physiology and medicine. *Genes Dev.* 2008;22(10):1276–1312.

24 Augustin HG, Young Koh G, Thurston G, Alitalo K. Control of vascular morphogenesis and homeostasis through the angiopoietin/tie system. *Nat Rev Mol Cell Biol.* 2009;10(3):165–177.

25 Huang H, Bhat A, Woodnutt G, Lappe R. Targeting the ANGPT/TIE2 pathway in malignancy. *Nat Rev Cancer.* 2010;10(8):575–585.

26 Dexter, JS. The analysis of a case of continuous variation in Drosophila by a study of its linkage relations. *Am Naturalist.* 1914;48(576): 712–758.

27 Morgan, TH. The theory of the gene. *Am Naturalist.* 1917;51(609):513–544.

28 Artavanis-Tsakonas S, Rand MD, Lake RJ. Notch signaling: cell fate control and signal integration in development. *Science.* 1999;284(5415): 7706.

29 Phng L, Gerhardt H. Angiogenesis: a team effort coordinated by notch. *Dev Cell.* 2009;16(2):196–208.

30 Desgrosellier JS, Cheresh DA. Integrins in cancer: biological implications and therapeutic opportunities. *Nat Rev Cancer.* 2010;10(1):9–22.

31 www.clinicaltrials.gov. Accessed March 23, 2013.

32 http://www.cancer.gov/clinicaltrials. Accessed March 23, 2013.

33 Shaked Y, Emmenegger U, Man S, et al. Optimal biologic dose of metronomic chemotherapy regimens is associated with maximum antiangiogenic activity. *Blood.* 2005;106:3058–3061.

34 Kerbel RS, Kamen BA. The anti-angiogenic basis of metronomic chemotherapy. *Nat Rev Cancer.* 2004;4:423–436.

35 Browder T, Butterfield CE, Kräling BM, et al. Antiangiogenic scheduling of chemotherapy improves efficacy against experimental drug-resistant cancer. *Cancer Res.* 2000;60:1878–1886.

36 Takahashi N, Haba A, Matsuno F, Seon BK. Antiangiogenic therapy of established tumors in human skin/severe combined immunodeficiency

mouse chimeras by anti-endoglin (CD105) monoclonal antibodies, and synergy between anti-endoglin antibody and cyclophosphamide. *Cancer Res.* 2001;61:7846–7854.

37 Hamano Y, Sugimoto H, Soubasakos MA, et al. Thrombospondin-1 associated with tumor microenvironment contributes to low-dose cyclophosphamide-mediated endothelial cell apoptosis and tumor growth suppression. *Cancer Res.* 2004;64:1570–1574.

38 Katsumata N, Yasuda M, Takahashi F, et al. Dose-dense paclitaxel once a week in combination with carboplatin every 3 weeks for advanced ovarian cancer: a phase 3, open-label, randomised controlled trial. *Lancet.* 2009;374:1331–1338.

39 Fujiwara K, Aotani E, Hamano T, et al. A randomized phase II/III trial of 3 weekly intraperitoneal versus intravenous carboplatin in combination with intravenous weekly dose-dense paclitaxel for newly diagnosed ovarian, fallopian tube and primary peritoneal cancer. *Jpn J Clin Oncol.* 2011;41:278–282.

40 Moebus V, Schneeweiss A, du Bois A, et al. Ten year follow-up analysis of intense dose-dense adjuvant ETC (epirubicin, paclitaxel and cyclophosphamide) confirms superior DFS and OS benefit in comparison to conventional dosed chemotherapy in high-risk breast cancer patients with ≥ 4 positive lymph nodes. Paper presented at: San Antonio Breast Cancer Symposium, December 6, 2012; Abstract S3–S4.

41 Chen HX, Cleck JN. Adverse effects of anticancer agents that target the VEGF pathway. *Nat Rev Clin Oncol.* 2009;6(8):465–477.

42 Maitland ML, Bakris GL, Black HR, et al. Initial assessment, surveillance, and management of blood pressure in patients receiving vascular endothelial growth factor signaling pathway inhibitors. *J Natl Cancer Inst.* 2010;102(9):596–604.

43 Ranpura V, Pulipati B, Chu D, Zhu X, Wu S. Increased risk of high-grade hypertension with bevacizumab in cancer patients: a meta-analysis. *Am J Hypertens.* 2010;23(5):460–468.

44 Wu S, Chen JJ, Kudelka A, Lu J, Zhu X. Incidence and risk of hypertension with sorafenib in patients with cancer: a systematic review and meta-analysis. *Lancet Oncol.* 2008;9:117–123.

45 Zhu X, Stergiopoulos K, Wu S. Risk of hypertension and renal dysfunction with an angiogenesis inhibitor sunitinib: systematic review and meta-analysis. *Acta Oncol.* 2009;48:9–17.

46 Steeghs N, Gelderblom H, Roodt JO, et al. Hypertension and rarefaction during treatment with telatinib, a small molecule angiogenesis inhibitor. *Clin Cancer Res.* 2008;14:3470–3476.

47 Stone RL, Sood AK, Coleman RL. Collateral damage: toxic effects of targeted antiangiogenic therapies in ovarian cancer. *Lancet Oncol.* 2010;11(5):465–475.

48 Scappaticci FA, Fehrenbacher L, Cartwright T, et al. Surgical wound healing complications in metastatic colorectal cancer patients treated with bevacizumab. *J Surg Oncol.* 2005;91:173.

49 Burger RA, Brady MF, Rhee J, et al. Prospective investigation of risk factors for gastrointestinal adverse events in a phase III randomized trial of bevacizumab in first-line therapy for advanced epithelial ovarian cancer, primary peritoneal cancer, or fallopian tube cancer: a Gynecologic Oncology Group study. Paper presented at: SGO 2011; Abstract 7.

50 Bergers G, Hanahan D. Modes of resistance to anti-angiogenic therapy. *Nat Rev Cancer.* 2008;8(8):592–603.

51 Bottsford-Miller JN, Coleman RL, Sood AK. Resistance and escape from antiangiogenesis therapy: clinical implications and future strategies. *J Clin Oncol.* 2012;30(32):4026–4034.

52 Pollard JW. Tumour-educated macrophages promote tumour progression and metastasis. *Nature Rev Cancer.* 2004;4:71–78.

53 Batchelor TT, Sorensen AG, di Tomaso E, et al. AZD2171, a pan-VEGF receptor tyrosine kinase inhibitor, normalizes tumor vasculature and alleviates edema in glioblastoma patients. *Cancer Cell.* 2007;11:83–95.

54 Ebos JM, Lee CR, Christensen JG, Mutsaers AJ, Kerbel RS. Multiple circulating proangiogenic factors induced by sunitinib malate are tumor-independent and correlate with antitumor efficacy. *Proc Natl Acad Sci U S A.* 2007;104:17069–17074.

55 Relf M, LeJeune S, Scott PA, et al. Expression of the angiogenic factors vascular endothelial cell growth factor, acidic and basic fibroblast growth factor, tumor growth factor β-1, platelet-derived endothelial cell growth factor, placenta growth factor, and pleiotrophin in human primary breast cancer and its relation to angiogenesis. *Cancer Res.* 1997;57:963–969.

56 Shojaei F, Wu X, Malik AK, et al. Tumor refractoriness to anti-VEGF treatment is mediated by CD11b+Gr1+ myeloid cells. *Nat Biotechnol.* 2007;25:911–920.

57 Siemann DW, Shi W. Dual targeting of tumor vasculature: combining Avastin and vascular disrupting agents (CA4P or OXi4503). *Anticancer Res.* 2008;28:2027–2031.

58 Blouw B, Song H, Tihan T, et al. The hypoxic response of tumors is dependent on their microenvironment. *Cancer Cell.* 2003;4:133–146.

59 Rubenstein JL, Kim J, Ozawa T, et al. Anti-VEGF antibody treatment of glioblastoma prolongs survival but results in increased vascular cooption. *Neoplasia.* 2000;2:306–314.

60 Du R, Lu KV, Petritsch C, et al. HIF1α induces the recruitment of bone marrow-derived vascular modulatory cells to regulate tumor angiogenesis and invasion. *Cancer Cell.* 2008;13:206–220.

61 Norden AD, Young GS, Setayesh K, et al. Bevacizumab for recurrent malignant gliomas: efficacy, toxicity, and patterns of recurrence. *Neurology.* 2008;70:779–787.

62 Jain RK, Duda DG, Willett CG, et al. Biomarkers of response and resistance to antiangiogenic therapy. *Nat Rev Clin Oncol.* 2009;6(6):327–338.

63 Rini BI, Cohen DP, Lu DR, et al. Hypertension as a biomarker of efficacy in patients with metastatic renal cell carcinoma treated with sunitinib. *J Natl Cancer Inst.* 2011;103(9):763–773.

64 Coleman RL, Duska LR, Ramirez PT, et al. Phase 1–2 study of docetaxel plus aflibercept in patients with recurrent ovarian, primary peritoneal, or fallopian tube cancer. *Lancet Oncol.* 2011;12(12):1109–1117.

65 Schneider BP, Wang M, Radovich M, et al. Association of vascular endothelial growth factor and vascular endothelial growth factor receptor-2 genetic polymorphisms with outcome in a trial of paclitaxel compared with paclitaxel plus bevacizumab in advanced breast cancer: ECOG 2100. *J Clin Oncol.* 2008;26:4672–4678.

66 Schultheis AM, Lurje G, Rhodes KE, et al. Polymorphisms and clinical outcome in recurrent ovarian cancer treated with cyclophosphamide and bevacizumab. *Clin Cancer Res.* 2008;14:7554–7563.

67 Spannuth WA, Sood AK, Coleman RL. Angiogenesis as a strategic target for ovarian cancer therapy. *Nat Clin Pract Oncol.* 2008;5(4):194–204. Available from: www.scopus.com Accessed March 23, 2015.

# CHAPTER 7

# Epigenetics and Epigenetic Therapy of Cancer

*Omotayo Fasan[1,2], Patrick Boland[1], Patricia Kropf[1], and Jean-Pierre J. Issa[3]*

[1]Department of Medicine, Temple University School of Medicine, Philadelphia, PA, USA
[2]Department of Hematologic Oncology and Blood Disorders, Levine Cancer Institute, Charlotte, NC, USA
[3]Fels Institute for Cancer Research and Molecular Biology, Temple University School of Medicine, Philadelphia, USA

## Structure of the Genetic Code

The human genetic code is made up of repeating sequence of deoxyribonucleic acids—adenine (A), cytosine (C), thymine (T), and guanine (G). It exists as a double-stranded helical structure. This simple code is packaged as a series of higher order structures with increasing complexity. The negatively charged double-stranded helical structure is folded by winding it around positively charged proteins called histones. Histones are grouped in octamers made of a pair of H2A-H2B dimers and a tetramer consisting of two H3 and two H4 histones. About 145–146 base pairs (bp) of DNA are wound around each histone octamer to make the structure called a nucleosome. The beaded string structure of histones is about 10–11 nm.

There is further aggregation of nucleosomes via linker histones (H1 or H5) into 30 nm structures called chromatin. Chromatin exists in two states—heterochromatin, which is closed and transcriptionally silent, and euchromatin, which is open and transcriptionally active.

Chromatin aggregates as a higher order structure in the form of chromosomes. Epigenetic alterations can occur at the level of cytosine nucleotides, histones, and chromatin.

## DNA Methylation

The common target of DNA methylation in mammalian cells is the cytosine nucleotide, primarily when it is followed by a guanosine (i.e., the Cytosine phospho Guanosine or CpG dinucleotide). Methylation is a covalent modification of the $5'$ position in the cytosine ring. DNA methylation occurs in S-phase and is catalyzed by DNA methyltransferases (DNMTs) with S-adenosyl methionine (SAM) serving as the methyl donor. CpG dinucleotides occur throughout the genome; however, there are certain regions where the CpG dinucleotides occur in greater abundance. These regions are called CpG islands (CGIs). CGIs are about 500–5000 bp long and occur at transcription start sites and promoter sites in about half of human genes. In normal tissues, about 70% of CpG dinucleotides are methylated and CGIs are relatively protected from methylation.

The opposite occurs in tumors where there is global hypomethylation of CpG dinucleotides and hypermethylation of promoter site CGIs.

Hypermethylation of promoter site CGIs leads to gene silencing. DNMT1 has a 5- to 30-fold preference for hemimethylated DNA and is present at a much higher concentration in adult cells than the other DNMTs. It is a housekeeping enzyme, which functions to maintain methylation patterns of the genome, ensuring stability throughout cell division. Though thought to be mainly functioning in maintaining already established methylation patterns, it may also function as a *de novo* methylator.[1,2] DNMT2 actually functions as an RNA methyltransferase and is not as a DNMT in humans.[3] DNMT3A and DNMT3B are classically known as the *de novo* methyltransferases, and their function is to methylate previously unmethylated DNA. Methylation of the CGIs by DNMT3A and DNMT3B leads to transcriptional repression while unmethylated CGI allows gene expression.

DNA methylation results in transcriptional repression by: (i) interfering with transcription factor binding, (ii) enhancing the binding of transcriptional repressors like methyl cytosine-binding proteins 1 and 2 (MeCP-1, MeCP-2), and (iii) altering chromatin structure resulting in stabilizing of the inactive state and blocks access to transcription factors.[4]

## DNA Demethylation

Global hypomethylation in tumors as compared to the normal surrounding tissue was one of the first epigenetic changes identified in malignancies. In fact, while DNA methylation and the significance of particular sets of hypermethylated genes has been an interest of research for quite sometime, hypomethylation is the predominant alteration seen in many malignancies. This hypomethylation is distributed across the genome at unique sequences, but particularly affects interspersed repetitive sequences (IRS), such as short interspersed nuclear elements (SINE) otherwise called Alu repeats, long interspersed nuclear elements (LINE), and gene promoters. LINE-1 hypomethylation correlates with tumor characteristics such as advanced stage metastases, progression, and higher grade. It also

*Targeted Therapy in Translational Cancer Research*, First Edition. Edited by Apostolia-Maria Tsimberidou, Razelle Kurzrock and Kenneth C. Anderson.
© 2016 John Wiley & Sons, Inc. Published 2016 by John Wiley & Sons, Inc.

correlates with increased chromosomal aberrations such as mutations, deletions, translocations, inversions, and amplifications.[5-7] DNA demethylation will occur naturally as a consequence of two rounds of DNA replication without maintenance of methylation, but the causes of global hypomethylation in cancer remain unclear. Hypomethylation can theoretically occur through loss of DNMT function or activation of demethylases. DNMT1 is most responsible for the maintenance of methylation, and disruption of its activity has been shown to promote tumorigenesis in human gliomas.[8] DNMT1 mutations can be found in some acute leukemias.

Demethylation of methylated CpGs can also occur following hydroxylation of 5-methylcytosine to 5-hydroxymethyl cytosine by the TET (Ten-Eleven Translocation) family of enzymes.[9,10]

## TET Proteins

Ten-Eleven Translocation (TET) proteins are so called because TET1 was first described as a partner for the MLL gene in the t(10;11) chromosomal fusion. There are three TET proteins in mammals which function as dioxygenases; they catalyze the oxidation of 5-methylcytosine in successive steps. The reaction requires ferrous iron and alpha ketoglutarate as cofactors and results in 5-hydroxymethylcytosine, an intermediary step in DNA demethylation. 5-hydroxymethylcytosine (5hmC) is oxidized to 5-formylcytosine (5fC), which is then oxidized to 5-carboxycytosine (5caC). 5caC is then excised by thymine-DNA glycosylase (TDG).[11] TET1 is located at chromosome 10q21.3, TET2 is at chromosome 4q24, and TET3 is at chromosome 2p13.1. TET proteins are mutated in several cancers; TET2 is frequently mutated in myeloid malignancies. TET2 mutations confer a poor prognosis in acute myeloid leukemia and may predict response to demethylating therapy with azacitidine.[12,13]

## Histone Modifications

Histone modification occurs at the N-terminal tails of histones. Modifications include lysine acetylation, lysine methylation, serine phosphorylation, serine ubiquitilation, SUMOylation, ADP ribosylation, and glycosylation. These modifications of the histone tails affect the stability of histones and their ability to attract other proteins, which may either result in formation of compact heterochromatin with resultant reduction of gene expression or the formation of open euchromatin, which allows access to transcription factors thus facilitating gene expression.[14]

Histone methyl transferase (HMT) is either lysine specific (KMT) or arginine specific (RMT). There are two types of lysine-specific HMT, one contains a protein domain called Su(var)3–9 Enhancer of Zeste, Trithorax (SET), while the other does not. Histone lysine trimethylation is catalyzed by histone methyl transferases (HMTs). When this occurs at H3K4, H3K36, and H3K79, it promotes gene expression; on the other hand when it occurs at H3K9, H3K27, and H3K40, it promotes the formation of heterochromatin and leads to transcriptional silencing. In particular, heterochromatin protein 1 (HP-1), a transcriptional repressor, binds to methylated H3K9 and promotes the formation of heterochromatin silencing gene transcription.[15] Histone (H3, H4) methylation at lysine or arginine residues are catalyzed by HMTs with SAM as the methyl donor.

Histone acetyl transferases (HATs) facilitate acetylation of histone tails resulting in gene expression, while histone deacetylation by histone deacetylase (HDAC) promotes the formation of heterochromatin and transcriptional repression.

## Noncoding RNA

Noncoding RNA are ribonucleic acid molecules that are not translated but rather regulate gene expression. About 97% of the output of the human genome is nonprotein-coding RNA. Some of this functions as regulators of genomic output either at the level of transcription or posttranscription. They function in both the nucleus and cytoplasm. They interact with the transcriptional machinery and are implicated in heterochromatin formation, transcriptional repression, and posttranscriptional gene silencing. Mechanisms of action include complementarity to the 3′ untranslated region leading to degradation of messenger RNA with resultant loss of gene expression. The three families of small noncoding RNA functional in eukaryotic cells are micro RNA (miRNA), small interfering RNA (siRNA), and piwi-interacting RNA (piRNA).[16] Mature miRNA are 21–23 nucleotides in length. Generation of miRNA involves processing of long RNA primary transcripts by the action of a microprocessor complex consisting of the nuclear endonuclease called DROSHA and a double-stranded RNA binding loop called PASHA (DGCR8). The product of the microprocessor complex is a short hairpin RNA called pre-miRNA. Further processing by the cytoplasmic nuclease called DICER forms the final mature miRNA.[16,17] The mature miRNA is then transported back to the nucleus as part of the RNA-induced silencing complex (RISC). They pair up with complementary sequences on messenger RNA resulting in degradation or translational silencing.

## Polycomb Repressive Complex

The polycomb group proteins (PcG) are multiprotein complexes that repress gene transcription. There are two complexes in this group: (i) Polycomb Repressive Complex 1 (PRC1) and (ii) Polycomb Repressive Complex 2 (PRC2). They function normally to regulate lineage choices during development and differentiation and, when deregulated, they contribute to tumorigenesis. PcG targeted genes are 12 times as likely to be methylated when compared to non-PcG genes in cancer cells. It has been noted that poorly differentiated and aggressive tumors are more likely to have methylated PcG target genes. It is thought that PcG cooperate with DNMTs to silence genes that promote differentiation and apoptosis skewing the phenotype toward a population of cells that, with additional hits, become poorly differentiated and aggressive tumors.[18]

PRC2 is made up of four subunits: (i) SUZ12, (ii) EED, (iii) the catalytic subunit Enhancer of Zeste homolog 2 (EZH2) or EZH1, and (iv) RbAp48. It essentially functions as a HMT that trimethylates histone H3 on lysine 27 (H3K27me3). Chromatin-containing H3K27me3 is transcriptionally silent (heterochromatin) and results in loss of gene expression. Interestingly, H3K27me3 also serves as an epigenetic mark that recruits DNMT and encourages *de novo* methylation of genes in cancer cells.[19] EZH2 functions in normal cells as a regulator of cellular differentiation while in tumor cells its dysfunction leads to lack of differentiation and tumor progression.[20,21] EZH2 silences several antimetastatic genes like E-cadherin and several tissue inhibitors of metalloproteinases. This inhibition favors cell invasion and anchorage-independent growth of tumor cells promoting metastases. Overexpression of EZH2 predicts for an aggressive phenotype with a poor prognosis in various tumor types.[22-25]

The ASXL1 (additional sex comb-like) gene is also a member of the PcG family of proteins. It functions normally in cells as a lysine deubiquitilator by associating with the calypso ortholog BAP1. This leads to deubiquitilation of H2AK119ub leading to gene repression. ASXL1 also interacts with EZH2 and SUZ12 (subunits of PRC2) to maintain PRC2 repression of transcription. Loss of function mutations of ASXL1 in tumor cells leads to loss of H3K27me3 histone marks which in turn leads to gene reexpression.[26,27] ASXL1 mutations are known to be associated with transformation and a poor prognosis in myeloid tumors.

## IDH1/2

Isocitrate dehydrogenase 1 (IDH1) and isocitrate dehydrogenase 2 (IDH2) enzymes normally function to catalyze the conversion of isocitrate generated from the Kreb's Cycle to alpha-ketoglutarate. The normal functioning enzyme is a homodimeric structure. Mutated IDH1/2 retains the ability to dimerize with its wild-type partner creating a neomorphic enzyme with abnormal conformation. This mutant dimer has an increased affinity for the substrate and catalyzes the reduction of alpha-ketoglutarate to the oncometabolite 2-hydroxyglutarate (2HG). Accumulation of 2HG in cells is associated with the alteration of methylome via inhibition of histone demethylases, hypoxia inducible factor (HIF), and prolyl hydoxylase.[28-30] IDH1 and IDH2 mutations lead to a global hypermethylated phenotype through inhibition of TET1/2-induced demethylation and may confer a poorer prognosis.[31]

## Epigenetic Perturbations in Hematologic Malignancies

Epigenetic abnormalities have been described as a frequent occurrence in myeloproliferative neoplasms (MPN), myelodysplastic syndromes (MDS), acute myeloid leukemia (AML), lymphoma, and multiple myeloma. The described abnormalities involve the entire epigenetic machinery including aberrant methylation, histone modifications, and miRNAs. Aberrant gene promoter hypermethylation is involved in the pathogenesis of MDS. Figueroa et al. analyzed the methylation status of 14,000 gene promoters in patients with MDS, secondary AML, and compared them to normal and *de novo* AML. They found an increase in methylation of promoters of genes involved in the WNT and MAPK signaling pathways in patients with MDS and secondary AML.[32] Aberrant DNA methylation can also be found in most hematologic malignancies examined.

Mutations in DNMT3A have been described in up to 20% of patients with *de novo* AML. These patients have typically intermediate-risk AML. When this occurs in MDS, it is associated with a rapid evolution to AML and a poor prognosis. In patients with AML, the median overall survival (OS) with a DNMT3A mutation is 12.3 months versus 41.1 months in patients without this mutation.[33] TET2 mutations have been described in patients with MDS, MPNs, and AML. It is thought to be a transformative lesion in MDS and MPN. TET2 mutations are prevalent in CMML and are associated with marked monocytosis. There have been differing reports on the effect of TET2 mutations on prognosis. Some authors report a poor prognosis, while others reported no impact on prognosis. IDH1/2 mutations in AML, MDS, and MPNs typically occur at the active site of the enzyme that is responsible for binding the substrate isocitrate. These heterozygous missense mutations are the likely gain of function mutations. As discussed above, the neomorphic enzyme catalyzes the formation of 2HG, which is associated with global hypermethylation via various mechanisms including inhibition of TET2.

Analysis of samples from 398 patients with AML enrolled in the ECOG E1900 study found that IDH mutant AML was associated with aberrant hypermethylation of genes involved in myeloid differentiation and leukemogenesis. TET2 mutations and IDH1/2 mutations are thought to be mutually exclusive. They likely represent a common pathway of leukemogenesis that involves deregulation of TET2 and global hypermethylation. EZH2 mutations have been described in myeloid malignancies where they are associated with a poor prognosis. In myeloid malignancies, the mutation is usually a missense mutation commonly affecting the SET catalytic domain of EZH2. This loss of function mutation suggests that EZH2 functions as a tumor suppressor in myeloid disorders. In lymphomas, EZH2 mutations result in a gain-of-function suggesting that it acts as an oncogene in these diseases. A particular recurrent monoallelic-activating EZH2 mutation at the Y641 residue is found in about a quarter of germinal center DLBCL and in some follicular lymphomas and may be a target for inhibitory therapy.

miRNAs have been shown to be dysregulated in hematological malignancies like MDS and myeloma. Overall, 10–15% of patients with MDS have EVI1 (ecotropic virus integration site 1) proto-oncogene activation; preclinical data suggest that the bone marrow failure that characterizes this subtype of MDS is due to failure to express miRNA-124 due to gene hypermethylation.[34] In myeloma, epigenetic gene silencing of the tumor suppressor miRNA-34B was found in 75% of cell lines analyzed by Wong et al. These investigators demonstrated that azacitidine therapy led to MIR34B/C demethylation and reexpression, and that in primary samples there was MIR34B/C hypermethylation in 5% of patients at diagnosis and in about 50% at disease relapse and progression.[35] Also currently used chemotherapy, such as melphalan and bortezomib, is associated with changes in epigenetic marks. Melphalan therapy was associated with a decrease in acetylation (gene silencing) at the c-myc and cyclin D1 gene loci and an increase in demethylation of H3K9 (gene silencing).[36]

## Epigenetic Perturbations in Breast Cancer

The several molecular subtypes of breast cancer based upon gene expression profiling correlate in part to hormonal receptor and HER2 expression. As with many other epithelial tumors, breast cancer is similarly characterized by global hypomethylation and promoter CpG island hypermethylation of genes such as BRCA-1, E-cadherin, TMS1, and the estrogen receptor. There is some evidence that patterns of DNA methylation correlate with the intrinsic breast cancer subtypes. The luminal A, luminal B, and the basal-like subtype appear to harbor-specific methylation profiles. Ras association domain-containing protein 1 gene a tumor suppressor (RASSF1) and glutathione S-transferase P1 gene (GSTP1) are significantly methylated in ER positive/luminal B, breast cancers.[37] Overall, basal-like breast cancers have a lower frequency of CpG methylation, potentially significant in light of the associated unstable genome and worsened outcomes in this subtype. In ER-negative tumors, however, hypermethylation is seen to cluster closer to the transcriptional start sites, suggesting increased transcriptional repression. As in ovarian cancer, the BRCA1 gene is frequently inactivated by methylation in up to 36.7% of triple negative breast cancers. This finding is associated with increased sensitivity to PARP inhibitors.[38] These findings have a direct translational potential that is currently under investigation.

## Epigenetic Perturbations in Lung Cancer

Epigenetic alterations could potentially serve as modulators between our environment and our genes. Interestingly, *in vitro* normal airway cells exposed to cigarette smoking condensate experience time and dose-dependent alterations in histone modifications, which is accompanied by a decrease in the expression of DNMT1 and an increase in DNMT3B; this is accompanied by an increase in MAGE-A3 expression and activation of WNT signaling as well as hypermethylation of tumor suppressor genes such as RASSF1A and RAR-beta. Sputum examination shows increased methylation of CDNK2A and MGMT in both smokers with lung cancer and chronic obstructive pulmonary disease (COPD) compared to healthy nonsmoking controls. Some studies have shown that cigarette smoking correlates with altered methylation patterns in former and current smokers, with similar patterns of methylation in nonsmokers exposed to second-hand smoke.[39] In general, lung cancers are characterized by the global hypomethylation and gene-specific promoter hypermethylation generally seen in neoplasia. Multiple genes have been shown to have abnormal methylation status in lung cancer, including p16, RASSF1A, APC, RARB-2, CDH1, CDH13, DAPK, MGMT, ASC/TMS1, FHIT, hSRBC, TSLC1, DAL-1, and PTEN.[39] Evidence suggests that these alterations have prognostic significance in pathogenesis of lung cancer. In stage I non-small cell lung cancer (NSCLC) methylation of the promoter regions of p16, CDH13, RASSF1A, and APC correlated with risk of early recurrence in multivariate analysis. A recent retrospective review of resected stage I and II NSCLC also revealed that methylation of PTEN, RASSF1, and DAPK was associated with shorter time to recurrence.[40] These alterations may eventually facilitate early diagnosis and more effective patient management strategies.

## Epigenetic Perturbations in Colon Cancer

As in lung cancer, a large proportion of colorectal cancers (CRCs) is characterized by global hypomethylation, associated with chromosomal instability. In colon cancer, it is recognized that a subset of patients, perhaps 30% of the entire population, is characterized by tumors with globally increased methylation of CGIs, the so-called CpG Island Methylator Phenotype (CIMP). CIMP CRCs are associated with older age, female sex, smoking history, family history, right-sided location, MSI, mucinous differentiation, and BRAF mutations. While the dominant cause of hypermethylation in colon cancer appears to be age-related and is present in normal tissues, there are additional loci of hypermethylation, which are predominantly restricted to the neoplastic tissues, with a three- to fivefold elevated frequency of altered gene methylation amongst the CIMP group of tumors.[41] The initial CIMP panel was described by Toyota et al. with an additional assortment of hypermethylated genes, which were also proposed by several other groups. Not long after microsatellite instability (MSI) was discovered in CRC, it was established that the majority of MSI-H patients have hypermethylation-related silencing of MLH1 rather than inactivation via somatic mutation.

While MSI-H patients have a better prognosis following surgical resection for early stage disease, results on the prognosis of the entire subset of patients with CIMP are conflicting. Generally, when CIMP is not associated with the MSI-H phenotype, the prognosis is worse. There is a suggestion of two distinct groups of CIMP in colon cancer (CIMP-high and CIMP-low or CIMP-1 and CIMP-2), charac-

terized by unique patterns of increased methylation and associated mutations. One group is closely associated with BRAF mutations and the other with a higher prevalence of KRAS mutations. In addition, there is evidence that some CRCs with CIMP begin as sessile serrated adenomas, further fueling the idea that these tumors represent a unique subtype of CRCs with a differing biologic behavior.[42] Across the spectrum of colon cancers, hypermethylation of genes is a prominent finding. In most colon cancers, multiple inhibitory members of the WNT pathway were epigenetically silenced, including SOX17, SFRP1, and WIF-1.

As in other cancers, RASSF1A (a negative effector of RAS signaling) and CDNK2A/P16 are frequently silenced by epigenetic mechanisms.[43] Other affected pathways include those that modulate epithelial–mesenchymal transition (EMT), transcriptional regulation, and DNA repair. Therefore, as in other malignancies, methylation-induced silencing is a regular occurrence at least in the majority of CRCs. Notably, IDH1, IDH2, MLL, UTX, and various other genes involved in the regulation of methylation were found to be mutated in a subset of CRCs. The significance of these mutations in CRC is still being investigated.

Alterations in modifiers of the chromatin structure are also abundant in CRCs. Multiple class I HDACs are upregulated, with HDAC1 in 36.4%, HDAC2 in 57.9%, and HDAC3 in 72.9% of patients. Increased expression is seen in poorly differentiated tumors and is associated with decreased survival. The class 3 HDAC SIRT1 is overexpressed in a large proportion of CRCs, associated, in part, with MSI-H and CIMP tumors.[42] Multiple miRNAs are noted to be upregulated or downregulated in colorectal adenomas and carcinomas. While miRNA regulation remains unclear in many cases, it is notable that a significant portion of colon cancers exhibits hypermethylation at the promoters of miRNA-137, miRNA-34-b, miRNA-34-c, miRNA-129-2, and miRNA-9-1. These are all embedded in CGIS, with methylation expectedly resulting in decreased expression.

## Epigenetics in Diagnostics

The use of DNA methylation as a diagnostic tool is very attractive because there is a clear difference in methylation status between normal and tumor tissues. Epigenetic changes like global DNA hypomethylation occur early in cancer, and high-level CGI methylation does not normally occur in normal tissue (with rare exceptions). Assay techniques like methylation-specific polymerase chain reaction (MSP) can detect 1 abnormal cell in 10,000, resulting in a very high sensitivity for the diagnostic test. MSP is a qualitative and semiquantitative method. Other utilized quantitative methods include real-time MSP, bisulfite-pyrosequencing and methylation-specific multiplex ligation dependent probe amplification (MS-MLPA).

Examples of diagnostic tests are: (i) glutathione S-transferase P1 gene (GSTP1) methylation status for diagnosis of prostate cancer utilizing prostate biopsies (sensitivity 91%, specificity 88%) or utilizing urine (sensitivity 75%, specificity 98%),[44] (ii) O6-methylguanine DNA methyltransferase gene (MGMT) methylation status assay for prediction of response to temozolamide in patients with glioblastomas utilizing tumor biopsy samples,[45] (iii) septin 9 gene (SEPT9) methylation status for CRC diagnosis utilizing plasma samples,[46] and (iv) vimentin methylation status for diagnosis of CRC utilizing stool samples.[47] Utilization of aberrantly methylated genes in the sputum of smokers for the diagnosis of lung cancer, aberrantly methylated genes in vaginal secretions for the diagnosis of endometrial cancer and many other examples are actively being investigated. MiRNAs may one day become a diagnostic tool as they are abundant in body fluids and they are differentially expressed between normal and cancer tissues.

## Role of Epigenetics in Therapeutics

### DNA Methyltransferase Inhibitors

DNA methyltransferase inhibitors (DNMTi) are either nucleoside analogs or non-nucleoside analogs. Nucleoside DNMT inhibitors are transported into the cell via nucleoside transporters. Once inside the cell they require phosphorylation to their active form. Nucleoside analog DNMTi include azacitidine, decitabine, zebularine, 5-fluoro-2-deoxycytidine, and SGI-110.

Notably, azacitidine diphosphate is converted to decitabine diphosphate by ribonuclease reductase, and SGI-110 is a dinucleotide that delivers decitabine with a prolonged half-life. Decitabine diphosphate is phosphorylated to decitabine triphosphate prior to incorporation into DNA. It forms irreversible covalent bonds with DNMTs yielding bulky DNA-protein adducts which are degraded, thus depleting DNMTs. Subsequent DNA synthesis leads to hypomethylation and reactivation of silenced genes. DNMTi as a therapeutic strategy has been successfully translated from the laboratory to the clinic. Azacitidine and decitabine were initially developed as cytosine analogs with the intention of being used as conventional cytotoxic agents, but they were found to induce multiple new phenotypes in cell lines treated *in vitro* as a consequence of the demethylating properties.[48] Not all cytosine analogs have this property rather only those with a 5′ modification of the cytosine ring. Zebularine, 5-fluoro-2-deoxycytidine, and SGI-110 also have this 5′ modification; of these zebularine is not being pursued for further clinical development because of toxicity in preclinical testing. 5-fluoro-2-deoxycytidine and SGI-110 are presently in clinical trials.[49]

Decitabine is FDA approved for the treatment of patients with *de novo*, untreated, and therapy-related MDS. There are two FDA-approved dose schedules: 15 mg/m$^2$ IV administered every 8 hours for 3 consecutive days and 20 mg/m$^2$ IV over 1 hour repeated daily for 5 days of a 28-day cycle. The most common adverse events include leukopenia, neutropenia, neutropenic fever, anemia, and thrombocytopenia. Although decitabine is not FDA approved for the treatment of AML, multiple phase II clinical trials have shown that it has clinical activity. A multicenter, randomized, open-label, phase III trial that compared the efficacy and safety of decitabine to supportive care or low-dose cytarabine (LDAC) 20 mg/m$^2$ daily subcutaneously for 10 days showed a statistically significant survival advantage for decitabine at 2 years. The median OS with decitabine was 7.7 months (6.2–9.2 months) versus 5 months for supportive care/LDAC. The CR + CRp rate was 17.8% versus 7.8%. The most common adverse events were hematologic with thrombocytopenia and neutropenia occurring in about 25% of patients.[50] Azacitidine was evaluated for the treatment of high-risk MDS in the landmark international multicenter phase III trial. Patients were randomized to receive azacitidine 75 mg/m$^2$ daily for 7 days every 28 days versus conventional care (best supportive care or LDAC or intensive therapy). The median OS was 24.5 months (9.9–not reached) versus 15 months (5.6–24.1 months). At 2 years, half of the patients treated with azacitidine were alive compared to about a quarter of the conventional care patients. A post hoc analysis of 113 patients with 20–30% blasts enrolled as high-risk MDS as per the FAB designation revealed a strong effect for treating with azacitidine. The 2-year survival in this cohort was 50% versus 16% for those treated with conventional care.[51]

Combinations of DNMTi and other agents are feasible and have been employed in the clinic, but caution is needed when combining these agents. The demethylating activity depends on being incorporated into the DNA and continued DNA synthesis; hence, agents that target the S-Phase of the cell cycle preventing cell division may be antagonistic to the demethylation that occurs in the daughter cells. In particular combinations with hydroxyurea a commonly employed agent used to lower high white blood cell counts in hematologic malignancies is contraindicated because it leads to cell cycle arrest in S phase. Also the inhibition of ribonucleotide reductase by hydroxyurea prevents the conversion of azacytidine diphosphate to decitabine diphosphate. Azacitidine and decitabine have been combined with histone deacetylase inhibitors like entinostat, vorinostat, and valproic acid. Studies in leukemias yielded promising response rates, but no randomized study has shown a survival advantage for the combination. Azacitidine in combination with entinostat was felt to result in chemosensitization in lung cancer, and decitabine has been successfully used in combination with carboplatin for the treatment of platinum-resistant ovarian cancer. It is believed that there is synergy in this combination as decitabine is able to resensitize ovarian cancer to platinum probably by demethylating hypermethylated genes. An unexpected adverse event of this combination was an increase in the occurrence of type I allergic reactions with this combination. Novel combinations and new indications for DNMTi also exist because of their immunomodulatory properties, which can be exploited in tumor vaccination and in breaking antitumor tolerance.

## Histone Deacetylase Inhibitors

The histone deacetylase inhibitors (HDACi) butyric acid was first discovered in the 1970s, when it was noted to induce cellular differentiation in erythroleukemic cells. Subsequently, it was demonstrated that growth inhibition appears to be related to cell cycle arrest, with the inhibitory concentrations being in the range of those concentrations required to produce histone hyperacetylation.[52] HDAC inhibition results in maintenance of acetylated histone tails promoting euchromatin formation and maintenance hence interaction with transcription factors leading to gene expression. The effects of HDACi are not limited to histone deacetylation, but rather include the acetylation and inactivation of various nuclear and cytoplasmic proteins as well. HDACi can initiate apoptosis via the intrinsic and extrinsic pathways, produce immune modulation via multiple mechanisms, and exert antiangiogenic effects, downregulating proangiogenic genes such as vascular endothelial factor (VEGF). Transcription factors such as p53, E2F-1, STAT1, and NF-KB may be acetylated directly. Multiple other cytoplasmic proteins may be acetylated, including Hsp90, Ku70, and α-tubulin. These events may have multiple downstream effects; for example, acetylated Hsp90 is maintained by HDACi-induced blockade of HDAC6, resulting in the release and destabilization of multiple client oncoproteins, including Akt, bcr-abl, c-kit, c-raf, ERBB1, and ERBB2.[53]

Several classes of HDACi are currently in clinical trials. They include the short-chain fatty acid derived HDACi, including butyrate and valproic acid (VPA). These have seen little clinical success to this point, possibly owing to their low *in vivo* potency.

Hydroxamate-based HDACi include the pan-HDACi vorinostat (SAHA), panobinostat (LBH589), belinostat (PXD101), and trichostatin A (TSA). They are among the most studied in the clinic, with class effects including fatigue, cytopenias, and GI toxicity. Cyclic tetrapeptides, such as depsipeptide, have a narrow spectrum of activity, and they affect only Class I HDACs (HDAC1, HDAC2). Notably, cardiotoxicity with QTc prolongation has been frequently observed with HDAC inhibition.[54] Based on favorable preliminary data regarding cardiotoxicity with the selective isoform entinostat, it is expected that the use of selective agents may be associated with reduced cardiotoxicity.

As single agents, HDACi have seen some success in hematologic malignancies, resulting in the approval of two agents for cutaneous T-cell lymphoma (CTCL) and accelerated approval of romidepsin for peripheral T-cell lymphoma (PTCL). Vorinostat was approved based on a study in the refractory setting, which demonstrated a response rate of 29.7% with a median time to progression of ≥299 days.

Romidepsin demonstrated activity in the same population with a 34% response rate with a median duration of response of 13.7 months.[55] A phase II trial in relapsed/refractory CTCL demonstrated an ORR of 38% and a PFS of 8.9 months.[56] Accelerated approval was granted based on these data and on further confirmatory data from a phase II trial in the same setting.[57] Other HDACi are being investigated for these diseases in earlier stages as well as in combination with other agents. When used as monotherapy, HDACi have shown limited activity other hematologic malignancies. However, recent reports have noted activity of panobinostat in refractory Hodgkin lymphoma with an anatomic response rate of 34% and a metabolic response rate of over 50%.[58] Preliminary activity has also been demonstrated in myelofibrosis, multiple myeloma, and B-cell lymphomas.[58] In contrast, minimal efficacy has been seen in solid tumors, with a few exceptions.[52]

Combinations of HDACi with multiple other agents have been piloted, with varying degrees of success. Given the panoply of effectors HDACs modulate, there is an enormous list of potential combinations, only a few of which will be reviewed here. One of the most fruitful approaches thus far stems from preclinical data suggesting synergy between HDAC and proteasome inhibition. Bortezomib inhibits class I HDACs and proteasome activity is deregulated by HDAC inhibition through a mechanism involving HR23B.[59,60] In relapsed and refractory multiple myeloma, this combination has shown some early promise. A small phase I trial utilizing romidepsin, bortezomib, and dexamethasone achieved a response rate of 72%, far greater than single agent activity of either romidepsin or bortezomib alone, with a median time to progression of 7.2 months.[59] Encouraging activity has also been published with the combinations of vorinostat and bortezomib, among other combinations.[61] Bortezomib and HDAC combinations in solid tumors, including colon cancer and primary brain tumors. However, a recent phase I trial in lung cancer demonstrated high levels of tumor necrosis in a third of patients utilizing preoperative bortezomib and vorinostat,[62] suggesting that these approaches merit further investigation.

Epigenetic mechanisms are believed to play a significant role in resistance to endocrine therapy in breast cancer as well as lack of hormone receptor expression in hormone receptor-negative disease. As a result, multiple epigenetic therapy studies are underway in breast cancer. Vorinostat has shown efficacy in patients with ER+ breast cancer resistant to hormone therapy. In a phase II trial, the combination of vorinostat and tamoxifen demonstrated a response rate of 19% (RECIST) and a clinical benefit rate (response or stable disease >24 weeks) of 40%. Reponses correlated with increased baseline HDAC2 expression and peripheral blood mononuclear hyperacetylation.[63] Combination therapy with other HDACi is being investigated with entinostat showing promising results in combination with exemestane. The strategy of mTOR inhibition combined with antihormonal therapy was recently proven to be beneficial in this setting, illuminating the notion that inhibition of the related protein AKT or hyperacetylation of other nonhistone targets may be responsible for the potential activity of HDACi. HDACi are being investigated with multiple other targeted agents based on preclinical work, including anti-HER2 antibodies and tyrosine kinase inhibitors (TKIs), mTOR inhibitors, EGFR inhibitors, and androgen blockade. A phase I study has shown promise in trastuzumab-refractory breast cancer.[64] Recently, a phase II trial of erlotinib +/− entinostat in patients with advanced lung cancer that progressed on prior chemotherapy produced intriguing results. PFS was poor in both arms, but the subset of patients with high E-cadherin levels who received both agents experienced a significantly improved OS compared to others (9.4 vs. 5.4 months, HR 0.35, $p = 0.03$). Induction of E-cadherin was previously demonstrated to sensitize EGFR-TKI resistant lung cancer cells to EGFR-TKIs. However, the subgroup with high E-cadherin levels did not derive greater benefit from erlotinib alone and the aforementioned benefit was maintained when patients with EGFR activating mutations were censored.[65] This strategy merits further investigation.

Combinations with traditional cytotoxic chemotherapy have generally been disappointing, with additive hematologic and gastrointestinal toxicities and minimal if any, additional signal of benefit. However, a recent phase I trial of pulsed high-dose vorinostat combined with RICE (rituximab, ifosfamide, carboplatin, etoposide) demonstrated high response rates (70%) in a refractory lymphoma population,[66] suggesting that the combination of HDACi with cytotoxic agents may be promising.

## EZH2 Inhibitors

As mentioned earlier, EZH2 is a HMT responsible for the trimethylation of H3K27, which leads to transcriptional repression. It is overexpressed or mutated in several tumors leading to tumor progression and an aggressive phenotype. EZH2 inhibitors are presently in preclinical development. For example, GSK 126 is a direct potent selective small molecule inhibitor of EZH2. It reversibly competes with SAM, the methyl donor to EZH2.

DLBCL cell lines with the Y641N, Y641F, and A677G mutations are the most sensitive with both cytostatic and cytotoxic responses.[67] A subset of follicular lymphoma also harbor the sensitive mutation Tyr641 (Y641N, Y641F) in the SET domain of EZH2 protein making them targets of EZH2 inhibition.[68]

EZH2 inhibitors will soon enter phase I trials for treatment of lymphomas with activating EZH2 mutations.

## Conclusions

Epigenetic processes are commonly deregulated in cancer and provide attractive targets for therapeutic intervention. Clinical trials have already established the efficacy of DNA methylation and histone HDACi in hematologic malignancies and numerous new targets are being tested in early phase studies.

# References

1 Okano M, Bell DW, Haber DA, Li E. DNA methyltransferases DNMT3a and DNMT3b are essential for de novo methylation and mammalian development. *Cell*. 1999;99:247–257.

2 Yoder JA, Soman NS, Verdine GL, Bestor TH. DNA (cytosine-5)-methyltransferases in mouse cells and tissues. Studies with a mechanism-based probe. *J Mol Biol*. 1997;270:385–395.

3 Jurkowski TP, Meusburger M, Phalke S, et al. Human DNMT2 methylates tRNA(Asp) molecules using a DNA methyltransferase-like catalytic mechanism. *RNA*. 2008;14:1663–1670.

4 Singal R, Ginder GD. DNA methylation. *Blood*. 1999;93:4059–4070.

5 Chen RZ, Pettersson U, Beard C, Jackson-Grusby L, Jaenisch R. DNA hypomethylation leads to elevated mutation rates. *Nature*. 1998;395:89–93.

6 Esteller M. Epigenetics in cancer. *N Engl J Med*. 2008;358:1148–1159.

7 Hoffmann MJ, Schulz WA. Causes and consequences of DNA hypomethylation in human cancer. *Biochem Cell Biol*. 2005;83:296–321.

8 Hervouet E, Lalier L, Debien E, et al. Disruption of Dnmt1/PCNA/UHRF1 interactions promotes tumorigenesis from human and mice glial cells. *PLoS One*. 2010;5:e11333.

9 Guo JU, Su Y, Zhong C, Ming GL, Song H. Hydroxylation of 5-methylcytosine by TET1 promotes active DNA demethylation in the adult brain. *Cell*. 2011;145:423–434.

10 Williams K, Christensen J, Helin K. DNA methylation: TET proteins-guardians of CpG islands? *EMBO Rep*. 2012;13:28–35.

11 Ko M, Rao A. TET2: epigenetic safeguard for HSC. *Blood*. 2011;118:4501–4503.

12 Abdel-Wahab O, Mullally A, Hedvat C, et al. Genetic characterization of TET1, TET2, and TET3 altcrations in myeloid malignancies. *Blood*. 2009;114:144–147.

13 Itzykson R, Kosmider O, Cluzeau T, et al. Impact of TET2 mutations on response rate to azacitidine in myelodysplastic syndromes and low blast count acute myeloid leukemias. *Leukemia*. 2011;25:1147–1152.

14 Bartova E, Krejci J, Harnicarova A, Galiova G, Kozubek S. Histone modifications and nuclear architecture: a review. *J Histochem Cytochem*. 2008;56:711–721.

15 Kouzarides T. Chromatin modifications and their function. *Cell*. 2007;128:693–705.

16 Murchison EP, Hannon GJ. miRNAs on the move: miRNA biogenesis and the RNAi machinery. *Curr Opin Cell Biol*. 2004;16:223–229.

17 Costa MC, Leitao AL, Enguita FJ. Biogenesis and mechanism of action of small non-coding RNAs: insights from the point of view of structural biology. *Int J Mol Sci*. 2012;13:10268–10295.

18 Bracken AP, Helin K. Polycomb group proteins: navigators of lineage pathways led astray in cancer. *Nat Rev Cancer*. 2009;9:773–784.

19 Schlesinger Y, Straussman R, Keshet I, et al. Polycomb-mediated methylation on Lys27 of histone H3 pre-marks genes for de novo methylation in cancer. *Nat Genet*. 2007;39:232–236.

20 Cao W, Ribeiro Rde O, Liu D. EZH2 promotes malignant behaviors via cell cycle dysregulation and its mRNA level associates with prognosis of patient with non-small cell lung cancer. *PLoS One*. 2012;7:e52984.

21 Chen YH, Hung MC, Li LY. EZH2: a pivotal regulator in controlling cell differentiation. *Am J Transl Res*. 2012;4:364–375.

22 Bachmann IM, HalvorsenOJ, Collett K, et al. EZH2 expression is associated with high proliferation rate and aggressive tumor subgroups in cutaneous melanoma and cancers of the endometrium, prostate, and breast. *J Clin Oncol*. 2006;24:268–273.

23 Bejar R, Stevenson KE, Caughey BA, et al. Validation of a prognostic model and the impact of mutations in patients with lower-risk myelodysplastic syndromes. *J Clin Oncol*. 2012;30:3376–3382.

24 Kleer CG, Cao Q, Varambally S, et al. EZH2 is a marker of aggressive breast cancer and promotes neoplastic transformation of breast epithelial cells. *Proc Natl Acad Sci U S A*. 2003;100:11606–11611.

25 Wagener N, Macher-Goeppinger S, Pritsch M, et al. Enhancer of zeste homolog 2 (EZH2) expression is an independent prognostic factor in renal cell carcinoma. *BMC Cancer*. 2010;10:524.

26 Abdel-Wahab O, Dey A. The ASXL-BAP1 axis: new factors in myelopoiesis, cancer and epigenetics. *Leukemia*. 2013;27:10–15.

27 Gelsi-Boyer V, Brecqueville M, Devillier R, Murati A, Mozziconacci MJ, Birnbaum D. Mutations in ASXL1 are associated with poor prognosis across the spectrum of malignant myeloid diseases. *J Hematol Oncol*. 2012;5:12.

28 Chowdhury R, Yeoh KK, Tian YM, et al. The oncometabolite 2-hydroxyglutarate inhibits histone lysine demethylases. *EMBO Rep*. 2011;12:463–469.

29 Dang L, White DW, Gross S, et al. Cancer-associated IDH1 mutations produce 2-hydroxyglutarate. *Nature*. 2009;462:739–744.

30 Ward PS, Patel J, Wise DR, et al. The common feature of leukemia-associated IDH1 and IDH2 mutations is a neomorphic enzyme activity converting alpha-ketoglutarate to 2-hydroxyglutarate. *Cancer Cell*. 2010;17:225–234.

31 Rakheja D, Konoplev S, Medeiros LJ, Chen W. IDH mutations in acute myeloid leukemia. *Human Pathol*. 2012;43:1541–1551.

32 Figueroa ME, Skrabanek L, Li Y, et al. MDS and secondary AML display unique patterns and abundance of aberrant DNA methylation. *Blood*. 2009;114:3448–3458.

33 Ley TJ, Ding L, Walter MJ, et al. DNMT3A mutations in acute myeloid leukemia. *N Eng J Med*. 2010;363:2424–2433.

34 Dickstein J, Senyuk V, Premanand K, et al. Methylation and silencing of miRNA-124 by EVI1 and self-renewal exhaustion of hematopoietic stem cells in murine myelodysplastic syndrome. *Proc Nat Acad Sci U S A*. 2010;107:9783–9788.

35 Wong KY, Yim RL, So CC, Jin DY, Liang R, Chim CS. Epigenetic inactivation of the MIR34B/C in multiple myeloma. *Blood*. 2011;118:5901–5904.

36 Krejci J, Harnicarova A, Streitova D, et al. Epigenetics of multiple myeloma after treatment with cytostatics and gamma radiation. *Leukemia Res*. 2009;33:1490–1498.

37 Holm K, Hegardt C, Staaf J, et al. Molecular subtypes of breast cancer are associated with characteristic DNA methylation patterns. *Breast Cancer Res*. 2010;12:R36.

38 Connolly R, Stearns V. Epigenetics as a therapeutic target in breast cancer. *J Mammary Gland Biol Neoplasia*. 2012;17:191–204.

39 Wen J, Fu J, Zhang W, Guo M. Genetic and epigenetic changes in lung carcinoma and their clinical implications. *Mod Pathol*. 2011;24:932–943.

40 Brzezianska E, Dutkowska A, Antczak A. The significance of epigenetic alterations in lung carcinogenesis. *Mol Biol Rep*. 2013;40:309–325.

41 Issa JP. CpG island methylator phenotype in cancer. *Nat Rev Cancer*. 2004;4:988–993.

42 Goel A, Boland CR. Epigenetics of colorectal cancer. *Gastroenterology*. 2012;143:1442.e1–1460.e1.

43 van Engeland M, Derks S, Smits KM, Meijer GA, Herman JG. Colorectal cancer epigenetics: complex simplicity. *J Clin Oncol*. 2011;29:1382–1391.

44 Woodson K, O'Reilly KJ, Hanson JC, Nelson D, Walk EL, Tangrea JA. The usefulness of the detection of GSTP1 methylation in urine as a biomarker

in the diagnosis of prostate cancer. *J Urol.* 2008;179:508–511; discussion 511–502.

45 Christians A, Hartmann C, Benner A, et al. Prognostic value of three different methods of MGMT promoter methylation analysis in a prospective trial on newly diagnosed glioblastoma. *PLoS One.* 2012;7: e33449.

46 Toth K, Sipos F, Kalmar A, et al. Detection of methylated SEPT9 in plasma is a reliable screening method for both left- and right-sided colon cancers. *PLoS One.* 2012;7:e46000.

47 Chen WD, Han ZJ, Skoletsky J, et al. Detection in fecal DNA of colon cancer-specific methylation of the nonexpressed vimentin gene. *J Natl Cancer Inst.* 2005;97:1124–1132.

48 Taylor SM, Jones PA. Multiple new phenotypes induced in 10T1/2 and 3T3 cells treated with 5-azacytidine. *Cell.* 1979;17:771–779.

49 Issa JP, Kantarjian HM. Targeting DNA methylation. *Clin Cancer Res.* 2009;15:3938–3946.

50 Kantarjian HM, Thomas XG, Dmoszynska A, et al. Multicenter, randomized, open-label, phase III trial of decitabine versus patient choice, with physician advice, of either supportive care or low-dose cytarabine for the treatment of older patients with newly diagnosed acute myeloid leukemia. *J Clin Oncol.* 2012;30:2670–2677.

51 Fenaux P, Mufti GJ, Hellstrom-Lindberg E, et al. Efficacy of azacitidine compared with that of conventional care regimens in the treatment of higher-risk myelodysplastic syndromes: a randomised, open-label, phase III study. *Lancet Oncol.* 2009;10:223–232.

52 Wagner JM, Hackanson B, Lubbert M, Jung M. Histone deacetylase (HDAC) inhibitors in recent clinical trials for cancer therapy. *Clin Epigenetics.* 2010;1:117–136.

53 Bolden JE, Peart MJ, Johnstone RW. Anticancer activities of histone deacetylase inhibitors. *Nat Rev Drug Discov.* 2006;5:769–784.

54 Shah MH, Binkley P, Chan K, et al. Cardiotoxicity of histone deacetylase inhibitor depsipeptide in patients with metastatic neuroendocrine tumors. *Clin Cancer Res.* 2006;12:3997–4003.

55 Gryder BE, Sodji QH, Oyelere AK Targeted cancer therapy: giving histone deacetylase inhibitors all they need to succeed. *Future Med Chem.* 2012;4:505–524.

56 Piekarz RL, Frye R, Prince HM, et al. Phase 2 trial of romidepsin in patients with peripheral T-cell lymphoma. *Blood.* 2011;117:5827–5834.

57 Coiffier B, Pro B, Prince HM, et al. Results from a pivotal, open-label, phase II study of romidepsin in relapsed or refractory peripheral T-cell lymphoma after prior systemic therapy. *J Clin Oncol.* 2012;30:631–636.

58 Deangelo DJ, Spencer A, Bhalla KN, et al. Phase Ia/II, 2-arm, open-label, dose-escalation study of oral panobinostat administered via 2 dosing schedules in patients with advanced hematologic malignancies. *Leukemia.* 2013;27(8):1628–1636.

59 Harrison SJ, Quach H, Link E, et al. A high rate of durable responses with romidepsin, bortezomib, and dexamethasone in relapsed or refractory multiple myeloma. *Blood.* 2011;118:6274–6283.

60 Khan O, Fotheringham S, Wood V, et al. HR23B is a biomarker for tumor sensitivity to HDAC inhibitor-based therapy. *Proc Natl Acad Sci U S A.* 2010;107:6532–6537.

61 Weber DM, Graef T, Hussein M, et al. Phase I trial of vorinostat combined with bortezomib for the treatment of relapsing and/or refractory multiple myeloma. *Clin Lymphoma Myeloma Leuk.* 2012;12:319–324.

62 Jones DR, Moskaluk CA, Gillenwater HH, et al. Phase I trial of induction histone deacetylase and proteasome inhibition followed by surgery in non-small-cell lung cancer. *J Thorac Oncol.* 2012;7:1683–1690.

63 Munster PN, Thurn KT, Thomas S, et al. A phase II study of the histone deacetylase inhibitor vorinostat combined with tamoxifen for the treatment of patients with hormone therapy-resistant breast cancer. *Br J Cancer.* 2011;104:1828–1835.

64 Thurn KT, Thomas S, Moore A, Munster PN. Rational therapeutic combinations with histone deacetylase inhibitors for the treatment of cancer. *Future Oncol.* 2011;7:263–283.

65 Witta SE, Jotte RM, Konduri K, et al. Randomized phase II trial of erlotinib with and without entinostat in patients with advanced non-small-cell lung cancer who progressed on prior chemotherapy. *J Clin Oncol.* 2012;30:2248–2255.

66 Budde LE, Zhang MM, Shustov AR, et al. A phase I study of pulse high-dose vorinostat (V) plus rituximab (R), ifosphamide, carboplatin, and etoposide (ICE) in patients with relapsed lymphoma. *Br J Haematol.* 2013;161(2):183–191.

67 McCabe MT, Ott HM, Ganji G, et al. EZH2 inhibition as a therapeutic strategy for lymphoma with EZH2-activating mutations. *Nature.* 2012;492:108–112.

68 Morin RD, Johnson NA, Severson TM, et al. Somatic mutations altering EZH2 (Tyr641) in follicular and diffuse large B-cell lymphomas of germinal-center origin. *Nat Genet.* 2010;42:181–185.

# CHAPTER 8

# The Role of microRNAs in Cancer

*Gianpiero Di Leva and Carlo M. Croce*

Department of Molecular Virology, Immunology and Medical Genetics, Comprehensive Cancer Center, Ohio State University, Columbus, OH, USA

## Introduction

Characterization of genes that control the timing of larval development in the worm *Caenorhabditis elegans* identified for the first time the importance of two small regulatory RNAs, named lin-4 and let-7, in gene expression regulation.[1] Homologs of let-7 were soon recognized in other animals, including mammals, and exhibited temporal expression resembling that is observed in worms, suggesting that let-7 might be playing orthologous roles in diverse metazoan lineages.[2] Soon thereafter, lin-4 and let-7 RNAs were reported to be part of a very large class of small endogenous RNAs found in worms, flies, and mammals which were named microRNAs (miRNAs).[3] miRNAs are single-stranded RNAs (ssRNAs) ~19–25 nucleotides in length that are generated from endogenous hairpin transcripts. They negatively regulate gene expression by base-pairing to partially complementary sites on the target messenger RNAs (mRNAs), usually in the 3′ untranslated region (UTR).[4] Binding of a miRNA to the target mRNA typically leads to translational repression and exonucleolytic mRNA decay.[5] In the latest version of the miRNA database (miRBase), released in August 2012, 2042 mature miRNAs were reported in humans, and approximately 1281 in mice. Many of the bilaterian animal miRNAs are phylogenetically conserved (Figure 8.1a); ~55% of worm miRNAs have homologs in humans, which indicates that miRNAs have had important roles throughout animal evolution. Most mammalian miRNA genes have multiple isoforms (paralogs) that are probably the result of gene duplications (Figure 8.1b). For instance, the human genome has 12 loci for let-7-family miRNAs. Paralogs often have identical sequences at nucleotide positions 2–7 relative to the 5′ end of the miRNA (Figure 8.1b). Because these six nucleotides (called seed) are crucial in base-pairing with the target mRNA, the paralogs are thought to act redundantly. However, because the 3′ sequences of miRNAs also contribute to target binding and because the expression patterns of these sister miRNAs are often different from each other, members of the same seed family might also have distinct roles *in vivo* and therefore more studies are needed to understand their differential function.

Most miRNA genes come from regions of the genome quite distant from previously annotated genes, implying that they represent independent transcription units.[4,6] Almost 50% of these independent miRNA genes are clustered in the genome and transcribed as a multicistronic primary transcripts (Figure 8.1c). Generally, miRNA clusters are related to each other and related miRNAs are, sometimes but not always, clustered (Figure 8.1c). In addition, about a quarter of the human miRNAs are located in the introns of other transcripts (Figure 8.1c). These miRNAs are preferentially in the same orientation as the predicted RNA transcripts, suggesting that they are not transcribed from their own promoters but are instead processed from the introns. In the canonical molecular framework of miRNA biogenesis (Figure 8.1d), primary (pri)-miRNA transcripts with stem–loop regions are usually produced by RNA polymerase II, but occasionally by RNA polymerase III.[6] The stem–loop precursor (pre)-miRNA is released by a cleavage event, which is catalyzed by the nuclear Microprocessor complex that contains the RNase III Drosha. Following this reaction, the precursor pre-miRNA is exported to the cytoplasm by using the shuffling system of XPO5/RanGTP. In the cytoplasm, a distinct RNase III, Dicer, subsequently produces a ~22 base-pair duplex RNA that is composed of the eventual mature miRNA, base-paired to the so-called miRNA* strand. In miRNA duplexes, the strand with the weakest 5′-end base-pairing is selected as the mature miRNA and loaded onto an Argonaute (Ago) proteins, whereas the miRNA* is degraded. Ago proteins are ubiquitous RNA-Induced-Silencing-Complex (RISC) components and provide the endonucleolytic RNase H activity of slicer-competent RISCs. Apart from canonical intronic miRNAs, a small group of miRNA-like RNAs have been discovered in introns of flies and mammals.[7] These small RNAs, mirtrons, do not require Drosha processing for their biogenesis (Figure 8.1c). Following completion of the splicing, the branch point of the lariat-shaped intron is resolved and the debranched intron, which forms a hairpin structure that resembles pre-miRNA, enter the export step and it is matured by Dicer into the cytoplasm.

The initial indications that miRNAs play important roles in human cancer came from studies of their functions in animal models and cancer cells.[8,9] Several factors contributed to an early appreciation of their significance in this pathologic setting. First, loss of lin-4 and let-7 in worm exhibited phenotypes that evoked some aspects of tumor biology, such as the failure to differentiate or reiterating cell divisions in adults—characteristic of earlier stages of embryonic development. Second, miRNAs were subsequently identified in Drosophila to regulate cell proliferation and apoptosis, further linking these regulatory RNAs to cancer-relevant pathways.[10] Finally, a seminal study by our laboratory showed that the miR-15a/16–1 cluster is frequently deleted in chronic lymphocytic

*Targeted Therapy in Translational Cancer Research*, First Edition. Edited by Apostolia-Maria Tsimberidou, Razelle Kurzrock and Kenneth C. Anderson.
© 2016 John Wiley & Sons, Inc. Published 2016 by John Wiley & Sons, Inc.

leukemia (CLL), implicating these miRNAs as tumor suppressor genes.[11] Together, these findings ignited an intensive decade of studies that highlighted a large involvement of miRNAs in all aspects of cancer biology.[8,12] In this chapter, we will discuss the pivotal role of miRNAs in tumor formation and progression and examine the current landscape for targeting miRNAs in cancer setting and the path from translating a miRNA lab discovery into a therapeutically useful modality.

## miRNAs Dysregulation in Cancer

miRNA expression profiling analyses have reported a general dysregulation of miRNA levels in all tumors.[13] A large majority of miRNA genes map to chromosomic regions that are known to be altered in human cancer, such as loss of heterozygosity regions (LOH) (e.g., miR-15a/16-1), amplified regions (e.g., miR-17-92 cluster, miR-155) and breakpoint regions and fragile sites (FRA) (e.g., let-7 family members).[14] Published studies have defined that elevated expression of some miRNAs (oncogenes: Table 8.1) as well as downregulation of others (tumor suppressors: Table 8.2) accompanies carcinogenesis and correlates with the development of cancer-associated phenotypes. As previously stated, the first evidence of miR involvement in cancer came from our laboratory in 2002. We identified that the miR-15 and miR-16 genomic locus is heterozygously deleted in 68% of all patients with B-cell chronic lymphocytic leukemia (B-CLL).[11] Loss of miR-15 and miR-16 reflects their tumor suppressor function via uncontrolled expression of their antiapoptotic target protein BCL2 in an *in vitro* model as well as specimens of patients with B-CLL.[15] Furthermore, a sequencing-based screen for miRNAs dysregulated in familial CLL patients identified a germ line mutation in the primary precursor of miR-15a/16-1 that impairs their processing, highlighting that not only deletions but also mutations may lead to miRNA loss of function.[16] The importance of genetic lesions reducing miR-15/16-1 cluster expression in CLL was furthermore confirmed by the identification of a point mutation located in the 3′ flanking region of miR-16 that reduces miR-16 expression in a naturally occurring CLL mouse model, the New Zealand black (NZB) mouse, that develops a hematological disorder similar to the human CLL.[17] Even more definitive genetic evidence of the tumor-suppressive effects of miR-15 and miR-16 came recently from the Dalla-Favera lab where miR-15/16 knockout mice were generated. Targeted deletion of miR-15 and miR-16 in mice at the age of 18 months recapitulates the spectrum of CLL-associated lymphoproliferations in humans, including CLL, CD5(+) monoclonal B-cell lymphocytosis, and CD5(−) non-Hodgkin lymphomas.[18] Specifically, miR-15a/16-1-deletion accelerates the proliferation of both human and mouse B cells by modulating the expression of genes controlling cell cycle progression like Cyclin D3, Cyclin E, CDK6, CHK1, and MCM5. Deletion of the miR-15/16-1 cluster also occurs in other form of tumors, such as multiple myeloma[19] and prostate cancer,[20] indicating that the loss of these miRNAs could be relevant to other pathogenic event. In this context, Bonci and coworkers demonstrated that, in prostate cancer, miR-15a/miR-16 levels are strongly downregulated in the vast majority of cases (up to 85% of the analyzed samples).[20] Interestingly, intraprostatic injection of miRNA antisense RNA oligonucleotide ("antagomirs") specific to miR-15a and miR-16 in a 6-week-old male BALB/c mice resulted in marked hyperplasia and knockdown of miR-15a and miR-16-promoted survival, proliferation, and invasiveness of untransformed prostate cells, which

became tumorigenic in immunodeficient NOD-SCID mice.[20] Furthermore, they also demonstrated that miR-15 and miR-16 are downregulated in fibroblasts surrounding the prostate tumors. Increased miR-15 and miR-16 expression in cancer-associated fibroblasts impaired tumor growth and expansion of prostate tumors in xenograft models through the reduced posttranscriptional repression of Fgf2 and its receptor Fgfr1.[21]

Similar to the downregulation of miR-15/16-1 cluster, another miRNA frequently lost in cancer is represented by the miR-34 family. This miRNA family, miR-34a on chromosome 1p36 and the miR-34b/c cluster on chromosome 11q23, is frequently deleted in neuroblastoma, breast, pancreas, hepatic, and colon carcinoma.[22] Loss of expression of the miR-34b/c cluster has also been associated with the hypermethylation of their CpG-associated promoter region in gastric cancer, while the same chromosomal region was not methylated in the normal gastric mucosa.[23] The miR-34 family has been shown to be transcriptionally activated by p53 and it represents one of the pivotal effectors of p53-induced apoptosis, senescence, and cell cycle arrest. These effects are achieved by repressing the expression of multiple oncogenes such as Notch-1,[24] Notch-2,[24] HMGA2,[24] Myc,[25] several cyclins and CDKs, CD44,[26] the antiapoptotic factor BCL2,[27] and the p-53 deacetylase, SIRT1.[28] Recently, miR-34-family knockout mice have been generated and no obvious developmental or pathological abnormalities have been observed at up to 12 months of age and, in contrast to p53-deficient mice, miR-34-deficient animals do not display increased susceptibility to spontaneous, irradiation-induced, or c-Myc-initiated tumorigenesis.[29,30] However, miR-34-deficient mouse embryonic fibroblasts accelerate the reprogramming by posttranscriptional derepression of pluripotency genes, such as Sox2, N-Myc, and Nanog.[29] Many other miRNAs have been reported to act as tumor suppressors (Table 8.2) by inhibiting tumor growth when expressed ectopically *in vitro* or *in vivo*; however, their bona fide tumor suppressor role is still missing. Examples include let-7 family,[31] miR-26,[32,33] miR-143/145 cluster,[34] miR-181 family,[35] miR-200 family,[36] and miR-31.[37]

Although there seems to be a general trend toward downregulation of miRNAs in cancer,[38] many different miRNAs follow the opposite pattern and, based on their ability to initiate or accelerate cancer, are named "oncomiRs." The first indication of oncogenic miRNA activity was presented in 2005 by Mendell and coworkers who showed that Myc can directly induce the expression of the polycistronic cluster miR-17/92.[39] By using a reconstituted mouse model of Myc-induced lymphoma expressing a truncated version of the miR-17/92 cluster in hematopoietic cells, the authors showed an accelerated tumor development probably due to an antiapoptotic mechanism associated with the suppression of their direct targets, such as inhibitors of proliferation CDKN1A,[40] direct regulators of the apoptosis PTEN,[41] and BCL2L11 (also known as BIM).[42] miR-17/92 cluster has been shown to be upregulated in many solid tumors such as breast, stomach, prostate, lung, and pancreatic tumors,[43] and genetic deletion of the miR-17/92 cluster in mice highlighted their importance in B-cell development as homozygous deletion of the cluster results in premature death of B cells at the pro-B and pre-B stages, resulting in lymphopenia.[44]

Another miRNA with oncogenic activity is represented by miR-21, which is highly expressed in the majority of human malignancies thus far analyzed including breast cancer,[45,46] glioblastoma,[47,48] hepatocellular carcinoma,[49] cholangiocarcinoma,[50] lung cancer,[51] tongue squamous cell carcinoma,[52] esophageal cancer,[53] stomach

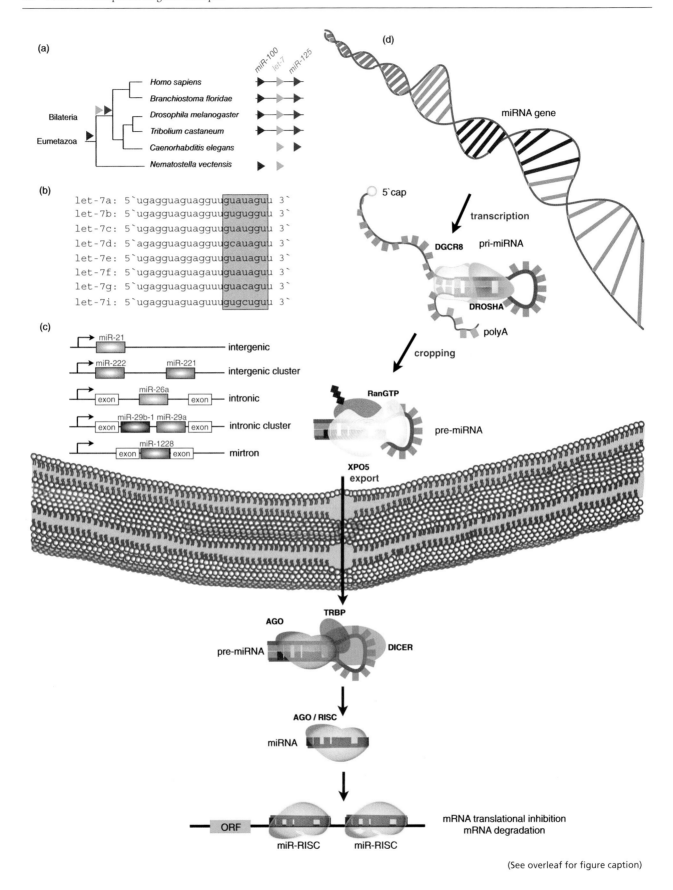

(a)

miR-100  let-7  miR-125

*Homo sapiens*
*Branchiostoma floridae*
*Drosophila melanogaster*
*Tribolium castaneum*
*Caenorhabditis elegans*
*Nematostella vectensis*

Bilateria
Eumetazoa

(b)

```
let-7a:  5`ugagguaguagguuguauaguu 3`
let-7b:  5`ugagguaguagguugugugguu 3`
let-7c:  5`ugagguaguagguuguaugguu 3`
let-7d:  5`agagguaguagguugcauaguu 3`
let-7e:  5`ugagguaggagguuguauaguu 3`
let-7f:  5`ugagguaguagauuguauaguu 3`
let-7g:  5`ugagguaguaguuuguacaguu 3`
let-7i:  5`ugagguaguaguuugugcuguu 3`
```

(c)

miR-21 — intergenic
miR-222    miR-221 — intergenic cluster
exon    miR-26a    exon — intronic
exon    miR-29b-1  miR-29a    exon — intronic cluster
exon    miR-1228    exon — mirtron

(d)

miRNA gene

5`cap

transcription

DGCR8    pri-miRNA

DROSHA

polyA

cropping

RanGTP

pre-miRNA

XPO5
export

AGO    TRBP

pre-miRNA    DICER

AGO / RISC

miRNA

ORF

miR-RISC    miR-RISC

mRNA translational inhibition
mRNA degradation

(See overleaf for figure caption)

cancer,[54] colorectal cancer,[55] chronic myelogeneous leukemia,[56] cervical cancer,[57] and prostate cancer.[58] Experimental data indicates that miR-21 plays a crucial role in tumor cell proliferation, apoptosis, and invasion consistent with miR-21's ability to repress important tumor suppressors such as PTEN,[49] PDCD4,[55] TPM-1,[59] Tap-63,[60] SPRY2,[61] and hMSH2.[62] Recently, the Slack lab generated the first conditional knock-in of miR-21 overexpressing mice that showed a 15- to 30-fold induction of miR-21.[63] The mice developed a severe pre-B-cell lymphoma but when miR-21 was reduced to endogenous levels, the mouse tumors completely disappeared, defining the concept of "oncomiR addiction."[63] Another *in vivo* evidence that miR-21 exerts an oncogenic function came from the DMBA-TPA skin carcinogenesis model used by Ma et al. on miR-21-null mice.[64] The miR-21 mice showed a significant reduction in papilloma formation compared with wild type mice, with miR-21-null mice exhibiting an increase in cellular apoptosis and decrease in cell proliferation that is explained by the upregulation of the miR-21 targets Spry1,[61] Pten,[49] and Pdcd4.[55]

Many other miRNAs have been reported to act as oncogenes (Table 8.1) by inducing tumor growth, aggressiveness, and resistance to chemotherapy when expressed ectopically *in vitro* or *in vivo*: miR-155, miR-221 and miR-222 cluster, and miR-106/363 clusters.

A particularly intriguing, but poorly understood aspect of the biology of miRNAs is their presence in numerous body fluids, including serum, plasma, saliva, and amniotic fluid.[65] miRNAs in serum correlate with the presence of hematologic malignancies and solid tumors and have been reported to be of value for early detection of various types of cancer, preceding diagnosis by conventional methods.[66] Many studies have systematically shown the remarkable stability of secretory miRNAs, despite the austere conditions they are subjected to in both the blood stream (RNase digestion) and during handling (e.g., extreme temperatures and pH values).[66] The secretory mechanism remains unclear, but three different possibilities have been suggested: a passive leakage from cells due to injury, chronic inflammation, apoptosis or necrosis, or from cells with short half-lives, such as platelets[67]; an active secretion via cell-derived membrane vesicles (nanovesicles), including exosomes, shedding vesicles, and apoptotic bodies[68,69]; an active secretion by a protein–miRNA complex such as lipoproteins (e.g., high-density lipoprotein—HDL) and proteins (e.g., Ago2).[70,71] Our laboratory recently contributed to the understanding of the function of circulatory miRNAs by showing that tumor-secreted miRNAs are able to interact with the Toll-like receptors of immune cells to stimulate the production of prometastatic inflammatory cytokines and inducing the protumor inflammatory processes.[72] In this scenario, circulating miRNAs can act as signals for receptor activation, a function that is completely independent of their conventional role in posttranscriptional gene regulation.

## miRNAs in Therapy

The most exciting fact that has emerged from our understanding of miRNA biology is the potential use of miRNA mimetics or antagonists as therapeutics. Because miRNA expression is dysregulated in cancer cells, agents that modulate miRNA activities could potentially produce antineoplastic-specific effects. Although the delivering of miRNAs for therapeutic purposes still represents a limitation, there are many reasons why miRNA modulation is attractive as a therapeutic approach. miRNA gain- and loss-of-function studies have highlighted that, if miRNA dysregulation is well tolerated in normal tissues, manipulation of miRNA levels profoundly influences the behavior of cells and tissues experiencing pathologic stress, such as malignant tissues.[9,73] Therefore, miRNA inhibition or delivery may provide a highly potent means to modulate a disease process while avoiding unwanted toxic effects in normal tissues. For endogenous aberrantly overexpressed oncogenic miRNAs (miR-21, miR-155, miR-17/92), this has been pursued by using either small antisense single-stranded oligonucleotides complementary to the miRNAs, functioning as miRNA antagonists/inhibitors, or mRNAs containing multiple target sites for a specific miRNA, acting as miRNA sponge that sequesters the oncogenic miRNAs. By contrast, tumor suppressor miRNAs (e.g., let-7 and miR-34 families, miR-15/16 and miR-143/145) are responsible for down-regulating oncogenes and are mostly underexpressed in cancer. In this case, miRNA replacement strategies are being developed to restore their normal cellular levels, via exogenous administration of short double-stranded miRNA mimics (functioning similarly to endogenous miRNAs) or DNA constructs coding for specific miRNAs.

The demonstration that oncogenic miRNAs are upregulated in cancer provided a rationale to investigate the use of antisense oligonucleotides to block their expression. Antisense oligonucleotides work as competitive inhibitors of miRNAs, presumably by annealing to the mature miRNA guide strand and inducing degradation or stoichiometric duplex formation.[74] To increase stability, binding affinity, and specificity of the oligonucleotides numerous modifications have been introduced into their chemical structure.[75] Among these modifications, we have to consider the introduction of $2'$-O-methyl groups that improve the nuclease resistance and binding affinities to the miRNAs. Oligonucleotides with $2'$-O-methyl groups have proved to be effective inhibitors of miRNA expression in several cancer cell lines. Another modification that have gained large attention at clinical level has been developed by Krutzfeldt et al. and consists in $2'$-O-methyl-modified cholesterol-conjugated single-stranded miRNA analogs, with phosphorothioate linkages, named "antagomirs."[76] In the original manuscript, antagomir complementary to miR-122, the most abundant miR in the liver, were injected into the tail vein of mice and the targeting of miR-122 in the liver was specific, efficient, and long-lasting with effects

---

**Figure 8.1** miRNAs biology. (a) Phylogenetic tree indicating conserved genomic clustering of miR-100, let-7, and miR-125/lin-4 microRNAs. Note that the human genome contains three miR-100, let-7, and miR-125/lin-4 clusters on chromosomes 9, 11, and 21 respectively. (b) Alignments of the human let-7 family members. The seed region of let-7 is highlighted in red: it is identical for all the paralogs. (c) Genomic organization of miRNA genes in human. Intergenic and intronic monocistronic or multicistronic miRNA genes are represented; miRtrons are also shown. (d) miRNAs are transcribed in the nucleus mainly by the RNA polymerase II producing a primary-miRNA (pri-miRNA). The primary step of miRNA biogenesis and

maturation is the nuclear cleavage of the pri-miRNA by a ribonuclease III enzyme called Drosha liberating a ~60–70 nt stem–loop intermediate known as the miRNA precursor called pre-miRNA (cropping). After this cleavage the pre-miRNA is transported into the cytoplasm by Exportin 5 (Exp 5), a Ran-GTP-dependent nucleo/citoplasmic cargo transporter (export). Once exported into the cytoplasm, pre-miRNAs are processed into short double-strand miRNA duplex by Dicer (dicing). Mature miRNA of 19–25 nt in length is incorporated into the RNA-induced silencing complex (RISC) where they target specific mRNAs for translational repression or mRNA cleavage therefore regulating gene expression.

**Table 8.1** Oncogenic miRNAs.

| miR | Chromosomic location | Tumor | Tumor | Impact on metastasis |
|---|---|---|---|---|
| miR-17–92 | chr 13 (q31.3) | TSP-1, CTGF | Colon | Promotes |
| | | E2F2, E2F3 | Prostate/Burkitt Lymphoma/testis carcinoma | |
| | | BIM | c-Myc-induced lymphoma | |
| | | PTEN | | |
| | | HIF1α | Lung cancer | |
| | | PTPRO | Cervix tumor cell line | |
| | | p63 | Myeloid cells | |
| | | BIM | T-cell acute lymphoblastic | |
| | | PTEN | Leukemia | |
| | | PRKAA1 | | |
| | | PPP2R5e | | |
| | | JAK1 | Endothelial cells | |
| | | HBP1 | Breast cancer | |
| | | p21(WAF1) | Ras-induced senescent fibroblasts | |
| | | TGFβII | Glioblastoma | |
| | | SMAD4 | | |
| | | MnSOD | Prostate cancer | |
| | | GPX2 | | |
| | | TRXR2 | | |
| miR-106a~363 | chr X (q26.2) | BIM, p21 | Gastric cancer | - |
| miR-106b~25 | chr 7 (q22.1) | E2F1 | Prostate cancer | |
| | | PTEN | Prostate cancer | |
| miR-21 | chr 17 (q23.1) | PTEN | Cholangiocarcinoma | Promotes |
| | | TPM1 | Breast cancer | |
| | | PDCD4 | Breast cancer | |
| | | SPRY1 | | |
| | | RECK, TIMP3 | Glioblastoma | |
| | | p63, JMY, TOPORS, TP53BP2, DAXX, HNRPK, TGFβRII | Glioblastoma | |
| | | MARKS | Prostate cancer | |
| | | ANP32A, SMARCA4 | Prostate cancer | |
| miR-155 | chr 21 (q21.3) | SOCS1 | Breast cancer | - |
| | | CEBPB, PU.1, CUTL1 | Breast cancer | |
| | | PICALM | | |
| | | BACH1, ZIC3 | | |
| | | ETS1, MEIS1 | Breast cancer | |
| | | C-MAF | Lymphocytes | |
| | | HGAL | Diffuse large B-cell lymphoma | |
| | | JMJD1A | Nasopharyngeal carcinoma | |
| | | WEE1 | Breast cancer | |
| | | TP53INP1 | Pancreatic cancer | |
| | | SMAD1, SMAD5, HIVEP2, CEBPB, RUNX2, MYO10 | | |
| | | FOXO3a | Breast cancer | |
| | | hMSH2, hMSH6, and hMLH1 | Colon cancer | |
| | | SMAD5 | Diffuse large B-cell lymphoma | |

still observed 23 days after injection. The authors also showed high bioavailability and silencing activity of the antagomirs in all the tissues tested except the brain tissue. Another important category of miRNA inhibitors is represented by the class of nucleic acid analogs in which the ribose ring is "locked" by a methylene bridge connecting the 2′-O atom and the 4′-C atom, known as LNAs.[77] By locking the molecule with the methylene bridge,

LNA oligonucleotides display unprecedented hybridization affinity toward complementary single-stranded RNAs, excellent mismatch discrimination and high aqueous solubility. "Anti-miR LNAs" have been used successfully in several *in vitro* studies to knock down specific miRNA expression. Systemic delivery of an unconjugated LNA anti-miR-122 has shown an effective antagonistic activity against liver-expressed miR-122 in nonhuman primates: by using

**Table 8.2** Tumor-suppressor miRNAs.

| miR | Chromosomic location | Tumor | Tumor | Impact on metastasis |
|---|---|---|---|---|
| miR-15/16 family | chr 13 (q14.2) | BCL2 | CLL | - |
| | chr 3 (q25.33) | COX-2 | Colon cancer | |
| | | COX-2 | Follicular lymphoma | |
| | | CEBPβ, CDC25a, CCNE1 | Fibroblast | |
| | | VEGF, VEGFR2, FGFR1 | Fibroblast | |
| | | FGF2, FGFR1 | Cancer-associated fibroblast | |
| | | CCNE1 | | |
| | | FGFR1, PI3KCa, MDM4, VEGFa | Multiple myeloma | |
| | | WIP1 | | |
| | | BMI-1 | Ovarian cancer | |
| | | CCND1, CCND2, CCNE1 | Lung cancer | |
| miR-31 | chr 9 (p21.3) | ITGA5, RDX, RhoA | Breast cancer | Suppresses |
| | | FZD3, M-RIP, MMP16 | | |
| | | SATB2 | Cancer-associated fibroblast | |
| miR-34 family | chr 1 (p36.22) | SIRT1 | Colon cancer | - |
| | chr 11 (q23.1) | BCL2, NOTCH, HMGA2 | | |
| | | MYC | Fibroblast | |
| | | AXL | Lung cancer | |
| | | MET | Ovarian cancer | |
| | | NANOG, SOX2, MYCN | Embryonic fibroblast | |
| | | SNAIL | Colon cancer | |
| Let-7 family | chr 9 (q22.32) | KRAS | Lung cancer | - |
| | chr 11 (q24.1) | HMGA2 | | |
| | chr 22 (q13.31) | MYC | Burkitt lymphoma | |
| | chr 21 (q21.1) | IMP-1 | | |
| | chr 19 (q13.41) | DICER | | |
| | chr X (p11.22) | CDC-34 | Fibroblast | |
| | chr 3 (p21.1) | Il6 | Breast cancer | |
| | chr 12 (q14.1) | E2F2, CCND2 | Prostate cancer | |
| | | BCL-XL | Liver cancer | |

three intravenous doses of 10 mg/kg in African green monkeys, the authors achieved an effective and long-lasting depletion of miR-122 in the liver without any evidence of LNA-associated toxicities or histopathological changes in the animals.[78] Elmen et al. also examined whether combining LNA anti-miR with phosphorothioate modifications could improve delivery of the compounds and silence miRNAs in mice without requiring additional chemical modifications. In a mouse model, intravenous injections of about 1–25 mg/kg of phosphorothioate-modified LNA anti-miR showed markedly improved efficiency in antagonizing miR-122 compared with cholesterol-conjugated antagomir-122, suggesting that phosphorothioate-modified LNAs are able to effectively silence their miRNA targets at much lower doses than cholesterol-based oligonucleotides.

A different methodology of miRNA inhibition is represented by the sponge mRNAs.[79] This is a dominant negative method in which the sponge mRNA contains multiple target sites complementary to the miRNA of interest. When the sponge is expressed at high levels, it specifically inhibits the activity of a family of miRNAs by sequestering the miRNAs from the endogenous targets. One of the best examples of the use of miRNA sponges in cancer research has been shown by Valastyan et al. in an effort to identify miRNAs with metastatic potential in a panel of breast cancer cell lines.[37] The

authors identified miR-31 as strongly downregulated in aggressive metastatic cancer. They set up an experimental model wherein human nonmetastatic breast cancer cells transduced with retroviral eGFP sponges for miR-31 or an irrelevant sequence were orthotopically implanted in mouse mammary fat pads. Primary tumor size was not significantly affected by the inhibition of miR-31, but, while the control sponge tumors did not metastasize, miR-31 sponge tumors metastasized to the lungs, forming ten times more lesions (easily identifiable by their GFP fluorescence). These results allowed the investigators to identify miR-31 as a suppressor of metastasis. A similar approach was also taken to show that miR-10b and miR-9 promote breast cancer metastasis.[80] A related experimental setting is represented by the application of a miRNA sponge to mimic the genetic state of patients with a genomic deletion of a particular miRNA or miRNA cluster. For example, miR-15a and miR-16 lentiviral GFP sponges were transduced in human prostate cancer cell lines and mir-15/16-inhibited cancer cells showed an enhanced tumor growth than their relative controls.[20] Although sponge technology has shown many positive aspects for discovery *in vitro* and *in vivo*, the antisense oligonucleotides technology is more promising from a therapeutic perspective, based on the development of new oligonucleotide chemistries and improvement in the delivery of antisense oligonucleotides to cells and tissues.

miRNA replacement represents the opportunity to explore the therapeutic potential of tumor suppressor miRNAs.[81] In the past, this therapeutic strategy has been already investigated for protein-coding tumor suppressor genes but a practical application of this approach is still far from the bedside. The logistic obstacles associated with the replacement gene therapy of protein-coding tumor suppressor genes usually involve the delivery of a relatively large DNA plasmid or viral vector that encodes the desired protein. In this scenario, miRNAs provide a new opportunity because—unlike proteins—miRNA mimics are substantially smaller, will merely have to enter the cytoplasm of target cells to be active and can be delivered systemically using modes and technologies that are also used for siRNAs. The most important aspect for exploring the therapeutic application of miRNAs is surely based on the ability of a single miRNA to control multiple oncogenes and oncogenic pathways that are commonly deregulated in cancer. In this way, even if the inhibitory effects induced by miRNAs on any particular target may be mild and may merely lead to a subtle reduction of protein expression, the simultaneous repression of a broad set of targets has far-reaching biological consequences that determine the course of the cellular phenotype. Another advantage of miRNA mimics consists in the sequence similarity between the miRNA mimic and the depleted tumor suppressor miRNA; therefore, it is expected that the miRNA mimic will target the same mRNAs pool that is also regulated by the natural miRNA.

The concept of miRNA replacement therapy is perhaps best exemplified by the *let-7* miRNA family. For example, the Slack laboratory demonstrated that let-7 is highly expressed in normal lung tissue, and overexpression of let-7 in cancer cell lines alters cell cycle progression and reduces cell division as well as the growth of lung cancer cell xenografts in immunodeficient mice. Using an established orthotopic mouse lung cancer model, the authors showed that intranasal let-7 administration reduces tumor formation *in vivo* in the lungs of animals expressing a G12D-activating mutation for the K-ras oncogene.[82,83] Another example that demonstrates the value of miRNA replacement is provided by miR-29 family. Garzon et al. found that enforced expression of miR-29a and -29b in AML cell lines and in primary AML blasts inhibited cell growth and induced apoptosis *in vitro* and *in vivo* through the downregulation of the Mcl-1 protein.[84] The data supported a tumor suppressor role for miR-29 and provide a rationale for the use of synthetic miR-29b oligonucleotides as a novel strategy to improve treatment response in AML.

Attacking multiple genes relevant to human disease at once is viewed as a powerful ability of therapeutic miRNA mimics. However, it also raises concerns about potential toxicity in normal tissues—especially under conditions where the therapeutic delivery of miRNA mimics will also lead to an accumulation of exogenous miRNA in normal cells. These toxic effects might be the result of overloading RISC with the exogenous miRNA, thereby competing with endogenous miRNAs necessary for normal cellular welfare, and/or hyperactivating cellular pathways that will also reduce the viability of normal cells. While these suppositions are well founded, *in vivo* evidence for toxicity induced by miRNA mimics is still lacking. Mouse studies that evaluated the therapeutic delivery of tumor suppressor miRNAs failed to reveal adverse events associated with miRNA and suggest that delivery of miRNA to normal tissues was well tolerated.[83,85] The miRNA sequences used in these studies are identical between the mouse and human species and, therefore, differences in homology will not account for the lack of toxicity in

normal tissues. Thus, therapeutic miRNA mimics may be better tolerated by normal cells than cancer cells because (i) pathways activated or repressed by the miRNA mimic are already activated or repressed by the endogenous miRNA; (ii) administration of therapeutic miRNA mimics is only an insignificant incremental increase of what is already present in normal cells; (iii) normal cells are not addicted to oncogenic pathways and manage to recover from the therapeutic dose used; or (iv) normal cells have the ability to regulate the activity or presence of the miRNA mimic while cancer cells do not. As therapeutic programs advance miRNAs closer to the clinic, it will become eminent to study miRNA-induced effects in normal cells and to assess potential toxicity in higher species.

## Conclusion

Studies from recent years have placed miRNAs as a critical class of regulator to protein-coding gene expression. As evolving evidence points out the importance of miRNA function during tumor development and progression, it is exciting to apply our knowledge and technology on miRNA into developing therapeutic reagents for treating cancer. Despite all advances that have been made in the new era of miRNA therapeutics there is still a significant gap between basic research on miRNAs and clinical application. Extensive pre-clinical and translational research is required to increase the efficacy and minimize the adverse effects of miRNA-based therapy. With better understanding of miRNA's function in tumor progression and more sophisticated design of miRNA-modulating molecules, miRNA-mediated therapy will give a new impetus to cure cancer.

## References

1 Grosshans H, Slack F. Micro-RNAs: small is plentiful. *J Cell Biol.* 2002;156(1):17–21.

2 Pasquinelli AE, Reinhart BJ, Slack F, et al. Conservation of the sequence and temporal expression of let-7 heterochronic regulatory RNA. *Nature.* 2000;408(6808):86–89.

3 Smallridge R. A small fortune. *Nat Rev Mol Cell Biol.* 2001;2(12): 867.

4 Bartel DP. MicroRNAs: genomics, biogenesis, mechanism, and function. *Cell.* 2004;116(2):281–297.

5 Eulalio A, Huntzinger E, Izaurralde E. Getting to the root of miRNA-mediated gene silencing. *Cell.* 2008;132(1):9–14.

6 Kim VN, Han J, Siomi MC. Biogenesis of small RNAs in animals. *Nat Rev Mol Cell Biol.* 2009;10(2):126–139.

7 Ruby JG, Jan CH, Bartel DP. Intronic microRNA precursors that bypass Drosha processing. *Nature.* 2007;448(7149):83–86.

8 Croce CM. Causes and consequences of microRNA dysregulation in cancer. *Nat Rev Genet.* 2009;10(10):704–714.

9 Mendell JT, Olson EN. MicroRNAs in stress signaling and human disease. *Cell.* 2012;148(6):1172–1187.

10 Ambros V. MicroRNA pathways in flies and worms: growth, death, fat, stress, and timing. *Cell.* 2003;113(6):673–676.

11 Calin GA. Dumitru CD, Shimizu M, et al. Frequent deletions and down-regulation of micro- RNA genes miR15 and miR16 at 13q14 in chronic lymphocytic leukemia. *Proc Natl Acad Sci U S A.* 2002;99(24):15524–15529.

12 Esquela-Kerscher A, Slack FJ. Oncomirs—microRNAs with a role in cancer. *Nat Rev Cancer.* 2006;6(4):259–269.

13 Calin GA, Croce CM. MicroRNA signatures in human cancers. *Nat Rev Cancer.* 2006;6(11):857–866.

14 Calin GA, Sevignani C, Dumitru CD, et al. Human microRNA genes are frequently located at fragile sites and genomic regions involved in cancers. *Proc Natl Acad Sci U S A*. 2004;101(9):2999–3004.

15 Cimmino A, Calin GA, Fabbri M, et al. miR-15 and miR-16 induce apoptosis by targeting BCL2. *Proc Natl Acad Sci U S A*. 2005;102(32):11755–11760.

16 Calin GA, Ferracin M, Cimmino A, et al. A microRNA signature associated with prognosis and progression in chronic lymphocytic leukemia. *N Engl J Med*. 2005;353(17):1793–1801.

17 Raveche ES, Salerno E, Scaglione BJ, et al. Abnormal microRNA-16 locus with synteny to human 13q14 linked to CLL in NZB mice. *Blood*. 2007;109(12):5079–5086.

18 Klein U, Lia M, Crespo M, et al. The DLEU2/miR-15a/16-1 cluster controls B cell proliferation and its deletion leads to chronic lymphocytic leukemia. *Cancer Cell*. 2010;17(1):28–40.

19 Roccaro AM, Sacco A, Thompson B, et al. MicroRNAs 15a and 16 regulate tumor proliferation in multiple myeloma. *Blood*. 2009;113(26):6669–6680.

20 Bonci D, Coppola V, Musumeci M, et al. The miR-15a-miR-16-1 cluster controls prostate cancer by targeting multiple oncogenic activities. *Nat Med*. 2008;14(11):1271–1277.

21 Musumeci M, Coppola V, Addario A, et al. Control of tumor and microenvironment cross-talk by miR-15a and miR-16 in prostate cancer. *Oncogene*. 2011;30(41):4231–4242.

22 Cannell IG, Bushell M. Regulation of Myc by miR-34c. *Cell Cycle*. 2010;9(14):2726–2730.

23 Suzuki H, Yamamoto E, Nojima M, et al. Methylation-associated silencing of microRNA-34b/c in gastric cancer and its involvement in an epigenetic field defect. *Carcinogenesis*. 2010;31(12):2066–2073.

24 Ji Q, Hao X, Nojima M, et al. MicroRNA miR-34 inhibits human pancreatic cancer tumor-initiating cells. *PLoS One*. 2009;4(8):e6816.

25 Christoffersen NR, Shalgi R, Frankel LB, et al. p53-independent upregulation of miR-34a during oncogene-induced senescence represses MYC. *Cell Death Differ*. 2008;17(2):236–245.

26 Liu C, Kelnar K, Liu B, et al. The microRNA miR-34a inhibits prostate cancer stem cells and metastasis by directly repressing CD44. *Nat Med*. 2011;17(2):211–215.

27 Cole KA, Attiyeh EF, Mosse YP, et al. A functional screen identifies miR-34a as a candidate neuroblastoma tumor suppressor gene. *Mol Cancer Res*. 2008;6(5):735–742.

28 Yamakuchi M, Ferlito M, Lowenstein CJ. miR-34a repression of SIRT1 regulates apoptosis. *Proc Natl Acad Sci U S A*. 2008;105(36):13421–13426.

29 Choi YJ, Lin C, Ho JJ, et al. miR-34 miRNAs provide a barrier for somatic cell reprogramming. *Nat Cell Biol*. 2011;13:1353–1360.

30 Concepcion CP, Han YC, Mu P, et al. Intact p53-dependent responses in miR-34-deficient mice. *PLoS Genet*. 2012;8(7):e1002797.

31 Johnson SM, Grosshans H, Shingara J. RAS is regulated by the let-7 microRNA family. *Cell*. 2005;120(5):635–647.

32 Kota J, Chivukula RR, O'Donnell KA, et al. Therapeutic microRNA delivery suppresses tumorigenesis in a murine liver cancer model. *Cell*. 2009;137(6):1005–1017.

33 Chen L, Zheng J, Zhang Y, et al. Tumor-specific expression of microRNA-26a suppresses human hepatocellular carcinoma growth via cyclin-dependent and -independent pathways. *Mol Ther*. 2011;19(8):1521–1528.

34 Kent OA, Chivukula RR, Mullendore M, et al. Repression of the miR-143/145 cluster by oncogenic Ras initiates a tumor-promoting feed-forward pathway. *Genes Dev*. 2010;24(24):2754–2759.

35 Pekarsky Y, Santanam U, Cimmino A, et al. Tcl1 expression in chronic lymphocytic leukemia is regulated by miR-29 and miR-181. *Cancer Res*. 2006;66(24):11590–11593.

36 Peter ME. Let-7 and miR-200 microRNAs: guardians against pluripotency and cancer progression. *Cell Cycle*. 2009;8(6):843–852.

37 Valastyan S, Reinhardt F, Benaich N, et al. A pleiotropically acting microRNA, miR-31, inhibits breast cancer metastasis. *Cell*. 2009;137(6):1032–1046.

38 Kumar MS, Lu J, Mercer KL, Golub TR, Jacks T. Impaired microRNA processing enhances cellular transformation and tumorigenesis. *Nat Genet*. 2007;39(5):673–677.

39 O'Donnell KA, Wentzel E, Zeller KI, Dang CV, Mendell JT. c-Myc-regulated microRNAs modulate E2F1 expression. *Nature*. 2005; 435(7043):839–843.

40 Ivanovska I, Ball AS, Diaz RL, et al. MicroRNAs in the miR-106b family regulate p21/CDKN1A and promote cell cycle progression. *Mol Cell Biol*. 2008;28(7):2167–2174.

41 Mu P, Han YC, Betel D, et al. Genetic dissection of the miR-17~92 cluster of microRNAs in Myc-induced B-cell lymphomas. *Genes Dev*. 2009;23(24):2806–2811.

42 Koralov SB, Muljo S, Galler GR, et al. Dicer ablation affects antibody diversity and cell survival in the B lymphocyte lineage. *Cell*. 2008; 132(5):860–874.

43 Volinia S, Calin GA, Liu CG, et al. A microRNA expression signature of human solid tumors defines cancer gene targets. *Proc Natl Acad Sci U S A*. 2006;103(7):2257–2261.

44 Ventura A, Young AG, Winslow MM, et al. Targeted deletion reveals essential and overlapping functions of the miR-17 through 92 family of miRNA clusters. *Cell*. 2008;132(5):875–886.

45 Huang GL, Zhang XH, Guo GL, Huang KT, Yang KY, Hu XQ. [Expression of microRNA-21 in invasive ductal carcinoma of the breast and its association with phosphatase and tensin homolog deleted from chromosome expression and clinicopathologic features]. *Zhonghua Yi Xue Za Zhi*. 2008;88(40):2833–2837.

46 Qian B, Katsaros D, Lu L, et al. High miR-21 expression in breast cancer associated with poor disease-free survival in early stage disease and high TGF-beta1. *Breast Cancer Res Treat*. 2009;117(1):131–140.

47 Corsten MF, Miranda R, Krichevsky AM, Weissleder R, Shah K. MicroRNA-21 knockdown disrupts glioma growth in vivo and displays synergistic cytotoxicity with neural precursor cell delivered S-TRAIL in human gliomas. *Cancer Res*. 2007; 67(19):8994–9000.

48 Gabriely G, Wurdinger T, Kesari S, et al. MicroRNA 21 promotes glioma invasion by targeting matrix metalloproteinase regulators. *Mol Cell Biol*. 2008;28(17):5369–5380.

49 Meng F, Henson R, Wehbe-Janek H, Ghoshal K, Jacob ST, Patel T. MicroRNA-21 regulates expression of the PTEN tumor suppressor gene in human hepatocellular cancer. *Gastroenterology*. 2007;133(2):647–658.

50 Selaru FM, Olaru AV, Kan T, et al. MicroRNA-21 is overexpressed in human cholangiocarcinoma and regulates programmed cell death 4 and tissue inhibitor of metalloproteinase 3. *Hepatology*. 2009;49(5):1595–1601.

51 Markou A, Tsaroucha EG, Kaklamanis L, Fotinou M, Georgoulias V, Lianidou ES. Prognostic value of mature microRNA-21 and microRNA-205 overexpression in non-small cell lung cancer by quantitative real-time RT-PCR. *Clin Chem*. 2008;54(10):1696–1704.

52 Li J, Huang H, Sun L, et al. MiR-21 indicates poor prognosis in tongue squamous cell carcinomas as an apoptosis inhibitor. *Clin Cancer Res*. 2009;15(12):3998–4008.

53 Hummel R, Hussey DJ, Michael MZ, et al. MiRNAs and their association with locoregional staging and survival following surgery for esophageal carcinoma. *Ann Surg Oncol.* 2011;18(1):253–260.

54 Zhang Z, Li Z, Gao C, et al. miR-21 plays a pivotal role in gastric cancer pathogenesis and progression. *Lab Invest.* 2008;88(12):1358–1366.

55 Asangani IA, Rasheed SA, Nikolova DA, et al. MicroRNA-21 (miR-21) post-transcriptionally downregulates tumor suppressor Pdcd4 and stimulates invasion, intravasation and metastasis in colorectal cancer. *Oncogene.* 2008;27(15):2128–2136.

56 Li Y, Zhu X, Gu J, et al. Anti-miR-21 oligonucleotide sensitizes leukemic K562 cells to arsenic trioxide by inducing apoptosis. *Cancer Sci.* 2010;101(4):948–954.

57 Yao Q, Xu H, Zhang QQ, Zhou H, Qu LH. MicroRNA-21 promotes cell prolifcration and down-regulates the expression of programmed cell death 4 (PDCD4) in HeLa cervical carcinoma cells. *Biochem Biophys Res Commun.* 2009;388(3):539–542.

58 Folini M, Gandellini P, Longoni N, et al. miR-21: an oncomir on strike in prostate cancer. *Mol Cancer.* 2010;9:12.

59 Zhu S, Si ML, Wu H, Mo YY. MicroRNA-21 targets the tumor suppressor gene tropomyosin 1 (TPM1). *J Biol Chem.* 2007;282(19):14328–14336.

60 Papagiannakopoulos T, Shapiro A, Kosik KS. MicroRNA-21 targets a network of key tumor-suppressive pathways in glioblastoma cells. *Cancer Res.* 2008;68(19):8164–8172.

61 Sayed D, Rane S, Lypowy J, et al. MicroRNA-21 targets Sprouty2 and promotes cellular outgrowths. *Mol Biol Cell.* 2008;19(8):3272–3282.

62 Valeri N, Gasparini P, Braconi C, et al. MicroRNA-21 induces resistance to 5-fluorouracil by down-regulating human DNA MutS homolog 2 (hMSH2). *Proc Natl Acad Sci U S A.* 2010;107(49):21098–21103.

63 Medina PP, Nolde M, Slack FJ. OncomiR addiction in an in vivo model of microRNA-21-induced pre-B-cell lymphoma. *Nature.* 2010;467(7311):86–90.

64 Ma X, Kumar M, Choudhury SN, et al. Loss of the miR-21 allele elevates the expression of its target genes and reduces tumorigenesis. *Proc Natl Acad Sci U S A.* 2011;108(25):10144–10149.

65 Cortez MA, Bueso-Ramos C, Ferdin J, et al. MicroRNAs in body fluids—the mix of hormones and biomarkers. *Nat Rev Clin Oncol.* 2011;8(8):467–477.

66 Boeri M, Verri C, Conte D, et al. MicroRNA signatures in tissues and plasma predict development and prognosis of computed tomography detected lung cancer. *Proc Natl Acad Sci U S A.* 2011;108(9):3713–3718.

67 Mitchell PS, Parkin RK, Kroh EM, et al. Circulating microRNAs as stable blood-based markers for cancer detection. *Proc Natl Acad Sci U S A.* 2008;105(30):10513–10518.

68 Valadi H, Ekström K, Bossios A, Sjöstrand M, Lee JJ, Lötvall JO. Exosome-mediated transfer of mRNAs and microRNAs is a novel mechanism of genetic exchange between cells. *Nat Cell Biol.* 2007;9(6):654–659.

69 Zernecke A, Bidzhekov K, Noels H, et al. Delivery of microRNA-126 by apoptotic bodies induces CXCL12-dependent vascular protection. *Sci Signal.* 2009;2(100):ra81.

70 Arroyo JD, Chevillet JR, Kroh EM, et al. Argonaute2 complexes carry a population of circulating microRNAs independent of vesicles in human plasma. *Proc Natl Acad Sci U S A.* 2011;108(12):5003–5008.

71 Turchinovich A, Weiz L, Langheinz A, Burwinkel B. Characterization of extracellular circulating microRNA. *Nucleic Acids Res.* 2011;39(16):7223–7233.

72 Fabbri M, Paone A, Calore F, et al. MicroRNAs bind to Toll-like receptors to induce prometastatic inflammatory response. *Proc Natl Acad Sci U S A.* 2012;109(31):E2120–E2126.

73 Leung AK, Sharp PA. MicroRNA functions in stress responses. *Mol Cell.* 2010;40(2):205–215.

74 Lennox KA, Behlke MA. A direct comparison of anti-microRNA oligonucleotide potency. *Pharm Res.* 2010;27(9):1788–1799.

75 Lennox KA, Behlke MA. Chemical modification and design of anti-miRNA oligonucleotides. *Gene Ther.* 2011;18(12):1111–1120.

76 Krützfeldt J, Rajewsky N, Braich R, et al. Silencing of microRNAs in vivo with 'antagomirs'. *Nature.* 2005;1438(7014):226–230.

77 Veedu RN, Wengel J. Locked nucleic acids: promising nucleic acid analogs for therapeutic applications. *Chem Biodivers.* 2010;7(3):536–542.

78 Elmen J, Lindow M, Schütz S, et al. LNA-mediated microRNA silencing in non-human primates. *Nature.* 2008;452(7189):896–899.

79 Ebert MS, Sharp PA. Emerging roles for natural microRNA sponges. *Curr Biol.* 2010;20(19):R858–R861.

80 Ma L, Young J, Prabhala H, et al. miR-9, a MYC/MYCN-activated microRNA, regulates E-cadherin and cancer metastasis. *Nat Cell Biol.* 2010;12(3):247–256.

81 Henry JC, Azevedo-Pouly AC, Schmittgen TD. MicroRNA replacement therapy for cancer. *Pharm Res.* 2011;28(12):3030–3042.

82 Johnson CD, Esquela-Kerscher A, Stefani G, et al. The let-7 microRNA represses cell proliferation pathways in human cells. *Cancer Res.* 2007;67(16):7713–7722.

83 Esquela-Kerscher A, Trang P, Wiggins JF, et al. The let-7 microRNA reduces tumor growth in mouse models of lung cancer. *Cell Cycle.* 2008;7(6):759–764.

84 Garzon R, Heaphy CE, Havelange V, et al. MicroRNA 29b functions in acute myeloid leukemia. *Blood.* 2009;114(26):5331–5341.

85 Castoldi M, Vujic Spasic M, Altamura S, et al. The liver-specific microRNA miR-122 controls systemic iron homeostasis in mice. *J Clin Invest.* 2011;121(4):1386–1396.

## CHAPTER 9

# Acute Myeloid Leukemia

*Ofir Wolach[1] and Richard M. Stone[2]*

[1]Adult Leukemia Program, Department of Medical Oncology, Dana-Farber Cancer Institute, Boston, MA, USA
[2]Department of Medical Oncology, Dana-Farber Cancer Institute, Boston, MA, USA

## Introduction

Acute myeloid leukemia (AML) represents a heterogeneous group of malignant hematopoietic stem cell disorders. It is the most common form of acute leukemia in adults with approximately 14,500 new cases reported in the United States in 2013. The incidence of AML significantly increases with age and the median age at diagnosis is approximately 70 years. Despite significant progress in our understanding of the pathogenetic processes associated with leukemogenesis, the outcome of patients with AML is still generally dismal and most patients die from their disease.[1,2] Recent data from a population-based registry in Sweden demonstrated a 5-year survival of 50–60% in younger adults up to the age of 44 years compared with less than 10% survival in patients over 65 years of age. While an improvement in survival was noted over the past decades in younger patients, a better outcome over time was not documented in the elderly population, mainly due to disease-related features associated with resistance to therapy and host-related factors such as age, functional status, and comorbidities.[3] Age, cytogenetics, and mutations in certain genes are the most powerful predictors of outcome and are used for prognostication and as means to guide therapy.[1,2] A detailed molecular description of AML was recently presented using whole-genome and whole-exome sequencing approaches. This study showed that there is an average of 13 mutations in an AML case, 5 of which are "drivers" which contribute to the pathophysiology, with at least one significant mutation in most patients.[4] While the prognostic relevance of some mutations such as FLT3-ITD and NPM1 are well established, the prognostic role of other mutations, as well as the complex interplay among the various mutations is still a matter of active research.[2,5]

Therapy for young and fit patients with AML involves intensive chemotherapy based on anthracycline and cytarabine followed by allogeneic stem cell transplantation (alloSCT) for most patients. Older and frail patients do not usually benefit from intensive cytotoxic approach in terms of survival; such therapies are frequently associated with significant treatment-related morbidity and mortality. Less intensive therapies such as hypomethylating agents (5-azacytidine and decitabine) and novel chemotherapeutic agents, such as clofarabine failed to convincingly prolong the survival of older patients with AML when tested in randomized controlled trials but are frequently used alone or in combination with other drugs in such patients.[1,2]

The abundance of genetic information and the growing understanding of survival and proliferation pathways in leukemic cells coupled with technological advancements in interventional capabilities such as production of monoclonal antibodies (mAb) or the assembly of chimeric T-cell receptors create many previously unavailable therapeutic opportunities to combat AML. Targeting specific elements of apoptotic pathways, kinase activation cascades and aspects of cellular metabolism, cell cycle regulation, nuclear transport of regulatory proteins, and the cross talk of leukemia cells with the microenvironment within the bone marrow (BM) niche are all active fields of pre-clinical and clinical research. Herein we summarize the main advancements and evolving approaches in the targeted therapy of AML (Table 9.1).

## Monoclonal Antibodies

Leukemic cells display a distinct set of surface molecules, which can be used to define lineage [AML vs. acute lymphoblastic leukemia (ALL)]. Since these moieties are accessible to circulating antibodies, the use of mAb to target these surface molecules represents an attractive therapeutic approach. "Naked" or simple antibodies usually kill the malignant target cell via Fc-mediated complement dependent cytotoxicity (CDC), antibody-dependent cell cytotoxicity (ADCC), or by direct toxicity.[6] Alternatively, engineered antibodies may be used as a means to deliver cytotoxic moieties (such as chemotherapy or a radioisotope) to the malignant cell. In addition, antibodies that target components of the immune system and promote an attack on leukemia cells are an evolving therapeutic approach.

### Antibodies Targeting CD33

CD33 is a 67-kDa transmembrane glycoprotein of unknown physiologic function that is predominantly found on cells of the myeloid lineage and is expressed on the surface of myeloid blasts in approximately 90% of AML cases.[7] Gemtuzumab ozogamicin (GO; Mylotarg) is a humanized anti-CD33 IgG4 mAb toxic conjugate which is linked to a semisynthetic derivative of calicheamicin, a potent cytotoxic anthracycline antibiotic.[7,8]

GO received accelerated FDA approval in 2000 as monotherapy for older patients with relapsed AML based on three phase II trials that enrolled 142 patients aged 43–73 years. The rates of

*Targeted Therapy in Translational Cancer Research*, First Edition. Edited by Apostolia-Maria Tsimberidou, Razelle Kurzrock and Kenneth C. Anderson.
© 2016 John Wiley & Sons, Inc. Published 2016 by John Wiley & Sons, Inc.

**Table 9.1** Targeted therapeutic approaches in AML.

| Compound | Class/mechanism | Stage of development/study | Clinical activity | Reference number |
|---|---|---|---|---|
| **Monocloncal antibodies** | | | | |
| Gemtuzumab ozogomicin | Anti-CD33 Ab conjugated to calicheamicin | Phase III RCT's | Active drug in favorable and intermediate risk AML and in APL | 7–19 |
| SGN-CD33A | Anti-CD33 Ab conjugated to a pyrrolobenzodiazepine dimer | Phase I ongoing | NA | 22, 23 |
| Lintuzumab-225 actinium | Alpha-particle nano-generator actinium-225 conjugated to lintuzumab, humanized anti-CD33 antibody | Phase I–II ongoing | Safe and tolerable; active in early phase clinical trials | 20, 21 |
| AMG 330 | BiTE with CD33 and CD3ε specifcity | Pre-clinical | NA | 25 |
| Brentuximab | Anti-CD30 monoclonal antibody linked to the anti-mitotic agent monomethyl auristatin E | Phase I ongoing | NA | |
| CSL360 | Chimeric anti-CD123 | Phase I | Safe and tolerable; no significant anti-leukemic activity in early phase clinical trials | 26 |
| IPH2101 | Anti-inhibitory KIR monoclonal antibody | Phase I | Safe and tolerable; encouraging preliminary results | 32 |
| CT-011 | Anti-PD-1 | Phase I ongoing for patients in remission in conjunction with a dendritic cell AML fusion vaccine | NA | |
| Ipilimumab | Anti-CTLA-4 | Phase I trial ongoing | NA | 37 |
| **Farnesyltransferase inhibitors** | | | | |
| Tipifarnib | Farnesyltransferase inhibitor | Phase III as monotherapy; phase II for combination regimens | Does not improve outcome as monotherapy; encouraging preliminary results in combination with other drugs | 40–44 |
| **Tyrosine kinase inhibitors** | | | | |
| Dasatinib | KIT inhibitor | Ongoing phase II trials | High remission rates when combined with chemotherapy; pending long-term results. Therapy for MRD positive CBF AML does not prevent relapse | 49–51 |
| Sorafenib | FLT3 inhibitor | Phase III trials ongoing/completed in combination with chemotherapy; phase II in combination with novel agents. | No overall survival benefit; improved EFS in younger patients | 56–64 |
| Lestaurtinib | FLT3 inhibitor | Phase III completed for combination therapy in the salvage setting; ongoing phase III in newly diagnosed | No benefit in combination with salvage chemotherapy in patients with relapsed AML | 65, 66 |
| Midostaurin | FLT3 inhibitor | Completed phase III—pending results | Blast and hematologic responses as monotherapy in phase II trials; pending results of phase III trial in combination with chemotherapy | 67–69 |
| Quizartinib | FLT3 inhibitor | Phase II | Significant responses in relapsed and refractory patients as single agent; one-third of patients salvaged to alloSCT | 71–76 |
| Crenolanib | FLT3 inhibitor | Phase II | Safe and tolerable; encouraging preliminary results | 77–79 |
| Selumetinib (AZD6244) | MEK inhibitor | Phase II | Modest responses in FLT3-ITD negative patients | 45 |
| GSK212 | MEK inhibitor | Phase I–II | Significant responses (including CR) in patients with RAS mutations | 46 |

**Table 9.1** (*Continued*)

| Compound | Class/mechanism | Stage of development/study | Clinical activity | Reference number |
|---|---|---|---|---|
| **Inhibitors of anti-apoptotoic pathways, cancer metabolism, and cellular signaling** | | | | |
| AG-120 | IDH1 inhibitor | Phase I ongoing | NA | |
| AG-221 | IDH2 inhibitor | Phase I ongoing | Safe and tolerable; encouraging preliminary results | 83 |
| OTX-015 | Bromodomain inhibitor | Phase I | Safe and tolerable; encouraging preliminary results | 84 |
| EPZ-5676 | DOT1L inhibitor | Phase I | Safe and tolerable; encouraging preliminary results in MLL rearranged leukemia | 85 |
| ABT-199 | BCL-2 inhibitor | Phase II ongoing | NA | 89, 90 |
| RG7112 | MDM2 inhibitor | Phase I | Promising preliminary results as monotherapy and in combination with cytarabine | 84, 85 |
| Selinexor (KPT-330) | Selective inhibitor of nuclear transport | Phase I ongoing | Manageable toxicity and apparent efficacy in phase I trial | 96 |
| Plerixafor | CXCR4 inhibitor | Phase I/II | Active in early phase clinical trials in combination with salvage chemotherapy | 99 |
| PF-04449913 | Hedgehog pathway inhibitor | Phase I | Safe and tolerable; encouraging preliminary results | 101 |
| **Chimeric antigen receptors and vaccines** | | | | |
| CAR T cells | Anti-CD123 CAR T cells | Pre-clinical | NA | 103 |
| CAR T cells | Anti-CD44v6 CAR T cells | Pre-clinical | NA | 104 |
| CAR T cells | Anti-LeY CAR T cells | Phase I ongoing | Manageable toxicity; encouraging preliminary results | 105 |
| WT1 vaccine | Peptide and DC–based vaccine targeting WT1 | Phase I/II | Manageable toxicity; clinical response in relapsed and refractory patients and as maintenance in CR | 108 |

RCTs – randomized controlled trials; NA – not available; MRD – minimal residual disease; alloSCT – allogeneic stem cell transplantation; DC – dendritic cells; EFS – event free survival.

complete remission (CR) were 16% and approached 30% when patients in remission with incomplete platelet recovery (CRp) were included in the analysis. The CR and CRp rates for patients over 60 years of age ($n = 80$) were 15% and 26%, respectively. Relapse-free survival (RFS) for patients over 60 was 17 months.[8] In 2010, GO was withdrawn from the market based on the results of the SWOG 0106 study,[9] in which 637 younger AML patients (18–60 years) were randomized to standard induction with cytarabine and daunorubicin (60 mg/m$^2$) or similar induction (albeit with daunorubicin 45 mg/m$^2$) with GO at 6 mg/m$^2$ on day 4 of induction. Patients in CR after consolidation with high-dose cytarabine were randomized to further GO versus observation. No difference between the two treatment arms was noted in CR rates or in the overall survival (OS) at 5 years (46% vs. 50% for the GO and control arms, respectively; $p = 0.85$). Treatment-related mortality in the GO arm was 5% compared with 1% in the control arm. The lack of GO efficacy and higher treatment-related mortality in SWOG 0106 coupled with reports of significant hepatotoxicity, notably sinusoidal obstructive syndrome[10] led to drug withdrawal. However, efficacy and safety data that emerged from several subsequent prospective trials challenged the decision to withdraw GO from the market. The MRC AML 15 trial randomized 1113 younger AML patients to GO 3 mg/m$^2$ on the first day of one of three induction arms. Patients were further randomized to an additional GO dose on one of three consolidation arms. While GO did not affect the rates of response or survival in the entire cohort, a predetermined analysis based on cyto-

genetic risk demonstrated a significant survival benefit for patients with favorable cytogenetics and a trend toward benefit in patients with intermediate-risk cytogenetics. No benefit was observed in patients with poor cytogenetics.[11] In the AML 16 trial, 1115 patients with a median age of 67 years (range, 51–84 years) were randomized to GO 3 mg/m$^2$ on day 1 with either daunorubicin/cytarabine or daunorubicin/clofarabine-based induction. While no difference was noted in CR/CRp rates (approximately 70% in both groups) or in treatment-related mortality, the addition of GO was associated with significant improvements in the 3-year cumulative incidence of relapse (68% and 76% in favor of the GO group) and in 3-year OS (25% and 20% for GO vs. no GO groups, respectively). In contrast to the AML15 trial, in this older population the benefit of GO was observed across all cytogenetic risk groups.[12] Another trial that favored the addition of GO was the ALFA-0701 French randomized phase III trial that enrolled 280 patients between the ages of 50 and 70 years (median, 62 years) to standard induction and consolidation or the same treatment with five doses of GO 3 mg/m$^2$ on days 1, 3, and 7 of induction and on day 1 of both consolidations. The use of this "fractionated" administration was associated with similar CR/CRp rates but demonstrated a dramatic increase in the 2-year event-free survival (EFS; 40.8% vs. 17.1%), OS (53.2% vs. 41.9%), and RFS (50.3% vs. 22.7%) in favor of the GO arm with no increase in the risk of toxic death.[13] Other trials failed to demonstrate an advantage for adding GO to chemotherapy. The United Kingdom LRF AML14 and NCRI AML 16 trials studied the utility of GO in the older, high-risk population who are ineligible for intensive therapy and randomized 495 patients to the addition of GO 5 mg/m$^2$ on day 1 of a low-dose cytarabine regimen for up to four cycles. GO improved the remission rates significantly (30% for the GO arm vs. 17% in the control arm) but this did not translate into a 1-year OS benefit (OS of approximately 25%).[14] A sequential treatment approach was recently reported by the EORTC and GIMEMA Consortium AML17 trial, in which 472 older patients (median age 67; range 61–75 years) were randomized to intensive induction and consolidation with or without GO at 6 mg/m$^2$ on days 1 and 15 administered up to 28 days before induction chemotherapy (depending on the response to initial GO). Patients randomized to GO at induction who achieved CR/CRp also received GO at 3 mg/m$^2$ with each consolidation. There was a trend toward reduced OS in the GO arm (median OS, 7.1 months vs. 10 months in the GO and control arms, respectively; $p = 0.07$) possibly related to the increased 30- and 60-day mortality rates in the GO arm (22% vs. 18% at 60 days) that was most prominent in patients older than 70 years.[15] The conflicting results in these various randomized trials suggest that the efficacy as well as toxicity of GO may be affected by patient-related factors such as disease risk and age, and by drug dose and timing of administration. Novel approaches which combine GO with newer agents such as epigenetic modifiers are an active area of clinical research.[16]

In APL, GO demonstrated significant activity in patients with molecular relapse[17] as well as in combination with arsenic trioxide (ATO) and all-trans retinoic acid (ATRA) for patients with hematologic relapse,[18] or as an adjuvant cytoreductive agent in the setting of upfront therapy for high-risk patients.[19]

Lintuzumab, a humanized anti-CD33 antibody, did not confer a survival benefit when added to MEC (mitoxantrone, etoposide, and cytarabine) chemotherapy in a phase III randomized trial involving 191 patients with relapsed/refractory AML (RR-AML).[20] Lintuzumab conjugated to the alpha-particle nano-generator actinium-225 is currently being tested in a phase I study in elderly patients with high-risk AML in combination with low-dose cytarabine with preliminary reports demonstrating safety and anti-leukemic activity.[21] SGN-CD33 A, a humanized anti-CD33 antibody conjugated to a novel synthetic DNA-linking pyrrolobenzodiazepine dimer, is a new compound that is currently being tested in a phase I study.[22] In pre-clinical models, this drug is more potent than GO and is active in multidrug-resistant cell lines.[23]

Another immunotherapeutic approach is to recruit the patients' own T cells and retarget them against the leukemic blasts. Bispecific T-cell engaging (BiTE) antibody is an antibody construct that physically approximates the cytotoxic T lymphocytes to tumor surface antigens. Such an approach with blinatumomab, a BiTE antibody with CD19 and CD3ε specificity, yielded encouraging early clinical results in acute lymphoblastic leukemia (ALL).[24] Recently, AMG330, a new BiTE compound directed against CD33 and CD3ε was shown to be effective in *ex vivo* primary AML blast cultures.[25]

## Non-CD33 Antibody Targets

CD123, the alpha subunit of interleukin 3 receptor (IL3R), has been shown to be aberrantly overexpressed on AML blasts, including in the CD34+ CD38– compartment of the leukemia stem cells (LSC).[6] Encouraging *in vitro* data was followed by phase I studies with several compounds including a chimeric, anti-CD123, "naked" antibody[26] and single chain variable antibody fragments conjugated to toxins such as the *diphtheria* toxin.[27] Dual affinity re-targeting molecules (DARTs) are engineered antibody constructs with speci-

ficity for both CD123 and CD3 that are made of two independent polypeptides comprised of the V$^H$ of one antibody in tandem with the V$^L$ of the other antibody. Encouraging data in AML mouse models were recently presented with this approach.[28]

Increasing interest in CD30 as a therapeutic target in AML recently emerged following the demonstration that CD30 was detected by flow cytometry in one-third of 135 samples of patients with AML and MDS[29] and was detected by immunohistochemistry in one-half of 26 bone-marrow biopsies of patients with AML with a strong association to FLT3 positivity in the latter study.[30] Brentuximab, an anti-CD30 mAB linked to the anti-mitotic agent monomethyl auristatin E, is FDA-approved for the treatment of Hodgkin's lymphoma and anaplastic large cell lymphoma. Brentuximab is currently being tested in an ongoing phase I trial in combination with salvage chemotherapy for patients with CD30-positive relapsed AML (NCT01830777).

## Antibodies to Target the Immune System

Another interesting approach to immunotherapy in AML is to augment the immunologic response against AML blasts by targeting non-leukemic antigens. Natural killer (NK) cells are members of the innate immune system and play a significant role in the eradication of cancer cells. NK recognition and cytotoxicity are regulated by a complex set of inhibitory and activating NK-cell receptors. When binding to their ligand, killer cell immunoglobulin-like receptors (KIRs) prevent NK-cell activation and it was previously suggested that KIR inhibition may be associated with an anti-leukemic effect.[31] IPH2101, an anti-inhibitory KIR mAB, was tested in a phase I trial in 23 elderly patients with AML in first remission. The use of IPH2101 was well tolerated and among the 20 evaluable patients, the median progression-free survival (PFS), RFS, and OS were 7.7, 10.8, and 12.7 months, respectively. A dose-dependent improvement in OS was observed.[32]

The interaction between programmed death-ligand 1 and 2 (PD-L1 and PD-L2) and PD-1 on activated T-cells represents a negative regulatory mechanism that represses T-cell activation. Tumors frequently express PD-L1 and PD-L2 as means to escape T-cell-mediated lysis.[33] Indeed, significant clinical responses were observed in patients with advanced cancer when treated with antibodies that block either PD-1 or PD-L1.[34] In one study, 18% of newly diagnosed patients with AML expressed high levels of PD-L1,[35] and the use of an antibody to block this ligand was shown in another study to reduce tumor burden and prolong survival in AML mouse models.[33] An ongoing phase I trial is assessing the safety of a dendritic cell (DC) AML fusion vaccine in combination with CT-011, a humanized mAb targeting PD-1 in patients with AML in remission (NCT01096602).

Another negative T-cell regulator that impairs T-cell response against leukemic cells is the cytotoxic T-lymphocyte associated antigen 4 (CTLA-4). Targeting this antigen with ipilimumab, a fully humanized mAB, demonstrated significant clinical activity in malignant melanoma.[36] Phase I trials are ongoing in patients with relapsed or refractory AML (NCT01757639, NCT00060372, NCT01822509[37]).

## Targeting Drivers of Proliferation in AML

The use of deep sequencing to study the molecular genomics of AML resulted in the identification of several classes of mutations that drive the process of leukemogenesis. Gene mutations that probably have relevance to the pathogenesis of AML can be categorized into nine groups: transcription-factor fusions, tumor suppressors, DNA-methylation-related genes, signaling genes, chromatin-modifying genes, myeloid transcription factor genes, cohesion complex genes, spliceosome complex genes, and NPM1.[4] Mutations in genes associated with constitutional activation of cell signaling and proliferation pathways in AML (e.g., RAS, FLT3, c-KIT) are the focus of many interventional efforts to combat AML and are discussed herein.

## RAS Inhibitors

The Ras/mitogen-activated protein kinase (MAPK) signaling pathway plays a central role in cell proliferation, differentiation, adhesion, and apoptosis. The Ras genes include H-ras, N-ras, and K-ras that encode small guanosine nucleotide-bound GTPases that are critical for intracellular signaling.[38] Activating mutations in the Ras genes are present in one-third of human tumors. In AML, mutations in N-ras can be found in approximately 10% of patients.[39] Farnesyltransferase (FT) is an enzyme involved in post-translational lipid modification of proteins that is critical for biological functionality of Ras-encoded proteins and inhibition of this enzyme by FT inhibitors (FTI), specifically tipifarnib, was the focus of many clinical trials in AML.[38] Phase I and II trials with tipifarnib in patients with high-risk AML demonstrated overall response rates (ORR) of 11–23% and remission rates of 4–14% that were interestingly unrelated to the mutational status of Ras.[40,41] Subsequently, a phase III trial randomized 457 elderly AML patients (over 70 years of age) to tipifarnib 600 mg bid for 21 of 28-day cycles or best supportive care (BSC). No difference in OS was noted between the groups (107 days vs. 109 days for the intervention and BSC groups, respectively).[42] The addition of tipifarnib to low-dose cytarabine in older patients with AML did not improve survival in the randomized British AML16 trial.[43] The combination of tipifarnib with etoposide may be synergistic and resulted in higher response rates in a phase II study (CR, 25%). This study also identified a 2-gene model based on the expression ratio of RASGRP1 to APTX that was able to predict response to tipifarnib.[44]

## MEK Inhibitors

Inhibition of TK targets downstream RAS in the RAS/RAF/MEK/ERK signaling pathway is an active area of clinical research in AML. Selumetinib (AZD6244) is a potent, selective, oral, non-ATP competitive mitogen-activated extracellular signal-related kinase (MEK) inhibitor that was investigated in 47 patients with high-risk AML in a phase II trial. This drug was administered at 100 mg bid in a continuous manner and was shown to be safe and well tolerated. Responses were modest (one PR and five blast responses) and were observed only in patients without FLT3-ITD mutations. Responses were correlated with a specific polymorphism in KIT.[45] In a phase I/II trial another MEK inhibitor, GSK212, was administered to 45 patients with relapsed/refractory myeloid malignancies, 42 of whom had AML. Rash and diarrhea were reported as the principle adverse events and myelosuppression did not occur. Significant responses were noticed in RAS-mutated patients ($n = 13$) with an ORR of 31% including three cases of CR/CRp, while RAS wild-type patients responded poorly (ORR 8% without CR).[46]

## KIT Inhibitors

KIT (CD117) plays an essential role in normal hematopoiesis. This protein is a member of the type III receptor tyrosine kinase (RTK) family. Normally, binding of the receptors' ligand, stem cell factor (SCF), will prompt dimerization of the receptor followed by autophosphorylation of KIT and subsequent activation of downstream signaling pathways such as Ras/MAPK, PI3K, Src kinase, and JAK/STAT. Activating mutations in KIT affect approximately one-third of patients with core binding factor AML (CBF-AML). Mutational clusters in KIT are found mainly in exon 17 (that encodes the activation loop) and exon 8 (that encodes an extracellular portion of the receptor). The prognostic effect of mutations in KIT was assessed in numerous retrospective analyses. KIT mutations seem to negatively impact outcome of patients with CBF-AML especially in patients with (8;21) translocation and exon 17 mutations.[47] The impact of the recognition of KIT mutation on clinical decision analysis is still unclear. According to the latest National Comprehensive Cancer Network (NCCN) consensus statement, the identification of KIT mutations will render a CBF-AML patient from favorable to intermediate-risk group.[1] Since KIT mutations seem to drive proliferation and affect outcome and since KIT is highly expressed even in non-mutated CBF-AML patients,[47] inhibition of KIT is an attractive therapeutic goal. Indeed, dasatinib, a potent KIT inhibitor, demonstrated efficacy in restricting growth of cells expressing wild-type and mutant KIT in vitro.[48] Anecdotal reports on the efficacy of dasatinib in CBF-AML with mutated KIT were also reported.[49] In the CALGB 10801 phase II trial, the safety and efficacy of dasatinib 100 mg/day combined with chemotherapy followed by dasatinib maintenance in patients with CBF-AML was assessed (regardless of KIT mutational status). Sixty-one patients (age, 19–85 years) received standard induction and consolidation chemotherapy with dasatinib administered immediately following every treatment cycle and 1 year of maintenance. The initial outcome and toxicity data were recently presented with very encouraging remission rates of 90% (93% and 79% for younger and older patients, respectively) and manageable toxicity.[50] In another report, dasatinib was administered as monotherapy to 26 patients with CBF AML in hematologic remission that had molecular evidence of disease or molecular relapse. Therapy with dasatinib did not prevent hematologic relapse in these patients and relapse rates were not reduced as compared to similar patients that did not receive dasatinib.[51] Clinical trials are ongoing to better define the role of KIT inhibition in CBF-AML.

## FLT3 Inhibitors

FLT3 receptor is a type III RTK that is expressed in normal hematopoietic cells and activates various downstream pathways associated with cell proliferation, differentiation, and survival. Activating mutations in FLT3 are found in approximately one-third of patients with AML. The most common activating mutation in FLT3 is an internal tandem duplication at the juxtamembrane domain (FLT3-ITD) and is associated with high relapse rates and poor patient outcome.[52] The allele burden of FLT3-ITD was shown to correlate with patient outcome,[53] while the effect of the ITD length on survival is still a matter of debate.[53,54] Single amino acid substitutions in the FLT3 tyrosine kinase (TK) domain (most commonly at codons D835 and I836) occur in AML at a frequency 4.8–7.7%[55] and their prognostic value is unclear.[52] Over the past years, numerous FLT3 inhibitors were introduced in pre-clinical and clinical research. Most of these compounds are structural mimics of the purine component of ATP and act by occupying the ATP-binding pocket of the TK. The various FLT3 inhibitors are oral agents that differ in their specificity, potency, and safety profile. Several reports describe their efficacy as monotherapy or in combination with other drugs in different AML disease settings.

Sorafenib is a multi-kinase inhibitor with inhibitory activity on FLT3, KIT, N-Ras, and RAF kinase, each of which may be useful in AML treatment. It is FDA-approved for advanced renal cell carcinoma and hepatocellular carcinoma; its activity in this setting is believed to be due to inhibition of vascular endothelial growth factor (VEGFR). Several trials demonstrated a clinically significant effect of sorafenib in patients with FLT3-ITD positive RR-AML. Metzelder et al. retrospectively studied 65 such patients, 29 of which relapsed after alloSCT. In this study, sorafenib monotherapy produced hematologic responses in 37%, CR/CRi in 23%, and complete molecular remissions in 15% of patients. Treatment of patients that relapsed after alloSCT was associated with less resistance and longer response durations to sorafenib therapy as compared to patients without prior alloSCT, suggesting that sorafenib may work synergistically to augment the graft versus leukemia effect.[56] Another study reported less encouraging results for sorafenib therapy in the setting of relapse after alloSCT with only 3 of 16 patients achieving PR without any CR reported.[57] A recent phase I trial demonstrated acceptable safety and encouraging efficacy signals for sorafenib when given as maintenance for patients with FLT3-ITD AML after alloSCT.[58] Sorafenib has also been tested in combination with other agents. Ravandi and colleagues studied the addition of sorafenib to idarubicin and cytarabine-based induction in 55 younger AML patients in a phase I–II trial. The addition of sorafenib to the induction regimen was safe with short-term outcomes comparable to historical controls. Of note, very high CR rates were achieved among patients that were FLT3-ITD positive (14 of 15 patients).[59] A phase III study of the European Study Alliance Leukemia randomized 201 older patients with newly diagnosed AML (age 60–80 years) regardless of their FLT3 mutation status to standard daunorubicin/cytarabine induction with either placebo or sorafenib given at 400 mg bid from 3 days after the end of chemotherapy until 3 days before the start of the next cycle. Patients in CR were randomized to 1 year of sorafenib maintenance. The addition of sorafenib did not confer an advantage in terms of EFS or OS. Moreover, the addition of sorafenib was associated with higher rates of early death (17% in the sorafenib arm vs. 7% in the control arm; $p = 0.052$).[60] Similarly, the addition of sorafenib to low-dose cytarabine in elderly high risk patients failed to demonstrate benefit.[61] Chemotherapy may elicit overexpression of FLT3 ligand that may interfere with FLT3 inhibition by sorafenib.[62,63] A recently reported large German phase III randomized placebo controlled trial studied the sequential addition of sorafenib to standard induction and consolidation chemotherapy in 267 younger patients with AML (age 18-60 years) regardless of their FLT3 mutational status. The addition of sorafenib was associated with similar remission rates but significantly better EFS (40% vs. 22%) and RFS (56% vs. 38%) at 3 years. Interestingly, these favorable results did not translate into an OS advantage, possibly reflecting the impact of alloSCT in first remission, offered to higher risk patients in this trial.[64] Encouraging results were reported with the combination of sorafenib with 5-azacytidine. In a phase II trial 43 patients with relapsed or refractory AML (93% harboring the FLT3-ITD mutation) were treated with repeated cycles of azacytidine 75 mg/m$^2$ for 7 days every 1–2 months combined with continuous sorafenib 400 mg bid. An ORR of 46% was observed with 43% achieving CR/CRi. The median duration of remission was 2.3 months with some patients having remissions lasting longer than a year. Interestingly, the FLT3 ligand surge that characterized the combination trials containing chemotherapy was blunted with this protocol.[62]

Lestaurtinib is another multi-kinase inhibitor with potent FLT3 receptor inhibition. Phase I and II trials of lestaurtinib demonstrated significant responses in patients with high-risk AML irrespective of FLT3 genotype.[65] A subsequent randomized trial assessed the addition of lestaurtinib to salvage chemotherapy in patients with FLT3-mutated relapsed AML. This study did not demonstrate a survival advantage for the addition of lestaurtinib.[66] Correlative studies demonstrated that most patients did not achieve FLT3 target inhibition, possibly due to the aforementioned FLT3 ligand surge.

Midostaurin (PKC412) is a FLT3 inhibitor that is currently evaluated in a large phase III randomized controlled trial. Midostaurin effectively inhibits various TKs, such as FLT3 (including FLT3 ITD and TKD), KIT and PDGFR and is currently evaluated in various hematologic clonal diseases such as AML and aggressive mastocytosis. In a phase IIB trial, 95 patients with relapsed/refractory or newly diagnosed (ineligible for chemotherapy) AML received midostaurin at either 50 mg or 100 mg bid as monotherapy. Reduction in blast counts were observed in more than two-thirds of patients with FLT3-ITD and in 42% of patients with unmutated FLT3 albeit with only one marrow remission.[67] Combining midostaurin with standard induction and consolidation was shown to be safe and potentially advantageous in a phase IB dose-finding trial that demonstrated a 14-day 50 mg bid schedule to be most tolerable with apparent efficacy.[68] The CALGB 10603 (RATIFY) trial is a randomized, placebo controlled study that randomized younger patients with newly diagnosed AML to standard induction and consolidation with either placebo or midostaurin at 50 mg bid for 14 of 28-day cycles followed by 1-year maintenance with the FLT3 inhibitor. This study recently completed accrual and results are eagerly anticipated.[69] As with other FLT3 inhibitors, early phase clinical studies demonstrate encouraging efficacy/toxicity profiles for the combination of midostaurin with novel drugs such as hypomethylating agents and mTOR inhibitors.

Some of the most exiting early clinical results are emerging with the non-protein bound potent FLT3 inhibitor quizartinib, a bis-aryl urea derivate.[70] A dose escalation phase I trial ($n = 76$) demonstrated that the maximum tolerated dose was 200 mg/day with grade III QT prolongation occurring at higher doses. Responses were observed at doses as low as 18 mg/day with 30% of all patients achieving remission or significant blast reduction (53% and 14% in the FLT3-ITD and wild type FLT3, respectively).[71] A large phase II trial included 333 patients and was composed of two patient cohorts that received oral quizartinib continuously at 90 mg/day for females and 135 mg/day for males. Cohort 1 comprised of 134 patients over 60 years of age with refractory AML or AML that relapsed within a year of first-line treatment. Cohort 2 included 137 patients over the age of 18 years that were either refractory to initial therapy or relapsed after second-line therapy, including after alloSCT. The composite remission (CRc = CR + Cri + CRp) rate in cohort 1 was 54% and 32% for ITD mutated and unmutated FLT3 patients, respectively; the median OS for patients with mutated and unmutated FLT3 was 25.3 and 19 weeks, respectively. In cohort 2, the CRc was 44% and 34% for ITD mutated and unmutated patients, respectively; the median OS for patients with mutated and unmutated FLT3 was 23.1 and 25.6 weeks, respectively. One-third of treated patients in cohort II were successfully bridged to alloSCT.[72,73] Further subgroup analysis of this cohort demonstrated that the 1-year OS of patients positive for FLT3-ITD that were transplanted after achieving at least a PR was 39%, regardless of the depth of remission prior to transplant. In contrast, patients that achieved CRc or PR that was not followed by alloSCT had 1-year OS of 25% and 5%, respectively. Among patients with unmutated FLT3 that were salvaged with quizartinib and alloSCT, the 1-year OS rates for patients achieving pre-transplant CRc or PR were 78% and 50%, respectively.[74] Furthermore it was demonstrated that patients over 70 years benefit from this therapy in terms of CRc rates with manageable toxicities.[75] Several phase I and II clinical trials are currently studying quizartinib in combination with chemotherapy or hypomethylating agents.[76]

A putative mechanism of resistance to quizartinib and other FLT3 inhibitors involves the emergence of kinase domain activating point mutations (namely D835 and F691L) that confer resistance to FLT3 inhibition. Most FLT3 inhibitors studied to date, including quizartinib, are type II TK inhibitors that can only bind to the inactive form of FLT3 receptor and are limited in efficacy when kinase domain mutations destabilize the inactive receptor configuration.[77] Recent *in vitro* studies demonstrated the efficacy of crenolanib in FLT3-inhibitor-resistant cell lines and xenograft models.[78] Crenolanib is a type I TK inhibitor that binds active as well as inactive forms of FLT3 receptor and thus may overcome resistance that stems from kinase domain activating mutations.[79]

## Targeting Apoptotic Pathways, Cell Cycle Regulation, and Cancer Cell Metabolism

Recent research has defined the critical role of cell cycle dysregulation and cancer cellular metabolism in maintaining and expanding malignant leukemic clones. These relevant intracellular pathways may serve as targets for novel anti-leukemic compounds.

Isocitrate dehydrogenase (IDH) is an enzyme that converts isocitrate into α-ketoglutarate (α-KG), an essential product that is involved in various cellular metabolic functions and also influences epigenetic cell regulation. Mutations in the genes encoding IDH1 and IDH2 occur in up to 20% of AML patients. These mutations, largely in critical arginine residues of the enzyme active site (R132 in IDH1; R140 and R172 in IDH2), alter the catalytic function of IDH. Mutated IDH enzyme converts α-KG to 2-hydroxyglutarate (2-HG), an "oncometabolite" that acts as a competitive inhibitor of dioxygenases. In order for IDH mutations to produce the oncometabolite, mutations must affect only one allele enabling α-KG production by wild-type enzyme and conversion of this substrate to 2-HG by the neo-enzyme encoded by the mutated IDH gene. The accumulation of 2-HG is associated with epigenetic dysregulation and the promotion of the leukemic phenotype.[80] Indeed, studies demonstrated that 2-HG levels in blood, marrow, and urine correlated well with IDH mutation status, and 2-HG levels decreased in response to chemotherapy.[81] Compounds that inhibit mutated IDH1 and IDH2 enzymes have been shown to retard the growth of IDH mutated cell cultures and reduce 2-HG levels.[82] Early phase clinical trials with AG-120, and AG-221, IDH1, and IDH2 inhibitors, are ongoing in patients with high risk advanced AML and significant single agent activity is preliminarily reported (NCT01915498, NCT02074839).[83] Several additional targeted approaches aimed at epigenetic regulators were recently reported in preclinical and early phase studies with encouraging preliminary data. These include bromodomain inhibitors (epigenetic 'readers' of acetylated histones)[84] and inhibitors of DOT1L, a histone methyltransferase implicated in the pathogenesis of MLL rearranged leukemia.[85]

Disruption of apoptotic pathways is a central theme in tumorigenesis and targeting this function represents an attractive strategy for therapeutic development. The B-cell lymphoma/leukemia 2 (BCL-2) family of proteins regulates the mitochondrial pathway that leads to apoptosis. The BCL-2 protein inhibits apoptosis by binding to pro-apoptotic proteins at its BH3 domain and prevents mitochondrial outer membrane permeabilization. This constitutes a major anti-apoptotic mechanism in hematologic malignancies.[86] ABT-199 is a potent selective BCL-2 inhibitor that has shown promise in non-Hodgkin's lymphoma[87] and in chronic lymphocytic leukemia (CLL) with tumor lysis syndrome as a reflection of drug efficacy in inducing apoptosis.[88] ABT-199 demonstrated considerable preclinical activity[89] and was recently reported to achieve 18% CR/CRi rates (5 of 28 patients) when administered as single agent to patients with advanced AML. Interestingly, the response group was enriched for patients with IDH mutations(NCT01994837).[90]

Another anti-apoptotic pathway that is emerging as a therapeutic target is the p53 pathway. P53 is a tumor suppressor that promotes apoptosis in the face of cellular DNA damage. While mutations in TP53 are present in a significant portion of human cancers, TP53 is inactivated by mutations in only 5–10% of AML cases. Murine double minute 2 (MDM2) is a protein that negatively regulates p53 activation via the promotion of p53-specific E3 ubiquitin degradation.[91] MDM2 overexpression is an important aspect of AML pathophysiology and MDM2 inhibitors such as nutlin-3 and MI219 promote apoptosis in human myeloblasts. This pro-apoptotic effect was noted almost exclusively in non-mutated TP53 samples; mutations in TP53 conferred resistance to MDM2 inhibition, although few responses were seen in p53 mutant AML.[91] MDM2 inhibition synergistically enhances the effect of cytotoxic drugs[91] and FLT3-ITD mutant blasts are exceptionally sensitive to MDM2 inhibition.[92] The MDM2 antagonist RG7112 was administered to 116 patients with advanced leukemia of various types (84 of which had relapsed/refractory AML) in a phase I study. In the AML cohort, 40% demonstrated hematologic improvement and 16% achieved CR. The majority of responders had an unmutated p53.[93] A phase IB study assessed the combination of cytarabine with RG7112. Sixteen patients ineligible for intensive chemotherapy were treated with RG7112 in combination with low-dose cytarabine and 27 patients with relapsed/refractory-AML were treated with RG7112 in combination with high-dose cytarabine. In the former group, the rates of overall response and CR were 43% and 21%, respectively while in the latter group the respective rates were 52% and 17%.[94]

P53 and other tumor suppressors as well as various other cell cycle proteins are shuttled between the nucleus and cytoplasm via a family of nuclear export receptors that recognize proteins bearing leucine-rich nuclear export signals. Exoportin-1 (also known as XPO1/CRM1) is a nuclear export receptor whose overexpression was shown to independently correlate with survival in AML. Inhibition of exoportin-1 in AML cell lines and in mouse models promotes p53-dependent apoptosis.[95] Selinexor (KPT-330) is a selective inhibitor of nuclear transport (SINE) that inhibits exoportin-1 and is currently being assessed in a phase I trial (NCT 01607892). Preliminary results in 48 patients with relapsed/refractory AML demonstrated manageable toxicity with 18% of patients achieving CR/Cri.[96]

The chemokine receptor CXCR4 and its substrate, stromal derived factor-1 (SDF-1/CXCR12), have a significant role in the interaction between leukemic blasts and the BM microenvironment. Elevated expression of CXCR4 on malignant cells promotes survival and retention of AML blasts within the BM niche and correlates with FLT3 expression and adverse patient outcome.[97] The small molecule CXC4 inhibitors such as plerixafor (AMD3100), AMD3465, and BKT140 were shown to inhibit blast proliferation via BM stomablast interaction. CXCR4 inhibition also partially abrogates the protective effects of the stroma on chemotherapy-induced apoptosis in AML cells, thus sensitizing cells to cytotoxic therapy.[97,98] This concept was tested in a phase I/II trial that involved 46 patients with relapsed/refractory AML treated with mitoxantrone, etoposide, and cytarabine in combination with the CXCR4 inhibitor plerixafor. This combination yielded a CR/CRi rate of 46%. Correlative studies demonstrated a twofold increase in blast mobilization into peripheral blood.[99] Several ongoing phase I and II trials are currently assessing plerixafor in combination with chemotherapy and other novel agents in high-risk AML.

The Hedgehog (Hh) signaling pathway is thought to have an important role in maintenance and expansion of the leukemic stem cell compartment as well as in AML resistance phenotype.[100] PF-04449913 is an oral compound that inhibits the Hh pathway by binding smoothened. Drug safety and tolerability were demonstrated in a phase I study that included 32 patients with various myeloid malignancies; two patients suffered from grade 3 toxicities (gastrointestinal bleeding and pulmonary toxicity); of 18 patients with AML in that study, 1 achieved a CR, and 5 demonstrated significant blast reduction.[101] PF-04449913 is currently tested in a phase II trial in combination with chemotherapy (NCT01546038) and in the setting of post alloSCT relapse of AML (NCT01841333).

## Chimeric Antigen Receptors and Vaccines

Chimeric antigen receptors (CARs) are artificial T-cell receptors that contain an extracellular antigen-binding domain composed of a single-chain variable-fragment antibody specific to a tumor antigen fused to a transmembrane domain and a T-cell signaling moiety, most commonly CD3-ζ. Second generation CARs also possess an endodomain from a T-cell co-stimulatory molecule (such as CD28, OX40, or 4-1BB).[102] The constructed receptor binds to the specified tumor antigen and initiates T-cell activation that results in target cell lysis. This technology, first implemented in CLL and later in ALL, holds promise in early phase studies. One report demonstrated that patient-derived T-cells can be modified to express anti-CD123 CARs and specifically lyse autologous blasts.[102] Pizzitola and colleagues studied CARs with anti-CD33 or anti-CD123 specificity introduced into cytokine-induced killer cells (a CD3+CD56+immune effector T-cell subpopulation) and demonstrated potent anti-leukemic activity in mouse models. They further demonstrated that targeting the CD123 antigen may be the preferred approach since it was associated with limited toxicity to normal hematopoietic stem cells as compared to anti-CD33 CARs.[103] Other relatively AML-specific antigens such as CD44v6 and LeY antigen were also assessed as CAR targets.[104,105] In an ongoing phase I study, LeY is targeted by CAR T-cells. Four patients were given anti-LeY antigen autologous CAR T-cells after fludarabine-based chemotherapy. Toxicity was manageable and significant clinical responses were observed with CAR T-cells persisting for several months.[105]

The development of endogenous T-cell immunity against antigens that are specific or associated with the leukemic phenotypes is frequently observed after alloSCT and is an essential part of the graft versus leukemia response. Induction of a T-cell response against such antigens using peptide or DC vaccines is an active field of investigation. In order to mount an effective and safe immunologic response against leukemia associated antigens the following criteria must be met: the antigen should be frequently and specifically expressed on leukemic blasts, the antigen should preferably have an oncogenic role in initiation and maintenance of the leukemic clone and a significant immunogenic response should be mounted.[106] Wilm's tumor 1 (WT1) is probably one of the most well characterized, relevant, and intensively studied antigens in that respect.[107] WT1 is a transcription factor that is associated with cell proliferation, differentiation, and apoptosis. It is relatively specific and highly expressed on leukemic cells, although expressed at low levels in healthy tissues (gonads, kidney, and spleen). WT1 is quite immunogenic and may mount CD8+, CD4+, and humoral responses.[108] Vaccine source is usually an antigen-derived peptide, a DC-loaded with a peptide or a DC-loaded with mRNA encoding full length WT1. Early phase trials in a variety of AML disease settings demonstrated the safety and potential efficacy of the WT1 vaccine strategy.[108]

## Summary

The past decade has been an exciting time for those caring for patients with AML. The delineation of the mutational landscape of AML, major advancements in our understanding of cancer cellular pathways, and the role of the immune system and microenvironment in initiating and maintaining the neoplastic clone will hopefully revolutionize our approach to AML in the near future. An abundance of new potentially druggable targets coupled with technological breakthroughs enable us to treat patients using a personalized approach based on specific genetic mutations and on leukemia-driving biological pathways. While these notions are promising, most of these new compounds are still in early clinical development. Moreover, current data suggest that even with these novel agents, resistance is still a major issue and that combination therapy may be needed to overcome this problem.

## References

1 National Comprehensive Cancer Network. Acute Myelois Leukemia (Version 1.2014). http://www.nccn.org/professionals/physician_gls/pdf/aml.pdf. Accessed February 16, 2014.

2 Dohner H, Estey EH, Amadori S, et al. Diagnosis and management of acute myeloid leukemia in adults: recommendations from an international expert panel, on behalf of the European LeukemiaNet. *Blood.* 2010;115(3):453–474.

3 Juliusson G, Lazarevic V, Horstedt AS, et al. Acute myeloid leukemia in the real world: why population-based registries are needed. *Blood.* 2012;119(17):3890–3899.

4 Cancer Genome Atlas Research Network. Genomic and epigenomic landscapes of adult de novo acute myeloid leukemia. *N Engl J Med.* 2013;368(22):2059–2074.

5 Patel JP, Gonen M, Figueroa ME, et al. Prognostic relevance of integrated genetic profiling in acute myeloid leukemia. *N Engl J Med.* 2012;366(12):1079–1089.

6 Gasiorowski RE, Clark GJ, Bradstock K, Hart DN. Antibody therapy for acute myeloid leukaemia. *Br J Haematol.* 2014;164(4):481–495.

7 Hutter ML, Schlenk RF. Gemtuzumab ozogamicin in non-acute promyelocytic acute myeloid leukemia. *Expert Opin Biol Ther.* 2011;11(10):1369–1380.

8 Bross PF, Beitz J, Chen G, et al. Approval summary: gemtuzumab ozogamicin in relapsed acute myeloid leukemia. *Clin Cancer Res.* 2001;7(6):1490–1496.

9 Petersdorf SH, Kopecky KJ, Slovak M, et al. A phase 3 study of gemtuzumab ozogamicin during induction and postconsolidation therapy in younger patients with acute myeloid leukemia. *Blood.* 2013;121(24):4854–4860.

10 Wadleigh M, Richardson PG, Zahrieh D, et al. Prior gemtuzumab ozogamicin exposure significantly increases the risk of veno-occlusive disease in patients who undergo myeloablative allogeneic stem cell transplantation. *Blood.* 2003;102(5):1578–1582.

11 Burnett AK, Hills RK, Milligan D, et al. Identification of patients with acute myeloblastic leukemia who benefit from the addition of gemtuzumab ozogamicin: results of the MRC AML15 trial. *J Clin Oncol.* 2011;29(4):369–377.

12 Burnett AK, Russell NH, Hills RK, et al. Addition of gemtuzumab ozogamicin to induction chemotherapy improves survival in older patients with acute myeloid leukemia. *J Clin Oncol.* 2012;30(32):3924–3931.

13 Castaigne S, Pautas C, Terre C, et al. Effect of gemtuzumab ozogamicin on survival of adult patients with de-novo acute myeloid leukaemia (ALFA-0701): a randomised, open-label, phase 3 study. *Lancet.* 2012;379(9825):1508–1516.

14 Burnett AK, Hills RK, Hunter AE, et al. The addition of gemtuzumab ozogamicin to low-dose Ara-C improves remission rate but does not significantly prolong survival in older patients with acute myeloid leukaemia: results from the LRF AML14 and NCRI AML16 pick-a-winner comparison. *Leukemia.* 2013;27(1):75–81.

15 Amadori S, Suciu S, Stasi R, et al.; UK National Cancer Research Institute AML Working Group. Sequential combination of gemtuzumab ozogamicin and standard chemotherapy in older patients with newly diagnosed acute myeloid leukemia: results of a randomized phase III trial by the EORTC and GIMEMA consortium (AML-17). *J Clin Oncol.* 2013;31(35):4424–4430.

16 Walter RB, Medeiros BC, Gardner KM, et al. Gemtuzumab ozogamicin in combination with vorinostat and azacitidine in older patients with relapsed or refractory acute myeloid leukemia: a phase I/II study. *Haematologica.* 2014;99(1):54–59.

17 Lo-Coco F, Cimino G, Breccia M, et al. Gemtuzumab ozogamicin (Mylotarg) as a single agent for molecularly relapsed acute promyelocytic leukemia. *Blood.* 2004;104(7):1995–1999.

18 Aribi A, Kantarjian HM, Estey EH, et al. Combination therapy with arsenic trioxide, all-trans retinoic acid, and gemtuzumab ozogamicin in recurrent acute promyelocytic leukemia. *Cancer.* 2007;109(7):1355–1359.

19 Ravandi F, Estey E, Jones D, et al. Effective treatment of acute promyelocytic leukemia with all-trans-retinoic acid, arsenic trioxide, and gemtuzumab ozogamicin. *J Clin Oncol.* 2009;27(4):504–510.

20 Feldman EJ, Brandwein J, Stone R, et al. Phase III randomized multicenter study of a humanized anti-CD33 monoclonal antibody, lintuzumab, in combination with chemotherapy, versus chemotherapy alone in patients with refractory or first-relapsed acute myeloid leukemia. *J Clin Oncol.* 2005;23(18):4110–4116.

21 Jurcic GH, Ravandi F, Pagel JM, et al. Phase I Trial Of The Targeted Alpha-Particle Nano-Generator Actinium-225 (225 Ac)-Lintuzumab (Anti-CD33) In Combination With Low-Dose Cytarabine (LDAC) For Older Patients With Untreated Acute Myeloid Leukemia (AML) [abstract]. *Blood.* 2013;122:1460.

22 Stein EM, Stein A, Walter RB, Fathi AT, Lancet JE, Kovacsovics TJ, Advani AS, DeAngelo DJ, O'Meara MM, Zhao B, Kennedy DA, Erba HP: Interim analysis of a phase 1 trial of sgn-cd33a in patients with cd33-positive acute myeloid leukemia (aml) [abstract]. *Blood* 2014; 124:623.

23 Kung Sutherland MS, Walter RB, Jeffrey SC, et al. SGN-CD33 A: a novel CD33-targeting antibody-drug conjugate using a pyrrolobenzodiazepine dimer is active in models of drug-resistant AML. *Blood.* 2013;122(8):1455–1463.

24 Topp MS, Kufer P, Gokbuget N, et al. Targeted therapy with the T-cell-engaging antibody blinatumomab of chemotherapy-refractory minimal residual disease in B-lineage acute lymphoblastic leukemia patients results in high response rate and prolonged leukemia-free survival. *J Clin Oncol.* 2011;29(18):2493–2498.

25 Laszlo GS, Gudgeon CJ, Harrington KH, et al. Cellular determinants for preclinical activity of a novel CD33/CD3 bispecific T-cell engager (BiTE) antibody, AMG 330, against human AML. *Blood.* 2014;123(4):554–561.

26 Roberts AW, He S, Ritchie D, et al. A phase I study of anti-CD123 monoclonal antibody (mAb) CSL360 targeting leukemia stem cells (LSC) in AML [abstract]. *J Clin Oncol.* 2010;28(15):e13012

27 Frankel A, Liu JS, Rizzieri D, Hogge D. Phase I clinical study of diphtheria toxin-interleukin 3 fusion protein in patients with acute myeloid leukemia and myelodysplasia. *Leuk Lymphoma.* 2008;49(3):543–553.

28 AL Hussaini MH, Ritchey J, Rettig MP, et al. Targeting CD123 in leukemic stem cells using dual affinity re-targeting molecules (DARTs®) [abstract]. *Blood.* 2013;122:360.

29 Zheng W, Medeiros LJ, Hu Y, et al. CD30 expression in high-risk acute myeloid leukemia and myelodysplastic syndromes. *Clin Lymphoma Myeloma Leuk.* 2013;13(3):307–314.

30 Fathi AT, Preffer FI, Sadrzadeh H, et al. CD30 expression in acute myeloid leukemia is associated with FLT3-internal tandem duplication mutation and leukocytosis. *Leuk Lymphoma.* 2013;54(4):860–863.

31 Lion E, Willemen Y, Berneman ZN, Van Tendeloo VF, Smits EL. Natural killer cell immune escape in acute myeloid leukemia. *Leukemia.* 2012;26(9):2019–2026.

32 Vey N, Bourhis JH, Boissel N, et al. A phase 1 trial of the anti-inhibitory KIR mAb IPH2101 for AML in complete remission. *Blood.* 2012;120(22):4317–4323.

33 Zhang L, Gajewski TF, Kline J. PD-1/PD-L1 interactions inhibit anti-tumor immune responses in a murine acute myeloid leukemia model. *Blood.* 2009;114(8):1545–1552.

34 Topalian SL, Hodi FS, Brahmer JR, et al. Safety, activity, and immune correlates of anti-PD-1 antibody in cancer. *N Engl J Med.* 2012;366(26):2443–2454.

35 Berthon C, Driss V, Liu J, et al. In acute myeloid leukemia, B7-H1 (PD-L1) protection of blasts from cytotoxic T cells is induced by TLR ligands and interferon-gamma and can be reversed using MEK inhibitors. *Cancer Immunol Immunother.* 2010;59(12):1839–1849.

36 Hodi FS, O'Day SJ, McDermott DF, et al. Improved survival with ipilimumab in patients with metastatic melanoma. *N Engl J Med.* 2010;363(8):711–723.

37 Davids MS, Kim HT, Costello CL, Avigan D, Chen Y-B, Armand P, Alyea EP, Hedlund J, McSweeney PA, Liguori R, Ritz J, Ball ED, Bashey A, Soiffer RJ: A multicenter phase i study of ctla-4 blockade with ipilimumab for relapsed hematologic malignancies after allogeneic hematopoietic cell transplantation [abstract]. *Blood* 2014; 124:3964.

38 Tsimberidou AM, Chandhasin C, Kurzrock R. Farnesyltransferase inhibitors: where are we now? *Expert Opin Investig Drugs.* 2010;19(12):1569–1580.

39 Bacher U, Haferlach T, Schoch C, Kern W, Schnittger S. Implications of NRAS mutations in AML: a study of 2502 patients. *Blood.* 2006;107(10):3847–3853.

40 Erba HP, Othus M, Walter RB, et al. Four different regimens of farnesyltransferase inhibitor tipifarnib in older, untreated acute myeloid leukemia patients: North American Intergroup phase II study SWOG S0432. *Leuk Res.* 2014;38(3):329–333.

41 Lancet JE, Gojo I, Gotlib J, et al. A phase 2 study of the farnesyltransferase inhibitor tipifarnib in poor-risk and elderly patients

with previously untreated acute myelogenous leukemia. *Blood.* 2007;109(4):1387–1394.

42 Harousseau JL, Martinelli G, Jedrzejczak WW, et al.; FIGHT-AML-301 Investigators. A randomized phase 3 study of tipifarnib compared with best supportive care, including hydroxyurea, in the treatment of newly diagnosed acute myeloid leukemia in patients 70 years or older. *Blood.* 2009;114(6):1166–1173.

43 Burnett AK, Russell NH, Culligan D, et al.; AML Working Group of the UK National Cancer Research Institute. The addition of the farnesyltransferase inhibitor, tipifarnib, to low dose cytarabine does not improve outcome for older patients with AML. *Br J Haematol.* 2012;158(4):519–522.

44 Karp JE, Vener TI, Raponi M, et al. Multi-institutional phase 2 clinical and pharmacogenomic trial of tipifarnib plus etoposide for elderly adults with newly diagnosed acute myelogenous leukemia. *Blood.* 2012;119(1):55–63.

45 Jain N, Curran E, Iyengar NM, et al. Phase II study of the oral MEK inhibitor selumetinib in advanced acute myelogenous leukemia: a University of Chicago phase II consortium trial. *Clin Cancer Res.* 2014;20(2):490–498.

46 Borthakur G, Popplewell L, Kirschbaum MH, et al. Phase I/II trial of the MEK1/2 inhibitor GSK1120212 (GSK212) in patients (pts) with relapsed/refractory myeloid malignancies: Evidence of activity in pts with RAS mutation [abstract]. *J Clin Oncol.* 2011;29(15): 6506.

47 Paschka P, Dohner K. Core-binding factor acute myeloid leukemia: can we improve on HiDAC consolidation? *Hematology Am Soc Hematol Educ Program.* 2013;2013:209–219.

48 Wang YY, Zhao LJ, Wu CF, et al. C-KIT mutation cooperates with full-length AML1-ETO to induce acute myeloid leukemia in mice. *Proc Natl Acad Sci U S A.* 2011;108(6):2450–2455.

49 Chevalier N, Solari ML, Becker H, et al. Robust in vivo differentiation of t(8;21)-positive acute myeloid leukemia blasts to neutrophilic granulocytes induced by treatment with dasatinib. *Leukemia.* 2010;24(10):1779–1781.

50 Marcucci G, Geyer S, Zhao J, et al. Adding the KIT inhibitor dasatinib (DAS) to standard induction and consolidation therapy for newly diagnosed patients (pts) with core binding factor (CBF) acute myeloid leukemia (AML): initial results of the CALGB 10801 (Alliance) study [abstract]. *Blood.* 2013;122:357.

51 Boissel N, Jourdan E, Pigneux A, et al. Single-agent dasatinib does not prevent hematological relapse in patients with core binding factor (CBF) acute myeloid leukemia (AML) in first complete remission, but persistent or re-appearing molecular minimal residual disease-results of the DASA-CBF trial from the French AML intergroup [abstract]. *Blood.* 2011;118:2608

52 Pratz KW, Luger SM. Will FLT3 inhibitors fulfill their promise in acute meyloid leukemia? *Curr Opin Hematol.* 2014;21(2):72–78.

53 Gale RE, Green C, Allen C, et al.; Medical Research Council Adult Leukaemia Working Party. The impact of FLT3 internal tandem duplication mutant level, number, size, and interaction with NPM1 mutations in a large cohort of young adult patients with acute myeloid leukemia. *Blood.* 2008;111(5):2776–2784.

54 Stirewalt DL, Kopecky KJ, Meshinchi S, et al. Size of FLT3 internal tandem duplication has prognostic significance in patients with acute myeloid leukemia. *Blood.* 2006;107(9):3724–3726.

55 Bacher U, Haferlach C, Kern W, Haferlach T, Schnittger S. Prognostic relevance of FLT3-TKD mutations in AML: the combination matters– an analysis of 3082 patients. *Blood.* 2008;111(5):2527–2537.

56 Metzelder SK, Schroeder T, Finck A, et al. High activity of sorafenib in FLT3-ITD-positive acute myeloid leukemia synergizes

with allo-immune effects to induce sustained responses. *Leukemia.* 2012;26(11):2353–2359.

57 Sharma M, Ravandi F, Bayraktar UD, et al. Treatment of FLT3-ITD-positive acute myeloid leukemia relapsing after allogeneic stem cell transplantation with sorafenib. *Biol Blood Marrow Transplant.* 2011;17(12):1874–1877.

58 Chen YB, Li S, Lane AA, Connolly C, Del Rio C, Valles B, Curtis M, Ballen K, Cutler C, Dey BR, El-Jawahri A, Fathi AT, Ho VT, Joyce A, McAfee S, Rudek M, Rajkhowa T, Verselis S, Antin JH, Spitzer TR, Levis M, Soiffer R: Phase i trial of maintenance sorafenib after allogeneic hematopoietic stem cell transplantation for fms-like tyrosine kinase 3 internal tandem duplication acute myeloid leukemia. *Biology of blood and marrow transplantation : journal of the American Society for Blood and Marrow Transplantation* 2014;20:2042-2048.

59 Ravandi F, Cortes JE, Jones D, et al. Phase I/II study of combination therapy with sorafenib, idarubicin, and cytarabine in younger patients with acute myeloid leukemia. *J Clin Oncol.* 2010;28(11):1856–1862.

60 Serve H, Krug U, Wagner R, et al. Sorafenib in combination with intensive chemotherapy in elderly patients with acute myeloid leukemia: results from a randomized, placebo-controlled trial. *J Clin Oncol.* 2013;31(25):3110–3118.

61 Macdonald DA, Assouline SE, Brandwein J, et al. A phase I/II study of sorafenib in combination with low dose cytarabine in elderly patients with acute myeloid leukemia or high-risk myelodysplastic syndrome from the National Cancer Institute of Canada Clinical Trials Group: trial IND.186. *Leuk Lymphoma.* 2013;54(4):760–766.

62 Ravandi F, Alattar ML, Grunwald MR, et al. Phase 2 study of azacytidine plus sorafenib in patients with acute myeloid leukemia and FLT-3 internal tandem duplication mutation. *Blood.* 2013;121(23):4655–4662.

63 Sato T, Yang X, Knapper S, et al. FLT3 ligand impedes the efficacy of FLT3 inhibitors in vitro and in vivo. *Blood.* 2011;117(12):3286–3293.

64 Röllig C, Müller-Tidow C, Hüttmann A, Noppeney R, Kunzmann V, Baldus CD, Brandts CH, Krämer A, Schäfer-Eckart K, Neubauer A, Krause SW, Giagounidis A, Aulitzky WE, Bornhäuser M, Schaich M, Parmentier SB, Thiede C, von Bonin M, Schetelig J, Kramer M, Serve H, Berdel WE, Ehninger G: Sorafenib versus placebo in addition to standard therapy in younger patients with newly diagnosed acute myeloid leukemia: Results from 267 patients treated in the randomized placebo-controlled sal-soraml trial [abstract]. *Blood* 2014; 124:6.

65 Knapper S, Burnett AK, Littlewood T, et al. A phase 2 trial of the FLT3 inhibitor lestaurtinib (CEP701) as first-line treatment for older patients with acute myeloid leukemia not considered fit for intensive chemotherapy. *Blood.* 2006;108(10):3262–3270.

66 Levis M, Ravandi F, Wang ES, et al. Results from a randomized trial of salvage chemotherapy followed by lestaurtinib for patients with FLT3 mutant AML in first relapse. *Blood.* 2011;117(12):3294–3301.

67 Fischer T, Stone RM, Deangelo DJ, et al. Phase IIB trial of oral Midostaurin (PKC412), the FMS-like tyrosine kinase 3 receptor (FLT3) and multi-targeted kinase inhibitor, in patients with acute myeloid leukemia and high-risk myelodysplastic syndrome with either wild-type or mutated FLT3. *J Clin Oncol.* 2010;28(28):4339–4345.

68 Stone RM, Fischer T, Paquette R, et al. Phase IB study of the FLT3 kinase inhibitor midostaurin with chemotherapy in younger newly diagnosed adult patients with acute myeloid leukemia. *Leukemia.* 2012;26(9):2061–2068.

69 Stone RM, Dohner H, Ehninger G, et al. CALGB 10603 (RATIFY): A randomized phase III study of induction (daunorubicin/cytarabine) and consolidation (high-dose cytarabine) chemotherapy combined with midostaurin or placebo in treatment-naive patients with FLT3 mutated AML [abstract]. *J Clin Oncol.* 2011;29(15):TPS199.

70 Pratz KW, Sato T, Murphy KM, et al. FLT3-mutant allelic burden and clinical status are predictive of response to FLT3 inhibitors in AML. *Blood.* 2010;115(7):1425–1432.

71 Cortes JE, Kantarjian H, Foran JM, et al. Phase I study of quizartinib administered daily to patients with relapsed or refractory acute myeloid leukemia irrespective of FMS-like tyrosine kinase 3-internal tandem duplication status. *J Clin Oncol.* 2013;31(29):3681–3687.

72 Cortes JE, Perl AE, Dombret H, et al. Final results of a Phase 2 open-label, monotherapy efficacy and safety study of quizartinib (AC220) in patients > = 60 years of age with FLT3 ITD positive or negative relapsed/refractory acute myeloid leukemia [abstract]. *Blood.* 2012;120:48.

73 Levis MJ, Perl AE, Dombret H, et al. Final results of a phase 2 open-label, monotherapy efficacy and safety study of quizartinib (AC220) in patients with FLT3-ITD positive or negative relapsed/refractory acute myeloid leukemia after second-line chemotherapy or hematopoietic stem cell transplantation [abstract]. *Blood.* 2012;120:673.

74 Cortes JE, Perl AE, Dombret H, et al. Response rate and bridging to hematopoietic stem cell transplantation (HSCT) with quizartinib (AC220) in patients with FLT3-ITD positive or negative relapsed/refractory AML after second-line chemotherapy or previous bone marrow transplant [abstract]. *J Clin Oncol.* 2013;31(15):7012.

75 Perl AE, Dohner H, Rousselot PH, et al. Efficacy and safety of quizartinib (AC220) in patients age ≥70 years with FLT3-ITD positive or negative relapsed/refractory acute myeloid leukemia (AML) [abstract]. *J Clin Oncol.* 2013;31(15):7023.

76 Borthakur G, Kantarjian HM, O'Brien S, Garcia-Manero G, Jabbour E, Daver N, Kadia TM, Gborogen R, Konopleva M, Andreeff M, Ravandi F, Cortes JE: The combination of quizartinib with azacitidine or low dose cytarabine is highly active in patients (pts) with flt3-itd mutated myeloid leukemias: Interim report of a phase i/ii trial [abstract]. *Blood* 2014; 124:388., 2014.

77 Fathi AT. Emergence of crenolanib for FLT3-mutant AML. *Blood.* 2013;122(22):3547–3548.

78 Zimmerman EI, Turner DC, Buaboonnam J, et al. Crenolanib is active against models of drug-resistant FLT3-ITD-positive acute myeloid leukemia. *Blood.* 2013;122(22):3607–3615.

79 Randhawa JK, Kantarjian HM, Borthakur G, Thompson PA, Konopleva M, Daver N, Pemmaraju N, Jabbour E, Kadia TM, Estrov Z, Ramachandran A, Paradela J, Andreef M, Levis M, Ravandi F, Cortes JE: Results of a phase ii study of crenolanib in relapsed/refractory acute myeloid leukemia patients (pts) with activating flt3 mutations [abstract]. *Blood* 2014; 124:389.

80 Levis M. Targeting IDH: the next big thing in AML. *Blood.* 2013;122(16):2770–2771.

81 Fathi AT, Sadrzadeh H, Borger DR, et al. Prospective serial evaluation of 2-hydroxyglutarate, during treatment of newly diagnosed acute myeloid leukemia, to assess disease activity and therapeutic response. *Blood.* 2012;120(23):4649–4652.

82 Emadi A, Jun SA, Tsukamoto T, et al. Inhibition of glutaminase selectively suppresses the growth of primary AML cells with IDH mutations. *Exp Hematol.* 2014;42(4):247–251.

83 Stein E, Tallman M, Pollyea DA, et al. Clinical safety and activity in a phase I trial of AG-221, a first in class, potent inhibitor of the IDH2-mutant protein, in patients with IDH2 mutant positive advanced hematologic malignancies [abstract]. *Blood* 2014;124:115.

84 Dombret H, Preudhomme C, Berthon C, Raffoux E, Thomas X, Vey N, Gomez-Roca C, Ethell M, Yee K, Bourdel F, Herait P, Michallet M, Recher C, Roumier C, Quesnel B: A phase 1 study of the bet-bromodomain inhibitor otx015 in patients with advanced acute leukemia [abstract]. *Blood* 2014; 124:117.

85 Stein EM, Garcia-Manero G, Rizzieri DA, Savona M, Tibes R, Altman JK, Jongen-Lavrencic M, Döhner H, Armstrong S, Pollock RM, Waters NJ, Legler M, Thomson B, Daigle S, McDonald A, Campbell C, Olhava E, Hedrick EE, Lowenberg B, Copeland RA, Tallman MS: The dot1l inhibitor epz-5676: Safety and activity in relapsed/refractory patients with mll-rearranged leukemia [abstract]. *Blood* 2014; 124: 387.

86 Davids MS, Letai A. ABT-199: taking dead aim at BCL-2. *Cancer Cell.* 2013;23(2):139–41.

87 Davids MS, Roberts AW, Anderson MA, et al. The BCL-2-specific BH3-mimetic ABT-199 (GDC-0199) is active and well-tolerated in patients with relapsed non-Hodgkin lymphoma: interim results of a phase I study [abstract]. *Blood.* 2012;120:304.

88 Souers AJ, Leverson JD, Boghaert ER, et al. ABT-199, a potent and selective BCL-2 inhibitor, achieves antitumor activity while sparing platelets. *Nat Med.* 2013;19(2):202–208.

89 Pan R, Hogdal LJ, Benito JM, et al. Selective BCL-2 inhibition by ABT-199 causes on target cell death in acute myeloid leukemia. *Cancer Discov.* 2014;4(3):362–375.

90 Konopleva M, Pollyea DA, Potluri J, et al. A Phase 2 Study of ABT-199 (GDC-0199) in Patients with Acute Myelogenous Leukemia (AML) [abstract]. *Blood.* 2014;124(21):118.

91 Kojima K, Konopleva M, Samudio IJ, et al. MDM2 antagonists induce p53-dependent apoptosis in AML: implications for leukemia therapy. *Blood.* 2005;106(9):3150–3159.

92 Long J, Parkin B, Ouillette P, et al. Multiple distinct molecular mechanisms influence sensitivity and resistance to MDM2 inhibitors in adult acute myelogenous leukemia. *Blood.* 2010;116(1):71–80.

93 Andreeff M, Kelly KR, Yee K, et al. Results of the phase 1 trial of RG7112, a small-molecule MDM2 antagonist, in acute leukemia [abstract]. *Blood.* 2012;120:675.

94 Martinelli G, Assouline S, Kasner M, et al. Phase 1b study of the MDM2 antagonist RG7112 in combination with 2 doses/schedules of cytarabine [abstract]. *Blood.* 2013;122:498.

95 Kojima K, Kornblau SM, Ruvolo V, et al. Prognostic impact and targeting of CRM1 in acute myeloid leukemia. *Blood.* 2013;121(20):4166–4174.

96 Yee k.W.L, savona m, sorensen m, et al. A phase 1 dose-escalation study of the oral selective inhibitor of nuclear export (sine) kpt-330 (selinexor) in patients (pts) with relapsed/refractory acute myeloid leukemia (aml) [abstract]. *J clin oncol* 2014; 32(15):7032

97 Peled A, Tavor S. Role of CXCR4 in the pathogenesis of acute myeloid leukemia. *Theranostics.* 2013;3(1):34–39.

98 Zhang Y, Patel S, Abdelouahab H, et al. CXCR4 inhibitors selectively eliminate CXCR4-expressing human acute myeloid leukemia cells in NOG mouse model. *Cell Death Dis.* 2012;3:e396.

99 Uy GL, Rettig MP, Motabi IH, et al. A phase 1/2 study of chemosensitization with the CXCR4 antagonist plerixafor in relapsed or refractory acute myeloid leukemia. *Blood.* 2012;119(17):3917–3924.

100 Irvine DA, Copland M. Targeting hedgehog in hematologic malignancy. *Blood.* 2012;119(10):2196–2204.

101 Jamieson C, Cortes JE, Oehler V, et al. Phase 1 dose-escalation study of PF-04449913, an oral hedgehog (Hh) inhibitor, in patients with select hematologic malignancies [abstract]. *Blood.* 2011;118:424.

102 Mardiros A, Brown CE, Budde LE, et al. Acute myeloid leukemia therapeutics: CARs in the driver's seat. *Oncoimmunology.* 2013;2(12):e27214.

103 Pizzitola I, Anjos-Afonso F, Rouault-Pierre K, et al. chimeric antigen receptors against CD33/CD123 antigens efficiently target primary acute myeloid leukemia cells in vivo. *Leukemia.* 2014. 28(8):1596–605.

104 Casucci M, Nicolis di Robilant B, Falcone L, et al. CD44v6-targeted T cells mediate potent antitumor effects against acute myeloid leukemia and multiple myeloma. *Blood.* 2013;122(20):3461–3472.

105 Ritchie DS, Neeson PJ, Khot A, et al. Persistence and efficacy of second generation CAR T cell against the LeY antigen in acute myeloid leukemia. *Mol Ther.* 2013;21(11):2122–2129.

106 Anguille S, Van Tendeloo VF, Berneman ZN. Leukemia-associated antigens and their relevance to the immunotherapy of acute myeloid leukemia. *Leukemia.* 2012;26(10):2186–2196.

107 Cheever MA, Allison JP, Ferris AS, et al. The prioritization of cancer antigens: a national cancer institute pilot project for the acceleration of translational research. *Clin Cancer Res.* 2009;15(17):5323–5337.

108 Van Driessche A, Berneman ZN, Van Tendeloo VF. Active specific immunotherapy targeting the Wilms' tumor protein 1 (WT1) for patients with hematological malignancies and solid tumors: lessons from early clinical trials. *Oncologist.* 2012;17(2):250–259.

# CHAPTER 10

# Targeted and Functional Imaging

*Jian Q. (Michael) Yu[1], Drew A. Torigian[2], and Abass Alavi[2]*

[1]Department of Diagnostic Imaging, Fox Chase Cancer Center, Philadelphia, PA, USA
[2]Department of Radiology, Hospital of the University of Pennsylvania, Philadelphia, PA, USA

## Introduction

Cancer is a major public health problem in the United States and many other parts of the world. Currently, one in four deaths in the United States is due to cancer.[1] Imaging plays a crucial role in oncology and is useful for screening, diagnosis and initial staging, prognosis assessment, treatment planning, treatment response assessment, restaging, and surveillance. As such, imaging may reduce cancer incidence and mortality and improve survival. Imaging technologies used to assess patients with cancer may be grossly subdivided into structural and functional imaging categories. Structural imaging entails the assessment of morphologic features or gross degree of contrast enhancement of normal tissues/organs of the body and of malignant lesions within these structures. Computed tomography (CT), magnetic resonance imaging (MRI), and ultrasonography (US) are the prototypical imaging technologies that are currently used for structural imaging in oncology.[2,3] However, functional or metabolic changes at the molecular, subcellular, or cellular level may occur well before gross structural or contrast enhancement changes become visible. Moreover, macroscopic abnormalities are nonspecific and often seen in non-neoplastic conditions. In addition, data regarding biological processes, physiology, and molecular characteristics of tumors are not available by structural-based imaging.

Thus, structural imaging lacks the necessary information to fully characterize or monitor lesions. In order to improve tumor evaluation, functional imaging is necessary for visualization and quantification of physiological and biochemical processes *in vivo*. Functional imaging can be performed via CT, MRI, and US, as well as through positron emission tomography (PET), single-photon emission computed tomography (SPECT), and optical imaging (OI), and is often performed in combination with structural imaging for optimal information gain.[2–6] Functional imaging modalities can grossly be divided into those that allow for evaluation of tumor physiology and those that allow for assessment of tumor molecular targets and processes. This chapter will review a selection of the wide variety of available functional imaging methods for non-invasive evaluation of tumor physiology and tumor molecular targets and processes.

The first two authors have contributed equally to this manuscript.

## Functional Imaging of Tumor Physiology

### Perfusion Imaging

Tumor angiogenesis is an essential process for the growth, proliferation, and metastasis of solid tumors.[7] Perfusion imaging allows for non-invasive *in vivo* assessment of functional aspects of tumor neovascularity. Of the imaging techniques capable of providing data regarding tumor vascularity, perfusion CT and dynamic contrast-enhanced MRI (DCE-MRI) have been widely investigated because they offer certain advantages. First, CT and MRI are already widely used in routine oncological imaging, so that perfusion studies can be incorporated with relative ease. Second, both CT and MRI offer good structural detail, such that reliable measurements can be obtained with high spatial resolution. Third, CT and MRI perfusional measurements have been shown to correlate with histologic markers of angiogenesis.[8,9]

Perfusion CT and DCE-MRI are performed by obtaining sequential images before, during, and after injection of a contrast agent (typically an iodine-based contrast agent for perfusion CT and a small molecular weight gadolinium-containing compound for DCE-MRI). There is a direct linear relationship between enhancement change on CT and iodine concentration, so that the arterial input, necessary for quantitative analysis, can be measured directly from an artery in the field of view. Thus, perfusion CT allows for absolute quantification of perfusion in terms of blood volume, blood flow, mean transit time, and permeability.[8] In contrast, the relation between MRI signal intensity change and paramagnetic contrast agent concentration is not as easily defined, since such contrast agents indirectly induce signal intensity changes by affecting the relaxation properties of surrounding water protons. Therefore, DCE-MRI quantification is technically more challenging. DCE-MRI can be performed via dynamic T2*-weighted or dynamic T1-weighted methods. Dynamic T2*-weighted methods are based on the phenomenon that the first pass of contrast through tissue causes a transient signal drop due to local magnetic susceptibility (T2*) effects (where T2*-weighting is due to combined T2-weighting and effects of magnetic field inhomogeneity) and can provide information about relative tumor perfusion, which may be related to tumor grade and vessel density.[8,9] Dynamic T1-weighted methods employ the T1 shortening effects of contrast, which lead to an increase in signal intensity as contrast passes from blood into extracellular space, and can provide information about blood vessel

*Targeted Therapy in Translational Cancer Research*, First Edition. Edited by Apostolia-Maria Tsimberidou, Razelle Kurzrock and Kenneth C. Anderson.
© 2016 John Wiley & Sons, Inc. Published 2016 by John Wiley & Sons, Inc.

permeability, capillary surface area, and leakage space, which may be related to microvessel density, tumor grade, and vascular endothelial growth factor expression.[8,9] Perfusion CT and DCE-MRI may be useful for tumor detection, characterization, grading and staging, prognosis assessment, response assessment, and restaging, as has been shown in many types of cancer, as well as for development of anti-angiogenic therapies.

## Diffusion Imaging

Diffusion-weighted imaging (DWI) is an MRI method that allows for non-invasive visualization and quantification of the random microscopic movement of water molecules (i.e., Brownian motion) within biologic tissues, without using contrast agents.[10] Pathologic processes that lead to changes in the diffusivity of water molecules can be evaluated using DWI. For example, an increase in tumor cellularity may lead to a decrease in extracellular volume, where increased tortuosity of the extracellular space leads to reduced water mobility. On the other hand, necrosis and apoptotic processes lead to loss of cell membrane integrity and decrease in cellularity, increasing the proportion of water molecules in the extracellular space where water mobility is less impeded.[11-13] Currently, the most common application of DWI is in the diagnosis of acute ischemic stroke, in which failure of the $Na^+K^+$ ATPase pump leads to a net displacement of water from the extracellular to intracellular compartment, where water mobility is relatively more impeded.[14] Thanks to technological advances, it is now possible to perform DWI outside of the brain, as a result of which the use of DWI in oncology is gaining widespread interest.[11-13] Since DWI suppresses many unwanted signals from background normal structures, lesions can be demonstrated to better effect. As such, DWI may be useful for purposes of tumor detection and staging. For example, recent studies report that the overall diagnostic performance of whole-body DWI (combined with conventional MRI sequences) was at least equal to that of 2-[18]F-fluoro-2-deoxy-D-glucose (FDG)-PET for regional nodal (N) staging[15] and distant metastasis (M) staging[16,17] in patients with non-small cell lung cancer.

Another important feature of DWI is that it allows for quantification of water molecule diffusivity in tissues by means of apparent diffusion coefficient (ADC) measurements, which may provide indirect information about tissue structure. ADC measurements may be useful for characterization of tumors and early detection of therapeutic response. For example, it has been reported that ADC measurements may facilitate grading of astrocytic brain tumors.[18] Other studies show that ADC measurements are at least equal to standardized uptake value (SUV) measurements from FDG-PET in differentiating benign from malignant pulmonary lesions.[19,20] Another recent study reports that preoperative lesional ADC, as well as maximum SUV obtained from FDG-PET, correlates with several prognostic factors and may have similar potential for predicting prognosis in patients with breast cancer.[21] Another promising application of DWI is in early response assessment. For example, a voxel-based quantitative DWI approach (called parametric response mapping of diffusion [$PRM_{ADC}$]), allows visualization and calculation of spatial tumor diffusion coefficient changes during treatment.[22,23] $PRM_{ADC}$ combined with traditional radiological response criteria 3 weeks after initiation of radiation therapy provides significantly improved prediction of therapeutic response in patients with high-grade gliomas relative to traditional size criteria or $PRM_{ADC}$ alone.[23] The $PRM_{ADC}$ approach is a considerable step forward towards more individualized treatment planning, although its application outside the brain is technologically more challenging. Nevertheless,

there are studies which have shown the feasibility of $PRM_{ADC}$ as an early biomarker for the prediction of therapeutic response in head and neck cancer, breast cancer, and bone marrow metastases from prostate cancer.[24-26] Overall, DWI is very promising with many potential applications in oncological imaging.

Interestingly, water molecule diffusivity in the body is not always isotropic. In particular, it is anisotropic in the nervous system since it is lowest perpendicular to and highest parallel to the course of nerve fibers.[27] This anisotropy can be exploited by diffusion tensor imaging (DTI), which is performed with diffusion-encoding gradients in six or more directions.[28] For example, DTI is useful for pretreatment assessment of white-matter tract involvement by tumor and for intraoperative visualization and localization of major white-matter tracts to decrease the chance of injury to normal tissues.[29-31]

## Elastography

Elastography involves imaging of tissue mechanical properties. Most elasticity imaging methods apply some sort of stress or mechanical excitation to tissue, measure tissue response, and calculate parameters that reflect the mechanical properties. Cross-sectional imaging modalities used for tissue response measurement include US and MRI. US-based elasticity imaging, however, is limited as it requires a suitable acoustic window and has a limited depth for measurements because of the limited penetration of ultrasound waves in tissue.[32]

Magnetic resonance elastography (MRE) involves induction of harmonic vibrations of acoustic-range frequencies in tissue and imaging of the propagation of these vibrations in tissue to calculate tissue mechanical parameters.[32,33] Currently, the most important clinical application of MRE is in non-invasive assessment of hepatic fibrosis and cirrhosis, where diseased liver stiffness is significantly higher than normal liver stiffness.[32,34] However, application of MRE may also be extended to tumor characterization. For example, the stiffness of malignant breast lesions is higher than that of benign lesions and normal breast tissue.[32,35] Similarly, MRE provides a significant diagnostic gain compared to dynamic contrast-enhanced MRI alone for evaluation of breast lesions, with an increase of about 20% in specificity at 100% sensitivity.[36] Oncological applications of MRE are very interesting, but more research is warranted before these are implemented in routine clinical practice.

## Functional Lymph Node Imaging

The accurate evaluation of lymph nodes is critical in the management of patients with cancer, because lymph node status has important therapeutic and prognostic implications. Current cross-sectional imaging modalities such as US, CT, and conventional MRI rely on insensitive and non-specific size criteria, which therefore lack the desired accuracy to characterize lymph nodes. Functional imaging techniques are under development to overcome these limitations.[37]

Sentinel lymph node mapping is currently the most frequently used method for functional lymph node imaging. The rationale for this method is that sentinel lymph nodes accurately reflect the status of the lymphatic basin draining the primary tumor. This assumption has been proven for malignant melanoma,[38] breast cancer,[39] and penile carcinoma.[40] Sentinel lymph node mapping is usually performed with radiotracers (e.g., [99m]Tc-sulfur colloid, [99m]Tc-antimony trisulfide colloid, or [99m]Tc-nanocolloid) and vital blue dyes. After intradermal injection around the tumor, the radioactive particles will become trapped in sentinel lymph nodes, whereas blue dyes typically pass into second echelon nodes.

Subsequently, sentinel lymph nodes can be identified by using pre-operative lymphoscintigraphy, an intraoperative gamma-detecting probe, and/or by using intraoperative visualization of blue-stained lymph nodes. Unfortunately, sentinel lymph node imaging does not allow for direct detection of involved lymph nodes, but instead directs surgical exploration to nodal sites that are potentially most vulnerable to cancer spread. Another drawback is that only lymph nodes in the vicinity of the primary tumor can be assessed. Furthermore, increasing tumor growth in the sentinel lymph node may obstruct its afferent lymphatic vessels, such that lymph flow through the node may be diverted to the next draining lymph node, leading to lack of depiction of the originally involved sentinel lymph node.[41–43] FDG-PET, which will be described in a later section, has an important advantage over sentinel lymph node mapping, in that it directly targets cancer cells in lymph nodes. Since intravenously administered FDG arrives in the lymph node through its arterial blood supply, lymphatic obstruction and subsequent reversal of lymph flow will not affect the performance of FDG-PET in diagnosing metastatic lymph nodes. Thus, in such settings, conventional sentinel lymph node imaging is complementary with whole-body FDG-PET nodal imaging.

Another functional imaging technique that allows for non-invasive detection of lymph node metastasis is ultrasmall super-paramagnetic iron oxide (USPIO)-enhanced MRI.[44] USPIO particles are non-targeted contrast agents that leak into the interstitium and reach lymph nodal reticuloendothelial cells via the lymphatic system, allowing for detection of micrometastases within normal-sized lymph nodes. Uptake of USPIO particles by normal lymph nodes creates local field inhomogeneities and turns them "black" (i.e., very low in signal intensity relative to that on precontrast images) on $T2^*$-weighted images. Metastatic lymph nodes, however, lack uptake of USPIO particles and stay "white" (i.e., intermediate in signal intensity relative to that on precontrast images) on $T2^*$-weighted images.[44] A meta-analysis including 38 studies investigating the diagnostic performance of USPIO-enhanced MRI for nodal staging in various tumors reports that overall (lymph node-based) sensitivity and specificity of USPIO-enhanced MRI (88% and 96%, respectively) were higher than those of unenhanced MRI (63% and 93%, respectively).[45] Although potentially useful, USPIO-enhanced MRI, unlike FDG-PET, indirectly reveals cancer sites in lymph nodes. Therefore, specificity may be suboptimal for evaluation of lymph nodes involved by non-neoplastic processes. Other important issues are that USPIO contrast agents are not approved for human use either by the Food and Drug Administration (FDA) or by the European Medicines Agency (EMEA), and that availability of these contrast agents is currently very limited. When USPIO contrast agents become more widely available, it would be of great interest to compare USPIO-enhanced MRI to FDG-PET for nodal staging in clinical studies.

DWI, which has been previously discussed, is another functional imaging technique that may be useful for lymph node characterization. Irrespective of their histological nature, lymph nodes are identified as high signal intensity structures at DWI, because of their relatively long T2 relaxation time and impeded water molecule diffusivity. Assessment of lymph node signal intensity at DWI or diffusivity by means of ADC measurements may aid in the characterization of lymph nodes, because different pathologic processes may lead to differences in diffusivity related to differences in cellularity, intracellular architecture, necrosis, and perfusion.[11] Several studies report that ADCs of metastatic lymph nodes are significantly lower than those of non-metastatic lymph nodes, independent of

size criteria.[46–48] This can be explained since malignant tissue generally exhibits hypercellularity, increased nucleus-to-cytoplasm ratios, and increased macromolecular proteins, resulting in decreased diffusivity in the extra- and intracellular compartments. Nevertheless, ADCs of metastatic and non-metastatic lymph nodes overlap.[46–48] Furthermore, some studies report that there is no significant difference between the ADCs of metastatic and non-metastatic lymph nodes.[49,50] Another issue is that ADC measurements of smaller lymph nodes may be less reliable due to insufficient spatial resolution, image distortion, and partial volume effects. Therefore, the value of ADC measurements in the assessment of lymph nodes is still questionable.

# Functional Imaging of Tumor Molecular Targets and Processes

## Molecular Imaging of Specific Receptor Targets

### Somatostatin Receptor Imaging

Receptor targeting is an attractive approach for non-invasive imaging including that of cancer. Somatostatin receptors (SSTRs) are overexpressed in many tumors (e.g., neuroendocrine, lung, and breast tumors and lymphomas), with subtype specificity for each histology. Five receptor subtypes (SSTR1–5), acting through transmembrane domain G proteins, have been identified. The most commonly used agent previously was [111]In-pentetreotide for SPECT imaging, although SSTR-targeted radiotracers have also been developed for PET, such as [68]Ga-DOTA-Phe$^1$-Tyr$^3$-octreotide ([68]Ga-DOTATOC) and Gluc-Lys([18]F-fluoropropionyl-TOCA). Such PET radiotracers are of substantial value for the evaluation of patients with SSTR-positive lesions such as neuroendocrine tumors, particularly carcinoid. [68]Ga-DOTATOC seems to be a very promising PET radiotracer for imaging SSTRs even in small meningiomas, offering excellent imaging properties and very high tumor-to-background ratio. Compared with [111]In-pentetreotide SPECT, Gluc-Lys([18]F-fluoropropionyl-TOCA)-PET revealed more than twice the number of lesions and resulted in near-perfect interobserver agreement.[51]

[68]Ga-DOTA-Tyr$^3$-Thr$^8$-octreotide ([68]Ga-DOTATATE) (an SSTR2-selective ligand) and [68]Ga-DOTA-1-NaI$_3$-octreotide ([68]Ga-DOTANOC) (with SSTR2, 3, and 5 affinity) are some newer SSTR PET imaging agents currently under clinical evaluation. A recent study demonstrates the utility of [68]Ga-DOTANOC to identify the primary lesion in patients with carcinoma of unknown origin of neuroendocrine type.[52] An additional prospective study from the same center also demonstrates that this radiotracer is also highly sensitive and specific for evaluation of patients with pheochromocytoma and paraganglioma, and seems to be superior to [131]I-MIBG scintigraphy.[53]

### Estrogen Receptor Imaging

Estrogen receptor (ER) expression in breast carcinoma is an indicator of patient prognosis and likelihood of tumor response to anti-estrogen therapy. Currently, treatment with anti-estrogen therapy depends on *in vitro* immunohistochemistry assays of biopsy material for ER expression in breast cancer. However, the *in vitro* assay cannot discriminate between functional and non-functional receptors. ER targeting radiotracers may therefore be useful to non-invasively assess the functional ER status of tumors *in vivo* through the use of [18]F-radiolabeled estrogen analogues for PET imaging, and 16α-[18]F-fluoroestradiol-17β (FES) is commonly used for this purpose due to its favorable biodistribution.[54] FES has shown the most promise for quantification of the functional ER status of breast cancer, both in the primary tumor and in metastatic sites. The amount of FES uptake in primary tumors correlates with ER expression measured by *in vitro* assays.[55] FES also provides sufficient image quality to image metastatic lesions with high sensitivity in patients with ER-positive tumors. In addition to aiding in selection of patients for anti-estrogen therapy, FES-PET may reveal a faster treatment response to tamoxifen than FDG-PET at 7–10 days after treatment initiation.[56,57]

## Molecular Imaging of Tumor Processes

Clinicians and scientists have been working to develop PET radiotracers to improve the diagnosis and monitoring of various cancers and to probe a wide multitude of biological or pathophysiological tumor processes *in vivo*. Many such radiotracers exist that are radiolabeled with short half-life radionuclides such as $^{11}$C (~20 minute half-life), $^{13}$N (~10 minute half-life), and $^{15}$O (~2 minute half-life), but require an onsite cyclotron. As such, such radiotracers are usually only available for research purposes at major academic institutions. However, given the availability of $^{18}$F (with a longer half-life of ~2 hours) for radiolabeling of compounds, $^{18}$F-radiolabeled radiotracers are generally available for delivery to PET centers around the world for routine clinical use. Various molecular targets (as discussed above), biological processes, and disease control points involved in cancer can be studied through use of some of the multitude of available PET radiotracers.[58] In the following sections, we will focus on some common tumor processes such as glucose and amino acid metabolism, cell proliferation, oxygenation/hypoxia, angiogenesis, and apoptosis that can be quantified *in vivo* with PET and other functional imaging techniques.

### Glucose Metabolism

FDG is the most commonly used PET radiotracer in the world and is FDA approved for clinical use in the United States. FDG-PET (typically performed as part of PET/CT and potentially in the future as part of PET/MRI) is often regarded as the "one-stop shop" technique for the evaluation of patients with cancer due to its versatility and high diagnostic performance for accurate localization of sites of disease with high sensitivity. It is a glucose analogue first tested in humans in 1976 at the Hospital of the University of Pennsylvania.[59] FDG is transported into cells via glucose transporters, such as GLUT-1, and subsequently phosphorylated by hexokinase, both of which are overexpressed in cancer cells. This protein overexpression, in combination with reduced or absent glucose-6-phosphatase levels in cancer cells, leads to the accumulation of the metabolic product 2-$^{18}$F-fluoro-2-deoxy-D-glucose-6-phosphate intracellularly, as it cannot undergo further metabolism through the glycolytic pathway. Persistent glucose uptake in cancer cells in a low serum insulin state makes FDG an ideal PET radiotracer for cancer imaging. As FDG-PET provides unique functional molecular information, it is complementary with structural imaging techniques for the management of patients with a wide variety of malignancies. Improved disease staging, treatment planning, and response monitoring are some of the most useful aspects of this powerful imaging technique.[60]

### Amino Acid Metabolism

PET imaging in conjunction with amino acid analogues, such as those of methionine, tyrosine, and L-dihydroxyphenylalanine (L-DOPA) allows for the assessment of more specific radiotracer uptake in tumors, since FDG-PET is known to show nonspecific

uptake in inflammatory cells and granulation tissue. For example, Rau et al. compare the tyrosine analogue O-(2-$^{18}$F-fluoroethyl)-L-tyrosine (FET) with $^{11}$C-methionine (MET) and FDG in animal models and demonstrate no uptake of FET in sites of acute or chronic inflammation.[61]

Advantages of imaging brain tumors with MET-PET are related to the low background uptake of MET in the brain. However, the major shortcoming of MET is the ~20-minute half-life of the $^{11}$C isotope, which requires an on-site cyclotron for imaging. Jacobs et al. showed a sensitivity of 91% for detecting gliomas, as well as larger detected tumor volumes compared to those detected with contrast-enhanced MRI, which may have an impact on radiation treatment planning.[62] In one of the earliest comparative studies between FET-PET and FDG-PET in peripheral tumors, it was observed that FET accumulated in squamous cell head and neck tumors, whereas adenocarcinomas and lymphomas exhibited no significant FET uptake.[63] $^{18}$F-6-fluorodihydroxyphenylalanine (FDOPA), an analogue of L-DOPA, accumulates in dopaminergic neurons in the basal ganglia and is useful to study patients with neuroendocrine tumors such as carcinoid tumor, islet cell tumor, and medullary thyroid cancer, melanoma, and brain tumors.[64] This radiotracer is also useful for evaluation of low-grade and recurrent brain tumors and for differentiation of low-grade tumors from necrosis.[65]

### Cell Proliferation Imaging

Cell proliferation is a hallmark of cancer, and 3′-deoxy-3′-$^{18}$F-fluorothymidine (FLT), a thymidine analogue, is one of the many PET radiotracers that has been developed to assess cell proliferation of tumors *in vivo* (Figure 10.1). Cellular FLT uptake reflects the activity of thymidine kinase-1 (TK1) (an enzyme involved in the salvage pathway of deoxyribonucleic acid (DNA) synthesis), is enhanced in proliferating cells, and correlates with Ki-67 assays of cell proliferation.[66,67] TK-1 then phosphorylates FLT to form negatively charged FLT monophosphate, resulting in intracellular trapping. FLT-PET has been utilized to evaluate various malignancies such as glioma, lung cancer, esophageal cancer, colorectal cancer, breast cancer, laryngeal cancer, melanoma, lymphoma, and soft-tissue sarcomas. Most data to date suggest that FLT is not a suitable biomarker for cancer staging because of the rather low fraction of tumor cells that undergo replication at a given time and the generally high FLT uptake in the liver and bone marrow. However, FLT-PET shows the most promise for early tumor response assessment purposes. Furthermore, in some settings, FLT-PET may have greater specificity for cancer than FDG-PET, as FDG also nonspecifically accumulates in sites of infection or inflammation.[66–69]

### Oxygenation Imaging

Tumor hypoxia is an important prognostic factor for cancer patients, and there is great interest for non-invasive quantification of the oxygenation status and presence of hypoxia in malignant tissues.[70] Hypoxic tumor cells are generally more radioresistant and chemoresistant than normoxic tumor cells.[70,71] Hence, detection and quantification of hypoxia in tumor with functional imaging may be useful to select and plan individualized treatments with radiotherapy and/or chemotherapy (Figure 10.2).[72]

There are currently many clinical trials in progress involving the use of hypoxia PET radiotracers such as $^{18}$F-fluoromisonidazole ($^{18}$F-FMISO), $^{18}$F-fluoroazomycin arabinoside ($^{18}$F-FAZA), $^{18}$F-radiolabeled 2-(2-nitro-$^{1}$H-imidazol-1-yl)-N-(2,2,3,3,3-pentafluoropropyl)-acetamide ($^{18}$F-EF5), $^{18}$F-HX4, $^{60}$Cu(II)-diacetyl-bis(N$^4$-methylthiosemicarbazone) ($^{60}$Cu-ATSM)

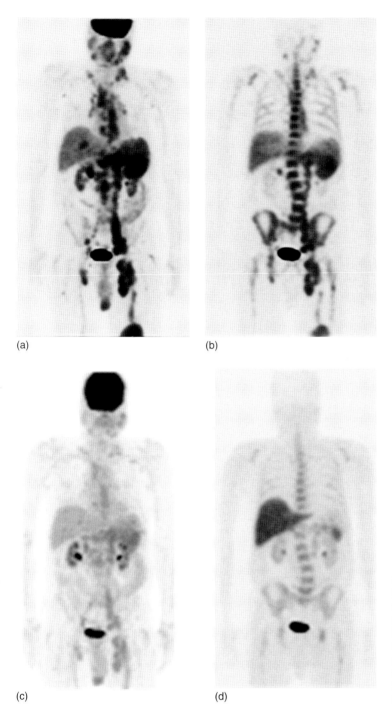

(a)

(b)

(c)

(d)

**Figure 10.1** Glucose metabolism and cell proliferation PET imaging. Whole-body FDG-PET and FLT-PET in 73-year-old man with mantle cell lymphoma for pre- and post-therapy evaluation. Coronal maximal intensity projection (MIP) images reveal multiple FDG and FLT avid lesions in lymph node chains. Pre-therapy FDG (a) and FLT (b) scans were performed within 24 hours of each other, as well as the post-therapy FDG (c) and FLT (d) scans. Note interval decrease in metabolism and cell proliferation in tumor sites following therapy.

or $^{64}$Cu-ATSM, and $^{124}$I-iodo-azomycin galactopyranoside ($^{124}$I-IAZGP), amongst others. $^{18}$F-FMISO is the most extensively studied radiotracer for PET assessment of tumor hypoxia, as it was the first radiolabeled nitroimidazole compound available for PET imaging.[73] Nitroimidazole compounds undergo intracellular chemical reduction; and under chronic hypoxic conditions, they covalently bind to macromolecules, mainly thiol-containing proteins, so that they are trapped in hypoxic tissues. These radiotracers have been utilized to evaluate malignancies including lung cancer, brain tumors, head and neck cancer, and cervical cancer, amongst others for purposes of treatment planning and outcome prediction. For example, uptake of $^{60}$Cu-ATSM in cervical cancer is inversely related to progression-free survival and overall survival and is useful to predict likelihood of tumor recurrence and locoregional nodal metastasis.[74]

Various functional MRI (fMRI) techniques are also available to non-invasively study oxygenation in tumors and to monitor changes in tumors related to therapy. These include blood oxygen level-dependent (BOLD) fMRI, overhauser-enhanced MRI, and electron paramagnetic resonance imaging (EPRI).[75]

### Angiogenesis Imaging

Angiogenesis is the physiological process that involves the growth of new blood vessels. Many tumors have increased angiogenic capability, and there are several available drugs that target this

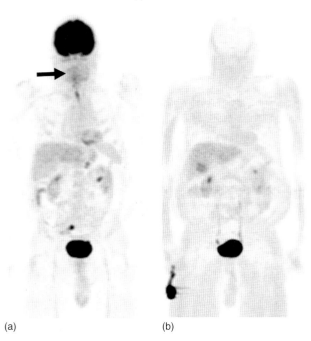

(a)                          (b)

**Figure 10.2** Glucose metabolism and hypoxia PET imaging. Whole-body FDG-PET (a) and whole-body $^{18}$F-HX4-PET (b) coronal images of 76-year-old man with laryngeal cancer status post combined chemoradiation therapy. Note mild FDG uptake in mid neck (arrow) due to post-treatment inflammation and lack of $^{18}$F-HX4 uptake indicating lack of tumor hypoxia. Patient is currently alive for approximately 3 years since PET imaging.

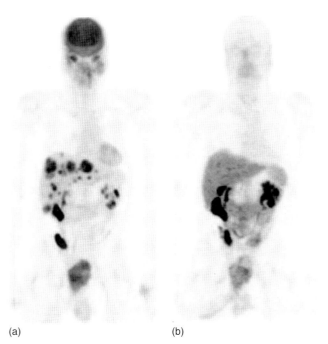

(a)                          (b)

**Figure 10.3** Glucose metabolism and angiogenesis PET imaging. Whole-body FDG-PET (a) and whole-body $^{18}$F-RGD-K5-PET (b) coronal MIP images of 60-year-old man with metastatic gastrointestinal stromal tumor to liver. Note multiple FDG avid hepatic metastases and lack of $^{18}$F-RGD-K5 uptake within metastatic lesions indicating lack of angiogenesis. The patient did not respond to anti-angiogenesis therapy and subsequently passed away several months after PET imaging due to tumor progression.

process in order to control or eradicate tumors. The most commonly studied angiogenesis PET radiotracers are related to the Arg–Gly–Asp peptide (RGD) and include $^{18}$F-galacto-RGD, $^{18}$F-RGD-K5, $^{64}$Cu-1,4,7,10-tetraazacyclododecane-N,N′,N″,N‴-tetraacetic acid-RGD ($^{64}$Cu-DOTA-RGD), and $^{68}$Ga-DOTA-RGD.[76] Peptides that contain RGD have a general affinity toward $\alpha_V\beta_3$ integrins on activated endothelial cells involved in angiogenesis. For example, $^{18}$F-galacto-RGD uptake correlates with $\alpha_V\beta_3$ expression, as well as microvessel density as observed at histology.[77] As such, these radiotracers may be useful for individualized treatment planning and anti-angiogenic therapy monitoring of malignancies, as activated endothelium is susceptible to anti-angiogenic therapy whereas quiescent endothelium is resistant to anti-angiogenic therapy (Figure 10.3).

One drawback of these radiotracers is that they bind to $\alpha_V\beta_3$ integrins present both on tumor cells and tumor-associated endothelial cells. In order to circumvent this problem and more specifically target vascular endothelial cells, imaging agents based on targeting of cell receptors such as vascular endothelial cell growth factor receptor, which are over-expressed on endothelial cells during angiogenesis, are currently under development.

### Apoptosis Imaging

Apoptosis is the process of programmed cell death, such that the cells that are deficient in this capability can become tumorigenic. There are several signal transduction pathways involved in apoptosis, and the major compounds used to non-invasively assess tumor apoptosis are Annexin V and its derivatives. Annexin V is a protein that binds with high affinity to phosphatidylserine on the exterior of cell membranes during early apoptosis, which can be radio-

labeled with either $^{99m}$Tc or with $^{124}$I, $^{18}$F or $^{64}$Cu in order to image early apoptosis *in vivo* using SPECT or PET, respectively.[78] These radiotracers have been studied in animal models and can accurately detect and quantify levels of apoptosis non-invasively, which may be useful for purposes of early treatment response assessment.[79,80] Caspases may also be suitable as targets for *in vivo* imaging of apoptosis, as they are involved in the cell death pathways.[78,81]

Superparamagnetic iron-based contrast agents and other paramagnetic contrast agents in conjunction with carrier nanoparticles that specifically target particular molecules or biologic processes of interest have also been studied using MRI.[82] For example, Schellenberger et al. used nanoparticles conjugated to Annexin V to target apoptosis for non-invasive MRI-based tumor monitoring.[83] However, limitations of such approaches using MRI include low signal-to-noise ratios (SNRs) with low sensitivity, lack of standardization of imaging sequences and parameters, lack of standardization of analysis methodologies for quantification, and potential toxicity of the contrast agents.

### Magnetic Resonance Spectroscopy

Magnetic resonance spectroscopy (MRS) is a molecular imaging method that allows for the separation of the MRI signal from a given tissue into its chemical components. This is possible since the magnetic field experienced by an atomic nucleus is minutely "shielded" or modified by the fields produced by neighboring atoms on the same molecule, which produces a "chemical shift" or small variation in the nuclear resonant frequency. A display of MRI signal amplitude as a function of nuclear resonance frequency forms a spectrum, with different chemical environments of a particular type of atomic nucleus within and between molecules forming peaks at characteristic chemical shift positions. As such, one can quantitatively assess the amount, type, and location of small molecular compounds within a tissue or organ of interest at the same time conventional MRI is performed.[84] The data are usually displayed as a grid of spectra of chemical compound abundances obtained at either single or multiple locations in a tissue or organ of interest. Such spectra are collected from spinning nuclei (spins), most often [1]H given the abundance of water in tissue.

[1]H MRS enables accurate quantitative assessment of the spatial distribution of tissue metabolites such as creatinine, amino acids, choline, nucleotides, lactate, and lipids.[85] Although nonspecific, there are several MRS findings that are more frequently seen in cancer. For example, increased concentrations of cell membrane metabolites such as phosphocholine may be present due to increased membrane synthesis, a higher concentration of lactate may be present due to increased metabolism through the glycolytic pathway, and lower concentrations of normal tissue metabolites (such as N-acetyl aspartate in cerebral tissue or citrate in prostatic tissue) may be encountered.[86,87]

In both research and clinical practice, [1]H MRS is most frequently applied in the brain, given the relative lack of motion in this location compared to other regions of the body. For example, [1]H MRS is useful for the characterization of brain tumors (including differentiation between pyogenic brain abscesses from cystic or necrotic brain tumors, and discrimination between gliomas and solitary brain metastases) and for grading of gliomas.[88–90] [1]H MRS also provides more accurate assessment of tumor cell infiltration than structural imaging alone, which has significant implications for treatment planning.[91,92] Furthermore, [1]H MRS may be useful to predict patient prognosis. For instance, patients with glioblastoma multiforme have significantly shorter median survival when a large volume of metabolic abnormality is seen at [1]H MRS.[93] [1]H MRS may be useful for the evaluation of extracranial tumors, including those involving the breast, pancreas, adrenal gland, cervix, prostate gland, bone, and soft-tissue.[94–99]

There is an increasing trend toward performing MRI at higher field strengths (>1.5 T), since SNR increases linearly with field strength.[100] Higher field strength may also be advantageous for MRS. First, more signal intensity is detectable from a given volume per unit of scan time, and, second, the frequency dispersion (chemical shift) that allows one to distinguish several lines in the spectra is also increased.[100] The increased chemical shift may not only improve the accuracy of determination of compounds, but may also allow detection of other compounds as useful tumor biomarkers. Although several technical challenges still have to be overcome, the first MRS studies at 7.0 T field strength are promising and confirm the theoretical advantages of performing MRS at higher field strengths.[101,102] For example, a volunteer study that compared brain [1]H MRS at 4.0–7.0 T reports that the spectral line width is increased by 50% at 7.0 T, resulting in a 14% increase in spectral resolution at 7.0 T relative to 4.0 T.[101] In addition, metabolite quantification at 7.0 T is less sensitive to reduced SNR than at 4.0 T, and precision of metabolite quantification and detectability of weakly represented metabolites are substantially increased at 7.0 T relative to 4.0 T. Because of the increased spectral resolution at 7.0 T, only one-half of the SNR of the 4.0 T spectrum was needed to obtain the same quantification precision.[101] Another study shows that prostate [1]H MRS is feasible at 7.0 T and allows detection of polyamines next to citrate, creatine, and choline, potentially improving *in vivo* detection, localization, and assessment of prostate cancer.[102] Other stud-

ies involving the application of 7.0 T [1]H MRS for the evaluation of tumors in other body regions are also currently ongoing.

Other nuclear candidates for MRS include [13]C, [19]F, [23]Na, and [31]P.[84] Phosphorus is fundamental to a number of cellular processes, including energy metabolism and membrane construction and may be studied via [31]P MRS, offering insight into processes such as cell energy metabolism, tissue oxygenation state, pH, and membrane turnover.[84] For example, [31]P MRS is useful to differentiate prostate carcinoma from benign prostatic hypertrophy.[103] It can also differentiate benign from malignant head and neck neoplasms, can predict treatment response, and demonstrate therapeutic effects in head and neck cancer.[104] One study reports that [31]P MRS pre-treatment measurement of phosphocholine and phosphoethanolamine content within non-Hodgkin's lymphoma predicts long-term response to treatment and time-to-treatment failure, particularly when combined with the international prognostic index.[105]

Another exciting development is the use of hyperpolarized contrast agents for molecular and metabolic MR imaging.[106,107] Hyperpolarization is the general term for a method of enhancing spin-polarization differences of nuclear populations in a magnetic field. Since signal intensity and SNR depend linearly upon polarization level, hyperpolarization makes it possible to visualize heteronuclei (i.e., atomic nuclei other than [1]H) that normally have a low abundance in the body. Although all heteronuclei can be hyperpolarized, at present only [13]C has been used for *in vivo* MRI experiments. This is due to its relatively high gyromagnetic ratio, which increases its sensitivity, and to the availability of dedicated coils tuned to the [13]C frequency. The highly increased signal intensity achievable through hyperpolarization makes it possible to detect newly formed [13]C compounds in very short times after injection of a hyperpolarized [13]C contrast agent without background signal. This makes visualization of molecules that represent key steps of cellular metabolism possible, providing direct access to physiological/pathological changes at the cellular level. Using chemical shift imaging sequences, more than one molecule may be visualized in the same anatomical region.[106,107] For example, animal studies show that it is possible to obtain maps of pyruvate, lactate, and alanine within a time frame of <1 minute after the intravenous administration of [13]C-hyperpolarized pyruvate, and report that tumors have a higher lactate concentration than normal tissue and that lactate SNR levels are correlated to histological grade.[108–110] The hyperpolarized [13]C-pyruvate technique may also be used for detecting tumor treatment response in *in vitro* and animal studies of lymphoma, as tumor conversion of pyruvate to lactate is reduced following treatment.[111] Several other hyperpolarized [13]C-molecules beyond [13]C-pyruvate that may enhance our understanding of tumor biology at the molecular level and that may improve the assessment of malignant lesions are currently being investigated.[106,107] However, an important prerequisite for MRS-based molecular imaging methods to be widely accepted in routine clinical practice is the standardization of acquisition and analysis protocols.

## Conclusion

A wide variety of functional imaging techniques is available for *in vivo* visualization and quantification of tumor physiology, molecular targets, and biological processes. In combination with structural imaging, functional imaging improves the efficiency and effectiveness of research in oncology, helps to characterize biomarkers of disease and new endpoints for assessment of tumor response, and can reduce cancer-related morbidity and mortality by improving the diagnostic performance of cancer screening, diagnosis, staging, prognosis assessment, treatment planning, response assessment, restaging, and surveillance. Familiarity with and use of functional imaging is therefore essential for optimal results in clinical oncology as well as for research purposes.

# References

1  Siegel R, Naishadham D, Jemal A. Cancer statistics. *CA Cancer J Clin.* 2012;62(1):10–29.

2  Kwee TC, Basu S, Saboury B, Alavi A, Torigian DA. Functional oncoimaging techniques with potential clinical applications. *Front Biosci (Elite Ed).* 2012;4:1081–1096.

3  Torigian DA, Huang SS, Houseni M, Alavi A. Functional imaging of cancer with emphasis on molecular techniques. *CA Cancer J Clin.* 2007;57(4):206–224.

4  Barentsz J, Takahashi S, Oyen W, et al. Commonly used imaging techniques for diagnosis and staging. *J Clin Oncol.* 2006;24(20):3234–3244.

5  Zaidi H, Montandon ML, Alavi A. The clinical role of fusion imaging using PET, CT, and MR imaging. *Magn Reson Imaging Clin N Am.* 2010;18(1):133–149.

6  Townsend DW. Dual-modality imaging: combining anatomy and function. *J Nucl Med.* 2008;49(6):938–955.

7  Folkman J. Tumor angiogenesis: therapeutic implications. *N Engl J Med.* 1971;285(21):1182–1186.

8  Brix G, Griebel J, Kiessling F, Wenz F. Tracer kinetic modelling of tumour angiogenesis based on dynamic contrast-enhanced CT and MRI measurements. *Eur J Nucl Med Mol Imaging.* 2010;37(Suppl 1):S30–S51.

9  Leach MO, Morgan B, Tofts PS, et al. Imaging vascular function for early stage clinical trials using dynamic contrast-enhanced magnetic resonance imaging. *Eur Radiol.* 2012;22(7):1451–1464.

10  Stejskal E, Tanner J. Spin diffusion measurements: spin echoes in the presence of a time-dependent field gradient. *J Chem Phys.* 1965;42:288–292.

11  Padhani AR, Liu G, Koh DM, et al. Diffusion-weighted magnetic resonance imaging as a cancer biomarker: consensus and recommendations. *Neoplasia.* 2009;11(2):102–125.

12  Kwee TC, Takahara T, Ochiai R, et al. Whole-body diffusion-weighted magnetic resonance imaging. *Eur J Radiol.* 2009;70(3):409–417.

13  Taouli B, Koh DM. Diffusion-weighted MR imaging of the liver. *Radiology.* 2010;254(1):47–66.

14  Merino JG, Warach S. Imaging of acute stroke. *Nat Rev Neurol.* 2010;6(10):560–571.

15  Nomori H, Mori T, Ikeda K, et al. Diffusion-weighted magnetic resonance imaging can be used in place of positron emission tomography for N staging of non-small cell lung cancer with fewer false-positive results. *J Thorac Cardiovasc Surg.* 2008;135(4):816–822.

16  Ohno Y, Koyama H, Onishi Y, et al. Non-small cell lung cancer: whole-body MR examination for M-stage assessment–utility for whole-body diffusion-weighted imaging compared with integrated FDG PET/CT. *Radiology.* 2008;248(2):643–654.

17  Takenaka D, Ohno Y, Matsumoto K, et al. Detection of bone metastases in non-small cell lung cancer patients: comparison of whole-body diffusion-weighted imaging (DWI), whole-body MR imaging without and with DWI, whole-body FDG-PET/CT, and bone scintigraphy. *J Magn Reson Imaging.* 2009;30(2):298–308.

18  Murakami R, Hirai T, Sugahara T, et al. Grading astrocytic tumors by using apparent diffusion coefficient parameters: superiority of a one- versus two-parameter pilot method. *Radiology.* 2009;251(3):838–845.

19  Mori T, Nomori H, Ikeda K, et al. Diffusion-weighted magnetic resonance imaging for diagnosing malignant pulmonary nodules/masses: comparison with positron emission tomography. *J Thorac Oncol.* 2008;3(4):358–364.

20  Ohba Y, Nomori H, Mori T, et al. Is diffusion-weighted magnetic resonance imaging superior to positron emission tomography with fludeoxyglucose F 18 in imaging non-small cell lung cancer? *J Thorac Cardiovasc Surg.* 2009;138(2):439–445.

21  Nakajo M, Kajiya Y, Kaneko T, et al. FDG PET/CT and diffusion-weighted imaging for breast cancer: prognostic value of maximum standardized uptake values and apparent diffusion coefficient values of the primary lesion. *Eur J Nucl Med Mol Imaging.* 2010;37(11):2011–2020.

22  Hamstra DA, Rehemtulla A, Ross BD. Diffusion magnetic resonance imaging: a biomarker for treatment response in oncology. *J Clin Oncol.* 2007;25(26):4104–4109.

23  Hamstra DA, Galban CJ, Meyer CR, et al. Functional diffusion map as an early imaging biomarker for high-grade glioma: correlation with conventional radiologic response and overall survival. *J Clin Oncol.* 2008;26(20):3387–3394.

24  Galban CJ, Mukherji SK, Chenevert TL, et al. A feasibility study of parametric response map analysis of diffusion-weighted magnetic resonance imaging scans of head and neck cancer patients for providing early detection of therapeutic efficacy. *Transl Oncol.* 2009;2(3):184–190.

25  Ma B, Meyer CR, Pickles MD, et al. Voxel-by-voxel functional diffusion mapping for early evaluation of breast cancer treatment. *Inf Process Med Imaging.* 2009;21:276–287.

26  Lee KC, Bradley DA, Hussain M, et al. A feasibility study evaluating the functional diffusion map as a predictive imaging biomarker for detection of treatment response in a patient with metastatic prostate cancer to the bone. *Neoplasia.* 2007;9(12):1003–1011.

27  Beaulieu C. The basis of anisotropic water diffusion in the nervous system—a technical review. *NMR Biomed.* 2002;15(7–8):435–455.

28  Hagmann P, Jonasson L, Maeder P, Thiran JP, Wedeen VJ, Meuli R. Understanding diffusion MR imaging techniques: from scalar diffusion-weighted imaging to diffusion tensor imaging and beyond. *Radiographics.* 2006;26(Suppl 1):S205–S223.

29  Nimsky C, Ganslandt O, Hastreiter P, et al. Preoperative and intraoperative diffusion tensor imaging-based fiber tracking in glioma surgery. *Neurosurgery.* 2005;56(1):130–137; discussion 138.

30  Nimsky C, Ganslandt O, Hastreiter P, et al. Intraoperative diffusion-tensor MR imaging: shifting of white matter tracts during neurosurgical procedures—initial experience. *Radiology.* 2005;234(1):218–225.

31  Nimsky C, Ganslandt O, Hastreiter P, et al. Preoperative and intraoperative diffusion tensor imaging-based fiber tracking in glioma surgery. *Neurosurgery.* 2007;61(Suppl 1):178–185; discussion 186.

32  Mariappan YK, Glaser KJ, Ehman RL. Magnetic resonance elastography: a review. *Clin Anat.* 2010;23(5):497–511.

33  Muthupillai R, Lomas DJ, Rossman PJ, Greenleaf JF, Manduca A, Ehman RL. Magnetic resonance elastography by direct visualization of propagating acoustic strain waves. *Science.* 1995;269(5232):1854–1857.

34  Huwart L, Sempoux C, Vicaut E, et al. Magnetic resonance elastography for the noninvasive staging of liver fibrosis. *Gastroenterology.* 2008;135(1):32–40.

35  Krouskop TA, Younes PS, Srinivasan S, Wheeler T, Ophir J. Differences in the compressive stress-strain response of infiltrating ductal carcinomas with and without lobular features—implications for mammography and elastography. *Ultrason Imaging.* 2003;25(3):162–170.

36  Sinkus R, Siegmann K, Xydeas T, Tanter M, Claussen C, Fink M. MR elastography of breast lesions: understanding the solid/liquid duality

can improve the specificity of contrast-enhanced MR mammography. *Magn Reson Med*. 2007;58(6):1135–1144.

37 Kwee TC, Basu S, Torigian DA, Saboury B, Alavi A. Defining the role of modern imaging techniques in assessing lymph nodes for metastasis in cancer: evolving contribution of PET in this setting. *Eur J Nucl Med Mol Imaging*. 2011;38(7):1353–1366.

38 Boland GM, Gershenwald JE. Sentinel lymph node biopsy in melanoma. *Cancer J*. 2012;18(2):185–191.

39 Cheng G, Kurita S, Torigian DA, Alavi A. Current status of sentinel lymph-node biopsy in patients with breast cancer. *Eur J Nucl Med Mol Imaging*. 2011;38(3):562–575.

40 Sadeghi R, Gholami H, Zakavi SR, Kakhki VR, Tabasi KT, Horenblas S. Accuracy of sentinel lymph node biopsy for inguinal lymph node staging of penile squamous cell carcinoma: systematic review and meta-analysis of the literature. *J Urol*. 2012;187(1):25–31.

41 Lam TK, Uren RF, Scolyer RA, Quinn MJ, Shannon KF, Thompson JF. False-negative sentinel node biopsy because of obstruction of lymphatics by metastatic melanoma: the value of ultrasound in conjunction with preoperative lymphoscintigraphy. *Melanoma Res*. 2009;19(2):94–99.

42 Goyal A, Douglas-Jones AG, Newcombe RG, Mansel RE. Effect of lymphatic tumor burden on sentinel lymph node biopsy in breast cancer. *Breast J*. 2005;11(3):188–194.

43 Leijte JA, van der Ploeg IM, Valdes Olmos RA, Nieweg OE, Horenblas S. Visualization of tumor blockage and rerouting of lymphatic drainage in penile cancer patients by use of SPECT/CT. *J Nucl Med*. 2009;50(3):364–367.

44 Weissleder R, Elizondo G, Wittenberg J, Lee AS, Josephson L, Brady TJ. Ultrasmall superparamagnetic iron oxide: an intravenous contrast agent for assessing lymph nodes with MR imaging. *Radiology*. 1990;175(2):494–498.

45 Will O, Purkayastha S, Chan C, et al. Diagnostic precision of nanoparticle-enhanced MRI for lymph-node metastases: a meta-analysis. *Lancet Oncol*. 2006;7(1):52–60.

46 Vandecaveye V, De Keyzer F, Vander Poorten V, et al. Head and neck squamous cell carcinoma: value of diffusion-weighted MR imaging for nodal staging. *Radiology*. 2009;251(1):134–146.

47 Kim JK, Kim KA, Park BW, Kim N, Cho KS. Feasibility of diffusion-weighted imaging in the differentiation of metastatic from non-metastatic lymph nodes: early experience. *J Magn Reson Imaging*. 2008;28(3):714–719.

48 Eiber M, Beer AJ, Holzapfel K, et al. Preliminary results for characterization of pelvic lymph nodes in patients with prostate cancer by diffusion-weighted MR-imaging. *Invest Radiol*. 2010;45(1):15–23.

49 Nakai G, Matsuki M, Inada Y, et al. Detection and evaluation of pelvic lymph nodes in patients with gynecologic malignancies using body diffusion-weighted magnetic resonance imaging. *J Comput Assist Tomogr*. 2008;32(5):764–768.

50 Lin G, Ho KC, Wang JJ, et al. Detection of lymph node metastasis in cervical and uterine cancers by diffusion-weighted magnetic resonance imaging at 3T. *J Magn Reson Imaging*. 2008;28(1):128–135.

51 Meisetschlager G, Poethko T, Stahl A, et al. Gluc-Lys([18F]FP)-TOCA PET in patients with SSTR-positive tumors: biodistribution and diagnostic evaluation compared with [111In]DTPA-octreotide. *J Nucl Med*. 2006;47(4):566–573.

52 Naswa N, Sharma P, Kumar A, et al. Ga-DOTANOC PET/CT in patients with carcinoma of unknown primary of neuroendocrine origin. *Clin Nucl Med*. 2012;37(3):245–251.

53 Naswa N, Sharma P, Nazar AH, et al. Prospective evaluation of Ga-DOTA-NOC PET-CT in phaeochromocytoma and paraganglioma: preliminary results from a single centre study. *Eur Radiol*. 2012;22(3):710–719.

54 Sundararajan L, Linden HM, Link JM, Krohn KA, Mankoff DA. 18F-Fluoroestradiol. *Semin Nucl Med*. 2007;37(6):470–476.

55 Eubank WB, Mankoff DA. Evolving role of positron emission tomography in breast cancer imaging. *Semin Nucl Med*. 2005;35(2):84–99.

56 Dehdashti F, Mortimer JE, Trinkaus K, et al. PET-based estradiol challenge as a predictive biomarker of response to endocrine therapy in women with estrogen-receptor-positive breast cancer. *Breast Cancer Res Treat*. 2008;113(3):509–517.

57 Linden HM, Stekhova SA, Link JM, et al. Quantitative fluoroestradiol positron emission tomography imaging predicts response to endocrine treatment in breast cancer. *J Clin Oncol*. 2006;24(18):2793–2799.

58 Chopra A, Shan L, Eckelman WC, et al. Molecular imaging and contrast agent database (MICAD): evolution and progress. *Mol Imaging Biol*. 2011;14(1):4–13.

59 Alavi A, Kung JW, Zhuang H. Implications of PET based molecular imaging on the current and future practice of medicine. *Semin Nucl Med*. 2004;34(1):56–69.

60 Hillner BE, Siegel BA, Shields AF, et al. The impact of positron emission tomography (PET) on expected management during cancer treatment: findings of the National Oncologic PET Registry. *Cancer*. 2009;115(2):410–418.

61 Rau FC, Weber WA, Wester HJ, et al. O-(2-[(18F]Fluoroethyl)- L-tyrosine (FET): a tracer for differentiation of tumour from inflammation in murine lymph nodes. *Eur J Nucl Med Mol Imaging*. 2002;29(8):1039–1046.

62 Jacobs AH, Thomas A, Kracht LW, et al. 18F-fluoro-L-thymidine and 11C-methylmethionine as markers of increased transport and proliferation in brain tumors. *J Nucl Med*. 2005;46(12):1948–1958.

63 Pauleit D, Stoffels G, Schaden W, et al. PET with O-(2-18F-fluoroethyl)-L-tyrosine in peripheral tumors: first clinical results. *J Nucl Med*. 2005;46(3):411–416.

64 Jager PL, Chirakal R, Marriott CJ, Brouwers AH, Koopmans KP, Gulenchyn KY. 6-L-18F-fluorodihydroxyphenylalanine PET in neuroendocrine tumors: basic aspects and emerging clinical applications. *J Nucl Med*. 2008;49(4):573–586.

65 Chen W, Silverman DH, Delaloye S, et al. 18F-FDOPA PET imaging of brain tumors: comparison study with 18F-FDG PET and evaluation of diagnostic accuracy. *J Nucl Med*. 2006;47(6):904–911.

66 Salskov A, Tammisetti VS, Grierson J, Vesselle H. FLT: measuring tumor cell proliferation in vivo with positron emission tomography and 3′-deoxy-3′-[(18)F]fluorothymidine. *Semin Nucl Med*. 2007;37(6):429–439.

67 Bading JR, Shields AF. Imaging of cell proliferation: status and prospects. *J Nucl Med*. 2008;49(Suppl 2):64S–80S.

68 Barwick T, Bencherif B, Mountz JM, Avril N. Molecular PET and PET/CT imaging of tumour cell proliferation using F-18 fluoro-L-thymidine: a comprehensive evaluation. *Nucl Med Commun*. 2009;30(12):908–917.

69 Soloviev D, Lewis D, Honess D, Aboagye E. [(18)F]FLT: an imaging biomarker of tumour proliferation for assessment of tumour response to treatment. *Eur J Cancer*. 2012;48(4):416–424.

70 Wilson WR, Hay MP. Targeting hypoxia in cancer therapy. *Nat Rev Cancer*. 2011;11(6):393–410.

71 Kirkpatrick JP, Cardenas-Navia LI, Dewhirst MW. Predicting the effect of temporal variations in PO2 on tumor radiosensitivity. *Int J Radiat Oncol Biol Phys*. 2004;59(3):822–833.

72 Krohn KA, Link JM, Mason RP. Molecular imaging of hypoxia. *J Nucl Med*. 2008;49(Suppl 2):129S–148S.

73 Rasey JS, Grunbaum Z, Magee S, et al. Characterization of radiolabeled fluoromisonidazole as a probe for hypoxic cells. *Radiat Res*. 1987;111(2):292–304.

74 Dehdashti F, Grigsby PW, Mintun MA, Lewis JS, Siegel BA, Welch MJ. Assessing tumor hypoxia in cervical cancer by positron emission tomography with 60Cu-ATSM: relationship to therapeutic response-a preliminary report. *Int J Radiat Oncol Biol Phys.* 2003;55(5):1233–1238.

75 Pacheco-Torres J, Lopez-Larrubia P, Ballesteros P, Cerdan S. Imaging tumor hypoxia by magnetic resonance methods. *NMR Biomed.* 2011;24(1):1–16.

76 Dobrucki LW, de Muinck ED, Lindner JR, Sinusas AJ. Approaches to multimodality imaging of angiogenesis. *J Nucl Med.* 2010;1:66S–79S.

77 Beer AJ, Haubner R, Sarbia M, et al. Positron emission tomography using [18F]Galacto-RGD identifies the level of integrin alpha(v)beta3 expression in man. *Clin Cancer Res.* 2006;12(13):3942–3949.

78 Reshef A, Shirvan A, Akselrod-Ballin A, Wall A, Ziv I. Small-molecule biomarkers for clinical PET imaging of apoptosis. *J Nucl Med.* 2010;51(6):837–840.

79 Hu S, Kiesewetter DO, Zhu L, et al. Longitudinal PET imaging of doxorubicin-induced cell death with (18)F-Annexin V. *Mol Imaging Biol.* 2012;14(6):762–770.

80 De Saint-Hubert M, Wang H, Devos E, et al. Preclinical imaging of therapy response using metabolic and apoptosis molecular imaging. *Mol Imaging Biol.* 2011;13(5):995–1002.

81 Nguyen QD, Smith G, Glaser M, Perumal M, Arstad E, Aboagye EO. Positron emission tomography imaging of drug-induced tumor apoptosis with a caspase-3/7 specific [18F]-labeled isatin sulfonamide. *Proc Natl Acad Sci U S A.* 2009;106(38):16375–16380.

82 Caruthers SD, Winter PM, Wickline SA, Lanza GM. Targeted magnetic resonance imaging contrast agents. *Methods Mol Med.* 2006;124:387–400.

83 Schellenberger EA, Hogemann D, Josephson L, Weissleder R. Annexin V-CLIO: a nanoparticle for detecting apoptosis by MRI. *Acad Radiol.* 2002;9(Suppl 2):S310–S311.

84 Aisen AM, Chenevert TL. MR spectroscopy: clinical perspective. *Radiology.* 1989;173(3):593–599.

85 Mountford C, Lean C, Malycha P, Russell P. Proton spectroscopy provides accurate pathology on biopsy and in vivo. *J Magn Reson Imaging.* 2006;24(3):459–477.

86 Sharma U, Mehta A, Seenu V, Jagannathan NR. Biochemical characterization of metastatic lymph nodes of breast cancer patients by in vitro 1H magnetic resonance spectroscopy: a pilot study. *Magn Reson Imaging.* 2004;22(5):697–706.

87 Kurhanewicz J, Vigneron DB, Nelson SJ. Three-dimensional magnetic resonance spectroscopic imaging of brain and prostate cancer. *Neoplasia.* 2000;2(1–2):166–189.

88 Hollingworth W, Medina LS, Lenkinski RE, et al. A systematic literature review of magnetic resonance spectroscopy for the characterization of brain tumors. *AJNR Am J Neuroradiol.* 2006;27(7):1404–1411.

89 Majos C, Aguilera C, Alonso J, et al. Proton MR spectroscopy improves discrimination between tumor and pseudotumoral lesion in solid brain masses. *AJNR Am J Neuroradiol.* 2009;30(3):544–551.

90 Stadlbauer A, Gruber S, Nimsky C, et al. Preoperative grading of gliomas by using metabolite quantification with high-spatial-resolution proton MR spectroscopic imaging. *Radiology.* 2006;238(3):958–969.

91 Laprie A, Catalaa I, Cassol E, et al. Proton magnetic resonance spectroscopic imaging in newly diagnosed glioblastoma: predictive value for the site of postradiotherapy relapse in a prospective longitudinal study. *Int J Radiat Oncol Biol Phys.* 2008;70(3):773–781.

92 Park I, Tamai G, Lee MC, et al. Patterns of recurrence analysis in newly diagnosed glioblastoma multiforme after three-dimensional conformal radiation therapy with respect to pre-radiation therapy magnetic resonance spectroscopic findings. *Int J Radiat Oncol Biol Phys.* 2007;69(2):381–389.

93 Oh J, Henry RG, Pirzkall A, et al. Survival analysis in patients with glioblastoma multiforme: predictive value of choline-to-N-acetylaspartate index, apparent diffusion coefficient, and relative cerebral blood volume. *J Magn Reson Imaging.* 2004;19(5):546–554.

94 Bartella L, Morris EA, Dershaw DD, et al. Proton MR spectroscopy with choline peak as malignancy marker improves positive predictive value for breast cancer diagnosis: preliminary study. *Radiology.* 2006;239(3):686–692.

95 Cho SG, Lee DH, Lee KY, et al. Differentiation of chronic focal pancreatitis from pancreatic carcinoma by in vivo proton magnetic resonance spectroscopy. *J Comput Assist Tomogr.* 2005;29(2):163–169.

96 Faria JF, Goldman SM, Szejnfeld J, et al. Adrenal masses: characterization with in vivo proton MR spectroscopy—initial experience. *Radiology.* 2007;245(3):788–797.

97 Mahon MM, Williams AD, Soutter WP, et al. 1H magnetic resonance spectroscopy of invasive cervical cancer: an in vivo study with ex vivo corroboration. *NMR Biomed.* 2004;17(1):1–9.

98 Swindle P, McCredie S, Russell P, et al. Pathologic characterization of human prostate tissue with proton MR spectroscopy. *Radiology.* 2003;228(1):144–151.

99 Wang CK, Li CW, Hsieh TJ, Chien SH, Liu GC, Tsai KB. Characterization of bone and soft-tissue tumors with in vivo 1H MR spectroscopy: initial results. *Radiology.* 2004;232(2):599–605.

100 Schick F. Whole-body MRI at high field: technical limits and clinical potential. *Eur Radiol.* 2005;15(5):946–959.

101 Tkac I, Oz G, Adriany G, Ugurbil K, Gruetter R. In vivo 1H NMR spectroscopy of the human brain at high magnetic fields: metabolite quantification at 4T vs. 7T. *Magn Reson Med.* 2009;62(4):868–879.

102 Klomp DW, Bitz AK, Heerschap A, Scheenen TW. Proton spectroscopic imaging of the human prostate at 7T. *NMR Biomed.* 2009;22(5):495–501.

103 Narayan P, Jajodia P, Kurhanewicz J, et al. Characterization of prostate cancer, benign prostatic hyperplasia and normal prostates using transrectal 31phosphorus magnetic resonance spectroscopy: a preliminary report. *J Urol.* 1991;146(1):66–74.

104 Shukla-Dave A, Poptani H, Loevner LA, et al. Prediction of treatment response of head and neck cancers with P-31 MR spectroscopy from pretreatment relative phosphomonoester levels. *Acad Radiol.* 2002;9(6):688–694.

105 Arias-Mendoza F, Smith MR, Brown TR. Predicting treatment response in non-Hodgkin's lymphoma from the pretreatment tumor content of phosphoethanolamine plus phosphocholine. *Acad Radiol.* 2004;11(4):368–376.

106 Viale A, Reineri F, Santelia D, et al. Hyperpolarized agents for advanced MRI investigations. *Q J Nucl Med Mol Imaging.* 2009;53(6):604–617.

107 Ross BD, Bhattacharya P, Wagner S, Tran T, Sailasuta N. Hyperpolarized MR imaging: neurologic applications of hyperpolarized metabolism. *AJNR Am J Neuroradiol.* 2010;31(1):24–33.

108 Golman K, Zandt RI, Lerche M, Pehrson R, Ardenkjaer-Larsen JH. Metabolic imaging by hyperpolarized 13C magnetic resonance imaging for in vivo tumor diagnosis. *Cancer Res.* 2006;66(22):10855–10860.

109 Albers MJ, Bok R, Chen AP, et al. Hyperpolarized 13C lactate, pyruvate, and alanine: noninvasive biomarkers for prostate cancer detection and grading. *Cancer Res.* 2008;68(20):8607–8615.

110 Larson PE, Bok R, Kerr AB, et al. Investigation of tumor hyperpolarized [1–13C]-pyruvate dynamics using time-resolved multiband RF excitation echo-planar MRSI. *Magn Reson Med.* 2010;63(3):582–591.

111 Day SE, Kettunen MI, Gallagher FA, et al. Detecting tumor response to treatment using hyperpolarized 13C magnetic resonance imaging and spectroscopy. *Nat Med.* 2007;13(11):1382–1387.

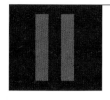

# PART II

# Targeted Therapy in Hematological Malignancies

# CHAPTER 11

# Targeted Therapies in Chronic Myeloid Leukemia

*Elias Jabbour and Jorge Cortes*
Department of Leukemia, The University of Texas MD Anderson Cancer Center, Houston, TX, USA

## Introduction

Advances in the genetic and molecular characterizations of leukemias have enhanced our capabilities to develop targeted therapies. The most dramatic example to date is chronic myeloid leukemia (CML). CML is a myeloproliferative neoplasm with an incidence of 1–2 cases per 100,000 adults, and accounts for approximately 15% of newly diagnosed cases of leukemia in adults.[1] Its incidence in the United States is about 5000 cases. Its prevalence is increasing annually (due to the low annual mortality rates of 1–2% since 2000); it is estimated to be about 80,000 cases in 2013, and will plateau at about 180,000 cases in 2030.[1] Central to the pathogenesis of CML is the fusion of the Abelson (ABL) gene on chromosome 9 with the breakpoint cluster region (BCR) gene on chromosome 22. This results in expression of an oncoprotein, BCR-ABL,[2] a constitutively active tyrosine kinase that promotes CML growth and replication through downstream pathways such as RAS, RAF, JUN kinase, MYC, and STAT.[3-9] This influences leukemogenesis by creating a cytokine-independent cell cycle with aberrant apoptotic signals.

Until 2000, therapy for CML was limited to nonspecific agents such as busulfan, hydroxyurea, and interferon-alpha (IFN-α).[10] IFN-α resulted in modest complete cytogenetic response (CCyR) rates (10–25%), and improved survival but was hindered by modest activity and significant toxicities. Allogeneic stem cell transplantation (alloSCT) was curative, but carried a high risk of morbidity and mortality, and was an option only for patients with good performance status and organ function, and with appropriate donors.

The landscape changed dramatically with the development of small-molecule tyrosine kinase inhibitors (TKIs) that was shown to potently interfere with the interaction between the BCR-ABL protein and adenosine triphosphate (ATP), blocking cellular proliferation of the malignant clone.[11] This "targeted" approach was found to dramatically alter the natural history of the disease, improving 10-year overall survival from approximately 20% to 80–90%.[1,12]

In this chapter, we will discuss front-line and salvage options for CML, and new compounds under investigation for the management of resistant disease.

## CML Frontline Treatment Options

Three TKIs are commercially available for the front-line treatment of CML: imatinib, dasatinib, and nilotinib. Current guidelines endorse all three as excellent options for the initial management of CML in the chronic phase (CML-CP) (Table 11.1).

### Imatinib

Imatinib mesylate (Gleevec, Novartis Pharmaceutical Corporation, NJ, USA), was the first TKI to receive approval by the Food and Drug Administration (FDA) for the treatment of patients with CML-CP. It acts via competitive inhibition at the ATP-binding site of the BCR-ABL oncoprotein, which results in the inhibition of phosphorylation of proteins involved in cell-signal transduction. It efficiently inhibits the BCR-ABL kinase activity, but also blocks the platelet-derived growth factor receptor (PGDFR), and the C-KIT tyrosine kinase.[11]

The International Randomized Study of IFN-α and STI571 (IRIS) study is considered a landmark clinical trial for TKIs and CML.[13] Investigators randomized 1106 patients to receive imatinib 400 mg/day or IFN-α plus subcutaneous low-dose cytarabine. After a median follow-up of 19 months, relevant outcomes for patients receiving imatinib were significantly better than for those treated with IFN plus cytarabine, notably the rate of CCyR (74% vs. 9%, $p < 0.001$), and freedom from progression to accelerated phase (AP) or blast phase (BP) at 12 months (99% vs. 93%, $p < 0.001$). The responses to imatinib were also durable, as shown in an 8-year follow-up of the IRIS study.[12] The estimated event-free survival (EFS) rate was 81%; the overall survival (OS) rate was 93% when only CML-related deaths were considered.

While the results using imatinib were impressive, only 55% of patients enrolled remained on therapy at the 8-year follow-up time. This underscores the need for additional options for patients who had failed or were intolerant to imatinib, and led to the rational development of second generation TKIs.

### Dasatinib

The DASISION trial was a phase III, randomized study comparing imatinib 400 mg once daily to dasatinib 100 mg once daily in newly diagnosed patients.[14] Dose escalations were allowed for

*Targeted Therapy in Translational Cancer Research*, First Edition. Edited by Apostolia-Maria Tsimberidou, Razelle Kurzrock and Kenneth C. Anderson.
© 2016 John Wiley & Sons, Inc. Published 2016 by John Wiley & Sons, Inc.

**Table 11.1** Summary of pivotal phase III trials of approved tyrosine kinase inhibitors for the treatment of front-line CML.

| Trial | Treatment | No. of patients | Primary endpoint | % MMR | Follow-up data | | |
|---|---|---|---|---|---|---|---|
| | | | | | % PFS | % OS | |
| IRIS | | | % PFS at 18 months | | 6 years/8 years | 6 years/8 years | |
| | Ima 400 mg qid | 553 | 97 | | 93/92 | 88/85 | |
| | IFN + ara-c | 553 | 91 (p < 0.001) | | | | |
| ENESTnd | | | % MMR at 12 months | | 5 years | | |
| | Nilo 300 mg bid | 282 | 44 | 77 | 92 | 93.6 | |
| | Nilo 400 mg bid | 281 | 43 | 77 | 95.3 (p = 0.03 vs. ima) | 96 (p = 0.04 vs. ima) | |
| | Ima 400 mg qid | 283 | 22 (p < 0.001 for both comparisons) | 60 (p < 0.0001 for both comparisons) | 91.1 | 91.6 | |
| DASISION | | | % CCyR at 12 months | | 4 years | | |
| | Dasa 100 mg qid | 259 | 77 | 74 | 90 | 92.9 | |
| | Ima 400 mg qid | 260 | Imatinib: 60 (p < 0.0001) Secondary endpoint: MMR at 12 months:Dasa: 46 Ima: 23 (p < 0.0001) | 46 | 90.2 | 92.1 | |

Free from progression to accelerated phase or blast crisis; ima, imatinib; nilo, nilotinib; dasa, dasatinib; ara-c, cytarabine; IFN, interferon; MMR, major molecular response; PFS, progression-free survival; OS, overall survival.

both drugs in the setting of suboptimal response as defined per protocol. The primary endpoint was confirmed complete cytogenetic response (cCCyR) at 12 months. A total of 519 patients were randomized in a 1:1 ratio. Patients assigned to dasatinib achieved cCCyR at 12 months more frequently than those on imatinib (77% vs. 66%, p = 0.007). Many of the secondary endpoints of interest were also significantly different between groups favoring the dasatinib arm. A 3-year follow-up of the trial was recently published and illustrated that dasatinib induces more rapid, deeper responses at early time points compared to imatinib.[15] For instance, at 3 months, a higher proportion of patients treated with dasatinib compared to imatinib achieved a BCR-ABL transcript level of less than or equal to 10% (84% vs. 64%, p < 0.0001). Meeting this threshold in either arm predicted for longer progression-free survival (PFS) and longer OS. As might be expected, pleural effusions occurred more frequently in the group receiving dasatinib (19% vs. <1%).

In another multicenter trial, several North American cooperative groups randomized patients with newly diagnosed CML to either dasatinib 100 mg once daily or imatinib 400 mg once daily.[16] Similar to the results of the DASISION study, dasatinib-treated patients achieved CCyR at a significantly higher rate compared to patients receiving imatinib (84% vs. 69%, p = 0.04). Of note, only a little more than 50% of patients had samples evaluable for the primary endpoint of cytogenetic response. This indicates that many clinicians are likely monitoring patients using molecular testing or assays that require only blood as opposed to bone marrow (see section Monitoring). Despite this possible shortcoming, the results for the patients that did have cytogenetic evaluation closely replicated what was found in DASISION. There was significantly more toxicity experienced in the dasatinib arm, as noted by the differences in rates of grades 3 or 4 adverse events experienced in each group (58% dasatinib, 35% imatinib). Much of the disparity was driven by more hematologic toxicity caused by dasatinib.

**Nilotinib**

Similar to the data with dasatinib, nilotinib has also been directly compared to imatinib in a large, international, randomized study (ENESTnd study).[17] The primary endpoint in this study was the rate of major molecular response (MMR) at 12 months. In a 3-arm randomized study, 846 patients received imatinib 400 mg daily (n = 283) nilotinib 400 mg twice a day (the approved dose for salvage therapy; n = 281), or nilotinib 300 mg twice daily (n = 282). The primary study endpoint, the incidence of major molecular response by 12 months of therapy, was significantly higher with nilotinib versus imatinib. With a minimum follow-up of 4 years, the two arms of nilotinib demonstrate better early results compared with imatinib.[18] The cumulative incidence of CCyR by 24 months was 87% with nilotinib 300 mg twice daily, 85% with nilotinib 400 mg twice daily, and 77% with imatinib 400 mg daily. The cumulative incidences of major molecular response by 48 months were 76%, 73%, and 56%, respectively (p < 0.0001%). The incidences of BCR-ABL transcripts <0.0032% (IS; roughly equivalent to a 4.5 log reduction of disease) by 48 months were 40%, 37%, and 23%, respectively (p < 0.0001%). The incidences of transformation to accelerated or blastic phases were 3.2%, 2.1%, and 6.7%, respectively (p < 0.02). The estimated 4-year EFS rates were 95%, 97%, and 93%, respectively. There was no difference in the estimated 4-year survival rates between the three arms (94%, 97%, 93%, respectively). Nilotinib therapy was associated with lower rates of fluid retention, diarrhea, headaches, muscle cramps, nausea and vomiting, and neutropenia compared to imatinib. However, nilotinib therapy was associated with higher rates of headaches, rashes, pruritus, and hyperglycemia, and with low but notable incidences of pancreatitis (less than 2%), ischemic heart disease (4–5% vs. 1% with imatinib), and peripheral arterial occlusive disease (1.4–1.8% vs. 0% with imatinib). Based on the results of the ENESTnd study, the FDA approved nilotinib 300 mg orally twice daily for front-line CML therapy in 2010.

## Bosutinib

A third TKI, bosutinib, was also recently compared to imatinib in newly diagnosed patients in chronic phase.[19] Investigators enrolled 502 patients to receive bosutinib 500 mg once daily or imatinib 400 mg once daily, with dose escalation possible for either group based on therapeutic benchmark attainment. The primary outcome was CCyR rate at 12 months, with similar secondary outcomes as the trials with other second generation TKIs. Unlike the previous studies, bosutinib was not superior to imatinib at 1 year, as rates of CCyR were similar between the groups (70% vs. 68%, $p = 0.60$). Despite failing to meet the primary endpoint, the bosutinib group did achieve a higher rate of MMR, making the results a bit difficult to interpret. A larger-than-expected number of patients were counted as nonresponders in both groups because they discontinued therapy prior to their first post-baseline assessment. This could potentially account for a lower CCyR rate in

## Other Strategies

Other strategies for front-line therapy include using higher doses of imatinib or combining a TKI with an additional agent, such as interferon. In the Tyrosine Kinase Inhibitor Optimization and Selectivity (TOPS) study, patients were randomized to take imatinib 400 mg once daily or twice daily (800 mg).[20] Patients in the 400 mg once daily group were able to have their doses escalated according to prespecified criteria of suboptimal response. MMR rate at 12 months was the primary endpoint, with cytogenetic response and time to such responses collected as secondary endpoints. While patients in the high-dose group did achieve CCyR and MMR faster, the rates were similar and not statistically significantly different at 12 months. Therefore, extended follow-up is necessary to determine whether the early surrogate markers have a long-term impact on the outcome.

Interferon has re-emerged as an intriguing therapeutic option for CML patients with the advent of pegylated formulations requiring less frequent administration and enhanced tolerability. In a phase III, randomized study conducted by the French, patients were assigned to one of four treatment arms (imatinib 400 mg once daily, imatinib 600 mg once daily, imatinib 400 mg once daily plus peginterferon alfa-2a, or imatinib 400 mg once daily plus subcutaneous cytarabine).[21] Patients were initially assigned to receive peginterferon alfa-2a at a dose of 90 mcg once weekly. However, there was a high rate of discontinuation due to toxicity, and the dose was later modified to 45 mcg once weekly. At 12 months, rates of CCyR were similar between all four groups. The peginterferon alfa-2a group did demonstrate higher rates of MMR and deeper molecular responses, but follow-up was not sufficient to determine whether this impacted longer-term outcomes. Other studies have found that cytogenetic and MMR rates are not significantly improved with the addition of interferon.[22,23]

## Choice of Frontline Therapy

Currently all three TKIs—imatinib, nilotinib, and dasatinib—are acceptable front-line therapies for CML. The choice of TKI may depend on the patient and physician preferences, and patient prior history and comorbidities (e.g., diabetes, pancreatitis, cardiac pulmonary conditions, pulmonary hypertension). Current drug price sensitivity and insurance coverage do not argue in favor of a particular TKI in the United States, although the oncology practice trends appear to increasingly favor nilotinib and dasatinib over imatinib

because of their better early results, particularly the lower early incidence of CML transformation. However, the high prices of TKIs may shift the treatment paradigms in some emerging nations to utilizing a particular TKI over others, or even to consider front-line alloSCT (total one time procedure cost of $30–$100,000) in situations where patients or the national healthcare system cannot afford the burden of the TKIs' economics. Imatinib may become available in generic formulations in 2015. The price of generic imatinib is unknown, but may be low ($2000–$10,000 per year). The choice of front-line TKI therapy may then depend on the differential pricing of generic imatinib versus dasatinib and imatinib, and the maturing long-term data (5–8 years) for survival, transformation-free survival (TFS), and EFS with the three TKIs. With an estimated 8-year survival rate of 93% with imatinib (considering only CML-related deaths) and the high efficacy of new generation TKIs as salvage therapies, the survival benefit with dasatinib or nilotinib may or may not be apparent compared with imatinib front-line therapy, careful monitoring for cytogenetic relapse, and rapid institution of second-line TKI therapies at that time.

## Management of TKI Resistance

A common mechanism of resistance to TKIs involves point mutations in the BCR-ABL kinase domain, which impair the activity of the particular TKIs. Second generation TKIs are able to overcome most of the mutations that confer resistance to imatinib, though novel mutations rendering the leukemia resistant to dasatinib and/or nilotinib have emerged. One important mutation, T315I, known as a "gatekeeper" mutation, displays resistance to all currently available TKIs except ponatinib.

Before defining a patient as having imatinib resistance and modifying therapy, treatment compliance and drug–drug interactions should be excluded. Rates of imatinib adherence range from 75% to 90%; lower adherence rates correlate with worse outcome.[24–26] In one study of 87 patients with CML-CP treated with imatinib 400 mg daily, an adherence rate of 90% or less resulted in MMR in only 28% versus 94% with greater than 90% adherence rates ($p < 0.001$).[26] Complete molecular response (CMR) rates were 0% versus 44% ($p = 0.002$); no molecular responses were observed when adherence rates were 80% or lower. Lower adherence rates have been described in younger patients, those with adverse effects to therapy, and those who have required dose escalation.[24]

## Second Generation TKI

Nilotinib and dasatinib were first approved for use as second-line CML salvage following prior therapy including imatinib. Results of second-line nilotinib, dasatinib, and bosutinib therapies following imatinib failure are summarized in Table 11.2. Several noteworthy observations emerged. First, second-line treatment can yield high rates of response in patients who have inadequate response to imatinib, including high rates of MMR. Second, dose escalation of imatinib can improve response rates in patients with inadequate response to standard-dose imatinib, but switching to second-line can be more effective.[27] Several studies that evaluated second-line nilotinib[28,29] or dasatinib[28–30] and high-dose imatinib (400 mg BID) have demonstrated significantly higher rates of complete hematologic response (CHR), CCyR, and MMR with the newer TKIs than with high-dose imatinib. PFS was also better with the newer TKIs. In addition, earlier change to second-line TKI may be more effective than later change.[31] In a retrospective pooled analysis of second-line

**Table 11.2** Summary of important phase II trials of 2nd and 3rd generation TKIs after prior TKI failure.

| Response | Dasatinib | | | | Nilotinib | | | | Bosutinib | | | Ponatinib | | |
|---|---|---|---|---|---|---|---|---|---|---|---|---|---|---|
| | CP $N=387$ | AP $N=174$ | MyBP $N=109$ | LyBP $N=48$ | CP $N=321$ | AP $N=137$ | MyBP $N=105$ | LyBP $N=31$ | CP $N=146$ | AP $N=51$ | BP $N=38$ | CP $N=271$ | AP $N=79$ | BP $N=6$ |
| Median follow-up (months) | 15 | 4 | 12+ | 12+ | 24 | 9 | 3 | 3 | 7 | 6 | 3 | 11 | 13 | 6 |
| % Resistant to imatinib | 74 | 93 | 91 | 88 | 70 | 80 | 82 | 82 | 69 | NR | NR | 96 | NR | NR |
| % Hematologic response | – | 79 | 50 | 40 | 94 | 56 | 22 | 19 | 85 | 54 | 36 | NR | NR | NR |
| CHR | 91 | 45 | 27 | 29 | 76 | 31 | 11 | 13 | 81 | 54 | 36 | NR | MaHR: 57 | MaHR: 34 |
| NEL | – | 19 | 7 | 6 | – | 12 | 1 | 0 | – | 0 | NR | NR | NR | NR |
| % Cytogenetic response | NR | 44 | 36 | 52 | NR | NR | NR | NR | – | NR | NR | NR | NR | NR |
| Complete | 49 | 32 | 26 | 46 | 46 | 20 | 29 | 32 | 34 | 27 | 35 | 46 | 55 | 36 |
| Partial | 11 | 7 | 7 | 6 | 15 | 12 | 10 | 16 | 13 | 20 | 18 | NR | NR | NR |
| % Survival (at 12 months) | 96 | 82 | 50 | 50 | 87 | 67 | 42 | 42 | 98 | 60 | 50 | 91 | 42 | 35 |

CP, chronic phase; AP, accelerated phase; MyBP, myeloid blast phase; LyBP, lymphoid blast phase; BP, blast phase; MaHR, major hematologic response; CHR, complete hematologic response; NEL, no evidence of leukemia; NR, not reported.

dasatinib in patients resistant to or intolerant of imatinib, an earlier change to dasatinib after the loss of major cytogenetic response (MCyR) (early intervention group) resulted in higher rates of CHR, CCyR, and MMR, and better 24-month EFS, TFS, and OS, than later change after the loss of CHR (late intervention group).[32]

Bosutinib was initially studied in patients that were resistant to or intolerant of imatinib.[33] After a dose escalation period, 500 mg once daily was selected to go forward as the phase II dose, with the potential for dose escalation to 600 mg once daily for patients not meeting prespecified benchmarks. There were 288 patients enrolled in the pivotal phase II trial, with more than two-thirds of the patients documented as having imatinib-resistant disease. The primary endpoint was MCyR at 6 months, and this was achieved in 31% of the patients treated. At any point during follow-up, 41% achieved a CCyR. Bosutinib appeared to retain activity across most known mutations that confer imatinib resistance, except for the T315I. Responses were independent of whether patients were resistant to or intolerant of imatinib. The most common toxicities noted were diarrhea, nausea, vomiting, and rash. Diarrhea occurred in 84% of the patients overall, with 9% experiencing an event classified as grade 3 (there were no grade 4 events documented). Other notable adverse events included myelosuppression and liver function test abnormalities.

### Third Generation TKI

Ponatinib is considered a third generation TKI, as it is the first compound in the class considered to exhibit activity against CML in the presence of a T315I mutation.[34] It is considered to be greater than 500 times as potent than imatinib at inhibiting BCR-ABL.[35] Evidence to support the approval of ponatinib was presented in the phase II PACE trial, where 449 patients with heavily pretreated CML or Philadelphia chromosome-positive acute lymphoblastic leukemia (ALL) were enrolled.[36] Patients were considered for this trial if they were resistant to or intolerant of dasatinib or nilotinib. Alternatively, any patient with a T315I mutation could be included. The dose of ponatinib was 45 mg once daily, and patients were stratified by phase of disease and whether or not there was a T315I mutation. Focusing on the 267 patients who received ponatinib in the chronic phase, 56% achieved an MCyR by 12 months, which included 70% of chronic phase patients with a T315I mutation ($n = 45$). Patients responded more favorably if they had received fewer TKIs. The most common adverse events were rash, dry skin, and abdominal pain. Other notable toxicities in the PACE study included hypertension and pancreatitis. Serious events possibly related to the drug included arterial thrombotic events, and the rate was reported to increase with longer durations of exposure to ponatinib. This led to a temporary suspension of the sale of ponatinib in the United States, as well as the modification or closure of several clinical trials. Revised labeling and a restricted access program were put in place allowing the manufacturer resume its marketing.

### Omacetaxine

Omacetaxine mepesuccinate, a semi-synthetic analogue of homoharringtonine, is a first-in-class cephalotaxine which acts as a protein synthesis inhibitor that induces apoptosis in leukemic cells by reducing levels of multiple oncoproteins, including BCR-ABL.[37] Data pooled from two phase II trials of subcutaneous omacetaxine, 1.25 mg/m$^2$ twice daily for 2 weeks every 4 weeks until response then for 1 week every 4 weeks, in 81 patients with chronic phase CML post-failure of $\geq 2$ TKIs resulted in a MCyR in 20% and CCyR

in 10%. The median response duration was 17.7 months and the median survival was 34 months.[38] Grade 3–4 side effects included cytopenias in 37–67% of patients, which were reversible. This led to the FDA approval of omacetaxine in 2012 for that indication.

## Definition of Response and Failure to TKI Therapy and Choice of Therapy

Monitoring response to TKI therapy in CML is a critical component of patients' outcomes. Responses to TKI treatment are described in terms of hematologic, cytogenetic, and molecular outcomes.[39, 40] Hematologic response is defined as normalization of white blood cell (WBC) count and splenomegaly. Cytogenetic response is determined by the percentage of cells with Philadelphia-positive (Ph+) metaphases, whereas assessment of molecular response relies on quantitative reverse-transcriptase polymerase chain reaction (qRT-PCR) to measure BCR-ABL transcripts, best expressed on the International Scale (IS).[41] On the IS, a MMR is defined as a BCR-ABL transcript level of 0.1% or less, which represents a 3-log reduction from a standardized baseline.[41] A CMR was defined in the European LeukemiaNet (ELN) recommendations and National Comprehensive Cancer Network Clinical Practice Guidelines in Oncology (NCCN Guidelines) as a BCR-ABL transcript level that is undetectable by qRT-PCR in an assay with adequate sensitivity (e.g., 4.5-logs).[39, 40] However, as more-sensitive PCR assays have been developed, 4-, 4.5-, and even 5-log reductions in BCR-ABL are now detectable, which raises the question of the true meaning of CMR and whether transcript-level changes below the level of MMR are meaningful.[39, 40]

Treatment failure is defined by the ELN and NCCN Guidelines recommendations as not achieving the specific milestones at defined time points.[39, 40] The main differences between these guidelines is the fact that ELN defines failure and suboptimal response and includes an additional response category (warnings), whereas the NCCN Guidelines do not formally define suboptimal response, but rather define target responses at specific time points. However, these recommendations continue to evolve. In our opinion, a simplified schema of response/failure would be more practical and less confusing (Table 11.3).

In several studies, the achievement of a CCyR (Ph-positive metaphases 0%; BCR-ABL transcripts (IS) $\leq 1\%$) at 12 months or later on TKI therapy was associated with significant survival benefit compared with achievement of lesser degrees of response.[15, 42] Therefore, achievement of CCyR is now the primary endpoint of TKI therapy. Achievement of BCR-ABL transcripts $\leq 0.1\%$ (IS) was associated with modest improvement in EFS rates, and with possible longer duration of CCyRs, but not with a survival benefit. The achievement of complete molecular response (nonmeasurable BCR-ABL transcripts) offers the possibility of treatment discontinuation in clinical trials only. Lack of achievement of major molecular response or of complete molecular response should not be interpreted as a need to change TKI therapy or to consider alloSCT. Response assessments at earlier times on front-line TKI therapy (3–6 months) have shown better outcomes with achievement of a MCyR by 3–6 months on imatinib therapy (pH-positive metaphases $\leq 35\%$, or BCR-ABL transcripts $\leq 10\%$). While this is interpreted to mean that a change to second TKI therapy may be considered if such outcome is not obtained, no studies have shown that changing therapy from imatinib to second TKIs has improved patients' outcomes.[43, 44] When nilotinib or dasatinib are used for front-line

**Table 11.3** Criteria for response/failure and change of therapy.

| Time (months) | Imatinib | Second generation TKI |
|---|---|---|
| 3–6 | MCyR; BCR-ABL transcript levels ≤10% (IS) | CCyR; BCR-ABL transcript levels ≤1% (IS) |
| 12 | CCyR; BCR-ABL transcript levels ≤1% (IS) | CCyR; BCR-ABL transcript levels ≤1% (IS) |
| Later | CCyR; BCR-ABL transcript levels ≤1% (IS) | CCyR; BCR-ABL transcript levels ≤1% (IS) |

MCyR, major cytogenetic response (pH ≤35%); CCyR, complete cytogenetic response (pH = 0%); IS, international scale
Note: MCyR roughly, BCR-ABL ≤10% (IS); CCyR roughly, BCR-ABL ≤1% (IS).

therapy, achievement of CCyR by 3–6 months of TKI therapy has been associated with improved outcomes.[45]

Currently, imatinib failure (requiring a change of therapy) should be strictly defined as failure to achieve a MCyR after 6 months of imatinib therapy and a CCyR after 12 months or cytogenetic or hematologic relapse at any later time, on an optimal imatinib dose schedule (adjusting dose for significant side effects or for intolerance; checking for treatment compliance). With second generation TKIs' use as front-line therapy, failure of TKI therapy has been suggested to be due to lack of achievement of CCyR or BCR-ABL transcript levels ≤1% by 3–6 months of therapy.[45] Such patients (<10% of the denominator) have a worse EFS, although their survival at 3–5 years remains in the range of 90%, better or equivalent to what would be achievable with alloSCT. Thus while the early surrogate response parameters at 3–6 months on front-line TKI therapy predict for differences in outcome, a change of therapy at that time point is not proven to improve long-term prognosis.

Patients with CML failure on imatinib therapy may be treated with newer generation TKIs as discussed earlier. Patients with CML and failure on front-line dasatinib or nilotinib therapy may possibly be salvaged with ponatinib if the CML clones exhibit a T315I mutation. If no such mutation is detected, they could be considered for other TKI therapies, alloSCT, treatment with omacetaxine, or combined-modality therapies including TKIs and older agents (hydroxyurea, cytarabine, decitabine).

## Can TKIs Be Safely Discontinued?

The Stop Imatinib (STIM) trial sought to investigate the risk of relapse in patients on imatinib with ongoing CMR for greater than two years who stopped treatment.[46,47] At the time of the most recent update, 100 patients had a median follow-up of 50 months and were monitored closely for evidence of molecular relapse. Overall, 61% experienced a molecular relapse, with 95% of the events occurring within 7 months of stopping imatinib. Almost all patients were able to re-achieve their CMR once imatinib therapy was restarted. One patient did have possible loss of cytogenetic response, necessitating a change in therapy to dasatinib. Having a low-risk Sokal score and duration of imatinib therapy greater than 60 months predicted for continued CMR after therapy cessation.

The results of the STIM trial have been confirmed by other large groups of CML researchers. The TWISTER study followed 40 patients who stopped imatinib after being without detectable minimal residual disease for greater than two years.[48] Patients were followed for a minimum of 15 months (median 43 months) from the time they stopped imatinib. Over the course of the study, 22 of 40 patients became molecularly positive. Nearly 70% of the molecular relapses occurred within the first 6 months of treatment cessation. Similarly, patients who resumed TKIs were able to recapture deep molecular responses. Interestingly, highly sensitive, patient-specific PCR was able to detect the original CML clone in several of the patients who remained off imatinib for several years. This indicates that it may not be necessary to completely eradicate the disease to allow patients to enjoy a functional cure.

The previous studies contained heterogeneous groups of patients, particularly ones exposed to interferon prior to the imatinib era. There have been conflicting results as to whether prior exposure to interferon plays a major role in sustaining deep molecular responses after TKI withdrawal. Therefore, the French group conducted a follow-up study to STIM enrolling patients who have only been exposed to imatinib as CML therapy (STIM2).[49] The inclusion criteria were similar to those used in STIM1. There were 124 patients identified who stopped imatinib therapy. With a median follow-up of 12 months, 48 patients had molecularly relapsed, 94% of which occurred within 6 months of TKI withdrawal. All patients remained sensitive to imatinib or a second generation TKI upon re-challenge. It has also been noted in this and other studies that patients with low-level positivity for BCR-ABL transcripts may be able to remain off therapy, with only close monitoring. This was recently addressed systematically by French investigators, where it appeared safe and effective to only resume patients on TKI therapy if their transcript level became greater than 0.1% (i.e., loss of MMR).[50]

Overall, these data indicate that stopping TKI therapy is feasible, and some patients may actually be cured of the disease. Nevertheless, at present, stopping TKI therapy should only be done in the context of a clinical trial.

## Conclusions and Future Perspectives

With the updates of the DASISION and ENESTnd trials, the question often arises as to the optimal choice for front-line management of CP-CML. Based on attainment of faster and higher rates of CCyR, MMR, and CMR, and a trend for lower progression rates to AP or BC, it is reasonable to use a second generation TKI for front-line management. For patients who progress to AP/BC, treatment options are limited, and the overall prognosis is poor. Therefore, a primary goal of first-line therapy is to prevent progression. However, second generation TKIs are expensive, serious adverse events are being reported, and by 2015, generic formulations of imatinib will be available. A large number of patients have optimal responses to imatinib therapy. Therefore, future research could identify baseline factors that may indicate which patients will benefit most from upfront treatment with a second generation TKI. New therapies will be tested alone and in combination with TKIs to continue to improve patient outcomes. The pursuit of a cure for all patients will continue, and the criteria for safe permanent discontinuation of TKIs will receive further attention.

# References

1 Huang X, Cortes J, Kantarjian H. Estimations of the increasing prevalence and plateau prevalence of chronic myeloid leukemia in the era of tyrosine kinase inhibitor therapy. *Cancer.* 2012;118(12):3123–3127.

2 Rowley JD. Letter: a new consistent chromosomal abnormality in chronic myelogenous leukaemia identified by quinacrine fluorescence and Giemsa staining. *Nature.* 1973;243(5405):290–293.

3 Mandanas RA, Leibowitz DS, Gharehbaghi K, et al. Role of p21 RAS in p210 Bcr-Abl transformation of murine myeloid cells. *Blood.* 1993;82(6):1838–1847.

4 Okuda K, Matulonis U, Salgia R, Kanakura Y, Druker B, Griffin JD. Factor independence of human myeloid leukemia cell lines is associated with increased phosphorylation of the proto-oncogene Raf-1. *Exp hematol.* 1994;22(11):1111–1117.

5 Raitano AB, Halpern JR, Hambuch TM. The Bcr-Abl leukemia oncogene activates Jun kinase and requires Jun for transformation. *Proceedings of the National Academy of Sciences of the United States of America.* 1995;92(25):11746–11750.

6 Sawyers CL, Callahan W, Witte ON. Dominant negative MYC blocks transformation by ABL oncogenes. *Cell.* 1992;70(6):901–910.

7 Shuai K, Halpern J, ten Hoeve J, Rao X, Sawyers CL. Constitutive activation of STAT5 by the BCR-ABL oncogene in chronic myelogenous leukemia. *Oncogene.* 1996;13(2):247–254.

8 Carlesso N, Frank DA, Griffin JD. Tyrosyl phosphorylation and DNA binding activity of signal transducers and activators of transcription (STAT) proteins in hematopoietic cell lines transformed by Bcr/Abl. *J Exp Med.* 1996;183(3):811–820.

9 Ilaria RL Jr, Van Etten RA. P210 and P190 (BCR/ABL) induce the tyrosine phosphorylation and DNA binding activity of multiple specific STAT family members. *J Biol Chem.* 1996;271(49):31704–31710.

10 Silver RT, Woolf SH, Hehlmann R, et al. An evidence-based analysis of the effect of busulfan, hydroxyurea, interferon, and allogeneic bone marrow transplantation in treating the chronic phase of chronic myeloid leukemia: developed for the American Society of Hematology. *Blood.* 1999;94(5):1517–1536.

11 Druker BJ, Tamura S, Buchdunger E, et al. Effects of a selective inhibitor of the Abl tyrosine kinase on the growth of Bcr-Abl positive cells. *Nat Med.* 1996;2:561–566.

12 Deininger M, O'Brien SG, Guilhot F, et al. International randomized study of interferon vs. STI571 (IRIS) 8-year follow up: sustained survival and low risk for progression of events in patients with newly diagnosed chronic myeloid leukemia in chronic phase (CML-CP) treated with imatinib. *Blood (ASH Annual Meeting Abstracts).* 2009;114: Abstract 1126.

13 O'Brien SG, Guilhot F, Larson RA, et al.; IRIS Investigators. Imatinib compared with interferon and low-dose cytarabine for newly diagnosed chronic-phase chronic myeloid leukemia. *N Engl J Med.* 2003;348(11):994–1004.

14 Kantarjian H, Shah NP, Hochhaus A, et al. Dasatinib versus imatinib in newly diagnosed chronic-phase chronic myeloid leukemia. *N Engl J Med.* 2010;362:2260–2270.

15 Jabbour E, Kantarjian HM, Saglio G, et al. Early response with dasatinib or imatinib in chronic myeloid leukemia: 3-year follow-up from a randomized phase 3 trial (DASISION). *Blood.* 2014;123(4):494–500.

16 Radich JP, Kopecky KJ, Appelbaum FR, et al. A randomized trial of dasatinib 100 mg versus imatinib 400 mg in newly diagnosed chronic-phase chronic myeloid leukemia. *Blood.* 2012;120(19):3898–3905.

17 Saglio G, Kim DW, Issaragrisil S, et al.; ENESTnd Investigators. Nilotinib versus imatinib for newly diagnosed chronic myeloid leukemia. *N Engl J Med.* 2010;362(24):2251–2259.

18 Larson RA, Hochhaus A, Clark RE, et al. Nilotinib vs imatinib in patients with newly diagnosed Philadelphia chromosome-positive chronic myeloid leukemia in chronic phase: ENESTnd 3-year follow up. *Leukemia.* 2012;26(10):2197–2203.

19 Cortes JE, Kim DW, Kantarjian HM, et al. Bosutinib versus imatinib in newly diagnosed chronic-phase chronic myeloid leukemia: results from the BELA trial. *J Clin Oncol.* 2012;30(28):3486–3492.

20 Cortes JE, Baccarani M, Guilhot F, et al. Phase III, randomized, open-label study of daily imatinib mesylate 400 mg versus 800 mg in patients with newly diagnosed, previously untreated chronic myeloid leukemia in chronic phase using molecular end points: tyrosine kinase inhibitor optimization and selectivity study. *J Clin Oncol.* 2010;28(3):424–430.

21 Preudhomme C, Guilhot J, Nicolini FE, et al.; SPIRIT Investigators; France Intergroupe des Leucémies Myéloïdes Chroniques (Fi-LMC). Imatinib plus peginterferon alfa-2 a in chronic myeloid leukemia. *N Engl J Med.* 2010;363(26):2511–2521.

22 Cortes J, Quintas-Cardama A, Jones D, et al. Immune modulation of minimal residual disease in early chronic phase chronic myelogenous leukemia: a randomized trial of frontline high-dose imatinib mesylate with or without pegylated interferon alpha-2b and granulocyte-macrophage colony-stimulating factor. *Cancer.* 2011;117(3):572–580.

23 Hehlmann R, Lauseker M, Jung-Munkwitz S, et al. Tolerability-adapted imatinib 800 mg/d versus 400 mg/d versus 400 mg/d plus interferon-alpha in newly diagnosed chronic myeloid leukemia. *J Clin Oncol.* 2011;29:1634–1642.

24 Marin D, Bazeos A, Mahon FX, et al. Adherence is the critical factor for achieving molecular responses in patients with chronic myeloid leukemia who achieve complete cytogenetic responses on imatinib. *J Clin Oncol.* 2010;28(14):2381–2388.

25 Darkow T, Henk HJ, Thomas SK, et al. Treatment interruptions and non-adherence with imatinib and associated healthcare costs: a retrospective analysis among managed care patients with chronic myelogenous leukaemia. *Pharmacoeconomics.* 2007;25(6):481–496.

26 Noens L, van Lierde MA, De Bock R, et al. Prevalence, determinants, and outcomes of nonadherence to imatinib therapy in patients with chronic myeloid leukemia: the ADAGIO study. *Blood.* 2009;113(22):5401–5411.

27 Jabbour E, Kantarjian HM, Jones D, et al. Imatinib mesylate dose escalation is associated with durable responses in patients with chronic myeloid leukemia after cytogenetic failure on standard-dose imatinib therapy. *Blood.* 2009;113(10):2154–2160.

28 Garcia-Gutierrez JV, Herrera P, Abalo LL, Rey MD, Calbacho M. Impact of second-generation tyrosine kinase inhibitors as second line treatment for patients with chronic myeloid leukemia. *Blood (ASH Annual Meeting Abstracts).* 2011;118: Abstract 3780.

29 Goh HG, Jootar S, Kim HJ, Sohn SK, Park JS, Kim SH. Efficacy of nilotinib versus high-dose imatinib in early chronic phase CML patients who have suboptimal molecular responses to standard-dose imatinib (RE-NICE multicenter study). *Blood (ASH Annual Meeting Abstracts).* 2011;118: Abstract 2765.

30 Kantarjian H, Pasquini R, Levy V, et al. Dasatinib or high-dose imatinib for chronic-phase chronic myeloid leukemia resistant to imatinib at a dose of 400 to 600 milligrams daily: two-year follow-up of a randomized phase 2 study (START-R). *Cancer.* 2009;115(18):4136–4147.

31 Yeung DT, Osborn M, White DL, Branford S, Kornhauser M, Slader C. Upfront imatinib therapy in CML patients with rapid switching to nilotinib for failure to achieve molecular targets or intolerance achieves high overall rates of molecular response and a low risk of progression—an update of the TIDEL-II trial. *Blood (ASH Annual Meeting Abstracts).* 2011;118: Abstract 451.

32 Quintas-Cardama A, Cortes JE, O'Brien S, et al. Dasatinib early intervention after cytogenetic or hematologic resistance to imatinib in patients with chronic myeloid leukemia. *Cancer.* 2009;115(13):2912–2921.

33 Cortes JE, Kantarjian HM, Brummendorf TH, et al. Safety and efficacy of bosutinib (SKI-606) in chronic phase Philadelphia chromosome-positive chronic myeloid leukemia patients with resistance or intolerance to imatinib. *Blood.* 2011;118(17):4567–4576.

34 O'Hare T, Shakespeare WC, Zhu X, et al. AP24534, a pan-BCR-ABL inhibitor for chronic myeloid leukemia, potently inhibits the T315I mutant and overcomes mutation-based resistance. *Cancer cell.* 2009;16(5):401–412.

35 Zhou T, Commodore L, Huang WS, et al. Structural mechanism of the pan-BCR-ABL inhibitor ponatinib (AP24534): lessons for overcoming kinase inhibitor resistance. *Chem Biol Drug Des.* 2011;77(1):1–11.

36 Cortes JE, Kim DW, Pinilla-Ibarz J, et al.; PACE Investigators. A phase 2 trial of ponatinib in Philadelphia chromosome-positive leukemias. *N Engl J Med.* 2013;369:1783–1796.

37 Quintas-Cardama A, Kantarjian H, Cortes J. Homoharringtonine, omacetaxine mepesuccinate, and chronic myeloid leukemia circa 2009. *Cancer.* 2009;115(23):5382–5393.

38 Wetzler M, Kantarjian H, Nicolini FE, et al. Pooled safety analysis of omacetaxine mepesuccinate in patients with chronic myeloid leukemia (CML) resistant to tyrosine-kinase inhibitors (TKIs). *J Clin Oncol.* 2012;30(suppl.): Abstract 6604.

39 Baccarani M, Deininger MW, Rosti G, et al. European LeukemiaNet recommendations for the management of chronic myeloid leukemia: 2013. *Blood.* 2013;122(6):872–884.

40 O'Brien S, Radich JP, Abboud CN, et al.; National comprehensive cancer network. Chronic myelogenous leukemia, Version 1.2014. *J Natl Compr Canc Netw.* 2013;11(11):1327–1340.

41 Hughes T, Deininger M, Hochhaus A, et al. Monitoring CML patients responding to treatment with tyrosine kinase inhibitors: review and recommendations for harmonizing current methodology for detecting BCR-ABL transcripts and kinase domain mutations and for expressing results. *Blood.* 2006;108(1):28–37.

42 Kantarjian H, Cortes J. Considerations in the management of patients with Philadelphia chromosome-positive chronic myeloid leukemia receiving tyrosine kinase inhibitors. *J Clin Oncol.* 2011;29:1512–1516.

43 Cortes JE, De Souza CA, Lopez JL, et al. Switching to nilotinib in patients with chronic myeloid leukemia in chronic phase with suboptimal cytogenetic response on imatinib: first results of the LASOR trial. *Blood (ASH Annual Meeting Abstracts).* 2013;122:95.

44 Leber B, Cervantes F, Spector N, et al. Achievement and maintenance of deeper molecular response by switching to nilotinib in patients with chronic myeloid leukemia in chronic phase with residual disease on long-term imatinib: ENESTcmr 36-month follow up. *Blood (ASH Annual Meeting Abstracts).* 2013;122:94.

45 Jabbour E, Kantarjian HM, O'Brien S, et al. Front-line therapy with second-generation tyrosine kinase inhibitors in patients with early chronic phase chronic myeloid leukemia: what is the optimal response? *J Clin Oncol.* 2011;29:4260–4265.

46 Mahon FX, Rea D, Guilhot J, et al.; Intergroupe Français des Leucémies Myéloïdes Chroniques. Discontinuation of imatinib in patients with chronic myeloid leukaemia who have maintained complete molecular remission for at least 2 years: the prospective, multicenter Stop Imatinib (STIM) trial. *Lancet Oncol.* 2010;11(11):1029–1035.

47 Mahon FX, Rea D, Guilhot J, et al. Long term follow-up after imatinib cessation for patients in deep molecular response: the updated results of the STIM1 study. *Blood (ASH Annual Meeting Abstracts).* 2013;122:255.

48 Ross DM, Branford S, Seymour JF, et al. Safety and efficacy of imatinib cessation for CML patients with stable undetectable minimal residual disease: results from the TWISTER study. *Blood.* 2013;122(4):515–522.

49 Mahon FX, Nicolini FE, Noel MP, et al. Preliminary report of the STIM2 study: a multicenter stop imatinib trial for chronic phase chronic myeloid leukemia de novo patients on imatinib. *Blood (ASH Annual Meeting Abstracts).* 2013;122:654.

50 Rousselot P, Charbonnier A, Cony-Makhoul P, et al. Loss of major molecular response as a trigger for restarting tyrosine kinase inhibitor therapy in patients with chronic-phase chronic myelogenous leukemia who have stopped imatinib after durable undetectable disease. *J Clin Oncol.* 2014;32(5):424–430.

## CHAPTER 12

# Targeted Therapy for Acute Lymphoblastic Leukemia

*Nitin Jain, Susan O'Brien, and Farhad Ravandi-Kashani*
Department of Leukemia, The University of Texas MD Anderson Cancer Center, Houston, TX, USA

## Introduction

Better understanding of molecular pathogenesis of acute lymphoblastic leukemia (ALL) has led to a variety of new treatment paradigms in ALL. Combination chemotherapy has been the cornerstone of ALL treatment. While currently employed induction regimens in adults with ALL routinely result in high complete remission (CR) rates of 80–90%, none of them have yet translated into the 80–85% disease-free survival (DFS) rates that are routinely achieved in pediatric ALL.[1] In adult ALL, the rates of DFS generally are 40–45% at 3 years and 30–35% at 5 years.[2] Thus, the main problem with the current treatment programs in adult ALL is disease relapse due to the emergence of resistant clones. Further intensification of chemotherapy has not proven to be effective.[3] The prognosis of patients with relapsed or refractory ALL is extremely poor. Outcome with further therapy is dependent on duration of first CR and the response to prior therapy. In patients with second relapse and beyond, achievement of a third CR is infrequent, occurring in less than 10% of the cases with the median survival being less than 6 months. Allogeneic stem cell transplantation (alloSCT) is the only potentially curative strategy after relapse, and in general, can only be performed if an adequate response to therapy (ideally a CR) is achieved. Durable responses that allow for sufficient time to identify a donor and proceed to alloSCT are infrequent even in first relapse (<25%). Novel therapeutic strategies are clearly needed.

## Prognostication in ALL

Prognostication based on clinical and biological risk factors has been useful in making informed decisions about post-remission therapy. Established adverse risk factors include age >60 years, elevated WBC count at diagnosis (>30,000/μL (B-cell ALL), >100,000/μL (T-cell ALL)), pro-B-cell or early T-cell immunophenotype, the presence of t(4;11)(q21;q23) and other MLL rearrangements, and hypodiploidy or complex karyotype).[4] Outcomes of patients with Philadelphia (Ph) chromosome, previously a very high-risk disease characteristic, have improved considerably with the use of tyrosine kinase inhibitors (TKIs). Minimal residual disease (MRD) at 3–6 months after initiation of therapy has been identified as a powerful prognostication tool.[5] Several of the recently described genetic aberrations (*IKAROS* deletion/mutation, *CRLF2*

overexpression, *JAK2* mutations, and Ph-like gene expression profile) are associated with poor prognosis and may further help classify patients.[6]

## Surface Antigen as a Therapeutic Target

Raponi et al. evaluated the expression level of surface markers on the B-cell ALL blasts by flow cytometry.[7] CD19 was expressed in all 451 cases of B-lineage ALL. CD20 expression increased with B-cell maturation with 0% positivity in pro-B cell cases, 30% in B-common ALL, 46% in pre-B ALL, and 100% in mature B-cell ALL. CD22 expression was noted in 93% of patients. Several of these surface antigens have now been exploited as a therapeutic target (Figure 12.1).

1 **CD20.** Thomas et al. were the first to report on the use of rituximab, an anti-CD20 monoclonal antibody in patients with ALL. In this study, rituximab was added for two doses with each of the first four hyper-CVAD cycles. In the younger cohort of patients (<60 years), incorporation of rituximab significantly improved the 3-year overall survival (OS) rates (75% vs. 47% in the historical controls, $p = 0.003$).[8] The German ALL study group (GMALL) have confirmed these results.[9] Traditionally, the cut-off for CD20 positivity has been >20% of CD20 expression in leukemic blasts. However, patients with a lower CD20 expression level may still benefit from the use of anti-CD20 monoclonal antibody as it is known that steroids (a routine part of ALL chemotherapy regimens) can upregulate CD20 expression. Dworzak et al. reported that CD20-positivity significantly increased from 45% in samples of childhood B-cell ALL at baseline to 81% at the end of induction therapy.[10] *In vitro*, CD20 upregulation significantly enhanced rituximab cytotoxicity. This concept merits further investigation.

Ofatumumab, another anti-CD20 monoclonal antibody, targets a different epitope of CD20 and has been found to be more potent than rituximab in promoting complement-dependent cytotoxicity (CDC) *in vitro*.[11] In a preliminary report, Jabbour et al. reported on 17 patients treated with hyper-CVAD plus ofatumumab who achieved a 94% CR rate.[12] The rates of 1-year CR duration and OS were 100% and 95%, respectively. These preliminary data are encouraging.

*Targeted Therapy in Translational Cancer Research*, First Edition. Edited by Apostolia-Maria Tsimberidou, Razelle Kurzrock and Kenneth C. Anderson.
© 2016 John Wiley & Sons, Inc. Published 2016 by John Wiley & Sons, Inc.

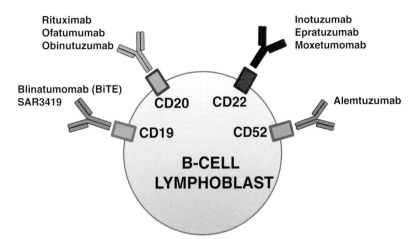

**Figure 12.1** Monoclonal antibodies in B-cell ALL.

Obinutuzumab (GA101), is a humanized type II CD20 monoclonal antibody with a glycoengineered Fc portion that leads to increased direct monoclonal antibody-induced leukemia cell death, enhanced antibody-dependent cellular cytotoxicity (ADCC), and lower CDC.[13] In preclinical studies, obinutuzumab was more effective than rituximab in B-cell depletion and in growth inhibition of human lymphomas in animal models.[13,14] In the recently reported CLL11 trial, treatment with obinutuzumab–chlorambucil as compared to rituximab–chlorambucil, resulted in a higher overall response rate (ORR) and improved progression-free survival (PFS) in patients with chronic lymphocytic leukemia (CLL).[15] Based on these data, obinutuzumab in combination with chlorambucil is now approved for patients with previously untreated CLL. Evaluation of obinutuzumab with chemotherapy for patients with CD20+ ALL would be of great interest.

2 **CD19.** CD19 is expressed uniformly in B-cell ALL. A novel approach to target B cells is through the use of a bispecific T-cell engager (BiTE) antibody.[16] Blinatumomab is a novel antibody (BiTE antibody) designed to target patient's T cells to CD19-expressing B cells resulting in a cytotoxic T-cell response. This was initially tested by the GMALL to eradicate MRD in ALL. Sixteen of the twenty evaluable patients achieved MRD-negativity.[17,18] Preliminary results of an ongoing phase II trial of single-agent blinatumomab in adult patients with relapsed/refractory B-cell ALL were recently reported.[19] Blinatumomab was administered by continuous intravenous infusion for 28 days followed by a 14-day treatment-free interval. Responding patients could receive three additional cycles of treatment or proceed to bone marrow transplantation. Seventeen of twenty-five evaluable patients (68%) reached a hematological CR/CR with incomplete recovery of platelets (CRp). Interestingly, six patients relapsed, of whom three were CD19-negative at the time of relapse. These data are particularly encouraging as a CR/CRp rate of 68% in the relapsed/refractory setting with a single-agent therapy is quite remarkable.

SAR3419 is an antibody–drug conjugate (ADC) that targets CD19. The ADC is created by conjugation of the IgG1 antibody huB4 to the maytansinoid DM4, a potent inhibitor of tubulin polymerization and microtubule assembly. In an initial phase I study, SAR3419 was administered every 3 weeks in patients with relapsed B-cell lymphoma.[20] The most common drug-related toxicity was ocular toxicity, which was noted in 44% of patients. The primary ocular symptom was blurred vision and the most common ocular finding was bilateral corneal epitheliopathy. Of 35 patients evaluable for efficacy, 26 (74%) patients demonstrated a reduction in their tumor size, including six patients who achieved partial or CR. A second phase I dose-escalation study was conducted to evaluate a once-weekly schedule of SAR3419 under the assumption that more frequent administrations at lower doses would improve antitumor activity and tolerance.[21] There was a lower incidence of ocular side effects and 55% of patients noticed tumor shrinkage. A phase II study with the weekly schedule of SAR3419 in patients with relapsed ALL is currently enrolling patients (NCT01440179).

3 **CD22.** CD22 expression occurs in >90% of patients with ALL. Inotuzumab ozogamicin is a CD22 monoclonal antibody bound to a toxin, calecheamicin, and has shown single-agent activity in relapsed/refractory ALL.[22] In a phase II study, patients were given inotuzumab ozogamicin (1.8 mg/m²) intravenously every 3–4 weeks. Forty-nine patients were treated. The median number of courses administered was two (range 1–5). The ORR was 57% (CR 18%, marrow CR 39%). Twenty-four percent of patients had grade 1–2 and 4% had grade 3 increases in bilirubin. Grade 1–2 elevations of serum aminotransferase were noted in 55% patients and grade 3 elevations in 2% patients. Based on higher *in vitro* efficacy with more frequent exposure, a weekly schedule (0.8 mg/m² on day 1, and 0.5 mg/m² on days 8 and 15, every 3–4 weeks) has been developed.[23] With the weekly schedule, the ORR was 53% (similar to 57% noted with the every 3 weeks schedule). With the weekly schedule, reversible grade 1–2 and 3–4 bilirubin elevations were observed in 3% and 0% patients, respectively. Reversible grade 1–2 and 3–4 liver enzyme elevations were observed in 21% and 6%, respectively with the weekly dose schedule. Thus, the weekly schedule has similar efficacy as the every 3-week schedule with an improved toxicity profile. A phase III trial of weekly inotuzumab ozogamicin versus investigator choice chemotherapy for patients with ALL in first or second relapse is currently in progress (NCT01564784). Inotuzumab ozogamicin has also been combined with lower intensity chemotherapy (mini-hyper-CVAD) for treatment of older patients with newly diagnosed B-cell ALL. Notably, anthracycline is omitted in this chemotherapy regimen and the dose of other cytotoxic drugs is reduced by 50% or greater. In the preliminary results reported by Jain et al., 15 patients were treated and the CR/CRp rate was 93%.[24] The 1-year DFS and OS were 83% and 93%, respectively. Treatment was well tolerated. These results appear to be better

than those achieved with chemotherapy alone in this patient population. Based on the preclinical evidence that the combination of inotuzumab ozogamicin with rituximab has additive activity,[25] a phase I/II study of inotuzumab ozogamicin with rituximab was conducted in patients with relapsed/refractory CD20+/CD22+ non-Hodgkin's lymphoma.[26] Patients with follicular lymphoma (FL) and diffuse large B-cell lymphoma (DLBCL) were treated with rituximab (375 mg/m$^2$ every 4 weeks) in combination with escalating doses of inotuzumab ozogamicin ranging from 0.8 to 1.8 mg/m$^2$ every 4 weeks. The maximum tolerated dose (MTD) of inotuzumab ozogamicin (in combination with rituximab) was 1.8 mg/m$^2$ every 4 weeks. The most common grade 3–4 adverse events were thrombocytopenia (31%) and neutropenia (22%). At the MTD, the objective response rates were 87% and 74% in patients with relapsed FL and DLBCL, respectively.

Epratuzumab, a humanized unconjugated monoclonal antibody targeting CD22, has activity in a subset of patients with ALL. In a Children's Oncology Group's pilot study, epratuzumab in combination with standard reinduction chemotherapy was evaluated in 15 pediatric patients with relapsed ALL.[27] There was rapid clearing of surface CD22 antigen and 9 of 15 patients achieved a CR. Advani et al. added epratuzumab to the combination of clofarabine and cytarabine in adults with relapsed/refractory B-cell ALL (Southwestern Oncology Group S0910).[28] The CR/CR with incomplete count recovery (CRi) rate was reported as 52%, significantly higher than their previous trial with clofarabine/cytarabine alone, where the response rate was only 17%.[29] Another form of epratuzumab (conjugated to SN-38, a topoisomerase I inhibitor that is derived from the prodrug, irinotecan) has also been developed.[30]

Moxetumomab pasudotox, is a recombinant immunotoxin composed of the Fv fragment of an anti-CD22 monoclonal antibody fused to a 38-kDa fragment of pseudomonas exotoxin A, called PE38.[31] Moxetumomab pasudotox is an improved, more active form of a predecessor recombinant immunotoxin, BL22, which produced CR in relapsed/refractory hairy cell leukemia (HCL). In a phase I study of moxetumomab pasudotox in patients with relapsed/refractory HCL, 28 patients were enrolled.[32] No DLT was observed. The ORR rate was 86%, with 46% achieving CR. In a phase I study in pediatric patients with relapsed/refractory CD22+ B-cell ALL, moxetumomab pasudotox was administered at doses of 5, 10, 20, 30, or 40 mcg/kg, every other day for 6 doses, every 21 days.[33] Twenty-one patients were treated. The most common treatment-related adverse events were increased weight, increased transaminases, and hypoalbuminemia. The ORR was 29% (CR, 24%). A phase I/II trial of moxetumomab pasudotox in adult patients with relapsed/refractory ALL is currently enrolling patients (NCT01891981).

4  **CD52.** CD52 is expressed on nearly all normal and malignant B lymphocytes and T lymphocytes, monocytes, and macrophages.[34] Granulocytes, platelets, erythrocytes, and hematopoietic stem cells typically lack CD52 expression. Alemtuzumab is a humanized, unconjugated monoclonal antibody directed against CD52. In a phase I/II study (CALGB 10102), alemtuzumab was administered to 24 patients with ALL in CR1 where it was given with an intent to eradicate MRD.[35] Serial assessment of MRD using clone-specific PCR was possible in 11 of 24 patients and a median 1-log decrease in MRD was noted in 8 patients. Viral infections, especially CMV reactivation, were common. Alemtuzumab, as a single-agent, has limited activity in relapsed/refractory pediatric and adult patients with ALL.[36,37] The combination of alem-

tuzumab and rituximab has been shown to be synergistic in a NOD-SCID mouse model.[38]

## BCR-ABL-Positive ALL

The Philadelphia chromosome [t(9;22)(q34;q11)] (Ph+), is the most common cytogenetic abnormality in adult patients with ALL and up to 50% of older patients with ALL carry the Ph+ chromosome.[2,39] Before the introduction of TKIs, Ph+ ALL was associated with a very poor prognosis with a median survival of less than 1 year.[40] TKI therapy has been the major treatment advance for patients with ALL in the last decade.[39] Thomas et al. combined imatinib with hyper-CVAD chemotherapy and reported significantly improved rates of 3-year CR duration and OS compared to historical controls treated with hyper-CVAD alone (68% vs. 24% and 54% vs. 15%, respectively, $p < 0.001$).[41,42] The second generation TKI, dasatinib, is a dual BCR-ABL and SRC kinase inhibitor with approximately 325-fold increased activity against BCR-ABL compared to imatinib. Unlike imatinib, dasatinib crosses the blood–brain barrier and thus may provide better CNS protection. Dasatinib has also been combined with hyper-CVAD chemotherapy with improved outcomes. Ravandi et al. treated 63 patients with newly diagnosed Ph+ ALL and 9 patients with 1 or 2 prior cycles of chemotherapy with dasatinib in combination with hyper-CVAD chemotherapy.[43,44] A total of 93% patients achieved a major molecular remission (MMR) and 65% achieved complete molecular remission (CMR). MRD negativity was achieved in 94% of the patients. The median DFS and OS were 31 months and 44 months, respectively. Several studies have confirmed these findings and early TKI therapy is now the standard treatment of Ph+ ALL.[2,4,45–48]

Nilotinib, a second generation TKI, has also been combined with multiagent chemotherapy for newly diagnosed patients with Ph+ ALL.[49] A total of 91 patients were enrolled. Complete hematologic response (CHR) was noted in 90% of patients and the cumulative major cytogenetic remission (MCR) rate was 84%. The estimated 2-year OS was 70%.

Ponatinib, a third generation TKI, is currently being investigated in combination with hyper-CVAD chemotherapy as front-line therapy for patients with ALL.[50] In a preliminary report, Jabbour et al. treated 30 patients with all patients achieving complete cytogenetic remission (CCyR) after one or two cycles with an MMR rate of 93% and a CMR rate of 70%. MRD negativity by flow cytometry was achieved in 90% of patients. Twenty percent of the patients experienced thromboembolic adverse events. These early data with hyper-CVAD plus ponatinib are encouraging, although increased thromboembolic complications have to be taken into account.

Dasatinib has also been investigated with low-intensity chemotherapy in older patients (≥55 years) with Ph+ ALL.[51] Induction consisted of dasatinib 140 mg once daily with weekly vincristine and dexamethasone. Consolidation consisted of dasatinib 100 mg once daily sequentially with methotrexate and asparaginase for cycles 1, 3, and 5 and cytarabine for cycles 2, 4, and 6. Seventy-one patients were treated with a median age of 69 years (range, 58–83 years). The CR rate after induction was 90% and MMR was achieved in 55.7% of the patients. The median RFS and OS were 22.1 and 27.1 months, respectively. Patients with additional cytogenetic abnormalities at diagnosis had an inferior RFS. Most relapses were associated with the T315I mutation.

## Ph-Like ALL

In 2009, a subgroup of pediatric patients with B-cell ALL was identified that had a gene expression signature similar to that of

BCR-ABL-positive ALL, but these patients did not carry the Philadelphia chromosome.[52,53] These patients had frequent deletion of transcription factor *IKZF1*, also common in BCR-ABL-positive ALL.[52–54] Such cases, categorized as "Ph-like ALL," comprise up to 15% of childhood B-cell ALL[55], 20–25% in adolescents and young adults, and a higher frequency of ALL in adults (up to 30%).[56] Patients with Ph-like ALL have a very high rate of disease relapse and short OS.[56–59]

In a study by the German and Dutch groups, 190 children with newly diagnosed ALL (154 B-cell ALL, 36 T-cell ALL) were evaluated by gene expression profiling using an Affymetrix chip assay.[52] A hierarchical clustering with a 110-gene probe set clustered major subtype of B-cell ALL into distinct groups (*ETV6-RUNX1* (*TEL-AML1*, t(12;21) (p13.1;q22)); hyperdiploid (>50 chromosomes); *TCF3* (*E2A*)-rearranged such as *TCF3–PBX1* (t(1;19)(q23;p13)); *MLL*-rearranged; *BCR-ABL1*). There were 44 patients who did not fit into any one of the known genetic subgroups and were classified as B other. Of these 44 patients, 30 patients (19% of the entire B-cell ALL cohort (30/154); 68% of B other (30/44)) had gene expression profile similar to patients with *BCR-ABL1*-positive ALL. These patients, referred to as Ph-like ALL, had very poor outcomes (5-year DFS 59% vs. 84% for remaining of B-cell ALL, $p = 0.01$).

Up to half of Ph-like ALL cases harbor a rearrangement of *CRLF2* located at the pseudoautosomal region of Xp22.3/Yp11.3, either as a translocation to the immunoglobulin heavy chain enhancer region at 14q32.33 (*IGH-CRLF2*), or a focal deletion proximal to *CRLF2* resulting in the expression of a *P2RY8-CRLF2* fusion transcript.[57,60–64] CRLF2 encodes cytokine-receptor-like factor 2 (also known as thymic stromal lymphopoietin (TSLP) receptor), a lymphoid-signaling receptor molecule that forms a heterodimeric complex with interleukin-7 receptor alpha (IL7R) and binds TSLP. The IL7-TSLP receptor signaling pathway is important in lymphoid development.[65] These two cytokine receptors are dimeric, share IL7R, and use IL2RG (interleukin-2 receptor gamma, which is a common gamma chain shared by the receptors of various cytokines, including interleukin 2, 4, 7, 9, and 15) and CRLF2, respectively, to form heterodimers. TSLP-CRLF2 signaling has important roles in T-cell and dendritic cell development, inflammation, and allergic disease and promotes B-lymphoid proliferation.[66] TSLP is produced by epithelial cells at sites of inflammation, where it activates myeloid dendritic cells and Th2 immune responses. Signaling from the TSLP receptor activates the signal transducer and activator of transcription (STAT5) by phosphorylation of JAK1 and JAK2 through association with IL-7R and CRLF2, respectively.[61,67,68]

Mulligan et al. initially identified deletion involving the pseudoautosomal region 1 (PAR1) of Xp22.3/Yp11.3 in B-cell ALL, including in several children with Down-syndrome-associated ALL (DS-ALL).[54,60,69] Further analysis showed that PAR1 deletion extended from immediately upstream of the *CRLF2* exon 1 to *P2RY8* intron 1 creating a fusion transcript *P2RY8-CRLF2*.[60] The breakpoints were identical in all patients and detectable by RT-PCR. These patients also had increased cell surface expression of *CRLF2*, detectable by flow cytometry. Overall 53% (40/75) of patients with DS-ALL had a *P2RY8-CRLF2* fusion. *IGH@-CRLF2* translocations, which also lead to increased CRLF2 expression, are rare in DS-ALL (only 1/75 patients in this study).[60] Importantly, *P2RY8-CRLF2* fusion was associated with JAK2 mutations (32% vs. 4% without the fusion), most commonly at the *JAK2* pseudokinase domain, *JAK2*R683. In contrast to myeloproliferative diseases, in which homozygous alteration of JAK2 V617F is common,

the JAK alterations in B-cell ALL are usually heterozygous and do not occur at JAK2 V617.[70–74] Coexpression of P2RY8-CRLF2 and JAK mutation resulted in constitutive JAK-STAT activation and cytokine-independent growth in Ba/F3-IL7R cells. Moreover, this transformation was attenuated by pharmacological JAK inhibition and knockdown of CRLF2 by shRNA.[60]

Harvey et al. evaluated 207 children with "high-risk" B-cell ALL enrolled in the COG P9906 study using the augmented BFM regimen.[57] Twenty-nine patients (14%) had CRLF2 overexpression (two-thirds were *IGH@-CRLF2* translocations; one-third was *P2RY8-CRLF2*). Notably, there is a higher rate (14%) of CRLF2 overexpression in this cohort of high-risk ALL patients, compared to 5% in unselected childhood B-cell ALL cases.[61] Patients with Hispanic ethnicity were more likely to have CRLF2 overexpression (35% vs. 7% in others, $p < 0.001$).[57] *IKZF1* alterations were more common in patients with CRLF2 overexpression (81% vs. 22% in non-CRLF2 overexpressed cases, $p < 0.001$). *JAK* mutations were more common in patients with CRLF2 overexpression (69% vs. 1% in non-CRLF2 overexpressed cases, $p < 0.001$). Patients with CRLF2 deregulation had a significantly inferior 4-year RFS rate compared to those with intact CRLF2 rate (35.3% vs. 71.3%, respectively; $p = 0.001$). There was no difference in the outcome according to the type of CRLF2 rearrangement (translocation vs. deletion). Approximately 62% of patients with CRLF2 deregulation were Ph-like on gene expression profiling.

Chen et al. evaluated a large cohort of pediatric patients with ALL ($n = 1061$), enrolled in the COG trials (P9905 and P9906).[75] A total of 186 of the 1061 patients (17.5%) were noted to have CRLF2 overexpression by quantitative RT-PCR. CRLF2 overexpression was noted in 19% of the high-risk (HR: age ≥10 years or initial WBC ≥ 50,000/μL) cohort and 16.2% of the standard risk (SR: age 1–9.99 years and initial WBC < 50,000/μL) cohort. The 186 ALL patients with high CRLF2 mRNA expression had higher rates of end-of-induction MRD (30% vs. 21.3%, $p = 0.016$) and higher rates of relapse (38.2% vs. 22.1%, $p < 0.001$). Cells from patients with high CRLF2 mRNA expression also contained all of the CRLF2 genomic lesions (*IGH@-CRLF2*, *P2RY8-CRLF2*, and CRLF2 F232C), virtually all of the JAK mutations (37 of 39), and a higher frequency of IKZF1 deletions and mutations (43.3% vs. 18.9%, $p < 0.001$). In addition, consistent with reports by other groups, high CRLF2-expressing ALL cases lacked common ALL-associated sentinel cytogenetic lesions. One surprising finding in this study was that only 53% of the cases with CRLF2 overexpression (9% of the entire ALL cohort) had genomic rearrangements of CRLF2 (ratio of *P2RY8-CRLF2:IGH@-CRLF2* = 2.1:1). In a multivariate model for RFS, four variables (NCI risk status, MRD, high *CRLF2* expression, and *IKZF1* deletions/mutations) retained independent prognostic significance.

Yoda et al. evaluated adults with B-cell ALL for CRLF2 overexpression and noted overexpression in 5.9% (15/254) cases.[64] As reported in the pediatric series, CRLF2 expression was restricted to patients without known recurrent chromosomal aberrations (12.5% (15/120) in those with lacking recurring chromosomal aberrations; none in 134 patients with recurrent chromosomal aberrations). They also reported a point mutation in the CRLF2 (CRLF2 F232C, CRLF2 711 T > G) in 3 of the 14 (21%) patients with CRLF2 overexpression. CRLF2 F232C, a gain of function mutation, leads to constitutive dimerization through the cysteine residues and thereby, signal transduction. They also reported that the CRLF2 F232C mutation was mutually exclusive with JAK mutations, suggesting that these mutations function within the same pathway. In this series, all patients with JAK mutations overexpressed CRLF2. They also screened patients with T-cell ALL and CLL, none of whom had CRLF2 overexpression.

In the UKALLXII/ECOG2993 trial, 454 patients (15- to 60-year old) with available samples were evaluated for CRLF2 dysregulation by fluorescence *in situ* hybridization (FISH) analysis.[76] The incidence of CRLF2 dysregulation was 5% (two-thirds were *IGH@-CRLF2* translocations; one-third were *P2RY8-CRLF2*). In most cases, CRLF2 dysregulation was not associated with other primary chromosomal abnormalities. Patients with CRLF2 deregulation had a higher WBC count, worse 5-year RFS (30% vs. 55% for all patients, $p = 0.02$) and worse 5-year OS (21% vs. 43% for all patients, $p = 0.03$).

*IL7R* is required for normal lymphoid development. Loss-of-function mutations in *IL7R* cause autosomal recessive severe combined immune deficiency by the complete absence of T lymphocytes and the presence of B and NK cells.[77] IL-7R heterodimerizes either with IL2RG to form a receptor for IL-7 or with CRLF2 to form a receptor for TSLP. Shochat et al. reported gain-of-function mutations in *IL7R* in 6% (8/133) of pediatric patients with B-cell ALL overexpressing CRLF2 compared to 0.6% (1/153) in the remaining of the B-cell ALL group.[78] They also showed that the presence of cysteine was critical for the gain-of-function phenotype. Biochemical and functional assays revealed that these *IL7R* mutations were activating mutations conferring cytokine-independent growth of progenitor lymphoid cells. A concomitant *JAK2* mutation was present in three out of eight samples. In contrast, Chen et al. reported *IL7R* mutations in 1.5% (5/335) patients with childhood B-cell ALL.[75] Surprisingly, only one of the five mutations was in the CRLF2 overexpression cohort, resulting in a frequency of 0.7% (1/141) for IL7R mutations in that cohort. Interestingly, *IL7R* mutations were also identified in 10.5% (30/295) of childhood T-ALL samples.[78] These alterations (*JAK* mutations, *CRLF2* overexpression, *IL7R* mutations) result in activation of JAK-STAT signaling and thus may be amenable to therapy with JAK inhibitors such as ruxolitinib.[79]

Transcriptome and whole genome sequencing of 15 Ph-like ALL cases, 12 of which lacked CRLF2 rearrangement, identified a set of genetic alterations activating cytokine receptor and tyrosine signaling.[62] These were most commonly rearrangements resulting in chimeric fusion genes deregulating tyrosine kinases (*NUP214-ABL1, ETV6-ABL1, RANBP2-ABL1, RCSD1-ABL1, BCR-JAK2, PAX5-JAK2, STRN3-JAK2,* and *EBF1-PDGFRB*) and cytokine receptors (*IGH-EPOR*). Up to 20% of Ph-like cases lack a chimeric fusion on mRNA-seq analysis, and sequence mutations (e.g., activating mutations of *FLT3* and *IL7R*) and structural alterations (e.g., focal deletions of *SH2B3*, also known as LNK, which suppresses JAK signaling)[80] activating signaling have been identified in fusion-negative cases.[78,81] These diverse genetic alterations activate specific signaling pathways, notably *ABL1* and *PDGFRB* (both of which may be inhibited with the TKI such as dasatinib) and JAK-STAT signaling (via *JAK* mutations and *JAK* fusions such as *BCR-JAK2, PAX5-JAK2, STRN3-JAK* which may be inhibited by *JAK* inhibitor such as ruxolitinib).[62,79] These rearrangements have been shown to activate signaling pathways in preclinical cell lines and xenograft models, and xenografts of Ph-like ALL are highly sensitive to TKIs *in vivo*.[62,79] Recent reports of patients with refractory *EBF1-PDGFRB*-positive ALL that were exquisitely sensitive to imatinib, and *RCSD1-ABL1*-positive ALL that was sensitive to dasatinib emphasizes the potential clinical utility of TKI therapy in Ph-like ALL.[82–86]

## PI3K/AKT/mTOR Signaling Pathway Inhibitors and B-Cell Receptor Inhibitors

Constitutive activation of the phosphatidylinositol 3-kinase (PI3K), Akt, and the mammalian target of rapamycin (mTOR) (PI3K/AKT/mTOR) signaling pathway is a feature of B-cell ALL.[87] Everolimus, an orally active inhibitor of mTOR, has been tested in combination with hyper-CVAD chemotherapy in patients with relapsed/refractory ALL.[88] Everolimus was administered at 5 or 10 mg continuously daily. Everolimus 5 mg daily was established as the MTD. In a preliminary report of 20 patients, a CR/CRi rate of 35% was noted.[88] Grade 3 mucositis was the dose-limiting toxicity (DLT). Ibrutinib, a B-cell receptor inhibitor, is also being explored in patients with relapsed/refractory B-cell ALL.[89]

## Chimeric Antigen Receptor Therapy

Immunotherapy with chimeric antigen receptors (CARs) is an active and exciting field of research. CARs are novel synthetic receptors composed of an antigen-binding domain (most commonly derived from the fused variable heavy- and light-chain domains of a tumor-targeted monoclonal antibody) fused to a transmembrane domain followed by one or more cytoplasmic signaling domains. The resultant receptor is then expressed on autologous (the most common strategy at this time) or allogeneic T cells. These T cells with CAR on their surface are infused into the patient where these T cells actively seek the tumor antigen and lyse the tumor cells. CD19 CARs have shown remarkable activity in B-cell ALL patients with >80% CR rate in a relapsed/refractory patient population.[90–92] Davila et al. reported on 16 patients with relapsed/refractory B-cell ALL who were treated with CD19-directed CAR T cells.[90] The overall CR rate was 88% with most of the patients transitioning to an alloSCT. Cytokine release syndrome remains a potential issue with CAR T-cell infusion. Targeting CD19 also leads to B-cell aplasia and these patients require monthly immunoglobulin replacement. Other novel surface receptors such as ROR1, expressed selectively on malignant B cells but not on normal B cells, are currently being studied in CLL.

## T-Cell ALL

Unlike B-cell ALL where several therapeutic targets are being investigated, only a limited number of drugs/targets are being investigated in T-cell ALL.

## Notch Inhibition in T-Cell ALL

Notch signaling is a highly conserved evolutional pathway and is required for commitment of stem cells to T-cell fate.[93] Notch proteins are synthesized as single precursor proteins, which are cleaved in the Golgi bodies into two subunits held together noncovalently by the N- and C-terminal subunits of the heterodimerization domains (HD).[94] Notch signaling is initiated by ligand receptor interaction, which induces a second cleavage at site S2 (close to the transmembrane domain) mediated by ADAM-type (A disintegrin and metalloprotease) metalloproteases followed by a third cleavage at S3 within the transmembrane domain mediated by the γ-secretase. This last proteolytic cleavage liberates the cytoplasmic domain of Notch receptors (NICD), which translocate to the nucleus and bind to the transcription factor CSL (CBF1, Suppressor of hairless, and Lag-1), converting it from a transcriptional repressor into a transcriptional activator by recruiting coactivators including mastermind-like proteins (MAML). NICD is polyubiquitinated by E3 ubiquitin ligases (including Fbw7), which marks NICD for proteosomal degradation. Ellisen et al. first reported Notch involvement in T-cell ALL when they described a translocation t(7;9)(q34;q34.3).[95] Weng et al. reported activating *NOTCH1* mutations in 56% of patients with T-cell ALL.[96] The majority of the mutations were in the HD domain. Asnafi et al. reported a 72% incidence of *NOTCH1* and *FBXW7* mutations (48% *NOTCH1* mutation alone; 9% *FBXW7* mutation alone; 15% both) in the GRAALL-2003 and LALA-894 trial.[97] They also reported better PFS and OS in patients with *NOTCH1/FBXW7* mutations. A phase I trial of an oral γ-secretase inhibitor MK-0752 in patients with relapsed/refractory T-cell ALL showed only minimal clinical activity but produced significant GI toxicities including diarrhea and colitis.[98] GI toxicity is an on-target effect of Notch inhibition in the small bowel where epithelial cells are skewed to goblet cell fate instead of enterocytes.[99] A phase I trial with an IV γ-secretase inhibitor, BMS-906024, given weekly, is currently underway (NCT01363817). Other inhibitors of the Notch pathway including an anti-Notch receptor antibody are in preclinical development.[100-102]

## Early T-Cell Precursor ALL

In 2009, the St. Jude's group reported on a subgroup of patients with T-cell ALL that had a myeloid signature based on gene expression profiling.[103] These were derived from early T-cell precursors (ETP), cells that recently arrived in the thymus from the bone marrow and retain multilineage differentiation potential. Approximately 10–15% of childhood cases of T-cell ALL and 7–10% of adult cases of T-cell ALL have the ETP phenotype.[103,104] ETP ALL is characterized by the following immunophenotype: (a) CD1a negative (<5%); (b) CD8 negative (<5%); (c) weak CD5 (<75%); and (d) presence of one or more of myeloid/stem cell marker (>25%) such as CD117, CD34, HLA-DR, CD13, CD33, CD11b, and CD65.[103] Patients with ETP ALL have significantly worse outcomes than those with non-ETP T-cell ALL (St. Jude's data—10-year OS, 19% for ETP ALL vs. 84% for non-ETP T-cell ALL, $p < 0.0001$; 10-year relapse rate, 72% for ETP ALL vs. 10% for non-ETP T-cell ALL, $p < 0.0001$).[103,105] Neumann et al. reported data in the adult patient population for the GMALL group.[104,106,107] ETP ALL cases comprise 7.4% of all adult T-cell ALL cases. They also reported a 35% incidence of FLT-3 mutation (D835 mutation two times more common than ITD) and a 14% incidence of a DNMT3A mutation. Given the high frequency of FLT3 mutation in ETP ALL, FLT3 inhibitors may be useful in this subgroup of T cell ALL. In addition, given the myeloid gene expression profile, a myeloid-based chemotherapy regimen could be considered for these patients. A distinct immunophenotype has been identified for patients with FLT-3 mutated ETP ALL: CD2+, CD5−, CD34+, CD117+, CD13+, and CD33−.[104,106,107]

## Conclusions

Significant advances in our understanding of ALL disease biology have led to several new and innovative treatment strategies. Clinical data with "targeted therapies" are very promising with several of these agents being investigated in phase III clinical trials (inotuzumab ozogamicin, blinatumomab). CAR therapies offer a promising approach and long-term follow-up data of this therapy are eagerly expected. Incorporation of these novel strategies into front-line programs, especially for adult patients, is a top research priority.

## References

1 Pui CH, Evans WE. A 50-year journey to cure childhood acute lymphoblastic leukemia. *Semin Hematol.* 2013;50(3):185–196.

2 Inaba H, Greaves M, Mullighan CG. Acute lymphoblastic leukaemia. *Lancet.* 2013;381(9881):1943–1955.

3 Faderl S, Thomas DA, O'Brien S, et al. Augmented hyper-CVAD based on dose-intensified vincristine, dexamethasone, and asparaginase in adult acute lymphoblastic leukemia salvage therapy. *Clin Lymphoma Myeloma Leuk.* 2011;11(1):54–59.

4 Faderl S, O'Brien S, Pui CH, et al. Adult acute lymphoblastic leukemia: concepts and strategies. *Cancer.* 2010;116(5):1165–1176.

5 Campana D. Minimal residual disease monitoring in childhood acute lymphoblastic leukemia. *Curr Opin Hematol.* 2012;19(4):313–318.

6 Mullighan CG. Genomic characterization of childhood acute lymphoblastic leukemia. *Semin Hematol.* 2013;50(4):314–324.

7 Raponi S, De Propris MS, Intoppa S, et al. Flow cytometric study of potential target antigens (CD19, CD20, CD22, CD33) for antibody-based immunotherapy in acute lymphoblastic leukemia: analysis of 552 cases. *Leuk Lymphoma.* 2011;52(6):1098–1107.

8 Thomas DA, O'Brien S, Faderl S, et al. Chemoimmunotherapy with a modified hyper-CVAD and rituximab regimen improves outcome in de novo Philadelphia chromosome-negative precursor B-lineage acute lymphoblastic leukemia. *J Clin Oncol.* 2010;28(24):3880–3889.

9 Hoelzer D, Huettmann A, Kaul F, et al. Immunochemotherapy with rituximab improves molecular CR rate and outcome in CD20+ B-lineage standard and high risk patients; results of 263 CD20+ patients studied prospectively in GMALL study 07/2003. *Blood (ASH Annual Meeting Abstracts).* 2010;116:Abstract 170.

10 Dworzak MN, Schumich A, Printz D, et al. CD20 up-regulation in pediatric B-cell precursor acute lymphoblastic leukemia during induction treatment: setting the stage for anti-CD20 directed immunotherapy. *Blood.* 2008;112(10):3982–3988.

11 Pawluczkowycz AW, Beurskens FJ, Beum PV, et al. Binding of submaximal C1q promotes complement-dependent cytotoxicity (CDC) of B cells opsonized with anti-CD20 mAbs ofatumumab (OFA) or rituximab (RTX): considerably higher levels of CDC are induced by OFA than by RTX. *J Immunol.* 2009;183(1):749–758.

12 Jabbour E, Hagop K, Thomas D, et al. Phase II study of the hyper-CVAD regimen in combination with ofatumumab as frontline therapy for adults with CD-20 positive acute lymphoblastic leukemia (ALL). *Blood.* 2013;122(21):2664.

13 Mossner E, Brunker P, Moser S, et al. Increasing the efficacy of CD20 antibody therapy through the engineering of a new type II anti-CD20 antibody with enhanced direct and immune effector cell-mediated B-cell cytotoxicity. *Blood.* 2010;115(22):4393–4402.

14 Herter S, Herting F, Mundigl O, et al. Preclinical activity of the type II CD20 antibody GA101 (obinutuzumab) compared with rituximab and ofatumumab in vitro and in xenograft models. *Mol Cancer Ther.* 2013;12(10):2031–2042.

15 Goede V, Fischer K, Busch R, et al. Obinutuzumab plus chlorambucil in patients with CLL and coexisting conditions. *N Engl J Med.* 2014;370(12):1101–1110.

16 Bargou R, Leo E, Zugmaier G, et al. Tumor regression in cancer patients by very low doses of a T cell-engaging antibody. *Science.* 2008;321(5891):974–977.

17 Topp MS, Kufer P, Gokbuget N, et al. Targeted therapy with the T-cell-engaging antibody blinatumomab of chemotherapy-refractory

minimal residual disease in B-lineage acute lymphoblastic leukemia patients results in high response rate and prolonged leukemia-free survival. *J Clin Oncol.* 2011;29(18):2493–2498.

18 Topp MS, Gokbuget N, Zugmaier G, et al. Long-term follow-up of hematologic relapse-free survival in a phase 2 study of blinatumomab in patients with MRD in B-lineage ALL. *Blood.* 2012;120(26): 5185–5187.

19 Topp M, Goekbuget N, Zugmaier G, et al. Effect of anti-CD19 BiTE blinatumomab on complete remission rate and overall survival in adult patients with relapsed/refractory B-precursor ALL. *American Society of Clinical Oncology Annual Meeting Abstracts.* 2012;30:6500a.

20 Younes A, Kim S, Romaguera J, et al. Phase I multidose-escalation study of the anti-CD19 maytansinoid immunoconjugate SAR3419 administered by intravenous infusion every 3 weeks to patients with relapsed/refractory B-cell lymphoma. *J Clin Oncol.* 2012;30(22):2776–2782.

21 Ribrag V, Dupuis J, Tilly H, et al. A dose-escalation study of SAR3419, an anti-CD19 antibody maytansinoid conjugate, administered by intravenous infusion once weekly in patients with relapsed/refractory B-cell non-Hodgkin lymphoma. *Clin Cancer Res.* 2014;20(1):213–220.

22 Kantarjian H, Thomas D, Jorgensen J, et al. Inotuzumab ozogamicin, an anti-CD22-calecheamicin conjugate, for refractory and relapsed acute lymphocytic leukaemia: a phase 2 study. *Lancet Oncol.* 2012;13(4):403–411.

23 O'Brien S, Thomas DA, Jorgensen JL, et al. Experience with 2 dose schedules of inotuzumab ozogamicin, single Dose, and weekly, in refractory-relapsed acute lymphocytic leukemia (ALL). *Blood (ASH Annual Meeting Abstracts).* 2012;120:671a.

24 Jain N, O'Brien S, Thomas DA, et al. Inotuzumab ozogamicin in combination with low-intensity chemotherapy (mini-hyper-CVD) as frontline therapy for older patients (≥60 years) with acute lymphoblastic leukemia (ALL). *Blood.* 2013;122(21):1432.

25 DiJoseph JF, Dougher MM, Kalyandrug LB, et al. Antitumor efficacy of a combination of CMC-544 (inotuzumab ozogamicin), a CD22-targeted cytotoxic immunoconjugate of calicheamicin, and rituximab against non-Hodgkin's B-cell lymphoma. *Clin Cancer Res.* 2006;12(1):242–249.

26 Fayad L, Offner F, Smith MR, et al. Safety and clinical activity of a combination therapy comprising two antibody-based targeting agents for the treatment of non-Hodgkin lymphoma: results of a phase I/II study evaluating the immunoconjugate inotuzumab ozogamicin with rituximab. *J Clin Oncol.* 2013;31(5):573–583.

27 Raetz EA, Cairo MS, Borowitz MJ, et al; Children's Oncology Group Pilot Study. Chemoimmunotherapy reinduction with epratuzumab in children with acute lymphoblastic leukemia in marrow relapse: a Children's Oncology Group Pilot Study. *J Clin Oncol.* 2008;26(22):3756–3762.

28 Advani AS, McDonough S, Coutre S, et al. SWOG S0910: a phase 2 trial of clofarabine/cytarabine/epratuzumab for relapsed/refractory acute lymphocytic leukaemia. *Br J Haematol.* 2014;165(4):504–509.

29 Advani AS, Gundacker HM, Sala-Torra O, et al. Southwest Oncology Group Study S0530: a phase 2 trial of clofarabine and cytarabine for relapsed or refractory acute lymphocytic leukaemia. *Br J Haematol.* 2010;151(5):430–434.

30 Sharkey RM, Govindan SV, Cardillo TM, Goldenberg DM. Epratuzumab-SN-38: a new antibody–drug conjugate for the therapy of hematologic malignancies. *Mol Cancer Ther.* 2012;11(1):224–234.

31 Alderson RF, Kreitman RJ, Chen T, et al. CAT-8015: a second-generation pseudomonas exotoxin A-based immunotherapy targeting CD22-expressing hematologic malignancies. *Clin Cancer Res.* 2009;15(3):832–839.

32 Kreitman RJ, Tallman MS, Robak T, et al. Phase I trial of anti-CD22 recombinant immunotoxin moxetumomab pasudotox (CAT-8015 or HA22) in patients with hairy cell leukemia. *J Clin Oncol.* 2012;30(15):1822–1828.

33 Wayne AS, Bhojwani D, Silverman LB, et al. A novel anti-CD22 immunotoxin, moxetumomab pasudotox: phase I study in pediatric acute lymphoblastic leukemia (ALL). *ASH Annual Meeting Abstracts.* 2011;118(21):248.

34 Ginaldi L, De Martinis M, Matutes E, et al. Levels of expression of CD52 in normal and leukemic B and T cells: correlation with in vivo therapeutic responses to Campath-1 H. *Leuk Res.* 1998;22(2):185–191.

35 Stock W, Sanford B, Lozanski G, et al. Alemtuzumab can be incorporated into front-line therapy of adult acute lymphoblastic leukemia (ALL): final phase I results of a cancer and leukemia group B study (CALGB 10102). *Blood.* 2009(114):838a.

36 Angiolillo AL, Yu AL, Reaman G, Ingle AM, Secola R, Adamson PC. A phase II study of Campath-1 H in children with relapsed or refractory acute lymphoblastic leukemia: a Children's Oncology Group report. *Pediatr Blood Cancer.* 2009;53(6):978–983.

37 Tibes R, Keating MJ, Ferrajoli A, et al. Activity of alemtuzumab in patients with CD52-positive acute leukemia. *Cancer.* 2006;106(12):2645–2651.

38 Nijmeijer BA, van Schie ML, Halkes CJ, Griffioen M, Willemze R, Falkenburg JH. A mechanistic rationale for combining alemtuzumab and rituximab in the treatment of ALL. *Blood.* 2010;116(26):5930–5940.

39 Liu-Dumlao T, Kantarjian H, Thomas DA, O'Brien S, Ravandi F. Philadelphia-positive acute lymphoblastic leukemia: current treatment options. *Curr Oncol Rep.* 2012;14(5):387–394.

40 Dombret H, Gabert J, Boiron JM, et al.; Groupe d'Etude et de Traitement de la Leucémie Aiguë Lymphoblastique de l'Adulte (GET-LALA Group). Outcome of treatment in adults with Philadelphia chromosome-positive acute lymphoblastic leukemia–results of the prospective multicenter LALA-94 trial. *Blood.* 2002;100(7): 2357–2366.

41 Kantarjian HM, Cortes JE, O'Brien S, et al. Long-term survival benefit and improved complete cytogenetic and molecular response rates with imatinib mesylate in Philadelphia chromosome-positive chronic-phase chronic myeloid leukemia after failure of interferon-alpha. *Blood.* 2004;104(7):1979–1988.

42 Thomas DA, Faderl S, Cortes J, et al. Treatment of Philadelphia chromosome-positive acute lymphocytic leukemia with hyper-CVAD and imatinib mesylate. *Blood.* 2004;103(12):4396–4407.

43 Ravandi F, O'Brien S, Thomas D, et al. First report of phase 2 study of dasatinib with hyper-CVAD for the frontline treatment of patients with Philadelphia chromosome-positive (Ph+) acute lymphoblastic leukemia. *Blood.* 2010;116(12):2070–2077.

44 Ravandi F, O'Brien S, Garris R, et al. Final report of single-center study of chemotherapy plus dasatinib for the initial treatment of patients with Philadelphia chromosome-positive acute lymphoblastic leukemia. *Blood (ASH Annual Meeting Abstracts).* 2013;122:3914a.

45 Bassan R, Rossi G, Pogliani EM, et al. Chemotherapy-phased imatinib pulses improve long-term outcome of adult patients with Philadelphia chromosome-positive acute lymphoblastic leukemia: Northern Italy Leukemia Group protocol 09/00. *J Clin Oncol.* 2010;28(22):3644–3652.

46 Fielding AK, Rowe JM, Buck G, et al. UKALLXII/ECOG2993: addition of imatinib to a standard treatment regimen enhances long-term outcomes in Philadelphia positive acute lymphoblastic leukemia. *Blood.* 2014;123(6):843–850.

47 Foa R, Vitale A, Vignetti M, et al.; GIMEMA Acute Leukemia Working Party. Dasatinib as first-line treatment for adult patients

with Philadelphia chromosome-positive acute lymphoblastic leukemia. *Blood.* 2011;118(25):6521–6528.

48 Lilly MB, Ottmann OG, Shah NP, et al. Dasatinib 140 mg once daily versus 70 mg twice daily in patients with Ph-positive acute lymphoblastic leukemia who failed imatinib: results from a phase 3 study. *Am J Hematol.* 2010;85(3):164–170.

49 Kim DY, Joo YD, Kim S, et al. Nilotinib combined with multi-agent chemotherapy for adult patients with newly diagnosed Philadelphia chromosome-positive acute lymphoblastic leukemia: final results of prospective multicenter phase 2 study. *Blood (ASH Annual Meeting Abstracts).* 2013;122:55a.

50 Jabbour E, Kantarjian H, Thomas DA, et al. Phase II study of combination of hyper-CVAD with ponatinib in front line therapy of patients (pts) with Philadelphia chromosome (Ph) positive acute lymphoblastic leukemia (ALL). *Blood (ASH Annual Meeting Abstracts).* 2013;122:2663a.

51 Rousselot P, Coudé MM, Huguet F, et al. Dasatinib (Sprycel®) and low intensity chemotherapy for first-line treatment in patients with de novo Philadelphia positive ALL aged 55 and over: final results of the EWALL-Ph-01 study. *Blood (ASH Annual Meeting Abstracts).* 2012;120:666a.

52 Den Boer ML, van Slegtenhorst M, De Menezes RX, et al. A subtype of childhood acute lymphoblastic leukaemia with poor treatment outcome: a genome-wide classification study. *Lancet Oncol.* 2009;10(2):125–134.

53 Mullighan CG, Su X, Zhang J, et al.; Children's Oncology Group. Deletion of IKZF1 and prognosis in acute lymphoblastic leukemia. *N Engl J Med.* 2009;360(5):470–480.

54 Mullighan CG, Miller CB, Radtke I, et al. BCR-ABL1 lymphoblastic leukaemia is characterized by the deletion of Ikaros. *Nature.* 2008;453(7191):110–114.

55 Loh ML, Zhang J, Harvey RC, et al. Tyrosine kinome sequencing of pediatric acute lymphoblastic leukemia: a report from the Children's Oncology Group TARGET Project. *Blood.* 2013;121(3):485–488.

56 Roberts KG, Li Y, Payne-Turner D, et al. Genomic characterization and experimental modeling of BCR-ABL1-like acute lymphoblastic leukemia. *ASH Annual Meeting Abstracts.* 2013(825a).

57 Harvey RC, Mullighan CG, Chen IM, et al. Rearrangement of CRLF2 is associated with mutation of JAK kinases, alteration of IKZF1, Hispanic/Latino ethnicity, and a poor outcome in pediatric B-progenitor acute lymphoblastic leukemia. *Blood.* 2010;115(26):5312–5321.

58 Harvey RC, Mullighan CG, Wang X, et al. Identification of novel cluster groups in pediatric high-risk B-precursor acute lymphoblastic leukemia with gene expression profiling: correlation with genome-wide DNA copy number alterations, clinical characteristics, and outcome. *Blood.* 2010;116(23):4874–4884.

59 Cario G, Zimmermann M, Romey R, et al. Presence of the P2RY8-CRLF2 rearrangement is associated with a poor prognosis in non-high-risk precursor B-cell acute lymphoblastic leukemia in children treated according to the ALL-BFM 2000 protocol. *Blood.* 2010;115(26):5393–5397.

60 Mullighan CG, Collins-Underwood JR, Phillips LA, et al. Rearrangement of CRLF2 in B-progenitor- and Down syndrome-associated acute lymphoblastic leukemia. *Nat Genet.* 2009;41(11):1243–1246.

61 Russell LJ, Capasso M, Vater I, et al. Deregulated expression of cytokine receptor gene, CRLF2, is involved in lymphoid transformation in B-cell precursor acute lymphoblastic leukemia. *Blood.* 2009;114(13):2688–2698.

62 Roberts KG, Morin RD, Zhang J, et al. Genetic alterations activating kinase and cytokine receptor signaling in high-risk acute lymphoblastic leukemia. *Cancer Cell.* 2012;22(2):153–166.

63 Hertzberg L, Vendramini E, Ganmore I, et al. Down syndrome acute lymphoblastic leukemia, a highly heterogeneous disease in which aberrant expression of CRLF2 is associated with mutated JAK2: a report from the International BFM Study Group. *Blood.* 2010;115(5):1006–1017.

64 Yoda A, Yoda Y, Chiaretti S, et al. Functional screening identifies CRLF2 in precursor B-cell acute lymphoblastic leukemia. *Proceedings of the National Academy of Sciences of the United States of America.* 2010;107(1):252–257.

65 Liu YJ, Soumelis V, Watanabe N, et al. TSLP: an epithelial cell cytokine that regulates T cell differentiation by conditioning dendritic cell maturation. *Annu Rev Immunol.* 2007;25:193–219.

66 Ziegler SF, Liu YJ. Thymic stromal lymphopoietin in normal and pathogenic T cell development and function. *Nat Immunol.* 2006;7(7):709–714.

67 Isaksen DE, Baumann H, Trobridge PA, Farr AG, Levin SD, Ziegler SF. Requirement for stat5 in thymic stromal lymphopoietin-mediated signal transduction. *J Immunol.* 1999;163(11):5971–5977.

68 Rochman Y, Kashyap M, Robinson GW, et al. Thymic stromal lymphopoietin-mediated STAT5 phosphorylation via kinases JAK1 and JAK2 reveals a key difference from IL-7-induced signaling. *Proceedings of the National Academy of Sciences of the United States of America.* 2010;107(45):19455–19460.

69 Mullighan CG, Goorha S, Radtke I, et al. Genome-wide analysis of genetic alterations in acute lymphoblastic leukaemia. *Nature.* 2007;446(7137):758–764.

70 Malinge S, Ben-Abdelali R, Settegrana C, et al. Novel activating JAK2 mutation in a patient with Down syndrome and B-cell precursor acute lymphoblastic leukaemia. *Blood.* 2007;109(5):2202–2204.

71 Bercovich D, Ganmore I, Scott LM, et al. Mutations of JAK2 in acute lymphoblastic leukaemias associated with Down's syndrome. *Lancet.* 2008;372(9648):1484–1492.

72 Gaikwad A, Rye CL, Devidas M, et al. Prevalence and clinical correlates of JAK2 mutations in Down syndrome acute lymphoblastic leukaemia. *Br J Haematol.* 2009;144(6):930–932.

73 Kearney L, Gonzalez De Castro D, Yeung J, et al. Specific JAK2 mutation (JAK2R683) and multiple gene deletions in Down syndrome acute lymphoblastic leukaemia. *Blood.* 2009;113(3):646–648.

74 Mullighan CG, Zhang J, Harvey RC, et al. JAK mutations in high-risk childhood acute lymphoblastic leukaemia. *Proceedings of the National Academy of Sciences of the United States of America.* 2009;106(23):9414–9418.

75 Chen IM, Harvey RC, Mullighan CG, et al. Outcome modeling with CRLF2, IKZF1, JAK, and minimal residual disease in pediatric acute lymphoblastic leukemia: a Children's Oncology Group study. *Blood.* 2012;119(15):3512–3522.

76 Moorman AV, Schwab C, Ensor HM, et al. IGH@ translocations, CRLF2 deregulation, and microdeletions in adolescents and adults with acute lymphoblastic leukemia. *J Clin Oncol.* 2012;30(25):3100–3108.

77 Puel A, Ziegler SF, Buckley RH, Leonard WJ. Defective IL7R expression in T(-)B(+)NK(+) severe combined immunodeficiency. *Nat Genet.* 1998;20(4):394–397.

78 Shochat C, Tal N, Bandapalli OR, et al. Gain-of-function mutations in interleukin-7 receptor-alpha (IL7R) in childhood acute lymphoblastic leukemias. *J Exp Med.* 2011;208(5):901–908.

79 Maude SL, Tasian SK, Vincent T, et al. Targeting JAK1/2 and mTOR in murine xenograft models of Ph-like acute lymphoblastic leukemia. *Blood.* 2012;120(17):3510–3518.

80 Bersenev A, Wu C, Balcerek J, et al. Lnk constrains myeloproliferative diseases in mice. *J Clin Invest.* 2010;120(6):2058–2069.

81 Tal N, Shochat C, Geron I, Bercovich D, Izraeli S. Interleukin 7 and thymic stromal lymphopoietin: from immunity to leukemia. *Cell Mol Life Sci.* 2014;71(3):365–378.

82 Lengline E, Beldjord K, Dombret H, Soulier J, Boissel N, Clappier E. Successful tyrosine kinase inhibitor therapy in a refractory B-cell precursor acute lymphoblastic leukemia with EBF1-PDGFRB fusion. *Haematologica.* 2013;98(11):e146–e148.

83 Weston BW, Hayden MA, Roberts KG, et al. Tyrosine kinase inhibitor therapy induces remission in a patient with refractory EBF1-PDGFRB-positive acute lymphoblastic leukemia. *J Clin Oncol.* 2013;31(25):e413–e416.

84 De Braekeleer E, Douet-Guilbert N, Rowe D, et al. ABL1 fusion genes in hematological malignancies: a review. *Eur J Haematol.* 2011;86(5):361–371.

85 Mustjoki S, Hernesniemi S, Rauhala A, et al. A novel dasatinib-sensitive RCSD1-ABL1 fusion transcript in chemotherapy-refractory adult pre-B lymphoblastic leukemia with t(1;9)(q24;q34). *Haematologica.* 2009;94(10):1469–1471.

86 Inokuchi K, Wakita S, Hirakawa T, et al. RCSD1-ABL1-positive B lymphoblastic leukemia is sensitive to dexamethasone and tyrosine kinase inhibitors and rapidly evolves clonally by chromosomal translocations. *Int J Hematol.* 2011;94(3):255–260.

87 Neri LM, Cani A, Martelli AM, et al. Targeting the PI3K/Akt/mTOR signaling pathway in B-precursor acute lymphoblastic leukemia and its therapeutic potential. *Leukemia.* 2014;28(4):739–748.

88 Daver N, Kantarjian HM, Thomas DA, et al. A phase I/II study of hyper-CVAD plus everolimus in patients with relapsed/refractory acute lymphoblastic leukemia. *Blood.* 2013;122(21):3916.

89 Kim E, Koehrer S, Rosin NY, et al. Bruton's tyrosine kinase inhibitor ibrutinib interferes with constitutive and induced pre-B cell receptor signaling in B-cell acute lymphoblastic leukemia. *Blood.* 2013;122(21):1399.

90 Davila ML, Riviere I, Wang X, et al. Efficacy and toxicity management of 19–28z CAR T cell therapy in B cell acute lymphoblastic leukemia. *Sci Transl Med.* 2014;6(224):224ra225.

91 Brentjens RJ, Davila ML, Riviere I, et al. CD19-targeted T cells rapidly induce molecular remissions in adults with chemotherapy-refractory acute lymphoblastic leukemia. *Sci Transl Med.* 2013;5(177):177ra138.

92 Grupp SA, Kalos M, Barrett D, et al. Chimeric antigen receptor-modified T cells for acute lymphoid leukemia. *N Engl J Med.* 2013;368(16):1509–1518.

93 Radtke F, Wilson A, Stark G, et al. Deficient T cell fate specification in mice with an induced inactivation of Notch1. *Immunity.* 1999;10(5):547–558.

94 Radtke F, Fasnacht N, Macdonald HR. Notch signaling in the immune system. *Immunity.* 2010;32(1):14–27.

95 Ellisen LW, Bird J, West DC, et al. TAN-1, the human homolog of the Drosophila notch gene, is broken by chromosomal translocations in T lymphoblastic neoplasms. *Cell.* 1991;66(4):649–661.

96 Weng AP, Ferrando AA, Lee W, et al. Activating mutations of NOTCH1 in human T cell acute lymphoblastic leukemia. *Science.* 2004;306(5694):269–271.

97 Asnafi V, Buzyn A, Le Noir S, et al. NOTCH1/FBXW7 mutation identifies a large subgroup with favorable outcome in adult T-cell acute lymphoblastic leukemia (T-ALL): a Group for Research on Adult Acute Lymphoblastic Leukemia (GRAALL) study. *Blood.* 2009;113(17):3918–3924.

98 Deangelo DJ, Stone RM, Silverman LB, et al. A phase I clinical trial of the notch inhibitor MK-0752 in patients with T-cell acute lymphoblastic leukemia/lymphoma (T-ALL) and other leukemias *American Society of Clinical Oncology Annual Meeting Abstracts.* 2006;24(18S):6585.

99 van Es JH, van Gijn ME, Riccio O, et al. Notch/gamma-secretase inhibition turns proliferative cells in intestinal crypts and adenomas into goblet cells. *Nature.* 2005;435(7044):959–963.

100 Wu Y, Cain-Hom C, Choy L, et al. Therapeutic antibody targeting of individual Notch receptors. *Nature.* 2010;464(7291):1052–1057.

101 Moellering RE, Cornejo M, Davis TN, et al. Direct inhibition of the NOTCH transcription factor complex. *Nature.* 2009;462(7270):182–188.

102 Groth C, Fortini ME. Therapeutic approaches to modulating Notch signaling: current challenges and future prospects. *Semin Cell Dev Biol.* 2012;23(4):465–472.

103 Coustan-Smith E, Mullighan CG, Onciu M, et al. Early T-cell precursor leukaemia: a subtype of very high-risk acute lymphoblastic leukaemia. *Lancet Oncol.* 2009;10(2):147–156.

104 Neumann M, Heesch S, Schlee C, et al. Whole-exome sequencing in adult ETP-ALL reveals a high rate of DNMT3A mutations. *Blood.* 2013;121(23):4749–4752.

105 Zhang J, Ding L, Holmfeldt L, et al. The genetic basis of early T-cell precursor acute lymphoblastic leukaemia. *Nature.* 2012;481(7380):157–163.

106 Neumann M, Coskun E, Fransecky L, et al. FLT3 mutations in early T-cell precursor ALL characterize a stem cell like leukemia and imply the clinical use of tyrosine kinase inhibitors. *PloS one.* 2013;8(1):e53190.

107 Neumann M, Heesch S, Gokbuget N, et al. Clinical and molecular characterization of early T-cell precursor leukemia: a high-risk subgroup in adult T-ALL with a high frequency of FLT3 mutations. *Blood Cancer J.* 2012;2(1):e55.

# CHAPTER 13

# Chronic Lymphocytic Leukemia

*Preetesh Jain and Susan O'Brien*
Department of Leukemia, The University of Texas MD Anderson Cancer Center, Houston, TX, USA

## Background

Advances in the understanding of the pathogenic pathways and biology of cancer cells ushered in the era of targeted anticancer therapies. Newer bioengineering and x-ray crystallographic techniques have helped in the development of targeted therapeutic agents. Since 1997, discovery of targeted agents such as the anti-CD20 mAb rituximab for lymphoid malignancies[1] and the BCR-ABL tyrosine kinase inhibitor (TKI) imatinib for chronic myeloid leukemia (CML)[2] have improved patient outcomes and changed the natural history of leukemias. In the context of chronic lymphocytic leukemia (CLL), commonly used targeted therapies include a combination of anti-CD20 mAbs with chemotherapy (chemoimmunotherapy (CIT))[3,4] and the recently approved Bruton's tyrosine kinase (BTK) inhibitor ibrutinib for relapsed patients.[5]

CLL is a disease of monoclonal B cells with a specific immunophenotype (CD5, CD19, and CD23 are strongly expressed while surface immunoglobulins (sIgs) CD22, CD79b, and FMC-7 are diminished or absent; kappa or lambda light chain restriction is present).[6] CLL predominantly affects the older population with a median age at diagnosis of 72 years.[7] Patients with CLL have a heterogeneous disease course. Clinical, immunophenotypic, cytogenetic, and molecular characteristics help in assessing the prognosis of patients with CLL. Recognition of the critical role played by the B-cell-receptor signaling (BCR) signaling pathway in the growth of CLL cells has propelled the development of novel agents targeting important kinases in this pathway including[8,9] BTK,[10–15] phosphatidylinositol 3-kinase (PI3K),[16–20] and spleen tyrosine kinase (SYK).[21–25] In addition to the BCR signaling pathway, other mechanisms of promoting CLL cell growth, survival, and chemotaxis include the overexpression of the antiapoptotic BCL-2 protein and microenvironmental factors such as chemokine–chemokine receptor interactions (CXCR4–CXCL12).[26]

## Biologic and Molecular Aspects of CLL

In addition to clinical staging of CLL, several factors can aid in predicting the prognosis of patients with CLL.[27] These factors included cytogenetic risk categories using fluorescent *in situ* hybridization (FISH) analysis,[28] mutation status of the immunoglobulin heavy chain variable (IGHV) region,[29,30] variable heavy chain (VH) gene usage patterns,[31] stereotypy of BCR,[32,33] expression of CD38[29] and Zap-70,[34] and serum levels of β2 microglobulin.[35]

In addition, whole exome sequencing of CLL cells has revealed that CLL cells exhibit recurrent gene mutations, for example, *TP53*, *NOTCH1*, *SF3B1*, *XPO-1*, and *BIRC3*.[36–42] A detailed discussion on various other prognostic factors is beyond the scope of this chapter and is reviewed elsewhere.[43] Here, we will present those biologic aspects of CLL cells, which have translated into targeted therapeutics.

## Mechanism of Action of mAbs Directed Against Surface Epitopes on CLL Cells

Antigens expressed on the CLL cell surface are potential targets for therapy. Some of these antigens include CD20, CD52, CD37, CD40, PD1, and CD200. Cytotoxicity by monoclonal antibodies (mAbs) can be mediated by different mechanisms:

**Complement-dependent cytotoxicity (CDC).**[44] Initiated by the activation of the complement cascade (C1q), development of the membrane attack complex (MAC) by antigen–antibody interaction, and ultimate lysis of the cells.[45]

**Antibody-dependent cellular cytotoxicity (ADCC).** Mediated by the attachment of mAb-coated cells to the effector immune cells (NK cells and macrophages) which causes cell lysis by release of the cytotoxic proteins, granzyme B, and perforin.[46]

**Direct cell death.** Mediated by the mobilization of cross-linked antibodies into the transmembrane protein and interaction with Src kinases which lead to direct cell death.[47–49]

**Adaptive immune response/vaccine effect.** Cross-presentation of CD20 to T cells (CD4 and CD8) and promotion of tumor uptake by dendritic cells create a passive and long-lasting antitumor cellular immune response.[50]

Anti-CD20 mAbs are the most commonly used mAbs in the treatment of CLL. Two types of CD20 mAbs have been described: type I and type II.[51,52] Table 13.1 shows the differences between type I and type II mAbs.[47,53–55]

**CD20 antigen.** CD20 antigen is a surface membrane protein expressed on normal B cells and in >90% of B-cell malignancies. CD20 antigen expression is dim on CLL B cells as compared to other B-cell malignancies and normal B cells.[56]

**CD52 antigen.** This is a glycosylated-membrane-bound glycoprotein strongly expressed on B and T lymphocytes, monocytes, eosinophil, macrophages, and dendritic cells and absent on granulocytes, platelets, red blood cells, and plasma cells.[56,57]

*Targeted Therapy in Translational Cancer Research*, First Edition. Edited by Apostolia-Maria Tsimberidou, Razelle Kurzrock and Kenneth C. Anderson.
© 2016 John Wiley & Sons, Inc. Published 2016 by John Wiley & Sons, Inc.

**Table 13.1** Difference among type I and type II mAbs.

| | Type I mAbs | Type II mAbs |
|---|---|---|
| Lipid rafts | Stabilize CD20 on lipid rafts and activate complement | No induction of CD20 into lipid rafts |
| Complement-dependent cytotoxicity (CDC) | High CDC | Less CDC |
| Antibody-dependent cellular cytotoxicity (ADCC) | Lesser | Greater |
| Cell–cell contact-lysosome-mediated direct cell death | Need cross-linking by antibody to cause apoptosis | Predominant mode of action |
| Depletion of B cells | Less potent | More potent |
| Examples | Rituximab, ofatumumab, veltuzumab, ocrelizumab, ocaratuzumab, and PRO-131921 | Obinutuzumab (GA-101) |

Other antigens which are under investigation for targeted therapies in CLL include:

**CD37 antigen.** This is a transmembrane protein expressed mainly on B cells (pre-B to mature B cells) and dimly on T cells, NK cells, and monocytes.[58]

**CD40 antigen.** This transmembrane protein is expressed on immature and mature B cells and is highly expressed on CLL cells.[59] CD40 belongs to the TNF receptor family protein. Binding of CD40 with CD40 ligand (CD40L) activates PI3K and the NFkB pathway in B cells and prevents the apoptosis of CLL cells.[60,61]

**PD-1/PD-L1 (programmed death-1 antigen and ligand)[62] and CD200 antigen.**[63] These proteins are expressed on CLL cells and T cells and induce suppression of antitumor immunity mediated by T cells by upregulation of regulatory T cells and suppressing the production of IFN-γ by CD8+ T cells.

## BCR Pathway in CLL

The relevance of chronic active BCR signaling for the growth of malignant B cells was initially reported for diffuse large B-cell lymphoma (DLBCL).[15] The presence of an active BCR signaling complex is vital for the growth and survival of CLL cells.[8] Figure 13.1 depicts the BCR signaling pathway kinases in CLL cells.

BCR is a transmembrane receptor complex consisting of an extracellular portion—sIg receptor comprising two heavy and two light chains which bind to the antigen (Ag) and a cytoplasmic portion comprised of a heterodimer of CD79a and CD79b (Ig alpha and beta, respectively). The sIg commonly belongs to the sIgM isotype, which has a strong stimulatory effect on CLL B cells as compared to other isotypes such as IgD, IgG, or IgE.[64] Stimulation of the BCR triggers a downstream signaling cascade through various kinases, which in turn activate NFkB and finally, CLL cell growth and proliferation.

Various combinations of variable (V), diversity (D), and joining (J) gene segments provide heterogeneity in the structure of the BCR. However, in CLL >20% cases exhibit identical sIg heavy and light chains (stereotypy)[65] which indicate the presence of a common antigen identified by CLL B cells.[33,66,67] Candidate antigens which can bind to CLL-derived antibodies include fungal antigen β-1-6-glucan,[68] oxidized low density lipoproteins (LDL),[69] viruses,[70] and exposed nonmuscle myosin heavy chain IIA (MYHIIA) from apoptotic cells.[71] Recently, two reports have shown that CLL cells can demonstrate autonomous BCR signaling via an interaction between an internal epitope on the framework region (FR2) of the VH gene segment with Ag-binding sites in a selected HCDR3 (complementarity determining region-3) sequence[72] and with the FR3 region as a self-recognition site of CLL BCR.[73] An alteration in the structural components of the sIg reliably predicts the clinical course of the disease. Somatic mutation status of the heavy chain of sIg segregates patients with CLL into mutated versus unmutated subgroups, which exhibit different clinical courses.[29] Furthermore, BCR signaling associated genes such as SYK and NFkB are overexpressed in the lymph node, considered as the site of CLL cell proliferation.[74]

**BCR signal propagation.** Cross-linking of BCR after engagement with an antigen leads to phosphorylation of ITAMs (immunoreceptor tyrosine-based activation motifs) on the CD79 heterodimer by SRC family kinases (LYN, FYN, and BLK). This in turn sequentially phosphorylates SYK via a docking protein 1 (DOK1) and SH2 domain containing inositol-5-phosphatase (SHIP1). Phosphorylated LYN also activates hematopoietic cell-specific LYN substrate-1 (HS1)[75] and cytoskeletal activators such as VAV1 which promote cytoskeletal organization, hematopoiesis, and BCR signaling.[8]

**SYK–BTK activation** (Figure 13.1). SYK is a nonreceptor tyrosine kinase[76] which shares a SH2 domain with Zap-70. Overexpression of Zap-70 in CLL cells is associated with enhanced BCR signaling and strongly correlates with unmutated IGHV status and a more aggressive clinical course.[34] Activation of SYK leads to recruitment of CIN-85 (cbl-interacting protein) and phosphorylation of an adaptor molecule B-cell linker protein (BLNK) otherwise known as SH2 domain containing leukocyte protein of 65 kDa (SLP65)[77]; this mini complex triggers intermediate enzymes—Bruton's tyrosine kinase (BTK) and phospholipase Cγ2 (PLCγ2).[78]

Activation of BTK requires the binding of BTK-PH domain (pleckstrin homology domain) to PIP3; subsequently BTK translocates to the cell membrane and is phosphorylated at tyrosine 551 in the BTK kinase domain and autophosphorylates at tyrosine 223 in the SH3 domain by LYN or SYK kinases. Activated BTK then phosphorylates PLCγ2 and promotes its lipase activity (PIP2 to IP3 and diacylglycerol (DAG)).[79] BTK belongs to a group of tyrosine kinase expressed in hepatocellular cancer (TEC) family of nonreceptor kinases present in the cytoplasm. Other members of the TEC family include TEC, bone marrow expressed kinase (BMX), IL-2 inducible T-cell kinase (ITK), and resting lymphocyte kinase (RLK). BTK inhibition by small interfering RNA (siRNA) promoted apoptosis of primary human CLL cells and delayed the development of CLL in a TCL-1 mouse model.[12] BTK can influence the biology of the CLL cells in different ways. BTK is involved in CLL cell homing and migration via CXCR4/CXCR5 receptors,[80,81] actin cytoskeleton organization, response to differentiation stimuli, cell adhesion, cytokine production, and promotion of toll-like receptor (TLR) signaling,[82] especially TLR9 activation, which promotes autoantibody production. BTK mutations and their implications in CLL will be discussed later in the chapter.

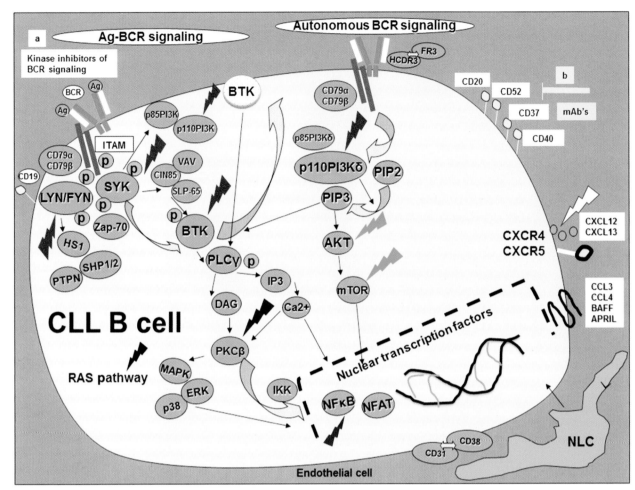

**Figure 13.1** B-cell receptor (BCR) signaling pathways and therapeutic targets in CLL B cell (shown with a lightning bolt symbol). BCR signaling pathways and therapeutic targets: BCR signaling in CLL can occur in the presence of an external antigen (Ag) or by recognizing an internal epitope on light chain FR3 with HCDR3 region on heavy chain of the surface immunoglobulin (sIg). Autonomous stimulation activates the phosphatidylinositol 3-kinase (PI3K) pathway directly while antigen-dependent signaling stimulates other signaling molecules as shown in the figure (see the main text for details). Chemokines, chemokine receptors, endothelial cells, and interactions of nurse-like cells (NLC) are shown. (a) Kinase inhibitors of BCR signaling. The lightning bolt symbol (pink) indicates major kinases LYN, SYK, BTK, p110PI3Kδ, and p110PI3K, and other isoforms (γ, α, β) as therapeutic targets across the BCR signaling pathway. Signaling cascade and specific inhibitors of each class are discussed in the main text. (b) Monoclonal antibodies (mAbs) (in yellow)—common surface epitopes used for developing therapeutic mAbs include CD20, CD52, CD37, and CD40. Other targets of potential relevance include inhibitors of mTOR/AKT pathway depicted in bolt (green), inhibitors of CXCR4 receptors depicted in bolt (white), inhibitors of RAS/MAP kinase pathway depicted in bolt (black), inhibitors of protein kinase C beta (PKCβ), and NFkB depicted in bolt (blue and brown, respectively).

**Downstream signaling PLCγ2 and PI3K.** After the activation of BTK and PLCγ2,[83] PLCγ2 cleaves PIP2 to IP3 (inositol triphosphate) and DAG which act as second messengers and mobilize intracellular calcium levels and trigger downstream RAS-RAF kinase, mitogen-activated protein (MAP) kinase, and protein kinase C beta (PKCβ) which in turn activate the nuclear transcription factor NFkB.[84] PIP3 accrues cytoplasmic kinases such as BTK, AKT, and PLCγ and forms a mini functional BCR signaling complex closer to the cell membrane.[85] An activated PI3Kδ also phosphorylates AKT. AKT can cause inhibition of GSK3 (glycogen synthase kinase 3), which degrades MCL1 (major antiapoptotic protein in CLL cells).[86] *PI3K* class IA isoforms are critical in CLL. The p85 regulatory subunit of PI3K activates the p110 catalytic subunit after association with phosphotyrosine motifs. The p110 delta isoform is expressed in leukocytes; it is the only p110 isoform with a lipid-binding domain and can promote cancerous transformation.[18] Both p110 alpha and delta isoforms are required for B-cell growth. Mutations or decreased expression of phosphatase and tensin homologue (PTEN) can cause sustained activation of the PI3K-AKT pathway and enhance B-cell growth.[87] In addition, activation of PI3K by other factors such as BAFF, CD40, and TLR can influence CLL cell proliferation, migration, and calcium mobilization.[19,88,89]

Activation of BCR can also occur in the absence of an antigen (Ag), known as tonic BCR signaling,[90] which is independent of LYN-SYK phosphorylation and is mediated via the PI3K pathway. Downstream binding of a Ras GTPase protein TC21 to nonphosphorylated CD79 heterodimer can activate PI3K.[91]

**Positive and negative regulation of BCR.** LYN kinases can upregulate PI3K directly by phosphorylation of tyrosine residues in the cytoplasmic tail of the CD19 molecule and can also downregulate BCR signaling via phosphorylation of inhibitory motifs on CD22, CD5, and FcγRIIB (low-affinity Fc receptor for IgG).[92,93]

**Table 13.2** Summary of kinases with therapeutic relevance in CLL.

| | *LYN* | *SYK* | *BTK* | *p110 PI3Kδ* |
|---|---|---|---|---|
| Type of kinase | SRC family TK | Nonreceptor TK close to Zap-70 | TEC family TK | Lipid kinase, catalytic subunit |
| Expression | Hematopoietic cells, neural, liver, and adipose tissue | Hematopoietic cells and other tissues | B cells and other hematopoietic cells except T cells | Leukocytes |
| Substrate | CD79a,Cd79b, SYK, CD22, phosphatases | CIN-85, SLP-65, or BLNK, BTK, PLCγ2, VAV1 | PLCγ2, PKCβ | PIP2 |
| Major pathways involved | BCR, CD40, CD19, FcγRIIB | BCR, BTK, PLCγ2 | BCR, NFkB, PI3K, CXCR4-CXCL12 axis | BCR, TLR, BAFF receptor, TNF receptor, CD40 |
| Functions | BCR signaling, positive and negative regulation, cytoskeletal organization with HS-1 | BCR signaling, chemokine, integrin signaling, TLR,C-type lectin signaling | BCR signaling, calcium release, NFkB activation, chemokine, integrin signaling | BCR signaling, homing, migration, and cell proliferation |
| Inhibitors | Bafetinib, dasatinib, bosutinib | Fostamatinib, GS-9973, PRT062607 | Ibrutinib, CC-292, ONO-4059, dasatinib, CG-1746 | Idelalisib, GS-9820, duvelisib (IPI-145; also blocks PI3Kγ) |

In addition, internalization of BCR and defective tyrosine phosphatase activity (SHP1, SHP2) can also abrogate BCR signaling.

The BCR signaling pathway is not an absolutely linear pathway. BTK, PI3K, LYN, and SYK kinases also participate in mediating chemokine–chemokine receptor interaction, integrin signaling, cell adhesion, and actin cytoskeleton activity (LYN-HS1 axis). Table 13.2 summarizes the major kinases in BCR signaling.[94] These signals are also affected by different microenvironmental factors in CLL and are more complex than was previously understood.

## Other Potential Therapeutic Targets in CLL

In addition to the BCR signaling pathway, CLL cells survive and grow under the influence of microenvironmental factors[95] and intrinsic defects in apoptosis.[96] Intervention in these pathologic mechanisms provides an opportunity to develop new, targeted therapeutics in CLL.

**Apoptotic pathway.** CLL cells exhibit defective apoptosis. An imbalance between proapoptotic proteins such as BH3-only proteins—BAX, BAK, BAD, BIM, NOXA, and PUMA, and anti-apoptotic proteins such as BCL-2, BCL-xL, and MCL1, aids in survival, drug resistance, and disease progression in CLL. Various factors promote antiapoptotic proteins in CLL cells—overexpression of BCL-2 proteins in CLL is attributed to the downregulation of microRNA15 and 16,[97] CD40L can increase MCL1 protein in the CLL lymph nodes and suppress proapoptotic proteins,[98] PI3K signaling can promote the levels of MCL1 by phosphorylation of AKT.[16] On the other hand, potentiation of death receptor ligand, TNF-related apoptosis inducing ligand (TRAIL), or inhibition of X-linked inhibitor of apoptosis (XIAP) by small molecules can induce apoptosis in CLL cells. Therefore, inhibition of antiapoptotic proteins (BCL-2, MCL1)[99] is considered a promising strategy to kill CLL cells.

**Chemokine–chemokine receptor interaction in CLL microenvironment.** CLL cells express chemokine and cytokine receptors and are surrounded by a network of monocyte-derived feeder cells, T cells, adhesion molecules, cytokines, and chemokines in their microenvironment. This intricate meshwork is responsible for the growth, maintenance, and drug resistance of CLL cells in various tissue compartments (peripheral blood, bone marrow, lymph nodes, and spleen). In addition, CLL cells also secrete chemokines such as CCL3 and CCL4, which protect CLL cells by promoting the adhesion molecules and growth of nurse-like cells (NLCs).[100] Chemokines and their receptors provide signals for CLL cell migration and trafficking to and from the tissues and peripheral blood. The chemokine CXCL12 is secreted by stromal cells and its receptor CXCR4 (CD184) is expressed on CLL cells. Activation of the CXCL12-CXCR4 axis can upregulate CLL cell growth by promoting adhesion to endothelial cells through actin polymerization, chemotaxis, and tissue homing. Intervention in any of these networks can significantly influence CLL cell growth.[101] Agents that inhibit CXCR4 receptors promote the egress of CLL cells from the protective tissue microenvironment into peripheral blood and also block the interaction of CLL cells with feeder NLCs.[102]

**Altered cell cycle in CLL.** Cell cycle in cancer cells is regulated by the presence of cyclin-dependent kinases (CDK). Some CDKs such as CDK 7, 8, and 9 can also regulate transcription and promote the levels of antiapoptotic proteins in cells. Inhibition of CDK is a potential therapeutic approach in patients with CLL.[103]

## Targeted Therapeutic Agents in the Treatment of CLL

### Results with Novel mAbs

Addition of the anti-CD20 mAb rituximab to FC (fludarabine and cyclophosphamide) (FCR chemoimmunotherapy) has significantly improved patient outcomes compared to chemotherapy (FC) alone.[3] Rituximab is a chimeric (mouse/human) anti-CD20 mAb. Administration of rituximab is associated with infusion-related toxicities and allergic reactions in some patients. Novel humanized anti-CD20 mAbs include ofatumumab and obinutuzumab (GA-101).[104–107] Results with rituximab are discussed in detail elsewhere.[108]

Ofatumumab is a fully human (IgG1κ) type I CD20 mAb, approved by the Food and Drug Administration (FDA) for the treatment of patients with CLL refractory to both fludarabine and alemtuzumab (FA-ref). Ofatumumab has features that may enhance its clinical efficacy, over rituximab. Ofatumumab binds to a distinct epitope on CD20 composed of amino acid residues 163–166 in the extracellular loop of CD20, closer to the cell membrane.[109] Binding to this site is thought to enhance lipid raft formation, which in turn could potentiate higher C1q activation and result in greater CDC. Laboratory studies have also demonstrated that ofatumumab is more potent than rituximab in mediating CDC, even in B cells that have dim CD20 expression (similar to CLL cells).[110,111] Ofatumumab has potent lytic activity against rituximab-resistant and -sensitive cell lines, lymphoma xenografts, and primary tumor cells from patients with B-cell NHL.[112,113]

### Results with Ofatumumab in CLL

**Pivotal 406 study.** This trial assessed the safety and efficacy of ofatumumab in patients with bulky (>5 cm lymph nodes) fludarabine refractory (bulky, fludarabine refractory (BFR); $n = 111$) or double-refractory (FA; $n = 95$) disease. Interim data were published[106] and final results were reported in 2010.[114] Ofatumumab was administered weekly via IV infusion for 8 weeks (dose 1, 300 mg; doses 2–8, 2000 mg), and then monthly until month 12 (2000 mg). Overall, 55% of patients in the BFR group and 59% of patients in the FA-refractory group were previously exposed to rituximab. The overall response rates (ORR) were 44% and 51%, respectively. Responses were partial and only one CR was noted in the BFR group. The median progression-free survival (PFS) was 5.5 months in both groups. The overall survival (OS) was 17.4 months in the BFR and 14.2 months in the FA-refractory group. Infusion reactions occurred in 63% of patients and most were grade 1–2. Ofatumumab was well tolerated and no unexpected toxicities or formation of human anti-human antibodies (HAHA) was noted.[115] Ofatumumab received FDA approval for use as a single agent in patients with FA-refractory CLL.

An *ad hoc* analysis of this study[116] evaluated the effect of prior rituximab. Rituximab-treated ($n = 117$; of whom 98 were rituximab-refractory) and rituximab-naïve ($n = 89$) patients were evaluated. The ORRs for rituximab-treated, rituximab-refractory, and rituximab-naïve patients were 43%, 44%, and 53%, respectively. The respective median PFS durations were 5.3, 5.5, and 5.6 months, and the median OS durations were 15.5, 15.5, and 20.2 months. A longer time period from the last rituximab regimen to initiation of ofatumumab was associated with longer median OS ($p = 0.024$). Toxicities were not different among the subgroups. In addition, ofatumumab was tested in combination with other TKIs, lenalidomide, and chemotherapy. Other trials with ofatumumab are summarized in Table 13.3. It is unclear whether ofatumumab can replace rituximab in routine clinical practice but ofatumumab appears to be more active and less toxic than rituximab as a single agent in the therapy of CLL.

### Results with Obinutuzumab (GA-101) in CLL

Obinutuzumab (GA-101) is a type II humanized IgG1 mAb, which is glycoengineered to lack a sugar moiety in the Fc region (fucosylated Fc), thus enhancing the ADCC of the mAb. It is potent in inducing direct cell death and phagocytosis and does not stabilize CD20 into lipid rafts (as does rituximab) (Table 13.1).[125] Obinutuzumab was shown to have activity in a phase I study in 13 relapsed or refractory patients with CLL (ORR 63% and rapid B-cell depletion) and was well tolerated.[126]

Recently, obinutuzumab combined with chlorambucil was compared with chlorambucil alone and chlorambucil with rituximab in older patients with previously untreated CLL in a phase III clinical trial in Germany (CLL11 trial).[105] The median age of the

patients was 73 years. Obinutuzumab was administered as an IV infusion of 1000 mg on days 1, 8, and 15 in cycle 1 and 1000 mg IV on day 1 in cycles 2–6. Obinutuzumab with chlorambucil ($n = 238$) significantly improved PFS and OS over that seen with chlorambucil alone ($n = 118$) (PFS—26.7 months vs. 11.1 months; OS—median not reached, hazard ratio for death, 0.41; 95% CI, 0.23–0.74; $p = 0.002$). Similarly, obinutuzumab with chlorambucil ($n = 333$) improved the PFS ($p < 0.001$) and the CR rate (21 vs. 7%) compared to those seen with rituximab and chlorambucil ($n = 330$). Obinutuzumab was approved by the FDA for use in combination with chlorambucil for the treatment of patients with previously untreated CLL. Obinutuzumab was combined with chemotherapy—fludarabine, cyclophosphamide (FC) ($n = 21$) or with bendamustine (B) ($n = 20$) in a phase I–II clinical trial in patients with relapsed CLL (Galton trial). The most common grade 3–4 adverse events in obinutuzumab-FC versus obinutuzumab-B were neutropenia (43/55%), infusion reactions (29/10%), and infections (19/5%). The ORR was 62/90%, and 2/4 achieved CR.[127] Obinutuzumab is also being investigated in combination with BCL-2 antagonists, BTK, and PI3Kδ inhibitors in lymphoid malignancies. Obinutuzumab has shown promising efficacy, especially in older patients with coexisting conditions.

### Other CD20 mAbs in Development

**Ublituximab.** A chimeric mAb with low fucose content in the Fc region, improved FcγRIIIa binding, and increased ADCC as compared to that seen with rituximab.[128] In a phase I trial it produced an ORR of 45% with manageable toxicity in relapsed or refractory patients with CLL ($n = 11$).[129]

**Veltuzumab.** A type I humanized IgG1 with a slower off-rate, that is, slower dissociation from targeted cells compared to rituximab.[130] It was shown to have similar activity (ORR 44%) to rituximab in a phase I/II trial for relapsed or refractory NHL at a lower dose and with similar toxicity.[131]

**Ocrelizumab.** A type I humanized mAb with enhanced CD16 binding and less CDC compared to rituximab. It has shown activity in a phase I/II trial for patients with relapsed or refractory follicular lymphoma.[132]

**Ocaratuzumab and PRO-131921.** These are type I humanized IgG1 glycoengineered mAbs with modified Fc domains. The modification enhances FcγRIIIa binding and ADCC.[133] These mAbs are in phase I/II trials in NHL and CLL.[134]

### Anti-CD52 mAb Alemtuzumab

This is a humanized mAb targeting the CD52 antigen, an antigen present on both B and T lymphocytes. Toxicities associated with alemtuzumab are significant. By virtue of T-cell depletion it predisposes to serious infections and reactivation of viruses such as cytomegalovirus. Patients with bulky disease do not respond well to alemtuzumab. It has been tested in the front-line setting as a single agent versus chlorambucil,[135] with FCR,[136] in low doses with FC,[137] and in the relapsed/refractory setting with glucocorticoids, lenalidomide, and chemotherapy.[138,139] Due to the toxicities and the more impressive responses seen with kinase inhibitors, this molecule is reserved for compassionate use in CLL.

### Anti-CD37 mAb Otlertuzumab (TRU-016)

This is a protein built on the modular protein technology. This protein is similar to a mAb but has a single chain without a constant heavy chain region-1. Due to this structural difference it has a

**Table 13.3** Clinical trials with ofatumumab in CLL.

| Regimen | N | ORR (%) | CR (%) | Comment |
|---------|---|---------|--------|---------|
| Single agent ofatumumab[117] | 33 | 44 | 0 | RR patients, 27/33 received 500 mg once in week 1, then 2000 mg weekly for weeks 2–4. Majority of the toxicities were grade 1–2, only three (9%) were grade 3–4. The median time-to-next treatment was 1 year and median PFS was 3.5 months. |
| Ofatumumab with high-dose glucocorticoids[118] | 10 | 20 | 0 | High-risk fludarabine refractory CLL (IV methylprednisolone (MP) 1 gm/m$^2$ every 28 days. High rate of infections. |
| Ofatumumab with dexamethasone[119] | 32 | 69 | 16 | RR patients. Cycles 1–6—dexamethasone (40 mg on days 1–4 and 15–18) with ofatumumab, 2000 mg cycle 1 and 1000 mg cycles 2–6. Grade 3/4 toxicity consisted of bacterial infections (25%), ofatumumab infusion-related side effects (9%), neutropenia (9%), hyperglycemia (6%), and anemia (3%). |
| Single agent ofatumumab[120] | 66 | 55 and 36 | 5 and 4 | Untreated CLL. Eight weekly doses of ofatumumab were administered to elderly ≥65 years or in patients aged 18–64 years who refused fludarabine-based regimen in two dose levels: 2000 mg (cohort 1) and 1000 mg (cohort 2). Responses—55% and 26% by iWCLL criteria with CR in 5% and 4% in cohort 1 and 2, respectively. Responders received maintenance ofatumumab for 2 years. Infrequent side effects. Neutropenia was the most common grade 3/4 hematologic adverse event (10 patients). |
| Ofatumumab with fludarabine and cyclophosphamide (O-FC) as front-line[107] | 61 | 77 and 73 | 32 and 50 | Ofatumumab at 500 mg ($n = 31$) or 1000 mg ($n = 30$) with FC for six cycles. Common toxicities among the total cohort were neutropenia (48%), infection (38%), nausea (41%), thrombocytopenia (26%), and rash (25%). Toxicities with O-FC were comparable to FCR. |
| Ofatumumab with pentostatin and cyclophosphamide (O-FC) as front-line[121] | 48 | 96 | 46 | Ofatumumab 300 mg on day 1 then 1000 mg on day 2 followed by 1000 mg on day 1 during cycles 2–6 every 3 weeks. Grade 3 hematologic toxicity was 27% and grade 3–4 nonhematologic toxicity was 23%. |
| Ofatumumab + chlorambucil vs. chlorambucil alone as front-line[122] | 221 226 | 82 vs. 69 | 14 vs. 1 | Addition of ofatumumab to chlorambucil, associated with improved response rate, PFS (22.1 vs. 13 months), and durable MRD-negative disease (12 vs. 4%), was tolerable regardless of age and minimal toxicity. Suitable for unfit patients. |
| Ofatumumab with ibrutinib in RR CLL[123] | 27 | 100 | 0 | Minimal side effects. Ofatumumab is added at a dose of 300 mg on day 1 of cycle 2, followed by 2000 mg every week in cycles 2 and 3, and on D1 of cycles 5–8 with ibrutinib 420 mg daily. Two patients progressed. |
| Ofatumumab or rituximab with idelalisib in RR CLL[124] | 39 | 83 | 8 | Idelalisib given at 150 mg bid in combination with total of 12 infusions of ofatumumab or rituximab. Durable tumor control in heavily pretreated patients. |

different pattern of BCR signaling.[140] It is considered a small modular immunopharmaceutical (SMIP) and has shown efficacy in a phase I trial in 83 patients with CLL, producing an ORR of 23% (all PRs). Higher response rates were seen in treatment-naïve patients. Otlertuzumab produces minimal toxicity.[141] It has also been combined with bendamustine and rituximab. Other anti-CD37 mAbs in development include 37.1, 37.2, IMGN-529, and the beta emitter [177]Lu-tetulomab.

## Other mAbs

Anti-CD40 mAb lucatumumab (HCD122) is a fully humanized mAb. In a phase I trial in relapsed CLL, lucatumumab demonstrated minimal activity as a single agent. Seventeen of twenty-six patients had stable disease.[142] Another example of anti-CD40 mAb is dacetuzumab (SGN-40) which showed minimal activity in a phase I trial.[143]

## Clinical Results with BCR Signaling Kinase Inhibitors

Development of BCR signaling kinase inhibitors in recent years is a paradigm change in the therapeutic landscape of CLL. These agents have minimal myelotoxicity, are orally available, and achieve remarkable responses in chemotherapy-resistant patients including those with del17p.

A common clinical observation with these drugs is "redistribution lymphocytosis" resulting in an increase in the absolute lymphocyte count within hours of starting therapy, which can persist for weeks accompanied by a rapid reduction in bulky adenopathy and splenomegaly. This phenomenon is due to rapid (<24 hours after drug intake) egress[144] and mobilization of CLL cells residing in the protective tissue niches of lymph nodes into the peripheral blood.[74,145] These agents interfere with the chemokine receptor interactions and homing of CLL cells, leading to lymphocytosis.[10,146] In one study[147] it was shown that patients with a mutated IGHV and bulky disease have a more pronounced and prolonged rise in lymphocyte counts after therapy with ibrutinib; redistribution lymphocytosis is not a sign of disease progression.

## Ibrutinib—A BTK Inhibitor

Currently, ibrutinib is the only BCR kinase inhibitor which is commercially available. Ibrutinib (previously known as PCI-32765) is an irreversible inhibitor, which binds to cysteine 481 within the ATP-binding site of the BTK kinase domain. Ibrutinib cross-reacts with other TEC kinases (BMX, ITK, and BLK).[14]

The phase II trial evaluated ibrutinib[5] in 85 patients (117 in a 2013 update)[148] with relapsed/refractory CLL/SLL. The majority of these patients had high-risk disease (unmutated IGHV and del17p cytogenetics). Patients received ibrutinib 420 mg ($n = 51$) or 840 mg ($n = 34$) orally daily. The ORR was 71% (88% in an update at ASH 2013) in both groups of patients. Responses were assessed according to the 2008 International Working Group of CLL (iWCLL) Guidelines[6] with the exception that lymphocytosis was not considered a sign of progression.[149] Responses were independent of high-risk features. Serum IgA levels increased while on therapy with ibrutinib.[5,150] Ibrutinib was well tolerated. The most common adverse effect was diarrhea, seen in 49 patients followed by upper respiratory tract infection and fatigue in 33 and 32 patients, respectively. Grade 3–4 hematological toxicity occurred in 6–15% patients. Thirty-six percent ($n = 31$) of patients discontinued therapy after a median follow-up of 21 months. At 26 months, the PFS was 75% and the OS was 83%. Ibrutinib 420 mg received an accelerated approval from the FDA in February 2014 for patients with CLL who have received at least one prior therapy. In July 2014, the FDA expanded the approval of ibrutinib to include the treatment of patients with CLL who harbor a 17p deletion.

Efficacy and safety of ibrutinib was also evaluated in previously untreated patients with CLL, aged ≥65 years. In 31 patients who received ibrutinib at 420 mg daily ($n = 27$) or at 840 mg daily ($n = 4$), the ORR was 71% (CR 13%, nodular PR 3%, and PR 55%) while 13% patients had PR with lymphocytosis and 10% had stable disease. Grade 3 diarrhea was seen in 13% of patients, grade 3 infections in 10% and grade 3–4 neutropenia and thrombocytopenia were noted in one patient each.[151]

The combination of ibrutinib and rituximab was studied in 40 patients with high-risk CLL in a phase II study. Among 39 evaluable patients, 87% achieved PR and 8% CR. The ORR in patients with del17p or TP53 mutation was 90%. The combination was well tolerated with six patients developing pneumonia. Patients had a significant improvement in quality of life and rapid resolution of lymphocytosis was noted with the addition of rituximab.[152]

Other trials with ibrutinib in patients with CLL include a combination of ibrutinib with bendamustine and rituximab (BR) (ORR, 93% in 30 relapsed patients with CLL).[153] The efficacy of ibrutinib ($n = 195$) was compared to that of ofatumumab ($n = 196$) in relapsed/refractory patients with CLL (RESONATE) trial. Ibrutinib significantly improved the response rate, PFS, and OS compared to that seen with ofatumumab.[154] Other ongoing trials include ibrutinib in patients with del17p, a randomized trial of ibrutinib compared with chlorambucil (RESONATE-2) in older patients, a randomized trial of ibrutinib with rituximab (IR) compared with FCR in patients with previously untreated CLL, and a randomized trial comparing IR versus BR versus ibrutinib alone in older patients with previously untreated CLL. Other trials in relapsed CLL are evaluating ibrutinib with lenalidomide or ofatumumab.

Potential advantages of ibrutinib over FCR could be due to significant activity in patients with del17p, minimal myelotoxicity, longer remission in the relapsed setting, and excellent tolerability in elderly patients with CLL. However, long-term follow-up with ibrutinib is limited as compared to FCR.

## BTK Mutations and Ibrutinib Resistance

BTK inhibitors (ibrutinib, CC-292) bind to cysteine 481 within the ATP-binding site. Recently, two groups have reported data on BTK mutations detected in patients with CLL who have progressed (without transformation) while receiving ibrutinib. Whole exome sequencing was done from peripheral blood samples at baseline and at the time of disease progression in six patients. Five of six patients demonstrated cysteine-to-serine substitution at position 481 of the BTK (C481S) gene. In the sixth patient a mutation involving the substitution of arginine to tryptophan (R665W) in PLCγ2, a substrate of BTK, was demonstrated.[155] None of the six patients had BTK mutations at baseline. In one of the six patients both C281S and PLCγ2 mutations (R665W, L845F, and S707Y) were detected. Functional experiments further demonstrated that these mutations prevent the irreversible binding of ibrutinib to BTK. In addition, this study showed that patients who develop prolonged lymphocytosis on ibrutinib therapy did not exhibit BTK mutations. In another report, three patients were evaluated: one patient showed a PLCγ2 mutation and two patients did not have evidence of C481S mutations.[156] Detection of BTK mutations in patients with CLL is significant, as the presence of these mutations not only explains the mechanism of resistance in some patients who progress on ibrutinib, but it further confirms the significance of the BCR signaling pathway in the pathophysiology of CLL.

## Other Novel BTK Inhibitors

**CC-292 (previously AVL-292).** CC-292 is a small molecule irreversible inhibitor of BTK at the C481 site. CC-292 was tested in a phase I trial[157] at four dose levels (750 mg od, 1000 mg od, 375 mg bid, 500 mg bid) in 83 patients with relapsed/refractory CLL. Nodal responses were more frequent in patients receiving bid dosing (375 mg: 67%; 500 mg: 62%) with an overall PR rate of 40%. CC-292 was well tolerated; side effects included grade 3–4 neutropenia (21%), thrombocytopenia (15%), pneumonia (10%), and anemia (8%). The most frequent treatment-related adverse events were diarrhea (60%), fatigue, and neutropenia. The combination of CC-292 with lenalidomide is under investigation.

**ONO-4059.** This agent is a reversible BTK inhibitor that acts by blocking autophosphorylation at the tyrosine 223 position. Results from a phase I trial (20–320 mg dose escalation study) showed an ORR of 89% in 19 patients with relapsed/refractory CLL. The ORR was 71% in seven patients with del17p. Nodal responses were seen in most of the patients. The drug was well tolerated with infrequent toxicities.[158]

**ACP-196.** This agent is a novel BTK inhibitor. A phase I trial is ongoing in patients with relapsed CLL (www.clinicaltrials.gov, NCT02029443).

**Other BTK inhibitors in preclinical studies.**[14] *CGI-1746* reversibly binds to the ATP-binding pocket of nonphosphorylated BTK and stabilizes it in an inactive form. It does not cross-react with other TEC family kinases suggesting that it may have less off-target effects and may not be affected by mutations in the C481 site of BTK. Other BTK inhibitors such as *GDC-0834, LFM-A13, and CNX-774* are under preclinical studies.

## Idelalisib—p110 PI3Kδ Inhibitor

This agent inhibits the p110 catalytic subunit of the PI3Kδ isoform. Inhibition of the p110 delta isoform of PI3K promotes the apoptosis of CLL cells,[16] blocks the relay of microenvironmental signals[17,159,160] and the secretion of prosurvival factors—CCL3 and CCL4, decreases AKT phosphorylation, and affects the chemotaxis of CLL cells. In a phase I trial[161] of 54 patients with relapsed/refractory CLL, various dose levels (50–350 mg once or twice daily) were tested. The ORR was 72% including 33% PR with lymphocytosis. The ORR in 13 patients with del17p was 54%. The median PFS for all patients was 15.8 months. Idelalisib did not influence serum immunoglobulin levels or T-cell numbers. The most common grade 3–4 adverse events were pneumonia (20%), neutropenic fever (11%), and diarrhea (6%).

The pivotal study of idelalisib was a phase III trial of idelalisib 150 mg bid combined with rituximab ($n = 110$) versus rituximab with placebo ($n = 110$) in high-risk patients with relapsed/refractory CLL.[162] The ORRs were 81% versus 13%, respectively, and the nodal response rates were 93% versus 4%, respectively. At 6 months, the PFS rates were 93% in the idelalisib and rituximab arm versus 46% in the rituximab and placebo arm. The median OS was significantly longer with idelalisib and rituximab versus rituximab alone (92% vs. 80% at 12 months). Grade 3–4 toxicities in the idelalisib and rituximab arm were neutropenia (34%), thrombocytopenia (10%), elevated transaminases (5%), diarrhea (4%), and pyrexia (3%). Other ongoing studies include idelalisib and ofatumumab; idelalisib, bendamustine, and rituximab; and idelalisib and rituximab or chlorambucil.

## IPI-145 (Duvelisib)—p110 PI3Kδ/γ Inhibitor

This agent was tested in a phase I dose escalation trial[163] in 52 patients with relapsed/refractory CLL and 15 previously untreated older patients with CLL. IPI-145 was administered as ≤25 mg bid orally in 28 patients or 75 mg bid in 24 patients with relapsed CLL or 25 mg bid in previously untreated patients (≥65 years or del17p/TP53 mutation). The ORR was 48% and nodal responses were observed in 89% of patients. Response was independent of del17p/TP53 status and dose of IPI-145. The drug was well tolerated—grade 3 neutropenia was seen in 17%, grade 3 anemia in 12%, and grade 3 diarrhea was observed in 6% of patients. IPI-145 is being tested in a phase III trial (25 mg bid) versus ofatumumab in patients with relapsed CLL.

## AMG-319—p110 PI3Kδ Inhibitor

This agent was tested in a phase I trial[164] involving 28 patients with relapsed/refractory CLL (42% with del17p). The drug was well tolerated up to a dose of 400 mg daily. Grade ≥3 treatment-related adverse events ($n > 1$) were colitis (11% of patients), neutropenia (11%), and leukocytosis (7%). One patient developed grade 3 hemolytic anemia at 25 mg. Rapid shrinkage of lymph nodes was observed at all dose levels.

## TGR-1202

This is a next generation PI3Kδ inhibitor. In a phase I trial in relapsed/refractory hematological malignancies *(ASCO 2014, Abstract 2513)*, TGR-1202 demonstrated a nodal response rate of 78% in relapsed/refractory patients with CLL at ≥800 mg po daily dose. Contrary to other PI3K inhibitors, TGR-1202 is not hepatotoxic and is administered daily in a single dose.

Similar to BTK inhibitors, PI3K isoenzyme inhibitors have advantages including oral bioavailability and remarkable nodal responses irrespective of high-risk prognostic features in patients with CLL. Of concern is the development of inflammatory colitis/diarrhea and/or pneumonitis in some patients receiving PI3K inhibitors. Colitis in these patients could be explained by data obtained from the PI3K delta deficient mouse model where colitis is attributed to an increase in Th1/Th17 associated proinflammatory cytokines and altered macrophage function.[165] Other PI3K inhibitors under investigation include GS-9820 and SAR-245408.

## Fostamatinib—SYK Inhibitor

The clinical trial of fostamatinib in relapsed CLL was the first one to be reported among the BCR kinase signaling inhibitors. Fostamatinib is an oral prodrug of the active metabolite R406, which is a competitive kinase inhibitor of SYK and other kinases. The phase I/II study[166] reported the efficacy of fostamatinib in 11 patients with relapsed CLL (ORR, 55%). Dose-limiting toxicities were grade 3 neutropenia (33%) and diarrhea (17%).

## GS-9973—A Selective SYK Inhibitor

This is an orally available selective SYK inhibitor, which was tested in a phase II trial in 44 patients with relapsed CLL. Nodal response was observed in 64% of patients. It was generally well tolerated.[167] GS-9973 was shown to have synergistic activity on CLL cells when combined with idelalisib.[168] A phase II study of GS-9973 with idelalisib was initiated but stopped early due to the high incidence of pneumonitis.[169]

## Other Kinase Inhibitors Tested in Clinical Trials in CLL

**mTOR (mammalian target of rapamycin) inhibitors (everolimus, temsirolimus).** Everolimus was tested in patients with relapsed CLL. Redistribution lymphocytosis was observed in these trials with nodal responses in 70% of patients.[170] However, immunosuppression, pneumonitis, and other infectious complications limited further testing of everolimus in patients with CLL.

**LYN kinase inhibitors (dasatinib, bafetinib).** Dasatinib is a dual inhibitor of ABL and SRC family kinases. Dasatinib was tested in 15 patients with relapsed/refractory CLL with an ORR of 20%; 27% patients had a nodal response.[171] Dasatinib was combined with fludarabine in 20 patients[172] and produced a PR rate of 16.7%. Myelosuppression was the main toxicity.

## Miscellaneous Kinase Inhibitors in Preclinical Research

**Proviral integration site for Moloney murine leukemia virus (PIM) kinase inhibitors.** These agents can induce apoptosis of CLL cells via MCL1 inhibition and block CXCR4 receptors.[173,174]

**AXL kinase inhibitor.** Preclinical data suggest that AXL kinase inhibitors can promote apoptosis and inhibit CLL cell migration.[175,176]

**Receptor tyrosine kinase-like orphan receptor (ROR1).** This molecule is overexpressed on CLL cells and is targeted by mAbs and immunotoxins.[177,178]

**PKCβ inhibitors.** Rottlerin and enzastaurin have been tested against CLL cells and have shown *in vitro* activity.[179,180]

**Casein kinase inhibitor CX-4945.** A selective CK inhibitor with preclinical data showing enhanced activity in CLL.[181]

## BCL-2 Antagonists

Various agents of this class have been tested in relapsed patients with CLL with modest efficacy. *Oblimersen* is a synthetic, 18-base, single-strand phorothioate DNA oligonucleotide designed to downregulate BCL-2 mRNA expression. Oblimersen was studied in relapsed patients with CLL. A significant 5-year survival benefit was observed in a subset of patients who had fludarabine-sensitive disease and those who achieved CR/PR with a combination of oblimersen with fludarabine and cyclophosphamide.[182] *Navitoclax (ABT-263) and obatoclax*[183] are pan-BCL-2 inhibitors. These agents inhibit BCL-2 and BCL-xL; obatoclax also inhibits MCL1. Navitoclax was evaluated in patients with relapsed CLL with modest response rates; preliminary results showed 70% responses when navitoclax was combined with rituximab and continued as maintenance therapy.[184] Since BCL-xL is inhibited by navitoclax, resulting in thrombocytopenia, further development of navitoclax was stopped. Structural changes in navitoclax and replacement of the indole ring led to the development of the orally bioavailable compound ABT-199.[185]

## ABT-199

An orally active and selective BCL-2 antagonist which spares platelets.[185] Recently, results of a phase I trial of ABT-199 in relapsed/refractory CLL (*n* = 67) were presented.[186] Fifty-two percent of patients were fludarabine-refractory and 37% had del17p. The ORR was 84% (CR, 23% and PR, 61%). Patients with del17p and those with fludarabine-refractory disease had an ORR of 82% and 89%, respectively. Some patients achieved a minimal residual disease (MRD) negative CR. Grade 3–4 tumor lysis syndrome (9%) is the toxicity of concern with this agent. Other grade 3–4 toxicities included neutropenia (36%), anemia (9%), and thrombocytopenia (9%). Another phase Ib trial combined ABT-199 with rituximab in relapsed/refractory CLL (*n* = 37). In 18 patients who completed therapy, the CR rate was 39% and the PR rate was 39%. MRD-negative CR was noted in five of seven patients achieving CR. The most common grade 3–4 toxicities included neutropenia (43%), thrombocytopenia (16%), and anemia (11%).[187]

Further investigations are continuing with ABT-199 to identify the optimal dose and minimize the toxicities. The efficacy of ABT-199 in combination with obinutuzumab is being assessed.

## Alvocidib (Flavopiridol), Dinaciclib—CDK Inhibitors

These agents have been tested in phase I and II clinical trials in relapsed/refractory CLL. Alvocidib is a pan-CDK inhibitor, which produces impressive nodal responses in patients with del17p and bulky disease, but is associated with significant hyperacute tumor lysis syndrome (48%) with 20% patients requiring dialysis; diarrhea and cytokine release syndrome were also seen. In a phase II study of relapsed patients with CLL (*n* = 64), the ORR was 53% (CR 1%, PR 47%, and nodular PR 5%).[188] Responses were independent of high-risk features (del17p and bulky disease). Another study combined alvocidib with cyclophosphamide and rituximab in nine patients with relapsed high-risk CLL. Seven of nine patients responded (CR, *n* = 3). The regimen was well tolerated with manageable toxicities.[189] *Dinaciclib* is a relatively selective CDK inhibitor (CDK, 1, 2, 5, and 9). A dose escalation trial included 52 patients with high-risk relapsed/refractory CLL. Common adverse events included leukopenia, anemia, thrombocytopenia, and metabolic evidence of tumor lysis (15% of patients). The ORR was 58% including patients

with del17p (57%).[190] Other CDK inhibitors under investigation include *seliciclib* and *SNS-032*.

## Plerixafor—CXCR4 Antagonist

These agents can abrogate the protective action of soluble factor CXCL12 emanating from NLCs on CLL cells, which express CD184 or CXCR4 receptors.[102,191] Plerixafor can mobilize the CLL cells from tissues into peripheral blood. In a phase I study of 14 patients with relapsed CLL, the addition of plerixafor to rituximab produced a 36% response rate (all PR).[192] A combination of lenalidomide (immunomodulatory agent) with plerixafor in patients with CLL is being investigated.

# Other Novel Therapeutic Agents in CLL

## Selinexor (KPT-330) Selective Inhibitor of Nuclear Export

Comprehensive analysis of the genome of CLL performed using whole exome sequencing was reported in 2011. In 363 patients with CLL, the presence of four recurrently mutated genes was noted (NOTCH1, MYD88, KLH-1, and XPO-1). The presence of XPO-1 (exportin-1) mutations was associated with unmutated IgVH. Exportin transports tumor suppressor proteins out of the nucleus. *Selinexor* is a selective oral inhibitor of exportin. *In vitro* data showed that selinexor can block BCR signaling and activation of CLL B cells.[193] In a phase I trial of 18 patients with relapsed/refractory NHL/CLL,[194] selinexor induced reduction in nodal size in 80% of patients. One patient with Richter's transformation responded to selinexor with a 60% nodal response and subsequently underwent stem cell transplantation. Further studies are ongoing with this molecule.

## IL-21 Cytokine

Interleukin-21 has a strong proapoptotic effect on CLL cells,[195] and CLL cells express IL-21 receptors. Recombinant IL-21 was combined with rituximab in 11 patients with relapsed CLL in a phase I trial.[196] The ORR was 40%. Toxicities were mild and manageable and included flu-like symptoms and fatigue.

# Conclusions

Recently, the treatment of CLL has undergone a paradigm shift with the discovery of targeted BCR kinase inhibitors such as ibrutinib and idelalisib. Oral bioavailability, excellent tolerability, and impressive responses, even in patients with high-risk prognostic markers, are the key advantages of ibrutinib and idelalisib. CIT with FCR has a limited role in patients with del17p/TP53 mutations and is myelotoxic. Since the majority of patients with CLL are older with concomitant comorbidities, the advent of kinase inhibitors is a significant improvement over conventional CIT particularly in elderly patients. However, only a few patients achieve CR with kinase inhibitors, therefore combination trials with rituximab and chemotherapeutic agents are ongoing to improve the depth of responses. As data thus far were derived from patients with relapsed CLL, ongoing clinical trials will evaluate whether BCR kinase inhibitors can replace CIT in the front-line setting. ABT-199 is a targeted BCL-2 antagonist. This agent has shown impressive activity in refractory CLL with some patients achieving MRD-negative CR. However, tumor lysis syndrome is a concern. Immunotherapeutic approaches with chimeric antigen receptor T cells are being studied in CLL. Future treatment of CLL appears promising and several preclinical and clinical studies are ongoing to discover additional targeted agents and improve patient outcome and quality of life.

# References

1 Maloney DG, Grillo-Lopez AJ, White CA, et al. IDEC-C2B8 (Rituximab) anti-CD20 monoclonal antibody therapy in patients with relapsed low-grade non-Hodgkin's lymphoma. *Blood*. 1997;90(6):2188–2195.

2 O'Brien SG, Guilhot F, Larson RA, et al. Imatinib compared with interferon and low-dose cytarabine for newly diagnosed chronic-phase chronic myeloid leukemia. *N Engl J Med*. 2003;348:994–1004.

3 Hallek M, Fischer K, Fingerle-Rowson G, et al. German Chronic Lymphocytic Leukaemia Study Group. Addition of rituximab to fludarabine and cyclophosphamide in patients with chronic lymphocytic leukaemia: a randomised, open-label, phase 3 trial. *Lancet*. 2010;376(9747):1164–1174.

4 Keating MJ, O'Brien S, Albitar M, et al. Early results of a chemoimmunotherapy regimen of fludarabine, cyclophosphamide, and rituximab as initial therapy for chronic lymphocytic leukemia. *J Clin Oncol*. 2005;23(18):4079–4088.

5 Byrd JC, Furman RR, Coutre SE, et al. Targeting BTK with ibrutinib in relapsed chronic lymphocytic leukemia. *N Engl J Med*. 2013;369(1):32–42.

6 Hallek M, Cheson BD, Catovsky D, et al. International Workshop on Chronic Lymphocytic Leukemia. Guidelines for the diagnosis and treatment of chronic lymphocytic leukemia: a report from the International Workshop on Chronic Lymphocytic Leukemia updating the National Cancer Institute-Working Group 1996 guidelines. *Blood*. 2008;111(12):5446–5456.

7 National Cancer Institute. SEER cancer statistics review (1975–2007). 2013. http://seer.cancer.gov/csr/1975_2007/. Accessed October 2, 2014.

8 Stevenson FK, Krysov S, Davies AJ, Steele AJ, Packham G. B-cell receptor signaling in chronic lymphocytic leukemia. *Blood*. 2011;118:4313–4320.

9 Young RM, Staudt LM. Targeting pathological B cell receptor signalling in lymphoid malignancies. *Nat Rev Drug Discov*. 2013;12:229–243.

10 Ponader S, Chen SS, Buggy JJ, et al. The Bruton tyrosine kinase inhibitor PCI-32765 thwarts chronic lymphocytic leukemia cell survival and tissue homing in vitro and in vivo. *Blood*. 2012;119:1182–1189.

11 Herman SE, Gordon AL, Hertlein E, et al. Bruton tyrosine kinase represents a promising therapeutic target for treatment of chronic lymphocytic leukemia and is effectively targeted by PCI-32765. *Blood*. 2011;117:6287–6296.

12 Woyach JA, Bojnik E, Ruppert AS, et al. Bruton's tyrosine kinase (BTK) function is important to the development and expansion of chronic lymphocytic leukemia (CLL). *Blood*. 2014;123(8):1207–1213.

13 Honigberg LA, Smith AM, Sirisawad M, et al. The Bruton tyrosine kinase inhibitor PCI-32765 blocks B-cell activation and is efficacious in models of autoimmune disease and B-cell malignancy. *Proc Natl Acad Sci U S A*. 2010;107(29):13075–13080.

14 Hendriks RW, Yuvaraj S, Kil LP. Targeting Bruton's tyrosine kinase in B cell malignancies. *Nat Rev Cancer*. 2014;14(4):219–232.

15 Davis RE, Ngo VN, Lenz G, et al. Chronic active B-cell-receptor signalling in diffuse large B-cell lymphoma. *Nature*. 2010;463(7277):88–92.

16 Herman SE, Gordon AL, Wagner AJ, et al. Phosphatidylinositol 3-kinase-delta inhibitor CAL-101 shows promising preclinical activity in chronic lymphocytic leukemia by antagonizing intrinsic and extrinsic cellular survival signals. *Blood*. 2010;116(12):2078–2088.

17 Hoellenriegel J, Meadows SA, Sivina M, et al. The phosphoinositide 3′-kinase delta inhibitor, CAL-101, inhibits B-cell receptor signaling and chemokine networks in chronic lymphocytic leukemia. *Blood*. 2011;118(13):3603–3612.

18 Kang S, Denley A, Vanhaesebroeck B, Vogt PK. Oncogenic transformation induced by the p110beta, -gamma, and -delta isoforms of class I phosphoinositide 3-kinase. *Proc Natl Acad Sci U S A*. 2006;103(5):1289–1294.

19 Srinivasan L, Sasaki Y, Calado DP, et al. PI3 kinase signals BCR-dependent mature B cell survival. *Cell*. 2009;139(3):573–586.

20 Clayton E, Bardi G, Bell SE, et al. A crucial role for the p110delta subunit of phosphatidylinositol 3-kinase in B cell development and activation. *J Exp Med*. 2002;196(6):753–763.

21 Cheng AM, Rowley B, Pao W, Hayday A, Bolen JB, Pawson T. Syk tyrosine kinase required for mouse viability and B-cell development. *Nature*. 1995;378(6554):303–306.

22 Gobessi S, Laurenti L, Longo PG, et al. Inhibition of constitutive and BCR-induced Syk activation downregulates Mcl-1 and induces apoptosis in chronic lymphocytic leukemia B cells. *Leukemia*. 2009;23:686–697.

23 Buchner M, Baer C, Prinz G, et al. Spleen tyrosine kinase inhibition prevents chemokine- and integrin-mediated stromal protective effects in chronic lymphocytic leukemia. *Blood*. 2010;115(22):4497–506.

24 Young RM, Hardy IR, Clarke RL, et al. Mouse models of non-Hodgkin lymphoma reveal Syk as an important therapeutic target. *Blood*. 2009;113(11):2508–2516.

25 Hoellenriegel J, Coffey GP, Sinha U, et al. Selective, novel spleen tyrosine kinase (Syk) inhibitors suppress chronic lymphocytic leukemia B-cell activation and migration. *Leukemia*. 2012;26(7):1576–1583.

26 Pleyer L, Egle A, Hartmann TN, Greil R. Molecular and cellular mechanisms of CLL: novel therapeutic approaches. *Nat Rev Clin Oncol*. 2009;6(7):405–418.

27 Cramer P, Hallek M. Prognostic factors in chronic lymphocytic leukemia-what do we need to know? *Nat Rev Clin Oncol*. 2011;8(1):38–47.

28 Dohner H, Stilgenbauer S, Benner A, et al. Genomic aberrations and survival in chronic lymphocytic leukemia. *N Engl J Med*. 2000;343(26):1910–1916.

29 Damle RN, Wasil T, Fais F, et al. Ig V gene mutation status and CD38 expression as novel prognostic indicators in chronic lymphocytic leukemia. *Blood*. 1999;94(6):1840–1847.

30 Hamblin TJ, Davis Z, Gardiner A, Oscier DG, Stevenson FK. Unmutated Ig V(H) genes are associated with a more aggressive form of chronic lymphocytic leukemia. *Blood*. 1999;94(6):1848–1854.

31 Tobin G, Thunberg U, Johnson A, et al. Chronic lymphocytic leukemias utilizing the VH3-21 gene display highly restricted Vlambda2-14 gene use and homologous CDR3s: implicating recognition of a common antigen epitope. *Blood*. 2003;101(12):4952–4957.

32 Messmer BT, Albesiano E, Efremov DG, et al. Multiple distinct sets of stereotyped antigen receptors indicate a role for antigen in promoting chronic lymphocytic leukemia. *J Exp Med*. 2004;200(4):519–525.

33 Stamatopoulos K, Belessi C, Moreno C, et al. Over 20% of patients with chronic lymphocytic leukemia carry stereotyped receptors: pathogenetic implications and clinical correlations. *Blood*. 2007;109(1):259–270.

34 Crespo M, Bosch F, Villamor N, et al. ZAP-70 expression as a surrogate for immunoglobulin-variable-region mutations in chronic lymphocytic leukemia. *N Engl J Med*. 2003;348(18):1764–1775.

35 Hallek M, Wanders L, Ostwald M, et al. Serum beta(2)-microglobulin and serum thymidine kinase are independent predictors of progression-free survival in chronic lymphocytic leukemia and immunocytoma. *Leuk Lymphoma*. 1996;22(5–6):439–447.

36 Stilgenbauer S, Schnaiter A, Paschka P, et al. Gene mutations and treatment outcome in chronic lymphocytic leukemia: results from the CLL8 trial. *Blood*. 2014;123(21):3247–3254.

37 Gaidano G, Foa R, Dalla-Favera R. Molecular pathogenesis of chronic lymphocytic leukemia. *J Clin Invest*. 2012;122(10):3432–3438.

38 Puente XS, Pinyol M, Quesada V, et al. Whole-genome sequencing identifies recurrent mutations in chronic lymphocytic leukaemia. *Nature*. 2011;475(7354):101–105.

39 Jeromin S, Weissmann S, Haferlach C, et al. SF3B1 mutations correlated to cytogenetics and mutations in NOTCH1, FBXW7, MYD88, XPO1 and TP53 in 1160 untreated CLL patients. *Leukemia*. 2014;28(1):108–117.

40 Quesada V, Ramsay AJ, Lopez-Otin C. Chronic lymphocytic leukemia with SF3B1 mutation. *N Engl J Med*. 2012;366(26):2530.

41 Rossi D, Rasi S, Spina V, et al. Integrated mutational and cytogenetic analysis identifies new prognostic subgroups in chronic lymphocytic leukemia. *Blood*. 2013;121(8):1403–1412.

42 Baliakas P, Hadzidimitriou A, Sutton LA, et al. Recurrent mutations refine prognosis in chronic lymphocytic leukemia. *Leukemia*. 2015;29(2):329–336.

43 Chiorazzi N. Implications of new prognostic markers in chronic lymphocytic leukemia. *Hematology Am Soc Hematol Educ Program*. 2012;2012:76–87.

44 Middleton O, Cosimo E, Dobbin E, et al. Complement deficiencies limit CD20 monoclonal antibody treatment efficacy in CLL. *Leukemia*. 2015;29(1):107–114.

45 Di Gaetano N, Cittera E, Nota R, et al. Complement activation determines the therapeutic activity of rituximab in vivo. *J Immunol*. 2003;171(13):1581–1587.

46 Uchida J, Hamaguchi Y, Oliver JA, et al. The innate mononuclear phagocyte network depletes B lymphocytes through Fc receptor-dependent mechanisms during anti-CD20 antibody immunotherapy. *J Exp Med*. 2004;199(12):1659–1669.

47 Ivanov A, Beers SA, Walshe CA, et al. Monoclonal antibodies directed to CD20 and HLA-DR can elicit homotypic adhesion followed by lysosome-mediated cell death in human lymphoma and leukemia cells. *J Clin Invest*. 2009;119(8):2143–2159.

48 Mossner E, Brunker P, Moser S, et al. Increasing the efficacy of CD20 antibody therapy through the engineering of a new type II anti-CD20 antibody with enhanced direct and immune effector cell-mediated B-cell cytotoxicity. *Blood*. 2010;115:4393–4402.

49 Honeychurch J, Alduaij W, Azizyan M, et al. Antibody-induced non-apoptotic cell death in human lymphoma and leukemia cells is mediated through a novel reactive oxygen species-dependent pathway. *Blood*. 2012;119(15):3523–3533.

50 Abes R, Gelize E, Fridman WH, Teillaud JL. Long-lasting antitumor protection by anti-CD20 antibody through cellular immune response. *Blood*. 2010;116(6):926–934.

51 Dalle S, Reslan L, Besseyre de Horts T, et al. Preclinical studies on the mechanism of action and the anti-lymphoma activity of the novel anti-CD20 antibody GA101. *Mol Cancer Ther*. 2011;10:178–185.

52 Beers SA, Chan CH, French RR, Cragg MS, Glennie MJ. CD20 as a target for therapeutic type I and II monoclonal antibodies. *Semin Hematol*. 2010;47:107–114.

53 Cragg MS, Morgan SM, Chan HT, et al. Complement-mediated lysis by anti-CD20 mAb correlates with segregation into lipid rafts. *Blood*. 2003;101(3):1045–1052.

54 Chan HT, Hughes D, French RR, et al. CD20-induced lymphoma cell death is independent of both caspases and its redistribution into triton X-100 insoluble membrane rafts. *Cancer Res*. 2003;63(17):5480–5489.

55 Ivanov A, Krysov S, Cragg MS, Illidge T. Radiation therapy with tositumomab (B1) anti-CD20 monoclonal antibody initiates extracellular signal-regulated kinase/mitogen-activated protein kinase-dependent cell death that overcomes resistance to apoptosis. *Clin Cancer Res*. 2008;14(15):4925–4934.

56 Rossmann ED, Lundin J, Lenkei R, Mellstedt H, Osterborg A. Variability in B-cell antigen expression: implications for the treatment of B-cell lymphomas and leukemias with monoclonal antibodies. *Hematol J*. 2001;2(5):300–306.

57 Ginaldi L, De Martinis M, Matutes E, et al. Levels of expression of CD52 in normal and leukemic B and T cells: correlation with in vivo therapeutic responses to Campath-1H. *Leuk Res*. 1998;22(2):185–191.

58 Schwartz-Albiez R, Dorken B, Hofmann W, Moldenhauer G. The B cell-associated CD37 antigen (gp40–52). Structure and subcellular expression of an extensively glycosylated glycoprotein. *J Immunol*. 1988;140(3):905–914.

59 Damle RN, Ghiotto F, Valetto A, et al. B-cell chronic lymphocytic leukemia cells express a surface membrane phenotype of activated, antigen-experienced B lymphocytes. *Blood*. 2002;99(11):4087–4093.

60 Romano MF, Lamberti A, Tassone P, et al. Triggering of CD40 antigen inhibits fludarabine-induced apoptosis in B chronic lymphocytic leukemia cells. *Blood*. 1998;92(3):990–995.

61 Cuni S, Perez-Aciego P, Perez-Chacon G, et al. A sustained activation of PI3K/NF-kappaB pathway is critical for the survival of chronic lymphocytic leukemia B cells. *Leukemia*. 2004;18(8):1391–1400.

62 Riches JC, Davies JK, McClanahan F, et al. T cells from CLL patients exhibit features of T-cell exhaustion but retain capacity for cytokine production. *Blood*. 2013;121(9):1612–1621.

63 Kretz-Rommel A, Bowdish KS. Rationale for anti-CD200 immunotherapy in B-CLL and other hematologic malignancies: new concepts in blocking immune suppression. *Expert Opin Biol Ther*. 2008;8(1):5–15.

64 Lanham S, Hamblin T, Oscier D, Ibbotson R, Stevenson F, Packham G. Differential signaling via surface IgM is associated with VH gene mutational status and CD38 expression in chronic lymphocytic leukemia. *Blood*. 2003;101(3):1087–1093.

65 Agathangelidis A, Darzentas N, Hadzidimitriou A, et al. Stereotyped B-cell receptors in one-third of chronic lymphocytic leukemia: a molecular classification with implications for targeted therapies. *Blood*. 2012;119(19):4467–4475.

66 Fais F, Ghiotto F, Hashimoto S, et al. Chronic lymphocytic leukemia B cells express restricted sets of mutated and unmutated antigen receptors. *J Clin Invest*. 1998;102(8):1515–1525.

67 Tobin G, Thunberg U, Karlsson K, et al. Subsets with restricted immunoglobulin gene rearrangement features indicate a role for antigen selection in the development of chronic lymphocytic leukemia. *Blood*. 2004;104(9):2879–2885.

68 Hoogeboom R, van Kessel KP, Hochstenbach F, et al. A mutated B cell chronic lymphocytic leukemia subset that recognizes and responds to fungi. *J Exp Med*. 2013;210(1):59–70.

69 Lanemo Myhrinder A, Hellqvist E, Sidorova E, et al. A new perspective: molecular motifs on oxidized LDL, apoptotic cells, and bacteria are targets for chronic lymphocytic leukemia antibodies. *Blood*. 2008;111(7):3838–3848.

70 Hwang KK, Trama AM, Kozink DM, et al. IGHV1-69 B cell chronic lymphocytic leukemia antibodies cross-react with HIV-1 and hepatitis C virus antigens as well as intestinal commensal bacteria. *PLoS One*. 2014;9:e90725.

71 Chu CC, Catera R, Zhang L, et al. Many chronic lymphocytic leukemia antibodies recognize apoptotic cells with exposed nonmuscle myosin heavy chain IIA: implications for patient outcome and cell of origin. *Blood*. 2010;115(19):3907–3015.

72 Duhren-von Minden M, Ubelhart R, Schneider D, et al. Chronic lymphocytic leukaemia is driven by antigen-independent cell-autonomous signalling. *Nature*. 2012;489(7415):309–312.

73 Binder M, Muller F, Frick M, et al. CLL B-cell receptors can recognize themselves: alternative epitopes and structural clues for autostimulatory mechanisms in CLL. *Blood*. 2013;121(1):239–241.

74 Herishanu Y, Perez-Galan P, Liu D, et al. The lymph node microenvironment promotes B-cell receptor signaling, NF-kappaB activation, and tumor proliferation in chronic lymphocytic leukemia. *Blood*. 2011;117(2):563–574.

75 ten Hacken E, Scielzo C, Bertilaccio MT, et al. Targeting the LYN/HS1 signaling axis in chronic lymphocytic leukemia. *Blood*. 2013; 121(12):2264–2273.

76 Mocsai A, Ruland J, Tybulewicz VL. The SYK tyrosine kinase: a crucial player in diverse biological functions. *Nat Rev Immunol*. 2010;10(6):387–402.

77 Oellerich T, Bremes V, Neumann K, et al. The B-cell antigen receptor signals through a preformed transducer module of SLP65 and CIN85. *EMBO J*. 2011;30(17):3620–3634.

78 Weber M, Treanor B, Depoil D, et al. Phospholipase C-gamma2 and Vav cooperate within signaling microclusters to propagate B cell spreading in response to membrane-bound antigen. *J Exp Med*. 2008;205(4):853–868.

79 Kim YJ, Sekiya F, Poulin B, Bae YS, Rhee SG. Mechanism of B-cell receptor-induced phosphorylation and activation of phospholipase C-gamma2. *Mol Cell Biol*. 2004;24(22):9986–9999.

80 de Gorter DJ, Beuling EA, Kersseboom R, et al. Bruton's tyrosine kinase and phospholipase Cgamma2 mediate chemokine-controlled B cell migration and homing. *Immunity*. 2007;26(1):93–104.

81 Spaargaren M, Beuling EA, Rurup ML, et al. The B cell antigen receptor controls integrin activity through Btk and PLCgamma2. *J Exp Med*. 2003;198(10):1539–1550.

82 Kubo T, Uchida Y, Watanabe Y, et al. Augmented TLR9-induced Btk activation in PIR-B-deficient B-1 cells provokes excessive autoantibody production and autoimmunity. *J Exp Med*. 2009;206(9):1971–1982.

83 Petro JB, Khan WN. Phospholipase C-gamma 2 couples Bruton's tyrosine kinase to the NF-kappaB signaling pathway in B lymphocytes. *J Biol Chem*. 2001;276(9):1715–1719.

84 Petro JB, Rahman SM, Ballard DW, Khan WN. Bruton's tyrosine kinase is required for activation of IkappaB kinase and nuclear factor kappaB in response to B cell receptor engagement. *J Exp Med*. 2000;191(10):1745–1754.

85 Nore BF, Vargas L, Mohamed AJ, et al. Redistribution of Bruton's tyrosine kinase by activation of phosphatidylinositol 3-kinase and Rho-family GTPases. *Eur J Immunol*. 2000;30(1):145–154.

86 Maurer U, Charvet C, Wagman AS, Dejardin E, Green DR. Glycogen synthase kinase-3 regulates mitochondrial outer membrane permeabilization and apoptosis by destabilization of MCL-1. *Mol Cell*. 2006;21(6):749–760.

87 Miletic AV, Anzelon-Mills AN, Mills DM, et al. Coordinate suppression of B cell lymphoma by PTEN and SHIP phosphatases. *J Exp Med*. 2010;207(11):2407–2420.

88 Baracho GV, Miletic AV, Omori SA, Cato MH, Rickert RC. Emergence of the PI3-kinase pathway as a central modulator of normal and aberrant B cell differentiation. *Curr Opin Immunol*. 2011;23(2):178–183.

89 Ramadani F, Bolland DJ, Garcon F, et al. The PI3K isoforms p110alpha and p110delta are essential for pre-B cell receptor signaling and B cell development. *Sci Signal*. 2010;3(134):ra60.

90 Lam KP, Kuhn R, Rajewsky K. In vivo ablation of surface immunoglobulin on mature B cells by inducible gene targeting results in rapid cell death. *Cell*. 1997;90(6):1073–1083.

91 Delgado P, Cubelos B, Calleja E, et al. Essential function for the GTPase TC21 in homeostatic antigen receptor signaling. *Nat Immunol*. 2009;10(8):880–888.

92 Contri A, Brunati AM, Trentin L, et al. Chronic lymphocytic leukemia B cells contain anomalous Lyn tyrosine kinase, a putative contribution to defective apoptosis. *J Clin Invest*. 2005;115(2):369–378.

93 Xu Y, Harder KW, Huntington ND, Hibbs ML, Tarlinton DM. Lyn tyrosine kinase: accentuating the positive and the negative. *Immunity*. 2005;22(1):9–18.

94 Rickert RC. New insights into pre-BCR and BCR signalling with relevance to B cell malignancies. *Nat Rev Immunol*. 2013;13:578–591.

95 Herishanu Y, Katz BZ, Lipsky A, Wiestner A. Biology of chronic lymphocytic leukemia in different microenvironments: clinical and therapeutic implications. *Hematol Oncol Clin North Am*. 2013;27:173–206.

96 Billard C. Apoptosis inducers in chronic lymphocytic leukemia. *Oncotarget*. 2014;5(2):309–325.

97 Calin GA, Dumitru CD, Shimizu M, et al. Frequent deletions and down-regulation of micro-RNA genes miR15 and miR16 at 13q14 in chronic lymphocytic leukemia. *Proc Natl Acad Sci U S A*. 2002;99(24):15524–15529.

98 Smit LA, Hallaert DY, Spijker R, et al. Differential Noxa/Mcl-1 balance in peripheral versus lymph node chronic lymphocytic leukemia cells correlates with survival capacity. *Blood*. 2007;109(4):1660–1668.

99 Campas C, Cosialls AM, Barragan M, et al. Bcl-2 inhibitors induce apoptosis in chronic lymphocytic leukemia cells. *Exp Hematol*. 2006;34(12):1663–1669.

100 Zucchetto A, Benedetti D, Tripodo C, et al. CD38/CD31, the CCL3 and CCL4 chemokines, and CD49 d/vascular cell adhesion molecule-1 are interchained by sequential events sustaining chronic lymphocytic leukemia cell survival. *Cancer Res*. 2009;69(9):4001–4009.

101 ten Hacken E, Burger JA. Molecular pathways: targeting the microenvironment in chronic lymphocytic leukemia–focus on the B-cell receptor. *Clin Cancer Res*. 2014;20(3):548–556.

102 Stamatopoulos B, Meuleman N, De Bruyn C, et al. AMD3100 disrupts the cross-talk between chronic lymphocytic leukemia cells and a mesenchymal stromal or nurse-like cell-based microenvironment: preclinical evidence for its association with chronic lymphocytic leukemia treatments. *Haematologica*. 2012;97(4):608–615.

103 Blachly JS, Byrd JC. Emerging drug profile: cyclin-dependent kinase inhibitors. *Leuk Lymphoma*. 2013;54(10):2133–2143.

104 Sehn LH, Assouline SE, Stewart DA, et al. A phase 1 study of obinutuzumab induction followed by 2 years of maintenance in patients with relapsed CD20-positive B-cell malignancies. *Blood*. 2012;119:5118–51125.

105 Goede V, Fischer K, Busch R, et al. Obinutuzumab plus chlorambucil in patients with CLL and coexisting conditions. *N Engl J Med*. 2014;370(12):1101–1110.

106 Wierda WG, Kipps TJ, Mayer J, et al. Hx-CD20-406 Study Investigators. Ofatumumab as single-agent CD20 immunotherapy in fludarabine-refractory chronic lymphocytic leukemia. *J Clin Oncol*. 2010;28:1749–1755.

107 Wierda WG, Kipps TJ, Durig J, et al. 407 Study Investigators. Chemoimmunotherapy with O-FC in previously untreated patients with chronic lymphocytic leukemia. *Blood*. 2011;117(24):6450–6458.

108 Jain P, O'Brien S. Anti-CD20 monoclonal antibodies in chronic lymphocytic leukemia. *Expert Opin Biol Ther*. 2013;13:169–182.

109 Teeling JL, Mackus WJ, Wiegman LJ, et al. The biological activity of human CD20 monoclonal antibodies is linked to unique epitopes on CD20. *J Immunol*. 2006;177(1):362–371.

110 Teeling JL, French RR, Cragg MS, et al. Characterization of new human CD20 monoclonal antibodies with potent cytolytic activity against non-Hodgkin lymphomas. *Blood*. 2004;104(6):1793–1800.

111 Rafiq S, Butchar JP, Cheney C, et al. Comparative assessment of clinically utilized CD20-directed antibodies in chronic lymphocytic leukemia cells reveals divergent NK cell, monocyte, and macrophage properties. *J Immunol*. 2013;190(6):2702–2711.

112 Barth MJ, Hernandez-Ilizaliturri FJ, Mavis C, et al. Ofatumumab demonstrates activity against rituximab-sensitive and -resistant cell lines, lymphoma xenografts and primary tumour cells from patients with B-cell lymphoma. *Br J Haematol*. 2012;156(4):490–498.

113 Li B, Zhao L, Guo H, et al: Characterization of a rituximab variant with potent antitumor activity against rituximab-resistant B-cell lymphoma. *Blood*. 2009;114(4):5007–5015.

114 Wierda WG, Kipps TJ, Mayer J, et al: Final analysis from the international trial of single-agent ofatumumab in patients with fludarabine-refractory chronic lymphocytic leukemia. *ASH Annual Meeting Abstracts*. 2010;116:921.

115 Wierda WG, Gupta IV, Lisby S, and Österborg A; On behalf of the Hx-CD20–406 Study Investigators. Pretreatment characteristics correlated with outcomes in patients with fludarabine-refractory CLL treated with ofatumumab: final response analysis. *Ann Oncol*. 22(suppl. 2):Abstract.

116 Wierda WG, Padmanabhan S, Chan GW, et al. Hx-CD20-406 Study Investigators. Ofatumumab is active in patients with fludarabine-refractory CLL irrespective of prior rituximab: results from the phase 2 international study. *Blood*. 2011;118(19):5126–5129.

117 Coiffier B, Lepretre S, Pedersen LM, et al. Safety and efficacy of ofatumumab, a fully human monoclonal anti-CD20 antibody, in patients with relapsed or refractory B-cell chronic lymphocytic leukemia: a phase 1–2 study. *Blood*. 2008;111(3):1094–1100.

118 Teichman ML, Ho Viet Q., Balducci, et al. Efficacy of ofatumumab and high-dose methylprednisolone for the treatment of relapsed or refractory chronic lymphocytic leukemia (CLL). *ASH Annual Meeting Abstracts*. 2011;118:4619.

119 Brychtova Y, Panovska A, Trizuljak J, et al. Ofatumumab added to dexamethasone in patients with relapsed or refractory chronic lymphocytic leukemia. Results from a phase II study of the Czech leukemia study group for life. *Blood*. 2013;122:2877.

120 Flinn IW, Harwin WN, Ward P, et al: Phase II Trial of ofatumumab (OFA) for older patients and patients who refuse fludarabine-based regimens with previously untreated chronic lymphocytic leukemia (CLL) or small lymphocytic lymphoma (SLL). *ASH Annual Meeting Abstracts*. 2012;120:719.

121 Shanafelt T, Lanasa MC, Call TG, et al. Ofatumumab-based chemoimmunotherapy is effective and well tolerated in patients with previously untreated chronic lymphocytic leukemia (CLL). *Cancer*. 2013;119(21):3788–3796.

122 Hillmen P, Robak T, Janssens A, et al. Chlorambucil plus ofatumumab versus chlorambucil alone in previously untreated patients with chronic lymphocytic leukaemia (COMPLEMENT 1): a randomised, multicentre, open-label phase 3 trial. *E Pub - Lancet*. 2015.

123 Jaglowski SM JJ, Flynn JM,Andritsos LA, Maddocks KJ, Blum KA. A phase Ib/II study evaluating activity and tolerability of BTK inhibitor PCI-32765 and ofatumumab in patients with chronic lymphocytic leukemia/small lymphocytic lymphoma (CLL/SLL) and related diseases. *J Clin Oncol*. 2012;30, suppl. ASCO Abstract 6508.

124 De Vos S, Leonard JP, Barrientos JC, et al. A phase 1 study of the selective PI3Kδ inhibitor Idelalisib (GS-1101) in combination with therapeutic anti-CD20 antibodies (Rituximab or Ofatumumab) in patients with relapsed or refractory chronic lymphocytic leukemia. *Blood*. 2013;122:4180.

125 Herter S, Herting F, Mundigl O, et al. Preclinical activity of the type II CD20 antibody GA101 (obinutuzumab) compared with rituximab and ofatumumab in vitro and in xenograft models. *Mol Cancer Ther*. 2013;12(10):2031–2042.

126 Mao Z, Quintanilla-Martinez L, Raffeld M, et al. IgVH mutational status and clonality analysis of Richter's transformation: diffuse large B-cell lymphoma and Hodgkin lymphoma in association with B-cell chronic lymphocytic leukemia (B-CLL) represent 2 different pathways of disease evolution. *Am J Surg Pathol*. 2007;31(10):1605–1614.

127 O'Brien S, Kingsley CD, Eradat H, et al: Safety and efficacy of obinutuzumab (GA101) with fludarabine/cyclophosphamide (G-FC) or bendamustine (G-B) in the initial therapy of patients with chronic lymphocytic leukemia (CLL): results from the phase 1b Galton trial (GAO4779g). *Blood*. 2013;122:523.

128 Le Garff-Tavernier M, Herbi L, de Romeuf C, et al. Antibody-dependent cellular cytotoxicity of the optimized anti-CD20 monoclonal antibody ublituximab on chronic lymphocytic leukemia cells with the 17p deletion. *Leukemia*. 2014;28:230–233.

129 Cazin B, Lepretre S, Coiffier B, et al: Multicentre phase I study with an 8-dose regimen of single agent anti-CD20 monoclonal antibody LFB-R603 in patients with relapsed chronic lymphocytic leukemia (CLL). *ASH Annual Meeting Abstracts*. 2011;118:2862.

130 Goldenberg DM, Rossi EA, Stein R, et al. Properties and structure-function relationships of veltuzumab (hA20), a humanized anti-CD20 monoclonal antibody. *Blood*. 2009;113(5):1062–1070.

131 Morschhauser F, Leonard JP, Fayad L, et al. Humanized anti-CD20 antibody, veltuzumab, in refractory/recurrent non-Hodgkin's lymphoma: phase I/II results. *J Clin Oncol*. 2009;27(5):3346–3353.

132 Morschhauser F, Marlton P, Vitolo U, et al. Results of a phase I/II study of ocrelizumab, a fully humanized anti-CD20 mAb, in patients with relapsed/refractory follicular lymphoma. *Ann Oncol*. 2010;21:1870–1876.

133 Cheney CM, Stephens DM, Mo X, et al. Ocaratuzumab, an Fc-engineered antibody demonstrates enhanced antibody-dependent cell-mediated cytotoxicity in chronic lymphocytic leukemia. *MAbs*. 2014;6:748–754.

134 Bowles JA, Wang SY, Link BK, et al. Anti-CD20 monoclonal antibody with enhanced affinity for CD16 activates NK cells at lower concentrations and more effectively than rituximab. *Blood*. 2006;108(8):2648–2654.

135 Hillmen P, Skotnicki AB, Robak T, et al. Alemtuzumab compared with chlorambucil as first-line therapy for chronic lymphocytic leukemia. *J Clin Oncol*. 2007;25(35):5616–5623.

136 Parikh SA, Keating MJ, O'Brien S, et al. Frontline chemoimmunotherapy with fludarabine, cyclophosphamide, alemtuzumab, and rituximab for high-risk chronic lymphocytic leukemia. *Blood*. 2011;118(8):2062–2068.

137 Geisler CH, van T'Veer MB, Jurlander J, et al. Frontline low-dose alemtuzumab with fludarabine and cyclophosphamide prolongs progression-free survival in high-risk chronic lymphocytic leukemia: a randomized trial. *Blood*. 2014;123(21):3255–3262.

138 Lozanski G, Heerema NA, Flinn IW, et al. Alemtuzumab is an effective therapy for chronic lymphocytic leukemia with p53 mutations and deletions. *Blood*. 2004;103(9):3278–3281.

139 Fiegl M, Stauder R, Steurer M, et al; Austrian Collaborative Study Group on Alemtuzumab in Chronic Lymphocytic Leukemia, in

cooperation with The Czech Leukemia Study Group for Life, CELL. Alemtuzumab in chronic lymphocytic leukemia: final results of a large observational multicenter study in mostly pretreated patients. *Ann Hematol.* 2014;93:267–277.

140 Robak T, Robak P. Anti-CD37 antibodies for chronic lymphocytic leukemia. *Expert Opin Biol Ther.* 2014;14(5):651–661.

141 Byrd JC, Pagel JM, Awan FT, et al. A phase 1 study evaluating the safety and tolerability of otlertuzumab, an anti-CD37 mono-specific ADAP-TIR therapeutic protein in chronic lymphocytic leukemia. *Blood.* 2014;123(9):1302–1308.

142 Byrd JC, Kipps TJ, Flinn IW, et al. Phase I study of the anti-CD40 humanized monoclonal antibody lucatumumab (HCD122) in relapsed chronic lymphocytic leukemia. *Leuk Lymphoma.* 2012;53(11):2136–2142.

143 Furman RR, Forero-Torres A, Shustov A, Drachman JG. A phase I study of dacetuzumab (SGN-40, a humanized anti-CD40 monoclonal antibody) in patients with chronic lymphocytic leukemia. *Leuk Lymphoma.* 2010;51(2):228–235.

144 Chang BY, Francesco M, De Rooij MF, et al. Egress of CD19(+)CD5(+) cells into peripheral blood following treatment with the Bruton tyrosine kinase inhibitor ibrutinib in mantle cell lymphoma patients. *Blood* 2013;122(14):2412–2424.

145 Woyach JA, Smucker K, Smith LL, et al. Prolonged lymphocytosis during ibrutinib therapy is associated with distinct molecular characteristics and does not indicate a suboptimal response to therapy. *Blood.* 2014;123(12):1810–1817.

146 de Rooij MF, Kuil A, Geest CR, et al. The clinically active BTK inhibitor PCI-32765 targets B-cell receptor- and chemokine-controlled adhesion and migration in chronic lymphocytic leukemia. *Blood.* 2012;119(11):2590–2594.

147 Herman SE, Niemann CU, Farooqui M, et al. Ibrutinib-induced lymphocytosis in patients with chronic lymphocytic leukemia: correlative analyses from a phase II study. *Leukemia.* 2014;28(11):2188–2196.

148 Furman RR, Fowler N, Coutre SE, et al. The Bruton's tyrosine kinase (BTK) inhibitor ibrutinib (PCI-32765) monotherapy demonstrates long-term safety and durability of response in chronic lymphocytic leukemia (CLL)/small lymphocytic lymphoma (SLL) patients in an open-label extension study. *Blood.* 2013;122(26):4163.

149 Cheson BD, Byrd JC, Rai KR, et al. Novel targeted agents and the need to refine clinical end points in chronic lymphocytic leukemia. *J Clin Oncol.* 2012;30(23):2820–2822.

150 Farooqui M, Jones J, Valdez J, et al. In patients with chronic lymphocytic leukemia (CLL) ibrutinib effectively reduces clonal IgM paraproteins and serum free light chains while increasing normal IgM, IgA serum levels, suggesting a nascent recovery of humoral immunity. *Blood.* 2013;122:4182.

151 O'Brien S, Furman RR, Coutre SE, et al. Ibrutinib as initial therapy for elderly patients with chronic lymphocytic leukaemia or small lymphocytic lymphoma: an open-label, multicentre, phase 1b/2 trial. *Lancet Oncol.* 2014;15:48–58.

152 Keating MJ, Wierda WG, Hoellenriegel J, et al. Ibrutinib in combination with Rituximab (iR) is well tolerated and induces a high rate of durable remissions in patients with high-risk chronic lymphocytic leukemia (CLL): new, updated results of a phase II trial in 40 patients. *Blood.* 2013;122:675.

153 Barrientos JC, Barr PM, Flinn I, et al. Ibrutinib in combination with bendamustine and rituximab is active and tolerable in patients with relapsed/refractory CLL/SLL: final results of a phase 1b study. *Blood.* 2013;122:525.

154 Byrd JC, Brown JR, O'Brien S, et al. RESONATE Investigators. Ibrutinib versus ofatumumab in previously treated chronic lymphoid leukemia. *N Engl J Med.* 2014;371(3):213–223.

155 Woyach JA, Furman RR, Liu TM, et al. Resistance mechanisms for the Bruton's tyrosine kinase inhibitor ibrutinib. *N Engl J Med.* 2014;370(24):2286–2294.

156 Landau D, Hoellenriegel J, Sougnez C, et al. Clonal evolution in patients with chronic lymphocytic leukemia (CLL) developing resistance to BTK inhibition. *Blood.* 2013;122(7):866.

157 Harb WA, Hill BT, Gabrilove J, et al. Phase 1 study of single agent CC-292, a highly selective bruton's tyrosine kinase (BTK) inhibitor, in relapsed/refractory chronic lymphocytic leukemia (CLL). *Blood.* 2013;122:1630.

158 Karlin L, Rule S, Shah N, et al: A phase I study of the oral btk inhibitor ONO-4059 in patients with relapsed/refractory and high risk chronic lymphocytic leukaemia (CLL). *Blood.* 2013;122:676.

159 Fiorcari S, Brown WS, McIntyre BW, et al. The PI3-kinase delta inhibitor idelalisib (GS-1101) targets integrin-mediated adhesion of chronic lymphocytic leukemia (CLL) cell to endothelial and marrow stromal cells. *PLoS One.* 2013;8:e83830.

160 Lannutti BJ, Meadows SA, Herman SE, et al. CAL-101, a p110delta selective phosphatidylinositol-3-kinase inhibitor for the treatment of B-cell malignancies, inhibits PI3K signaling and cellular viability. *Blood.* 2011;117(2):591–594.

161 Brown JR, Byrd JC, Coutre SE, et al. Idelalisib, an inhibitor of phosphatidylinositol 3-kinase p110delta, for relapsed/refractory chronic lymphocytic leukemia. *Blood.* 2014;123:3390–3397.

162 Furman RR, Sharman JP, Coutre SE, et al. Idelalisib and rituximab in relapsed chronic lymphocytic leukemia. *N Engl J Med.* 2014;370(11):997–1007.

163 Patel M, Kahl BS, Horwitz SM, et al. Preliminary safety and efficacy of IPI-145, a potent inhibitor of phosphoinositide-3-Kinase-δ,γ, in patients with chronic lymphocytic leukemia. *Blood.* 2013;122:677.

164 Glenn M, Mato AR, Allgood SD, et al. First-in-human study of AMG 319, a highly selective, small molecule inhibitor of PI3Kδ, in adult patients with relapsed or refractory lymphoid malignancies. *Blood.* 2013;122:678.

165 Uno JK, Rao KN, Matsuoka K, et al. Altered macrophage function contributes to colitis in mice defective in the phosphoinositide-3 kinase subunit p110δ. *Gastroenterology.* 2010;139(5):1642–1653.

166 Friedberg JW, Sharman J, Sweetenham J, et al. Inhibition of Syk with fostamatinib disodium has significant clinical activity in non-Hodgkin lymphoma and chronic lymphocytic leukemia. *Blood.* 2010;115(13):2578–2585.

167 Sharman JP, KLM, Boxer M, et al. Phase 2 trial of GS-9973, a selective Syk inhibitor, in chronic lymphocytic leukemia (CLL). *J Clin Oncol.* 2014;32:5s (suppl.; abstract 7007).

168 Burke RT, Meadows S, Loriaux MM, et al. A potential therapeutic strategy for chronic lymphocytic leukemia by combining Idelalisib and GS-9973, a novel spleen tyrosine kinase (Syk) inhibitor. *Oncotarget.* 2014;5(4):908–915.

169 Barr PM, Saylors GB, Spurgeon SEF, et al. Phase 2 trial of GS-9973, a selective syk inhibitor, and idelalisib (idela) in chronic lymphocytic leukemia (CLL) and non-Hodgkin lymphoma (NHL). *J Clin Oncol.* 2014;32:5s (suppl.; abstract 7059).

170 Zent CS, LaPlant BR, Johnston PB, et al. The treatment of recurrent/refractory chronic lymphocytic leukemia/small lymphocytic lymphoma (CLL) with everolimus results in clinical responses and mobilization of CLL cells into the circulation. *Cancer.* 2010;116(9):2201–2207.

171  Amrein PC, Attar EC, Takvorian T, et al. Phase II study of dasatinib in relapsed or refractory chronic lymphocytic leukemia. *Clin Cancer Res.* 2011;17(9):2977–2986.

172  Kater AP, Spiering M, Liu RD, et al. Dasatinib in combination with fludarabine in patients with refractory chronic lymphocytic leukemia: a multicenter phase 2 study. *Leuk Res.* 2014;38(1):34–41.

173  Decker S, Finter J, Forde AJ, et al. PIM kinases are essential for chronic lymphocytic leukemia cell survival (PIM2/3) and CXCR4-mediated microenvironmental interactions (PIM1). *Mol Cancer Ther.* 2014;13(5):1231–1245.

174  Chen LS, Redkar S, Bearss D, Wierda WG, Gandhi V. Pim kinase inhibitor, SGI-1776, induces apoptosis in chronic lymphocytic leukemia cells. *Blood.* 2009;114(19):4150–4157.

175  Ghosh AK, Secreto C, Boysen J, et al: The novel receptor tyrosine kinase Axl is constitutively active in B-cell chronic lymphocytic leukemia and acts as a docking site of nonreceptor kinases: implications for therapy. *Blood.* 2011;117(6):1928–1937.

176  Boysen J, Sinha S, Price-Troska T, et al. The tumor suppressor axis p53/miR-34a regulates Axl expression in B-cell chronic lymphocytic leukemia: implications for therapy in p53-defective CLL patients. *Leukemia.* 2014;28(2):451–455.

177  Daneshmanesh AH, Hojjat-Farsangi M, Khan AS, et al. Monoclonal antibodies against ROR1 induce apoptosis of chronic lymphocytic leukemia (CLL) cells. *Leukemia.*2012; 26(6):1348–1355.

178  Hudecek M, Schmitt TM, Baskar S, et al. The B-cell tumor-associated antigen ROR1 can be targeted with T cells modified to express a ROR1-specific chimeric antigen receptor. *Blood.* 2010;116(22):4532–4541.

179  Lutzny G, Kocher T, Schmidt-Supprian M, et al. Protein kinase c-beta-dependent activation of NF-kappaB in stromal cells is indispensable for the survival of chronic lymphocytic leukemia B cells in vivo. *Cancer Cell.* 2013;23(1):77–92.

180  Ringshausen I, Oelsner M, Weick K, Bogner C, Peschel C, Decker T. Mechanisms of apoptosis-induction by rottlerin: therapeutic implications for B-CLL. *Leukemia.* 2006;20(3):514–520.

181  Prins RC, Burke RT, Tyner JW, Druker BJ, Loriaux MM, Spurgeon SE. CX-4945, a selective inhibitor of casein kinase-2 (CK2), exhibits anti-tumor activity in hematologic malignancies including enhanced activity in chronic lymphocytic leukemia when combined with fludarabine and inhibitors of the B-cell receptor pathway. *Leukemia.* 2013;27(10):2094–2096.

182  O'Brien S, Moore JO, Boyd TE, et al. 5-year survival in patients with relapsed or refractory chronic lymphocytic leukemia in a randomized, phase III trial of fludarabine plus cyclophosphamide with or without oblimersen. *J Clin Oncol.* 2009;27(31):5208–5212.

183  O'Brien SM, Claxton DF, Crump M, et al. Phase I study of obatoclax mesylate (GX15–070), a small molecule pan-Bcl-2 family antagonist, in patients with advanced chronic lymphocytic leukemia. *Blood.* 2009;113(2):299–305.

184  Eradat H, Grosicki S, Catalono J, et al. Preliminary results of a phase II open-Label, randomized study of the BH3 mimetic protein navitoclax (ABT-263) with or without rituximab for treatment of previously untreated B-Cell chronic lymphocytic leukemia. *ASH Annual Meeting Abstracts.* 2012;120:190.

185  Souers AJ, Leverson JD, Boghaert ER, et al. ABT-199, a potent and selective BCL-2 inhibitor, achieves antitumor activity while sparing platelets. *Nat Med.* 2013;19(2):202–208.

186  Davids MS, Pagel JM, Kahl BS, et al. Bcl-2 Inhibitor ABT-199 (GDC-0199) monotherapy shows anti-tumor activity including complete remissions in high-risk relapsed/refractory (R/R) chronic lymphocytic leukemia (CLL) and small lymphocytic lymphoma (SLL). *Blood.* 2013;122:872.

187  Ma S. SJF, Lanasa MC, Kipps TJ, Barrientos JC, Davids MS. et al. ABT-199 (GDC-0199) combined with rituximab (R) in patients (pts) with relapsed/refractory (R/R) chronic lymphocytic leukemia (CLL): interim results of a phase 1b study. *J Clin Oncol.* 2014;32:5s (suppl.; abstract 7013).

188  Lin TS, Ruppert AS, Johnson AJ, et al. Phase II study of flavopiridol in relapsed chronic lymphocytic leukemia demonstrating high response rates in genetically high-risk disease. *J Clin Oncol.* 2009;27(35):6012–6018.

189  Stephens DM, Ruppert AS, Maddocks K, et al. Cyclophosphamide, alvocidib (flavopiridol), and rituximab, a novel feasible chemoimmunotherapy regimen for patients with high-risk chronic lymphocytic leukemia. *Leuk Res.* 2013;37(10):1195–1199.

190  Andritsos LA, Jones JA, Johnson AJ, et al. Dinaciclib (SCH 727965) is a novel cyclin-dependent kinase (CDK) inhibitor that exhibits activity in patients with relapsed or refractory chronic lymphocytic leukemia (CLL). *Blood.* 2013;122:871.

191  Burger M, Hartmann T, Krome M, et al. Small peptide inhibitors of the CXCR4 chemokine receptor (CD184) antagonize the activation, migration, and antiapoptotic responses of CXCL12 in chronic lymphocytic leukemia B cells. *Blood.* 2005;106(5):1824–1830.

192  Andritsos L, Byrd J, Hewes B, Kipps T, Johns D, Burger J. Preliminary results from a phase I dose escalation study to determine the maximum tolerated dose of plerixafor in combination with rituximab in patients with relapsed chronic lymphocytic leukemia. *Haematologica.* 2010;95(suppl. 2):321, Abstracts 0772, 2010.

193  Zhong Y, El-Gamal D, Dubovsky JA, et al. Selinexor suppresses downstream effectors of B-cell activation, proliferation and migration in chronic lymphocytic leukemia cells. *Leukemia.* 2014;28(5):1158–1163.

194  Gutierrez M, Shah BD, Gabrail NY, et al. Preliminary evidence of anti tumor activity of selinexor (KPT-330) in a phase I trial of a first-in-class oral selective inhibitor of nuclear export (SINE) in patients (pts) with relapsed/refractory non Hodgkin's lymphoma (NHL) and chronic lymphocytic leukemia (CLL). *Blood.* 2013;122:90.

195  Gowda A, Roda J, Hussain SR, et al. IL-21 mediates apoptosis through up-regulation of the BH3 family member BIM and enhances both direct and antibody-dependent cellular cytotoxicity in primary chronic lymphocytic leukemia cells in vitro. *Blood.* 2008;111:4723–4730.

196  Timmerman JM, Byrd JC, Andorsky DJ, et al. A phase I dose-finding trial of recombinant interleukin-21 and rituximab in relapsed and refractory low grade B-cell lymphoproliferative disorders. *Clin Cancer Res.* 2012;18(20):5752–5760.

## CHAPTER 14

# Multiple Myeloma

*Giada Bianchi and Kenneth C. Anderson*

LeBow Institute for Myeloma Therapeutics and Jerome Lipper Myeloma Center, Department of Medical Oncology,
Dana-Farber Cancer Institute, Harvard Medical School, Boston, MA, USA

## MM as a Neoplastic Factory of Immunoglobulins: Biologic and Clinical Implications

### The Importance of Protein Synthesis in MM Oncogenesis

Multiple myeloma (MM) is the second most common hematologic cancer in the United States, with 26,850 new cases and 11,240 deaths estimated for the year 2015, typically affecting the elderly with a median age at diagnosis of 69 years.[1] MM evolves from monoclonal gammopathy of undetermined significance (MGUS), a common premalignant condition characterized by 1% per year risk of evolution into MM or a related malignancy.[2] The final oncogenic events in the transformation from MGUS and MM appear to take place in the postgerminal center stage of B lymphopoiesis within the bone marrow (BM) microenvironment (Figure 14.1).[3] Specifically, MM is the malignant transformation of BM-resident, long-lived plasma cells (PC) and retains the capability of synthesizing large amounts of monoclonal immunoglobulin (Ig) or light chain only, detectable via serum and/or urine protein electrophoresis, immunofixation, and/or serum-free light chain assay.[4] The transcription factor X-box binding protein 1 (XBP-1) is necessary for proper Ig-secreting PC differentiation during physiologic B lymphopoiesis.[5] The spliced form of XBP-1 (sXBP-1) is the terminal effector of the inositol-requiring transmembrane kinase/endonuclease 1α (IRE-1α) branch of the unfolded protein response (UPR), a phylogenetically highly conserved, tripartite, and adaptive response of eukaryotic cells to stress derived from increased *de novo* protein synthesis and/or misfolding.[6]

The observation that forced expression of sXBP-1 in B-cell precursors led to the development of an MM-like disease in a murine model, and that sXBP-1 is highly expressed in primary MM cells and correlates with poor overall survival (OS), raised interest in this molecule as a therapeutic target in MM.[7]

Quality control mechanisms involved in DNA replication, RNA transcription, and protein translation are novel molecular targets for cancer therapy.[8] Since MM represents the paradigm of secretory cancers, an intact endoplasmic reticulum (ER) quality control including UPR branches, molecular chaperones, and ER-associated degradation (ERAD), is necessary to ensure adequate folding and/or disposal of newly synthesized proteins as well as avoidance of proteotoxic stress.[9] As discussed in the following sections, several molecular targets of anti-MM therapy have been identified among proteins mediating these processes (Figure 14.2).

### Disrupting the UPR and ER Quality Control

XBP-1 is the only known substrate of IRE-1α endoribonuclease activity, while its kinase activity is necessary for trans-autophosphorylation and activation of the c-Jun N-terminal kinase (JNK) pathway.[10] Efforts have been directed to develop specific pharmacologic inhibitors of IRE-1α endoribonuclease activity while sparing the kinase activity, in order to avoid a paradoxical antiapoptotic effect due to JNK inhibition. IRE-1α endoribonuclease activity inhibitors STF-083010 and MKC-3946 showed significant activity in a murine model of MM, alone and in combination with bortezomib, and are promising molecules for further clinical development.[11,12]

Inhibitors of molecular chaperones, particularly heat shock protein 90 (HSP90), have also been examined in MM. Since HSP90 is implicated in the conformation and signaling of oncogenes, including tyrosine kinase receptors, cell cycle molecules, transcription factors, and antiapoptotic proteins, blockade of HSP90 may inhibit multiple targets at the same time.[13] Clinical development of the HSP90 inhibitor tanespimycin (17-AAG, KOS-953), did not achieve objective clinical responses as a single agent in MM and solid malignancies. However, a 27% overall response rate (ORR) was observed when combined with bortezomib.[14] The development of second-generation, geldanamycin-derived HSP90 inhibitors was discontinued due to intolerable toxicities, in particular transaminitis and liver failure.[15] The resorcinol derivatives NVP-AUY922 (VER52296) and KW-2478 showed promising anti-MM activity alone or in combination with bortezomib *in vitro*, and are currently being evaluated in phase I/II clinical trials in combination with bortezomib.[16,17]

### Blocking the Ubiquitin-Proteasome System

Native proteins incapable of achieving a stable tertiary/quaternary conformation represent a danger for cell homeostasis and are quickly disposed of.[18] In eukaryotic cells, the ubiquitin-proteasome system (UPS) accounts for the bulk of degradation of these misfolded proteins (Figure 14.2).[19] The proteasome is an ATP-dependent, multicatalytic complex organized in a 20S core composed of two outer heptameric α rings and two inner heptameric β rings containing the catalytic activities and one 19S regulatory cap at

*Targeted Therapy in Translational Cancer Research*, First Edition. Edited by Apostolia-Maria Tsimberidou, Razelle Kurzrock and Kenneth C. Anderson.
© 2016 John Wiley & Sons, Inc. Published 2016 by John Wiley & Sons, Inc.

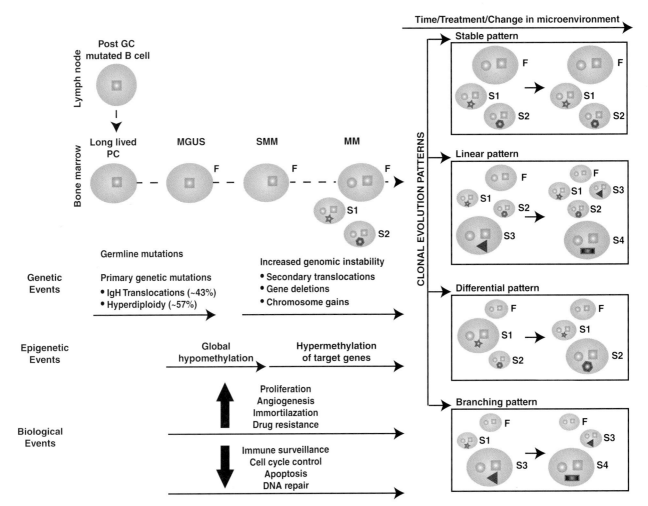

**Figure 14.1** Pathogenesis of MM. MM is the cancer transformation of BM-resident long-lived PC and evolves from the premalignant conditions MGUS and smoldering MM. Initial oncogenic events are hypothesized to take place during the process of immunoglobulin isotype switch and somatic hypermutation in the GC. Genetic, epigenetic, and biologic events are outlined along with the neoplastic evolution. Diverse patterns of clonal evolution have been recently identified in MM and are outlined here and are overall characterized by a progressive increase in genomic complexity culminating at the leukemic stage of MM.[105] Abbreviations: GC: germinal center; PC: plasma cell; MGUS: monoclonal gammopathy of undetermined significance; SMM: smoldering MM; MM: multiple myeloma; F: founder clone; S: subclone. Modified with permission from Reference 106.

each side. The caspase-like (C-L, β-1); trypsin-like (T-L, β-2); and chymotrypsin-like (CT-L β-5) proteolytic sites can be replaced by their respective inducible subunits (β1i or LMP2, β2i or MECL-1, and β5i or LMP7) in an interferon-γ driven process, thus forming the immunoproteasome, abundantly expressed in MM cells.[20]

Initially implemented as biochemistry tools to study proteolysis, proteasome inhibitors (PIs) were discovered to be powerful antineoplastic *in vitro*, particularly against MM cells.[21] Despite initial concerns regarding PI therapeutic index, bortezomib, the first clinically implemented PI, proved remarkably active in heavily pretreated MM patients with tolerable toxicity, mainly in the form of peripheral neuropathy and cyclic thrombocytopenia.[22] Bortezomib reversibly inhibits the chymotrypsin-like and caspase-like activities of the proteasome.[23] In MM, it induces apoptosis and cell cycle arrest via multiple mechanisms, including cleavage of caspase 8 and 9; inhibition of canonical nuclear factor-κB (NF-κB) signaling via stabilization of inhibitor of NF-κB (IκB); and induction of JNK and the terminal branches of the UPR.[24] Recently, accumulation of polyubiqui-

tinated proteins was shown to correlate *in vitro* with sensitivity to PIs, consistent with proteotoxic stress as a molecular mechanism of effectiveness of PIs in MM.[25]

The APEX trial, a randomized, phase III study of bortezomib versus dexamethasone in relapsed/refractory MM patients showed a 43% ORR and a 6-month increment in median OS (29.8 months vs 23.7 months) for patients receiving the PI, despite significant crossover from the control to the treatment arm.[26] As front-line therapy in combination with melphalan and prednisone, bortezomib increased median OS from 43.1 to 56.4 months.[27] Bortezomib was FDA-approved as first-line therapy for MM in 2008 and in combination with immunomodulatory drugs (IMiDs) and steroids it is a mainstay of front-line treatment for both transplant eligible and ineligible patients.[28]

Having established the critical role of an intact UPS for survival of MM cells, second generation PIs have been developed aiming at broader or deeper inhibition of catalytic subunits, increased potency, improved side effect profile, and/or oral bioavailability

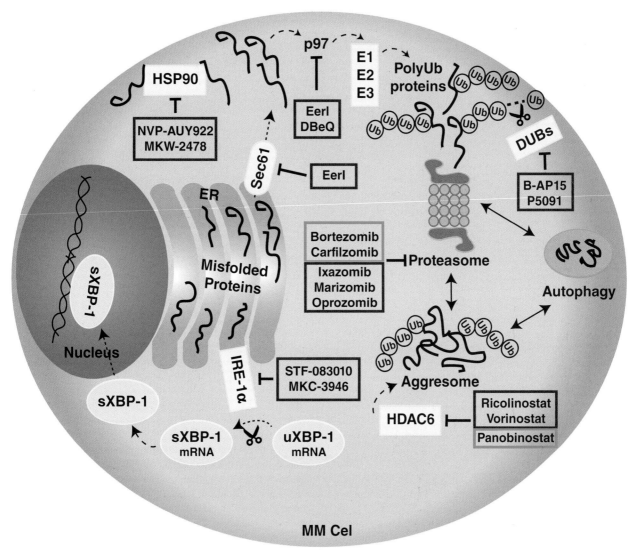

**Figure 14.2** Molecular targets in MM involved in protein synthesis, folding and disposal. The cartoon synthesizes the molecular targets identified along the processes of protein synthesis, folding and disposal, in particular along the ubiquitin-proteasome pathway and alternative proteolytic pathways. Green boxes outline FDA-approved while red boxes signify drugs currently being evaluated in clinical trials. Abbreviations: E1: ubiquitin-activating enzymes; E2: ubiquitin-conjugating enzymes; E3: ubiquitin ligase enzymes; Ub: ubiquitin; DUBs: deubiquitinating enzymes.

(Table 14.1).[29] Among these, carfilzomib was FDA-approved under the accelerated program in 2012 for treatment of MM patients who have progressed after at least two lines of therapy, including bortezomib and an IMiD. Carfilzomib is a peptide epoxyketone, irreversibly inhibiting the β5 and β5i proteasome subunits.[30] Approval was granted based on the results of an open-label, single-arm phase II study in relapsed/refractory MM patients showing an ORR of 23.7% and median OS of 15.6 months.[31] Peripheral neuropathy was negligible for rate (12.4%) and severity (mostly grade 1–2), however rare, but severe and occasionally fatal cardiac events, including congestive heart failure, cardiac arrest, and myocardial infarction were noted. Four phase III clinical trials are ongoing to confirm phase II results.[32]

Oprozomib is an orally bioavailable, carfilzomib-derived, PI, currently being evaluated in phase I/II trials in combination with IMiDs and dexamethasone. Oprozomib recapitulates carfilzomib for potency and spectrum of inhibition of proteasome activity and displayed a similar pattern of cytotoxicity in preclinical studies.[33]

MLN9708, an orally available PI, chemically related to bortezomib, is a reversible, specific inhibitor of chymotrypsin- and caspase-like activity.[34] After successful evaluation in the preclinical setting, phase I/II trials proved MLN9708 effective alone or in combination with lenalidomide and dexamethasone in newly diagnosed and relapsed/refractory MM patients.[35,36] A phase III trial, TOURMALINE-MM1, is currently evaluating the benefit of adding MLN9708 to lenalidomide and dexamethasone in relapsed/refractory MM patients.[32]

NPI-0052, a β-lactone-γ-lactam PI targeting all three catalytic subunits of the proteasome showed promising activity in preclinical studies even in primary MM cells derived from bortezomib-resistant patients.[38] Several phase I studies in solid and hematologic malignancies proved NPI-0052 to be well tolerated with no evidence

**Table 14.1** A comparison of proteasome inhibitors approved or in advanced clinical development.

| Name | Alternative names | Manufacturer | Chemical structure | Target subunits | Pattern of inhibition | Route of administration | Clinical development |
|---|---|---|---|---|---|---|---|
| Bortezomib | PS-341 Velcade | Millennium: The Takeda Oncology Co, Cambridge, MA | Boronic acid | CT-L, C-L | Reversible | IV/SC | FDA-approved, first line |
| Carfilzomib | PX-171 Kyprolis | Onyx Pharmaceuticals, South San Francisco, CA | Epoxyketone | CT-L | Irreversible | IV | FDA-approved, third line |
| Ixazomib | MLN-9708 | Millennium: The Takeda Oncology Co, Cambridge, MA | Boronic acid | CT-L, C-L | Reversible | IV/PO | Phase III |
| Marizomib | NPI-0052 salinosporamide A | Triphase Accelerator Co, San Diego, CA | Lactam/ β-lactone | CT-L, T-L, C-L | Irreversible | IV | Phase I/II |
| Oprozomib | ONX-0912 PR-047 | Onyx Pharmaceuticals, South San Francisco, CA | Epoxyketone | CT-L | Irreversible | PO | Phase I/II |

The table provides a comparison of chemical and pharmacologic characteristics of FDA-approved PIs and those in advanced clinical development.
CT-L, chymotrypsin-like; C-L, caspase-like; T-L, trypsin-like; IV, intravenous; SC, subcutaneous; PO, per os (oral).

of peripheral neuropathy.[37] It is currently evaluated in phase I and I/II clinical trials alone or in combination with pomalidomide and dexamethasone in patients with refractory/relapsed MM.[32]

Deubiquitinating enzymes (DUBs) are key for UPS homeostasis by removing ubiquitin from protein substrates, thus regulating proteasome-mediated degradation and ubiquitin-mediated signaling.[39] Deregulation in DUBs have been recognized in several pathogenic processes, including cancer.[40] Around 100 DUBs, with different client protein specificity, have been identified in humans, making them attractive molecular targets in oncology. B-AP15, a selective inhibitor of USP14 and UCHL5 DUBs, and P5091, a USP7 inhibitor, proved effective anti-MM drugs in preclinical studies.[41,42] Both drugs induced apoptosis in a broad range of MM cell lines and primary MM cells, including those derived from bortezomib-resistant patients, and both synergized with dexamethasone, the histone deacetylase (HDAC) inhibitor vorinostat (SAHA) and lenalidomide *in vitro*.

Another appealing target for MM is pharmacologic blockade of the ERAD. Eeyarestatin I (EerI) is a small molecule inhibitor of Sec61, thus blocking retrotranslocation of proteasome client-proteins from the ER. It also inhibits deubiquitination by targeting PAD and ATX3, thus providing another molecular mechanism of effectiveness in cancer. EerI induced apoptosis in various histologic cancer subtypes and synergized with bortezomib, arguing for its potential implementation in MM.[43]

### Blocking Alternative Proteolytic Pathways as a Strategy to Overcome PI Resistance

Eukaryotic cells are equipped with alternative proteolytic pathways that work in cooperation with the proteasome to dispose of misfolded/aged proteins and thus avoid proteotoxicity (Figure 14.2).[44]

In MM, proteasome inhibition results in induction of autophagy and aggresome formation, potentially representing a mechanism of PI-resistance.[45,46] The microtubule-associated protein HDAC6, a class II HDAC, is necessary for proper aggresome formation in face of proteotoxic stress.[47] The HDAC6-selective inhibitor ACY-1215 blocked aggresome formation in MM cells and synergized with bortezomib in preclinical studies.[48] Preliminary results of phase I/II trials of ACY-1215 alone or in combination with bortezomib/dexamethasone or lenalidomide/dexamethasone showed

good therapeutic index and promising activity in heavily pretreated MM patients.[49,50] HDACs are a family of enzymes mediating deacetylation of core histones, resulting in epigenetic inhibition of gene expression, and of other nonhistone proteins involved in crucial cellular processes. HDACs are often overexpressed in cancer, thus making them an appealing drug target.[51]

The pan-HDAC inhibitor panobinostat (LBH-589) and the class I and IIb inhibitor vorinostat (SAHA) have been evaluated in combination with PIs and IMiDs. A phase III, randomized, multicenter clinical trial comparing vorinostat/bortezomib versus bortezomib alone showed a modest, but statistically significant progression-free survival (PFS) benefit in the treatment arm (7.6 months vs 6.8 months, respectively, $p = 0.0100$). Significant adverse, hematologic events, in particular grade 3–4 thrombocytopenia (45% of patients) were noted in individuals receiving vorinostat.[52] A phase I trial of vorinostat in combination with lenalidomide and dexamethasone reported similar toxicity profile with optimistic preliminary data regarding clinical effectiveness.[53]

Panobinostat showed a similar side-effect profile with cytopenias, particularly thrombocytopenia, diarrhea, and fatigue, in a phase Ib clinical trial in combination with bortezomib and a phase II study with bortezomib/dexamethasone. Both studies showed a promising ORR (73.3% in the former and 34.5% in the latter), including responses in bortezomib-refractory patients.[54,55] In a phase III clinical study, the combination of panobinostat plus bortezomib resulted in a 4-month improvement in PFS (12 versus 8 months, respectively, $p < 0.0001$) and a near CR (nCR) rate of 28% compared to 16% ($p = 0.00006$) for patients receiving bortezomib alone.[56] Based on these results, panobinostat was granted FDA approval as a third line agent in combination with bortezomib and dexamethasone in MM patients who had previously received bortezomib and IMiDs.

The role of autophagy in MM remains controversial. Macroautophagy is a nonapoptotic death pathway and a proteolytic apparatus especially relevant for clearance of aggresomes.[57] Predicated on the former mechanism, inhibitors of the mTOR pathway, in particular mTORC1, an inducer of autophagy, have been studied in MM but clinical results have been largely disappointing.[58] The focus has now moved to autophagy inhibitors as a tool to further exacerbate proteotoxicity in MM cells.[59]

# A Broader View: MM in the Context of the BM Niche

## The Role of BM Microenvironment in the Pathogenesis of MM and Support of MM Progression

A prime role for cancer microenvironment in promoting neoplastic progression and metastasis has been recognized over the past decade.[60] MM cells preferentially home and are retained within a specialized BM niche via the chemokine axis CXCR4/SDF-1α.[61] The baseline hypoxic BM environment and the evidence of increased expression of hypoxia-inducible factor 1α (HIF-1α) in MM, linked to cancer cell survival, trafficking, and neoangiogenesis provided the framework to evaluate HIF and its downstream signaling molecule inhibitors in MM.[62] Direct and paracrine interaction with cellular elements as well as contact with extracellular matrix are crucial for MM survival, proliferation, and treatment resistance (Figure 14.3).[63]

Cancer-cell-induced imbalance in bone metabolism, with exuberant osteoclast (OC) and decreased osteoblast (OB) activity, plays a major role in MM-related morbidity due to skeletal events, and pathogenesis by supporting MM cell survival and proliferation.[64] An imbalance between the pro-osteoclastic factor, receptor activator of NF-κB ligand (RANKL), and the pro-osteoblastic one, osteoprotegerin (OPG), is one of the mechanisms responsible for MM-related bone imbalance.[65]

Similar to other malignancies, immunosurveillance is impaired in MM due to functional defects in cytotoxic lymphocytes and dendritic cells (DCs), including BM-resident plasmacytoid DC, and increased regulatory T ($T_{reg}$) and T-helper 17 cells ($T_{H17}$), overall resulting in tumor tolerance, proliferation, and survival.[66-68]

## Immunomodulatory Drugs

Initially pursued as anti-MM therapy predicated on its antiangiogenic properties, thalidomide soon proved to have more complex molecular mechanisms of effectiveness within the BM niche, in particular, modulation of the immune system.[69] Second-generation thalidomide derivatives, lenalidomide, and pomalidomide have even more pronounced immunomodulatory activity, thus the name IMiDs.

Among their pleiotropic effects, IMiDs elicit direct caspase 8-mediated cytotoxic and cell cycle arrest; disrupt MM–BM stromal cell interaction; inhibit pro-survival cytokines and growth factor production; and restore immunosurveillance via activation of natural killer (NK) and CD8+ T cells. Cereblon (CRBN), a component of an E3, ubiquitin-ligase complex was identified as the molecular target responsible for thalidomide-induced phocomelia.[70] Recent studies showed that the anti-MM effect of lenalidomide is mediated by the degradation of the transcription factors Ikaros (IKZF1) and Aiolos (IKZF3). Lenalidomide binds to damage-specific DNA-binding protein 1 (DDB1) and CRBN and modulates the activity of their E3 ubiquitin-ligase complex, causing ubiquitination and proteasome-mediated degradation of IKZF1 and IKZF3[71,72] Depletion of the same transcription factors appears responsible for lenalidomide immunomodulatory properties by inducing IL-2 production in T lymphocytes.

IMiDs are highly effective drugs in MM and typically included in first-line regimens with bortezomib/dexamethasone.[73] In combination with dexamethasone, thalidomide is FDA-approved as first-line and lenalidomide as second-line treatment for MM (Table 14.2). Pomalidomide was granted accelerated approval in December 2013

for patients progressing after two lines of treatment, including bortezomib and lenalidomide, on the base of a phase II clinical trial of pomalidomide alone or in combination with low-dose dexamethasone showing ORR of 18% and 33%, respectively, even in patients resistant to both lenalidomide and bortezomib, with an OS of 13.6 and 16.5 months, respectively.[74] A phase III trial of pomalidomide plus low-dose dexamethasone versus dexamethasone alone confirmed safety and effectiveness of pomalidomide in relapsed/refractory MM patients.[75] Recently the FIRST trial showed continuos lenalidomide/dexamethasone to be superior to 72 weeks of lenalidomide/dexamethasone or melphalan/prednisone/thalidomide for PFS and OS in transplant ineligible patients, with no increased adverse events, leading to the FDA approval of this combination as first line in transplant ineligible MM patients.[76]

Beyond its use for induction and consolidation, lenalidomide was shown to prolong survival when used as maintenance therapy both in patients post autologous stem cell transplant (ASCT) and those undergoing conventional therapy.[77,78] An increased incidence of second primary malignancies, in particular hematologic, was observed in patients receiving lenalidomide. A recent metanalysis showed that such increased risk involved mainly patients receiving oral melphalan/lenalidomide treatment, suggesting that this combination should be avoided.[79]

## Molecular Targets in Immunotherapy

The proof of concept of increased immunosurveillance being effective as anti-MM therapy is the prolonged disease-free survival observed in patients post allogeneic hematopoietic stem cell transplant (HSCT) and donor lymphocyte infusion.[80] As treatment-related mortality remains significant in the face of alternative, effective pharmacologic therapies, allogeneic HSCT is not routinely pursued in MM. However, cellular-based immunotherapies, in particular those based on antigen-presenting cells such as DC vaccination and/or modulation of T-cell subsets in the myeloma microenvironment have been investigated.[81]

The activation of cytotoxic T cells is complex and typically requires both an antigen-mediated stimulatory signal via the T-cell receptor and a co-stimulatory signal transmitted by a variety of surface molecules.[82] This process can be modulated through the engagement of different surface co-receptors with either stimulatory or inhibitory function. CTLA-4 and PD-1 are two such co-receptors with inhibitory function for which drugs have been developed and successfully implemented, mostly in solid malignancies. Similar to other tumors, MM cells overexpress the ligand of PD-1, PD-L1, while BM T cells have increased expression of PD-1.[83,84] Several inhibitors of CTLA-4, PD-1, and PD-L1 are being evaluated in clinical trials alone or in combination with other immunotherapies such as DC vaccine.[85]

## Molecular Targets Within the BM Microenvironment

Initially developed for the mobilization of stem cells from the BM, the selective SDF-1α antagonist AMD3100 (plerixafor) has been evaluated as an anti-MM therapy given the role of the CXCR4/SDF-1α axis in retaining MM cells in the BM niche and supporting their proliferation and trafficking.[86] Preclinical studies showed AMD3100 to sensitize MM cells to bortezomib and standard chemotherapy agents (dexamethasone, melphalan, doxorubicin).[87] A phase I/II study of plerixafor in combination with bortezomib in relapsed/refractory MM patients is ongoing.

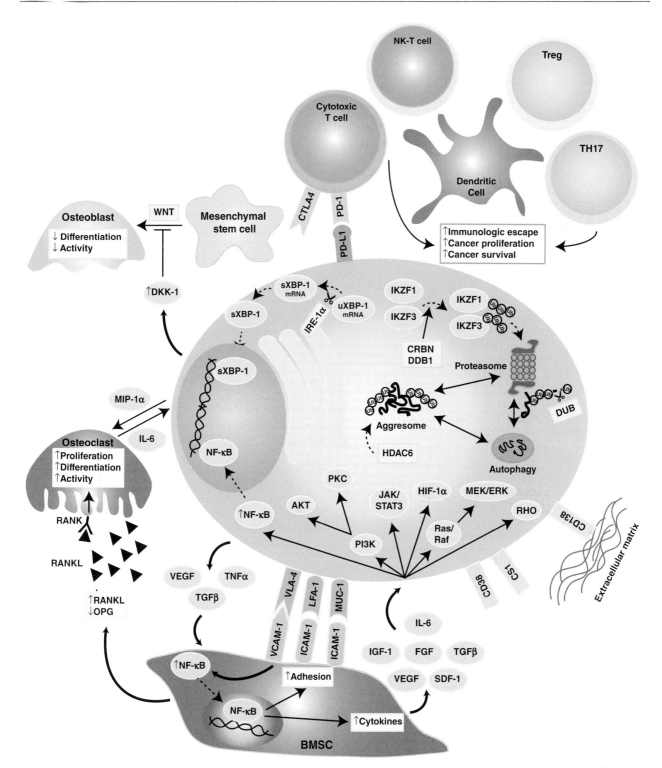

**Figure 14.3** The large blue cell in the center is a MM cell with nucleus, endoplasmic reticulum and proteolytic pathways outlined. The close interplay with bone marrow stromal cells (BMSC) in light brown, osteoclasts (in red) and osteblasts (in green) is outlined. Immune cells relevant for immunologic escape of MM are also represented. Key signaling molecules and cytokines are represented in pale pink ovals while in pale pink squares are molecules targeted by currently approved therapies. Modified with permission from Reference 106.

**Table 14.2** FDA-approved targeted therapies in MM.

| Name | Drug class | Route of administration | Significant side effects | Notes | FDA-approved indications in MM |
|---|---|---|---|---|---|
| Bortezomib (PS-341, Velcade) | PI | IV/SC | • Peripheral neuropathy<br>• Cytopenia<br>• Fatigue | • Avoidance of pregnancy should be advised<br>• Renal adjustment not required<br>• SC administration significantly reduces the incidence of peripheral neuropathy | First line (2008) |
| Thalidomide (Thalomid) | IMiD | PO | • Peripheral neuropathy<br>• Increased VTE risk in combination regimens<br>• Somnolence<br>• Rash<br>• Constipation<br>• Teratogenicity | • VTE prophylaxis indicated in combination regimens<br>• Two adequate birth control methods or abstinence required<br>• No need for renally adjusted dosing | First line in combination with dexamethasone (2006) |
| Lenalidomide (Revlimid) | IMiD | PO | • Myelosuppression<br>• Fatigue<br>• Increased VTE risk in combination regimens<br>• Increased risk of second primary malignancies<br>• Likely teratogenicity | • VTE prophylaxis indicated in combinatory regimens<br>• Two adequate birth control methods or abstinence required<br>• Renally adjusted dosing for CrCl <60 mL/min/m2<br>• Combination with oral melphalan to be avoided due to increased risk of secondary cancer | Second line in combination with dexamethasone (2006) |
| Carfilzomib (PX-171, Kyprolis) | PI | IV | • Cardiac arrest<br>• Congestive heart failure<br>• Myocardial ischemia<br>• Pneumonia<br>• Acute renal failure<br>• Pyrexia<br>• Fatigue<br>• Potential teratogenicity | • Avoidance of pregnancy should be advised<br>• Renal adjustment not required | Third line after bortezomib and an IMiD (2012) |
| Pomalidomide (Pomalyst) | IMiD | PO | • Myelosuppression<br>• Fatigue<br>• Nausea<br>• Diarrhea<br>• Likely increased VTE risk in combination regimens<br>• Likely teratogenicity | • VTE prophylaxis indicated<br>• Two adequate birth-control methods or abstinence required<br>• Renal adjustment not established | Third line after bortezomib and an IMiD (2013) |
| Panobinostat | HDACi | PO | • Diarrhea<br>• Fatigue<br>• Nausea<br>• Peripheral edema<br>• Cytopenias<br>• Hepatotoxicity<br>• Cardiac arrhythmias | • Pregnancy category D. Avoidance of pregnancy is recommended<br>• Approved with a Risk Evaluation and Mitigation Strategy (REMS): a plan of communication to help inform health care professionals of severe, potential side effects | Third line after bortezomib and IMiD (2015) |

The table summarizes the most significant side effects and clinically relevant considerations for the six FDA-approved molecular therapeutics in MM.

**Table 14.3** Molecular targeted therapies in phase III clinical trials.

| Drug class | Drug | ClinicalTrials.gov identifier | Trial name | Study design | Primary end point | Expected completion date |
|---|---|---|---|---|---|---|
| PI | Ixazomib (MLN9708) | NCT01564537 | TOURMALINE-MM1 | Ixazomib/Len/Dex vs. Placebo/Len/Dex in relapsed/refractory MM patients | PFS | June 2014 |
| | | NCT01850524 | C16014 | Ixazomib/Len/Dex vs. Placebo/Len/Dex in transplant-ineligible, newly diagnosed MM patients | PFS | June 2018 |
| | Oprozomib (ONX-0912) | NCT01999335 | OPZ007 | Oprozomib/Pom/Dex vs. Placebo/Pom/Dex in relapsed/refractory MM patients | PFS | June 2016 |
| | Carfilzomib (PX-171) | NCT01568866 | ENDEAVOR | Carfilzomib/Dex vs. Bortezomib/Dex in relapsed MM patients | PFS | Jan 2016 |
| | | NCT01818752 | CLARION | Carfilzomib/Mel/Pred vs. Bortezomib/Mel/Pred in transplant-ineligible, newly diagnosed MM patients | PFS | April 2016 |
| | | NCT01080391 | ASPIRE | Carfilzomib/Len/Dex vs. Len/Dex in relapsed/refractory MM patients | PFS | Dec 2014 |
| | | NCT01302392 | FOCUS | Carfilzomib vs. best supportive care in patients with relapsed/refractory MM who have exhausted all therapeutic options | PFS | June 2014 |
| | | NCT01863550 | E1A11 | Carfilzomib/Len/Dex vs. Bortezomib/Len/Dex followed by limited vs. indefinite Len maintenance in patients with newly diagnosed MM | OS | May 2016 |
| IMiD | Pomalidomide | NCT01311687 | NIMBUS | Pomalidomide/loDex vs. high-dose Dex in patients with refractory/relapsed MM | PFS | March 2013 |
| | | NCT01734928 | OPTIMISM | Pomalidomide/Bortezomib/Dex vs. Bortezomib/Dex in patients with relapsed/refractory MM | PFS | Jan 2015 |
| Signaling inhibitors | Masitinib | NCT01470131 | AB06002 | Masitinib/Bortezomib/Dex vs. Placebo/Bortezomib/Dex as second line therapy in patients with relapsing MM | PFS | April 2013 |
| | Aplidin | NCT01102426 | ADMYRE | Aplidin/Dex vs. Dex alone in patients with relapsed/refractory MM | PFS | June 2014 |
| MoAb | Elotuzumab | NCT01239797 | ELOQUENT-2 | Elotuzumab/Len/Dex vs. Placebo/Len/Dex in patients with relapsed/refractory MM | PFS | Aug 2017 |
| | Daratumumab | NCT02076009 | CR103663 | Daratumumab/Len/Dex vs. Placebo/Len/Dex in patients with relapsed/refractory MM | PFS | May 2017 |

PI, proteasome inhibitor; IMiD, immunomodulatory drug; HDAC, histone deacetylase; MoAb, monoclonal antibody; Dex, dexamethasone; Len, lenalidomide; PFS, progression-free survival; OS, overall survival.

The hypoxia-activated prodrug TH-302 proved effective in an MM mouse model by reducing MM proliferation and neo-angiogenesis, thus prompting evaluation of a phase I/II trial in combination with dexamethasone and bortezomib.[88]

The inhibition of MM–OC interaction has attracted interest as a tool to not only halt bone-related events but also arrest MM proliferation and survival. Recently, bisphosphonates have been shown to improve survival in MM, suggesting direct anti-MM effect via interruption of the maladaptive OC–MM interaction.[89] On the opposite front, stimulation of OB differentiation and activity via BHQ-880, a blocking antibody against Dickkopf-1 (DKK-1), caused inhibition of MM growth in preclinical models and this molecule is currently being evaluated in phase I/II clinical trials in combination with zoledronic acid.[90]

## Distinct Molecular Targets of MM Cells

### Surface Molecular Targets for Immunotherapy

Several surface molecules highly expressed in MM have been evaluated as targets for the development of monoclonal antibodies (MoAb). The most advanced in clinical development is elotuzumab, an MoAb targeting the glycoprotein CS1, highly expressed by MM cells. *In vitro*, elotuzumab causes antibody-dependent cell-mediated cytotoxicity (ADCC), directly enhances NK cell function, inhibits interaction with BMSC and synergizes with lenalidomide.[91] While its activity as monotherapy proved modest in clinical trials, the combination with lenalidomide/dexamethasone or bortezomib/dexamethasone was highly effective in phase I/II studies. In particular, the ORR to elotuzumab/lenalidomide/dexamethasone was 82% with a median time to progression not yet reached after 16.4 months follow-up in refractory/relapsed MM patients.[92,93] These results provided the framework for a phase III trial of such combination.

The MoAb daratumumab, targeting CD38, has anti-MM activity via ADCC, complement-dependent cytotoxicity (CDC), and direct cytotoxic effect and proved highly effective in preclinical studies[94] Preliminary data of phase I/II trial of daratumumab in combination with lenalidomide/dexamethasone are highly encouraging with all patients achieving at least a partial response with 50% very good partial response or better.[95]

Immunoconjugated drugs, such as BT062, a CD138 MoAb conjugated to maytansinoid DM4, and BB10901 (huN901), an anti-CD56 MoAb conjugated to DM1, release the highly cytotoxic chemotherapy agent only after antigen binding and internalization, thus selectively targeting MM cells.[96,97] They are currently being evaluated in phase I clinical trials alone or in combination with lenalidomide/dexamethasone.

### Signaling Molecules Critical for MM Survival and Proliferation

Several signaling pathways are altered in MM and have been the focus of development of targeted therapies. Among these, inhibitors of the AKT and the c-JUN pathways are the most advanced in clinical development (Table 14.3).

Signaling through AKT is constitutively active in MM cells, contributing to cancer proliferation and drug resistance via a number of downstream effectors such as mTOR and NF-κB.[98] Contact with BMSC and exposure to certain compounds, including bortezomib, cause increased activation of AKT, representing a mechanism of drug resistance.[99] The AKT inhibitor perifosine caused significant cytotoxicity against MM and synergized with both conventional drugs and bortezomib. Beyond downregulation of AKT pathway, induction of JNK and downregulation of survivin have also been reported as mechanisms of perifosine effectiveness. A phase II clinical trial of perifosine/bortezomib showed encouraging data with responses seen in 32% of bortezomib-refractory and 65% bortezomib-relapsed patients, posing the frame for a phase III clinical trial of such combination.[100]

The marine-derived molecule, plitidepsin (Aplidin) caused significant anti-MM cytotoxicity *in vitro* via activation of p38 and JNK signaling.[101] A phase II study of plitidepsin showed limited activity when used as monotherapy (ORR 13%) which was significantly improved by combination with dexamethasone (ORR 22%), thus prompting evaluation of plitidepsin/dexamethasone in a phase III clinical trial currently ongoing.

Also being evaluated in phase III clinical trial in combination with bortezomib/dexamethasone, is the tyrosine kinase inhibitor masitinib (AB1010). Masitinib targets a broad spectrum of key oncogenes, including c-Kit, platelet-derived growth factor receptor (PDGFR), fibroblast growth factor receptor (FGFR) 3, and Lyn which have all being implicated in MM proliferation and survival.[102]

Among other attractive targets in clinical development are musculoaponeurotic fibrosarcoma oncogene homolog (MAF), a B-ZIP transcription factor frequently overexpressed in MM; Janus-associated kinase 2 (JAK2) and its downstream transcription factor signal transducer and activator of transcription 3 (STAT3); aurora kinase A and B; kinesin spindle (KSP); nuclear transport, and cyclin dependent kinases (CDKs) and Bruton's kinase (BTK), found to have direct anti-MM and OC activity.[103,104]

## Conclusions and Future Perspective

The past two decades have been an exciting time for patients with MM with the introduction of nine new, FDA-approved treatment and a two- to threefolds prolongation in OS. The clinical implementation of DNA sequencing techniques now provides the opportunity to uncover the genetic asset of cancer cells and develop more specific therapies guided by the pattern of mutations. Novel targets have also been identified in MM providing the framework for the development of novel targeted therapies.[105] As we move forward, the goal is to further understand the etiopathogenic mechanisms behind the evolution of MM from MGUS and identify the key molecules in this process in order to provide effective, specific therapies to render MM a chronic, if not a curable disease.

## References

1 Siegel RL, Miller KD, Jemal A. Cancer statistics, 2015. *CA Cancer J Clin.* 2015.

2 Kyle RA, Therneau TM, Rajkumar SV, et al. A long-term study of prognosis in monoclonal gammopathy of undetermined significance. *N Engl J Med.* 2002;346(8):564–569.

3 Martinez-Lopez J, Fulciniti M, Barrio S, et al. Deep sequencing reveals oligoclonality at the immunoglobulin locus in multiple myeloma patients. American Society of Hematology (ASH) Annual Meeting. *Blood.*2013;401.

4 Anderson KC, Carrasco RD. Pathogenesis of myeloma. *Annu Rev Pathol.* 2011;6:249–274.

5 Reimold AM, Iwakoshi NN, Manis J, et al. Plasma cell differentiation requires the transcription factor XBP-1. *Nature.* 2001;412(6844):300–307.

6 Iwakoshi NN, Lee AH, Vallabhajosyula P, Otipoby KL, Rajewsky K, Glimcher LH. Plasma cell differentiation and the unfolded protein response intersect at the transcription factor XBP-1. *Nat Immunol.* 2003;4(4):321–329.

7 Carrasco DR, Sukhdeo K, Protopopova M, et al. The differentiation and stress response factor XBP-1 drives multiple myeloma pathogenesis. *Cancer Cell.* 2007;11(4):349–360.

8 Sontag EM, Vonk WI, Frydman J. Sorting out the trash: the spatial nature of eukaryotic protein quality control. *Curr Opin Cell Biol.* 2014;26:139–146.

9 Cenci S, van Anken E, Sitia R. Proteostenosis and plasma cell pathophysiology. *Curr Opin Cell Biol.* 2011;23(2):216–222.

10 Walter P, Ron D. The unfolded protein response: from stress pathway to homeostatic regulation. *Science.* 2011;334(6059):1081–1086.

11 Papandreou I, Denko NC, Olson M, et al. Identification of an Ire1alpha endonuclease specific inhibitor with cytotoxic activity against human multiple myeloma. *Blood.* 2011;117(4):1311–1314.

12 Mimura N, Hideshima T, Gorgun G, et al. Targeting IRE1 alpha-XBP1 pathway is a novel therapeutic strategy in multiple myeloma. *Blood.* 2010;116(21):1659.

13 Hartl FU, Bracher A, Hayer-Hartl M. Molecular chaperones in protein folding and proteostasis. *Nature.* 2011;475(7356):324–332.

14 Richardson PG, Chanan-Khan AA, Lonial S, et al. Tanespimycin and bortezomib combination treatment in patients with relapsed or relapsed and refractory multiple myeloma: results of a phase 1/2 study. *Br J Haematol.* 2011;153(6):729–740.

15 Garcia-Carbonero R, Carnero A, Paz-Ares L. Inhibition of HSP90 molecular chaperones: moving into the clinic. *Lancet Oncol.* 2013;14(9):e358–e369.

16 Stuhmer T, Zollinger A, Siegmund D, et al. Signalling profile and anti-tumour activity of the novel Hsp90 inhibitor NVP-AUY922 in multiple myeloma. *Leukemia.* 2008;22(8):1604–1612.

17 Nakashima T, Ishii T, Tagaya H, et al. New molecular and biological mechanism of antitumour activities of KW-2478, a novel nonansamycin heat shock protein 90 inhibitor, in multiple myeloma cells. *Clin Cancer Res.* 2010;16(10):2792–2802.

18 Yewdell JW, Anton LC, Bennink JR. Defective ribosomal products (DRiPs): a major source of antigenic peptides for MHC class I molecules? *J Immunol.* 1996;157(5):1823–1826.

19 Goldberg AL. Functions of the proteasome: the lysis at the end of the tunnel. *Science.* 1995;268(5210):522–523.

20 Neefjes J, Jongsma ML, Paul P, Bakke O. Towards a systems understanding of MHC class I and MHC class II antigen presentation. *Nat Rev Immunol.* 2011;11(12):823–836.

21 Adams J. The proteasome: a suitable antineoplastic target. *Nat Rev Cancer.* 2004;4(5):349–360.

22 Orlowski RZ, Stinchcombe TE, Mitchell BS, et al. Phase I trial of the proteasome inhibitor PS-341 in patients with refractory hematologic malignancies. *J Clin Oncol.* 2002;20(22):4420–4427.

23 Kisselev AF, Goldberg AL. Proteasome inhibitors: from research tools to drug candidates. *Chem Biol.* 2001;8(8):739–758.

24 Hideshima T, Mitsiades C, Akiyama M, et al. Molecular mechanisms mediating antimyeloma activity of proteasome inhibitor PS-341. *Blood.* 2003;101(4):1530–1534.

25 Bianchi G, Oliva L, Cascio P, et al. The proteasome load versus capacity balance determines apoptotic sensitivity of multiple myeloma cells to proteasome inhibition. *Blood.* 2009;113(13):3040–3049.

26 Richardson PG, Sonneveld P, Schuster M, et al. Extended follow-up of a phase 3 trial in relapsed multiple myeloma: final time-to-event results of the APEX trial. *Blood.* 2007;110(10):3557–3560.

27 San Miguel JF, Schlag R, Khuageva NK, et al. Persistent overall survival benefit and no increased risk of second malignancies with bortezomib-melphalan-prednisone versus melphalan-prednisone in patients with previously untreated multiple myeloma. *J Clin Oncol.* 2013;31(4):448–455.

28 Kumar SK, Mikhael JR, Buadi FK, et al. Management of newly diagnosed symptomatic multiple myeloma: updated mayo stratification of myeloma and risk-adapted therapy (mSMART) consensus guidelines. *Mayo Clin Proc.* 2009;84(12):1095–1110.

29 Orlowski RZ. Novel agents for multiple myeloma to overcome resistance in phase III clinical trials. *Semin Oncol.* 2013;40(5):634–651.

30 Kuhn DJ, Chen Q, Voorhees PM, et al. Potent activity of carfilzomib, a novel, irreversible inhibitor of the ubiquitin-proteasome pathway, against preclinical models of multiple myeloma. *Blood.* 2007;110(9):3281–3290.

31 Siegel DS, Martin T, Wang M, et al. A phase 2 study of single-agent carfilzomib (PX-171-003-A1) in patients with relapsed and refractory multiple myeloma. *Blood.* 2012;120(14):2817–2825.

32 clinicaltrials.gov [Internet].

33 Chauhan D, Singh AV, Aujay M, et al. A novel orally active proteasome inhibitor ONX 0912 triggers in vitro and in vivo cytotoxicity in multiple myeloma. *Blood.* 2010;116(23):4906–4915.

34 Avet-Loiseau H, Attal M, Moreau P, et al. Genetic abnormalities and survival in multiple myeloma: the experience of the Intergroupe Francophone du Myelome. *Blood.* 2007;109(8):3489–3495.

35 Richardson PG, Hofmeister CC, Rosenbaum CA, et al. Twice-weekly oral MLN9708 (ixazomib citrate), an investigational proteasome inhibitor, in combination with lenalidomide (Len) and dexamethasone (Dex) in patients (Pts) with newly diagnosed multiple myeloma (MM): final phase 1 results and phase 2 data. American Society of Hematology (ASH) Annual Meeting. *Blood.*2013;535.

36 Kumar SK, Roy V, Reeder C, et al. Phase 2 trial of single agent MLN9708 in patients with relapsed multiple myeloma not refractory to bortezomib. American Society of Hematology (ASH) Annual Meeting. *Blood.*2013;1944.

37 Millward M, Price T, Townsend A, et al. Phase 1 clinical trial of the novel proteasome inhibitor marizomib with the histone deacetylase inhibitor vorinostat in patients with melanoma, pancreatic and lung cancer based on in vitro assessments of the combination. *Invest New Drugs.* 2012;30(6):2303–2317.

38 Chauhan D, Catley L, Li G, et al. A novel orally active proteasome inhibitor induces apoptosis in multiple myeloma cells with mechanisms distinct from Bortezomib. *Cancer Cell.* 2005;8(5):407–419.

39 Komander D, Clague MJ, Urbe S. Breaking the chains: structure and function of the deubiquitinases. *Nat Rev Mol Cell Biol.* 2009;10(8):550–563.

40 Fraile JM, Quesada V, Rodriguez D, Freije JM, Lopez-Otin C. Deubiquitinases in cancer: new functions and therapeutic options. *Oncogene.* 2012;31(19):2373–2388.

41 Tian Z, D'Arcy P, Wang X, et al. A novel small molecule inhibitor of deubiquitylating enzyme USP14 and UCHL5 induces apoptosis in multiple myeloma and overcomes bortezomib resistance. *Blood.* 2014;123(5):706–716.

42 Chauhan D, Tian Z, Nicholson B, et al. A small molecule inhibitor of ubiquitin-specific protease-7 induces apoptosis in multiple myeloma cells and overcomes bortezomib resistance. *Cancer Cell.* 2012;22(3):345–358.

43 Wang Q, Mora-Jensen H, Weniger MA, et al. ERAD inhibitors integrate ER stress with an epigenetic mechanism to activate BH3-only protein NOXA in cancer cells. *Proc Natl Acad Sci U S A.* 2009;106(7):2200–2205.

44 Driscoll JJ, Chowdhury RD. Molecular crosstalk between the proteasome, aggresomes and autophagy: translational potential and clinical implications. *Cancer Letters.* 2012;325(2):147–154.

45 Hoang B, Benavides A, Shi Y, Frost P, Lichtenstein A. Effect of autophagy on multiple myeloma cell viability. *Mol Cancer Ther.* 2009;8(7):1974–1984.

46 Catley L, Weisberg E, Kiziltepe T, et al. Aggresome induction by proteasome inhibitor bortezomib and alpha-tubulin hyperacetylation by tubulin deacetylase (TDAC) inhibitor LBH589 are synergistic in myeloma cells. *Blood.* 2006;108(10):3441–3449.

47 Kawaguchi Y, Kovacs JJ, McLaurin A, Vance JM, Ito A, Yao TP. The deacetylase HDAC6 regulates aggresome formation and cell viability in response to misfolded protein stress. *Cell.* 2003;115(6):727–738.

48 Santo L, Hideshima T, Kung AL, et al. Preclinical activity, pharmacodynamic and pharmacokinetic properties of a selective HDAC6 inhibitor,

ACY-1215, in combination with bortezomib in multiple myeloma. *Blood.* 2012.

49 Yee A, Vorhees P, Bensinger WI, et al. ACY-1215, a selective histone deacetylase (HDAC) 6 inhibitor, in combination with lenalidomide and dexamethasone (dex), is well tolerated without dose limiting toxicity (DLT) in patients (Pts) with multiple myeloma (MM) at doses demonstrating biologic activity: interim results of a phase 1b trial. American Society of Hematology (ASH) Annual Meeting. *Blood*;2013. 3190.

50 Raje N, Vogl DT, Hari PN, et al. ACY-1215, a selective histone deacetylase (HDAC) 6 inhibitor: interim results of combination therapy with bortezomib in patients with multiple myeloma (MM). American Society of Hematology (ASH) Annual Meeting. *Blood*;2013. 759.

51 Bolden JE, Peart MJ, Johnstone RW. Anticancer activities of histone deacetylase inhibitors. *Nat Rev Drug Discov.* 2006;5(9):769–784.

52 Dimopoulos M, Siegel DS, Lonial S, et al. Vorinostat or placebo in combination with bortezomib in patients with multiple myeloma (VANTAGE 088): a multicentre, randomised, double-blind study. *Lancet Oncol.* 2013;14(11):1129–1140.

53 Siegel DS, Richardson P, Dimopoulos M, Moreau P, Mitsiades C, Weber D, et al. Vorinostat in combination with lenalidomide and dexamethasone in patients with relapsed or refractory multiple myeloma. *Blood Cancer J.* 2014;4:e202.

54 Richardson PG, Schlossman RL, Alsina M, et al. PANORAMA 2: panobinostat in combination with bortezomib and dexamethasone in patients with relapsed and bortezomib-refractory myeloma. *Blood.* 2013;122(14):2331–2337.

55 San-Miguel JF, Richardson PG, Gunther A, Sezer O, Siegel D, Blade J, et al. Phase Ib study of panobinostat and bortezomib in relapsed or relapsed and refractory multiple myeloma. *J Clin Oncol.* 2013;31(29):3696–3703.

56 San-Miguel JF, Hungria VT, Yoon SS, Beksac M, Dimopoulos MA, Elghandour A, et al. Panobinostat plus bortezomib and dexamethasone versus placebo plus bortezomib and dexamethasone in patients with relapsed or relapsed and refractory multiple myeloma: a multicentre, randomised, double-blind phase 3 trial. *Lancet Oncol.* 2014;15(11):1195–1206.

57 Puissant A, Robert G, Auberger P. Targeting autophagy to fight hematopoietic malignancies. *Cell Cycle.* 2010;9(17):3470–3478.

58 Gera J, Lichtenstein A. The mammalian target of rapamycin pathway as a therapeutic target in multiple myeloma. *Leuk Lymphoma.* 2011;52(10):1857–1866.

59 Yuko M, Santo L, Cirstea DD, et al. Inhibition of autophagy by ACY-1215, a selective HDAC6 inhibitor accelerates carfilzomib-induced cell death in multiple myeloma. American Society of Hematology (ASH) Annual Meeting. *Blood*;2013. 4431.

60 Quail DF, Joyce JA. Microenvironmental regulation of tumor progression and metastasis. *Nat Med.* 2013;19(11):1423–1437.

61 Aggarwal R, Ghobrial IM, Roodman GD. Chemokines in multiple myeloma. *Exp Hematol.* 2006;34(10):1289–1295.

62 Martin SK, Diamond P, Gronthos S, Peet DJ, Zannettino AC. The emerging role of hypoxia, HIF-1 and HIF-2 in multiple myeloma. *Leukemia.* 2011;25(10):1533–1542.

63 Hideshima T, Mitsiades C, Tonon G, Richardson PG, Anderson KC. Understanding multiple myeloma pathogenesis in the bone marrow to identify new therapeutic targets. *Nat Rev Cancer.* 2007;7(8):585–598.

64 Abe M, Hiura K, Wilde J, et al. Osteoclasts enhance myeloma cell growth and survival via cell-cell contact: a vicious cycle between bone destruction and myeloma expansion. *Blood.* 2004;104(8):2484–2491.

65 Giuliani N, Bataille R, Mancini C, Lazzaretti M, Barille S. Myeloma cells induce imbalance in the osteoprotegerin/osteoprotegerin ligand system in the human bone marrow environment. *Blood.* 2001;98(13):3527–3533.

66 Brown RD, Pope B, Murray A, et al. Dendritic cells from patients with myeloma are numerically normal but functionally defective as they fail to up-regulate CD80 (B7–1) expression after huCD40LT stimulation because of inhibition by transforming growth factor-beta1 and interleukin-10. *Blood.* 2001;98(10):2992–2998.

67 Chauhan D, Singh AV, Brahmandam M, et al. Functional interaction of plasmacytoid dendritic cells with multiple myeloma cells: a therapeutic target. *Cancer Cell.* 2009;16(4):309–323.

68 Favaloro J, Brown R, Aklilu E, et al. Myeloma skews regulatory T and pro-inflammatory T helper 17 cell balance in favor of a suppressive state. *Leuk Lymphoma.* 2014;55(5):1090–1098.

69 Davies F, Baz R. Lenalidomide mode of action: linking bench and clinical findings. *Blood Rev.* 2010;24(suppl. 1):S13–S19.

70 Ito T, Ando H, Suzuki T, et al. Identification of a primary target of thalidomide teratogenicity. *Science.* 2010;327(5971):1345–1350.

71 Kronke J, Udeshi ND, Narla A, et al. Lenalidomide causes selective degradation of IKZF1 and IKZF3 in multiple myeloma cells. *Science.* 2014;343(6168):301–305.

72 Lu G, Middleton RE, Sun H, et al. The myeloma drug lenalidomide promotes the cereblon-dependent destruction of Ikaros proteins. *Science.* 2014;343(6168):305–309.

73 Stewart AK, Richardson PG, San-Miguel JF. How I treat multiple myeloma in younger patients. *Blood.* 2009;114(27):5436–5443.

74 Richardson PG, Siegel DS, Vij R, et al. Pomalidomide alone or in combination with low-dose dexamethasone in relapsed and refractory multiple myeloma: a randomized phase 2 study. *Blood.* 2014;123(12):1826–1832.

75 San Miguel J, Weisel K, Moreau P, et al. Pomalidomide plus low-dose dexamethasone versus high-dose dexamethasone alone for patients with relapsed and refractory multiple myeloma (MM-003): a randomised, open-label, phase 3 trial. *Lancet Oncol.* 2013;14(11):1055–1066.

76 Benboubker L, Dimopoulos MA, Dispenzieri A, et al. Lenalidomide and dexamethasone in transplant-ineligible patients with myeloma. *N Engl J Med.* 2014;371(10):906–917.

77 Attal M, Lauwers VC, Marit G, Caillot D, Facon T, Hulin C, et al. Maintenance treatment with lenalidomide after transplantation for myeloma: final analysis of the IFM 2005–02. *Blood.* 2010;116(21):141.

78 Palumbo A, Hajek R, Delforge M, et al. ;MM-015 Investigators. Continuous lenalidomide treatment for newly diagnosed multiple myeloma. *N Engl J Med.* 2012;366(19):1759–1769.

79 Palumbo A, Bringhen S, Kumar SK, et al. Second primary malignancies with lenalidomide therapy for newly diagnosed myeloma: a meta-analysis of individual patient data. *Lancet Oncol.* 2014;15(3):333–342.

80 Cook G, Bird JM, Marks DI. In pursuit of the allo-immune response in multiple myeloma: where do we go from here? *Bone Marrow Transplant.* 2009;43(2):91–99.

81 Arnason J, Avigan D. Evolution of cellular immunotherapy: from allogeneic transplant to dendritic cell vaccination as treatment for multiple myeloma. *Immunotherapy.* 2012;4(10):1043–1051.

82 Baxter AG, Hodgkin PD. Activation rules: the two-signal theories of immune activation. *Nat Rev Immunol.* 2002;2(6):439–446.

83 Gorgun G, Samur MK, Cowens KB, et al. Lenalidomide enhances immune checkpoint blockade induced immune response in multiple myeloma. *Clin Cancer Res.* 2015;CCR-15-0200.

84 Pardoll DM. The blockade of immune checkpoints in cancer immunotherapy. *Nat Rev Cancer.* 2012;12(4):252–264.

85 Rosenblatt J, Glotzbecker B, Mills H, et al. PD-1 blockade by CT-011, anti-PD-1 antibody, enhances ex vivo T-cell responses to autologous

dendritic cell/myeloma fusion vaccine. *J Immunother.* 2011;34(5): 409–418.

86 Hideshima T, Chauhan D, Hayashi T, et al. The biological sequelae of stromal cell-derived factor-1alpha in multiple myeloma. *Mol Cancer Ther.* 2002;1(7):539–544.

87 Azab AK, Runnels JM, Pitsillides C, et al. CXCR4 inhibitor AMD3100 disrupts the interaction of multiple myeloma cells with the bone marrow microenvironment and enhances their sensitivity to therapy. *Blood.* 2009;113(18):4341–4351.

88 Hu J, Handisides DR, Van Valckenborgh E, et al. Targeting the multiple myeloma hypoxic niche with TH-302, a hypoxia-activated prodrug. *Blood.* 2010;116(9):1524–1527.

89 Raje N, Roodman GD. Advances in the biology and treatment of bone disease in multiple myeloma. *Clin Cancer Res.* 2011;17(6):1278–1286.

90 Fulciniti M, Tassone P, Hideshima T, et al. Anti-DKK1 mAb (BHQ880) as a potential therapeutic agent for multiple myeloma. *Blood.* 2009;114(2):371–379.

91 Lonial S, Kaufman J, Laubach J, Richardson P. Elotuzumab: a novel anti-CS1 monoclonal antibody for the treatment of multiple myeloma. *Expert Opin Biol Ther.* 2013;13(12):1731–1740.

92 Jakubowiak AJ, Benson DM, Bensinger W, et al. Phase I trial of anti-CS1 monoclonal antibody elotuzumab in combination with bortezomib in the treatment of relapsed/refractory multiple myeloma. *J Clin Oncol.* 2012;30(16):1960–1965.

93 Lonial S, Vij R, Harousseau JL, Facon T, Moreau P, Mazumder A, et al. Elotuzumab in combination with lenalidomide and low-dose dexamethasone in relapsed or refractory multiple myeloma. *J Clin Oncol.* 2012;30(16):1953–1959.

94 de Weers M, Tai YT, van der Veer MS, et al. Daratumumab, a novel therapeutic human CD38 monoclonal antibody, induces killing of multiple myeloma and other hematological tumors. *J Immunol.* 2011;186(3):1840–1848.

95 Plesner T, Arkenau T, Lokhorst H, et al. Preliminary safety and efficacy data of daratumumab in combination with lenalidomide and dexamethasone in relapsed or refractory multiple myeloma. American Society of Hematology (ASH) Annual Meeting. *Blood;*2013. 1986.

96 Ikeda H, Hideshima T, Fulciniti M, et al. The monoclonal antibody nBT062 conjugated to cytotoxic Maytansinoids has selective cytotoxicity against CD138-positive multiple myeloma cells in vitro and in vivo. *Clin Cancer Res.* 2009;15(12):4028–4037.

97 Tassone P, Gozzini A, Goldmacher V, et al. In vitro and in vivo activity of the maytansinoid immunoconjugate huN901-N2′-deacetyl-N2′-(3-mercapto-1-oxopropyl)-maytansine against CD56 +multiple myeloma cells. *Cancer Res.* 2004;64(13):4629–4636.

98 Harvey RD, Lonial S. PI3 kinase/AKT pathway as a therapeutic target in multiple myeloma. *Future Oncol.* 2007;3(6):639–647.

99 Hideshima T, Catley L, Yasui H, et al. Perifosine, an oral bioactive novel alkylphospholipid, inhibits Akt and induces in vitro and in vivo cytotoxicity in human multiple myeloma cells. *Blood.* 2006;107(10):4053–4062.

100 Richardson PG, Wolf J, Jakubowiak A, et al. Perifosine plus bortezomib and dexamethasone in patients with relapsed/refractory multiple myeloma previously treated with bortezomib: results of a multicenter phase I/II trial. *J Clin Oncol.* 2011;29(32):4243–4249.

101 Mitsiades CS, Ocio EM, Pandiella A, et al. Aplidin, a marine organism-derived compound with potent antimyeloma activity in vitro and in vivo. *Cancer Res.* 2008;68(13):5216–5225.

102 Dubreuil P, Letard S, Ciufolini M, et al. Masitinib (AB1010), a potent and selective tyrosine kinase inhibitor targeting KIT. *PloS one.* 2009;4(9):e7258.

103 Tai YT, Chang BY, Kong SY, et al. Bruton tyrosine kinase inhibition is a novel therapeutic strategy targeting tumor in the bone marrow microenvironment in multiple myeloma. *Blood.* 2012;120(9):1877–1887.

104 Ramakrishnan V, Kimlinger T, Haug J, et al. TG101209, a novel JAK2 inhibitor, has significant in vitro activity in multiple myeloma and displays preferential cytotoxicity for CD45+ myeloma cells. *Am J Hematol.* 2010;85(9):675–686.

105 Bolli N, Avet-Loiseau H, Wedge DC, et al. Heterogeneity of genomic evolution and mutational profiles in multiple myeloma. *Nat Commun.* 2014;5:2997.

106 Bianchi G and Anderson KC. Understanding biology to tackle the disease: Multiple myeloma from bench to bedside, and back. *CA Cancer J Clin.* 2014;64(6):422–444.

**CHAPTER 15**

# The Impact of Genomics on Targeted Therapy in Multiple Myeloma and Lymphomas

*Jens G. Lohr*[1,3] *and Birgit Knoechel*[1,2,3]

[1] Dana-Farber Cancer Institute, Boston, MA, USA
[2] Boston Children's Hospital, Boston, MA, USA
[3] Harvard Medical School, Boston, MA, USA

## Genomics of Hematologic Neoplasms and Their Potential to Inform Rationale Therapies

The success of targeted therapy with imatinib in chronic myelogenous leukemia (CML) has spurred much interest in the development of rational treatments with defined molecular targets,[1] and targeting the BCR-ABL translocation is often regarded as a blueprint for linking a defined genetic aberration to a specific therapeutic intervention. Since the initial advent of imatinib therapy in CML, certain mutations have been described to confer resistance to imatinib (e.g., T315I) and to occur with treatment over time, and as a consequence several newer tyrosine kinase inhibitors have been developed, with potency even in patients with resistant disease.

Therefore, in principle, the genotype of a tumor represents a sophisticated biomarker that may predict the response to a particular therapy. Modern genotyping technology such as deep sequencing[2] now allows us to determine somatic mutations, translocations, and copy number variations in a comprehensive fashion. Since the first human genome was decoded over a decade ago, "next-generation" sequencing technologies have led to a massive increase in available genetic data in many types of cancer, including multiple myeloma (MM) and diffuse large B cell lymphoma (DLBCL).[3–8] DLBCL is an aggressive Non-Hodgkin lymphoma that affects ~20,000 new patients in the United States every year. While the majority of patients can be cured with chemo-immunotherapy, the treatment success of patients with relapsed and refractory disease is generally poor.[9] Multiple myeloma affects over 25,000 new patients every year in the United States (http://seer.cancer.gov). Traditionally, treatment of MM with conventional antiproliferative drugs has yielded little success. Since the development of the proteasome inhibitor bortezomib and its integration into clinical trials, a substantial improvement in overall survival has been seen in patients with MM.[10] This has led to the development of other proteasome inhibitors, such as carfilzomib and other drugs listed in Table 15.1. Immunomodulatory drugs such as thalidomide, lenalidomide, and more recently pomalidomide belong to another major drug class that is currently used as standard treatment in MM. Interestingly, although immunomodulatory drugs have long been known to be effective in MM, their molecular targets have only been described recently.[11–13] Combination therapy with proteasome inhibitors, immunomodulatory drugs, and corticosteroids has been reported to lead to impressive response rates of 80% and greater in patients with MM.[14]

Despite these improvements, MM remains an incurable disease, and drug resistance develops eventually. This may be explained by the outgrowth of MM clones with somatic resistance mutations, which is well known to mediate resistance to particular drugs in other types of cancer. In some malignancies, resistance mutations emerge within genes that are known drug targets (e.g., EGFR, BCR-ABL), but any genetic event that confers a competitive advantage to a cancer cell represents a candidate resistance gene. Therefore, a deep understanding of the genomics of cancer may identify new oncogenes as well as resistance genes, and thus point to novel therapeutic targets. Given the suboptimal clinical outcomes in MM and DLBCL, there is a great medical need to define the underlying genetic abnormalities that are associated with these diseases and translate them into rational novel therapeutic strategies.

Deep sequencing studies performed in patients with DLBCL or MM identified many novel significantly mutated genes.[3–8] Substantial overlap exists between mutations that were defined by independent groups of investigators, suggesting that the identified mutations are recurrent and reproducible and thus are highly likely to represent "drivers" of the tumor. Multiple computational methods have been developed to recognize which mutated genes confer a competitive advantage to the tumor cell and thus represent putative therapeutic targets. These methods take into account the prevalence of particular mutations among patients, the enrichment of mutations in genes that belong to experimentally validated key signaling pathways, and identification of mutational hotspots in conserved genomic regions. While traditionally the anti-neoplastic capacity of a compound has often been discovered before a target was

---

*Targeted Therapy in Translational Cancer Research*, First Edition. Edited by Apostolia-Maria Tsimberidou, Razelle Kurzrock and Kenneth C. Anderson.
© 2016 John Wiley & Sons, Inc. Published 2016 by John Wiley & Sons, Inc.

**Table 15.1** Molecular targets and associated therapeutic strategies in patients with MM and DLBCL currently under investigation in clinical trials.

**Multiple myeloma**

| Target | Small molecule inhibitors | | | |
|---|---|---|---|---|
| Akt | Afuresertib | GSK2141795 | | |
| BET | GSK525762 | CPI-0610 | | |
| BRAF | Vemurafenib | | | |
| BTK | ACP-196 | | | |
| MET, RET, VEGFR, KIT, FLT-3, TIE-2, AXL, TRKB | Cabozantinib | | | |
| CDKs | Dinaciclib | Palbociclib | | |
| CK2 | Silmitasertib | | | |
| Dual HDAC / PI3K | CUDC-907 | | | |
| HDAC | ACY-1215 | AR-42 | CXD101 | Panobinostat |
| Hsp 90 | Ganetespib | | | |
| STAT3 | OPB-31121 | | | |
| MEK1/MEK2 | Trametinib | | | |
| mTOR | CC-223 | Everolimus | | |
| pan-Pim kinase | LGH447 | | | |
| PI3K | BYL719 | | | |
| Proteasome | Ixazomib | Marizomib | Oprozomib | |
| IGF1R | Linsitinib | | | |

| Target | Antibodies | |
|---|---|---|
| CD138 | BT-062 | |
| CD38 | Daratumumab | MOR03087 |
| CS1 | Elotuzumab | |
| DKK1 | DKN-01 | |
| ICAM-1 (CD54) | BI-505 | |
| PD-1 | Pembrolizumab | Pidilizumab |
| IL-6 | Siltuximab | |

**Diffuse large B cell lymphoma**

| Target | Small molecule inhibitors | | |
|---|---|---|---|
| Akt | MK2206 | | |
| Bcl-2 | GDC-0199 | | |
| BTK | ACP-196 | CC-292 | Ibrutinib |
| HDAC | Belinostat | Panobinostat | AR-42 |
| EZH2 | E7438 | GSK2816126 | |
| mTOR | CC-223 | Everolimus | |
| PI3K | BKM120 | | |
| Syk | GS-9973 | TAK-659 | |
| Dual ALK / EGFR | AP26113 | | |
| PARP | Veliparib | | |

| Target | Antibodies | | |
|---|---|---|---|
| CD20 | Obinutuzumab | Ofatumumab | Veltuzumab |
| PD-L1 | MEDI4736 | | |
| PD-1 | Nivolumab | | |
| CTLA4 | Ipilimumab | | |

| Target | CARs |
|---|---|
| CD19 | Anti-CD19-CAR vector-transduced T cells |
| CD20 | Anti-CD20-CAR vector-transduced autologous T cells |

As of August 2014 there were more than 500 clinical trials listed in the National Institutes of Health registry, as either actively recruiting or in the process of opening for accrual, for patients with multiple myeloma, plasma cell dyscrasias or related disorders. DLBCL was the subject of more than 250 clinical trials (www.clinicaltrials.gov). A large number of these trials were focused on small molecule inhibitors with defined molecular targets or antibodies targeting cell surface molecules as single agent or in combination therapy. There is substantial overlap between therapeutic approaches that are used in MM and DLBCL. Only a small selection of the strategies that are currently pursued in clinical trials is listed. Several of the listed inhibitors may target more than one protein, and some antibodies may be linked to cytotoxic agents. The listed target names either represent Hugo Gene Nomenclature Committee-approved names or commonly used protein family names.

identified (often as a coincidence),[15] the increasing understanding of the genomic basis of neoplasms has paved the way for developing targeted therapeutic agents based on specific genetic aberrations.

## Targeted Agents in Clinical Trials for Patients with MM and DLBCL

As of August 2014 there were 568 clinical trials listed in the National Institutes of Health registry, either actively recruiting or about to open for accrual, with a focus on or including patients with MM or other plasma cell dyscrasias (www.clinicaltrials.gov) and 261 clinical trials including patients with DLBCL. A substantial fraction of these included drugs with defined molecular targets, based on the identification of recurrent genetic aberrations in tumor cells or the characterization of oncogenic signaling pathways in tumor cells (Table 15.1). In addition to small molecule inhibitors, antibodies represent an important class of therapeutics with defined targets (Table 15.1). Such rationally designed drugs with defined targets will likely increase in number over the next few years based on our expanding knowledge of the genetic and molecular basis of disease. In the following we will describe several examples.

### BTK Inhibition in DLBCL

Chronic active B cell receptor signaling in the activated B cell-like (ABC) subtype of DLBCL engages the SRC-family kinases SYK and BTK to activate downstream NF-κB and PI3K pro-survival pathways.[16] Somatic mutations in the *SYK* tyrosine kinase have been identified in DLBCL, inhibition of which has activity in patients with DLBCL.[17] The BTK inhibitor ibrutinib has been tested in clinical trials for patients with DLBCL with promising results, preferentially for patients with ABC DLBCL refractory to other chemotherapy regimens. Responses were more frequent among ABC DLBCLs with a *CD79B* ITAM mutation, including cases with a *MYD88* L265P mutation, but not in patients with tumors that only harbored a *MYD88* L265P mutation or *CARD11* mutations.[18,19] These data illustrate that recurrent mutations can be useful either as a positive or a negative predictive biomarker for the response to BTK inhibition. Several different BTK inhibitors are currently under investigation in clinical trials.

### BRAF and MEK Inhibition in MM

Recurrent somatic mutations in the *BRAF* oncogene in MM were discovered by a next-generation sequencing effort and have since been validated in several MM cohorts.[6-8] Many of these are V600E missense mutations or mutations which are clustered in close proximity to each other at other sites, occurring in about 6% of MM patients. Preclinical data suggest that MM cell lines with *BRAF* mutations are more susceptible to BRAF inhibitors than cell lines without *BRAF* mutations, and treatment with a BRAF inhibitor of an MM patient who harbored a *BRAF* V600E mutation resulted in a rapid and durable response.[20] This patient had previously become refractory to several lines of standard therapy. Patients with *BRAF*-mutated MM were also found to have a higher incidence of extramedullary disease and shorter overall survival. These data implicate mutated *BRAF* as a predictive biomarker as well as a promising target in patients with MM. Other data suggest that the BRAF/MEK/ERK signaling pathway is often activated in MM, even in the absence of *BRAF* mutations.[21] Therefore MEK inhibitors are actively pursued in clinical trials for the treatment of MM, but genetic alterations that can be used as reliable predictive biomarkers to inform these treatments remain to be defined.

### EZH2 Inhibition in DLBCL

EZH2 is recurrently mutated in DLBCL resulting in gain of function.[3-5] Although EZH2 mutations have not been described in multiple myeloma to date, EZH2 is overexpressed in multiple myeloma cells in contrast to normal plasma cells and has been implicated in increasing proliferation of multiple myeloma cells *in vitro*.[22] EZH2 is a member of the polycomb repressive complex 2 (PRC2) that methylates histone H3 on lysine 27 (H3K27). EZH2 exerts an important role in lymphoma initiation. It is highly expressed in normal germinal center B cells, where it causes the formation of bivalent chromatin domains at the promoters of genes required for exit of B cells from the germinal center state. Thus, by repressing the expression of these genes, germinal center B cells are kept in a physiologic dedifferentiated state. In mouse models of the germinal center B cell like (GCB) subtype of DLBCL, *EZH2* mutations cause differentiation blockade, resulting in germinal center hyperplasia and ultimately accelerated lymphomagenesis in the presence of BCL2 overexpression.[23]

Two EZH2 inhibitors have recently been developed, GSK126 and EPZ-6438 (E7438), and are now under investigation in early phase clinical trials. GSK126, a small-molecule inhibitor of the EZH2 methyltransferase activity, inhibits the proliferation of *EZH2*-mutant lymphoma cell lines *in vitro* and in xenograft models *in vivo*.[24] EPZ-6438 inhibits H3K27 methylation in *EZH2*-mutated and nonmutated lymphoma cells. It has cytotoxic effects and causes apoptosis in mutant cell lines. Treatment of *EZH2*-mutant lymphomas in murine xenografts with EPZ-6438 resulted in strong and sustained effects on tumor growth even after treatment was stopped.[25] Based on these data, the translation of these EZH2 inhibitors holds great therapeutic promise toward improving treatment efficacy for patients with gain of function *EZH2* mutations.

### CDK Inhibitors in MM

Cell cycle regulators, including cyclin-dependent kinases (CDKs), have also been investigated for their effects in MM. For example, inhibition of CDK4/6 has been shown to mediate growth arrest, but not death of MM cells *in vitro*, in contrast to seliciclib, a multitarget CDK inhibitor that also elicits cell death, suggesting that multiple cell cycle targets need to be inhibited to overcome redundancy of oncogenic "driver" pathways.[26,27] Accordingly, two CDK inhibitors currently in clinical trials for patients with MM (dinaciclib, palbociclib, Table 15.1) are investigated as part of combination therapies together with bortezomib and lenalidomide, respectively. Notably, as a group of genes, cell cycle regulators, including Cyclin D1 (*CCND1*) and Cyclin-dependent kinase inhibitor 1B (*CDKN1B,* p27[Kip1]), are the most significantly mutated gene set in patients with MM.[7] It is an attractive hypothesis that MM patients, who harbor mutations in one or more of these genes, may be more responsive to CDK inhibition. Careful analysis of responses of genetically defined subgroups in MM patients treated with these drugs will elucidate this question.

### Other Targeted Therapies

As outlined in Table 15.1, many more small molecules are currently explored in the context of clinical trials. Some of them target an underlying genetic alteration such as *BCL2/JH* rearrangements which leads to increased expression of BCL2 and survival of DLBCL cells, as an underlying rationale for Bcl-2 inhibitors. Other compounds target hyperactive signaling pathways, which drive cell growth in many types of cancer, including inhibitors of PI3K, AKT, mTOR, for which genetic defects associated with activation of these pathways are largely unknown in DLBCL and MM. In addition to genetic defects, epigenetically defined targets and biomarkers are gaining attention. For example, the inhibition of bromodomain and extra-terminal domain (BET) proteins has recently been explored experimentally in DLBCL.[28] BET inhibitors are under investigation for a number of different hematologic malignancies. Defining the relationship between targeted therapeutic agents and genetic or epigenetic alterations will be essential for future clinical trials.

## Immunological Therapies

In addition to small molecules with defined targets, therapeutic antibodies have had a huge impact on the treatment of lymphoid neoplasms. Rituximab, a chimeric antibody targeting the CD20 epitope on B cells, has been a successful part of standard treatment in various B lymphocytic malignancies. Therapeutic antibodies currently explored in MM or DLBCL are either directed against a surface epitope that is specific (or overexpressed) on the tumor cells or the lineage they are derived from. For example, CD138 and CD38 are highly expressed on malignant plasma cells, and CD20 and CD19 are expressed on B cells, including DLBCL. Other strategies targeting these epitopes include chimeric antigen receptor (CAR) T cells.[29] Non-specific stimulation of the immune system through inhibition of molecules, which physiologically downregulate immune responses, is another treatment strategy that is under investigation in both MM and DLBCL, with the goal of promoting an anti-tumor immune response. It is easily conceivable that responses of the tumor to these treatments are determined by the genetic profile of the particular tumor cells in an individual patient. To date, the specific genetic defects that regulate whether any of these therapies are successful are largely unknown.

## New Therapeutic Challenges Revealed by Genomics

Therapeutic responses as dramatic and sustained as in CML treated with tyrosine kinase inhibitors are uncommon for single agent treatment in MM or DLBCL, which may be explained by several reasons. First, more than one genetic abnormality that confers a growth advantage to the tumor cells exist in an individual patient with MM or DLBCL. Genetic driver events can occur together in the same tumor cells. Co-occurrence in the same cell can activate alternative pathways with similar downstream effects, ultimately promoting cell growth and thus drug resistance. Alternatively, driver mutations can occur in different cells in the same patient. For instance, MM cells which harbor gain of function mutations in the *BRAF* gene can co-occur in the same patient who harbors mutations in either the *KRAS* or *NRAS* gene, but in different tumor cells.[7] In these cases, the success of treatment with a BRAF inhibitor is difficult to predict, as treatment may successfully target the *BRAF*-mutated subclone, but may not reduce the cell number of *KRAS*- or *NRAS*-mutated subclones. This intra-individual genetic heterogeneity and the co-existence of drug-susceptible and drug-resistant clones complicate targeted therapy.

Second, compounds targeting individual molecules are rarely completely specific, and off-target effects lead to side effects in normal tissue limiting the tolerated dose and thus resulting in only partial inhibition of the target. Third, as is true for the mutational landscape in other cancers, therapeutic targeting of individual mutations in patients with MM and DLBCL may only be feasible in some cases, given the multitude of recurrent genes with mutations and structural alterations. It would therefore be desirable to classify genetic alterations into distinct pathways. Targeting a few pathways rather than many individual mutations would be a much more feasible therapeutic approach.

"Precision medicine" based on high-resolution genotyping is complicated further by the fact that resistant subclones can already be present at the time of treatment initiation but only become detectable after reaching a detection threshold over time. In addition, nongenetic resistance mechanisms may exist, which are mediated through epigenetic changes or by survival signals from the tumor microenvironment, like cytokines or cell–cell interaction. For MM and DLBCL and most other malignant diseases, a combination of resistance mechanisms is likely responsible for the poor response rates of treatment with single drugs and relapse after standard treatment.

Strategies to increase initial response rates and reduce drug resistance are under active investigation. MM is preceded in many, if not all, cases by a premalignant monoclonal gammopathy of undetermined significance (MGUS) phase, which then transitions to smoldering myeloma. It is therefore conceivable that early treatment in the MGUS or smoldering myeloma state may reduce the outgrowth of resistant subclones, and this is currently explored in clinical trials. Furthermore, combination therapy with several targeted drugs may inhibit redundant oncogenic signaling pathways at the same time, and thus may increase efficacy.

Understanding the genomic basis of MM and DLBCL, as well as the genetic evolution that leads to the development of drug resistance, is an important research focus in order to connect genomic data to the mechanism of action of a particular drug. Data addressing these questions will likely accumulate in the near future and will be essential for successful targeted therapy. In a few cases, a direct relation between a genetic alteration and a corresponding drug already exists (e.g., *BRAF V600E*–BRAF inhibition), but such relations remain to be elucidated more comprehensively in MM and DLBCL. The success of "precision medicine" will depend on our ability to establish robust predictive biomarkers based on the available genomic data.

## References

1 Druker BJ. Translation of the Philadelphia chromosome into therapy for CML. *Blood*. 2008;112(13):4808–4817.

2 Koboldt DC, Steinberg KM, Larson DE, Wilson RK, Mardis ER. The next-generation sequencing revolution and its impact on genomics. *Cell*. 2013;155(1):27–38.

3 Morin RD, Mendez-Lago M, Mungall AJ, et al. Frequent mutation of histone-modifying genes in non-Hodgkin lymphoma. *Nature*. 2011;476(7360):298–303.

4 Lohr JG, Stojanov P, Lawrence MS, et al. Discovery and prioritization of somatic mutations in diffuse large B-cell lymphoma (DLBCL) by whole-exome sequencing. *Proc Natl Acad Sci U S A*. 2012;109(10):3879–3884.

5 Zhang J, Grubor V, Love CL, et al. Genetic heterogeneity of diffuse large B-cell lymphoma. *Proc Natl Acad Sci U S A*. 2013;110(4):1398–1403.

6 Chapman MA, Lawrence MS, Keats JJ, et al. Initial genome sequencing and analysis of multiple myeloma. *Nature*. 2011;471(7339):467–472.

7 Lohr JG, Stojanov P, Carter SL, et al. Widespread genetic heterogeneity in multiple myeloma: implications for targeted therapy. *Cancer Cell*. 2014;25(1):91–101.

8 Bolli N, Avet-Loiseau H, Wedge DC, et al. Heterogeneity of genomic evolution and mutational profiles in multiple myeloma. *Nat Commun*. 2014;5:2997.

9 Roschewski M, Staudt LM, Wilson WH. Diffuse large B-cell lymphoma-treatment approaches in the molecular era. *Nat Rev Clin Oncol.* 2014;11(1):12–23.

10 Palumbo A, Anderson K. Multiple myeloma. *N Engl J Med.* 2011;364(11):1046–1060.

11 Lu G, Middleton RE, Sun H, et al. The myeloma drug lenalidomide promotes the cereblon-dependent destruction of Ikaros proteins. *Science.* 2014;343(6168):305–309.

12 Ito T, Ando H, Suzuki T, et al. Identification of a primary target of thalidomide teratogenicity. *Science.* 2010;327(5971):1345–1350.

13 Krönke J, Udeshi ND, Narla A, et al. Lenalidomide causes selective degradation of IKZF1 and IKZF3 in multiple myeloma cells. *Science.* 2014;343(6168):301–305.

14 Richardson PG, Weller E, Lonial S, et al. Lenalidomide, bortezomib, and dexamethasone combination therapy in patients with newly diagnosed multiple myeloma. *Blood.* 2010;116(5):679–686.

15 Chabner BA, Roberts TG. Timeline: chemotherapy and the war on cancer. *Nat Rev Cancer.* 2005;5(1):65–72.

16 Young RM, Staudt LM. Targeting pathological B cell receptor signalling in lymphoid malignancies. *Nat Rev Drug Discov.* 2013;12(3):229–243.

17 Friedberg JW, Sharman J, Sweetenham J, et al. Inhibition of Syk with fostamatinib disodium has significant clinical activity in non-Hodgkin lymphoma and chronic lymphocytic leukemia. *Blood.* 2010;115(13):2578–2585.

18 Chavez JC, Sahakian E, Pinilla-Ibarz J. Ibrutinib: an evidence-based review of its potential in the treatment of advanced chronic lymphocytic leukemia. *Core Evid.* 2013;8:37–45.

19 Fowler N, Davis E. Targeting B-cell receptor signaling: changing the paradigm. *Hematology Am Soc Hematol Educ Prog.* 2013;2013:553–560.

20 Andrulis M, Lehners N, Capper D, et al. Targeting the BRAF V600E mutation in multiple myeloma. *Cancer Discov.* 2013;3(8):862–869.

21 Chang-Yew Leow C, Gerondakis S, Spencer A. MEK inhibitors as a chemotherapeutic intervention in multiple myeloma. *Blood Cancer J.* 2013;3:e105.

22 Croonquist PA, Van Ness B. The polycomb group protein enhancer of zeste homolog 2 (EZH 2) is an oncogene that influences myeloma cell growth and the mutant ras phenotype. *Oncogene.* 2005;24(41):6269–6280.

23 Béguelin W, Popovic R, Teater M, et al. EZH2 is required for germinal center formation and somatic EZH2 mutations promote lymphoid transformation. *Cancer Cell.* 2013;23(5):677–692.

24 McCabe MT, Ott HM, Ganji G, et al. EZH2 inhibition as a therapeutic strategy for lymphoma with EZH2-activating mutations. *Nature.* 2012;492(7427):108–112.

25 Knutson SK, Kawano S, Minoshima Y, et al. Selective inhibition of EZH2 by EPZ-6438 leads to potent antitumor activity in EZH2-mutant non-Hodgkin lymphoma. *Mol Cancer Ther.* 2014;13(4):842–854.

26 Huang X, Di Liberto M, Jayabalan D, et al. Prolonged early G(1) arrest by selective CDK4/CDK6 inhibition sensitizes myeloma cells to cytotoxic killing through cell cycle-coupled loss of IRF4. *Blood.* 2012;120(5):1095–1106.

27 Raje N, Kumar S, Hideshima T, et al. Seliciclib (CYC202 or R-roscovitine), a small-molecule cyclin-dependent kinase inhibitor, mediates activity via down-regulation of Mcl-1 in multiple myeloma. *Blood.* 2005;106(3):1042–1047.

28 Chapuy B, McKeown MR, Lin CY, et al. Discovery and characterization of super-enhancer-associated dependencies in diffuse large B cell lymphoma. *Cancer Cell.* 2013;24(6):777–790.

29 Maus MV, Grupp SA, Porter DL, June CH. Antibody-modified T cells: CARs take the front seat for hematologic malignancies. *Blood.* 2014;123(17):2625–2635.

# 16

# CHAPTER 16

# Targeted Therapy in Myelodysplastic Syndromes

*Guillermo Montalbán-Bravo[1] and Guillermo García-Manero[2]*

[1] Department of Hematology, Hospital Universitario La Paz, Madrid, Spain

[2] Department of Leukemia, The University of Texas MD Anderson Cancer Center, Houston, TX, USA

## Biological Hallmarks of Myelodysplasia

### Myelodysplasia as a Disease of the Hematopoietic Stem Cell

Increasing evidence has supported the idea that myelodysplastic syndromes (MDS) are essentially a stem cell disease, with most of the genetic and epigenetic alterations leading to myelodysplasia occurring in an early progenitor that will, due to a progressive accumulation of mutations, ultimately evolve to a leukemic clone. Several murine models have been developed to try to prove this concept with encouraging results. Nilsson et al. were able to determine a likelihood in expression profiles between hematopoietic stem cells (HSC) from del(5q) MDS cases and normal HSC.[1] Pellagati et al.[2] determined the existence of deregulation of different pathways in CD34+ MDS cells some of which are known to be important regulators of stem cell biology (such as Wnt/β-catenine, EVI-1 and thrombopoietin signaling). In their study, they were also able to characterize the existence of distinct pathway patterns in different cytogenetic subgroups of CD34+ MDS cells, some of which were associated with apoptosis signaling. This is consistent with both morphologic and molecular data that highlight the existence of increased apoptosis in MDS pathogencsis. Similar to this group, Will et al. also studied genetic and epigenetic alterations in MDS HSCs showing distinctive methylation patterns in different cellular pathways.[3] It is clear that increased proliferation of clonal progenitors with impaired differentiation and increased apoptosis is a hallmark of myelodysplasia.[4] Despite the fact that we do not yet fully understand the molecular reasoning behind this phenomenon, the origin of increased apoptosis in MDS seems complex and related to different mechanisms[5] including stem cell aging (due to oxidative stress and impaired cytokine regulation), decreased quiescence of normal HSC with increased myeloid skewing, decreased global methylation and overexpression of Fas ligand (FasL), and TNF-related apoptosis-inducing ligand (TRAIL) in MDS HSCs. Microenvironment also seems to be an important factor in this proapoptotic state through Interleukin 6 (IL-6) and tumor necrosis factor α (TNF-α) secretion and increased expression of calreticulin (a prophagocytic surface molecule) in HSCs.

## Recurrently Mutated Pathways in MDS and Disease Evolution to AML

Many groups have studied the mutational landscape of myelodysplasia in the last decades, and much information is now available regarding the different pathways recurrently involved in disease initiation and progression. Table 16.1 summarizes the different frequently mutated genes in MDS and their impact on disease evolution. Up to 89.5% of MDS cases harbor at least one mutation with some cases accumulating up to 12 different coexisting mutations.[6] Despite the importance of isolated mutations in MDS pathogenesis, clonality and hierarchy of mutational acquisition has risen as an essential hallmark of disease initiation and progression. Current evidence suggests that a progressive acquisition of mutations is the key to disease spectrum and ultimate transformation to AML. Initial founder mutations affecting spliceosome genes (SF3B1, SRSF2, U2AF1, ZRSR2), present in 45–85% patients,[9] and DNA methylation regulators (TET2, IDH, DNMT3A), present in 10–30% cases,[7] occur in HSCs with self-renewal and proliferation potential. These mutations seem to confer a biological advantage to the clone that can expand in the bone marrow and develop myelodysplastic features and cytopenias due to impaired differentiation and increased apoptosis. Some of these subclones will continue to accumulate additional hits[10] in chromatin and transcription regulators (EZH2, ASXL1), further impairing differentiation, along with cytogenetic alterations and mutations in transcription factors (RUNX1, ETV6), kinase pathways (FLT3, RAS), and cell-cycle regulators (TP53) leading to increased proportion of blasts, proliferation, and ultimate transformation to leukemia. There is increasing evidence supporting this model of leukemogenesis with regard to the acquisition of these somatic mutations present in MDS. Mutations in DNMT3A and TET2 and their resulting leukemogenic potential (impaired differentiation and increased self-renewal capacity) in mouse models suggest the existence of pre-leukemic HSCs harboring these mutations, which, in fact, can also be identified in healthy population using high-throughput sequencing technology.[11] In fact, the existence of some of these mutations, such as EZH2, ASXL1 and those affecting the spliceosome, are highly specific of secondary AML and

*Targeted Therapy in Translational Cancer Research*, First Edition. Edited by Apostolia-Maria Tsimberidou, Razelle Kurzrock and Kenneth C. Anderson.
© 2016 John Wiley & Sons, Inc. Published 2016 by John Wiley & Sons, Inc.

**Table 16.1** Frequently mutated genes in MDS.

| Molecular pathway | Gene | Frequency (%) | Clinical phenotype and associated mutations | Prognostic impact |
| --- | --- | --- | --- | --- |
| RNA splicing | SF3B1 | 10–30 | Associated with RARS/RARS-T (80%) Coexistence of DNMT3A$_{mt}$ | Good OS and low risk of evolution to AML |
| | SRSF2 | 10–20 | Male gender, advanced age, associated with RCMD or RAEB Comutation with TET2 in CMML | Poor OS and high risk of evolution to AML |
| | U2AF1 | 5–10 | Associated with RCMD and RAEB Enriched in patients with del(20q) and ASXL1$_{mt}$ | High risk of evolution to AML |
| | ZRSR2 | 3–10 | Male predominance, isolated neutropenia Associated with TET2 mutations | Unknown |
| DNA methylation | TET2 | 20–30 | All MDS subtypes. Generally a founding mutation High frequency in CMML (50–60%) | Response to hypomethylating agents No impact on OS |
| | IDH1/IDH2 | 5–10 | Mutually exclusive to TET2$_{mt}$ Associated with normal karyotype, RCMD, or RAEB | Unfavorable prognosis |
| | DNMT3A | 3–13 | All MDS subtypes Founding mutation Co-mutation with SF3B1 in RARS | Unfavorable prognosis and risk of leukemic evolution (mitigated by SF3B1$_{mt}$ in RARS) |
| Histone modification | ASXL1 | 10–20 | RCMD or RAEB with high mutation frequency in CMML (40%) | Unfavorable prognosis and evolution to AML |
| | EZH2 | 6–8 | Associated with RCMD or RAEB UPD of 7q in MDS/MPN | Unfavorable prognosis |
| Transcription factors and cell-cycle regulators | RUNX1 | ~10 | Associated with thrombocytopenia, RCMD, RAEB, and tMDS | Unfavorable prognosis and increased risk of transformation to AML |
| | BCOR | <5 | Associated with RAEB and RCMD | Unfavorable prognosis |
| | ETV6 | 1–3 | Not defined | Unfavorable prognosis |
| | TP53 | 5–10 | Association with advanced disease, isolated del(5q) (20%), and complex cytogenetics | Poor OS and high risk of transformation to AML Poor response to lenalidomide in del(5q) MDS |
| Kinase signaling | NRAS | 6–17 | Present in different MDS subtypes with higher frequency in CMML | Associated with evolution to AML |
| | CBL | 1–3 | Frequent in CMML and MDS/MPN | Not defined |
| | FLT3-ITD | 1–3 | MDS progressing to AML | Associated with leukemic transformation |
| | JAK2 | <5 | High frequency in RARS-T (50–70%) and CMML (10%) | Not defined |
| | KIT | <1 | High-risk MDS | Associated with leukemic transformation |
| | NF1 | <5 | Found in different MDS subtypes | Not defined |
| DNA replication | SETBP1 | <5 | Advanced MDS or CMML | Associated with poor OS and high risk of evolution to AML |

*Source:* Data from References 6, 7, and 8.
RARS, refractory anemia with ring sideroblasts; RARS-T, refractory anemia with ring sideroblasts and thrombocytosis; RCMD, refractory cytopenia with multilineage dysplasia; RAEB, refractory anemia with excess blasts; CMML, chronic myelomonocytic leukemia.

virtually absent in de novo AML further supporting this conception of MDS evolution and progression to AML.[12] It is therefore essential to view molecular pathway alterations in MDS as an interrelated process and not as isolated events due to the distinct biological advantages each different pathway can confer to the leukemic clone, and its potential to generate myelodysplasia in any of its forms.

## Epigenetic Deregulation in Myelodysplasia

Epigenetic modulation of gene expression through DNA methylation, histone modifications, posttranscriptional modification of proteins (alternative splicing), and miRNA modulation represents an increasingly important group of mechanisms in MDS pathogenesis.[13] Alteration of methylation patterns in MDS CD34+ cells, characterized by aberrant hypermethylation in 3–5% of promoter-associated C—phosphate—G (CpG) islands, can occur in initial stages of the disease mainly due to the early appearance of mutations in epigenetic regulators (such as TET2 and DNMT3A), and represent a risk factor of leukemic evolution. This increase in promoter methylation seems to induce a genomic shift leading to a decrease in cell differentiation and maturation along with a progressive increased expression of genes related to myeloid proliferation and expansion (such as the HOX group of genes). Disruption of TET2 through loss-of-function mutations and inhibition by 2-hydroxyglutarate produced by mutant IDH has been associated with increased methylation and upregulation of HOXA genes with resultant myeloid expansion.[14,15] Similar events are known to appear with DNMT3A mutations[16] and through mutation of histone regulators such as ASXL1, a member of the Polycomb Repressor Complex 1 (PRC 1),[17] and EZH2,[18] a member of PRC 2, resulting in impaired myeloid differentiation, derepression of proliferation and induction of stem cell expansion. It therefore seems clear that deregulation of the normal epigenetic processes responsible for cell differentiation and regulation of proliferation is an essential hallmark of the initiation and development of myelodysplasia and is related to disease progression and transformation.

## Current Standard of Care in MDS

Treatment strategies in MDS have evolved in the last years since the appearance of hypomethylating agents. Prior to the development of these drugs, very few available therapies existed

and management of the disease was extremely limited. Disease risk determination is essential prior to initiation of therapy. Several prognostic scores exist with the International Prognostic Scoring System (IPSS)[19] being the most commonly used. This highly reproducible system allows stratification of patients into four major groups: low risk, intermediate-I, intermediate-II, and high risk depending on the bone marrow blast count, cytogenetic alterations, and number of cytopenias. Its recently revised version (IPSS-R)[20] further stratifies patients into five risk categories. Despite this four-group classification of the IPSS, patients with MDS are generally classified as either low risk (including low and intermediate-I IPSS cases) or high risk (including intermediate-II and high IPSS cases) when treatment strategy decisions have to be made. Treatment is summarized in Figure 16.1.

In lower-risk patients, treatment objectives have been generally focused in controlling cytopenias and overcoming transfusion dependency mainly through growth factor support using G-CSF and erythroid-stimulating agents (ESAs) and lenalidomide in cases harboring del(5q), with hypomethylating agents playing a role after the failure of prior therapies. The use of ESAs in low-risk MDS, especially in those with low endogenous erythropoietin levels and low transfusion burden, has allowed to decrease transfusion dependence. Addition of G-CSF in patients not responding initially to ESAs has been shown to increase response rates to these agents and is therefore a reasonable option if no improvement is observed after 8 weeks of therapy.[21,22] However, in the last years, reducing progression to higher-risk MDS in low-risk patients with poor prognostic

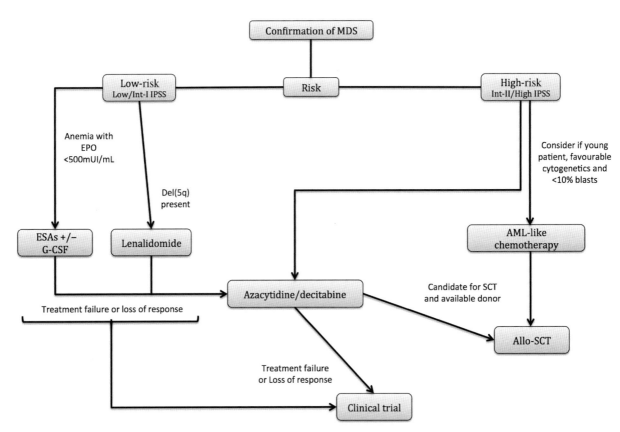

**Figure 16.1** Treatment algorithm for the current standard of care in MDS. **Low-risk MDS:** Consider ESAs +/− G-CSF if EPO levels predict possibility of response (<500 mUI/mL). In patients with del(5q) treatment with lenalidomide should be initiated. If loss of response appears, consider treatment with hypomethylating agents or inclusion in clinical trial. **High-risk MDS:** Standard treatment should involve HMA treatment followed by alloSCT if candidate to transplantation. Inclusion in a clinical trial if relapse or loss of response should be considered if available.

features has become an area of interest, and therefore several trials analyzing the possible impact of low doses of azacitidine and decitabine are currently under development. Lenalidomide has been associated with an increase in hemoglobin levels and acquisition of transfusion independency (the most important prognostic factor for overall survival (OS) in low-risk MDS) in patients with MDS with del(5q), and improved OS among responders.[23,24] Different groups have recurrently tried to elucidate the mechanism of action of this drug, with interesting results. Reduced erythropoiesis in del(5q) MDS appears due to haploinsufficiency of RPS14 (a ribosomal protein) which leads to accumulation of free ribosomes, MDM2 inhibition, increased free p53 and subsequent apoptosis of erythroid progenitors. Haploinsufficiency of miR-145 and miR-146a induce upregulation of TRAF6 and IL-6R inducing thrombocytosis, neutropenia, and megakaryocytic dysplasia. Loss of several tumor suppressor genes such as EGR1, APC, SPARC, and DIAPH grant proliferation and survival advantage to the MDS clone. Lenalidomide has the potential to target and revert these different molecular processes.[25]

Allogeneic stem cell transplantation (alloSCT) is not generally recommended in lower-risk patients due to a decreased OS associated with transplant (due to high TRM) compared to the long expected survival of patients with lower-risk MDS,[26] even when applying reduced conditioning regimens.[27]

Treatment of higher-risk patients is, however, focused on repression of the leukemic clone in order to control cytopenias, improve a compromised OS and prevent leukemic transformation. Hypomethylating agents have risen as a key therapeutic weapon in this subset of patients and have shown to induce responses, decrease the risk of transformation to AML and improve OS compared to best supportive care or AML-type chemotherapy.[28] These drugs have been consistently studied in higher-risk MDS[29,30] and have therefore been approved as the standard of care in these patients. Both azacitidine and decitabine seem to exert this effect through DNMT1 depletion and hypomethylation inducing differentiation and p53-independent apoptosis.[31] Despite the revolution that these drugs have introduced in high-risk MDS, eventual loss of response to therapy remains a major challenge.[32] Regardless of the efforts being made in the understanding of the biological processes behind this phenomenon, there is still much improvement to be made in this field. AML-like chemotherapy remains a treatment option in these patients; however, it is associated with lower complete response (CR) rates and shorter duration of responses. Due to its increased toxicity, it is generally considered as an option for younger patients with >10% blasts and favorable cytogenetics, who are candidates for alloSCT. Allogeneic transplantation remains the only curative option in MDS, with prolonged disease-free survival (DFS) in up to 50% of patients,[33] and is therefore a standard treatment in higher-risk patients who are candidates for transplant and have an available donor. The optimal time for transplantation is, nevertheless, a challenge and a topic under discussion. There is evidence to suggest early transplantation in patients with high-risk MDS is ideal in order to prevent transformation to AML prior to transplant. However, controlling the clone and achieving cytogenetic responses prior to transplantation with several cycles of therapy can lower the risk of relapse specifically in MDS with unfavorable cytogenetics.[34] Individual assessment of each patient's risk, cytogenetics, donor availability, and response to therapy should be taken into account when deciding the ideal timing for transplantation. Exploring the use of azacitidine after transplant in order to reduce disease relapse is currently an area of research with encouraging results.[35,36]

## New Therapeutic Targets in MDS

Due to the advances in the last decades in the pathogenesis of MDS, a number of targeted therapies have been developed in order to try to improve the therapeutic armamentarium at our disposal. In the current section, we describe some of the molecules currently under development in low- and high-risk MDS (Figure 16.2).

### p38 MAPK Inhibition: SCIO-469 and ARRY-614

The p38 mitogen-activated protein kinase (MAPK) pathway participates in several important cellular mechanisms including apoptosis, transcriptional regulation, cytokine production and cell cycle progression.[37,38] This pathway is normally activated by a variety of cytokines and growth factors including IFNs, TNF-α and TGF-β.[39] Altered p38 MAPK signaling consisting in over-activation of this pathway leading to increased apoptosis through BCL-XL inhibition and cytokine overproduction has also been found in myelodysplasia.[40,41] Inhibition of this overactivation of p38 MAPK has been shown to restore normal hematopoiesis of MDS progenitors.[42] Due to this observation, several inhibitors of this pathway have been developed. SCIO-469 was the first molecule to be tested in patients with low- and intermediate-I MDS in a phase 1–2 multicenter study with modest results.[43] ARRY-614 is another dual inhibitor of p38 MAPK and Tie2 with potential activity. Results from a phase 1–2 trial evaluating the potential of this drug in patients with low- or intermediate-I MDS with failure to prior therapy with ESAs, lenalidomide, or hypomethylating agents were promising.[44]

### TGF-β Modulation: Sotatercept or ACE-11

TGF-β is known to play a major role in cell proliferation and growth control. Increased levels of this cytokine in the bone marrow of patients with MDS are well established,[45] with evidence of constitutive activation and overexpression in MDS precursors leading to inhibition of erythropoiesis and induction of apoptosis of erythroid precursors through SMAD2 signaling. Different efforts have been made in order to block this pathway, and activin receptor ligand traps represent the most promising compounds. Sotatercept (ACE-11) is a fusion protein of Activin receptor type-IIA and the Fc portion of human IgG1 that binds to the activin receptor blocking TGF-β union and inhibiting SMAD2 activation. A clinical trial is currently underway in order to explore the efficacy of this agent in low-risk MDS patients (NCT01736683).

### NF-κβ Inhibition: Bortezomib

Activation of the NF-κβ signaling pathway is involved in the pathogenesis of both low-risk and high-risk MDS. Bone marrow microenvironment signals through different cytokines such as IL-8, chronic inflammation, and toll-like receptors (TLRs), through TRAF6 and MYD88, induce activation of NF-κβ impairing erythropoiesis via JMJD3 in low-risk MDS.[46,47] This has led to the initiation of a trial evaluating the potential effect of Bortezomib, a proteasome inhibitor, in low-risk MDS patients with p65 activation (NCT01891968). Higher activation of NF-κβ pathway is seen in high-risk MDS and AML in which the p65/p50 complex induces proliferation and upregulation of an array of anti-apoptotic proteins such as BCL2, BIRC2/BIRC3, and CFLAR.[5] An ongoing trial is evaluating the potential of this drug in combination with Belinostat, a histone deacetylase (HDAC) inhibitor, in refractory AML and high-risk MDS (NCT01075425).

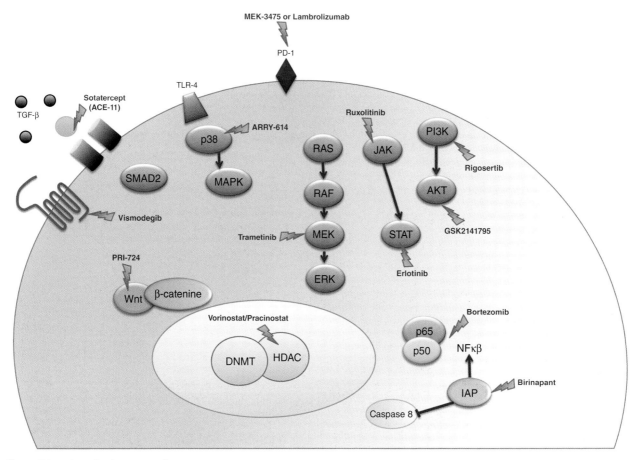

**Figure 16.2** Main molecular targets of new transduction inhibitors in MDS.

## Multikinase Inhibition: Rigosertib

Rigosertib is an inhibitor of Polo-like kinase and PI3K/AKT kinase pathways with *in vitro* activity in MDS CD34+ cells harboring trisomy 8[48] with modest activity in monotherapy. Two trials are currently evaluating its potential in combination with azacitidine in patients with MDS and AML (NCT01926587) and in patients with MDS with excess blasts progressing after hypomethylating therapy (NCT01928537).

## Farnesyltransferase Inhibition: Tipifarnib

Many protein substrates involved in cell proliferation and differentiation suffer posttranslational regulation through farnesyltransferase. This is the case of RAS which is mutated in up to 6–17% of patients with MDS.[8] Tipifarnib was the first inhibitor to be developed and has been studied in both MDS and AML. A phase II study in 82 patients with high-risk MDS showed 15% CR (17/82) with long-term responses of 11.5 months and acceptable tolerability.[49]

## SMAC Activation: Birinapant

Despite the existence of increased apoptosis in low-risk MDS, progressive evasion of apoptosis with increased proliferation remains an important hallmark of high-risk MDS and evolution to AML. Deregulation of inhibitor of apoptosis proteins (IAP) is one of the mechanisms behind evasion of apoptosis in cancer. IAPs are regulated by SMAC, an endogenous antagonist. Birinapant is a SMAC mimetic that inhibits IAP activity by blocking TRAF2-mediated NF-κβ activation through TNF inhibition, therefore, restoring caspase-8-dependent apoptosis.[50] An ongoing phase I–II trial is evaluating the possible activity of this compound in combination with azacitidine for patients with MDS with or without prior treatment or failure to hypomethylating agents (NCT01828346).

## MEK Inhibition: GSK1120212 or Trametinib

As previously stated, RAS mutations appear in up to 17% of patients with MDS. Activation of the Ras/Raf/MEK/ERK pathway leads to increased proliferation in these cases. Trametinib is a MEK inhibitor that has been evaluated in monotherapy in patients with $RAS_{mt}$ MDS with 31% overall response rate (ORR) and 23% CR. It is currently being explored in combination with GSK2141795 (an AKT inhibitor) in patients with $RAS_{mt}$ MDS (NCT01907815).

## JAK Inhibition: Ruxolitinib

Only 5% of patients with MDS harbor JAK2 mutations. This frequency increases up to 50–70% in RARS-T and to 10% in patients with CMML.[8] Due to the potential driver effect of JAK2 in this subgroup of patients with MDS, one can speculate a potential effect of JAK inhibition. An exploratory trial is evaluating the possible benefit of combining Ruxolitinib with azacitidine in MDS/MPN patients with frequent JAK mutations (NCT01787487).

## HDAC Inhibition: Vorinostat and Pracinostat

HDAC inhibitors represent a well-explored therapy in AML and MDS. Vorinostat has shown to be active *in vitro* by promoting cell-cycle arrest, growth inhibition, apoptosis, and differentiation of AML and MDS blasts.[51] Results from a recent phase II trial of vorinostat in combination with azacitidine in patients with MDS were encouraging[52] with 70% ORR and 20% CR. Pracinostat is another HDAC inhibitor that was initially studied in a phase II trial in combination with azacitidine in nine patients with high-risk MDS showing 89% ORR with 78% CR + CRi, including complete cytogenetic responses in 56% patients.[53] These results have led to the initiation of a phase II study in combination with azacitidine in patients with high-risk MDS and AML (NCT01912274).

### PD-1 Inhibition: MK-3475 or Lambrolizumab

Programmed death-1 protein (PD-1) and its ligand PDL-1 are membrane proteins that participate in lymphocyte function. PD-1 enrichment by demethylation was noted in patients with MDS after exposure and failure to hypomethylating agents,[54] suggesting a possible implication in treatment failure. In order to try and elucidate the potential of PD-1 inhibition in this context, a trial with an anti-PD1 antibody, MK-3475, or lambrolizumab, is currently ongoing in patients with MDS, which failed to respond to azacitidine or decitabine (NCT01953692).

### EGFR Inhibition: Erlotinib

EGFR inhibition resulted in induction of apoptosis and inhibition of proliferation in AML and MDS cell lines in preclinical studies. This led to the development of a phase II study of erlotinib in MDS patients, which resulted in an ORR of 17% (CR, 13%).[55] An ongoing trial is evaluating its effect in AML including AML evolving from MDS after failure to azacitidine (NCT01664897).

### Wnt and Hedgehog Inhibition: PRI-724 and Vismodegib

Targeting the leukemic stem cell through inhibition of several essential pathways, including Wnt/β-catenine and Hedgehog, is a novel area of research.[56] This has led to the development of several compounds that are being explored in various types of cancers including MDS. Two trials are currently evaluating the potential of Wnt inhibitor PRI-724 (NCT01606579) and Hedgehog inhibitor Vismodegib (NCT01880437) in patients with AML and MDS.

## Conclusions

Knowledge regarding the underlying molecular processes of MDS pathogenesis has expanded in the last decades with important advances in therapy development. Nevertheless, there are still many unanswered questions regarding the mechanisms of interrelation between the different hallmarks of the disease, and an appropriate understanding of this molecular communication is paramount if we are to be able to design optimal therapeutic strategies. Regardless of these facts, it is clear that MDS has risen as an extraordinarily diverse disease with an array of possible molecular pathways that will ultimately require a personalized approach and selection of therapy in the coming years.

## References

1 Nilsson L, Edén P, Olsson E, et al. The molecular signature of MDS stem cells supports a stem-cell origin of 5q myelodysplastic syndromes. *Blood*. 2007;110(8):3005–3014.

2 Pellagatti A, Cazzola M, Giagounidis A, et al. Deregulated gene expression pathways in myelodysplastic syndrome hematopoietic stem cells. *Leukemia*. 2010;24(4):756–764.

3 Will B, Zhou L, Vogler TO, et al. Stem and progenitor cells in myelodysplastic syndromes show aberrant stage-specific expansion and harbor genetic and epigenetic alterations. *Blood*. 2012;120(10):2076–2086.

4 Raza A, N Galili. The genetic basis of phenotypic heterogeneity in myelodysplastic syndromes. *Nat Rev Cancer*. 2012;12(12):849–859.

5 Karlic H, Herrmann H, Varga F, et al. The role of epigenetics in the regulation of apoptosis in myelodysplastic syndromes and acute myeloid leukemia. *Crit Rev Oncol Hematol*. 2014;90(1):1–16.

6 Haferlach T, Nagata Y, Grossmann V, et al. Landscape of genetic lesions in 944 patients with myelodysplastic syndromes. *Leukemia*. 2014;28(2):241–247.

7 Cazzola M, Della Porta MG, Malcovati L. The genetic basis of myelodysplasia and its clinical relevance. *Blood*. 2013;122(25):4021–4034.

8 Kulasekararaj AG, Mohamedali AM, GJ Mufti. Recent advances in understanding the molecular pathogenesis of myelodysplastic syndromes. *Br J Haematol*. 2013;162(5):587–605.

9 Yoshida K, Sanada M, Shiraishi Y, et al. Frequent pathway mutations of splicing machinery in myelodysplasia. *Nature*. 2011;478(7367):64–69.

10 Papaemmanuil E, Gerstung M, Malcovati L, et al.; Chronic Myeloid Disorders Working Group of the International Cancer Genome Consortium. Clinical and biological implications of driver mutations in myelodysplastic syndromes. *Blood*. 2013;122(22):3616–3627; quiz 3699.

11 Corces-Zimmerman MR, Majeti R. Pre-leukemic evolution of hematopoietic stem cells: the importance of early mutations in leukemogenesis. *Leukemia*. 2014; 28(12):2276–2282.

12 Lindsley RC, et al. Acute myeloid leukemia ontogeny is defined by distinct somatic mutations. *Blood*. 2015. 125(9):1367–1376.

13 Issa JP. The myelodysplastic syndrome as a prototypical epigenetic disease. *Blood*. 2013;121(19):3811–3817.

14 Li Z, Cai X, Cai CL, et al. Deletion of Tet2 in mice leads to dysregulated hematopoietic stem cells and subsequent development of myeloid malignancies. *Blood*. 2011;118(17):4509–4518.

15 Moran-Crusio K, Reavie L, Shih A, et al. Tet2 loss leads to increased hematopoietic stem cell self-renewal and myeloid transformation. *Cancer Cell*. 2011;20(1):11–24.

16 Jost E, Lin Q, Weidner CI, et al. Epimutations mimic genomic mutations of DNMT3A in acute myeloid leukemia. *Leukemia*. 2014;28(6):1227–1234.

17 Wang J, Li Z, He Y, et al. Loss of Asxl1 leads to myelodysplastic syndrome-like disease in mice. *Blood*. 2014;123(4):541–553.

18 Kamminga LM, Bystrykh LV, de Boer A, et al. The Polycomb group gene Ezh2 prevents hematopoietic stem cell exhaustion. *Blood*. 2006;107(5):2170–2179.

19 Greenberg P, Cox C, LeBeau MM, et al. International scoring system for evaluating prognosis in myelodysplastic syndromes. *Blood*. 1997;89(6):2079–2088.

20 Greenberg PL, Tuechler H, Schanz J, et al. Revised international prognostic scoring system for myelodysplastic syndromes. *Blood*. 2012;120(12):2454–2465.

21 Garcia-Manero G. Myelodysplastic syndromes: 2014 update on diagnosis, risk-stratification, and management. *Am J Hematol*. 2014;89(1):97–108.

22 Malcovati, L, et al. Diagnosis and treatment of primary myelodysplastic syndromes in adults: recommendations from the European LeukemiaNet. *Blood*. 2013;122(17):2943–2964.

23 List A, Dewald G, Bennett J, et al.; Myelodysplastic Syndrome-003 Study Investigators. Lenalidomide in the myelodysplastic syndrome with chromosome 5q deletion. *N Engl J Med*. 2006;355(14):1456–1465.

24 List AF, Bennett JM, Sekeres MA, et al.; MDS-003 Study Investigators. Extended survival and reduced risk of AML progression in erythroid-responsive lenalidomide-treated patients with lower-risk del(5q) MDS. *Leukemia* 2014;28(5):1033–1040.

25 Giagounidis A, Mufti GJ, Fenaux P, Germing U, List A, MacBeth KJ. Lenalidomide as a disease-modifying agent in patients with del(5q) myelodysplastic syndromes: linking mechanism of action to clinical outcomes. *Ann Hematol.* 2014;93(1):1–11.

26 Cutler CS, Lee SJ, Greenberg P, et al. A decision analysis of allogeneic bone marrow transplantation for the myelodysplastic syndromes: delayed transplantation for low-risk myelodysplasia is associated with improved outcome. *Blood.* 2004;104(2):579–585.

27 Koreth J, Pidala J, Perez WS, et al. Role of reduced-intensity conditioning allogeneic hematopoietic stem-cell transplantation in older patients with de novo myelodysplastic syndromes: an international collaborative decision analysis. *J Clin Oncol.* 2013;31(21):2662–2670.

28 Fenaux P, Mufti GJ, Hellstrom-Lindberg E, et al. International Vidaza High-Risk MDS Survival Study Group. Efficacy of azacitidine compared with that of conventional care regimens in the treatment of higher-risk myelodysplastic syndromes: a randomised, open-label, phase III study. *Lancet Oncol.* 2009;10(3):223–232.

29 Silverman LR, Demakos EP, Peterson BL, et al. Randomized controlled trial of azacitidine in patients with the myelodysplastic syndrome: a study of the cancer and leukemia group B. *J Clin Oncol.* 2002;20(10):2429–2440.

30 Steensma DP, Baer MR, Slack JL, et al. Multicenter study of decitabine administered daily for 5 days every 4 weeks to adults with myelodysplastic syndromes: the alternative dosing for outpatient treatment (ADOPT) trial. *J Clin Oncol.* 2009;27(23):3842–3848.

31 Hollenbach PW, Nguyen AN, Brady H, et al. A comparison of azacitidine and decitabine activities in acute myeloid leukemia cell lines. *PLoS One.* 2010;5(2):e9001.

32 Jabbour E, Garcia-Manero G, Batty N, et al. Outcome of patients with myelodysplastic syndrome after failure of decitabine therapy. *Cancer.* 2010;116(16):3830–3834.

33 Chang C, Storer BE, Scott BL, et al. Hematopoietic cell transplantation in patients with myelodysplastic syndrome or acute myeloid leukemia arising from myelodysplastic syndrome: similar outcomes in patients with de novo disease and disease following prior therapy or antecedent hematologic disorders. *Blood.* 2007;110(4):1379–1387.

34 Van Gelder M, Schetelig J, Volin L, et al. Monosomal karyotype predicts poor outcome for MDS/sAML patients with chromosome 7 abnormalities after allogeneic stem cell transplantation for MDS/sAML. A study of the MDS subcommittee of the chronic leukemia working party of the European group for blood and marrow transplantation (EBMT). *ASH Annual Meeting Abstracts.* 2009;114(22):293.

35 de Lima M, Giralt S, Thall PF, et al. Maintenance therapy with low-dose azacitidine after allogeneic hematopoietic stem cell transplantation for recurrent acute myelogenous leukemia or myelodysplastic syndrome: a dose and schedule finding study. *Cancer.* 2010;116(23):5420–5431.

36 Schroeder T, Czibere A, Platzbecker U, et al. Azacitidine and donor lymphocyte infusions as first salvage therapy for relapse of AML or MDS after allogeneic stem cell transplantation. *Leukemia.* 2013;27(6):1229–1235.

37 Chang L, Karin M. Mammalian MAP kinase signalling cascades. *Nature.* 2001;410(6824):37–40.

38 Schaeffer HJ, Weber MJ. Mitogen-activated protein kinases: specific messages from ubiquitous messengers. *Mol Cell Biol.* 1999;19(4):2435–2444.

39 Kitagawa M, et al. Overexpression of tumor necrosis factor (TNF)-alpha and interferon (IFN)-gamma by bone marrow cells from patients with myelodysplastic syndromes. *Leukemia.* 1997;11(12):2049–2054.

40 Katsoulidis E, et al. Role of the p38 mitogen-activated protein kinase pathway in cytokine-mediated hematopoietic suppression in myelodysplastic syndromes. *Cancer Res.* 2005;65(19):9029–9037.

41 Peng H, et al. A systematic modeling study on the pathogenic role of p38 MAPK activation in myelodysplastic syndromes. *Mol Biosyst.* 2012;8(4):1366–1374.

42 Navas TA, Mohindru M, Estes M, et al. Inhibition of overactivated p38 MAPK can restore hematopoiesis in myelodysplastic syndrome progenitors. *Blood.* 2006;108(13):4170–4177.

43 Sokol L, Cripe L, Kantarjian H, et al. Randomized, dose-escalation study of the p38alpha MAPK inhibitor SCIO-469 in patients with myelodysplastic syndrome. *Leukemia.* 2013;27(4):977–980.

44 Garcia-Manero G, Sekeres MA, List AF, et al. Phase 1 dose-escalation/expansion study of ARRY-614 in patients with IPSS low/int-1 risk myelodysplastic syndromes. *Blood.* 2013;122(21):387.

45 Wang Z, Tang X, Xu W, et al. The different immunoregulatory functions on dendritic cells between mesenchymal stem cells derived from bone marrow of patients with low-risk or high-risk myelodysplastic syndromes. *PLoS One.* 2013;8(3):e57470.

46 Wei Y, Dimicoli S, Bueso-Ramos C, et al. Toll-like receptor alterations in myelodysplastic syndrome. *Leukemia.* 2013;27(9):1832–1840.

47 Wei, Y, Chen R, Dimicoli S, et al. Global H3K4me3 genome mapping reveals alterations of innate immunity signaling and overexpression of JMJD3 in human myelodysplastic syndrome CD34+ cells. *Leukemia.* 2013;27(11):2177–2186.

48 Olnes MJ, Shenoy A, Weinstein B, et al. Directed therapy for patients with myelodysplastic syndromes (MDS) by suppression of cyclin D1 with ON 01910.Na. *Leuk Res.* 2012;36(8):982–989.

49 Fenaux P, Raza A, Mufti GJ, et al. A multicenter phase 2 study of the farnesyltransferase inhibitor tipifarnib in intermediate- to high-risk myelodysplastic syndrome. *Blood.* 2007;109(10):4158–4163.

50 Benetatos CA, Mitsuuchi Y, Burns JM, et al. Birinapant (TL32711), a bivalent SMAC mimetic, targets TRAF2-associated cIAPs, abrogates TNF-induced NF-kappaB activation, and is active in patient-derived xenograft models. *Mol Cancer Ther.* 2014;13(4):867–879.

51 Silva G, doso BA, Belo H, Almeida AM. Vorinostat induces apoptosis and differentiation in myeloid malignancies· genetic and molecular mechanisms. *PLoS One.* 2013;8(1):e53766.

52 Silverman LR, Verma A, Odchimar-Reissig R, et al. A phase II trial of epigenetic modulators vorinostat in combination with azacitidine (azaC) in patients with the myelodysplastic syndrome (MDS): initial results of study 6898 of the New York Cancer Consortium. *Blood.* 2013;122(21):386.

53 Quintas-Cardama, A., Kantarjian HM, Ravandi F, et al. Very high rates of clinical and cytogenetic response with the combination of the histone deacetylase inhibitor pracinostat (SB939) and 5-azacitidine in high-risk myelodysplastic syndrome. *ASH Annual Meeting Abstracts.* 2012;120(21):3821.

54 Yang H, Bueso-Ramos C, DiNardo C, et al. Expression of PD-L1, PD-L2, PD-1 and CTLA4 in myelodysplastic syndromes is enhanced by treatment with hypomethylating agents. *Leukemia.* 2014;28(6):1280–1288.

55 Komrokji RS, Padron E, Yu D, et al. Erlotinib for treatment of myelodysplastic syndromes: a phase II clinical study. *ASH Annual Meeting Abstracts.* 2010;116(21):1854.

56 Chen K, Huang YH, Chen JL. Understanding and targeting cancer stem cells: therapeutic implications and challenges. *Acta Pharmacol Sin.* 2013;34(6):732–740.

# CHAPTER 17

# Lymphoma and Targeted Therapies

*Sonali M. Smith[1] and Julie M. Vose[2]*

[1]Department of Medicine, The University of Chicago, Chicago, IL, USA
[2]Division of Hematology/Oncology, University of Nebraska Medical Center, Omaha, NE, USA

## Overview

Hodgkin's and non-Hodgkin's lymphomas (NHLs) are a complex set of lymphoproliferative malignancies of mature B and T cells. The current World Health Organization (WHO) recognizes several dozen categories of lymphomas with approximately 60 unique clinicopathologic subtypes. The prognosis and management of any individual patient relies heavily on the precise diagnosis, yet much of the therapeutic approach continues to depend on chemotherapy, which is typically considered a nontargeted and generalized approach. However, the past decade has witnessed a dramatic increase in the understanding of lymphomagenesis, leading to the identification of new targets leading toward individualized approaches.

The current repertoire of agents in development addresses both targets that are broadly relevant across subtypes (i.e., proteasome inhibition, PI3K/Akt/mTOR) and several that are specific to unique subsets of lymphomas (B-cell receptor (BCR) signaling, CD20, ALK). This review will focus on a selected subset of targets based on promising clinical potential.

## Surface Antigens as a Target in Lymphomas

For decades, knowledge regarding surface antigens in lymphoma was widely used as a classification and diagnostic tool. CD20, for example, was simply a marker for a mature B cell and delineated the progression from an immature B cell and prior to terminal differentiation into a plasma cell.

## Rituximab

This genetically engineered anti-CD20 monoclonal antibody was the first therapeutic monoclonal antibody approved for the treatment of cancer. It was approved by the Food and Drug Administration (FDA) in 1997 for the treatment of relapsed CD20-positive indolent lymphoma. It is now used not only for indolent lymphoma, but also for aggressive lymphomas, and for some nonmalignant conditions such as rheumatoid arthritis. Many studies have now demonstrated that it can be combined with multiple chemotherapeutic agents and more recently with other monoclonal antibodies and targeted agents.

## Brentuximab Vedotin

This is an antibody-drug conjugate comprised of an anti-CD30 antibody conjugated by a protease-cleavable linker to monomethyl auristatin E (MMAE) which is a potent antitubulin agent (Figure 17.1)[1]. This agent was tested in a phase I study of patients with C30-expressing lymphomas and showed a response rate of 38%[2] Two phase II studies in relapsed Hodgkin's lymphoma or anaplastic large-cell lymphoma (ALCL) demonstrated overall response rates (ORRs) of 75% and 86%, respectively[3,4] This agent is now in further trials in combination with standard chemotherapy in the relapsed and first-line settings for CD30+ lymphoma therapy.

Multiple other unconjugated or conjugated antibodies are under current clinical development including targets of CD19, CD22, CD40, and CD79a. Another promising approach is the development of bispecific antibodies that simultaneously target a tumor antigen (i.e., CD19) and an effector cell (i.e., a T cell) in order to bring the target and the immune system in physical proximity. These "bispecific T-cell engaging (BiTE)" molecules are made by combining the fragment, antigen-binding (Fab) portions of two separate antibodies into a complex without an Fc portion, and studies in lymphoid malignancies are ongoing.[5]

## Signal Transduction Pathways

### B-Cell Receptor Signaling

BCR is critically important for both normal and malignant B-cell survival, and has recently been identified as a rational target in lymphoma. The BCR is a complex that includes membrane-bound immunoglobulin (either IgD or IgM), a short, intracellular domain, and a set of noncovalently attached signaling proteins (Igα/Igβ heterodimer) (reviewed in References 6 and 7). Igα and Igβ are also known as CD79a and CD79b, respectively. An intact BCR is required for both survival and entry into the germinal center.[8–10] Tonic (nonligand-dependent) BCR signaling is critical to survival in this process, as reflected by the elimination of all B cells in mouse models where the BCR is conditionally deleted[11]; furthermore, a defective BCR marks that cell for an apoptotic death.[8]

Although tonic BCR signaling is required for survival, B-cell *activation* generally requires ligand binding by an antigen, thus triggering a series of intracellular events requiring several kinases, including SRC-family members LYN and SYK.[7,12] A number of downstream kinases are recruited and assembled, with the three main signaling cascades involving Bruton's tyrosine kinase (BTK), phospholipase C-γ2 (PLCγ2), and phosphatidylinositol-3-kinase (PI3K).[13] PI3K appears particularly important since introduction of

*Targeted Therapy in Translational Cancer Research*, First Edition. Edited by Apostolia-Maria Tsimberidou, Razelle Kurzrock and Kenneth C. Anderson.
© 2016 John Wiley & Sons, Inc. Published 2016 by John Wiley & Sons, Inc.

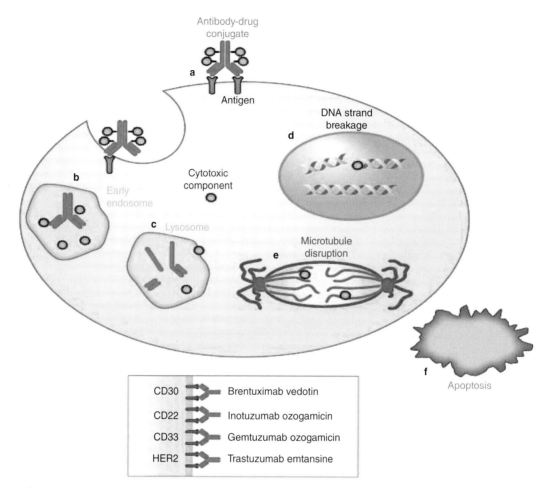

**Figure 17.1** Antibody-drug conjugates (ADC). *Source:* Reproduced from Sievers and Senter 2013, Reference 1 with permission of Annual Reviews.

constitutive PI3K signaling can rescue B cells with a defunct or absent BCR.[14]

Malignant B cells accentuate this dependence on an intact BCR, thus forming the basis for several new targeted agents entering clinical trials. In particular, agents against SYK, BTK, and PI3K are in active development with exciting early data. This pathway with potential targets is outlined in Figure 17.2.[15]

## SYK Inhibitors

The central role of Syk in maintaining the BCR signal in lymphomas is apparent in numerous preclinical models[16,17] and is relevant in many lymphoma subtypes including diffuse large B-cell lymphoma (DLBCL), mantle cell lymphoma (MCL), and follicular lymphoma (FL). Src-family kinases are constitutively expressed in several lymphoma cell lines and murine models, and SYK is important for both DLBCL and FL cell survival in preclinical models.[18–21] Syk expression patterns vary among lymphoma subtypes.[22]

Fostamatinib disodium (R788) is an orally bioavailable and highly specific Syk inhibitor. In the first-in-man phase 1/2 trial, neutropenia, diarrhea, and thrombocytopenia were the dose-limiting toxicities.[23] Among 68 heavily pretreated lymphoma patients included in the phase II portion, the ORR varied by histology and ranged from 10% in FL patients to 55% in chronic lymphocytic leukemia (CLL) patients. This latter finding is interesting, particularly since others have shown that Syk expression is actually lowest in CLL and typically countered by an increase in Lyn expression.[24]

Dasatinib (BMS-354825) is an oral kinase inhibitor that is much less specific than fostamatinib, instead inhibiting a range of kinase families including BCR-ABL, SRC, c-KIT, PDGF receptors, and ephrin (EPH) receptor kinases. It has activity against both Syk and Lyn in nanomolar ranges, and is active in murine lymphoma models.[18,25] Vose et al. reported an ORR of 32% in a very heavily pretreated subset of lymphoma patients, including both B- and T-cell lymphomas.[26] The most common toxicities were myelosuppression and pleural effusion.

## BTK Inhibitors

An early downstream component of BCR signaling is the Tec (tyrosine-protein kinase) kinase, BTK. Its central relevance to B-cell maturation is underscored by inherited gene mutations resulting in the virtual absence of mature B cells and low immunoglobulin levels as part of the X-linked agammaglobulinemia syndrome.[27] Similar to Syk, BTK also amplifies the BCR signal.[28–30] BTK activation leads to autophosphorylation, phosphorylation, and activation of PI3K/Akt pathway, and IkB kinase activation.[31] Unbiased screening of activated B-cell subsets of DLBCL identified BTK as an important component.[32] There are at least two BTK inhibitors in development, including PCI-32765 and AVL-292, although most mature data are available with the former compound.

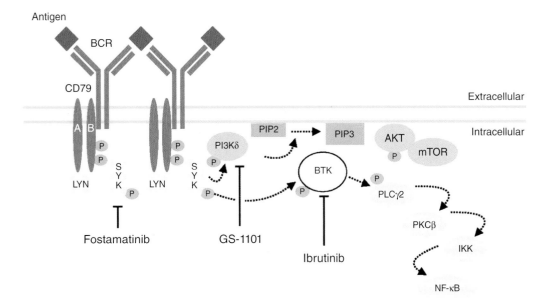

**Figure 17.2** Antigen-dependent B-cell receptor (BCR) signaling and its targeting by small-molecule inhibitors. Antigen binding induces the aggregation of the BCR with its co-receptors CD79 A and B, which become phosphorylated by the tyrosine kinases LYN and SYK. SYK activates phosphoinositide 3–kinase (PI3Kδ), which in turn converts phosphatidylinositol 4,5-bisphosphate (PIP2) to phosphatidylinositol 3,4,5-triphosphate PIP3. PIP3 serves as a docking site for the cytoplasmic kinases Bruton's tyrosine kinase (BTK) and AKT. BTK phosphorylates and thereby activates phospholipase C gamma 2 (PLCγ2), which in turn generates a set of second messengers to activate protein kinase C beta (PKCβ). PKCβ phosphorylates IκB kinase (IKK) to activate nuclear factor κB (NF-κB) transcription factors that regulate gene expression of several survival factors. The kinases inhibited by small molecules with promising clinical activity are indicated. *Source:* Reproduced from Wiester 2013, © 2013, Reference 15 with permission of the American Society of Clinical Oncology.

PCI-32765 (ibrutinib) is the first BTK inhibitor in development, with an exciting and promising activity profile. Ibrutinib was selected for development among several potential BTK inhibitors based on its specificity and potency in chemical screens.[33] A phase I trial utilized a unique design of dose level escalation based on a goal of proceeding to three dose levels above the group achieving over 90% BTK occupancy using this probe, as long as no dose-limiting toxicities occurred.[34] Among 47 heavily pretreated patients with a variety of lymphoma subtypes, the ORR was over 40%, with several complete responses. Toxicity was mild, and no cumulative hematologic toxicity or other safety concerns were identified. Seven out of nine MCL patients responded, prompting a subsequent phase II open label trial in this subset. Overall, 111 heavily pretreated MCL patients were treated with 560 mg of ibrutinib daily and stratified by prior bortezomib exposure.[35] The ORR was 68%, and with a median follow-up of 15 months, the median response duration was 17.5 months.

Despite the enthusiasm over the BCR as a target, however, it is clear that some lymphomas are "BCR-dependent" and others are not.[36] A recent quantitative immunofluorescence assay on paraffin-embedded tissue shows encouraging ability to identify DLBCL subsets reliant on activated BCR signaling, which may further allow individualized application of these agents.[37]

A final note on components of BCR signaling is that several downstream kinases may also be important therapeutic targets in T-cell lymphomas, which clearly do not possess a BCR. In particular, Syk is overexpressed in T-cell lymphoma preclinical models, and inhibition of Syk leads to apoptosis and decreased proliferation.[38] This may be due to a unique fusion oncogene (ITK–SYK),[39,40] and underscores the variability of potential therapeutic targets in etiology and genesis among the lymphomas.

### PI3K/Akt/mTOR Pathway Inhibitors

Similar to BTK, PI3K is a proximal node within the BCR signaling network, but also has important roles independent of the BCR affecting cellular proliferation, motility, metabolism, and cell growth versus cell survival.[41] The gene for PI3K, *PIK3CA*, is somatically mutated in many cancers, establishing this as an important oncogene. There are four isoforms (alpha, beta, gamma, and delta) but it is the delta isoform that is expressed in human leukocytes.

GS-1101 (formerly called CAL-101), or idelalisib, is an orally bioavailable PI3K inhibitor that is highly selective for the p110 delta isoform.[42] The IC50 for idelalisib is significantly higher for other PI3K isoforms and against a panel of nearly 100 other kinases (including the mammalian target of rapamycin (mTOR) kinase). *In vitro* testing against a variety of human-derived cell lines established higher activity in B-cell malignancies as compared to myeloid cell lines. Furthermore, idelalisib successfully downregulates pAkt in both CLL and MCL models.

Idelalisib has promising single-agent activity in B-cell malignancies, including MCL and other histologies.[43–45] In a phase I trial of indolent MCLs (*n* = 51) and CLL (*n* = 54), idelalisib was sequentially escalated from 50 mg bid to 350 mg bid on continuous 28-day cycles, and an additional cohort of once daily dosing (300 mg) was also evaluated. These were heavily pretreated patients with a median of five prior regimens. Seventy-six percent of MCL patients had received prior bortezomib, which is currently FDA-approved for relapsed MCL. In this setting, single-agent idelalisib demonstrated remarkable activity, with 17 of 21 MCL patients showing a tumor response and 10 of 21 patients (48%) achieving a complete or partial response with a median progression-free survival (PFS) of four cycles. The most common grade 3 or 4 adverse event was transient elevation of hepatic enzymes, occurring in 27% of patients.

There are now a number of studies underway combining idelalisib with both chemotherapy (bendamustine), immunotherapy (rituximab), and immunomodulatory agents (lenalidomide).

Downstream of PI3K is another important kinase, mTOR, which regulates cell size and metabolism via control over mRNA translational initiation.[46,47] In lymphomas, mTOR signaling is frequently aberrant and is an important potential therapeutic target across histologies.[48,49] First generation mTOR inhibitors (MTI) are primarily rapamycin prodrugs or analogs, and have been tested in MCL (based on control over Cyclin D1 mRNA translation) as well as other lymphoma subtypes. Both temsirolimus and everolimus produce response rates of approximately 30–50%, with strongest activity in MCL and FL.[50–53] Based on a phase III trial comparing "low-dose" and "high-dose" temsirolimus versus investigator's choice, temsirolimus is now approved in Europe for the treatment of relapsed MCL.[51] A major challenge in the development of MTIs is the relatively short response duration, and a number of mechanistic explanations are available. In particular, there is a feedback loop involving paradoxical Akt activation that is an important means of resistance to MTIs.[54] In addition, mTOR kinase exists in two mutually exclusive pools (termed mTORC1 and mTORC2); inhibition of mTORC1 by first generation MTIs leads to an increase in mTORC2, which activates Akt. This has led to a second generation of MTIs of small molecule ATP inhibitors of sites within the mTOR protein itself.

## Proteasome Inhibitors

The ubiquitin proteasome system is a highly conserved means of managing intracellular protein levels and protein turnover.[55] Polyubiquitinated proteins are shuttled into the proteasome, where a variety of proteolytic enzymes mediate degradation into oligopeptides, effectively eliminating that protein. Inhibiting this system has an important impact on anticancer therapies by modifying levels of cell cycle proteins, apoptotic, and anti-apoptotic proteins, among others.

Bortezomib is the first proteasome inhibitor and is currently FDA-approved for the treatment of relapsed or refractory MCL. Based on hints of activity in a phase I trial, four subsequent phase II trials in relapsed MCL have established bortezomib's response rate of 30–35% and a median PFS of 6–10 months.[56–60] Although generally well tolerated, the main adverse effect of bortezomib limiting long-term use is sensorimotor neuropathy, occurring in half the patients enrolled on the largest trial to date, the PINNACLE trial.[57,61] A correlative analysis of the MCL specimens in the PINNACLE trial suggests that elevated NFkB p65 and low PSMA expression may predict for higher rates of response, time to progression, or overall survival, perhaps identifying a subgroup of patients with a favorable benefit–risk ratio.[62]

In several studies, bortezomib has been added to other biologic agents, such as rituximab, or to chemotherapy, including bendamustine.[63,64] A phase III trial of approximately 700 patients with relapsed FL showed an improvement of PFS from 11 months for rituximab alone to 12.8 months for rituximab plus bortezomib; although it was statistically significant, this difference was not considered clinically meaningful.[64] Most recently, bortezomib has been integrated into chemotherapy regimens[65–68] and combinations with bendamustine and rituximab are now being prospectively tested in cooperative group studies. Newer proteasome inhibitors have several potential advantages, including irreversible binding to the proteasome, more convenient dosing, and different toxicity profiles which might facilitate incorporation into existing NHL regi-

mens. Carfilzomib, a second generation proteasome inhibitor, has an excellent activity spectrum in multiple myeloma.[69] Importantly, peripheral neuropathy was uncommon and typically mild in severity. The development of proteasome inhibitors in lymphoma continues to evolve with numerous ongoing trials.

Although the proteasome pathway appears to be an important component of lymphomagenesis in several subtypes, the strongest link to pathogenesis is in the activated B-cell type of DLBCL (ABC-DLBCL). Gene expression profiling clearly identifies that ABC-DLBCL is molecularly distinct and characterized by upregulation of NFkB target genes[70]. The unique dependence on NFkB signaling is underscored by selective toxicity to ABC-DLBCL cell lines using small interfering RNAs.[71] Based on these observations, several studies are evaluating bortezomib specifically in ABC-DLBCL.

## Epigenetic Targeting in Lymphoma

Although targeting the epigenome is highly successful in myeloid malignancies, it has only recently been appreciated that cytosine methylation patterns contribute greatly to lymphomagenesis. There are recurrent and abnormal methylation patterns that not only distinguish benign from malignant lymphoproliferation, but also can identify unique lymphoma subsets.[72–74] In MCL, for example, methylation status of five genes (SOX9, HOXA9, AHR, NR2F2, ROBO1) correlates with both histologic proliferation and clinical outcomes.[75] The ability to potentially reverse and/or modify acquired methylation profiles using clinically available hypomethylating agents and histone deacetylase inhibitors (HDACi) has led to a number of new trials in lymphoma.

The most successful approach has been the application of HDACi in both cutaneous and systemic T-cell lymphomas. Romidepsin is a potent bicyclic class 1 selective HDACi, which is FDA-approved for treatment of relapsed peripheral T-cell lymphoma (PTCL). It was evaluated in 130 patients with relapsed PTCL and found to have an ORR of 25%.[76] Vorinostat is an orally bioavailable HDACi that is approved for the treatment of mycosis fungoides.[77] The most common adverse events of HDACi are fatigue, cytopenias, and nausea. These agents are currently in multiple combination trials.

## Lymphoma Microenvironment as a Target

### Lenalidomide

This agent has various antitumor effects including inhibition of angiogenesis, enhancement of T cell and NK cell functions, and immunomodulatory effects (Figure 17.3).[78] It has been tested in several trials for treatment of NHL. In a trial for patients with relapsed aggressive NHL, the ORR was 35% with a median PFS of 4 months.[79] The pivotal MCL-001 trial evaluated single-agent lenalidomide in patients with relapsed MCL. The ORR was 28% (37/134) (CR, 8%). The median duration of response was 16.6 months.[80] This trial resulted in the FDA approval of lenalidomide for the treatment of relapsed MCL. The major toxicities of lenalidomide are cytopenias, thrombosis, fatigue, diarrhea, and rarely secondary malignancies. Lenalidomide is often combined with rituximab, chemotherapy, and/or targeted agents. Other immunomodulatory drugs have also been developed to attack the microenvironment, but none of these drugs are currently approved for NHL.

## Specific Oncogenes

### Anaplastic Lymphoma Kinase

In 1994, Morris et al. first described a unique translocation between the anaplastic lymphoma kinase (ALK) gene and the

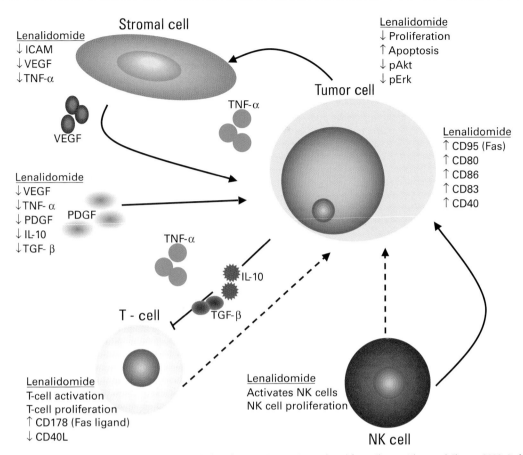

**Figure 17.3** Potential effects of immunomodulatory agents in lymphomas. *Source:* Reproduced from Chanan-Khan and Cheson 2008, Reference 78 with permission of the American Society of Clinical Oncology.

nucleophosmin (NPM) gene in an uncommon subset of PTCLs called anaplastic large cell lymphoma (ALCL).[81] ALK is actually a promiscuous gene with multiple genetic partners. Its transforming potential in both lymphomas and solid tumors including non-small cell lung cancer and neuroblastoma, is clearly established.[82] In addition to ALK-positive ALCL, ALK occurs in a rare and particularly aggressive variant of large B-cell lymphoma (LBCL).[83,84] There are important biologic and clinical associations that differ between ALK-positive ALCL and ALK-positive LBCL. The major genetic lesion in ALK positive ALCL is t(2;5), and the outcome of most patients is relatively favorable compared to other T-cell lymphomas.[85] In contrast, the genetic lesion in ALK-positive LBCL is t(2;17)(p23;q23) involving the clathrin gene; this rare condition has a grim prognosis with profound chemoresistance and a median survival less than 1 year.

Crizotinib is an oral inhibitor of ALK and c-MET that was recently approved for use in ALK-rearranged non-small cell lung cancer. To date, there are only case reports of crizotinib in lymphomas, with intriguing response in some patients with refractory disease.[86] A handful of clinical trials further evaluating crizotinib in lymphomas are ongoing.

## Summary

A number of targets have been recently identified in lymphomas, spurring a new generation of agents in clinical trial settings. The vast majority of new agents are rationally selected and/or designed based on a greater understanding of lymphomagenesis. There are many challenges in incorporating new targeted agents into existing treatment paradigms, including differing relevance among lymphoma subtypes, high degrees of redundancy and thus potential resistance, and noncrossover toxicity with existing agents. Ideally, a system of identifying which pathways and targets are relevant within individual patients should be developed, but this has thus far been elusive in most NHL categories. Nevertheless, ongoing development of new agents promises to broaden treatment options for lymphoma patients, with the hope of eventually offering personalized and targeted therapy to all patients.

## References

1 Sievers EL, Senter PD. Antibody-drug conjugates in cancer therapy. *Annu Rev Med.* 2013;64:15–29. doi: 10.1146/annurev-med-050311-201823.

2 Younes A, Bartlett NL, Leonard JP, et al. Brentuximab vedotin (SGN-35) for relapsed CD30-positive lymphomas. *N Engl J Med.* 2010;363(19):1812–1821.

3 Pro B, Advani R, Brice P, et al. Brentuximab vedotin (SGN-35) in patients with relapsed or refractory systemic anaplastic large cell lymphoma: Results of a phase II study. *J Clin Onc.* 2012;30(19):2190–2196.

4 Younes A, Gopal AK, Smith SE, et al. Results of a pivotal phase II study of Brentuximab vedotin for patients with relapsed or refractory Hodgkin's lymphoma. *J Clin Onc.* 2012;30(18):2183–2189.

5 Nagorsen D, Bargou R, Ruttinger D, Kufer P, Baeuerle PA, Zugmaier G. Immunotherapy of lymphoma and leukemia with T-cell engaging BiTE antibody blinatumomab. *Leuk Lymphoma.* 2009;50(6):886–891.

6 Treanor B. B-cell receptor: from resting state to activate. *Immunology.* 2012;136(1):21–27

7 Monroe JG. ITAM-mediated tonic signalling through pre-BCR and BCR complexes. *Nat Rev Immunol.* 2006;6(4):283–294.

8 Kraus M, Alimzhanov MB, Rajewsky N, Rajewsky K. Survival of resting mature B lymphocytes depends on BCR signaling via the Iglalpha/beta heterodimer. *Cell.* 2004;117(6):787–800.

9 Patterson HC, Kraus M, Kim YM, Ploegh H, Rajewsky K. The B cell receptor promotes B cell activation and proliferation through a non-ITAM tyrosine in the Igalpha cytoplasmic domain. *Immunity.* 2006;25(1):55–65.

10 Reichlin A, Gazumyan A, Nagaoka H, et al. A B cell receptor with two Igalpha cytoplasmic domains supports development of mature but anergic B cells. *J Exp Med.* 2004;199(6):855–865.

11 Lam KP, Kuhn R, Rajewsky K. In vivo ablation of surface immunoglobulin on mature B cells by inducible gene targeting results in rapid cell death. *Cell.* 1997;90(6):1073–1083.

12 Saijo K, Schmedt C, Su IH, et al. Essential role of Src-family protein tyrosine kinases in NF-kappaB activation during B cell development. *Nat Immunol.* 2003;4(3):274–279.

13 Woyach JA, Johnson AJ, Byrd JC. The B-cell receptor signaling pathway as a therapeutic target in CLL. *Blood.* 2012;120(6):1175–1184.

14 Srinivasan L, Sasaki Y, Calado DP, et al. PI3 kinase signals BCR-dependent mature B cell survival. *Cell.* 2009;139:573–586.

15 Wiestner A. Targeting B-Cell receptor signaling for anticancer therapy: the Bruton's tyrosine kinase inhibitor ibrutinib induces impressive responses in B-cell malignancies. *J Clin Oncol.* 2013;31(1):128–130.

16 Young RM, Hardy IR, Clarke RL, et al. Mouse models of non-Hodgkin lymphoma reveal Syk as an important therapeutic target. *Blood.* 2009;113(11):2508–2516.

17 Chen L, Monti S, Juszczynski P, et al. SYK-dependent tonic B-cell receptor signaling is a rational treatment target in diffuse large B-cell lymphoma. *Blood.* 2008;111(4):2230–2237.

18 Ke J, Chelvarajan RL, Sindhava V, et al. Anomalous constitutive Src kinase activity promotes B lymphoma survival and growth. *Mol Cancer.* 2009;8:132.

19 Cheng S, Coffey G, Zhang XH, et al. SYK inhibition and response prediction in diffuse large B-cell lymphoma. *Blood.* 2011;118(24):6342–6352.

20 Fruchon S, Kheirallah S, Al Saati T, et al. Involvement of the Syk-mTOR pathway in follicular lymphoma cell invasion and angiogenesis. *Leukemia.* 2012;26(4):795–805.

21 Leseux L, Hamdi SM, Al Saati T, et al. Syk-dependent mTOR activation in follicular lymphoma cells. *Blood.* 2006;108(13):4156–4162.

22 Ponzoni M, Uccella S, Mian M, et al. Syk expression patterns differ among B-cell lymphomas. *Leuk Res.* 2010;34(9):e243–e245.

23 Friedberg JW, Sharman J, Sweetenham J, et al. Inhibition of Syk with fostamatinib disodium has significant clinical activity in non-Hodgkin lymphoma and chronic lymphocytic leukemia. *Blood.* 2010;115(13):2578–2585.

24 Contri A, Brunati AM, Trentin L, et al. Chronic lymphocytic leukemia B cells contain anomalous Lyn tyrosine kinase, a putative contribution to defective apoptosis. *J Clin Invest.* 2005;115(2):369–378.

25 Dargart JL, Fish K, Gordon LI, Longnecker R, Cen O. Dasatinib therapy results in decreased B cell proliferation, splenomegaly, and tumor growth in a murine model of lymphoma expressing Myc and Epstein-Barr virus LMP2 A. *Antiviral Res.* 2012;95(1):49–56.

26 William BM, Hohenstein M, Loberiza FR, et al. Phase I/II Study of Dasatinib In Relapsed or Refractory Non-Hodgkin's Lymphoma (NHL). *Blood.* 2010;116.

27 Satterthwaite AB, Willis F, Kanchanastit P, et al. A sensitized genetic system for the analysis of murine B lymphocyte signal transduction pathways dependent on Bruton's tyrosine kinase. *Proc Natl Acad Sci U S A.* 2000;97(12):6687–6692

28 Tsukada S, Saffran DC, Rawlings DJ, et al. Deficient expression of a B cell cytoplasmic tyrosine kinase in human X-linked agammaglobulinemia. *Cell.* 1993;72(2):279–290.

29 Vetrie D, Vorechovsky I, Sideras P, et al. The gene involved in X-linked agammaglobulinaemia is a member of the src family of protein-tyrosine kinases. *Nature.* 1993;361(6409):226–233.

30 Khan WN, Alt FW, Gerstein RM, et al. Defective B cell development and function in Btk-deficient mice. *Immunity.* 1995;3(3):283–299.

31 Petro JB, Rahman SM, Ballard DW, et al. Bruton's tyrosine kinase is required for activation of IkappaB kinase and nuclear factor kappaB in response to B cell receptor engagement. *J Exp Med.* 2000;191(10):1745–1754.

32 Davis RE, Ngo VN, Lenz G, et al. Chronic active B-cell-receptor signalling in diffuse large B-cell lymphoma. *Nature.* 2010;463(7277):88–92.

33 Honigberg LA, Smith AM, Sirisawad M, et al. The Bruton tyrosine kinase inhibitor PCI-32765 blocks B-cell activation and is efficacious in models of autoimmune disease and B-cell malignancy. *Proc Natl Acad Sci U S A.* 2010;107(29):13075–13080.

34 Fowler N, Sharman J, Smith SM, et al. The Btk inhibitor, PCI-32765, induces durable responses with minimal toxicity in patients with relapsed/refractory B-cell malignancies: results from a phase I study. *Blood.* 2010;116.

35 Wang ML, Rule S, Martin P, et al. Targeting BTK with Ibruitinib in relapsed or refractory mantle-cell lymphoma. *N Engl J Med.* 2013;369:507–516.

36 Juszczynski P, Chen L, O'Donnell E, et al. BCL6 modulates tonic BCR signaling in diffuse large B-cell lymphomas by repressing the SYK phosphatase, PTPROt. *Blood.* 2009;114(26):5315–5321

37 Bogusz AM, Baxter RH, Currie T, et al. Quantitative Immunofluorescence Reveals the Signature of Active B Cell Receptor Signaling in Diffuse Large B Cell Lymphoma. *Clin Cancer Res.* 2012;18(22):6122–6135.

38 Wilcox RA, Sun DX, Novak A, et al. Inhibition of Syk protein tyrosine kinase induces apoptosis and blocks proliferation in T-cell non-Hodgkin's lymphoma cell lines. *Leukemia.* 2010;24(1):229–232.

39 Pechloff K, Holch J, Ferch U, et al. The fusion kinase ITK-SYK mimics a T cell receptor signal and drives oncogenesis in conditional mouse models of peripheral T cell lymphoma. *J Exp Med.* 2010;207(5):1031–1044.

40 Dierks C, Adrian F, Fisch P, et al. The ITK-SYK fusion oncogene induces a T-cell lymphoproliferative disease in mice mimicking human disease. *Cancer Res.* 2010;70:6193–6204.

41 Yuan TL, Cantley LC. PI3 K pathway alterations in cancer: variations on a theme. *Oncogene.* 2008;27:5497–5510.

42 Lannutti BJ, Meadows SA, Herman SE, et al. CAL-101, a p110delta selective phosphatidylinositol-3-kinase inhibitor for the treatment of B-cell malignancies, inhibits PI3 K signaling and cellular viability. *Blood.* 2011;117(2):591–594

43 Furman R BJ, Brow JR, et al. CAL-101, an isoform-selective inhibitor of phosphatidylinositol 3-kinase P110, demonstrates clinical activity and pharmacodynamic effects in patients with relapsed or refractory chronic lymphocytic leukemia. *Blood (ASH Annual Meeting Abstracts).* 2010;116.

44 Kahl BS, Byrd JC, Flinn IW, et al. Clinical safety and activity in a phase 1 study of CAL-101, an isoform-selective inhibitor of phosphatidylinositol 3-kinase P110, in patients with relapsed or refractory non-Hodgkin lymphoma. *Blood.* 2010;116.

45 Webb H, Chen H, Yu HS, et al. Clinical pharmacokinetics of CAL-101, a p110 isoform-selective PI3 K inhibitor, following single- and multiple-dose administration in healthy volunteers and patients with hematological malignancies. *Blood.* 2010;116.

46 Fingar DC, Blenis J. Target of rapamycin (TOR): an integrator of nutrient and growth factor signals and coordinator of cell growth and cell cycle progression. *Oncogene*. 2004;23(18):3151–3171.

47 Laplante M, Sabatini DM. mTOR signaling in growth control and disease. *Cell*. 2012;149(2):274–293.

48 Smith SM, van Besien K. mTOR inhibition in lymphoma: a rational and promising strategy. *Letters in Drug Design and Discovery*. 2007;4:224–231.

49 Smith SM. Targeting mTOR in mantle cell lymphoma: current and future directions. *Best Pract Res Clin Haematol*. 2012;25:175–183.

50 Ansell SM, Geyer SM, Kurtin P, et al. Anti-tumor activity of mTOR inhibitor temsirolimus for relapsed mantle cell lymphoma: A phase II trial in the North Central Cancer Treatment Group. *J Clin Oncol*. 2006;18:A7532.

51 Hess G, Herbrecht R, Romaguera J, et al. Phase III study to evaluate temsirolimus compared with investigator's choice therapy for the treatment of relapsed or refractory mantle cell lymphoma. *J Clin Oncol*. 2009;27(23):3822–3829.

52 Witzig TE, Geyer SM, Ghobrial I, et al. Phase II trial of single-agent temsirolimus (CCI-779) for relapsed mantle cell lymphoma. *J Clin Oncol*. 2005;23(23):5347–5356.

53 Smith SM, van Besien K, Karrison T, et al. Temsirolimus has activity in non-mantle cell non-Hodgkin's lymphoma subtypes: The University of Chicago phase II consortium. *J Clin Oncol*. 2010;28:4740–4746.

54 Petrich AM, Leshchenko V, Kuo PY, et al. Akt inhibitors MK-2206 and nelfinavir overcome mTOR inhibitor resistance in diffuse large B-cell lymphoma. *Clin Cancer Res*. 2012;18(9):2534–2544.

55 Orlowski RZ, Kuhn DJ. Proteasome inhibitors in cancer therapy: lessons from the first decade. *Clin Cancer Res*. 2008;14(6):1649–1657.

56 Belch A, Kouroukis CT, Crump M, et al. A phase II study of bortezomib in mantle cell lymphoma: the National Cancer Institute of Canada Clinical Trials Group trial IND.150. *Ann Oncol*. 2007;18(1):116–121

57 Fisher RI, Bernstein SH, Kahl BS, et al. Multicenter phase II study of bortezomib in patients with relapsed or refractory mantle cell lymphoma. *J Clin Oncol*. 2006;24(30):4867–4874.

58 Goy A, Bernstein SH, Kahl BS, et al. Bortezomib in patients with relapsed or refractory mantle cell lymphoma: updated time-to-event analyses of the multicenter phase 2 PINNACLE study. *Ann Oncol*. 2009;20(3):520–525.

59 Goy A, Younes A, McLaughlin P, et al. Phase II study of proteasome inhibitor bortezomib in relapsed or refractory B-cell non-Hodgkin's lymphoma. *J Clin Oncol*. 2005;23(4):667–675

60 O'Connor OA, Wright J, Moskowitz C, et al. Phase II clinical experience with the novel proteasome inhibitor bortezomib in patients with indolent non-Hodgkin's lymphoma and mantle cell lymphoma. *J Clin Oncol*. 2005;23(4):676–684

61 Kane RC, Farrell AT, Sridhara R, Pazdur R. United States Food and Drug Administration approval summary: bortezomib for the treatment of progressive multiple myeloma after one prior therapy. *Clin Cancer Res*. 2006;12(10):2955–2960

62 Goy A, Bernstein SH, McDonald A, et al. Potential biomarkers of bortezomib activity in mantle cell lymphoma from the phase 2 PINNACLE trial. *Leuk Lymphoma*. 2010;51:1269–1277.

63 De Vos S, Dakhil SR, McLaughlin P, et al. Bortezomib plus rituximab in patients with indolent non-hodgkin's lymphoma (NHL): a phase 2 study. *Blood*. 2005;106:17 Abstract.

64 Coiffier B, Osmanov EA, Hong Xiaonan, et al.; LYM-3001 study investigators. Bortzomib plus rituximab versus rituximab alone in pateints with relapsed, rituximab-naïve or rituximab-sensitve, follicular lymphoma: a randomised phase 3 trial. *Lancet Onc*. 2011;12(8):773–784.

65 Fowler N, Kahl BS, Lee P, et al. Bortezomib, bendamustine, and rituximab in patients with relapsed or refractory follicular lymphoma: the phase II VERTICAL study. *J Clin Oncol*. 2011;29(25):3389–3395.

66 Friedberg JW, Vose JM, Kelly JL, et al. The combination of bendamustine, bortezomib, and rituximab for patients with relapsed/refractory indolent and mantle cell non-Hodgkin lymphoma. *Blood*. 2011;117(10):2807–2812.

67 Sehn LH, MacDonald D, Rubin S, et al. Bortezomib ADDED to R-CVP is safe and effective for previously untreated advanced-stage follicular lymphoma: a phase II study by the National Cancer Institute of Canada Clinical Trials Group. *J Clin Oncol*. 2011;29(25):3396–3401.

68 Chang JE, Peterson C, Choi S, et al. VcR-CVAD induction chemotherapy followed by maintenance rituximab in mantle cell lymphoma: a Wisconsin Oncology Network study. *Br J Haematol*. 2011;155(2):190–197.

69 Siegel DS, Martin T, Wang M, et al. A phase 2 study of single-agent carfilzomib (PX-171-003-A1) in patients with relapsed and refractory multiple myeloma. *Blood*. 2012;120(14):2817–2825.

70 Rui L, Schmitz R, Ceribelli M, Staudt LM. Malignant pirates of the immune system. *Nat Immunol*. 2011;12(10):933–940.

71 Lam LT, Davis RE, Pierce J, et al. Small molecule inhibitors of IkappaB kinase are selectively toxic for subgroups of diffuse large B-cell lymphoma defined by gene expression profiling. *Clin Cancer Res*. 2005;11(1):28–40.

72 Shaknovich R, Melnick A. Epigenetics and B-cell lymphoma. *Curr Opin Hematol*. 2011;18(4):293–299.

73 Shaknovich R, Geng H, Johnson NA, et al. DNA methylation signatures define molecular subtypes of diffuse large B-cell lymphoma. *Blood*. 2010;116(20):e81–e89.

74 Eberle FC, Rodriguez-Canales J, Wei L, et al. Methylation profiling of mediastinal gray zone lymphoma reveals a distinctive signature with elements shared by classical Hodgkin's lymphoma and primary mediastinal large B-cell lymphoma. *Haematologica*. 2011;96(4):558–566.

75 Enjuanes A, Fernandez V, Hernandez L, et al. Identification of methylated genes associated with aggressive clinicopathological features in mantle cell lymphoma. *PLoS One*. 2011;6(5):e19736.

76 Coiffer B, Pro B, Prince HM, et al. Results from a Pivotal, Open-label, phase II study of romidepsin in relapsed or refractory peripheral T-cell lymphoma after prior systemic therapy. *J Clin Onc*. 2012;30(6):631–636.

77 Olsen EA, Kim YH, Kuzel TM, et al. Phase IIB Multicenter trial of vorinostat in patients with persistent, progressive, or treatment refractory cutaneous T-cell lymphoma. *J Clin Onc*. 2007;25(21):3109–3115.

78 Chanan-Khan AA, Cheson BD. Lenalidomide for the treatment of B-cell malignancies. *J Clin Oncol*. 2008;26(9):1544–1552.

79 Wiernik PH, Lossos, IS, Tuscano JM, et al. Lenalidomide monotherapy in relapsed or refractory aggressive non-Hodgkin lymphoma. *J Clin Onc*. 2008;26:4952–4957.

80 Goy A, Sinha R, Williams ME, et al. Phase II multicenter study of single-agent lenalidomide in subjects with mantle cell lymphoma who relapsed or progressed after or were refractory to bortezomib: The MCL-001 "EMERGE" study. *J Clin Onc*. 2013;31(29):3688–3695.

81 Morris SW, Kirstein MN, Valentine MB, et al. Fusion of a kinase gene, ALK, to a nucleolar protein gene, NPM, in non-Hodgkin's lymphoma. *Science*. 1994;263(5151):1281–1284.

82 Morales La Madrid A, Campbell N, Smith S, Cohn SL, Salgia R. Targeting ALK: a promising strategy for the treatment of non-small cell lung cancer, non-Hodgkin's lymphoma, and neuroblastoma. *Target Oncol*. 2012;V(3):199–210.

83 Laurent C, Do C, Gascoyne RD, et al. Anaplastic lymphoma kinase-positive diffuse large B-cell lymphoma: a rare clinicopathologic entity with poor prognosis. *J Clin Oncol*. 2009;27(25):4211–4216.

84 Gascoyne RD, Lamant L, Martin-Subero JI, et al. ALK-positive diffuse large B-cell lymphoma is associated with Clathrin-ALK rearrangements: report of 6 cases. *Blood*. 2003;102(7):2568–2573.

85 Vose J, Armitage J, Weisenburger D: International T-Cell Lymphoma Project. International peripheral T-cell and natural killer/T-cell lymphoma study: pathology findings and clinical outcomes. *J Clin Oncol*. 2008;26(25):4124–4130.

86 Gambacorti-Passerini C, Messa C, Pogliani EM. Crizotinib in anaplastic large-cell lymphoma. *N Engl J Med*. 2011;364(8):775–776.

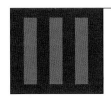

# PART III

# Targeted Therapy in Solid Tumors

## CHAPTER 18

# Targeted Therapy in Solid Tumors: Brain

*Shiao-Pei Weathers, Barbara J. O'Brien, John F. de Groot, and W. K. Alfred Yung*

Department of Neuro-Oncology, The University of Texas MD Anderson Cancer Center, Houston, TX, USA

## Introduction

Although rare in contrast to other solid tumors, primary brain tumors are among the top 10 in cancer-related deaths and cause a disproportionate amount of cancer morbidity and mortality. Gliomas represent approximately 30% of all brain tumors but account for 80% of malignant primary brain tumors.[1] Gliomas comprise astrocytomas, ependymomas, and oligodendrogliomas. Astrocytomas are characteristically infiltrative in nature rendering them surgically incurable. The World Health Organization (WHO) classification of brain tumors classifies four major entities of astrocytic gliomas based on histologic features associated with biological aggressiveness (i.e., mitotic figures, necrosis, vascular proliferation): pilocytic astrocytoma (WHO grade I), diffuse astrocytoma (WHO grade II), anaplastic astrocytoma (WHO grade III), and glioblastoma (WHO grade IV).[2]

Glioblastomas are categorized as either primary or secondary. Primary glioblastomas represent 95% of all glioblastomas and present as advanced tumors while secondary glioblastomas result from malignant progression from an antecedent lower-grade tumor and account for approximately 5% of all glioblastomas.[3] Primary and secondary glioblastomas are characterized by different sets of molecular genetic aberrations.[4] Despite optimal multimodality treatment which typically includes surgery, radiotherapy, and cytotoxic chemotherapy, recent clinical trials have reported a median survival of only 14–16 months with a 26–33% 2-year survival rate.[5,6] The lethality of glioblastoma, despite conventional therapies, has resulted in a pressing need to devise innovative therapeutic approaches to improve outcomes in patients with the disease. The lack of effective therapies to date can be attributed to the fact that glioblastoma is a dynamic, molecularly heterogeneous tumor which presents major challenges in the development of novel treatments that can block essential tumor survival and growth factor pathways.

## Predictive and Prognostic Factors

The identification of markers predictive of survival in gliomas could optimize and potentially aid in the personalization of therapy by identifying those patients more likely to respond to standard therapy versus those individuals who are refractory and may benefit from alternate approaches. For this latter group of patients,

molecular profiling would aid in the identification of potential actionable targets. Although molecular factors predictive of outcome have been difficult to identify, recent research in gliomas has yielded several significant molecular predictive factors.

In anaplastic oligodendrogliomas, allelic losses of chromosomes 1p and 19q (1p19q LOH) have emerged as markers of chemotherapeutic response and longer survival,[7,8] qualifying 1p19q loss as a prognostic factor. In addition, recent studies now confirm that 1p19q LOH is also predictive of response to chemotherapy. In seminal studies by both the EORTC and RTOG, patients with anaplastic oligodendrogliomas harboring the 1p19q LOH fared significantly better when treated with combined radiation and chemotherapy compared to radiotherapy alone. Tumors without 1p19q LOH were found to not incur a survival benefit from the combined treatment.

In patients with glioblastoma, a true predictive factor has not been fully established. However, two molecular markers have been identified as important prognostic factors. O-6-methylguanine-DNA methyltransferase (MGMT) is a DNA repair protein that reverses the damage induced by alkylating agents such as temozolomide and has been implicated as a major mechanism of resistance to alkylating agents.[9] Methylation of the *MGMT* gene promoter results in decreased expression of the enzyme, potentially rendering tumor cells more susceptible to alkylating agents. In retrospective analyses, this phenomenon has been observed to translate into a striking survival benefit for those patients treated with radiotherapy and temozolomide.[10] Large prospective studies validating these results are currently lacking and patients with tumors that lack *MGMT* promoter methylation also appear to benefit from temozolomide.

Isocitrate dehydrogenase (IDH) mutations in gliomas are now known to be a positive prognostic factor with an increase in overall survival noted in patients harboring an IDH mutation over those with wild-type IDH, but to date specific treatments based on this finding have not been established.[11] IDH mutations have a significant positive statistical association with overall survival. In low-grade gliomas, anaplastic gliomas, and glioblastoma, IDH mutation status appears to be the most important prognostic factor.[3,12] Targeting this mutation or its molecular or metabolic effects may be feasible. Small-molecule IDH1 mutant-specific inhibitors are under current investigation. All of these findings serve as clues that a molecular diagnosis is trending towards significantly influencing the clinical management of patients.

*Targeted Therapy in Translational Cancer Research*, First Edition. Edited by Apostolia-Maria Tsimberidou, Razelle Kurzrock and Kenneth C. Anderson.
© 2016 John Wiley & Sons, Inc. Published 2016 by John Wiley & Sons, Inc.

## Molecular Profiling

In recent years, our understanding of glioma tumor biology has grown significantly as a result of large-scale molecular profiling efforts. Glioblastoma was selected as one of the first three cancers to be profiled by the National Institutes of Health's The Cancer Genome Atlas (TCGA) and is now one of the most molecularly profiled of all human cancers. These molecular profiling efforts have resulted in the identification of molecular prognostic factors and molecular vulnerabilities that could be potentially targeted in the development of novel treatments in gliomas. TCGA has

established a comprehensive catalog of the genomic alterations driving gliomagenesis. Furthermore, TCGA has attempted to catalog the spectrum of molecular abnormalities seen in glioblastoma resulting in the identification of molecular subclasses each characterized by its own genomic signature. These analyses yielded identification of four subclasses termed proneural, neural, classical, and mesenchymal grouped based on shared genomic, epigenomic, and transcriptional features.[13] Figure 18.1 highlights the molecular subclasses of glioblastoma and their genomic molecular correlates.[14]

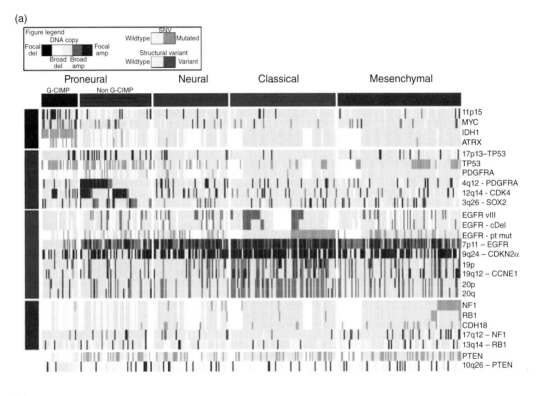

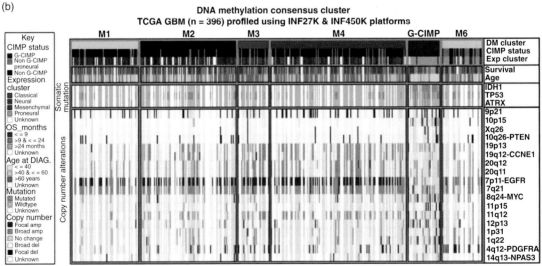

**Figure 18.1** Molecular subclasses of GBM and their genomic molecular correlates. Genomic alterations and survival associated with five molecular subtypes of GBM. Expression and DNA methylation profiles were used to classify 332 GBMs with available (native DNA and whole genome amplified DNA) exome sequencing and DNA copy-number levels.

The most significant genomic associations were identified through Chi-Square tests, with p-values corrected for multiple testing using the Benjamini-Hochberg method. Reproduced from Brennan et al., 2013, Reference 14 with permission from Elsevier.

The proneural subtype is more frequently seen in younger patients and is predominantly grade II and grade III gliomas. This subtype is commonly associated with platelet-derived growth factor receptor (PDGFR) amplification and IDH1 mutation.[13] The mesenchymal subtype is associated with neurofibromatosis 1 (NF1) gene loss or mutation, frequent TP53 loss, ink4a/arf loss, and mesenchymal markers including MET.[13] The classical subtype is seen in association with PTEN loss, absence of a TP53 mutation, and amplification and activating mutations of epidermal growth factor receptor (EGFR).[15] TCGA profiling efforts have additionally identified a subset of glioblastoma with characteristic promoter DNA methylation alterations referred to as the glioma-CpG island methylator phenotype (G-CIMP). G-CIMP tumors belong to the proneural subgroup. They harbor distinct molecular features including a high frequency of IDH1 mutations and display characteristic copy-number alterations. Patients with G-CIMP tumors are typically younger at diagnosis and experience improved survival.[16]

Although subclass does not play a role in treatment decisions, the recognition of molecular subclasses has piqued interest that tumor profiling in gliomas may translate into stratification of treatment and the development of therapies targeting these subgroups. Improving patient outcomes will require the development of therapies directed against the molecular aberrations within a patient's tumor.

### Signaling Pathways Driving Disease Progression

Molecular analysis of glioblastoma has aided in the understanding of the underlying biology of tumorigenesis and the drivers leading to oncogenesis and sustained tumor growth. The genomic analyses described by TCGA have uncovered that glioblastomas are associated with alterations in three core overlapping pathways: receptor tyrosine kinase/RAS/phosphatidylinositol 3 kinase (RTK/RAS/PI3K) signaling (altered in 88% of glioblastomas), TP53 signaling (altered in 87% of glioblastomas), and RB signaling (altered in 78% of glioblastomas).[15] These signaling alterations were noted in the majority of tumor samples analyzed and are postulated to be keys to gliomagenesis and potentially clinically actionable. In the TCGA cohort, inactivation of the TP53 pathway was seen in the form of ARF deletions, MDM amplifications, and mutations of TP53 itself. In the RTK/PI3K pathway, PTEN deletions and mutations were frequent, as were aberrations in EGFR, ERBB2, PDGFRA, and MET. Dysregulation of the RB pathway most commonly occurred with deletion of CDKN2A/CDKN2B locus on chromosome 9p21, followed by CDK4 locus amplification.[15] These pathways are undoubtedly biologically informative and likely to be just a few of many other alterations which will likely be uncovered with further sequencing.

### Molecular Targets in Gliomas

The development of molecular targeted therapy for gliomas has been accelerated by the profiling advances made in the identification of tumor-specific molecular aberrations and the key intracellular signaling pathways driving disease progression. A multitude of molecular alterations have been identified in gliomas resulting in a number of potential actionable targets. Pathway alterations in glioblastoma are highlighted in Figure 18.2.

Targets for therapy should harbor certain characteristics. Ideally, the target should be highly expressed and specific to tumor cells, differentially expressed on tumor tissue in contrast to normal tissue, essential to tumor survival, proliferation, and invasion, and

involved in gliomagenesis. Although most targets do not harbor all of these ideal characteristics, there have been several key regulators of cell growth and invasion which have been identified as potential actionable targets in glioma. The development of effective targeted therapies is further complicated by the difficulty in penetrating the blood–brain barrier in therapeutic concentrations without resulting in significant systemic and/or central nervous system toxicity.

Tumors are capable of utilizing multiple cellular pathways in a redundant fashion rendering therapies targeted to a single molecule or pathway likely to be ineffective if used alone. These critical pathways are so vital to tumor cells that they have developed numerous ways to maintain signal flux to their core downstream effectors. The challenge moving forward is identifying which collateral pathways require inhibition as overlapping pathways provide a multitude of escape mechanisms to overcome targeted therapy. Therapeutic molecular targets are summarized in Table 18.1.

## Targets for Therapy

### Cell Surface Growth Factor Receptors

In gliomas, several growth factor receptors are found to be frequently overexpressed and are suspected to drive gliomagenesis and progression. These growth factor receptors are hence appealing targets in drug development.[17,18] These receptors predominantly act through receptor tyrosine kinases and are found on the cell surface where they interact with effector molecules, second messengers, and other intracellular signaling pathway mediators, including the Ras/Raf/mitogen-activated protein kinase (MAPK) and phosphatidylinositol 3-kinase (PI3K) pathways.[17] As a result, secondary pathways then activate additional downstream effectors culminating in enhanced cell survival, proliferation, migration and invasion, evasion of apoptosis, angiogenesis, and resistance to treatment.[17] The core growth factor pathways involved in glioma formation and progression include those mediated by the EGFR, PDGFR, vascular endothelial growth factor (VEGF), transforming growth factor receptor (TGFR)—alpha and beta, and fibroblast growth factor receptor (FGFR).[18] In addition, glioma cells are also known to secrete growth factors for these receptors which are typically overexpressed on the cell surface, resulting in the establishment of autocrine and paracrine loops which ultimately stimulate and sustain growth. The critical role these growth factors exhibit and their overexpression on glial tumors have made them attractive targets.

### Epidermal Growth Factor Receptor

The most common oncogenic aberration in gliomas is alterations (overexpression, amplification, or mutation) in epidermal growth factor receptor (EGFR), which is seen in approximately 60% of patients with primary glioblastoma.[19,20] EGFR is a receptor tyrosine kinase which plays a critical role in the growth and transformation of glioblastoma. EGFR expression has been linked to increased tumor cell proliferation, increased cellular migration and invasion, and resistance to chemotherapy. The EGFR pathway in gliomas can be activated by multiple mechanisms via initiation of signal transduction through major pathways including MAPK cascade and PI3K/Akt ultimately promoting cell proliferation and survival.[19] Some glioblastomas are also capable of secreting ligands EGF and TGF-α which results in autocrine and paracrine loops that effect the constitutive activation of the receptor and downstream pathways.

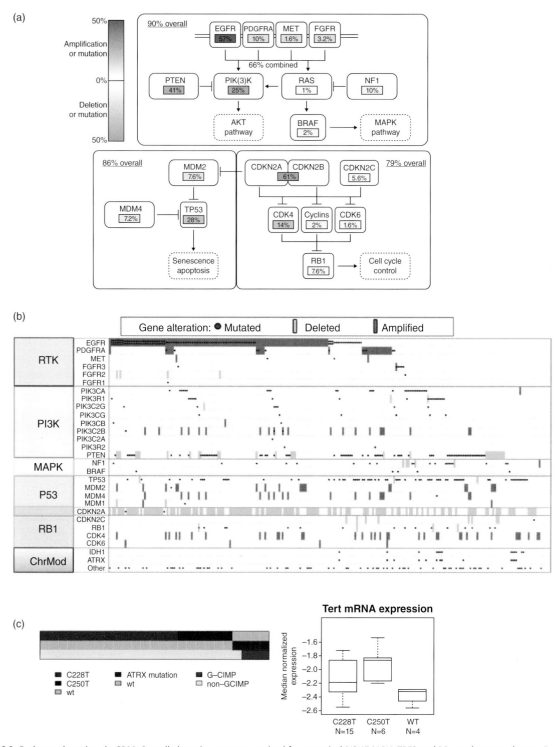

**Figure 18.2** Pathway alterations in GBM. Overall alteration rate summarized for canonical PI3K/MAPK, TP53 and RB regulatory pathways. Reproduced from Brennan et al., 2013, Reference 14 with permission from Elsevier.

Amplification or overexpression of EGFR is most common but a relatively high percent of tumors also demonstrate a unique mutation designated EGFRvIII. EGFRvIII mutation represents a partial deletion of exons 2–7 resulting in loss of the extracellular ligand-binding domain that constitutively activates the receptor of the ligand.[21,22] EGFRvIII mutation is seen in approximately 40% of tumors with EGFR amplification.[18,20] The relatively high frequency of EGFR amplification, EGFRvIII mutation, and other EGFR extra-cellular domain mutations make EGFR and its downstream pathways compelling targets in glioma therapy for several reasons. EGFR is found widely expressed in gliomas. EGFR overexpression is cor-related with poorer prognosis (decreased overall survival time and shorter time to progression), and EGFR plays no role in critical physiological role in otherwise healthy adults.

**Table 18.1** Therapeutic molecular targets.

| Target | Drug | Phase of clinical development |
|---|---|---|
| EGFR | Gefitinib | I/II |
| | Erlotinib | I/II |
| | Lapatinib | I/II II |
| | Cetuximab | I/II |
| | (125) I-mAb 425 | I/II |
| | Nimotuzamab EMD 55,900 | I/II |
| PDGF | Imatinib | II/III |
| | Sunitinb | I |
| | Vandetanib | I |
| PKC | Enzataurin | I/II/III |
| PI3K | BKM120 | I/II |
| Farneysl transferase | Tipifarnib | I |
| | Lonafarnib | I |
| MAPK cascade/Raf | Sorafenib | II |
| | TLN-4601 | II |
| mTOR | Everolimus | I |
| | Temsirolimus | I/II |
| | Rapamycin | I |
| SRC | Dasatinib | I/II |
| VEGF | Bevacizumab | II |
| VEGFR | Pazopanib | II |
| | Vatalanib | I |
| | Cediranib | II |
| Integrin | Cilengitide | II |
| HDACs | Vorinostat | I/II |
| | Romidepsin | I/II |
| Proteasome | Bortezomib | I |
| Endothelin A receptor | Atrasentan | I |
| Matrix metallo-protease | Marimastat | II |

Reversible and irreversible inhibitors of EGFR exist with the latter agents being more able to effectively bind and inhibit the inactive conformation adopted by EGFR extracellular domain mutants.[23] Unfortunately, the first-generation single-agent small-molecule tyrosine kinase inhibitors used in clinical trials targeting EGFR in glioblastoma, gefitinib (ZD1839;Iressa) and erlotinib (OSI-779;Tarceva), have been largely unsuccessful even in patients with tumors in which the gene is overexpressed or the EGFRvIII mutation is present.[24–27] Although well-tolerated, these agents disappointingly did not result in a treatment benefit. Limited efficacy was also observed with cetuximab (Erbitux, ImClone Systems), a monoclonal antibody against EGFR likely related to its inadequate penetration across the blood–brain barrier translating to limited clinical activity.

The lack of success seen with the first-generation EGFR inhibitors in glioma may relate to inadequate drug levels of the tumor, inability to inhibit the receptor for a sufficient period of time, and the rapid activation of resistance pathways. Therapies that inhibit EGFR have led to an improved understanding of the mechanism(s) mediating resistance along this important pathway. Constitutively active mutant EGFRvIII expression sensitizes tumors to EGFR inhibitors *in vitro* and clinically, but only if the PTEN tumor suppressor protein is intact.[28] PTEN is an important factor in determining EGFR tyrosine kinase inhibitor response. EGFRvIII expression and loss

of PTEN result in resistance to EGFR tyrosine kinase inhibitors in glioblastoma patients and preclinical models as signal flux through the PI3K signaling pathway is maintained.[28] PDGFRα and c-MET are receptor tyrosine kinases that contribute to PI3K pathway activation which can be coactivated in EGFR-amplified tumors.[29] Next generation tyrosine kinase inhibitors such as afatinib, dacomitinib, and nimotuzumab which have reversible EGFR inhibition are under current development and testing.[30]

Preclinical studies have identified lapatinib (GW572016, GlaxoSmithKline, USA) as an irreversible inhibitor of EGFR suggesting a possible therapeutic advantage in contrast to prior tyrosine kinase inhibitors such as erlotinib. Recent studies examining potential EGFR pathway inhibition suggest that agents that target the intracellular component, such as lapatinib, may have greater efficacy.[23] A phase I/II study evaluating the combination of the antiangiogenic agent pazopanib and lapatinib in patients with glioblastoma and known EGFRvIII status found limited antitumor activity. The pharmacokinetic data indicated that exposure to lapatinib was subtherapeutic in the phase II evaluation.[31] The subtherapeutic levels of lapatinib were concluded to have likely contributed to the poor outcome observed underscoring the need to improve dosing strategies to achieve better intratumoral lapatinib concentrations. Studies are presently underway evaluating pulsatile, intermittent scheduling of lapatinib at higher dose levels.

### Platelet-Derived Growth Factor Receptor

Platelet-derived growth factor receptor (PDGFR) is another important growth pathway believed to drive gliomagenesis. Stimulation of PDGFR results in activation of downstream signaling cascades involving the Ras/Raf/MAPK and PI3K/Akt pathways. These effects translate to promotion of cell survival, proliferation, invasion, and resistance to apoptosis. PDGF was originally identified as a potent mitogen for fibroblasts, glial cells, and smooth muscle and was found to stimulate tumor growth and angiogenesis in preclinical studies.[32] Both the ligand (PDGF) and the receptor (PDGFR) are found to be overexpressed in primary brain tumors which is a similar phenomenon seen in other receptor tyrosine kinases. This suggests that autocrine and paracrine growth stimulatory loops result in the constitutive activation of this receptor.[33] Overexpression of PDGF and PDGFR is seen in both low and high-grade astrocytomas suggesting the overall critical role they have in the development of gliomas. Furthermore, the proneural subtype of glioblastoma is commonly associated with PDGFR amplification[13] which could potentially allow for this patient population to be specifically selected for clinical trials with PDGFR inhibitors.

There have been a number of PDGFR inhibitors under investigation. Imatinib (STI-571, Gleevec, Novartis Pharmaceuticals), is an inhibitor of PDGFR, c-Kit, and BCR-ABL. Its inhibition of the BCR-ABL tyrosine kinase revolutionized the treatment of Ph(+) CML and emerged as a paradigm for the development of targeted therapy in cancer.[34] Although imatinib showed some activity in preclinical testing in glioma cell lines, it has shown only minimal activity in both single-agent and combination therapy. A phase II trial of ramucirumab, an anti-PDGFR alpha monoclonal antibody IMC-3G3, is currently being evaluated in the setting of recurrent glioblastoma (ClinicalTrials.gov NCT00895180). Second generation multi-tyrosine kinase inhibitors such as tandutinib and dasatinib recently underwent evaluation in clinical trials and the results have not been encouraging suggesting that PDGFR may be a challenging target in glioblastoma.

## Fibroblast Growth Factor Receptor

Fibroblast growth factor receptor (FGFR) signaling has received recent attention as a potential actionable target. Inhibition of FGFR signaling may block angiogenesis.[35] FGFR dysregulation ultimately leads to upregulation of both the (Ras-dependent) Ras/MAPK pathway and the (Ras-independent) PI3K/Akt pathway.[35] Although FGFR seems like a reasonable therapeutic target, FGFR is intimately involved in many normal biologic processes raising concern for potential toxicity.[35] Recent work has identified that a small subset of glioblastomas harbor an oncogenic chromosomal translocation that fuse in-frame the tyrosine kinase coding domains of FGFR genes (FGFR1 or FGFR3) to the transforming acidic coiled-coil (TACC) coding domains of TACC1 or TACC3, respectively. The FGFR-TACC fusion protein was found to display oncogenic activity in the mouse brain. In preclinical studies, oral administration of an FGFR inhibitor was found to prolong the survival of mice harboring the intracranial FGFR3-TACC3-initiated glioma suggesting that targeted FGFR kinase inhibition may benefit the small subset of glioblastoma patients with FGFR-TACC fusions.[36] Clinical trials specifically targeting this unique fusion protein have recently opened for patients with recurrent glioblastoma. However, the very low incidence (approximately 3%) will present a challenge in identifying appropriate patients to complete protocol accrual.

## Ras/MAPK

The Ras/MAPK (mitogen-activated protein kinase) pathway is a key pathway activated by the receptor tyrosine kinases EGFR and PDGFR. Ras is a second-messenger protein which is an important signal transduction effector. In 25% of cancers, oncogenic mutations in Ras result in its overactivation.[37] The increased Ras activity observed in a large proportion of glioblastomas (~88%)[38] is felt to be attributable to the downstream effects of activation of the receptor tyrosine kinases, mutation or homozygous deletion of NF1 (~18%), mutation or homozygous deletion of PTEN (~35%), mutation of PIK3CA (~15%), RAS mutation (2%), amplification of AKT (~2%) and mutation of FOXO (~1%).[15] These observations suggest that inhibiting Ras-dependent signaling could be a useful therapeutic strategy.[18] Several steps are required in the activation of Ras. Ras must be farnesylated and then catalyzed by the farnesyltransferase enzyme to be active and then recruited to the plasma membrane. Ras subsequently then activates a number of downstream molecules including Raf which activates several MAPKs. This Ras/MAPK pathway enhances cell proliferation and plays a role in cell migration.

Ras has emerged as a potential actionable target in glioma therapeutics for a several reasons. Foremost, Ras is activated by many receptor tyrosine kinases. Ras is activated in gliomas, and inhibition of Ras results in a dramatic reduction in glioma growth.[38] The approach to pharmacologically inhibit Ras activity is indirect. Farnesyltransferase rather than Ras itself can be inhibited; two farnesyltransferase inhibitors (FTIs) of Ras farnesylation, tipifarnib (R111577, Zarnestra, Johnson and Johnson) and lonafarnib (SCH66336, SARASAR, Schering-Plough) have been studied as potential therapies in patients with gliomas. The initial studies of tipifarnib seemed promising, but unfortunately the results have demonstrated only modest activity against glioblastoma.[18] The initial studies of lonafarnib have demonstrated some promising results but will require further evaluation in terms of its efficacy against gliomas.[39,40] The vital role Ras plays in signal transduction and glioma growth, renders it a very appealing target in glioma therapy, and ongoing efforts to target Ras are warranted.

The MAPK cascade involves multiple protein kinases including Raf which phosphorylates and activates MEK which then subsequently activates MAPK.[18,41] Sorafenib (BAY43–9006, Bayer) is both a Raf kinase inhibitor and VEGFR inhibitor. As a single agent, very little activity has been noted but it continues to be evaluated in drug combination studies.[42,43] Although the results from clinical trials targeting Raf have not been promising, there are several new MEK inhibitors in development that may effectively inactivate this pathway in patients with glioblastoma. The MEK inhibitor MSC1936369B in combination with SAR245409 Pi3K/mTOR inhibitor is currently being evaluated (ClinicalTrials.gov NCT01390818).

## PI3K/Akt

Activation of receptor tyrosine kinases additionally results in the activation of the PI3K pathway via a complex second-messenger signaling cascade to activate several molecules, including Akt and mammalian target of rapamycin (mTOR). The PI3K pathway plays a critical role in the regulation of cancer cell growth, proliferation, and apoptosis. PI3K pathway-activating genetic alterations occur in almost 90% of glioblastomas arising due to amplification and/or mutation in EGFR or other RTKs, PIK3CA or PIK3RA mutation, or PTEN loss. Activation of the PI3K pathway is associated with poor prognosis in glioma.[18,44,45] Akt phosphorylation is commonly observed[46] and is a major pathway in growth factor receptor signaling.[18] The tumor suppressor phosphatase and tensin homolog (PTEN) is an important regulator of the EGFR pathway and can antagonize PI3K. PTEN function loss results in constitutive activation of the PI3K pathway and is seen in at least 35% of glioblastomas.[18] In addition, PTEN loss is associated with higher activated Akt levels in glioma cell. Higher Akt levels subsequently activates downstream targets essential to cell survival and growth signaling.[18]

Recognition that PI3K/AKT signaling is hyperactivated has made PI3K and its key downstream effector AKT appealing targets for therapy in glioblastoma. PI3K and AKT inhibitors are currently under investigation. Although the PI3K pathway remains an intriguing therapeutic target, early studies have been complicated by unacceptable toxicities, likely related to the importance of these pathways in normal cellular homeostasis making it difficult to inhibit Akt in cancer treatment without affecting numerous other biologic processes. Perifosine (keryx) is an Akt inhibitor and LY294002, a PI3K inhibitor, are being evaluated but unfortunately have had poor toxicity profiles.[18] More selective inhibitors are currently in early phase clinical trials for glioblastoma including agents inhibiting upstream and downstream targets within the PI3K/Akt pathway and inhibitors directly targeting PI3K and mTOR. Blood–brain-barrier penetrant inhibitors of PI3K have also recently been developed including BKM120 (Novartis) and GDC-0084 (Genentech) and are under evaluation in phase I and II clinical trials in patients with recurrent glioblastoma.

mTOR is activated by both the Akt and Ras pathways and is an important downstream target in the promotion of cell survival and growth signaling. mTOR transduces proliferative signals mediated by PI3K/Akt activating downstream effectors. The overexpression of growth factors or deletion of PTEN increases mTOR activation. mTOR inhibitors include rapamycin (sirolimus, Rapamune, Wyeth), temsirolimus (CCI-779, Wyeth), AP23573 (ariad), and everolimus (Rad-001, Certican, Novartis). These agents inhibit glioblastoma proliferation in glioma cell lines.[18]

In a phase I trial of neoadjuvant rapamycin in patients with recurrent PTEN-deficient glioblastoma, rapamycin was orally administered to patients prior to a scheduled tumoral resection with the primary goal of defining the dose required for mTOR target inhibition and assessing the anti-proliferative effects on tumor cells. At recurrence, patients with PTEN-deficient tumors received a 10-day course of rapamycin at 1 of 3 dosages (2, 5, or 10 mg/kg bid.) followed by surgical resection. Intratumoral rapamycin concentrations that were sufficient to inhibit mTOR *in vitro* were achieved in all patients, but the magnitude of mTOR inhibition varied substantially from patient to patient, irrespective of dose. Reduced tumor cell proliferation *in vivo* was significantly related to the degree of inhibition of mTORC1 signaling. mTORC1 inhibition of more than 50% resulted in significantly inhibited tumor cell proliferation while inhibition of less than 50% did not result in a cytostatic response.[47]

mTOR inhibitors have been administered as single agents as well as in combination with EGFR inhibitors in patients with glioblastoma and have been found to be ineffective.[18,48,49] Although these results are discouraging, mTOR inhibitors may benefit a subpopulation of patients with glioblastoma who possess high tumor levels of a downstream activator of mTOR signaling.[30,48] Mechanisms of escape from mTOR inhibition also warrant further clinical study to enhance our understanding of mTOR signaling in glioblastoma.

## Protein Kinase C

Protein kinase C (PKC) is another important signaling pathway in glioma. PKC is a family of protein tyrosine kinases that are downstream signaling pathway components of several receptor tyrosine kinases including EGFR and PDGFR. The overactivity of PKC is not secondary to mutations in PKC but rather activation of upstream kinases which is a similar phenomenon seen with Ras. It has been demonstrated that PKC is important in glioma growth as well as angiogenesis.[50–52] The activation of PKC results in the phosphorylation of other effectors including Raf and MAPK in addition to Ras activation.[18,50,53] PKC activation can induce signaling through the Ras/extracellular signal-regulated Ras/MAPK pathway which plays an important role in cellular survival, proliferation, and invasion. The ability to target PKC in glioblastoma has been limited. Tamoxifen, an estrogen receptor antagonist, inhibits PKC but failed to demonstrate any benefit in clinical studies.[18,54,55] Enzastaurin (LY317615, Eli Lilly and Company) is a PKC inhibitor with antiangiogenic and anti-tumor activity in glioma cell lines[56] inhibiting signaling through the PI3K/Akt pathway. Although the initial results seemed promising, a Phase III study was terminated due to lack of clinical efficacy.[18]

## TP53

TP53 is yet another key signaling pathway recognized in glioblastoma. The loss of TP53 function via either mutation or homozygous deletion provides a tumor growth advantage resulting in clonal expansion of glioma cells and brain tumor progression.[57] Inactivation of the TP53 pathway can occur as mutation of TP53 itself, or as ARF deletion (55%), or amplifications of MDM2 (11%) and MDM4 (4%).[15] The TP53 tumor-suppressor gene encodes a protein that causes cell-cycle arrest in the G1 and/or G2 phase of the cell cycle, and promotes apoptosis following DNA damage.[57,58] At this time, there are no effective therapies that can restore TP53 protein and its function making TP53 not a molecule for targeting.

## Rb Signaling

Rb constitutes another key signaling pathway in glioblastoma. The cell cycle is kept in check by the RB protein until phosphorylated by cyclin D, CDK4, and CDK 66.[30] The RB pathway is altered in 77% of glioblastoma predominantly through amplification of CDK4 or CDK6 (14%) or deletion of CDKN2 A/CDKN2B (55% and 53%) respectively.[15] Novel agents that interfere with downstream molecules are currently under investigation. For example PD 0332991 and LY83583 are CDK4/6 inhibitors under evaluation in recurrent glioblastomas that harbor known Rb-pathway alterations.

## Vascular Endothelial Growth Factor Receptor and Angiogenesis

Rapidly growing tumors rely on the ability to release growth factors in order to promote new blood vessel formation, a process termed angiogenesis. Angiogenesis plays a vital role in the development and maintenance of solid tumors, and endothelial cell proliferation is a pathologic hallmark of glioblastoma. The expression of VEGF among other pro-angiogenic cytokines is one of the most important regulators of angiogenesis in glioblastoma.[59] Genetic aberrations resulting in upregulation of proangiogenic factors and downregulation of antiangiogenic inhibitors are seen in glioblastoma.[60,61] The expression of VEGF and other proangiogenic cytokines in glioblastoma results in the development of abnormal tumor vasculature characterized by tortuous, hyperpermeable vessels, increased vessel diameter, and abnormally thickened basement membranes. This aberrant tumor vasculature is believed to enhance tumor hypoxia and impair the delivery of cytotoxic chemotherapy. VEGF is released by glioma cells in the tumor microenvironment which then activates VEGF tyrosine kinase receptors on vascular endothelial cells. This results in the activation of an intracellular signaling cascade via stimulation of the PI3K/Akt and Ras/MAPK pathways resulting in endothelial cell proliferation, migration, and survival.[30,62]

VEGF is an essential regulator of angiogenesis which has rendered it an appealing target in cancer therapeutics.[63] Several studies have demonstrated that VEGF and its receptors can be antagonized by monoclonal antibodies to VEGF and small-molecule inhibitors of VEGFR-2.[64–66] Other mediators of angiogenesis in glioblastoma include PDGF, the angiopoietins (ang1 and ang2) and their receptor (Tie-2), bFGH, HIF-1alpha, and HGF[30,67] and the Notch signaling pathway.[30,68]

Bevacizumab (Avastin, Genentech/Roche) is a recombinant, humanized neutralizing monoclonal antibody which binds to VEGF preventing its interaction with VEGFRs resulting in suppression of VEGF signaling. Bevacizumab received accelerated FDA approval in May 2009 for use as a single agent in patients with glioblastoma with progressive disease following front-line therapy consisting of surgical resection, radiotherapy, and temozolomide. Bevacizumab is the only antiangiogenic agent currently approved for the treatment of glioblastoma. In the early, uncontrolled clinical studies, impressive radiographic responses and prolongation of progression-free survival were noted. The results of single-arm phase II clinical trials, the pan-VEGF receptor (VEGFR)-2 tyrosine kinase inhibitor cediranib (AZD2171, AstraZeneca) and the anti-VEGF-A antibody bevacizumab (Avastin, Genentech/Roche) seemed promising. These agents then entered phase III clinical trials for recurrent (cediranib) and newly diagnosed (bevacizumab) glioblastoma with no effect on overall patient survival.

Two recently completed large randomized phase III trials, AVAglio and RTOG 0825 demonstrated that the addition of bevacizumab to upfront treatment with radiation and temozolomide conferred no benefit in terms of overall survival in patients with newly diagnosed glioblastoma when compared to the standard treatment arm, although some prolongation of progression-free survival was documented.[69,70] VEGF inhibitors have failed to demonstrate enduring clinical and radiographic responses in multiple cancer types including glioblastoma with response rates measured only on the order of months. The clinical and radiographic responses seen initially are likely the results of the anti-permeability effects of anti-VEGF agents. The sobering realization that VEGF pathway inhibitors result in only transitory clinical and radiographic response on the order of months prior to inevitable progression has prompted the effort to better understand the mechanistic basis underlying resistance to antiangiogenic therapy. The rapid and robust radiographic response of angiogenesis inhibitors suggests that they have little intrinsic antitumor activity and that the main benefit is derived from the indirect effects secondary to reduction in cerebral edema and the potential to enhance the efficacy of other therapies.

The lack of a durable response seen with the use of antiangiogenic agents has been disappointing. Complicating factors warranting consideration of using bevacizumab in the treatment of gliomas include the difficulty of assessing tumor response and the unknown optimal biologic dosing schedule and length of treatment. Efforts are underway to better understand the mechanisms underlying the resistance to anti-VEGF therapy in order to improve our current therapeutic approaches. Adaptive (evasive) resistance and intrinsic (pre-existing) non-responsiveness have emerged as the modes of resistance to antiangiogenic therapy with multiple mechanisms believed to underlie each type.[71] Adaptive mechanisms described have included activation and/or upregulation of alternative pro-angiogenic signaling pathways within the tumor, recruitment of bone marrow derived pro-angiogenic cells, increased pericyte coverage of the tumor vasculature, and activation and enhancement of invasion and metastasis.[71] It has also been proposed that some glioblastoma-associated blood vessels are inherently resistant to antiangiogenic therapy based on the observation of patients on clinical trials with VEGF pathway inhibitors who had no discernible reduction in contrast enhancement on MRI after treatment with antiangiogenic therapy. A subset of patients in clinical trials for bevacizumab, sorafenib, and sunitinib was identified who did not demonstrate any transitory radiographic response or clinical benefit[72] characterized by no evidence of reduction in vascular permeability, no cessation of tumor growth or retardation of growth rate, no observed quality of life benefit, and no evidence of increased survival.[71] This lack of response is speculated to be related to tumor expression of high levels of multiple pro-angiogenic growth factors such as placental growth factor, in addition to VEGF or because the tumor angiogenesis is completely VEGF-independent.

Although the results to date regarding the use of antiangiogenic therapies have been largely disappointing and unfortunately have not translated into improved patient survival, there is likely a role for angiogenesis inhibitors in the treatment of high grade gliomas. Future efforts will need to be directed towards broadening our understanding of the mechanisms of action of VEGF inhibitors, determining the optimal biologic dose, and identifying the patient subsets most likely to derive a durable benefit. The present lack of a durable response to antiangiogenic therapies highlights the need

for a better understanding of how best to incorporate antiangiogenic therapy into our treatment paradigm in order to optimize radiation and chemotherapy.

## Histone Deacetylase Inhibition

Alterations of gene expression by epigenetic changes may influence tumor growth. Histone proteins organize DNA into units called nucleosomes. The acetylation (by histone acetyltransferases) and deacetylation (by histone deacetylases [HDACs]) play a key role in the regulation of gene expression.[18,73] Histone processing may be altered in gliomas. Inhibition of histone deacetylases has been another target being evaluated in glioma therapy. HDAC inhibitors, including LBH589, valproic acid, depsipeptide, and suberolylanilide hydroxamic acid (SAHA) (vorinostat), are under investigation.[18]

## Combination Therapy

To date, single-agent molecularly targeted therapies have been largely ineffective despite promising preclinical data.[18] The molecular heterogeneity of gliomas has made the development of targeted therapy challenging. This heterogeneity is both intertumoral and intratumoral, further complicated by continued molecular changes over time. Recurrence in glioblastoma is inevitable, and there is a present lack of effective salvage therapies. The molecular profile of the tumor tissue obtained at time of diagnosis is distinctly different from tissue at time of recurrence as a result of accumulated genomic alterations. This phenomenon is evidenced by a recent mutational analysis of paired glioma samples. Exomes of 23 initial low-grade gliomas of predominantly astrocytic histology and recurrent tumors resected from the same patients were analyzed. In 43% of the cases, at least half of the tumors in the initial tumor were undetected at recurrence including driver mutations in *TP53, ATRX, SMARCA4,* and *BRAF.*[74] The effect of temozolomide on the mutational profile of recurrent tumors was also examined revealing hypermutated tumors harboring driver mutations in the RB and Akt-mTOR pathways.[74] These findings of an evolving genomic landscape from the time of diagnosis to recurrence highlight the difficulty in the development of targeted therapies in the setting of progressive disease.

The development of targeted therapy is further complicated by the complexity and redundancy of signaling pathways. The lack of effectiveness of single agent therapies is likely attributable to the tumor's capability to utilize multiple cellular pathways in a redundant fashion underscoring the need to investigate the combination of targeted therapies and other agents both targeted and less targeted. Use of multi-agent drug combinations may result in less resistance to treatment.

## Future Perspectives

### Personalized Medicine

In oncology, there has been a movement towards personalized medicine or, tailoring treatment to the individual patient. Ideally, tumor and patient evaluations would lead to the selection of the best treatment (based on tumor characterization) and the right dosing schedule (based on patient characterization). This comprehensive understanding of tumor biology and patient characteristics will lead to the design of optimally effective treatments. However, this concept is challenged by our increasing recognition of the heterogeneity of the disease (glioblastoma) and the patients. This challenge is further compounded by the relative rarity of glioblastoma in contrast to other cancers, slowing progress by limited accrual to clinical trials.

The ability to develop targeted therapy in glioblastoma will require a large-scale molecular profiling effort to be able to identify targets for therapy. Even if an actionable target is identified, success will be contingent upon these agents being administered to a properly selected group of patients harboring the correct molecular target or pathway of interest.

Patients with glioblastoma are far from a homogenous patient group with only a subset of these patients demonstrating a response to standard therapy. The molecular intragroup heterogeneity among patients with glioblastoma is vast resulting in very small numbers of patients with similar molecular aberrations. A myriad of genetic alterations have been described in glioblastoma with many of these mutations seen only in a small percentage of patients. Even the most common mutations in glioblastoma, such as EGFR amplification, are seen in less than half of all glioblastomas.

## Implementing Targeted Therapy into Clinical Trials

The known disease heterogeneity of glioblastoma must be met with creative clinical trial designs that incorporate both clinical and molecular factors. The integration of these factors into clinical trial designs may help accelerate our progress towards the development of targeted therapy in glioblastoma. There should be a collaborative movement on a multi-institutional level to make prospective collection of blood for genomic testing and tumor tissue from patients on clinical trials a standard of care.

Small sample sizes will pose a significant challenge in the evaluation of targeted therapies in glioblastoma. As mentioned above, the rarity of specific molecular aberrations among patients with glioblastoma underscores the need for the molecular profiling of as many patients as possible. Although the number of patients with a selected molecular aberration will result in a small pool of eligible candidates for accrual in a clinical trial, small numbers of patients may suffice in demonstrating a clinical benefit if the patient population is appropriately selected.

## Concluding Remarks

Glioblastoma is one of the most lethal human cancers. They are surgically incurable secondary to their infiltrative nature and are one of the most resistant to radiation and chemotherapy among all cancers. The current standard multimodality treatment results in only a modest survival benefit at best for a subset of patients with glioblastoma. The challenges in developing effective treatments for patients with glioblastoma are attributed to the relative rarity of the tumor and its molecular heterogeneity. Glioblastoma is now one of the most molecularly characterized of all human cancers. Genomic analyses have furthered our understanding of the complex molecular landscape of glioblastomas and have accelerated our understanding of this molecularly heterogeneous disorder providing insight into potential actionable targets in the development of targeted therapeutics. Pharmacologic inhibitors and modulators are currently under active investigation. Future efforts should focus on the use of combination therapies. Transformation of the treatment of patients with glioblastoma will require furthering our understanding of this heterogeneous disease, devising innovative therapies to exploit identified molecular vulnerabilities, and designing creative clinical trials. A collaborative effort between investigators and clinicians on a multi-institutional level will also be necessary.

## References

1 Dolecek TA, Propp JM, Stroup NE, Kruchko C. CBTRUS statistical report: primary brain and central nervous system tumors diagnosed in the United States in 2005–2009. *Neuro Oncol.* 2012; 14(Suppl 5):v1–49.

2 Louis DN, Ohgaki H, Wiestler OD, et al. The 2007 WHO classification of tumours of the central nervous system. *Acta Neuropathol.* 2007;114(2):97–109.

3 Parsons DW, Jones S, Zhang X, et al. An integrated genomic analysis of human glioblastoma Multiforme. *Science.* 2008;321(5897):1807–1812.

4 Ohgaki H, Kleihues P. The definition of primary and secondary glioblastoma. *Clin Cancer Res.* 2013;19(4):764–772.

5 Stupp R, Mason WP, van den Bent MJ, et al.; National Cancer Institute of Canada Clinical Trials Group. Radiotherapy plus concomitant and adjuvant temozolomide for glioblastoma. *N Engl J Med.* 2005;352(10):987–996.

6 Gilbert M, Wang M, Aldape KD, et al. Dose-dense temozolomide for newly diagnosed glioblastoma: a randomized phase III clinical trial. *J Clin Oncol.* 2013;31(32):4085–4091.

7 Cairncross JG, Ueki K, Zlatescu MC, et al. Specific genetic predictors of chemotherapeutic response and survival in patients with anaplastic oligodendrogliomas. *J Natl Cancer Inst.* 1998;90(19):1473–1479.

8 Ino Y, Betensky RA, Zlatescu MC, et al. Molecular subtypes of anaplastic oligodendroglioma: implications for patient management at diagnosis. *Clin Cancer Res.* 2001;7(4):839–845.

9 Esteller M, Garcia-Foncillas J, Andion E, et al. Inactivation of the DNA-repair gene MGMT and the clinical response of gliomas to alkylating agents. *N Engl J Med.* 2000;343(23):1350–1354.

10 Hegi ME, Diserens AC, Gorlia T, et al. MGMT gene silencing and benefit from temozolomide in glioblastoma. *N Engl J Med.* 2005;352(10):997–1003.

11 Yan H, Parsons DW, Jin G, et al. IDH1 and IDH2 mutations in gliomas. *N Engl J Med.* 2009;360(8):765–773.

12 Hartmann C, Hentschel B, Wick W, et al. Patients with IDH1 wild type anaplastic astrocytomas exhibit worse prognosis than IDH1-mutated glioblastomas, and IDH1 mutation status accounts for the unfavorable prognostic effect of higher age: implications for classification of gliomas. *Acta Neuropathol.* 2010;120(6):707–718.

13 Verhaak RG, Hoadley KA, Purdom E, et al.; Cancer Genome Atlas Research Network. Integrated genomic analysis identifies clinically relevant subtypes of glioblastoma characterized by abnormalities in PDGFRA, IDH1, EGFR, and NF1. *Cancer Cell.* 2010;17(1):98–110.

14 Brennan CW, Verhaak RG, McKenna A, et al.; TCGA Research Network. The somatic genomic landscape of glioblastoma. *Cell.* 2013;155(2):462–477.

15 The Cancer Genome Atlas Research Network. Comprehensive genomic characterization defines human glioblastoma genes and core pathways. *Nature.* 2008;455(7216):1061–1068.

16 Noushmehr H, Weisenberger DJ, Diefes K, et al.; Cancer Genome Atlas Research Network. Identification of a CpG island methylator phenotype that defines a distinct subgroup of glioma. *Cancer Cell.* 2010;17(5):510–522.

17 Kleihues P, W.K. Cavenee, and International Agency for Research on Cancer. *Pathology and Genetics of Tumours of the Nervous System.* World Health Organization Classification of Tumours. Lyon: IARC Press; 2000:314 p.

18 Thaker NG, Pollack IF, Molecularly targeted therapies for malignant glioma: rationale for combinatorial strategies. *Expert Rev Neurother.* 2009;9(12):1815–1836.

19 Hegi ME, Rajakannu P, Weller M. Epidermal growth factor receptor: a re-emerging target in glioblastoma. *Curr Opin Neurol*. 2012;25(6):774–779.

20 Wong AJ, Bigner SH, Bigner DD, Kinzler KW, Hamilton SR, Vogelstein B. Increased expression of the epidermal growth-factor receptor gene in malignant gliomas is invariably associated with gene amplification. *Proc Natl Acad Sci U S A*. 1987;84(19):6899–6903.

21 Libermann TA, Nusbaum HR, Razon N, et al. Amplification, enhanced expression and possible rearrangement of Egf receptor gene in primary human-brain tumors of glial origin. *Nature*. 1985;313(5998):144–147.

22 Sugawa N. Ekstrand AJ, James CD, Collins VP. Identical Splicing of Aberrant Epidermal Growth-Factor Receptor Transcripts from Amplified Rearranged Genes in Human Glioblastomas. *Proc Natl Acad Sci U S A*. 1990;87(21):8602–8606.

23 Vivanco I, Robins HI, Rohle D, et al. Differential sensitivity of glioma-versus lung cancer-specific EGFR mutations to EGFR kinase inhibitors. *Cancer Discov*. 2012;2(5):458–471.

24 Raizer JJ, Abrey LE, Lassman AB, et al. A phase II trial of erlotinib in patients with recurrent malignant gliomas and nonprogressive glioblastoma multiforme postradiation therapy. *Neuro Oncol*. 2010;12(1):95–103.

25 Yung WK Vredenburgh JJ, Cloughesy TF, et al. Safety and efficacy of erlotinib in first-relapse glioblastoma: a phase II open-label study. *Neuro Oncol*. 2010;12(10):1061–1070.

26 Kesavabhotla K, Schlaff CD, Shin B, et al. Phase I/II study of oral erlotinib for treatment of relapsed/refractory glioblastoma multiforme and anaplastic astrocytoma. *J Exp Ther Oncol*. 2012;10(1):71–81.

27 Franceschi E, Cavallo G, Lonardi S, et al., Gefitinib in patients with progressive high-grade gliomas: a multicentre phase II study by Gruppo Italiano Cooperativo di Neuro-Oncologia (GICNO). *Br J Cancer*. 2007;96(7):1047–1051.

28 Mellinghoff IK, Wang MY, Vivanco I, et al. Molecular determinants of the response of glioblastomas to EGFR kinase inhibitors. *N Engl J Med*. 2005;353(19):2012–2024.

29 Furnari FB. Fenton T, Bachoo RM, et al. Malignant astrocytic glioma: genetics, biology, and paths to treatment. *Genes Dev*. 2007;21(21):2683–2710.

30 Tanaka S, Louis DN, Curry WT, Batchelor TT, Dietrich J. Diagnostic and therapeutic avenues for glioblastoma: no longer a dead end? *Nat Rev Clin Oncol*. 2013;10(1):14–26.

31 Reardon DA, Groves MD, Wen PY, et al. A Phase I/II trial of pazopanib in combination with lapatinib in adult patients with relapsed malignant glioma. *Clin Cancer Res*. 2013;19(4):900–908.

32 Pollack IF, Randall MS, Kristofik MP, Kelly RH, Selker RG, Vertosick FT Jr. Response of low-passage human-malignant gliomas in vitro to stimulation and selective-inhibition of growth factor-mediated pathways. *J Neurosurg*. 1991;75(2):284–293.

33 Hermanson M, Funa K, Hartman M, et al. Platelet-derived growth-factor and its receptors in human glioma tissue: expression of messenger-RNA and protein suggests the presence of autocrine and paracrine loops. *Cancer Res*. 1992;52(11):3213–3219.

34 Druker BJ, Talpaz M, Resta DJ, et al. Efficacy and safety of a specific inhibitor of the BCR-ABL tyrosine kinase in chronic myeloid leukemia. *N Engl J Med*. 2001;344(14):1031–1037.

35 Brooks AN, Kilgour E, Smith PD. Molecular pathways: fibroblast growth factor signaling: a new therapeutic opportunity in cancer. *Clin Cancer Res*. 2012;18(7):1855–1862.

36 Singh D, Chan JM, Zoppoli P, et al. Transforming fusions of FGFR and TACC genes in human glioblastoma. *Science*. 2012;337(6099):1231–1235.

37 Burgart LJ, Robinson RA, Haddad SF, Moore SA. Oncogene abnormalities in astrocytomas: Egf-R gene alone appears to be more frequently amplified and rearranged compared with other protooncogenes. *Modern Pathol*. 1991;4(2):183–186.

38 Guha A, Feldkamp MM, Lau N, Boss G, Pawson A. Proliferation of human malignant astrocytomas is dependent on Ras activation. *Oncogene*. 1997;15(23):2755–2765.

39 Sharma S, Kemeny N, Kelsen DP, et al., A phase II trial of farnesyl protein transferase inhibitor SCH 66336, given by twice-daily oral administration, in patients with metastatic colorectal cancer refractory to 5-fluorouracil and irinotecan. *Ann Oncol*. 2002;13(7):1067–1071.

40 Kim ES, Kies MS, Fossella FV, et al. Phase II study of the farnesyltransferase inhibitor lonafarnib with paclitaxel in patients with taxane-refractory/resistant nonsmall cell lung carcinoma. *Cancer*. 2005;104(3):561–569.

41 Freed E, Symons M, Macdonald SG, McCormick F, Ruggieri R. Binding of 14–3–3-proteins to the protein-kinase Raf and effects on its activation. *Science*. 1994;265(5179):1713–1716.

42 Jane EP, Premkumar DR, Pollack IF, Coadministration of sorafenib with rottlerin potently inhibits cell proliferation and migration in human malignant glioma cells. *J Pharmacol Exp Ther*. 2006;319(3):1070–1080.

43 Wilhelm SM, Carter C, Tang L, et al. BAY 43–9006 exhibits broad spectrum oral antitumor activity and targets the RAF/MEK/ERK pathway and receptor tyrosine kinases involved in tumor progression and angiogenesis. *Cancer Res*. 2004;64(19):7099–7109.

44 Chakravarti A, Zhai G, Suzuki Y, et al. The prognostic significance of phosphatidylinositol 3-kinase pathway activation in human gliomas. *J Clin Oncol*. 2004;22(10):1926–1933.

45 Newton HB. Molecular neuro-oncology and the development of targeted therapeutic strategies for brain tumors. Part 3: brain tumor invasiveness. *Expert Rev Anticancer Ther*. 2004;4(5):803–821.

46 Riemenschneider MJ, Betensky RA, Pasedag SM, Louis DN. AKT activation in human glioblastomas enhances proliferation via TSC2 and S6 kinase signaling. *Cancer Res*. 2006;66(11):5618–5623.

47 Cloughesy TF, Yoshimoto K, Nghiemphu P, et al. Antitumor activity of rapamycin in a Phase I trial for patients with recurrent PTEN-deficient glioblastoma. *PLoS Med*. 2008;5(1):e8.

48 Galanis E, Buckner JC, Maurer MJ, et al.; North Central Cancer Treatment Group. Phase II trial of temsirolimus (CCI-779) in recurrent glioblastoma multiforme: a North Central Cancer Treatment Group Study. *J Clin Oncol*. 2005;23(23):5294–5304.

49 Kreisl TN, Lassman AB, Mischel PS, et al., A pilot study of everolimus and gefitinib in the treatment of recurrent glioblastoma (GBM). *J Neurooncol*. 2009;92(1):99–105.

50 Couldwell WT, Uhm JH, Antel JP, Yong VW, et al. Enhanced protein kinase C activity correlates with the growth rate of malignant gliomas in vitro. *Neurosurgery*. 1991;29(6):880–886; discussion 886–887.

51 Yoshiji H, Kuriyama S, Ways DK, et al. Protein kinase C lies on the signaling pathway for vascular endothelial growth factor-mediated tumor development and angiogenesis. *Cancer Res*. 1999;59(17):4413–4418.

52 da Rocha AB, Mans DR, Regner A, Schwartsmann G. Targeting protein kinase C: new therapeutic opportunities against high-grade malignant gliomas? *Oncologist*. 2002;7(1):17–33.

53 Marais R, Light Y, Mason C, Paterson H, Olson MF, Marshall CJ. Requirement of Ras-GTP-Raf complexes for activation of Raf-1 by protein kinase C. *Science*. 1998;280(5360):109–112.

54 Brandes AA, Ermani M, Turazzi S, et al. Procarbazine and high-dose tamoxifen as a second-line regimen in recurrent high-grade gliomas: a phase II study. *J Clin Oncol*. 1999;17(2):645–650.

55 Spence AM, Peterson RA, Scharnhorst JD, Silbergeld DL, Rostomily RC. Phase II study of concurrent continuous Temozolomide (TMZ) and

Tamoxifen (TMX) for recurrent malignant astrocytic gliomas. *J Neurooncol.* 2004;70(1):91–95.

56 Graff JR, McNulty AM, Hanna KR, et al. The protein kinase Cbeta-selective inhibitor, Enzastaurin (LY317615.HCl), suppresses signaling through the AKT pathway, induces apoptosis, and suppresses growth of human colon cancer and glioblastoma xenografts. *Cancer Res.* 2005;65(16):7462–7469.

57 Sidransky D, Mikkelsen T, Schwechheimer K, Rosenblum ML, Cavanee W, Vogelstein B. Clonal expansion of p53 mutant cells is associated with brain tumour progression. *Nature.* 1992;355(6363):846–847.

58 Vousden KH, Lane DP. p53 in health and disease. *Nat Rev Mol Cell Biol.* 2007;8(4):275–283.

59 Carmeliet P. VEGF as a key mediator of angiogenesis in cancer. *Oncology.* 2005;69(Suppl 3):4–10.

60 Kieran MW, Anti-angiogenic chemotherapy in central nervous system tumors. *Cancer Treat Res.* 2004;117:337–349.

61 Purow B, Fine HA. Antiangiogenic therapy for primary and metastatic brain tumors. *Hematol Oncol Clin North Am.* 2004;18(5):1161–1181, x.

62 Gomez-Manzano C,Fueyo J, Jiang H, et al. Mechanisms underlying PTEN regulation of vascular endothelial growth factor and angiogenesis. *Ann Neurol.* 2003;53(1):109–117.

63 Ebos JM, Kerbel RS. Antiangiogenic therapy: impact on invasion, disease progression, and metastasis. *Nat Rev Clin Oncol.* 2011;8(4):210–221.

64 Grunwald V, Hidalgo M. Development of the epidermal growth factor receptor inhibitor Tarceva (OSI-774). *Adv Exp Med Biol.* 2003;532:235–246.

65 Prewett M, Huber J, Li Y, et al. Antivascular endothelial growth factor receptor (fetal liver kinase 1) monoclonal antibody inhibits tumor angiogenesis and growth of several mouse and human tumors. *Cancer Res.* 1999;59(20):5209–5218.

66 Viloria-Petit A, Crombet T, Jothy S, et al. Acquired resistance to the antitumor effect of epidermal growth factor receptor-blocking antibodies in vivo: a role for altered tumor angiogenesis. *Cancer Res.* 2001;61(13):5090–5101.

67 Norden AD, Drappatz J, Wen PY. Antiangiogenic therapies for high-grade glioma. *Nat Rev Neurol.* 2009;5(11):610–620.

68 Kerbel RS, Tumor angiogenesis. *N Engl J Med.* 2008;358(19):2039–2049.

69 Gilbert MR, Dignam JJ, Armstrong TS, et al. A randomized trial of bevacizumab for newly diagnosed glioblastoma. *N Engl J Med.* 2014;370(8):699–708.

70 Chinot OL, Wick W, Mason W, et al. Bevacizumab plus radiotherapy-temozolomide for newly diagnosed glioblastoma. *N Engl J Med.* 2014;370(8):709–22.

71 Bergers G, Hanahan D. Modes of resistance to anti-angiogenic therapy. *Nat Rev Cancer.* 2008;8(8):592–603.

72 Batchelor TT, Sorensen AG, di Tomaso E, et al. AZD2171, a pan-VEGF receptor tyrosine kinase inhibitor, normalizes tumor vasculature and alleviates edema in glioblastoma patients. *Cancer Cell.* 2007;11(1):83–95.

73 Gray SG, Ekstrom TJ. The human histone deacetylase family. *Exp Cell Res.* 2001;262(2):75–83.

74 Johnson BE, Mazor T, Hong C, et al. Mutational analysis reveals the origin and therapy-driven evolution of recurrent glioma. *Science.* 2014;343(6167):189–193.

# CHAPTER 19

# Targeted Therapy for Breast Cancer

*Harold J. Burstein[1,2]*
[1]Dana-Farber Cancer Institute, Harvard Medical School Boston, MA, USA
[2]Brigham and Women's Hospital, Harvard Medical School, Boston, MA, USA

Breast cancer remains the "original" solid tumor for which targeted therapy proved clinically useful. Characterization of biomarker targets, estrogen receptor (ER), progesterone receptor (PR) and HER2 is essential for appropriate management of breast cancer. In many models of solid tumor therapy, molecular targets are identified as having acquired point mutations or chromosomal rearrangements. In breast cancer, the key known targets are functional growth factors. Expression of the receptors is the *sine qua non* for clinical activity of targeted treatments. For this reason, high-quality pathology for ER and HER2 testing is also essential to patient management.

## Targeting ER in Breast Cancer

Hormonal therapy for ER positive breast cancer constitutes both the original use of targeted therapy in oncology, and the paradigm for the subsequent development of targeted therapies in cancer care. The utilization of ovarian resection as treatment for advanced breast cancer dates to the late 19th century, and through the 1960s, hormonal ablation of ovarian, pituitary and adrenal reserve constituted the only known medical therapies for breast cancer. These interventions were deployed without consideration of tumor biomarker status, and were known to be effective—that is, causing a remission—in about one-third to one-half of women with advanced breast cancer.[1]

Treatment toward "targeted" therapy evolved rapidly in the 1970s with the characterization of ER and PR expression in breast cancers, and the recognition that hormone receptor expression was the sine qua non for effective treatment with hormonal therapy.[2] In advanced breast cancer, response rates and time to tumor progression were entirely dependent on quantitative levels of ER and/or PR expression; the higher the expression of ER, the higher were tumor response rates and time to tumor progression. Response rates among tumors that were hormone-receptor-negative were so rare as to suggest testing artifact. Based on these data, it became increasingly routine to test breast cancers for hormone-receptor expression. This kind of "hand-and-glove" approach to cancer therapeutics—relying on individual tumor testing of a specific biomarker for determining whether to offer a specific therapy—has become the hallmark for all successful targeted therapies in oncology, and was first demonstrated of value in breast cancer.

A second paradigmatic lesson from advanced breast cancer was that, having established a targeted pathway as important, multiple lines of therapy against that pathway could be proven of value. The mechanisms of resistance to endocrine therapy remain poorly understood despite decades of research. While many tumors lose PR expression during exposure to anti-estrogen treatments, most still retain expression of ER, suggesting that signaling pathway modulation is a key component of treatment resistance. Recently, specific acquired mutations in ER have been identified that emerge during anti-estrogen treatment.[3] These mutations may be clinically relevant as they affect the hormone binding site on the receptor. However, they have only been found to date in a small percentage of tumors; for most ER positive breast cancers, ER signaling remains operational despite overt clinical progression, and subsequent lines of endocrine treatment can still be clinically effective. While the yield for each subsequent line of treatment declines, on average, there nonetheless remains clinically valuable benefit with second, third, and in some cases, additional lines of endocrine treatment. Based on these clinical observations, a number of novel hormonal therapies for breast cancer including tamoxifen, aromatase inhibitors, progestational agents, and fulvestrant have become common for use in advanced disease.[1]

The success of endocrine therapy for advanced breast cancer enabled clinical trials of adjuvant therapy for early stage disease, another example of how targeted therapy in breast cancer has served as the model for the development of targeted agents in oncology. While the earliest studies of adjuvant tamoxifen therapy did not specifically select for tumors that were ER positive, subsequent retrospective analyses showed that, as with treatment in the advanced setting, ER expression was essential for realizing benefits of adjuvant treatment with tamoxifen.[4] Also in parallel with the experience in metastatic disease, quantitative levels of ER are potent predictors of benefit from adjuvant endocrine treatment.

Current guidelines for adjuvant endocrine therapy recommend a minimum of 5 years of adjuvant treatment with either tamoxifen, an aromatase inhibitor (if postmenopausal) or a sequence of tamoxifen followed by an aromatase inhibitor. The demonstration that durations of treatment beyond 5 years of tamoxifen with either continued tamoxifen therapy for a total of 10 years, or extended therapy with 5 years of an aromatase inhibitor after 5 years of tamoxifen, is shifting practice toward longer treatment patterns for many patients.[5]

*Targeted Therapy in Translational Cancer Research*, First Edition. Edited by Apostolia-Maria Tsimberidou, Razelle Kurzrock and Kenneth C. Anderson.

## Targeting HER2 in Breast Cancer

ER-targeted therapy for breast cancer emerged from decades worth of clinical observations among women offered endocrine treatment, and retrospective analyses that deciphered the relationship between ER and endocrine treatment outcomes. By contrast, the development of anti-HER2 therapies was prompted by the recognition of gene amplification and overexpression of the HER2 oncogene as a poor prognostic factor in breast cancer.[6] HER2 overexpression arises in approximately 15–20% of early stage breast cancer, and historically carried higher risk of recurrence, with relative resistance to standard endocrine therapy and chemotherapy. The development of targeted treatments for HER2 was by rational design, with the creation of humanized anti-HER2 antibodies. Preclinical studies provided evidence that anti-HER2 antibodies would only have potency in tumors that overexpressed HER2. This finding prompted the development of a robust clinical assay for HER2 expression to enable tumor and patient selection for clinical trials of anti-HER2 therapy. Subsequently, the trastuzumab antibody was shown to have substantial clinical activity in advanced breast cancer when combined with standard chemotherapy.[7] Five years later, trastuzumab became a standard adjuvant option for early stage, HER2 overexpressing breast cancer.[8]

There remains minor controversy as to whether anti-HER2 therapy may have clinical effects in HER2 "normal" or non-overexpressing breast cancers. Studies in the metastatic setting have not demonstrated compelling clinical benefit. Retrospective analyses of the pivotal adjuvant trials have suggested that even tumors that, upon central review, lack HER2 overexpression, may benefit from adjuvant trastuzumab.[9] Ongoing prospective studies are assessing the value of trastuzumab in HER2 "normal" breast cancers.

HER2 overexpression is frequently characterized as a "driver" mutation in breast cancer. Ongoing trastuzumab therapy beyond progression has been shown to be clinically beneficial, suggesting that clinical resistance to anti-HER2 therapies is a relative term. At present, there are no established markers of specific tumor changes that are linked to resistance to anti-HER2 therapy. Indeed, in current practice, most women with advanced HER2 positive breast cancer will receive multiple lines of anti-HER2 treatment.[10]

As with the experience in ER targeted therapy for breast cancer, the success of the initial anti-HER2 treatment, trastuzumab, engendered development of multiple anti-HER2 therapies.[11] Lapatinib, a dual kinase inhibitor of the EGFR and HER2 tyrosine kinases, has activity in trastuzumab-refractory breast cancer. The antibody–drug conjugate, ado-trastuzumab emtansine (TDM-1), is a unique therapy in which the original trastuzumab antibody has been modified by covalent linkage to a potent maytansanoid chemotherapy.[12] TDM1 has major clinical activity in trastuzumab-resistant breast cancer, and in first-line treatment, has clinical efficacy comparable to the combination of taxane chemotherapy and trastuzumab. A different anti-HER2 antibody, pertuzumab, also binds HER2 but unlike trastuzumab, blocks the heterodimer interactions between HER2 and HER2. Pertuzumab has little single-agent activity but when added to trastuzumab, can overcome clinical resistance to trastuzumab.[13] Based on improvement in response rate, time to progression, and overall survival, pertuzumab in combination with chemotherapy and trastuzumab is a standard first-line treatment for HER2 positive advanced breast cancer.[14] Adjuvant trials are evaluating the addition of pertuzumab, and separately, TDM1, to standard chemotherapy-trastuzumab-based treatment for early stage breast cancer.

The US Food and Drug administration has recently outlined a pathway by which breast cancer treatments could receive accelerated approval based on improvements in the rate of complete pathological response when given as neoadjuvant therapy.[15] This pathway is designed to streamline truly innovative products into the management of early stage breast cancer at a faster pace. Traditionally, drugs approved based on activity in advanced breast cancer have then been advanced into trials of adjuvant therapy, a process that can demand thousands of patients and multiple years of study development and analysis. Neoadjuvant therapy offers the potential to evaluate and approve drugs based on the short-term endpoint of pathological response in the breast, requiring, in theory, trials of fewer patients and less time to accrue and analyze. As part of the approval process, the FDA requires a confirmatory experience—either adjuvant or based on neoadjuvant treatment—that demonstrates improvement in disease-free and overall survival in order to achieve full approval.

Based on the improved rate of complete pathological response when pertuzumab was added to chemotherapy and trastuzumab,[16] the FDA granted accelerated approval for use of pertuzumab as part of neoadjuvant treatment for HER2 positive breast cancer. It remains to be determined whether pertuzumab will otherwise impact the natural history of early stage, HER2 positive disease.

## Novel Targeted Treatments in ER Positive Breast Cancer

Cell regulatory pathways including the PI3K / mTOR / AKT have been implicated in the regulation of growth of ER positive breast cancers.[17] Genomic sequencing has identified mutations in this pathway in a large percentage of luminal (ER-positive) breast cancers. For these reasons, a variety of clinical trials have analyzed the addition of mTOR inhibitors and PI3-kinase inhibitors for treatment of advanced breast cancer. The mTOR inhibitor, everolimus, has been shown to have mild effects at overcoming resistance to endocrine therapy in aromatase inhibitor-refractory tumors.[18] However, mutations in the PI3K / mTOR paths were not predictive of clinical benefit for everolimus-based therapy.

Current drug discovery is focusing on the cyclin-dependent kinases 4 and 6, critical mediators of cell cycle control in many cancer cells.[19] Recent randomized phase II trials have suggested that CDK4/6 inhibition when added to first-line endocrine treatment of ER positive metastatic breast cancer can improve progression-free survival. These findings await confirmation in larger trials but may open a new class of pathway-targeted treatment in advanced breast cancer.

The androgen receptor (AR) is expressed in the vast majority of ER-positive breast cancers. Interestingly, a subset of ER negative tumors also expresses AR.[20] The clinical significance of AR as a target in breast cancer is unknown but ongoing clinical trials are examining androgen deprivation and androgen receptor blockade as targeted treatments in ER-positive and ER-negative tumors.

## BRCA-Associated Tumors and PARP Inhibitors

Hereditary BRCA1 and BRCA2 mutations give rise to high risks of developing breast and ovarian cancer.[21] These two genes are the most common and highly penetrant of genes known to give rise to hereditary breast cancer. The underlying mechanism of tumorigenesis caused by BRCA1/2 mutations is thought to be due to the role these proteins play in normal DNA repair. In cells with BRCA1/2 deficiency, the PARP enzyme complex takes on additional roles in DNA repair.[22] This invites the possibility of achieving "synthetic lethality" by PARP inhibitors in BRCA-associated breast cancers, rendering the cells unable to fundamentally repair DNA and vulnerable to apoptosis.

Phase II studies have shown that PARP inhibitors can yield clinical responses in BRCA-associated breast cancer, but not in non-BRCA-associated breast cancers.[23] Studies designed for drug approval are now comparing PARP inhibitors against standard chemotherapy as treatment for advanced breast cancer in women with hereditary BCA1/2 tumors. Should PARP inhibitors prove clinically valuable in breast cancer, there would be a rationale for widespread testing of breast cancers or patients for hereditary mutations.

## Genomic Profiling

Multiple academic centers have conducted large-scale sequencing studies of breast cancers.[24] These studies have suggested certain prevalent mutations in breast cancers, including mutations in PIK3CA, TP53, MAP kinase, FGFR, and multiple other pathways, with sufficient frequency so as to enable clinical trials of targeted therapies. Many of these markers have existing targeted agents, or possible targeted agents. The availability of sequence profiling and targeted therapies lend themselves to straightforward clinical studies to evaluate targeted agents in well-defined and selected tumors. Large-scale clinical trial platforms are now integrating genomic sequencing of human breast tumors for targeted mutations, in coordination with clinical trials looking at pools of targeted therapies aligned for many mutations. It is hoped that this advancement of linking carefully the mutated tumor pathway with the targeted agent will enable rapid assessment of clinical activity and molecular predictors of outcome.

## References

1 Schiavon G, Smith IE. Endocrine therapy for advanced/metastatic breast cancer. *Hematol Oncol Clin North Am*. 2013;27(4):715–736.

2 McGuire WL. Hormone receptors: their role in predicting prognosis and response to endocrine therapy. *Semin Oncol*. 1978;5(4):428–433.

3 Jeselsohn R, Yelensky R, Buchwalter G, et al. Emergence of constitutively active estrogen receptor-α mutations in pretreated advanced estrogen receptor-positive breast cancer. *Clin Cancer Res*. 2014;20(7):1757–1767.

4 Early Breast Cancer Trialists' Collaborative Group, Davies C, Godwin J. Relevance of breast cancer hormone receptors and other factors to the efficacy of adjuvant tamoxifen: patient-level meta-analysis of randomised trial. *Lancet*. 2011;378:771–784.

5 Burstein HJ, Temin S, Anderson H, et al. Adjuvant endocrine therapy for women with hormone receptor-positive breast cancer: American Society of Clinical Oncology Clinical Practice Guideline Focused Update. *J Clin Oncol*. 2014;32(21):2255–2269. doi:10.1200/JCO.2013.54.2258.

6 Slamon DJ, Clark GM, Wong SG, Levin WJ, Ullrich A, McGuire WL. Human breast cancer: correlation of relapse and survival with amplification of the HER-2/neu oncogene. *Science*. 1987;235(4785):177–182.

7 Slamon DJ, Leyland-Jones B, Shak S, et al. Use of chemotherapy plus a monoclonal antibody against HER2 for metastatic breast cancer that overexpresses HER2. *N Engl J Med*. 2001;344(11):783–792.

8 Romond EH, Perez EA, Bryant J, et al. Trastuzumab plus adjuvant chemotherapy for operable HER2-positive breast cancer. *N Engl J Med*. 2005;353(16):1673–1684.

9 Paik S, Kim C, Wolmark N. HER2 status and benefit from adjuvant trastuzumab in breast cancer. *N Engl J Med*. 2008;358(13):1409–1411. doi:10.1056/NEJMc0801440.

10 Deah SH, Luis IV, Macrae E, et al. Use and duration of chemotherapy in patients with metastatic breast cancer according to tumor subtype and line of therapy. *J Natl Compr Canc Netw*. 2014;12(1):71–80.

11 Pegram MD. Treating the HER2 pathway in early and advanced breast cancer. *Hematol Oncol Clin North Am*. 2013;27:751–766.

12 Verma S, Miles D, Gianni L, et al.; EMILIA Study Group. Trastuzumab emtansine for HER2-positive advanced breast cancer. *N Engl J Med*. 2012 ;367(19):1783–1791.

13 Baselga J, Gelmon KA, Verma S, et al. Phase II trial of pertuzumab and trastuzumab in patients with human epidermal growth factor receptor 2-positive metastatic breast cancer that progressed during prior trastuzumab therapy. *J Clin Oncol*. 2010;28(7):1138–1144.

14 Baselga J, Cortés J, Kim SB, et al.; CLEOPATRA Study Group. Pertuzumab plus trastuzumab plus docetaxel for metastatic breast cancer. *N Engl J Med*. 2012;366(2):109–119.

15 Prowell TM, Pazdur R. Pathological complete response and accelerated drug approval in early breast cancer. *N Engl J Med*. 2012;366(26):2438–2441.

16 Gianni L, Pienkowski T, Im YH, et al. Efficacy and safety of neoadjuvant pertuzumab and trastuzumab in women with locally advanced, inflammatory, or early HER2-positive breast cancer (NeoSphere): a randomised multicentre, open-label, phase 2 trial. *Lancet Oncol*. 2012;13(1):25–32.

17 Rugo HS, Keck S. Reversing hormone resistance: have we found the golden key? *J Clin Oncol*. 2012;30(22):2707–2709.

18 Baselga J, Campone M, Piccart M, et al. Everolimus in postmenopausal hormone-receptor positive advanced breast cancer. *N Engl J Med*. 2012;366(6):520–529.

19 Dickson MA. Molecular Pathways: CDK4 Inhibitors for Cancer Therapy. *Clin Cancer Res*. 2014;20(13):3379–3383. doi:10.1158/1078-0432.CCR-13—1551.

20 Lehmann BD, Bauer JA, Chen X, et al. Identification of human triple-negative breast cancer subtypes and preclinical models for selection of targeted therapies. *J Clin Invest*. 2011;121(7):2750–2767.

21 Robson M, Offit K. Clinical practice. Management of an inherited predisposition to breast cancer. *N Engl J Med*. 2007;357(2):154–162.

22 Do K, Chen AP. Molecular pathways: targeting PARP in cancer treatment. *Clin Cancer Res*. 2013;19(5):977–984.

23 Tutt A, Robson M, Garber JE, et al. Oral poly(ADP-ribose) polymerase inhibitor olaparib in patients with BRCA1 or BRCA2 mutations and advanced breast cancer: a proof-of-concept trial. *Lancet*. 2010;376(9737):235–244.

24 Cancer Genome Atlas Network. Comprehensive molecular portraits of human breast tumours. *Nature*. 2012;490(7418):61–70.

# CHAPTER 20

# Targeted Therapy in Solid Tumors: Colorectal Cancer

*Maen Abdelrahim[1], Scott Kopetz[2], and David Menter[2]*

[1]Department of Internal Medicine, Baylor College of Medicine, Houston, TX, USA
[2]Department of Gastrointestinal Medical Oncology, The University of Texas MD Anderson Cancer Center, Houston, TX, USA

## Overview

### Epidemiology, Encouraging Trends, and Young-Onset Cohorts

The incidence and mortality rates of colorectal cancer (CRC) vary significantly by geographic area. The highest incidence rates are in Australia, New Zealand, Europe, and North America, and the lowest rates are in Africa and South-Central Asia.[1] Globally, CRC is the third most commonly diagnosed cancer in men and the second most commonly diagnosed cancer in women. Encouragingly, both the incidence and mortality rates of CRC in the United States have slowly decreased.[2] CRC incidence rates have decreased by 2–3% per year over the past 15 years. Approximately 142,820 new cases of CRC are diagnosed annually; of these, 102,480 are colon cancers, and the remaining are rectal cancers.[3] Approximately 50,830 Americans die of CRC annually. This accounts for nearly 9% of all cancer deaths. Although the incidence of CRC is decreasing among all age groups older than 50 years, the incidence is increasing in younger individuals who are not routinely screened.[4]

### Mutations, Next Generation Sequencing, Key Genes, and Tumorigenesis

Most CRCs grow from pre-existing adenomas that harbor certain genetic malignant fingerprints.[5] Different gene mutations are linked to colorectal carcinogenesis.[6] Only a limited number of these genes, mainly adenomatous polyposis coli (*APC*), *K-ras*, and *p53*, are commonly altered in a major proportion of CRCs.[7] One report noted that the combination of these mutations in the same cancer, however, is uncommon.[8] More recently, The Cancer Genome Atlas consortium also found this panel of frequently mutated genes.[9] This study involved next-generation sequencing (NGS) of 97 samples and the authors categorized the observed mutation frequencies into either non-hypermethylated or hypermethylated subtypes. Significant mutation frequencies occurred in the commonly reported *APC*, *TP53*, *SMAD4*, *PIK3CA*, and *KRAS* along with 24 other genes that often segregated according to methylation status. Frequent mutations were also found in *ARID1A*, *SOX9*, and *FAM123B*. A high frequency of mutations in these commonly found pathways is likely to drive CRC, depending on the accompanying epigenetic background.

The most commonly mutated gene in CRC is *APC*.[9] It is mutated in 81% of non-hypermethylated CRCs and 53% of hypermethylated CRCs. APC is a scaffold protein that brings multiple transducing proteins together and functions as a tumor suppressor gene.[10, 11] The majority of the mutations in the *APC* gene are frameshift or nonsense mutations that lead to premature truncation of protein synthesis.[12] The APC protein is an important regulator of epithelial homeostasis, predominantly through the mediation of ubiquitination and subsequent degradation of cytoplasmic β-catenin.[13] APC and β-catenin are components of the Wnt signaling pathway. When *APC* is mutated, cytoplasmic β-catenin fails to ubiquitinate or degrade and accumulates in the nucleus. Once in the nucleus, β-catenin binds to T-cell transcription factors, altering the expression of various genes affecting proliferation, differentiation, migration, apoptosis, cell cycle progression, and microtubule and chromosome stability.[14] Truncations in APC interfere with microtubule-associated protein RP/EB family member 1 (MAPRE1/EB-1) along with plus-end microtubule attachments during polymerization that leads to mitotic abnormalities.[15, 16] Truncated APC scaffolds with an inability to effectively mediate attachments between microtubules and kinetochores during cell division are likely to influence genetic instability.[17]

The early association of MAPRE1/EB-1 as a circulating biomarker with CRC was observed in the plasma of women preceding a diagnosis of CRC.[18] Early changes in APC, in concert with early elevation of MAPRE1/EB-1 levels in plasma prior to the onset of CRC, supports the notion of a potential link.

Proto-oncogene activation is an important driver of CRC. K-ras is a key proto-oncogene that is frequently mutated in 30–60% of CRCs and large adenomas.[19] Activated K-ras often plays an important role in the transition from adenoma to carcinoma through the activation of downstream targets including *BCL-2*, *H2AFZ*, *RAP1B*, *TBX19*, *E2F4*, and *MMP1*.[20] Ras activation affects multiple cellular pathways that control cellular growth, differentiation, survival, apoptosis, cytoskeleton organization, motility, proliferation, and inflammation.[21] The *K-ras* gene product is a GTPase that is involved in signal transduction and is activated in response to extracellular signals. Once Kras binds to guanosine triphosphate (GTP), Kras becomes activated and recruits and stimulates other signaling factors. In concert with the activation of Kras, GTPase

*Targeted Therapy in Translational Cancer Research*, First Edition. Edited by Apostolia-Maria Tsimberidou, Razelle Kurzrock and Kenneth C. Anderson.
© 2016 John Wiley & Sons, Inc. Published 2016 by John Wiley & Sons, Inc.

activity very slowly cleaves GTP to guanosine diphosphate to gradually inactivate itself. The rate of GTP conversion is increased by GTPase-activating protein cofactors. Kras is reactivated through guanine nucleotide exchange factors that enhance guanosine diphosphate release in exchange for GTP binding. The mutated protein is locked in the active form, and most activating mutations are found not only in codons 12 and 13 of exon 1 but also 61 and 146.[22] These mutation clusters have been graphically modeled around common structural regions of the Kras protein.[23] Structurally, single point mutations affecting residue G12 or Q61 of H-Ras abolish p120 GTPase-activating protein-induced GTP hydrolysis through steric or van der Waals alterations.[24] Some ongoing efforts to identify Kras inhibitors are focused on RAS-guanine nucleotide exchange factor interactions with activated KRAS$^{G12D}$ mutant structures, among other structural sites.[25] Despite these intensive efforts, no small-molecule therapy capable of specifically and effectively targeting mutant KRAS is currently available.

The loss of tumor suppressor function is another key driver of CRC tumorigenesis. The p53 protein was the first factor identified to validate the tumor suppressor hypothesis.[26] It maintains genomic stability and guards against the accumulation of mutations. It senses DNA damage and initiates G1/S cell cycle arrest by stimulating p21 synthesis and activating DNA repair.[27] The stability of p53 and transport from the nucleus to the cytoplasm involves the E3 ubiquitin ligase mouse double minute 2 homolog.[28] Once DNA repair is complete, p53 reactivates the cell cycle; however, if repair is unsuccessful, apoptosis is triggered to eliminate damaged cells. With numerous complex biological roles, p53 protein can interact with as many as 106 other proteins within the cell. It is among the most frequently mutated genes in cancer as a target for both inactivating point mutations and chromosomal loss of heterozygosity.[29] It can also incur gain-of-function mutations that promote cancer.[30] Mutations in TP53 result in compensatory overexpression of the gene product, which is readily detectable via immunohistochemical analysis.[31]

In addition to the aforementioned activities, p53 dysfunction can influence genetic instability.[32] This occurs through abnormal centrosome hyperamplification,[33] deregulation of the centrosome duplication cycle, and cytokinesis failure, leading to aneuploidy.[34,35] p53 also influences centrosome clustering, thereby preventing multipolar mitosis in tetraploid cells.[36] Thus, loss or mutation of p53 increases the risk of genomic instability owing to breakdown in centrosomal function during mitosis. In effect, p53 loss or dysfunction contributes to higher mutation rates that manifest in distal colon and rectal tumors and is also associated with a poorer prognosis after adjuvant therapy.[37] However, research findings have been mixed, and the clinical significance of p53 mutation remains unclear.[38]

Using NGS, we continue to make new breakthroughs and confirm the existence of high-frequency mutations in *APC*, *TP53*, *SMAD4*, *PIK3CA*, and *KRAS* genes that influence CRC tumorigenesis. At the same time, NGS is facilitating the discovery of epigenetic processes that influence genomic stability and gene expression in CRC.

## Genomic Instability, Microsatellites, and Epigenetics

Genomic instability and epigenetically regulated gene expression play critical roles in the CRC transformation process.[39] Currently, three distinct and non-mutually exclusive molecular pathways to CRC are recognized: chromosomal instability (CIN), microsatellite instability (MSI), and CpG island methylator phenotype (CIMP) pathways.[40]

CIN is the most common cause of genomic instability in CRC and accounts for 65–70% of sporadic CRCs.[41] CIN results from defective spindle pole geometry, defective chromosome segregation, or telomere dysfunction that is often accompanied by defects in DNA damage response mechanisms.[42,43] The consequences include an imbalance in the chromosome number (aneuploidy), chromosomal genomic amplifications, and a high frequency of loss of heterozygosity.[42,43] Analyses of DNA copy number variation have revealed that deletions often occur in chromosomes 4, 8, 15, 17, and 18.[44] In the same study, chromosomal duplications occurred in more than 50% of cases in chromosomes 7, 8, 13, 20, and X.[44] In addition, focal gains or losses are found in regions containing important cancer genes such as vascular endothelial growth factor (*VEGF*), *MYC*, *MET*, *LYN*, and phosphatase and tensin homolog (*PTEN*).[45] The most common single genetic alterations are mutations in the *APC* and *K-ras* genes. As previously mentioned in the case of APC, truncations interfere with MAPRE1/EB-1 and microtubule attachments during polymerization and contribute to these mitotic abnormalities.[16] As also mentioned, p53 dysfunction increases the risk of genomic instability owing to the breakdown in centrosomal function during mitosis.[32]

*Microsatellites* are short repeat nucleotide sequences throughout the genome that are prone to errors in shortening or lengthening due to DNA mismatch repair (MMR).[46] The DNA MMR system recognizes and repairs base-pair mismatches that occur during DNA replication. Members of the MMR system include MSH2, MLH1, MSH6, PMS2, MLH3, MSH3, PMS1, and Exo1.[47] The instability of microsatellites reflects the inability of the MMR system to correct these errors. The linkage of MSI to hereditary nonpolyposis colorectal cancer (HNPCC) and the subsequent cloning of MMR genes implicate MSI as an alternative pathway in colorectal carcinogenesis.[48] Germline mutations in MMR genes result in HNPCC, whereas somatic mutations or hypermethylation silencing of MMR genes accounts for about 15% of sporadic CRCs.[49] Other genes associated with high MSI include cyclooxygenase-2 as a rate-limiting enzyme that initiates the synthesis of proinflammatory bioactive lipids.[50]

CIMP is the concordant methylation of the CpG dinucleotides in the promoter region of multiple genes. CIMP can be independently associated with significantly poorer prognosis in patients with CRC.[51] CIMP is also frequently associated with the activating BRAF$^{V600E}$ mutation.[52] In studies involving activated KRAS-positive human CRC cell lines and tumors, a zinc-finger DNA-binding protein, ZNF304, was revealed to bind promoters of INK4-ARF and other CIMP genes.[53] Promoter-bound ZNF304 recruits a corepressor complex that includes the DNA methyltransferase DNMT1, resulting in DNA hypermethylation and transcriptional silencing. KRAS can thereby promote CIMP silencing through the upregulation of ZNF304.[53] Proinflammatory prostaglandin E$_2$ can also silence certain tumor suppressor genes and DNA repair genes through DNA methylation by upregulating DNA methyltransferases to promote tumor growth.[54] Patients with CIMP tumors have distinct clinical and pathologic characteristics.[55–57] Classifying CRC based on the presence of CIMP (and MSI) was suggested by Jeremy Jass[58] and is summarized elsewhere in this chapter (Table 20.1).

Genetic instability in concert with commonly identified mutations can heighten the selective Darwinian pressures on tumor evolution.[59] The concept of tumor evolution has been validated through single-cell sequencing efforts.[60,61] The tumor evolution process is

**Table 20.1** Molecular subtypes classification of colorectal cancer. Classifying colorectal cancer based on the presence of MSI, CIMP and BRAF. The classification describes five molecular subtypes, each with a different molecular profile and clinico-pathological features.

| Molecular subtypes | CIMP | MSI | BRAF | Percentage of colorectal cancer | Adenoma type | Characteristics |
|---|---|---|---|---|---|---|
| I | High | Microsatellite instability | Mut | 12% | Serrated | BRAF mutation MLH1 methylation associated with MSI |
| II | High | Microsatellite stable | Mut | 8% | Serrated | BRAF mutation Methylation of multiple genes |
| III | Low | Microsatellite stable | Wt | 20% | Tubular Tubulovillus Serrated | Chromosomal instability Higher rate of Kras mutation |
| IV | Negative | Microsatellite stable | Wt | 57% | Traditional | Chromosomal instability |
| V | Negative | Microsatellite instability | Wt | 2–3% | Low- and high-grade dysplastic | Negative for BRAF mutations High rates of HNPCC |

Mut, Mutant; Wt, Wild type.

thought to proceed through punctuated clonal expansions driven by a few persistent intermediates.[60] The evolution of tumor heterogeneity and clonal selection in response to targeted therapies can influence treatment sensitivity, acquired resistance, and clinical outcomes.[60] The notion that this evolution occurs through the selection of pre-existing clones remains controversial.[61,62] One of the best clinical model systems to demonstrate this type of evolving tumor heterogeneity is found in patients with metastatic colorectal cancer (mCRC) treated with epidermal growth factor receptor (EGFR) inhibitors.[63] The emergence of high-sensitivity sequencing technology coupled with noninvasive blood-based assays can now facilitate the detection of evolving tumor heterogeneity and ultimately improve outcomes through better selection of patients for EGFR inhibitor therapy.[64]

## Familial Predisposition, Autosomal Dominance, and Adenomas

Rapid progress is being made in the characterization of the molecular pathogenesis of CRC. Several specific inherited genetic autosomal dominant disorders occur in humans and are associated with a high risk of developing CRC. Familial adenomatous polyposis (FAP) and HNPCC are the two most common familial CRC syndromes.[65]

Classic FAP and its variants—Gardner syndrome, Turcot syndrome, and attenuated adenomatous polyposis—collectively account for less than 1% of CRCs.[66] In classic FAP, more than 100 colonic adenomas typically appear during childhood. Patients usually develop symptoms at an average age of 16 years, and colonic cancer occurs in 90% of untreated individuals by age 45.[67] Multiple germline mutations in the APC gene that lead to truncations are found in FAP.[68] Experimentally, the use of reporter plasmids in CRC cells demonstrated that several aminoglycosides and tylosin, a member of the macrolide family, induced read-through of nonsense mutations that cause truncation of the APC gene.[69] Gardner syndrome is characterized by extracolonic symptoms that include osteomas and desmoid tumors.[70] Turcot syndrome is generally characterized by the association of FAP with a primary central nervous system tumor involving APC mutations,[71] although some cases have been reported to have mutations in the MMR genes MSH-2 and MSH-6.[72] Finally, attenuated FAP is characterized by

fewer than 100 colorectal polyps and a later age at onset of the cancer that exhibits a variety of APC mutations.[73,74] Most often, prophylactic total colectomy is recommended for these collective cohorts of FAP patients,[75] and nonsteroidal anti-inflammatory drugs are thought to reduce adenoma development.[76]

HNPCC (also known as Lynch syndrome) is more common than FAP and accounts for approximately 3–5% of all colonic adenocarcinomas.[77] High MSI is a genetic hypermutability feature of HNPCC.[78,79] Patients with MSI are frequent carriers of MMR gene mutations with a high lifetime risk for CRCs and endometrial cancers, among other malignancies.[79] MLH1 and MSH2 are the most commonly defective MMR genes, although MSH6, PMS2, and EPCAM can be defective as well.[80,81] In contrast with sporadic CRCs, most HNPCC tumors occur in the transverse or right colon, and yearly colonoscopy is recommended beginning at age 20–25 years.[82] We now know that extracolonic cancers also include cancers of the ovary, small bowel, hepatobiliary system, renal pelvis or ureter, and possibly breast and prostate in addition to gastric and endometrial carcinoma.[83]

In nearly 10–15% of Lynch syndrome cases, MMR mutation analyses are incongruent with high MSI and abnormal immunohistochemical analysis results.[84] This recessive form of adenomatous polyposis results from biallelic germline mutations in the base excision repair gene MUTYH.[84] MUTYH is a DNA glycosylase that corrects mismatches resulting from a faulty replication of the oxidized base 8-hydroxyguanine (8-oxodG).[85,86] Removal of adenosine-inserted 8-oxodG mispairs by MUTYH promotes error-free base excision repair by faithfully incorporating cytosine opposite 8-oxo-G, thereby correcting this genetic lesion.[85] MUTYH-associated polyposis occurs in a small proportion of patients with more than 100 colorectal adenomas.[87] The APC gene is frequently involved[88] but with a more favorable prognosis in the MUTYH-associated polyposis setting.[89]

## Targeted Therapy, Receptors, and Signaling Networks

CRC is a prime example of successfully merging molecular biology with advances in targeted therapy to optimize outcomes: the

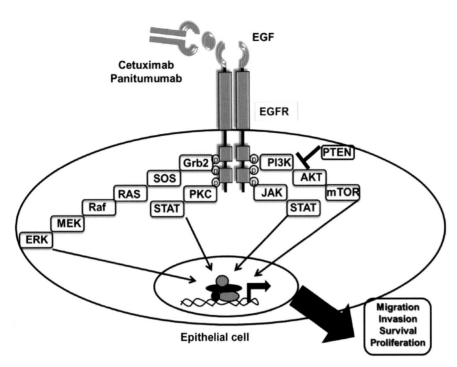

**Figure 20.1** Epidermal growth factor receptor (EGFR) targeting using monoclonal antibodies (mAbs), cetuximab and panitumumab. Epithelial cells are stimulated by EGF to activate multiple signaling cascades that initiate mRNA transcription and translation to protein that leads to migration, invasion, survival and proliferation. EGFR is inhibited by these mAbs. The proteins in these signaling cascades are defined as folows: (1) growth factor receptor-bound protein 2 (Grb2) → son of sevenless (SOS) → rat sarcoma (Ras) → rapidly accelerated fibrosarcoma (RAF) → microtubule-associated protein kinase (MAPK)-extracellular signal regulated kinase (ERK and MEK); (2) sarcoma (Src) → signal transducer and activator of transcription (STAT); (3) Janus kinase (JAK) → STAT; (4) phosphatidylinositol-4, 5-bisphosphate 3-kinase (PI3K) → v-akt murine thymoma viral oncogene homolog 1 (AKT) → mammalian target of rapamycin (mTOR) that is inhibited by phosphatase and tensin homolog (PTEN).

EGFR and VEGF pathways are the targets of several U.S. Food and Drug Admnistration (FDA)-approved drugs or investigational therapeutics.

## Targeting the EGFR Pathway

EGFR mutation and overexpression occur at high frequency in patients with CRC.[90] This overexpression is commonly associated with shorter survival and poor response to cytotoxic chemotherapies.[91] EGFR ligands include epidermal growth factor, transforming growth factor alpha, and others.[91] Receptor–ligand complex formation initiates EGFR homodimerization or heterodimerization with other members of the Her family of receptors followed by autophosphorylation.[91] Downstream signaling is activated through Grb2/SOS/Ras/Raf/MEK and either MAPK or ERK.[91] The activation of the alternate pathways PI3K/AKT/mTOR, Src/STAT, and PLC/PKC can occur, among other signaling cascades.[91-93] Monoclonal antibodies (mAB) such as cetuximab or panitumumab inhibit EGFR by blocking ligand binding to the extracellular receptor domain.[91] This increases EGFR turnover by internalization and degradation, complement-mediated cytotoxicity, and immune cell-mediated cytotoxicity (Figure 20.1).[91]

## EGFR mAB: Cetuximab

Cetuximab is a chimeric mouse–human immunoglobulin (IgG)1 anti-hEGFR antibody.[91] The efficacy of cetuximab was initially demonstrated when it was administered as third-line treatment. The BOND1 study helped secure the FDA approval of cetuximab for use in combination with irinotecan in irinotecan-refractory disease or as a single agent in patients intolerant to irinotecan.[90] Cetuximab induced a response in 11% of patients who had disease progression while receiving irinotecan-containing regimens or had refractory disease to prior irinotecan-containing regimens, with a median time to progression of 1.5 months when used alone. Furthermore, when cetuximab was combined with irinotecan, 23% of patients responded with a median time to progression of 4.1 months. In a separate third-line setting trial, single-agent cetuximab also resulted in a 10% response rate.[94]

Cetuximab was shown to confer a significant survival benefit in a randomized international phase III trial as monotherapy versus best supportive care (BSC) in patients with refractory metastatic disease.[95] The overall survival (OS) increased from 4.6 months to 6.1 months.[95] The survival benefit of cetuximab as first-line therapy for mCRC was confirmed in the randomized phase III trial CRYSTAL (cetuximab combined with irinotecan)[96] and the randomized phase II trial OPUS (oxaliplatin and cetuximab).[97] The CRYSTAL trial specifically investigated the efficacy and safety of treating mCRC with irinotecan in combination with fluorouracil and leucovorin (FOLFIRI) plus cetuximab.[96] In this case, combining cetuximab plus FOLFIRI, compared with FOLFIRI alone, reduced the risk of disease progression by 15%. In addition, adding cetuximab to FOLFIRI improved the response rate by nearly 10% but showed no significant difference in OS between the treatment groups. Subgroup analysis demonstrated that cetuximab benefits were limited to patients with *KRAS* wild-type (WT) tumors.[96] Additional phase 1 and 2 studies also showed that cetuximab was active as first-line treatment when added to irinotecan-based therapy[98] or oxaliplatin-based therapy.[97,99]

Cetuximab also improved survival and quality of life in patients with advanced CRC in studies conducted by the National Cancer Institute of Canada Clinical Trials Group and Australian Gastro-Intestinal Trials Group (CO-17 study).[95] In this case, cetuximab prolonged OS (median, 6.1 months vs. 4.6 months) and progression-free survival (PFS; hazard ratio [HR], 0.68) and improved disease control rate (31.4% vs. 10.9%) compared with BSC alone in patients with advanced and chemotherapy-refractory CRC.

## EGFR mAB: Panitumumab

Panitumumab is a fully humanized IgG2 anti-hEGFR antibody with clinical benefit.[91] Panitumumab as a single agent along with BSC in patients with chemorefractory CRC was shown to confer a benefit versus BSC alone.[100] Panitumumab significantly improved PFS with manageable toxicity. The rate of disease progression based on the HR was approximately half in the panitumumab group versus the BSC group. Statistically, HR excluded a PFS rate reduction of less than 33%, which was the hypothesized treatment effect. Although the absolute effect of panitumumab was relatively small, the magnitude of the improvement in PFS as measured by the HR of PFS for panitumumab relative to the BSC control was significant. This compares favorably with recent trials leading to important advances in the treatment of mCRC, including those testing novel agents as earlier lines of therapy.[90, 101]

Patients with WT KRAS tend to benefit from anti-EGFR therapy. The predictive role of KRAS was assessed in panitumumab monotherapy with BSC.[102] The primary objective was to assess the effect of panitumumab monotherapy on PFS in patients with mutant (43%) versus WT *KRAS* tumors. PFS was significantly greater in the WT *KRAS* group (HR, 0.45) than in the mutant group (HR, 0.99). The median PFS in the WT *KRAS* group was 12.3 weeks for those who received panitumumab and 7.3 weeks for those who received BSC. The response rates to panitumumab were 17% and 0%, for the WT and mutant groups, respectively. Generally, WT *KRAS* patients with mCRC had longer OS (HR, 0.67) with panitumumab monotherapy. Thus, WT *KRAS* status should be considered when selecting patients with mCRC as candidates for panitumumab monotherapy.

## Biomarkers, KRAS, NRAS, BRAF, and Other Targets

Although mutant KRAS status is the best predictor of poor activity of EGFR-targeted mAbs, other factors may be involved. Other factor involvement was suggested by the finding that response rates only rose from about 15% in an unselected patient population to about 30% in those with KRAS-WT tumors.[103] Potential factors/biomarkers of response and resistance to EGFR-targeted therapy are summarized in the following sections and listed in Table 20.2.

## KRAS

Cancer-related EGFR changes and downstream signal transduction prompted the development of EGFR-targeted mAbs.[91] Mutant KRAS-related failure of responses to EGFR-targeted mAbs is a key assessment for treating mCRC.[91] KRAS gene mutations constitutively activate downstream signaling that confers a lack of response to treatment.[91] Patients with KRAS mutations who are unlikely

to benefit can now be identified before treatment or predicted to exhibit an adverse prognosis.[137] Patients with KRAS-mutant tumors receiving an EGFR-targeted mAb combined with oxaliplatin-based therapy have poorer responses than those receiving oxaliplatin-based therapy alone.[104] However, retrospective data suggest that patients with KRAS-mutant CRC respond better than patients with KRAS-WT CRC when treated with oxaliplatin-based regimens such as FOLFOX6 alone.[138] Activating mutations in *RAS* (*KRAS* or *NRAS*) in addition to *KRAS* mutations in exon 2 are negative predictive biomarkers for anti-EGFR therapy. *KRAS* and *NRAS* are closely related *RAS* oncogene family members, and mutations in either gene at codons 12, 13, 61, 117, and 146 increase the levels of guanosine triphosphate-bound RAS proteins.[139, 140] In addition, *KRAS* and *NRAS* mutations at these codons tend to be mutually exclusive, which suggests they are functionally redundant.[141] In a randomized phase 3 study of panitumumab monotherapy[142] and other studies,[143, 144] most patients with mCRC tumors harbored a mutation in *KRAS* or *NRAS* and did not respond to anti-EGFR therapy. In contrast, mutations in *HRAS* are infrequent in CRC.[145]

A recent trial (AIO KRK-0306)[146] compared the efficacy of infusional FOLFIRI plus cetuximab to FOLFIRI plus bevacizumab as first-line treatment of mCRC. This trial was amended in October 2008 to exclude patients with KRAS-mutated tumors.[147] A subsequent subgroup analysis compared treatment efficacy and survival in patients with KRAS codon 12- or KRAS codon 13-mutated tumors treated with FOLFIRI plus cetuximab versus FOLFIRI plus bevacizumab. Interestingly, there was no significant difference in the response rate when cetuximab was compared with bevacizumab in combination with chemotherapy. FOLFIRI plus cetuximab induced an overall response rate (ORR) of 44%. This was higher than that previously observed in the CRYSTAL trial (ORR = 31%)[148] but similar to that in a phase II study by the CECOG group (ORR = 41%)[149] as well as the German AIO KRK-0104 study (ORR = 49%)[150] that used capecitabine and irinotecan plus cetuximab. Furthermore, pooled analyses of the CRYSTAL and OPUS trials[151] point to a similar conclusion. Therefore, cumulative evidence supports KRAS mutations as mandatory exclusion criteria for anti-EGFR therapy.

## Extended RAS

The treatment effect of the *RAS* mutation spectrum (*KRAS* and *NRAS*) on PFS and OS was recently analyzed in a prospective–retrospective biomarker study. This randomized phase 3 study

**Table 20.2** Biomarkers for EGFR-targeted therapy. Clinical values and incidence of EGFR-targeted therapy biomarkers.

| Biomarker | Value | Incidence% | References |
|---|---|---|---|
| KRAS mutation | Prognostic value is controversial | 35–45 | 96, 104–114 |
|  | Main predictor of resistance to anti-EGFR mAbs |  |  |
| BRAF mutations | Identifies patients with poor prognosis | 4–15 | 104, 115–119 |
|  | Predictive value is controversial |  |  |
| PIK3CA mutations | Prognostic value is controversial | 10–20 | 107, 109, 110, 120–126 |
|  | Predictive value is controversial |  |  |
| PTEN status | Prognostic value is controversial | 19–42 | 120–122, 127, 128 |
|  | Predictive value is controversial |  |  |
| Epiregulin/amphiregulin expression | Prognostic value in WT KRAS | Unreported | 129–133 |
|  | Associated with clinical benefit to anti-EGFR therapies |  |  |
| EGFR protein expression | No prognostic value | 80–85 | 104, 134–136 |
|  | No predictive value |  |  |

of panitumumab plus FOLFOX-4 (oxaliplatin and infused 5-FU/leucovorin) compared with FOLFOX4 alone was conducted in patients with previously untreated mCRC.[152] Among patients without *RAS* mutations, the median PFS was 10.1 months in the panitumumab-FOLFOX4 arm versus 7.9 months in the FOLFOX4 arm. The median OS was 26.0 months in the panitumumab–FOLFOX4 arm versus 20.2 months in the FOLFOX4 arm. When the patients were substratified, 17% of those with WT *KRAS* had other *RAS* mutations with inferior PFS and OS after panitumumab–FOLFOX4 treatment, which was similar to patients with *KRAS* mutations in exon 2. Therefore, additional *RAS* mutations could predict a lack of response to panitumumab–FOLFOX4. These findings are currently being confirmed in other studies and regimens, and it is anticipated that expanded RAS testing, including codons 12, 13, 59, 61, 117, 146 of both KRAS and NRAS will be required prior to administration of EGFR monoclonal antibodies.

## BRAF

Research continues to emerge on biomarkers other than KRAS that influence the activity of EGFR-targeted mAbs. For example, BRAF V600E-activating mutations are currently under consideration for use as a prognostic biomarker of EGFR-targeted mAbs. Occurring in approximately 10% of CRCs, they are generally mutually exclusive to KRAS mutations.[103] BRAF V600E mutations are more prevalent in older females with WT KRAS in right-sided colon cancers (50%) compared with unselected patients (10%).[153] These clinicopathologic characteristics and the BRAF V600E mutation may help identify mCRC patients with a poorer prognosis.

The impact of BRAF status on treatment efficacy is not well defined, owing to the low occurrence rate of BRAF mutations and their lack of prior consideration.[154,155] The CRYSTAL trial showed improvements in median PFS and OS (not statistically significant) with the addition of cetuximab to FOLFIRI in patients with WT KRAS/BRAF-mutant disease.[148] Emerging evidence indicates that the BRAF V600E mutation helps identify patients with a poor prognosis. This is regardless of the treatment regimen or the addition

of EGFR-targeted therapy.[104,115–117] Thus, the prognostic value of the BRAF V600E mutation could override any predictive values. For example, in a cohort of 173,200 patients enrolled in the Nurses' Health Study and the Health Professional Followup study, 17% had a BRAF mutation.[116,129] In this study, BRAF mutations were associated with increased colon cancer-specific mortality with an HR of 1.97 in multivariate analyses.

Additional biomarkers under investigation (Table 20.2) include PIK3CA mutations and loss of PTEN expression or activity.[120,127,155–157] Similarly, the overexpression or amplification of EGFR and its ligands are key biomarkers.[117,158,159] Their use as predictive markers of response remain inconsistent, and validation tests are necessary before their use in clinical practice is considered.

## Targeting the VEGFR Pathway

The first biological targeted therapy to be used in mCRC was the vascular endothelial growth factor-A (VEGF-A)-targeted agent, bevacizumab.[160] Bevacizumab is a chimeric mouse–human IgG1 anti-hVEGF-A antibody.[161,162] It binds to all biologically active isoforms of VEGF-A and blocks binding to its receptors VEGFR 1 and 2 (Figure 20.2).[161]

Bevacizumab was initially combined with standard chemotherapy in a phase III setting to treat patients with mCRC. Specifically, irinotecan plus weekly bolus of 5-fluorouracil (5-FU)/leucovorin (IFL) plus bevacizumab was compared to IFL alone. The addition of bevacizumab resulted in no serious adverse events and improved OS and PFS.[101] It is typically used in combination with basic chemotherapeutic regimens,[163] primarily in a metastatic setting.[164] Anti-VEGF agents are commonly used without anti-EGFR agents since no benefit is conferred when these agents are combined.[105,164] In fact, this combination may be associated with poorer survival in CRC.

The efficacy and safety of bevacizumab plus capecitabine compared with capecitabine alone was assessed in a phase III trial of elderly patients with previously untreated mCRC.[165] The PFS was significantly longer with bevacizumab and capecitabine than with capecitabine alone (median, 9.1 months vs. 5.1 months, HR 0.53).

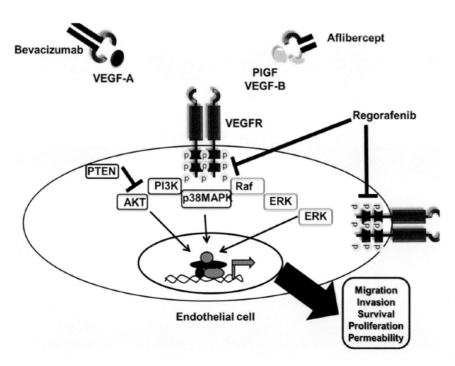

**Figure 20.2** Vascular endothelial growth factor (VEGF) targeting uses monoclonal antibodies (mAbs), bevacizumab and aflibercept. Vascular endothelial cells are stimulated by VEGF to activate multiple signaling cascades that initiate mRNA transcription and translation to protein that initiate migration, invasion, survival and proliferation and alter vascular permeability along with angiogenesis. The key signaling cascades are defined in Figure 20.1. Regorafenib is a potent multi-target kinase inhibitor that prevents the phosphorylation and activation of multiple VEGFR isoforms 1–3 along with numerous other targets.

Treatment-related adverse events of grade 3 or worse occurred in 40% of patients in the combination group compared to 22% in the capecitabine group and mainly included hand-and-foot syndrome, diarrhea, and venous thromboembolic events. Based on this trial, the combination of bevacizumab and capecitabine is currently considered an effective and well-tolerated regimen for elderly patients with mCRC.

Bevacizumab was evaluated further in a first-line setting with oxaliplatin-based regimens. In the NO16966 trial,[166] patients who were naïve to chemotherapy and bevacizumab were randomly assigned to oxaliplatin-based regimens (FOLFOX-4 or capecitabine plus oxaliplatin) and then to either placebo or bevacizumab. A statistically significant 9.4-month PFS advantage was observed in the bevacizumab group versus 8.0 months in the placebo group (HR 0.83), but the difference in OS between the two groups was not statistically significant. Contrasting this finding in a second-line setting, the Eastern Cooperative Oncology Group-3200 trial[163] evaluated the use of bevacizumab in combination with the FOLFOX-4 regimen for patients who were naïve to bevacizumab treatment and for whom irinotecan and 5-FU had failed. OS, PFS, and ORR were higher in the group that received FOLFOX-4 plus bevacizumab than in the group that received FOLFOX-4 alone. This trial was the first to provide safety data for the combination of bevacizumab and FOLFOX-4, leading to its acceptability as a first-line option in the United States. Bevacizumab improves survival in patients with mCRC, as first- or second-line therapy, and is approved for use with regimens combining 5-FU with either irinotecan or oxaliplatin as well as with 5-FU alone for patients unable to receive irinotecan or oxaliplatin. In another phase III trial, ML18147,[167] bevacizumab plus standard second-line chemotherapy was investigated in patients with mCRC that progressed after standard first-line bevacizumab-based treatment. Maintaining VEGF inhibition with bevacizumab plus standard second-line chemotherapy beyond disease progression provided clinical benefit in patients with mCRC. The median OS was 11.2 months in patients who received bevacizumab plus chemotherapy compared with 9.8 months in the patients who received chemotherapy alone (HR 0.81). This approach has also been investigated in other tumor types, including metastatic breast cancer and non-small cell lung cancer.

Another VEGF targeted agent used in mCRC is aflibercept, known as VEGF Trap or zivaflibercept in the United States. It is a recombinant fusion protein containing VEGF-binding portions from the extracellular domains of human VEGF receptors 1 and 2 fused to the Fc portion of human IgG1. Aflibercept blocks the activity of VEGFA, VEGFB, and placental growth factor by acting as a high-affinity ligand trap (Figure 20.2). Phase I and phase II trials have investigated aflibercept as a single agent and in combination with a number of chemotherapy regimens, including irinotecan, FU, and leucovorin.[168,169] Aflibercept was approved by the FDA in August 2012 based on the phase III VELOUR trial.[170] In patients previously treated with an oxaliplatin-containing regimen on this trial, the median survival was significantly improved from 12 months to 13.5 months with an 18% relative risk reduction by adding aflibercept to FOLFIRI. A significant improvement in PFS from 4.6 months to 6.9 months with a 24% relative risk reduction was also observed. The ORR in the aflibercept plus FOLFIRI arm was 19.8% versus 11.1% for in the FOLFIRI arm. Aflibercept is now indicated for treating mCRC in combination with FOLFIRI in patients whose disease is resistant to or has progressed following an oxaliplatin-based regimen.

## Multityrosine Kinase Inhibitors

The overall experience with the mAbs bevacizumab, aflibercept, cetuximab, and panitumumab indicates the importance of targets for therapy. Multiple signaling pathways have been implicated in the development and progression of CRC, involving receptor tyrosine kinases (e.g., EGFR, VEGFR, and others) and downstream signaling cascades (Grb2/SOS/RAS-RAF/MEK and PI3K-PTEN-AKT-mTOR).[171] Multi-tyrosine kinase inhibitors are an attractive approach for refractory disease. Regorafenib is the first small-molecule multikinase inhibitor with survival benefits in mCRC, which has progressed after all standard therapies. The structure of regorafenib is similar to that of sorafenib; however, regorafenib has a wider spectrum of activity and more potent action. As a potent multi-target kinase inhibitor, it targets VEGFR-1–3, PDGFRβ, Kit, RET, and Raf-1 along with IgG and epidermal growth factor homology domain 2 (TIE2) activity.[172]

Preclinically, regorafenib has had antitumor activity in CRC models.[172] In a phase 1B clinical trial, oral regorafenib had a tolerable toxicity profile, and preliminary evidence showed antitumor activity in patients with progressive CRC.[173] Subsequently, the CORRECT phase 3 trial[174] assessed the efficacy and safety of regorafenib as third-line treatment. Specifically, the study enrolled patients whose disease progressed after oxaliplatin-, fluoropyrimidine-, and irinotecan-based chemotherapy, anti-VEGF therapy, or anti-EGFR therapy. Patients had mCRC that progressed after standard cytotoxic and targeted treatments. Regorafenib significantly prolonged survival compared with placebo. The median OS was 6.4 months in the regorafenib group versus 5.0 months in the placebo group (HR, 0.77). The most common significant treatment-related adverse events were hand and foot skin reaction, fatigue, diarrhea, and hypertension. The CORRECT trial led to the approval of regorafenib by the FDA in September 2012 for treatment-refractory WT KRAS mCRC.

## Conclusion

In the past decade, the OS for patients diagnosed with mCRC has improved significantly.[175] Survival improvements began in 2004 when new EGFR- and VEGF-targeted drugs became available for use in the United States for treating mCRC. Rapid increases in bevacizumab (2004) and cetuximab (2004) usage helped initiate these improvements. Confirmation of this temporal trend was based on the analysis of the National Cancer Institute Surveillance, Epidemiology, and End Results data set.[175] Further improvements in patient survival are expected to be achieved through continued advances in targeted therapy combined with the optimization of current chemotherapy regimens.

The growing acceptance of KRAS testing as a diagnostic tool for selecting patients prior to EGFR-targeted treatment is an excellent example of fine tuning targeted therapy. This process may seem daunting considering emerging evidence that complex signaling pathways and crosstalk between them drive disease. As such, analysis of single marker is unlikely to fully predict disease progression. Therefore, concomitant analysis of multiple genetic and epigenetic events involved in the EGFR-initiated signaling cascade among other oncogenic signaling cascades is likely to enhance the prediction ability of the biomarkers used individually. A future challenge is standardizing, implementing, and validating promising molecular marker subsets in large prospective clinical trials. Other challenges include identifying potential mechanisms and pathways involved in acquired resistance to anti-EGFR therapies to more effectively target effectors downstream of EGFR.

Each CRC patient can be considered to have unique disease characteristics that are driven by discrete genetic/epigenetic events requiring better understanding prior to treatment. Molecular classification that accurately reflects these underlying patient-centric characteristics responsible for carcinogenesis is essential for better success in the clinic. In leukemia and lymphoma for example, molecular classification considerably advanced the field over the past couple of decades.[176] Molecular classification of CRC continues to evolve and improve. On a larger scale, global genomic and epigenetic status plays a significant role in determining clinical, pathological, and biological characteristics of CRC. One can theoretically divide tumors into different groups by the presence or absence of any molecular event(s). Molecular subsets can be useful classifiers, in particular, for predicting response to targeted therapies.

# References

1 Jemal A, Bray F, Center MM, Ferlay J, Ward E, Forman D. Global cancer statistics. *CA Cancer J Clin*. 2011;61(2):69–90.

2 Jemal A, Simard EP, Dorell C, et al. Annual Report to the Nation on the Status of Cancer, 1975–2009, featuring the burden and trends in human papillomavirus(HPV)-associated cancers and HPV vaccination coverage levels. *J Natl Cancer Inst*. 2013;105(3):175–201.

3 Siegel R, Naishadham D, Jemal A. Cancer statistics, 2013. *CA Cancer J Clin*. 2013;63:11–30.

4 Ahnen DJ, Wade SW, Jones WF, et al. The increasing incidence of young-onset colorectal cancer: a call to action. *Mayo Clini Proc*. 2014;89(2):216–224.

5 Winawer SJ, Zauber AG, Fletcher RH, et al.; US Multi-Society Task Force on Colorectal Cancer; American Cancer Society. Guidelines for colonoscopy surveillance after polypectomy: a consensus update by the US Multi-Society Task Force on Colorectal Cancer and the American Cancer Society. *Gastroenterology*. 2006;130(6):1872–1885.

6 Starr TK, Allaei R, Silverstein KA, et al. A transposon-based genetic screen in mice identifies genes altered in colorectal cancer. *Science*. 2009;323(5922):1747–1750.

7 Fearon ER, Vogelstein B. A genetic model for colorectal tumorigenesis. *Cell*. 1990;61(5):759–767.

8 Smith G, Carey FA, Beattie J, et al. Mutations in APC, Kirsten-ras, and p53—alternative genetic pathways to colorectal cancer. *Proc Natl Acad Sci U S A*. 2002;99(14):9433–9438.

9 Cancer Genome Atlas Network. Comprehensive molecular characterization of human colon and rectal cancer. *Nature*. 2012;487(7407):330–337.

10 Lui C, Mills K, Brocardo MG, Sharma M, Henderson BR. APC as a mobile scaffold: regulation and function at the nucleus, centrosomes, and mitochondria. *IUBMB life*. 2012;64(3):209–214.

11 Kinzler KW, Nilbert MC, Su LK, et al. Identification of FAP locus genes from chromosome 5q21. *Science*. 1991;253(5020):661–665.

12 Beroud C, Soussi T. APC gene: database of germline and somatic mutations in human tumors and cell lines. *Nucleic Acids Res*. 1996;24(1):121–124.

13 Goss KH, Groden J. Biology of the adenomatous polyposis coli tumor suppressor. *J Clin Oncol*. 2000;18(9):1967–1979.

14 Galiatsatos P, Foulkes WD. Familial adenomatous polyposis. *Am J Gastroenterol*. 2006;101(2):385–398.

15 Su LK, Burrell M, Hill DE, et al. APC binds to the novel protein EB1. *Cancer Res*. 1995;55(14):2972–2977.

16 Draviam VM, Shapiro I, Aldridge B, Sorger PK. Misorientation and reduced stretching of aligned sister kinetochores promote chromosome missegregation in EB1- or APC-depleted cells. *EMBO J*. 2006;25(12):2814–2827.

17 Bakhoum SF, Genovese G, Compton DA. Deviant kinetochore microtubule dynamics underlie chromosomal instability. *Curr Biol*. 2009;19(22):1937–1942.

18 Ladd JJ, Busald T, Johnson MM, et al. Increased plasma levels of the APC-interacting protein MAPRE1, LRG1, and IGFBP2 preceding a diagnosis of colorectal cancer in women. *Cancer Prev Res (Phila)*. 2012;5(4):655–664.

19 McGrath JP, Capon DJ, Smith DH, et al. Structure and organization of the human Ki-ras proto-oncogene and a related processed pseudogene. *Nature*. 1983;304(5926):501–506.

20 Wang JY, Wang YH, Jao SW, et al. Molecular mechanisms underlying the tumorigenesis of colorectal adenomas: correlation to activated K-ras oncogene. *Oncol Rep*. 2006;16(6):1245–1252.

21 Pino MS, Chung DC. The chromosomal instability pathway in colon cancer. *Gastroenterology*. 2010;138(6):2059–2072.

22 Brink M, de Goeij AF, Weijenberg MP, et al. K-ras oncogene mutations in sporadic colorectal cancer in The Netherlands Cohort Study. *Carcinogenesis*. 2003;24:703–710.

23 Ryslik GA, Cheng Y, Cheung KH, Modis Y, Zhao H. A graph theoretic approach to utilizing protein structure to identify non-random somatic mutations. *BMC Bioinformatics*. 2014;15:86.

24 Scheffzek K, Ahmadian MR, Kabsch W, et al. The Ras-RasGAP complex: structural basis for GTPase activation and its loss in oncogenic Ras mutants. *Science*. 1997;277(5324):333–338.

25 Wang Y, Kaiser CE, Frett B, Li HY. Targeting mutant KRAS for anticancer therapeutics: a review of novel small molecule modulators. *J Med Chem*. 2013;56(13):5219–5230.

26 Baker SJ, Fearon ER, Nigro JM, et al. Chromosome 17 deletions and p53 gene mutations in colorectal carcinomas. *Science*. 1989;244(4901):217–221.

27 Maltzman W, Czyzyk L. UV irradiation stimulates levels of p53 cellular tumor antigen in nontransformed mouse cells. *Mol Cell Biol*. 1984;4(9):1689–1694.

28 el-Deiry WS, Tokino T, Velculescu VE, et al. WAF1, a potential mediator of p53 tumor suppression. *Cell*. 1993;75:817–825.

29 Leroy B, Anderson M, Soussi T. TP53 Mutations in Human Cancer: Database Reassessment and Prospects for the Next Decade. *Hum Mutat*. 2014;35(6):672–688.

30 Liu J, Zhang C, Feng Z. Tumor suppressor p53 and its gain-of-function mutants in cancer. *Acta Biochim Biophys Sin (Shanghai)*. 2014;46(3):170–179.

31 Rodrigues NR, Rowan A, Smith ME, et al. p53 mutations in colorectal cancer. *Proc Natl Acad Sci U S A*. 1990;87(19):7555–7559.

32 Rao CV, Yamada HY. Genomic instability and colon carcinogenesis: from the perspective of genes. *Front Oncol*. 2013;3:130.

33 Carroll PE, Okuda M, Horn HF, et al. Centrosome hyperamplification in human cancer: chromosome instability induced by p53 mutation and/or Mdm2 overexpression. *Oncogene*. 1999;18(11):1935–1944.

34 Tarapore P, Fukasawa K. Loss of p53 and centrosome hyperamplification. *Oncogene*. 2002;21(40):6234–6240.

35 Tomasini R, Mak TW, Melino G. The impact of p53 and p73 on aneuploidy and cancer. *Trends Cell Biol*. 2008;18(5):244–252.

36 Yi Q, Zhao X, Huang Y, et al. p53 dependent centrosome clustering prevents multipolar mitosis in tetraploid cells. *PloS one*. 2011;6(11):e27304.

37 Russo A, Bazan V, Iacopetta B, et al.; TP53-CRC Collaborative Study Group. The TP53 colorectal cancer international collaborative study on

the prognostic and predictive significance of p53 mutation: influence of tumor site, type of mutation, and adjuvant treatment. *J Clin Oncol.* 2005;23(30):7518–7528.

38 Neal CP, Garcea G, Doucas H, et al. Molecular prognostic markers in resectable colorectal liver metastases: a systematic review. *Eur J Cancer.* 2006;42(12):1728–1743.

39 Lao VV, Grady WM. Epigenetics and colorectal cancer. *Nat Rev Gastroenterol Hepatol.* 2011;8(12):686–700.

40 Goel A, Arnold CN, Niedzwiecki D, et al. Characterization of sporadic colon cancer by patterns of genomic instability. *Cancer Res.* 2003;63(7):1608–1614.

41 Hawthorn L, Lan L, Mojica W. Evidence for field effect cancerization in colorectal cancer. *Genomics.* 2014;103(2–3):211–221.

42 Heng HH, Bremer SW, Stevens JB, et al. Chromosomal instability (CIN): what it is and why it is crucial to cancer evolution. *Cancer Metastasis Rev.* 2013;32(2–4):325–240.

43 Burgess RJ, Zhang Z. Histone chaperones in nucleosome assembly and human disease. *Nat Struct Mol Biol.* 2013;20(1):14–22.

44 Ashktorab H, Schaffer AA, Daremipouran M, Smoot DT, Lee E, Brim H. Distinct genetic alterations in colorectal cancer. *PloS one.* 2010;5(1):e8879.

45 Sheffer M, Bacolod MD, Zuk O, et al. Association of survival and disease progression with chromosomal instability: a genomic exploration of colorectal cancer. *Proc Natl Acad Sci U S A.* 2009;106(17):7131–7136.

46 Kim TM, Laird PW, Park PJ. The landscape of microsatellite instability in colorectal and endometrial cancer genomes. *Cell.* 2013;155(4):858–868.

47 Boland CR, Goel A. Microsatellite instability in colorectal cancer. *Gastroenterology.* 2010;138(6):2073–2087 e3.

48 Drost M, Lutzen A, van Hees S, et al. Genetic screens to identify pathogenic gene variants in the common cancer predisposition Lynch syndrome. *Proc Natl Acad Sci U S A.* 2013;110(23):9403–9408.

49 Boland CR, Thibodeau SN, Hamilton SR, et al. A National Cancer Institute Workshop on Microsatellite Instability for cancer detection and familial predisposition: development of international criteria for the determination of microsatellite instability in colorectal cancer. *Cancer Res.* 1998;58(22):5248–5257.

50 Baba Y, Nosho K, Shima K, et al. PTGER2 overexpression in colorectal cancer is associated with microsatellite instability, independent of CpG island methylator phenotype. *Cancer Epidemiol Biomarkers Prev.* 2010;19(3):822–831.

51 Juo YY, Johnston F, Zhang D, et al. Prognostic Value of CpG Island Methylator Phenotype among Colorectal Cancer Patients: A Systematic Review and Meta-Analysis. *Ann Oncol.* 2014;25(12):2314–2327.

52 Chen D, Huang JF, Liu K, et al. BRAFV600E Mutation and Its Association with Clinicopathological Features of Colorectal Cancer: A Systematic Review and Meta-Analysis. *PloS one.* 2014;9:e90607.

53 Serra RW, Fang M, Park SM, Hutchinson L, Green MR. A KRAS-directed transcriptional silencing pathway that mediates the CpG island methylator phenotype. *ELife.* 2014;3:e02313.

54 Xia D, Wang D, Kim SH, Katoh H, DuBois RN. Prostaglandin E2 promotes intestinal tumor growth via DNA methylation. *Nature medicine.* 2012;18(2):224–226.

55 Remo A, Pancione M, Zanella C, Vendraminelli R. Molecular pathology of colorectal carcinoma. A systematic review centred on the new role of the pathologist. *Pathologica.* 2012;104(6):432–441.

56 Ang PW, Loh M, Liem N, et al. Comprehensive profiling of DNA methylation in colorectal cancer reveals subgroups with distinct clinicopathological and molecular features. *BMC Cancer.* 2010;10:227.

57 Tanaka H, Deng G, Matsuzaki K, et al. BRAF mutation, CpG island methylator phenotype and microsatellite instability occur more frequently and concordantly in mucinous than non-mucinous colorectal cancer. *Int J Cancer.* 2006;118(11):2765–2771.

58 Jass JR. Classification of colorectal cancer based on correlation of clinical, morphological and molecular features. *Histopathology.* 2007;50(1):113–130.

59 Cahill DP, Kinzler KW, Vogelstein B, Lengauer C. Genetic instability and darwinian selection in tumours. *Trends Cell Biol.* 1999;9(12):M57–60.

60 Navin N, Kendall J, Troge J, et al. Tumour evolution inferred by single-cell sequencing. *Nature.* 2011;472(7341):90–94.

61 Navin NE. Tumor evolution in response to chemotherapy: phenotype versus genotype. *Cell Rep.* 2014;6(3):417–419.

62 Ding L, Ley TJ, Larson DE, et al. Clonal evolution in relapsed acute myeloid leukaemia revealed by whole-genome sequencing. *Nature.* 2012;481(7382):506–510.

63 Montagut C, Dalmases A, Bellosillo B, et al. Identification of a mutation in the extracellular domain of the Epidermal Growth Factor Receptor conferring cetuximab resistance in colorectal cancer. *Nat Med.* 2012;18(2):221–223.

64 Crowley E, Di Nicolantonio F, Loupakis F, Bardelli A. Liquid biopsy: monitoring cancer-genetics in the blood. *Nat Rev Clin Oncol.* 2013;10(8):472–484.

65 Lynch HT, Smyrk TC, Watson P, et al. Genetics, natural history, tumor spectrum, and pathology of hereditary nonpolyposis colorectal cancer: an updated review. *Gastroenterology.* 1993;104(5):1535–1549.

66 Garber JE, Offit K. Hereditary cancer predisposition syndromes. *J Clin Oncol.* 2005;23(2):276–292.

67 Burt RW, DiSario JA, Cannon-Albright L. Genetics of colon cancer: impact of inheritance on colon cancer risk. *Annu Rev Med.* 1995;46:371–379.

68 De Queiroz Rossanese LB, De Lima Marson FA, Ribeiro JD, Coy CS, Bertuzzo CS. APC germline mutations in families with familial adenomatous polyposis. *Oncol Rep.* 2013;30(5):2081–2088.

69 Zilberberg A, Lahav L, Rosin-Arbesfeld R. Restoration of APC gene function in colorectal cancer cells by aminoglycoside- and macrolide-induced read-through of premature termination codons. *Gut.* 2010;59(4):496–507.

70 Casper M, Petek E, Henn W, et al. Multidisciplinary treatment of desmoid tumours in Gardner's syndrome due to a large interstitial deletion of chromosome 5q. *QJM.* 2014;107(7):521–527.

71 Cazorla A, Viennet G, Uro-Coste E, Valmary-Degano S. Mucoepidermoid carcinoma: A yet unreported cancer associated with familial adenomatous polyposis. *J Craniomaxillofac Surg.* 2014;42(3):262–264.

72 Grandhi R, Deibert CP, Pirris SM, Lembersky B, Mintz AH. Simultaneous Muir-Torre and Turcot's syndrome: A case report and review of the literature. *Surg Neurol Int.* 2013;4:52.

73 Schlussel AT, Donlon SS, Eggerding FA, Gagliano RA. Identification of an APC Variant in a Patient with Clinical Attenuated Familial Adenomatous Polyposis. *Case Rep Med.* 2014;2014:432324.

74 Cheah PY, Wong YH, Koh PK, Loi C, Chew MH, Tang CL. A novel indel in exon 9 of APC upregulates a 'skip exon 9' isoform and causes very severe familial adenomatous polyposis. *Eur J Hum Genet.* 2013;22(6):833–836.

75 Guillem JG, Wood WC, Moley JF, et al. ASCO/SSO review of current role of risk-reducing surgery in common hereditary cancer syndromes. *Ann Surg Oncol.* 2006;13(10):1296–1321.

76 Giardiello FM, Yang VW, Hylind LM, et al. Primary chemoprevention of familial adenomatous polyposis with sulindac. *N Engl J Med.* 2002;346(14):1054–1059.

77  Lynch HT, Lynch J. Lynch syndrome: genetics, natural history, genetic counseling, and prevention. *J Clin Oncol.* 2000;18(21 Suppl):19S–31S.

78  Jenkins MA, Baglietto L, Dowty JG, et al. Cancer risks for mismatch repair gene mutation carriers: a population-based early onset case-family study. *Clin Gastroenterol Hepatol.* 2006;4(4):489–498.

79  Steinke V, Holzapfel S, Loeffler M, et al. Evaluating the performance of clinical criteria for predicting mismatch repair gene mutations in Lynch syndrome: A comprehensive analysis of 3,671 families. *Int J Cancer.* 2014;135(1):69–77.

80  Kastrinos F, Stoffel EM. History, genetics, and strategies for cancer prevention in lynch syndrome. *Clin Gastroenterol Hepatol.* 2014;12(5):715–727.

81  Tutlewska K, Lubinski J, Kurzawski G. Germline deletions in the EPCAM gene as a cause of Lynch syndrome—literature review. *Hered Cancer Clin Pract.* 2013;11(1):9.

82  Lindor NM, Petersen GM, Hadley DW, et al. Recommendations for the care of individuals with an inherited predisposition to Lynch syndrome: a systematic review. *JAMA.* 2006;296(12):1507–1517.

83  See WA. Commentary on "Risks of primary extracolonic cancers following colorectal cancer in Lynch syndrome." Win AK, Lindor NM, Young JP, Macrae FA, Young GP, Williamson E, Parry S, Goldblatt J, Lipton L, Winship I, Leggett B, Tucker KM, Giles GG, Buchanan DD, Clendenning M, Rosty C, Arnold J, Levine AJ, Haile RW, Gallinger S, Le Marchand L, Newcomb PA, Hopper JL, Jenkins MA, Centre for Molecular, Environmental, Genetic and Analytic Epidemiology, Melbourne School of Population Health, The University of Melbourne, Victoria, Australia: J Natl Cancer Inst 2012;104(18):1363–72 [Epub 2012 Aug 28]. *Urol Oncol.* 2013;31(5):716.

84  Morak M, Heidenreich B, Keller G, et al. Biallelic MUTYH mutations can mimic Lynch syndrome. *Eur J Hum Genet.* 2014;22(11):1334–1337.

85  Mazzei F, Viel A, Bignami M. Role of MUTYH in human cancer. *Mutat Res.* 2013;743–744:33–43.

86  Markkanen E, Dorn J, Hubscher U. MUTYH DNA glycosylase: the rationale for removing undamaged bases from the DNA. *Front Genet.* 2013;4:18.

87  Sieber OM, Lipton L, Crabtree M, et al. Multiple colorectal adenomas, classic adenomatous polyposis, and germ-line mutations in MYH. *N Engl J Med.* 2003;348(9):791–799.

88  Sampson JR, Dolwani S, Jones S, et al. Autosomal recessive colorectal adenomatous polyposis due to inherited mutations of MYH. *Lancet.* 2003;362(9377):39–41.

89  Nielsen M, van Steenbergen LN, Jones N, et al. Survival of MUTYH-associated polyposis patients with colorectal cancer and matched control colorectal cancer patients. *J Natl Cancer Inst.* 2010;102(22):1724–1730.

90  Cunningham D, Humblet Y, Siena S, et al. Cetuximab monotherapy and cetuximab plus irinotecan in irinotecan-refractory metastatic colorectal cancer. *N Engl J Med.* 2004;351(4):337–345.

91  Chong CR, Janne PA. The quest to overcome resistance to EGFR-targeted therapies in cancer. *Nat Med.* 2013;19(11):1389–1400.

92  Mendelsohn J, Baselga J. Epidermal growth factor receptor targeting in cancer. *Semin Oncol.* 2006;33(4):369–385.

93  Goffin JR, Zbuk K. Epidermal growth factor receptor: pathway, therapies, and pipeline. *Clin Ther.* 2013;35:1282–1303.

94  Saltz LB, Meropol NJ, Loehrer PJ, Sr., Needle MN, Kopit J, Mayer RJ. Phase II trial of cetuximab in patients with refractory colorectal cancer that expresses the epidermal growth factor receptor. *J Clin Oncol.* 2004;22:1201–1208.

95  Jonker DJ, O'Callaghan CJ, Karapetis CS, et al. Cetuximab for the treatment of colorectal cancer. *N Engl J Med.* 2007;357(20):2040–2048.

96  Van Cutsem E, Kohne CH, Hitre E, et al. Cetuximab and chemotherapy as initial treatment for metastatic colorectal cancer. *N Engl J Med.* 2009;360(14):1408–1417.

97  Bokemeyer C, Bondarenko I, Makhson A, et al. Fluorouracil, leucovorin, and oxaliplatin with and without cetuximab in the first-line treatment of metastatic colorectal cancer. *J Clin Oncol.* 2009;27(5):663–671.

98  Folprecht G, Lutz MP, Schoffski P, et al. Cetuximab and irinotecan/5-fluorouracil/folinic acid is a safe combination for the first-line treatment of patients with epidermal growth factor receptor expressing metastatic colorectal carcinoma. *Ann Oncol.* 2006;17(3):450–456.

99  Arnold D, Hohler T, Dittrich C, et al. Cetuximab in combination with weekly 5-fluorouracil/folinic acid and oxaliplatin (FUFOX) in untreated patients with advanced colorectal cancer: a phase Ib/II study of the AIO GI Group. *Ann Oncol.* 2008;19(8):1442–1449.

100 Van Cutsem E, Peeters M, Siena S, et al. Open-label phase III trial of panitumumab plus best supportive care compared with best supportive care alone in patients with chemotherapy-refractory metastatic colorectal cancer. *J Clin Oncol.* 2007;25(13):1658–1664.

101 Hurwitz H, Fehrenbacher L, Novotny W, et al. Bevacizumab plus irinotecan, fluorouracil, and leucovorin for metastatic colorectal cancer. *The New England journal of medicine.* 2004;350:2335–2342.

102 Amado RG, Wolf M, Peeters M, et al. Wild-type KRAS is required for panitumumab efficacy in patients with metastatic colorectal cancer. *N Engl J Med.* 2008;26(23):1626–1634.

103 Pritchard CC, Grady WM. Colorectal cancer molecular biology moves into clinical practice. *Gut.* 2011;60(1):116–129.

104 Maughan TS, Adams RA, Smith CG, et al. MRC COIN Trial Investigators. Addition of cetuximab to oxaliplatin-based first-line combination chemotherapy for treatment of advanced colorectal cancer: results of the randomised phase 3 MRC COIN trial. *Lancet.* 2011;377(9783):2103–2114.

105 Tol J, Koopman M, Cats A, et al. Chemotherapy, bevacizumab, and cetuximab in metastatic colorectal cancer. *N Engl J Med.* 2009;360(6):563–572.

106 Douillard JY, Siena S, Cassidy J, et al. Randomized, phase III trial of panitumumab with infusional fluorouracil, leucovorin, and oxaliplatin (FOLFOX4) versus FOLFOX4 alone as first-line treatment in patients with previously untreated metastatic colorectal cancer: the PRIME study. *J Clin Oncol.* 2010;28(31):4697–4705.

107 Lievre A, Bachet JB, Le Corre D, et al. KRAS mutation status is predictive of response to cetuximab therapy in colorectal cancer. *Cancer Res.* 2006;66(8):3992–3995.

108 Lievre A, Bachet JB, Boige V, et al. KRAS mutations as an independent prognostic factor in patients with advanced colorectal cancer treated with cetuximab. *J Clin Oncol.* 2008;26(3):374–379.

109 Bokemeyer C, Bondarenko I, Hartmann JT, et al. Efficacy according to biomarker status of cetuximab plus FOLFOX-4 as first-line treatment for metastatic colorectal cancer: the OPUS study. *Ann Oncol.* 2011;22(7):1535–1546.

110 De Roock W, Claes B, Bernasconi D, et al. Effects of KRAS, BRAF, NRAS, and PIK3CA mutations on the efficacy of cetuximab plus chemotherapy in chemotherapy-refractory metastatic colorectal cancer: a retrospective consortium analysis. *Lancet Oncol.* 2010;11(8):753–762.

111 Karapetis CS, Khambata-Ford S, Jonker DJ, et al. K-ras mutations and benefit from cetuximab in advanced colorectal cancer. *N Engl J Med.* 2008;359(17):1757–1765.

112 Esteller M, Gonzalez S, Risques RA, et al. K-ras and p16 aberrations confer poor prognosis in human colorectal cancer. *N Engl J Med.* 2001;19(17):299–304.

113 Ogino S, Meyerhardt JA, Irahara N, et al. Cancer and Leukemia Group B; North Central Cancer Treatment Group; Canadian Cancer Society Research Institute; Southwest Oncology Group. KRAS mutation in stage III colon cancer and clinical outcome following intergroup trial CALGB 89803. *Clin Cancer Res*. 2009;15(23):7322–7329.

114 Roth AD, Tejpar S, Delorenzi M, et al. Prognostic role of KRAS and BRAF in stage II and III resected colon cancer: results of the translational study on the PETACC-3, EORTC 40993, SAKK 60–00 trial. *J Clin Oncol*. 2010;28(3):466–474.

115 Tveit KM, Guren T, Glimelius B, et al. Phase III trial of cetuximab with continuous or intermittent fluorouracil, leucovorin, and oxaliplatin (Nordic FLOX) versus FLOX alone in first-line treatment of metastatic colorectal cancer: the NORDIC-VII study. *J Clin Oncol*. 2012;30(15):1755–1762.

116 Ogino S, Nosho K, Kirkner GJ, et al. CpG island methylator phenotype, microsatellite instability, BRAF mutation and clinical outcome in colon cancer. *Gut*. 2009;58(1):90–96.

117 Tol J, Dijkstra JR, Klomp M, et al. Markers for EGFR pathway activation as predictor of outcome in metastatic colorectal cancer patients treated with or without cetuximab. *Eur J Cancer*. 2010;46(11):1997–2009.

118 Di Nicolantonio F, Martini M, Molinari F, et al. Wild-type BRAF is required for response to panitumumab or cetuximab in metastatic colorectal cancer. *J Clin Oncol*. 2008;26(35):5705–5712.

119 Richman SD, Seymour MT, Chambers P, et al. KRAS and BRAF mutations in advanced colorectal cancer are associated with poor prognosis but do not preclude benefit from oxaliplatin or irinotecan: results from the MRC FOCUS trial. *J Clin Oncol*. 2009;27(35):5931–5937.

120 Sartore-Bianchi A, Martini M, Molinari F, et al. PIK3CA mutations in colorectal cancer are associated with clinical resistance to EGFR-targeted monoclonal antibodies. *Cancer Res*. 2009;69(5):1851–1857.

121 Perrone F, Lampis A, Orsenigo M, et al. PI3KCA/PTEN deregulation contributes to impaired responses to cetuximab in metastatic colorectal cancer patients. *Ann Oncol*. 2009;20(1):84–90.

122 Laurent-Puig P, Cayre A, Manceau G, et al. Analysis of PTEN, BRAF, and EGFR status in determining benefit from cetuximab therapy in wild-type KRAS metastatic colon cancer. *J Clin Oncol*. 2009;27(35):5924–5930.

123 Samowitz WS, Sweeney C, Herrick J, et al. Poor survival associated with the BRAF V600E mutation in microsatellite-stable colon cancers. *Cancer Res*. 2005;65(14):6063–6069.

124 Souglakos J, Philips J, Wang R, et al. Prognostic and predictive value of common mutations for treatment response and survival in patients with metastatic colorectal cancer. *Br J Cancer*. 2009;101(3):465–472.

125 Prenen H, De Schutter J, Jacobs B, et al. PIK3CA mutations are not a major determinant of resistance to the epidermal growth factor receptor inhibitor cetuximab in metastatic colorectal cancer. *Clin Cancer Res*. 2009;15(9):3184–3188.

126 Jhawer M, Goel S, Wilson AJ, et al. PIK3CA mutation/PTEN expression status predicts response of colon cancer cells to the epidermal growth factor receptor inhibitor cetuximab. *Cancer Res*. 2008;68(6):1953–1961.

127 Razis E, Briasoulis E, Vrettou E, et al. Potential value of PTEN in predicting cetuximab response in colorectal cancer: an exploratory study. *BMC Cancer*. 2008;8:234.

128 Loupakis F, Pollina L, Stasi I, et al. PTEN expression and KRAS mutations on primary tumors and metastases in the prediction of benefit from cetuximab plus irinotecan for patients with metastatic colorectal cancer. *J Clin Oncol*. 2009;27(16):2622–2629.

129 Khambata-Ford S, Garrett CR, Meropol NJ, et al. Expression of epiregulin and amphiregulin and K-ras mutation status predict disease control in metastatic colorectal cancer patients treated with cetuximab. *J Clin Oncol*. 2007;25(22):3230–3237.

130 Jacobs B, De Roock W, Piessevaux H, et al. Amphiregulin and epiregulin mRNA expression in primary tumors predicts outcome in metastatic colorectal cancer treated with cetuximab. *J Clin Oncol*. 2009;27(30):5068–5074.

131 Tabernero J, Cervantes A, Rivera F, et al. Pharmacogenomic and pharmacoproteomic studies of cetuximab in metastatic colorectal cancer: biomarker analysis of a phase I dose-escalation study. *J Clin Oncol*. 2010;28(7):1181–1189.

132 Saridaki Z, Tzardi M, Papadaki C, et al. Impact of KRAS, BRAF, PIK3CA mutations, PTEN, AREG, EREG expression and skin rash in >/ = 2 line cetuximab-based therapy of colorectal cancer patients. *PloS one*. 2011;6(1):e15980.

133 Kuramochi H, Nakajima G, Kaneko Y, et al. Amphiregulin and Epiregulin mRNA expression in primary colorectal cancer and corresponding liver metastases. *BMC Cancer*. 2012;12:88.

134 Rao S, Starling N, Cunningham D, et al. Matuzumab plus epirubicin, cisplatin and capecitabine (ECX) compared with epirubicin, cisplatin and capecitabine alone as first-line treatment in patients with advanced oesophago-gastric cancer: a randomised, multicentre open-label phase II study. *Ann Oncol*. 2010;21(11):2213–2219.

135 Chung KY, Shia J, Kemeny NE, et al. Cetuximab shows activity in colorectal cancer patients with tumors that do not express the epidermal growth factor receptor by immunohistochemistry. *J Clin Oncol*. 2005;23(9):1803–1810.

136 Lenz HJ, Van Cutsem E, Khambata-Ford S, et al. Multicenter phase II and translational study of cetuximab in metastatic colorectal carcinoma refractory to irinotecan, oxaliplatin, and fluoropyrimidines. *J Clin Oncol*. 2006;24(30):4914–4921.

137 Andreyev HJ, Norman AR, Cunningham D, Oates JR, Clarke PA. Kirsten ras mutations in patients with colorectal cancer: the multicenter "RASCAL" study. *J Natl Cancer Inst*. 1998;90(9):675–684.

138 Basso M, Strippoli A, Orlandi A, et al. KRAS mutational status affects oxaliplatin-based chemotherapy independently from basal mRNA ERCC-1 expression in metastatic colorectal cancer patients. *Br J Cancer*. 2013;108(1):115–120.

139 Karnoub AE, Weinberg RA. Ras oncogenes: split personalities. *Nat Rev Mol Cell Biol*. 2008;9(7):517–531.

140 Janakiraman M, Vakiani E, Zeng Z, et al. Genomic and biological characterization of exon 4 KRAS mutations in human cancer. *Cancer Res*. 2010;70(14):5901–5911.

141 Fernandez-Medarde A, Santos E. Ras in cancer and developmental diseases. *Genes Cancer*. 2011;2(3):344–358.

142 Peeters M, Oliner KS, Parker A, et al. Massively parallel tumor multigene sequencing to evaluate response to panitumumab in a randomized phase III study of metastatic colorectal cancer. *Clin Cancer Res*. 2013;19(7):1902–1912.

143 De Roock W, Jonker DJ, Di Nicolantonio F, et al. Association of KRAS p.G13D mutation with outcome in patients with chemotherapy-refractory metastatic colorectal cancer treated with cetuximab. *JAMA*. 2010;304(16):1812–1820.

144 Peeters M, Douillard JY, Van Cutsem E, et al. Mutant KRAS codon 12 and 13 alleles in patients with metastatic colorectal cancer: assessment as prognostic and predictive biomarkers of response to panitumumab. *J Clin Oncol*. 2013;31(6):759–765.

145 Forbes SA, Bindal N, Bamford S, et al. COSMIC: mining complete cancer genomes in the Catalogue of Somatic Mutations in Cancer. *Nucleic Acids Res*. 2011;39:D945–D950.

146 Heinemann V, Fischer von Weikersthal L, Decker T, et al. Randomized comparison of FOLFIRI plus cetuximab versus FOLFIRI plus

bevacizumab as first-line treatment of KRAS wild-type metastatic colorectal cancer: German AIO study KRK-0306 (FIRE-3). *J Clin Oncol.* 2013;31(suppl.): Abstract LBA3506.

147 Stintzing S, Fischer von Weikersthal L, Decker T, et al. FOLFIRI plus cetuximab versus FOLFIRI plus bevacizumab as first-line treatment for patients with metastatic colorectal cancer-subgroup analysis of patients with KRAS: mutated tumours in the randomised German AIO study KRK-0306. *Ann Oncol.* 2012;23(7):1693–1699.

148 Van Cutsem E, Kohne CH, Lang I, et al. Cetuximab plus irinotecan, fluorouracil, and leucovorin as first-line treatment for metastatic colorectal cancer: updated analysis of overall survival according to tumor KRAS and BRAF mutation status. *J Clin Oncol.* 2011;29(15):2011–2019.

149 Ocvirk J, Brodowicz T, Wrba F, et al. Cetuximab plus FOLFOX6 or FOLFIRI in metastatic colorectal cancer: CECOG trial. *World J Gastroenterol.* 2010;16(25):3133–3143.

150 Moosmann N, von Weikersthal LF, Vehling-Kaiser U, et al. Cetuximab plus capecitabine and irinotecan compared with cetuximab plus capecitabine and oxaliplatin as first-line treatment for patients with metastatic colorectal cancer: AIO KRK-0104–a randomized trial of the German AIO CRC study group. *J Clin Oncol.* 2011;29(8):1050–1058.

151 Tejpar S, Celik I, Schlichting M, Sartorius U, Bokemeyer C, Van Cutsem E. Association of KRAS G13D tumor mutations with outcome in patients with metastatic colorectal cancer treated with first-line chemotherapy with or without cetuximab. *J Clin Oncol.* 2012;30(29):3570–3577.

152 Douillard JY, Oliner KS, Siena S, et al. Panitumumab-FOLFOX4 treatment and RAS mutations in colorectal cancer. *N Engl J Med.* 2013;369(11):1023–1034.

153 Tie J, Gibbs P, Lipton L, et al. Optimizing targeted therapeutic development: analysis of a colorectal cancer patient population with the BRAF(V600E) mutation. *Int J Cancer.* 2011;128(9):2075–2084.

154 Mao C, Liao RY, Qiu LX, Wang XW, Ding H, Chen Q. BRAF V600E mutation and resistance to anti-EGFR monoclonal antibodies in patients with metastatic colorectal cancer: a meta-analysis. *Mol Biol Rep.* 2011;38(4):2219–2223.

155 De Roock W, De Vriendt V, Normanno N, Ciardiello F, Tejpar S. KRAS, BRAF, PIK3CA, and PTEN mutations: implications for targeted therapies in metastatic colorectal cancer. *Lancet Oncol.* 2011;12(6):594–603.

156 Sood A, McClain D, Maitra R, et al. PTEN gene expression and mutations in the PIK3CA gene as predictors of clinical benefit to anti-epidermal growth factor receptor antibody therapy in patients with KRAS wild-type metastatic colorectal cancer. *Clin Colorectal Cancer.* 2012;11(2):143–150.

157 Mao C, Liao RY, Chen Q. Loss of PTEN expression predicts resistance to EGFR-targeted monoclonal antibodies in patients with metastatic colorectal cancer. *Br J Cancer.* 2010;102(5):940.

158 Di Fiore F, Sesboue R, Michel P, Sabourin JC, Frebourg T. Molecular determinants of anti-EGFR sensitivity and resistance in metastatic colorectal cancer. *Br J Cancer.* 2010;103(12):1765–1772.

159 Heinemann V, Stintzing S, Kirchner T, Boeck S, Jung A. Clinical relevance of EGFR- and KRAS-status in colorectal cancer patients treated with monoclonal antibodies directed against the EGFR. *Cancer Treat Rev.* 2009;35(3):262–271.

160 Kabbinavar F, Hurwitz HI, Fehrenbacher L, et al. Phase II, randomized trial comparing bevacizumab plus fluorouracil (FU)/leucovorin (LV) with FU/LV alone in patients with metastatic colorectal cancer. *J Clin Oncol.* 2003;21(1):60–65.

161 Gerber HP, Ferrara N. Pharmacology and pharmacodynamics of bevacizumab as monotherapy or in combination with cytotoxic therapy in preclinical studies. *Cancer Res.* 2005;65(3):671–680.

162 Presta LG, Chen H, O'Connor SJ, et al. Humanization of an anti-vascular endothelial growth factor monoclonal antibody for the therapy of solid tumors and other disorders. *CancerRes.* 1997;57(20):4593–4599.

163 Giantonio BJ, Catalano PJ, Meropol NJ, et al.; Eastern Cooperative Oncology Group Study E3200. Bevacizumab in combination with oxaliplatin, fluorouracil, and leucovorin (FOLFOX4) for previously treated metastatic colorectal cancer: results from the Eastern Cooperative Oncology Group Study E3200. *J Clin Oncol.* 2007;25(12):1539–1544.

164 Allegra CJ, Yothers G, O'Connell MJ, et al. Initial safety report of NSABP C-08: A randomized phase III study of modified FOLFOX6 with or without bevacizumab for the adjuvant treatment of patients with stage II or III colon cancer. *J Clin Oncol.* 2009;27:3385–3390.

165 Cunningham D, Lang I, Marcuello E, et al. Bevacizumab plus capecitabine versus capecitabine alone in elderly patients with previously untreated metastatic colorectal cancer (AVEX): an open-label, randomised phase 3 trial. *Lancet Oncol.* 2013;14(11):1077–1085.

166 Saltz LB, Clarke S, Diaz-Rubio E, et al. Bevacizumab in combination with oxaliplatin-based chemotherapy as first-line therapy in metastatic colorectal cancer: a randomized phase III study. *J Clin Oncol.* 2008;26(12):2013–2019.

167 Bennouna J, Sastre J, Arnold D, et al.; ML18147 Study Investigators. Continuation of bevacizumab after first progression in metastatic colorectal cancer (ML18147): a randomised phase 3 trial. *Lancet Oncol.* 2013;14(1):29–37.

168 Lockhart AC, Rothenberg ML, Dupont J, et al. Phase I study of intravenous vascular endothelial growth factor trap, aflibercept, in patients with advanced solid tumors. *J Clin Oncol.* 2010;28(2):207–214.

169 de Groot JF, Lamborn KR, Chang SM, et al. Phase II study of aflibercept in recurrent malignant glioma: a North American Brain Tumor Consortium study. *J Clin Oncol.* 2011;29(19):2689–2695.

170 Van Cutsem E, Tabernero J, Lakomy R, et al. Addition of aflibercept to fluorouracil, leucovorin, and irinotecan improves survival in a phase III randomized trial in patients with metastatic colorectal cancer previously treated with an oxaliplatin-based regimen. *J Clin Oncol.* 2012;30(28):3499–3506.

171 Chu E. An update on the current and emerging targeted agents in metastatic colorectal cancer. *Clin Colorectal Cancer.* 2012;11(1):1–13.

172 Wilhelm SM, Dumas J, Adnane L, et al. Regorafenib (BAY 73–4506): a new oral multikinase inhibitor of angiogenic, stromal and oncogenic receptor tyrosine kinases with potent preclinical antitumor activity. *Int J Cancer.* 2011;129(1):245–255.

173 Strumberg D, Scheulen ME, Schultheis B, et al. Regorafenib (BAY 73–4506) in advanced colorectal cancer: a phase I study. *Br J Cancer.* 2012;106(11):1722–1727.

174 Grothey A, Van Cutsem E, Sobrero A, et al.; CORRECT Study Group. Regorafenib monotherapy for previously treated metastatic colorectal cancer (CORRECT): an international, multicentre, randomised, placebo-controlled, phase 3 trial. *Lancet.* 2013;381(9863):303–312.

175 Kopetz S, Chang GJ, Overman MJ, et al. Improved survival in metastatic colorectal cancer is associated with adoption of hepatic resection and improved chemotherapy. *J Clin Oncol.* 2009;27(22):3677–3683.

176 Bagg A, Kallakury BV. Molecular pathology of leukemia and lymphoma. *Am J Clin Pathol.* 1999;112:S76–S92.

# CHAPTER 21

# Endometrial Cancer

*Jessica L. Bowser[1], Russell R. Broaddus[1], Robert L. Coleman[2,3], and Shannon N. Westin[2]*

[1]Department of Pathology, The University of Texas MD Anderson Cancer Center, Houston, TX, USA

[2]Department of Gynecologic Oncology and Reproductive Medicine, The University of Texas MD Anderson Cancer Center Houston, TX, USA

[3]Center for RNA Interference and Non-Coding RNA, The University of Texas MD Anderson Cancer Center Houston, TX, USA

## Endometrial Cancer

Endometrial cancer is the most common gynecologic malignancy and the fourth most common cancer diagnosis in women.[1] The incidence of endometrial cancer has continued to increase over the past decade. This rise has been attributed to the current obesity epidemic, as obesity, diabetes, and insulin resistance are strongly associated with endometrial cancer.[2] Approximately 72% of endometrial cancer cases are diagnosed at early stage (stages I, II), whereas regional disease (stage III) occurs in 20% and distant disease (stage IV) in 8% of cases.[3] For women diagnosed with early-stage disease, the prognosis is favorable and surgery alone or in combination with local therapy is generally curative. Five-year survival rates for stage I and stage II disease are 97% and more than 80%, respectively.[4] However, the prognosis for patients with advanced or recurrent disease is quite poor; thus, need for novel therapies in this population is great.

Similarities in histology, clinical, and molecular characteristics have led to the sub-classification of endometrial cancers. Endometrioid type is the most common (80%) and is strongly associated with the presence of exogenous and endogenous unopposed estrogen and may arise from complex atypical hyperplasia.[5] The non-endometrioid type includes serous, clear cell, and carcinosarcoma histologies. This aggressive type represents the minority of endometrial cancer cases (20%); however, it accounts for a large portion of endometrial cancer mortalities.[6] Non-endometrioid carcinomas occur in older women, are unrelated to estrogen, and may be associated with endometrial intraepithelial carcinoma (EIC) as a precursor lesion.[5]

## Molecular Alterations in Endometrial Cancer

The molecular alterations found in endometrial cancers generally coincide with the histologic subtype. Table 21.1 summarizes the known molecular alterations among endometrioid and non-endometrioid tumors. The most common molecular alteration in endometrial carcinomas is the loss of tumor suppressor PTEN, occurring in approximately 80% of endometrioid carcinomas.[7] PTEN is a phosphatase widely known for its role in opposing PI3K activity by mediating the dephosphylation of $PIP_3$ to $PIP_2$, which normally inhibits AKT signaling, but also has involvement in cell cycle arrest and proapoptotic responses.[8] In endometrial cancer, PTEN loss occurs primarily by mutation.[9] Other common alterations affecting the activity of PI3K include activating mutations in $PIK3CA$,[10] and $PIK3R1$.[11] Microsatellite instability (MSI),[12] IGF-1R overexpression,[13] and mutations in $K$-$Ras$,[14] $FGFR2$,[15] and $CTNNB1$ (β-catenin),[16] are also commonly found in endometrioid carcinomas. In endometrioid carcinomas, $PI3K$ pathway mutations, $K$-$Ras$ mutations, and MSI often coexist, whereas mutations in $CTNNB1$ usually occur alone. In contrast to endometrioid carcinomas, non-endometrioid carcinomas frequently show alterations, including $p53$ mutations,[17] inactivation of cyclin-dependent kinase inhibitor 2A ($CDKN2A$, p16),[18] and E-cadherin,[19] as well as amplification and overexpression of human epidermal growth factor receptor 2 (ErbB-2, HER2),[20] and chromosomal instability.[21]

## Opportunities for Targeted Therapy in Endometrial Cancer

Although the majority of endometrial cancers present at early stage and are effectively cured by surgery with or without adjuvant radiotherapy, approximately 15–20% of these cases will recur and have limited response to therapy. Current therapy approaches include hormone therapy, radiation, and chemotherapy. Great effort has gone into improving clinical responses by using combination approaches with these modalities. Response rates, however, have only been modest and efficacy of second-line therapy is considerably limited. Moreover, progression-free survival (median, 6–14 months) and overall survival (median, 12 months) for women with advanced stage or recurrent endometrial cancer has not significantly improved despite years of investigation.[22]

The use of agents that target the molecular alterations in tumor cells has been a major advance in the treatment of cancer. This surge has been the result of important advances made in understanding the molecular alterations that are important to cancer cell growth and survival. The attractiveness of targeted agents is their potential to be more selective against cancer cells compared to conventional chemotherapy. Such specificity may provide less toxicity to patients and, in some cases, improved benefit over conventional chemotherapy. The use of targeted therapy in endometrial cancer has lagged

*Targeted Therapy in Translational Cancer Research*, First Edition. Edited by Apostolia-Maria Tsimberidou, Razelle Kurzrock and Kenneth C. Anderson.
© 2016 John Wiley & Sons, Inc. Published 2016 by John Wiley & Sons, Inc.

**Table 21.1** Molecular alterations in endometrial cancer.

| Alterations | Endometrioid (%) | Non-endometrioid (%) |
|---|---|---|
| PIK3CA mutation | 30–40 | 20 |
| PIK3CA amplification | 2–4 | 46 |
| PIK3R1 mutation | 43 | 12 |
| K-Ras mutation | 10–30 | 0–10 |
| AKT mutation | 2–3 | 0 |
| PTEN mutation | 30–50 | 0–11 |
| PTEN loss of function | 80 | 5 |
| E-cadherin loss | 5–50 | 60–90 |
| P53 mutation | 20 | 90 |
| EGFR overexpression | 46 | 34 |
| HER2 overexpression | 3–10 | 32 |
| HER2 amplification | 1 | 17 |
| IGF-1R overexpression | 78 | – |
| FGFR2 mutation | 12–16 | 1 |
| CTNNB1 mutation | 16–45 | 0 |
| Microsatellite instability | 15–25 | 0–5 |

PIK3CA, phosphalidylinosilol 3 kinase, catalytic, a polypeptide; PIK3RI, phosphatidylinositol 3 kinase regulatory polypeptide; K-Ras, V-Ki-ras2 Kirsten rat sarcoma viral oncogene homolog; AKT, v-akt murine thymoma viral oncogene homolog 1; PTEN. phosphatase and tensin homolog deleted on chromosome 10; EGFR, epidermal growth factor receptor HER2, epidermal growth factor 2 receptor IGF-1R, insulin-like growth factor 1 receptor; FGFR2, fibroblast growth factor receptor 2.

far behind that of other common cancers in light of the growing understanding of the molecular alterations in this disease.

## Molecular Pathways of Therapeutic Interest in Endometrial Cancer

Given the myriad of molecular alterations in endometrial cancer, there is a real opportunity for targeted therapies to become mainstay treatment for patients with advanced or recurrent stage disease. The pathways and molecular targets discussed in this chapter represent those that are the most developed for targeted therapy in endometrial cancer, including the PI3K/AKT and Ras/Raf/MEK pathways, RTKs, EGFR and HER2, and VEGFR. A schematic of these relevant pathways and targets in endometrial cancer is represented in Figure 21.1. Additionally, the benefit of exploiting PARP inhibitors and the use of metformin in endometrial cancer is discussed along with brief discussion on targeting challenging yet prevalent molecular alterations of p53 and E-cadherin.

## PI3K/PTEN/AKT/mTOR

The constitutive activation of the PI3K/AKT pathway in endometrial cancer occurs at many levels and includes activating mutations in PI3K catalytic and regulatory subunits genes, PIK3CA, PIK3R1, and PIK3R2, activating mutations in AKT1, PTEN loss of function, and receptor tyrosine kinase (RTK) amplification. PTEN loss of function and activating PIK3CA mutations are the most common events in endometrial cancer and a considerable frequency of coexisting PTEN and PIK3CA mutations is seen.[10] An important node in the PI3K/AKT pathway is the mammalian target of rapamycin (mTOR). mTOR is an atypical serine/threonine kinase and member of the phosphoinositide3-kinase (PI3K)-related kinase family. mTOR interacts with several proteins to form two distinct com-

plexes, mTORC1 and mTORC2, which differ in their activation of further downstream effectors.[23] A myriad of preclinical studies have provided evidence for mTOR activity in endometrial cancer following PTEN loss of function or PIK3CA mutation, and accordingly, have supported the potential clinical benefit of rapalogs and PI3K or AKT inhibitors.[24] Additionally, compelling associations between PTEN loss, mTOR activity, and inactivation of mTOR translational inhibitor, 4EBP1, are seen in human endometrial cancer.[25] Hence, targeting the PI3K/AKT pathway via the mTOR node is the subject of many recent and ongoing clinical trials in endometrial cancer.

Preliminary results and those from recently completed early phase trials evaluating the mTORC1 inhibitors, everolimus,[26] ridaforlimus,[27–29] and temsirolimus,[30, 31] as single agents in endometrial cancer have been reported. Clinical response rates have been modest, but encouraging; temsirolimus has shown the most promise. Responses in chemotherapy naïve patients were 14% and 69% for partial response (PR) and stable disease (SD), respectively.[31] A less dramatic benefit of 4% PR and 28% SD occurred in patients with one prior chemotherapy.[31] With all rapalogs, chemotherapy naïve patients tend to fare better. Chemotherapy naïve patients that received ridaforlimus achieved PR and SD rates of 7.7% and 58%, respectively.[32] However, these rates dropped to 7% PR and 26% SD in patients with prior treatment.[27]

While the data from these studies and others show promise for the use of rapalogs in endometrial cancer, they have fallen short of the high expectations held for such a frequently altered pathway. The limited efficacy of single-agent rapalogs may be related, in part, to the activation of feedback pathways resulting from the inhibition of mTORC1. One possibility is that the negative regulation of mTORC2 by mTORC1 via S6K is relieved by rapalogs allowing for mTORC2-mediated AKT activation.[33] Another possibility is the relief of autoinhibitory pathways controlled by mTORC1 that inhibit activation of RTKs, which subsequently act to induce PI3K/AKT pathway activity.[34] In addition, mTORC1 activation of S6K in normal cells abrogates insulin growth factor receptor (IGF-R)-mediated activity of PI3K by causing the degradation of IGF-R docking protein, insulin receptor substate-1 (IRS-1).[35] Accordingly, treatment of cancer cells with rapamycin or rapalogs is shown to cause the loss of this autoinhibitory pathway on IGF-R signaling, leading to PI3K activation and counteracting the anti-tumor response.[34] Other potential causes for low efficacy with rapalogs include the PI3K-dependent activation of the Ras/Raf/MEK pathway, and the general observation that rapalogs are cytostatic rather than cytotoxic in animal models and human cancers.[36]

Given these issues, there is a great enthusiasm for agents that target multiple PI3K/AKT pathway nodes. Studies are currently underway evaluating the efficacy of inhibitors which effectively inhibit both mTORC1 and mTORC2 or mTOR and other PI3K pathway targets. The combination of rapalogs and chemotherapy agents, cisplatin or paclitaxel, in endometrial cells has shown synergistic effects.[37] As a result, everolimus, ridaforolimus, and temsirolimus are being evaluated in combination with different chemotherapy agents in the upfront and recurrent endometrial cancer settings.

Along with mTOR, other PI3K/AKT pathway nodes are being explored in early phase studies in endometrial cancer and include inhibitors directed at AKT and PI3K. As with rapalogs, there is reason to believe that PI3K or AKT as single agents will potentially activate feedback pathways that diminish clinical response rates. In vitro studies and animal models have shown AKT inhibition to increase the expression and phosphorylation of RTKs,

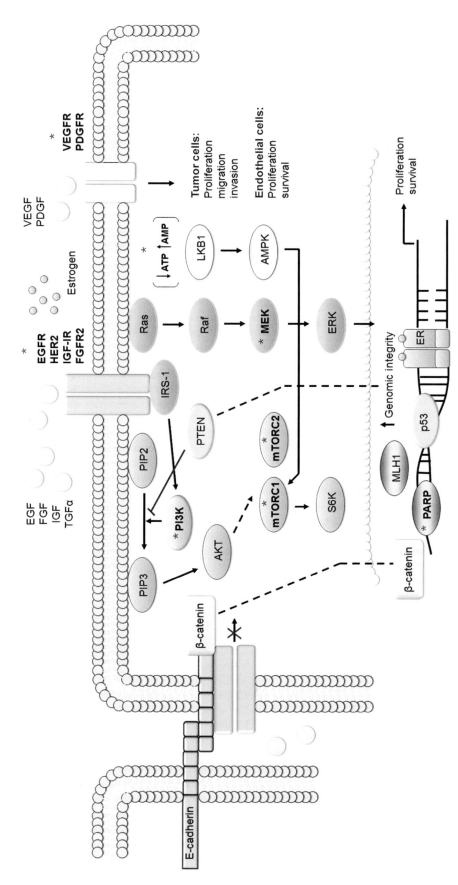

**Figure 21.1** Relevant pathways and druggable targets in endometrial cancer. Abbreviations: PIP2, phosphatidylinositol 4,5-bisphosphate; PIP3, phosphatidylinositol 3,4,5-triphosphate; PI3K, phosphatidylinositol 3 kinase; PTEN, phosphatase and tensin homolog deleted on chromosome 10; AKT, v-akt murine thymoma viral oncogene homolog 1; mTORC1, mammalian target of rapamycin complex 1; mTORC2, mammalian target of rapamycin complex 2; S6K, ribosomal protein S6kinase beta-1; Ras, rat sarcoma gene; Raf, v-raf-1 murine leukemia viral oncogene homolog 1; MEK, mitogen activated protein kinase kinase; ERK, mitogen activated protein kinase; IRS-1, insulin receptor substrate 1; LKB1, liver kinase B1; AMPK, adenosine monophosphate kinase; ATP, adenosine triphosphate; AMP, adenosine, monophosphate; EGFR, epidermal growth factor receptor; HER2, epidermal growth factor 2 receptor; IGF-1R, insulin-like growth factor 1 receptor; FGFR2, fibroblast growth factor receptor 2; VEGFR, vascular endothelial growth factor receptor; PDGFR, platelet-derived growth factor receptor; EGF, epidermal growth factor; FGF, fibroblast growth factor; IGF, insulin-like growth factor; TGFα, transforming growth factor α; VEGF, vascular endothelial growth factor; PDGF, platelet-derived growth factor; MLH1, mutL homolog 1; PARP, poly ADP-ribose polymerase; ER, estrogen receptor. Asterisks indicate druggable targets that have been or are currently being evaluated in clinical trials for the treatment of endometrial cancer. Highly prevalent alterations, such as p53 and E-cadherin, remain major obstacles for conventional drug design.

HER3 and IGF-R1, and insulin receptor (IR).[38] The AKT-mediated increase of RTK expression is shown to be independent of mTORC1 activity.[38]

For the most part, ongoing clinical trials evaluating AKT or PI3K inhibitors in endometrial cancer are being examined as single agents. Consistent with the idea of greater benefit with combination strategies, there are accumulating data that strongly indicate that cancer cells survive chemotherapy treatment by activating the PI3K/AKT pathway.[39] Likewise, it is shown that the cytotoxic effects of chemotherapy agents on various cancer cell types are strongly correlated to reduced activity of AKT.[39] Similar results have been reported in endometrial cancer cells treated with cisplatin and pacitaxel,[40] which are among the most active chemotherapy agents in this disease.[41] Additional studies have reported high levels of AKT2 and AKT3 in endometrial cancer cells which are resistant to cisplatin.[42] Accordingly, the cisplatin resistance of these cells was overcome following siRNA knockdown of AKT2 and AKT3.[42] Though these studies represent only initial observations, it is possible that the use of AKT and/or PI3K inhibitors in patients resistant to chemotherapy may provide benefit given this chemotherapy-induced PI3K/AKT-mediated survival response. Such an approach would be irrespective of the common assumption that patients will only benefit from PI3K/AKT/mTOR inhibitors based on the molecular profile of their tumor. Interestingly, this may provide an alternative rationale for responses seen in early rapalog studies, as no associations were seen between the molecular status of the primary tumor and clinical response when *PTEN* mutation, PTEN loss, or phosphorylation of mTOR, AKT, or S6K were assessed.[31,43,44]

## Ras/Raf/MEK—Mitogen-Activated Protein Kinase

Raf and MEK are two pivotal kinases of the mitogen-activated protein kinase (MAPK) pathway. The upstream GTPase, Ras, serves as a link between cell surface signaling and Raf/MEK activation of downstream extracellular signal-related kinases (ERKs).[45] Activating mutations in *K-Ras* are relatively frequent in endometrial cancer, occurring in 10–30% of endometrioid cases.[46] *K-Ras* mutations are also seen in 6–16% of endometrial atypical hyperplasia and thus, are considered one of the earliest molecular events in endometrial cancer.[47] *H-Ras* mutations have been reported in approximately 7% of endometrial carcinomas.[48] Mutations of other primary Ras/Raf/MEK nodes, such as *B-Raf*, are rare.

Due to the frequency of Ras mutations in many cancer types, Ras emerged as a major target of interest for the development of novel anti-cancer agents. This enthusiasm, however, has declined in recent years as attempts targeting Ras proteins, specifically the use of farnesyltransferase inhibitors (FTIs), have failed in show clinical benefit in Ras mutant tumors.[49] Recently, studies using endometrial cancer cell lines have shown that two FDA-approved drugs, metformin, a drug used for treatment of diabetes mellitus, and fendiline, a now-clinically obsolete L-type calcium channel blocker, displace K-Ras from the membrane. Metformin, which is discussed later in this chapter and is currently in early phase trials, decreased tumor growth in xenograft models of endometrial cancer, with the greatest response being observed in mutant K-Ras cells.[50] Accordingly, treatment of K-Ras mutant cells with metformin resulted in the displacement of K-Ras from the plasma membrane, which subsequently uncoupled MAPK signaling.[50] Similarly, fendiline was found to displace K-Ras from the membrane and inhibit K-Ras signaling.[51] Consistent with this, fendiline significantly inhibited the proliferation of endometrial, pancreatic, colon, and lung cancer cell lines expressing mutant K-Ras.[51] How metformin displaces K-Ras is not currently known. However, the effects of fendiline on K-Ras displacement are found to be independent of the prenylation process.[51] This finding has been exciting and merits further consideration as an anti-Ras therapy.

Given that targeting Ras has been widely unsuccessful, strategies for targeting Ras/Raf/MEK signaling have moved to downstream targets, Raf and MEK. The Gynecologic Oncology Group (GOG) recently reported on a Phase II trial of AZD6244, a selective MEK1/2 inhibitor, in recurrent endometrial cancer. Results were modest, achieving an objective response rate of 6% and a stable disease rate of 26%.[52] There is potential to improve on this modest activity by moving MEK inhibition earlier in the disease process and in combination with cytotoxic chemotherapy.

Combination approaches of MEK and PI3K/AKT inhibitors have gained clinical interest given that AKT or mTOR inhibition results in Ras/Raf/MEK activity and due to the high frequency of coexisting *K-Ras* mutations and PI3K/AKT pathway mutations in cancer cells. Activation of Ras/Raf/MEK following mTOR inhibition involves IRS-1 and its activation of PI3K, which leads to PI3K activation of Ras and ERK activity.[53] The presence of such a feedback loop has been supported by the findings of ERK activity in prostate cancer animal models and biopsies of advanced cancer patients receiving everolimus.[53] In endometrial cancer, *K-Ras* mutations are found to coexist with mutations in *PTEN*, *PIK3CA*, and *PIK3R1*, suggesting that *K-Ras* mutations are not functionally redundant.[54] Accordingly, functional synergy has been seen between mutant *K-Ras* and mutant *PIK3CA* in transformed HMLE cells.[55] In cancer cells, *K-Ras* mutations segregate with reduced sensitivity to the mTOR inhibitor, everolimus,[56] and dual PI3K/mTOR inhibitor, NVP-BEZ23[57]; and in a conditional mouse model of endometrial cancer, which PTEN was ablated and K-Ras activated, tumor development was accelerated as compared to mice with only a single gene alteration.[58] Thus, K-Ras down-stream targets, such as Raf and RalGDS, provide a "workaround" in tumorigenesis in the presence of PI3K pathway blockade. These results and others have strongly supported that the combined use of PI3K/AKT/mTOR and Ras/Raf/MEK pathway inhibitors are more likely to provide greater clinical benefit than targeting either pathway alone, as well as, identifying patients who may be best matched for specific therapy or combination of therapies. Indeed, preliminary results have shown that in most endometrial cancer cell lines, a synergistic inhibition of cell growth is observed when a MEK inhibitor (GDC-097) is combined with either an AKT inhibitor (GDC-0068) or a PI3K inhibitor (GDC-0941).[59] Moreover, in a recent study, the combined use of MEK inhibitors, PD98059 or UO126, were shown to sensitize K-Ras mutant endometrial cancer cells to NVP-BEZ235.[60] Accordingly, the GOG has recently activated a trial of trametinib (MEK inhibitor) alone or in combination with GSK2141795 (AKT inhibitor; NCT 01935973).

## Receptor Tyrosine Kinases

The constitutive activation of PI3K/AKT and Ras/Raf/MEK pathways occurs at various nodal levels in endometrial cancer. In addition to mutations in resident kinases, these pathways can also be driven by growth factor stimulation of overexpressed RTKs or by activating mutations in RTKs. RTKs of therapeutic interest in endometrial cancer include epidermal growth factor receptor 1 (EGFR; ErbB-1; HER1) and 2 (ErbB-2; HER2), IGF-1R, and fibroblast growth factor receptor 2 (FGFR2). Activity of these RTKs in cancer cells results in a wide range of events, including proliferation, avoidance of apoptosis, migration and invasion, therapy resistance, and tumor angiogenesis.

## EGFR and HER2

EGFR (ErbB-1; HER1) and HER2 (ErbB-2) are two members of the epidermal growth factor receptor family that also includes the receptors HER3 (ErbB-3) and HER4 (ErbB-4). EGFR ligands, such as epidermal growth factor (EGF), transforming growth factor-α (TGF-α), and amphiregulin, bind EGFR and cause receptor dimerization and subsequent autophosphorylation, leading to downstream kinase activity. Overexpression of EGFR occurs in approximately 60% of endometrial cancers and is unrelated to a specific histotype. Amphiregulin and TGF-α are also reported to be overexpressed in endometrial cancer.[61]

Despite considerable activity of EGFR inhibition in other cancer types, studies evaluating tyrosine kinase inhibitors of EGFR, erlotinib,[62] or gefitinib[63] in patients with recurrent and/or advanced endometrial cancer have been disappointing. Erlotinib has shown the most promising results with 12.5% PR and 47% SD rates in chemotherapy naïve patients.[62] Response rates for patients who have received 1–2 prior regimens treated with gefitinib were low with 3% complete response (CR) and 24% SD.[63] Similar low response rates, 5% PR and 10% SD, were reported with cetuximab, a humanized monoclonal antibody to EGFR, in endometrial cancer patients who had received prior chemotherapy treatment.[64] This low efficacy may be explained by what is known about anti-EGFR therapies in cancer types which benefit the most from these inhibitors. Clinical studies in non-small cell lung cancer have shown EGFR overexpression alone is not sufficient for predicting response to EGFR inhibitors and the response to EGFR therapies is strongly related to sensitizing *EGFR* mutations, *EGFR* amplification, PTEN expression, and absence of *K-Ras* mutations.[65] Studies in colon cancer also show PTEN loss of function[66] and *K-Ras* mutations[67] to be strongly related to the lack of clinical response to anti-EGFR therapy. The frequency of mutations in *EGFR* in endometrial cancer has not been explored in detail, but in limited phase II trials of EGFR inhibitors among women with recurrent, previously treated endometrial cancers, the frequency was between 5 and 10% in exons 18–21.[63,68] In serous carcinomas[69] and carcinosarcomas[70] *EGFR* mutations are rare. In a clinical study evaluating gefitinib in endometrial cancer patients, no correlations were found between *EGFR* mutation, EGFR expression, phosphorylation of EGFR, or phosphorylation of ERK and patient response.[63]

HER2 overexpression and amplification is commonly seen among non-endometrioid cancers of serous histology.[20] Results of a study of the HER2 humanized antibody, trustuzumab, in recurrent and advanced stage endometrial cancer patients were disappointing, despite inclusion criteria including only patients whose tumors overexpressed or had amplified *HER2*. A 40% SD rate was seen, but no clinical responses were reported.[71] Similarly, a study evaluating lapatinib, a dual tyrosine kinase inhibitor of EGFR and HER2, had only one response (PR, 3%). Interestingly, this patient had a mutation in exon 18, E690 K of *EGFR* indicating potential benefit in selected cases.[68] The combination of trastuzumab and chemotherapy agents has proven to be superior to chemotherapy alone in patients with metastatic breast cancer that overexpressed or has amplified HER2.[72] A clinical study is underway in recurrent and advanced stage serous endometrial cancers which will evaluate the benefit of paclitaxel and carboplatin with or without the addition of trustuzumab in patients with tumors overexpressing or having amplified *HER2* (NCT01367002).

## IGF-1R

IGF-1R belongs to a family of RTKs which include the insulin receptor and insulin-like growth factor 2 receptor (IGF-2R). IGF-1R is overexpressed in endometrial cancer, as well as the endometrioid precursor lesion, atypical hyperplasia. IGF-1R ligands, insulin-like growth factor-1 (IGF-1), IGF-2, and insulin act as powerful mitogens that activate both PI3K/AKT and Ras/Raf/MEK pathways. In contrast to HER2, high levels of IGF-1R alone do not trigger its activation, and gene amplification or activating mutations for IGF-1R are considerably rare. Clinical and epidemiological evidence shows an association between circulating insulin and/or IGF-1 levels and poor prognosis, providing the reasoning for IGF-1R targeting in many cancer types, especially those related to obesity.

Humanized antibodies, including cixutumumab and ganitumab, and small molecules intended on inhibiting the tyrosine kinase activity of the receptor have been developed for IGF-1R. *In vitro* studies of endometrial cancer cells have shown cixutumumab[73] and ganitumab[74] to inhibit proliferation and disrupt both PI3K/AKT and Ras/Raf/MEK signaling. Additional studies have shown similar findings in endometrial cancer cells with NVP-AEW541, an inhibitor of IGF-1R tyrosine kinase activity, as both PI3K/AKT and Ras/Raf/MEK signaling pathways were inactivated.[75] These results, combined with the fact that IGF-1R is induced after treatment with PI3K/AKT/mTOR inhibitors, provide rationale to explore the combination of IGF-1R and mTOR inhibitors in endometrial cancer. Dual targeting of the IGF and PI3K axes is currently under clinical investigation in solid tumors (NCT01243762, NCT01234857). Endometrial cancer patients may additionally benefit from IGF-1R inhibitors given that there is a substantial interplay between IGF and estrogen signaling, and that estrogen receptor α (ERα) plays a key role in increasing IGF-1R expression.

## FGFR2

Like IGF-1R, FGFR2 represents an emerging target in endometrial cancer. FGFR2 is one of the four members of the fibroblast growth factor receptor family including FGFR1, FGFR3, and FGFR4. FGFRs have important roles in cancer cell proliferation, migration, and survival as well as angiogenesis.[76] Activating *FGFR2* mutations are found most often in endometrial cancers that are endometrioid histology (16%) and appear to be mutually exclusive with *K-Ras* mutations, whereas *FGFR2* mutations occur in the presence of PTEN loss of function.[77] *In vitro* studies have shown that endometrial cancer cells with activating *FGFR2* mutations are selectively sensitive to pan-FGFR inhibitors, and that this sensitivity is independent of mutations that are ligand-dependent or ligand-independent.[78] Further, loss of PTEN function in endometrial cancer cells does not affect the sensitivity of the cells to FGFR2 inhibitors.[77] Based on these studies, there is strong reason to believe that targeting FGFR2 may be beneficial. Several clinical studies are underway to evaluate FGFR2 inhibitors in endometrial cancer patients including cedirinib (NCT01132820),[79] an inhibitor of VEGFR2, VEGFR3, PDGFR, and FGFR2; brivanib (NCT00888173),[80] a dual inhibitor of VEGFR2 and FGFR2, and FP-1039 (NCT01244438),[81] a soluble fusion protein that binds FGF ligands. Further, a trial using dovitinib, an FGFR3-inhibitor, in endometrial cancer which stratifies for FGFR2 mutation prior to treatment is ongoing (NCT01379534).

## Vascular Endothelial Growth Factor

Vascular Endothelial Growth Factor (VEGF) is most associated with tumor angiogenesis, a hallmark of tumorigenesis in which the tumor generates dysfunctional yet adequate vasculature by stimulating endothelial cell proliferation.[82] In addition to endothelial cells, stromal, tumor, and immune progenitor cells of the microenvironment also express functional VEGF receptors and benefit from VEGF synthesis and release. VEGF activity on tumor cells leads to proliferation, survival, and metastasis, which is predominantly, but not exclusively, related to angiogenesis.[83] Thus, targeting VEGF and/or VEGFRs may provide added benefit in addition to its impact on tumor angiogenesis.

In endometrial cancer, VEGFR expression is correlated with microvessel density and endothelial cell proliferation and is associated with poor prognostic factors, such as vascular invasion, and poor overall survival.[84,85] Accordingly, in orthotopic mouse models using patient samples or endometrial carcinoma cell lines, bevacizumab, a humanized monoclonal antibody targeting VEGF-A, markedly reduced tumor size.[85] Approaches to target VEGF activity include humanized monoclonal antibodies to VEGF or VEGFRs, soluble decoy VEGF receptors, and small molecule tyrosine kinase inhibitors to VEGFRs. Several early phase studies evaluating bevacizumab,[86] suntinib,[87] or sorafenib[88] as single agents in patients with recurrent and/or advanced endometrial cancer have been completed or have reported early results. Bevacizumab has been the most successful, with 2% CR, 11.5% PR, and 40.4% SD reported in pretreated patients.[86] A recent trial evaluating aflibercept (VEGF-Trap), a fusion protein that serves as a decoy receptor for VEGF isoforms, in endometrial cancer patients who have received prior therapy has shown beneficial effects with 7% PR and 32% SD.[89] However, significant toxicity was seen in this study, and the authors caution that dose and schedule should be carefully considered prior to the future development of VEGF-Trap therapy in this patient population.[89]

Recently, inhibition of VEGF/VEGFR signaling in xenograft models of endometrial cancer was studied, which aimed to identify molecular markers of sensitivity or resistance to bevacizumab.[90] The downregulation of Rho-Type GTPase-Activating Protein 6 (ARHGAP6) and MMP15 transcripts indicated sensitivity to bevacizumab, whereas inhibition of PKCδ- or S6K-dependent signaling and upregulation of TNFRS4 or MMP13 and MMP14 mark a developing resistance to bevacizumab therapy. The activation of oncogene, c-Jun in bevacizumab-treated tumors also suggests that c-Jun-mediated pathways may contribute to bevacizumab resistance in endometrial cancer.[90] Given the need of identifying biomarkers that predict response, it would be interesting to examine these newly identified markers in tissues of patients receiving anti-VEGF therapy.

Like other targeted therapies, a growing amount of data have indicated added benefit from combining VEGFR targeted approaches with chemotherapy, even in situations where VEGFR inhibiting agents had low activity as a single agent. The principle behind this approach is based on the study by Klement et al. which demonstrated that in combination with low dose chemotherapy, a VEGFR antibody induced sustained tumor regression.[91] With this combination it was found that chemotherapy inhibited the proliferation of endothelial cells, while the VEGFR antibody diminished survival signaling.[91] Consistent with this, *in vivo* models of endome-

trial cancer show that the combination of anti-vascular therapy and chemotherapy is highly effective.[85] A clinical study is currently underway in patients with endometrial cancer combining of bevacizumab with cisplatin (NCT01005329).

## Poly (ADP-Ribose) Polymerase

Poly (ADP-Ribose) Polymerase (PARP) enzymes are nuclear enzymes that facilitate DNA repair by recognizing and binding single-strand breaks (SSB) and synthesizing pol(ADP-ribose) polymers. When unrepaired, SSB can lead to double-strand breaks (DSB) and cell death following replication. Accordingly, PARP inhibitors have shown to be particularly beneficial in patients with hereditary breast and ovarian cancer syndrome related to *BRCA* mutation, a gene involved in homologous recombination (HR) and subsequent DSB repair.[92] The hypersensitivity of this patient population is considered to be the result of SSB accumulation, due to PARP inhibition, and defective HR and DSB repair, due to *BRCA* mutation.[93] A recent study, however, has indicated a critical role of non-homologous end joining (NHEJ), a second mechanism of DSB repair, in the hypersensitivity of cells to PARP inhibitors.[94] Accordingly, PARP inhibition enhances error-prone NHEJ activity, by releasing PARP's control on NHEJ genes, which ensures the genomic instability and eventual lethality in HR-deficient cells.[94] Alternatively, disabling NHEJ renders PARP inhibitors useless on HR-deficient cells.[94] With this, NHEJ activity in tumors may need to be taken into consideration when evaluating PARP inhibitor efficiency, as low NHEJ activity may predict less responsive tumors to PARP inhibitors in light of genetic alterations that would suggest HR defects.[94]

The excitement of PARP inhibitors as a more comprehensive cancer therapy has come from studies indicating that cells having other genetic alterations affecting HR, such as PTEN loss of function, are highly sensitive to PARP inhibitors.[95] Accordingly, PARP inhibitors are reasoned to provide potential benefit in endometrial cancer due to the high frequency of PTEN loss. Along with the function of PTEN to oppose PI3K/AKT pathway signaling, PTEN also maintains genomic stability.[93] *In vitro* studies, in endometrial cancer cells, have shown PTEN loss of function to result in HR defects, resulting in an increased sensitivity to PARP inhibitors.[96] In the United Kingdom, the PTEN and Olaparib in Endometrial Cancer Treatment (POEM) study is underway, which is evaluating the PARP inhibitor olaparib as a single agent in comparison to standard of care. Further combinations of PARP inhibitors and agents that target the PI3K/AKT pathway are underway (NCT01623349).

## Protein 53

TP53 has a major role in cellular differentiation and senescence, cell cycle arrest, inhibition of angiogenesis, and DNA repair. Inactivation of TP53 in cancer cells occurs primarily by mutation, but also occurs via defective post-translational modification or abrogation of TP53 interacting proteins. Studies have indicated that TP53 inactivation is necessary to maintain the tumor phenotype, thus there is a great need and interest in the development of approaches that can restore wild-type TP53 function in tumors.[97] In endometrial cancer, TP53 aberrations are common in non-endometrioid cases, occurring in approximately 90% of serous carcinomas[98] and up to 80% of carciosarcomas.[99] Aberrant accumulation of inactivated TP53 is almost always absent in grade 1 or 2 endometrioid cases; however, it may be found in up to 50% of grade 3 endometrioid cases.[100] Agents that capitalize on TP53 aberrations have a significant potential in this disease, however, development of these agents has been challenging.

TP53 is a key cell cycle regulator, acting at the G1 checkpoint.[101] Many tumors with TP53 aberrations demonstrate subsequent loss of function of the G1 checkpoint, placing additional dependence on the G2 and S-phase checkpoints.[102] MK-1775 is a highly selective, small molecule inhibitor of Wee 1, a tyrosine kinase that mediates the G2 cell cycle checkpoint. Thus, TP53 deficient tumors may be particularly sensitive to checkpoint abrogation caused by Wee-1 inhibitors.[103] This drug is being explored in ovarian cancer, but has not yet been employed against non-ovarian cancers.

### Metformin

Metformin is a biquanide drug used in the treatment of type II diabetes that has received attention as a possible cancer therapy due to its association with reducing cancer risk and its inhibition of cancer cell proliferation in several cancer types.[104] The anti-cancer effects of metformin on cancer cells are the result of both direct (insulin-independent) and indirect (insulin-dependent) effects, which include the activation of AMP-activated protein kinase (AMPK) to inhibit mTOR activity and the reduction of circulating insulin, which acts as a mitogen.[105]

The use of metformin as a therapy in endometrial cancer has been an area of interest, given the role of obesity and high prevalence of insulin resistance in women with this disease.[106] Studies in cancer cells, including endometrial, have shown metformin to induce a range of events, including cell-cycle arrest, decrease hTERT expression, reduction in mTOR activity, induction of apoptosis, and increase the expression of cyclin-dependent kinase inhibitor, p27.[105] Enrollment is currently underway for a phase 0 study that intends to evaluate endometrial cancer patients receiving metformin as a neoadjuvant therapy in non-diabetics (NCT01205672). Combination approaches have also gathered a certain amount of interest following *in vitro* data which indicate progesterone resistance can be overcome by metformin treatment,[107, 108] and that paclitaxel-induced mTOR activity can be inhibited when combined with metformin.[109] A study evaluating metformin in combination with standard chemotherapy in primary advanced endometrial cancer is planned. More studies will be necessary to further evaluate the potential benefit of combination approaches involving metformin.

### Combination Approaches to Overcome Hormone Therapy Resistance

Hormone therapy is the only FDA-approved therapy for recurrent endometrial cancer and is used for the nonsurgical treatment of early grade endometrial cancer; however, resistance is an issue. The response to progestins, such as medroxyprogestrone acetate (MPA) and megestrol acetate, is often low (25%) and short-lived, with progression-free survival ranging from 2.5 to 8.5 months in the recurrent setting.[110] There is growing evidence that suggests endometrial cancers cells resistant to hormone therapy have active survival pathways,[107, 108] including PI3K/AKT/mTOR.[111]

The loss of progesterone receptor by the cancer cells is another cause of progestin resistance. Interestingly, the inhibition of the PI3K/AKT pathway has been shown to increase progesterone receptor expression.[111] Further, in response to combining MPA with a PI3K inhibitor, resistance has been overcome *in vitro* and *in vivo* in endometrial cancer models.[111] In a similar study, metformin combined with MPA increased progesterone receptor expression in progestin resistant endometrial cancer cells, which was related to AMPK-directed reduction of S6K.[108] Thus, combi-

nation approaches that include PI3K, AKT, mTOR inhibitors, or metformin along with progestins may represent an opportunity to improve the clinical response rates in endometrial cancer patients who receive hormonal therapy.

### E-cadherin

E-cadherin is a cell–cell adhesion protein and its downregulation in tumors is associated with epithelial-to-mesenchymal transition (EMT) and tumor cell migration and invasion. In addition, the loss of E-cadherin also impacts cancer cell proliferation, transcriptional control, oncogenic receptor activity and signaling, and sensitivity to chemotherapy. The re-expression of E-cadherin in cancer cells has shown to increase the sensitivity of cancer cells to chemotherapy[112] and targeted therapy[113] agents. E-cadherin directly binds to important RTKs, EGFR, IGF-1R, and the cMET receptor.[114] The homeotypic interaction of E-cadherin between cells prevents the activity of these RTKs. This inactivity potentially could alter tumor cells that are dependent on over-expressed RTKs or additionally, negatively impact the activity of feedback pathways activated by PI3K inhibitors.[114] *CTNNB1* (β-catenin) mutations occur in approximately 16–45% of endometrioid carcinomas.[46] Accumulation of mutant β-catenin in the nucleus is related to oncogenic Wnt/β-catenin signaling. In colon cancer cells, recombinant E-cadherin can outcompete Wnt/β-catenin signaling factor, lymphocyte-enhancer factor-1 (LEF-1), and recruit β-catenin to the cell membrane, preventing its nuclear accumulation.[115] In endometrial cancer, β-catenin mutations occur in exon 3, a region outside of the binding site for E-cadherin.[45] Thus, it can be speculated that re-expression of E-cadherin may act as a biological sponge for soaking up mutant β-catenin. Given that E-cadherin loss occurs in up to 50% of endometrioid cases and up to 90% of non-endometrioid cases, this would be an ideal target to explore. However, similar to other challenging targets, such as p53, the ability to target E-cadherin by conventional drug approaches remains a major obstacle for this highly prevalent alteration.

Histone deacetylase inhibitors (HDACIs) can indirectly induce E-cadherin expression. HDACI use in non-small lung cancer cells is shown to induce E-cadherin expression, which subsequently increases the sensitivity of cells to EGFR-inhibitors.[113] In endometrial cancer cells, HDACIs have also been reported to induce the expression of E-cadherin along with cyclin-dependent kinase inhibitors, p21 and p27, and decrease the expression of cyclin D1, cyclin D2, and anti-apoptotic factor, bcl-2.[116] A main concern with HDACIs is the possibility of inducing gene expression that promotes tumor progression alongside the induced expression of anti-tumor genes. More studies are needed to determine the overall clinical benefit of restoring E-cadherin in endometrial cancer. Irrespective of the induction of E-cadherin, *in vitro* studies of HDACIs in endometrial cancer have shown promising anti-tumor effects. These results are encouraging and provide support for consideration of HDACIs in endometrial cancer.

### Conclusions

Our understanding of the molecular alterations in endometrial cancer and their potential as therapeutic targets has advanced considerably over the last few decades, which has come from the relentless efforts of dedicated clinicians, scientists, and their teams of professionals. A significant challenge that remains is the implementation and success of targeted agents into the clinical practice of this disease. Given the plethora of information from early phase trials and preclinical studies and the increasing efforts of moving newly found targets closer to clinical consideration, this challenge will soon be met. At the forefront of the most likely candidates for targeted therapy in endometrial cancer are combination approaches involving PI3K/AKT/mTOR inhibitors. Importantly, as we move ahead, we must continue to explore and advance new targets and known aberrations that remain difficult to successfully target. Though these represent a significant challenge, their translation to the clinic will surely make a significant impact on the lives of those that suffer from this disease.

# References

1 Siegel R, Naishadham D, Jemal A. Cancer statistics, 2013. *CA Cancer J Clin*. 2013;63:11–30.

2 Soliman PT, Wu D, Tortolero-Luna G, et al. Association between adiponectin, insulin resistance, and endometrial cancer. *Cancer*. 2006;106:2376–2381.

3 Surveillance Epidemiology and End Results Program. *SEER Cancer Statistics Review 1957–2007*; 2013.

4 Fujimoto T, Nanjyo H, Fukuda J, et al. Endometrioid uterine cancer: histopathological risk factors of local and distant recurrence. *Gynecol Oncol*. 2009;112:342–347.

5 Hecht JL, Mutter GL. Molecular and pathologic aspects of endometrial carcinogenesis. *J Clin Oncol*. 2006;24:4783–4791.

6 Hamilton CA, Cheung MK, Osann K, et al. Uterine papillary serous and clear cell carcinomas predict for poorer survival compared to grade 3 endometrioid corpus cancers. *Br J Cancer*. 2006;94:642–646.

7 Mutter GL, Lin MC, Fitzgerald JT, et al. Altered PTEN expression as a diagnostic marker for the earliest endometrial precancers. *J Natl Cancer Inst*. 2000;92:924–930.

8 Song MS, Salmena L, Pandolfi PP. The functions and regulation of the PTEN tumour suppressor. *Nat Rev Mol Cell Biol*. 2012;13:283–296.

9 Kong D, Suzuki A, Zou TT, et al. PTEN1 is frequently mutated in primary endometrial carcinomas. *Nat Genet*. 1997;17:143–144.

10 Oda K, Stokoe D, Taketani Y, McCormick F. High frequency of coexistent mutations of PIK3CA and PTEN genes in endometrial carcinoma. *Cancer Res*. 2005;65:10669–10673.

11 Urick ME, Rudd ML, Godwin AK, Sgroi D, Merino M, Bell DW. PIK3R1 (p85alpha) is somatically mutated at high frequency in primary endometrial cancer. *Cancer Res*. 2011;71, 4061–4067.

12 MacDonald ND, Salvesen HB, Ryan A, Iversen OE, Akslen LA, Jacobs IJ. Frequency and prognostic impact of microsatellite instability in a large population-based study of endometrial carcinomas. *Cancer Res*. 2000;60:1750–1752.

13 McCampbell AS, Broaddus RR, Loose DS, Davies PJ. Overexpression of the insulin-like growth factor I receptor and activation of the AKT pathway in hyperplastic endometrium. *Clin Cancer Res*. 2006;12:6373–6378.

14 Boyd J, Risinger JI. Analysis of oncogene alterations in human endometrial carcinoma: prevalence of ras mutations. *Mol Carcinog*. 1991;4:189–195.

15 Pollock PM, Gartside MG, Dejeza LC, et al. Frequent activating FGFR2 mutations in endometrial carcinomas parallel germline mutations associated with craniosynostosis and skeletal dysplasia syndromes. *Oncogene*. 2007;26:7158–7162.

16 Fukuchi T, Sakamoto M, Tsuda H, Maruyama K, Nozawa S, Hirohashi S. Beta-catenin mutation in carcinoma of the uterine endometrium. *Cancer Res*. 1998;58:3526–3528.

17 Lax SF, Kendall B, Tashiro H, Slebos RJ, Hedrick L. The frequency of p53, K-ras mutations, and microsatellite instability differs in uterine endometrioid and serous carcinoma: evidence of distinct molecular genetic pathways. *Cancer*. 2000;88:814–824.

18 Salvesen HB, Das S, Akslen LA. Loss of nuclear p16 protein expression is not associated with promoter methylation but defines a subgroup of aggressive endometrial carcinomas with poor prognosis. *Clin Cancer Res*. 2000;6:153–159.

19 Holcomb K, Delatorre R, Pedemonte B, McLeod C, Anderson L, Chambers J. E-cadherin expression in endometrioid, papillary serous, and clear cell carcinoma of the endometrium. *Obstet Gynecol*. 2002;100:1290–1295.

20 Slomovitz BM, Broaddus RR, Burke TW, et al. Her-2/neu overexpression and amplification in uterine papillary serous carcinoma. *J Clin Oncol*. 2004;22:3126–3132.

21 Sonoda G, du Manoir S, Godwin AK, et al. Detection of DNA gains and losses in primary endometrial carcinomas by comparative genomic hybridization. *Genes Chromosomes Cancer*. 1997;18:115–125.

22 Miller D, Filiaci V, Fleming G, et al. Randomized phase III noninferiority trial of first line chemotherapy for metastatic or recurrent endometrial carcinoma: a Gynecologic Oncology Group study. *Gynecol Oncol*. 2012;125:771.

23 Laplante M, Sabatini DM. mTOR signaling in growth control and disease. *Cell*. 2012;149:274–293.

24 Slomovitz BM, Coleman RL. The PI3K/AKT/mTOR pathway as a therapeutic target in endometrial cancer. *Clin Cancer Res*. 2012;18:5856–5864.

25 Castellvi J, Garcia A, Ruiz-Marcellan C, et al. Cell signaling in endometrial carcinoma: phosphorylated 4E-binding protein-1 expression in endometrial cancer correlates with aggressive tumors and prognosis. *Hum Pathol*. 2009;40:1418–1426.

26 Slomovitz BM, Lu KH, Johnston T, et al. A phase 2 study of the oral mammalian target of rapamycin inhibitor, everolimus, in patients with recurrent endometrial carcinoma. *Cancer*. 2010;116:5415–5419.

27 Colombo N, McMeekin S, Schwartz P, et al. A phase II trial of the mTOR inhibitor AP23573 as a single agent in advanced endometrial cancer. *J Clin Oncol*. 2007;25(suppl.). Abstract 5516.

28 Mackay H, Welch S, Tsao MS, et al. Phase II Study of Oral Ridaforolimus in Patients with Metastatic and/or Locally Advanced Recurrent Endometrial Cancer: NCIC CTG IND 192. *J Clin Oncol*. 2011;29(suppl.). Abstract 5013.

29 Oza AM, Poveda A, Clamp AR, et al. Phase II (RP2) Trial of Ridaforolimus (R) Compared with Progestin (P) or Chemotherapy (C) in Female Adult Patients with Advanced Endometrial Carcinoma. *J Clin Oncol*. 2011;29(suppl.). Abstract 5009.

30 Oza AM, Elit L, Provencher D, et al. Phase II study of temsirolimus (CCI-779) in patients with metastatic and/or locally advanced recurrent endometrial cancer previously treated with chemotherapy. *J Clin Oncol*. 2008;26(suppl.). Abstract 5516.

31 Oza AM, Elit L, Tsao MS, et al. Phase II study of temsirolimus in women with recurrent or metastatic endometrial cancer: a trial of the NCIC Clinical Trials Group. *J Clin Oncol*. 2011;29:3278–3285.

32 Mackay H, Welch S, Tsao MS, et al. Phase II study of oral ridaforolimus in patients with metastatic and/or locally advanced recurrent endometrial cancer: NCIC CTG IND 192. *J Clin Oncol*. 2011;29(suppl.). Abstract 5013

33 Sarbassov DD, Guertin DA, Ali SM, Sabatini DM. Phosphorylation and regulation of Akt/PKB by the rictor-mTOR complex. *Science*. 2005;307:1098–1101.

34 O'Reilly KE, Rojo F, She QB, et al. mTOR inhibition induces upstream receptor tyrosine kinase signaling and activates Akt. *Cancer Res.* 2006;66:1500–1508.

35 Haruta T, Uno T, Kawahara J, et al. A rapamycin-sensitive pathway down-regulates insulin signaling via phosphorylation and proteasomal degradation of insulin receptor substrate-1. *Mol Endocrinol.* 2000;14:783–794.

36 Meric-Bernstam F, Gonzalez-Angulo AM. Targeting the mTOR signaling network for cancer therapy. *J Clin Oncol.* 2009;27:2278–2287.

37 Shafer A, Zhou C, Gehrig PA, Boggess JF, Bae-Jump VL. Rapamycin potentiates the effects of paclitaxel in endometrial cancer cells through inhibition of cell proliferation and induction of apoptosis. *Int J Cancer.* 2010;126:1144–1154.

38 Chandarlapaty S, Sawai A, Scaltriti M, et al. AKT inhibition relieves feedback suppression of receptor tyrosine kinase expression and activity. *Cancer Cell.* 2011;19:58–71.

39 West KA, Castillo SS, Dennis PA. Activation of the PI3K/Akt pathway and chemotherapeutic resistance. *Drug Resist Updat.* 2002;5:234–248.

40 Hoekstra AV, Ward EC, Hardt JL, et al. Chemosensitization of endometrial cancer cells through AKT inhibition involves FOXO1. *Gynecol Oncol.* 2008;108:609–618.

41 Moxley KM, McMeekin DS. Endometrial carcinoma: a review of chemotherapy, drug resistance, and the search for new agents. *Oncologist.* 2010;15:1026–1033.

42 Gagnon V, Mathieu I, Sexton E, Leblanc K, Asselin E. AKT involvement in cisplatin chemoresistance of human uterine cancer cells. *Gynecol Oncol.* 2004;94:785–795.

43 Meyer LA, Slomovitz BM, Djordjevic B, et al. The search continues: looking for predictive biomarkers for response mTOR inhibition in endometrial cancer. *J Clin Oncol.* 2011;29(suppl.): Abstract 5016.

44 Mackay HJ, Eisenhauer EA, Kamel-Reid S, et al. Molecular determinants of outcome with mammalian target of rapamycin inhibition in endometrial cancer. *Cancer.* 2013;120(4):603–610.

45 Montagut C, Settleman J. Targeting the RAF-MEK-ERK pathway in cancer therapy. *Cancer Lett.* 2009;283:125–134.

46 Samarnthai N, Hall K, Yeh IT. Molecular profiling of endometrial malignancies. *Obstet Gynecol Int.* 2010;2010:162363.

47 Sasaki H, Nishii H, Takahashi H, et al. Mutation of the Ki-ras protooncogene in human endometrial hyperplasia and carcinoma. *Cancer Res.* 1993;53:1906–1910.

48 Varras MN, Koffa M, Koumantakis E, et al. Ras gene mutations in human endometrial carcinoma. *Oncology.* 1996;53:505–510.

49 Gysin S, Salt M, Young A, McCormick F. Therapeutic strategies for targeting ras proteins. *Genes Cancer.* 2011;2:359–372.

50 Iglesias D, Yates MS, van der Hoeven D, et al. Another Surprise from Metformin: novel mechanism of action via K-Ras influences endometrial cancer response to therapy. *Mol Cancer Ther.* 2013;12(12):2847–2856.

51 van der Hoeven D, Cho KJ, Ma X, Chigurupati S, Parton RG, Hancock JF. Fendiline inhibits K-Ras plasma membrane localization and blocks K-Ras signal transmission. *Mol Cell Biol.* 2013;33:237–251.

52 Coleman R, Sill M, Thaker P, et al. A phase II evaluation of AZD6244, a selective MEK-1/2 inhibitor in the treatment of recurrent or persistent endometrial cancer: a Gynecologic Oncology Group study. *Gynecol Oncol.* 2013;130(1):e12-e13.

53 Carracedo A, Ma L, Teruya-Feldstein J, et al. Inhibition of mTORC1 leads to MAPK pathway activation through a PI3K-dependent feedback loop in human cancer. *J Clin Invest.* 2008;118:3065–3074.

54 Cheung LW, Hennessy BT, Li J, et al. High frequency of PIK3R1 and PIK3R2 mutations in endometrial cancer elucidates a novel mechanism

55 Oda K, Okada J, Timmerman L, et al. PIK3CA cooperates with other phosphatidylinositol 3′-kinase pathway mutations to effect oncogenic transformation. *Cancer Res.* 2008;68:8127–8136.

56 Di Nicolantonio F, Arena S, Tabernero J, et al. Deregulation of the PI3K and KRAS signaling pathways in human cancer cells determines their response to everolimus. *J Clin Invest.* 2010;120:2858–2866.

57 Engelman JA, Chen L, Tan X, et al. Effective use of PI3K and MEK inhibitors to treat mutant Kras G12D and PIK3CA H1047R murine lung cancers. *Nat Med.* 2008;14:1351–1356.

58 Kim TH, Wang J, Lee KY, et al. The synergistic effect of conditional pten loss and oncogenic K-ras mutation on endometrial cancer development occurs via decreased progesterone receptor action. *J Oncol.* 2010;2010:139087.

59 Wongchenko MJ, Guan Y, Wagle M, et al. Sensitivity of endometrial cancer cells to inhibitors targeting different nodes of the PI3K pathway and their combination with a MEK inhibitor. *Cancer Res.* 2013;73 (8 suppl. 1):Abstract 3479.

60 Shoji K, Oda K, Kashiyama T, et al. Genotype-dependent efficacy of a dual PI3K/mTOR inhibitor, NVP-BEZ235, and an mTOR inhibitor, RAD001, in endometrial carcinomas. *PLoS One.* 2012;7:e37431.

61 Pfeiffer D, Spranger J, Al-Deiri M, et al. mRNA expression of ligands of the epidermal-growth-factor-receptor in the uterus. *Int J Cancer.* 1997;72:581–586.

62 Oza AM, Eisenhauer EA, Elit L, et al. Phase II study of erlotinib in recurrent or metastatic endometrial cancer: NCIC IND-148. *J Clin Oncol.* 2008;26:4319–4325.

63 Leslie KK, Sill MW, Darcy KM, et al. Efficacy and safety of gefitinib and potential prognostic value of soluble EGFR, EGFR mutations, and tumor markers in a Gynecologic Oncology Group phase II trial of persistent or recurrent endometrial cancer. *J Clin Oncol.* 2009;27(suppl.): Abstract e16542.

64 Slomovitz B, Schmeler K, Miller D, et al. Phase II study of cetuximab (Erbitux) in patients with progressive or recurrent endometrial cancer. *Gynecol Oncol.* 2010;116(suppl.): Abstract 13.

65 Langer CJ. Roles of EGFR and KRAS Mutations in the Treatment Of Patients With Non-Small-Cell Lung Cancer. *P T.* 2011;36:263–279.

66 Frattini M, Saletti P, Romagnani E, et al. PTEN loss of expression predicts cetuximab efficacy in metastatic colorectal cancer patients. *Br J Cancer.* 2007;97:1139–1145.

67 Di Fiore F, Blanchard F, Charbonnier F, et al. Clinical relevance of KRAS mutation detection in metastatic colorectal cancer treated by Cetuximab plus chemotherapy. *Br J Cancer.* 2007;96:1166–1169.

68 Leslie KK, Sill MW, Lankes HA, et al. Lapatinib and potential prognostic value of EGFR mutations in a Gynecologic Oncology Group phase II trial of persistent or recurrent endometrial cancer. *Gynecol Oncol.* 2012;127(2):345–350.

69 Hayes MP, Douglas W, Ellenson LH. Molecular alterations of EGFR and PIK3CA in uterine serous carcinoma. *Gynecol Oncol.* 2009;113:370–373.

70 Biscuola M, Van de Vijver K, Castilla MÁ, et al. Oncogene alterations in endometrial carcinosarcomas. *Hum Pathol.* 2013;44:852–859.

71 Fleming GF, Sill MW, Darcy KM, et al. Phase II trial of trastuzumab in women with advanced or recurrent, HER2-positive endometrial carcinoma: a Gynecologic Oncology Group study. *Gynecol Oncol.* 2010;116:15–20.

72 Dang CT, Hudis CA (eds.) *New Treatment Paradigms in Metastatic Breast Cancer.* CMPMedica; 2008.

73 Attias-Geva Z, Bentov I, Ludwig DL, Fishman A, Bruchim I, Werner H. Insulin-like growth factor-I receptor (IGF-IR) targeting with

monoclonal antibody cixutumumab (IMC-A12) inhibits IGF-I action in endometrial cancer cells. *Eur J Cancer*. 2011;47:1717–1726.

74  Mendivil A, Zhou C, Cantrell LA, et al. AMG 479, a novel IGF-1-R antibody, inhibits endometrial cancer cell proliferation through disruption of the PI3K/Akt and MAPK pathways. *Reprod Sci*. 2011;18:832–841.

75  Attias-Geva Z, Bentov I, Fishman A, Werner H, Bruchim I. Insulin-like growth factor-I receptor inhibition by specific tyrosine kinase inhibitor NVP-AEW541 in endometrioid and serous papillary endometrial cancer cell lines. *Gynecol Oncol*. 2011;121:383–389.

76  Haugsten EM, Wiedlocha A, Olsnes S, Wesche J. Roles of fibroblast growth factor receptors in carcinogenesis. *Mol Cancer Res*. 2010;8:1439–1452.

77  Byron SA, Gartside MG, Wellens CL, et al. Inhibition of activated fibroblast growth factor receptor 2 in endometrial cancer cells induces cell death despite PTEN abrogation. *Cancer Res*. 2008;68:6902–6907.

78  Dutt A, Salvesen HB, Chen TH, et al. Drug-sensitive FGFR2 mutations in endometrial carcinoma. *Proc Natl Acad Sci U S A*. 2008;105:8713–8717.

79  Brave SR, Ratcliffe K, Wilson Z, et al. Assessing the Activity of Cediranib, a VEGFR-2/3 Tyrosine Kinase Inhibitor, against VEGFR-1 and Members of the Structurally Related PDGFR Family. *Mol Cancer Ther*. 2011;10:861–873.

80  Marathe PH, Kamath AV, Zhang Y, D'Arienzo C, Bhide R, Fargnoli J. Preclinical pharmacokinetics and in vitro metabolism of brivanib (BMS-540215), a potent VEGFR2 inhibitor and its alanine ester prodrug brivanib alaninate. *Cancer Chemother Pharmacol*. 2009;65:55–66.

81  Marshall ME, Hinz TK, Kono SA, et al. Fibroblast growth factor receptors are components of autocrine signaling networks in head and neck squamous cell carcinoma cells. *Clin Cancer Res*. 2011;17:5016–5025.

82  Hanahan D, Weinberg RA. Hallmarks of cancer: the next generation. *Cell*. 2011;144:646–674.

83  Ellis LM, Hicklin DJ. VEGF-targeted therapy: mechanisms of antitumour activity. *Nat Rev Cancer*. 2008;8:579–591.

84  Stefansson IM, Salvesen HB, Akslen LA. Vascular proliferation is important for clinical progress of endometrial cancer. *Cancer Res*. 2006;66:3303–3309.

85  Kamat AA, Merritt WM, Coffey D, et al. Clinical and biological significance of vascular endothelial growth factor in endometrial cancer. *Clin Cancer Res*. 2007;13:7487–7495.

86  Aghajanian C, Sill MW, Darcy KM, et al. Phase II trial of bevacizumab in recurrent or persistent endometrial cancer: a Gynecologic Oncology Group study. *J Clin Oncol*. 2011;29:2259–2265.

87  Correa R, Mackay H, Hirte HW, et al. A phase II study of sunitinib in recurrent or metastatic endometrial carcinoma: a trial of the Princess Margaret Hospital, The University of Chicago, and California Cancer Phase II Consortia. *J Clin Oncol*. 2010;28(suppl. 15): Abstract 5038.

88  Nimeiri HS, Oza AM, Morgan RJ, et al. Sorafenib (SOR) in patients (pts) with advanced/recurrent uterine carcinoma (UCA) or carcinosarcoma (CS): a phase II trial of the University of Chicago, PMH, and California Phase II Consortia. *J Clin Oncol*. 2008;26(suppl.): Abstract 5585.

89  Coleman RL, Sill MW, Lankes HA, et al. A phase II evaluation of aflibercept in the treatment of recurrent or persistent endometrial cancer: a Gynecologic Oncology Group study. *Gynecol Oncol*. 2012;127:538–543.

90  Davies S, Dai D, Pickett G, Thiel KW, Korovkina VP, Leslie KK. Effects of bevacizumab in mouse model of endometrial cancer: defining the molecular basis for resistance. *Oncol Rep*. 2011;25:855–862.

91  Klement G, Baruchel S, Rak J, et al. Continuous low-dose therapy with vinblastine and VEGF receptor-2 antibody induces sustained tumor regression without overt toxicity. *J Clin Invest*. 2000;105:R15–24.

92  Fong PC, Boss DS, Yap TA, et al. Inhibition of poly(ADP-ribose) polymerase in tumors from BRCA mutation carriers. *N Engl J Med*. 2009;361:123–134.

93  Dedes KJ, Wilkerson PM, Wetterskog D, Weigelt B, Ashworth A, Reis-Filho JS. Synthetic lethality of PARP inhibition in cancers lacking BRCA1 and BRCA2 mutations. *Cell Cycle*. 2011;10:1192–1199.

94  Patel AG, Sarkaria JN, Kaufmann SH. Nonhomologous end joining drives poly(ADP-ribose) polymerase (PARP) inhibitor lethality in homologous recombination-deficient cells. *Proc Natl Acad Sci U S A*. 2011;108:3406–3411.

95  Mendes-Pereira AM, Martin SA, Brough R, et al. Synthetic lethal targeting of PTEN mutant cells with PARP inhibitors. *EMBO Mol Med*. 2009;1:315–322.

96  Dedes KJ, Wetterskog D, Mendes-Pereira AM, et al. PTEN deficiency in endometrioid endometrial adenocarcinomas predicts sensitivity to PARP inhibitors. *Sci Transl Med*. 2010;2:53ra75.

97  Ventura A, Kirsch DG, McLaughlin ME, et al. Restoration of p53 function leads to tumour regression in vivo. *Nature*. 2007;445:661–665.

98  Tashiro H, Isacson C, Levine R, Kurman RJ, Cho KR, Hedrick L. p53 gene mutations are common in uterine serous carcinoma and occur early in their pathogenesis. *Am J Pathol*. 1997;150:177–185.

99  Kounelis S, Jones MW, Papadaki H, Bakker A, Swalsky P, Finkelstein SD. Carcinosarcomas (malignant mixed mullerian tumors) of the female genital tract: comparative molecular analysis of epithelial and mesenchymal components. *Hum Pathol*. 1998;29:82–87.

100  Zannoni GF, Vellone VG, Arena V, et al. Does high-grade endometrioid carcinoma (grade 3 FIGO) belong to type I or type II endometrial cancer? A clinical-pathological and immunohistochemical study. *Virchows Arch*. 2010;457:27–34.

101  Kuerbitz SJ, Plunkett BS, Walsh WV, Kastan MB. Wild-type p53 is a cell cycle checkpoint determinant following irradiation. *Proc Natl Acad Sci U S A*. 1992;89:7491–7495.

102  Nigro JM, Baker SJ, Preisinger AC, et al. Mutations in the p53 gene occur in diverse human tumour types. *Nature*. 1989;342:705–708.

103  Wang Y, Li J, Booher RN, et al. Radiosensitization of p53 mutant cells by PD0166285, a novel G(2) checkpoint abrogator. *Cancer Res*. 2001;61:8211–8217.

104  Li D. Metformin as an antitumor agent in cancer prevention and treatment. *J Diabetes*. 2011;3:320–327.

105  Dowling RJ, Goodwin PJ, Stambolic V. Understanding the benefit of metformin use in cancer treatment. *BMC Med*. 2011;9:33.

106  Burzawa JK, Schmeler KM, Soliman PT, et al. Prospective evaluation of insulin resistance among endometrial cancer patients. *Am J Obstet Gynecol*. 2011;204:355.e1–7.

107  Zhang Z, Dong L, Sui L, et al. Metformin reverses progestin resistance in endometrial cancer cells by downregulating GloI expression. *Int J Gynecol Cancer*. 2011;21:213–221.

108  Xie Y, Wang YL, Yu L, et al. Metformin promotes progesterone receptor expression via inhibition of mammalian target of rapamycin (mTOR) in endometrial cancer cells. *J Steroid Biochem Mol Biol*. 2011;126:113–120.

109  Hanna RK, Zhou C, Malloy KM, et al. Metformin potentiates the effects of paclitaxel in endometrial cancer cells through inhibition of cell proliferation and modulation of the mTOR pathway. *Gynecol Oncol*. 2012;125:458–469.

110  Bender D, Buekers T, Leslie K. Hormones and receptors in endometrial cancer. *Proc Obstet Gynecol*. 2011;2:1–25.

111 Gu C, Zhang Z, Yu Y, et al. Inhibiting the PI3K/Akt pathway reversed progestin resistance in endometrial cancer. *Cancer Sci.* 2011;102:557–564.

112 Fricke E, Hermannstädter C, Keller G, et al. Effect of wild-type and mutant E-cadherin on cell proliferation and responsiveness to the chemotherapeutic agents cisplatin, etoposide, and 5-fluorouracil. *Oncology.* 2004;66:150–159.

113 Witta SE, Gemmill RM, Hirsch FR, et al. Restoring E-cadherin expression increases sensitivity to epidermal growth factor receptor inhibitors in lung cancer cell lines. *Cancer Res.* 2006;66:944–950.

114 Qian X, Karpova T, Sheppard AM, McNally J, Lowy DR. E-cadherin-mediated adhesion inhibits ligand-dependent activation of diverse receptor tyrosine kinases. *EMBO J.* 2004;23:1739–1748.

115 Orsulic S, Huber O, Aberle H, Arnold S, Kemler R. E-cadherin binding prevents beta-catenin nuclear localization and beta-catenin/LEF-1-mediated transactivation. *J Cell Sci.* 1999;112(Pt 8):1237–1245.

116 Takai N, Narahara H. Preclinical studies of chemotherapy using histone deacetylase inhibitors in endometrial cancer. *Obstet Gynecol Int.* 2010;2010:923824.

# CHAPTER 22

# Targeted Therapy in Solid Tumors: Head and Neck

*Marcus M. Monroe[1] and Jeffrey N. Myers[2]*

[1]Department of Otolaryngology, University of Utah School of Medicine, Salt Lake City, UT

[2]Department of Head and Neck Surgery, The University of Texas MD Anderson Cancer Center, Houston, TX, USA

## Introduction

Head and neck squamous cell carcinoma (HNSCC) encompasses a heterogenous group of squamous epithelial malignancies arising from the mucosal lining of the upper aerodigestive tract that includes cancers of the sinonasal tract, oral cavity, nasopharynx, oropharynx, hypopharynx, and larynx. With over 680,000 estimated cases yearly, HNSCC is the seventh leading cause of cancer-related deaths worldwide.[1] As a whole, the incidence of HNSCC has been declining in the United States, attributed to declining rates of tobacco use.[2] However, incidence rates are increasing for certain subsets of HNSCC. Most striking of these is the rise in squamous cell carcinoma of the oropharynx attributed to oncogenic human papilloma virus (HPV) infection.[3–5] While the age-adjusted incidence rates of smoking-related cancers in the oral cavity continue to decline by approximately 2% annually, the incidence of HPV-related oropharyngeal cancer has risen by an estimated 5% annually.[2]

The overall survival for HNSCC across all stages has changed little over the past decades and remains in the range of 60% at 5 years.[6] Despite trends towards intensification of treatment, the gains in survival outcomes have been modest, with most differences in survival in contemporary cohorts coming as the result of improved survival of HPV-induced malignancies compared to those related to tobacco use.[7] It is clear that there remains a desperate need for improved therapies in HNSCC.

## Genetic Alterations in Head and Neck Squamous Cell Carcinoma

Large-scale studies aimed at identifying the genetic alterations in HNSCC have now been completed.[8–10] Using next generation sequencing technology to illuminate the genetic changes in large cohorts of HNSCCs, the frequent genetic drivers of HNSCC have been largely uncovered. Historically noted genetic alterations including a high frequency of TP53 mutations, cyclin D amplifications and deletions and/or mutations in CDKN2A, among others, have been confirmed from these studies. The most frequently encountered mutations in these series include alterations in TP53 (47-72%), CDKN2A (9-22%), PIK3CA (6-21%), FAT1 (12-23%) and NOTCH1 (14-19%; Table 22.1). Focal amplifications and deletions have also been a common finding in HNSCC, while structural rearrangements such as gene–gene fusions have not been consistently identified. The most common amplifications include regions containing CCND1, EGFR, FGFR, MYC, PIK3CA and ERBB2 among others.[9,11] Frequently deleted regions containing CDKN2A, PTEN, LRP1B and FAT1 among many others are thought to be a common method for loss of tumor suppressor function in addition to somatic mutations.[9,11]

Some of the most interesting findings coming from these recent large-scale analyses have been the finding of previously unidentified inactivating Notch1 mutations in a significant percentage of HNSCCs[8] as well as the considerable differences in the mutational spectrum of HPV-positive and HPV-negative HNSCC. As a whole, HPV-induced HNSCCs carry less genetic alterations than HPV-negative tumors, although certain mutations, such as PIK3CA, appear to occur with increased frequency in HPV-positive tumors.[9]

The genomic alterations in HNSCC are predominantly characterized by a loss of tumor suppressor activity. Frequent loss of TP53, CKDN2A, FAT1 and/or NOTCH1 activity occur in a high percentage of HNSCCs. Oncogenic gain-of-function mutations are uncommon, while gene amplification and increased expression occur in a wide variety of growth promoting pathways, making targeted therapy challenging given the vast array of potential targets.[12]

## Current Treatment for Head and Neck Squamous Cell Carcinoma

Current management paradigms for HNSCC involve multiple treatment modalities, including surgery, radiotherapy and systemic chemotherapy. To a significant degree, the selection of therapeutic modalities differs by the anatomic site of the primary tumor as well as the disease stage. For early stage disease (stage I/II), single-modality therapy with either radiation or surgery alone is typically sufficient, with the choice between the two being guided by the anatomic site, tumor characteristics, in addition to patient and physician preferences. For locoregionally advanced disease (stage III/IV), local therapy with surgery and/or radiotherapy is frequently combined with systemic therapy. For metastatic disease and unresectable locoregional recurrence following previous radiotherapy, the goals of therapy shift to palliation and systemic therapy is frequently given alone, with surgery and/or radiation reserved for locoregional palliation.

*Targeted Therapy in Translational Cancer Research*, First Edition. Edited by Apostolia-Maria Tsimberidou, Razelle Kurzrock and Kenneth C. Anderson.
© 2016 John Wiley & Sons, Inc. Published 2016 by John Wiley & Sons, Inc.

**Table 22.1** Frequent genetic alterations in head and neck squamous cell carcinoma.

| Frequent genetic alterations in head and neck squamous cell carcinoma | |
| --- | --- |
| **Mutations** | **Estimated frequency** |
| TP53 | 47–72% |
| FAT1 | 12–23% |
| CDKN2A | 9–22% |
| PIK3CA | 6–21% |
| SYNE1 | 20% |
| NOTCH1 | 14–19% |
| MLL2 | 11–18% |
| NSD1 | 10% |
| CASP8 | 8–9% |
| TP63 | 7% |
| PTEN | 7% |
| JUB | 6% |
| MED1 | 5% |
| IRF6 | 5% |
| SYNE2 | 5% |
| EZH2 | 5% |
| NOTCH2 | 5% |
| FBXW7 | 5% |
| HRAS | 4–5% |
| **Regions of frequent amplification** | **Selected genes in peak** |
| 11q13.3 | CCND1 |
| 3q26.33 | SOX2, PIK3CA |
| 7p11.2 | EGFR |
| 8p11.23 | FGFR |
| 8q24.21 | MYC, POU5F1B |
| 13q22.1 | KLF5 |
| 12q15 | MDM2 |
| 17q12 | ERBB2, GRB7 |
| 11p13 | CD44 |
| 9p24.1 | JAK2 |
| **Regions of frequent deletion** | **Selected genes in peak** |
| 9p21.3 | CDKN2A |
| 8p23.2 | CSMD1 |
| 2q22.1 | LRP1B |
| 4q35.2 | FAT1 |
| 19p13.3 | LKB1 |
| 2q37.3 | ING5, SP100, SP110, HDAC4, SP140 |
| 18q23 | GALR1, MBP, NFATC1 |
| 1p13.2 | NRAS, NOTCH2, BCL9, CHD1L |
| 7q36.1 | MLL3 |
| 9p24.1 | PTPRD |
| 11q23.1 | ATM, MLL, CXCR5 |
| 13q14.11 | BRCA2, RB1, FOXO1, SMAD9 |
| 9q34.3 | NOTCH1 |
| 10q23.31 | PTEN, KLLN |
| 18q21.2 | SMAD4, BCL2, DCC |

Chemotherapy given as part of multimodal therapy for locoregionally advanced disease can be delivered in both the neoadjuvant (induction) or adjuvant (concurrent or post-operative) setting. Platinum-based agents (cisplatin and carboplatinum) remain the backbone of both the induction and concurrent regimens, with frequent concomitant use of taxanes and fluorouracil. Chemotherapy given concurrently with radiation may be delivered postoperatively following surgery or as definitive therapy without prior surgical intervention. In the post-operative setting, meta-analyses have demonstrated a survival benefit for the addition of cisplatin-based chemotherapy to radiation when pathologic review of the surgical specimen reveals positive resection margins or extracapsular extension in regional lymph nodes.[13–15]

Induction chemotherapy regimens typically include multiple cytotoxic chemotherapeutics at higher doses than those delivered during concurrent chemoradiation. Meta-analyses of induction chemotherapy trials for head and neck cancer suggest that induction chemotherapy decreases the rate of distant metastatic disease but does not improve overall survival or locoregional control.[16] Recently attempted phase III trials failed to show a survival advantage for induction chemotherapy followed by concurrent chemoradiation versus concurrent chemoradiation alone.[17,18]

Despite intense multimodal therapy, survival rates for advanced-stage disease remain poor. For patients with recurrent or metastatic disease, short-term responses to systemic therapy can often be achieved but long-term disease control is rare and significant treatment related toxicity is common. There is a pressing need for systemic agents with improved activity and less toxicity.

## Targeted Therapy in Head and Neck Squamous Cell Carcinoma

Although a number of targeted agents have been evaluated in HNSCC (Table 22.2), only cetuximab, the monoclonal antibody against the epidermal growth factor receptor (EGFR), has been approved by the FDA for use in HNSCC. To date, the effect of most targeted agents tested in HNSCC has been modest at best, although they have frequently been tested in heavily pretreated patients without biomarker selection.

## Targeting the Epidermal Growth Factor Receptor

Overexpression of the epidermal growth factor receptor (EGFR) is a frequent finding in HNSCC, with up to 80–90% of tumors demonstrating elevated levels of EGFR expression.[40] Activating mutations in the EGFR gene are relatively infrequent,[41] while an increase in EGFR copy number occurs in a significant percentage of HNSCCs.[9] Overexpression of EGFR is associated with decreased survival in patients with head and neck cancer undergoing treatment,[42] as are elevated EGFR gene copy numbers.[43,44] Furthermore, elevated EGFR gene copy numbers are associated with progression of oral premalignant lesions to invasive carcinoma,[45] highlighting the importance of this pathway in oral cancer.

Monoclonal antibodies targeting the extracellular domain of the EGFR and small-molecule inhibitors of the intracellular tyrosine kinase domain are the two current approaches to targeting EGFR in HNSCC. Only the monoclonal antibody cetuximab has demonstrated a significant overall survival advantage in combination with cytotoxic chemotherapy and radiation, leading to its approval by the FDA for use in HNSCC. To date, small-molecule inhibition of the EGFR receptor has been disappointing, with only modest clinical effect evident and no significant survival advantage being demonstrated.

**Table 22.2** Selected phase II and III targeted therapy trials in HNSCC.

| Trial | Agent | Phase | Population | Treatment | No. of patients | Outcome |
|---|---|---|---|---|---|---|
| **EGFR targeted therapy** | | | | | | |
| Bonner et al.[19] | Cetuximab | III | LRA HNSCC | RT +/− cetuximab | 424 | Improved LRC (14.9 vs. 24.4, HR 0.68, $p = 0.005$) |
| | | | | | | Improved OS (29.3 vs. 49 mos, HR 0.7, $p = 0.006$) |
| EXTREME Trial Vermorken et al.[20] | Cetuximab | III | R/M HNSCC | CDDP, 5FU +/− cetuximab | 442 | Improved RR (20 vs. 36%) |
| | | | | | | Improved PFS (3.3 vs. 5.6 mos, HR 0.54, $p < 0.001$) |
| | | | | | | Improved OS (7.4 vs. 10.1 mos, HR 0.8, $p = 0.04$) |
| ECOG 1395 Burtness et al.[21] | Cetuximab | III | R/M HNSCC | CDDP +/− cetuximab | 117 | Improved RR (10 vs. 26%, $p = 0.03$) |
| | | | | | | No difference in PFS (2.7 vs. 4.2 mos, HR 0.78, $p = 0.09$) |
| | | | | | | No difference in OS (7.9 vs. 9.2 mos, $p = 0.21$) |
| SPECTRUM Trial Vermorken et al.[22] | Panitumumab | III | R/M HNSCC | CDDP, 5FU +/− panitumumab | 657 | Improved PFS (3.6 vs. 5.8 mos, HR 0.78, $p = 0.0036$) |
| | | | | | | No difference in OS (9 vs. 11.1, HR 0.873, $p = 0.14$) |
| Machiels et al.[23] | Zalatumumab | III | R/M HNSCC | Best supportive care +/− zalatumumab | 286 | Improved PFS (8.4 vs. 9.9 mos, HR 0.63, $p = 0.0012$) |
| | | | | | | No difference in OS (5.2 vs. 6.7 mos, HR 0.77, $p = 0.0648$) |
| Stewart et al.[24] | Gefitinib | III | R/M HNSCC | Methotrexate vs. gefitinib (250/500 mg/d) | 486 | No difference in RR (3.9 vs. 2.7/7.6%, $p = 0.57/0.17$) |
| | | | | | | No difference in OS (6.7 vs. 5.6/6.0 mos, HR 1.22/1.12, $p = 0.12/0.39$) |
| ECOG 1302 Argiris et al.[25] | Gefitinib | III | R/M HNSCC | Docetaxel +/− gefitinib | 270 | No difference in RR (6.2 vs. 12.5%, $p = 0.13$) |
| | | | | | | No difference in PFS (2.1 vs. 3.5 mos, HR = 0.81, $p = 0.19$) |
| | | | | | | No difference in OS (6.0 vs. 7.3 mos, HR 0.93, $p = 0.6$) |
| Martins et al.[26] | Erlotinib | II | LRA HNSCC | Cisplatin, RT +/− erlotinib | 204 | No difference in CRR (40 vs. 52%, $p = 0.08$) |
| | | | | | | No difference in PFS (HR = 0.9, $p = 0.71$) |
| **VEGFR targeted therapy** | | | | | | |
| RTOG 0615 Lee et al.[27] | Bevacizumab | II | LRA NPC | Cisplatin, RT + bevacizumab | 44 | 2 yr LRPFS 83.7% (95% CI, 72.6–94.9) |
| | | | | | | 2 yr PFS 74.7% (95% CI, 61.8–87.6) |
| | | | | | | 2 yr OS 90.9% (95% CI, 82.3–99.4) |
| Argiris et al.[28] | Bevacizumab | II | R/M HNSCC | Pemetrexed + bevacizumab | 40 | RR 30% (95% CI, 17–42) |
| | | | | | | Median PFS 5 mos (90% CI, 4–7) |
| | | | | | | Median OS 11.3 mos (90% CI, 8.7–16.8) |
| Fury et al.[29] | Bevacizumab | II | LRA HNSCC | RT + bevacizumab | 42 | 2 yr PFS 75.9% (95% CI, 63.9–90.1) |
| | | | | | | 2 yr OS 88% (95% CI, 78.6–98.4) |
| **Multi-kinase inhibition** | | | | | | |
| Argiris et al.[30] | Bevacizumab Cetuximab | II | R/M HNSCC | Cetuximab + bevacizumab | 46 | RR 16% (95% CI, 7–24) |
| | | | | | | Median PFS 2.8 mos (95% CI, 2.7–4.2) |
| | | | | | | Median OS 7.5 mos (95% CI, 5.7–9.6) |
| Cohen et al.[31] | Bevacizumab Gefitinib | I/II | R/M HNSCC | Erlotinib + bevacizumab | 48 | RR 15% (95% CI, 6–28) |
| | | | | | | Median PFS 4.1 mos (95% CI, 2.8–4.4) |
| | | | | | | Median OS 7.1 mos (95% CI, 5.7–9.0) |
| GORTEC 2006-01 Machiels et al.[32] | Sunitinib | II | R/M HNSCC | Sunitinib | 38 | RR 2.6% |
| | | | | | | Median PFS 2 mos (95% CI, 1.3–2.7) |
| | | | | | | Median OS 3.4 mos (95% CI, 2.7–4.1) |
| SWOG S0420 Williamson et al.[33] | Sorafenib | II | R/M HNSCC | Sorafenib | 41 | RR 2% (95% CI, 0–13) |
| | | | | | | Median PFS 4 mos (95% CI, 2–4) |
| | | | | | | Median OS 9 mos (95% CI, 7–14) |

**Table 22.2** (Continued)

| Trial | Agent | Phase | Population | Treatment | No. of patients | Outcome |
|---|---|---|---|---|---|---|
| **Proteasome targeted therapy** | | | | | | |
| Chung et al.[34] | Bortezomib | II | R/M HNSCC | Docetaxel + bortezomib | 21 | RR 5%, Median OS 6.6 mos<br>Trial terminated early |
| Argiris et al.[35] | Bortezomib | I | Stage IV, R/M HNSCC | RT, cetuximab + bortezomib | 7 | Median PFS 4.8 mos (95% CI, 2.6–6.9)<br>Trial terminated early |
| ECOG 1304 Gilbert et al.[36] | Bortezomib | II | R/M HNSCC | Bortezomib +/– irinotecan | 61 | RR (2.6 vs. 13.1%)<br>No difference in PFS (1.5 vs. 1.6 mos) |
| **TP53 targeted therapy** | | | | | | |
| Yoo et al.[37] | INGN 201 | II | LRA HNSCC | Surgery + INGN 201 +/– chemoradiation | 13 | 1 yr PFS 90% (95% CI, 56–100) |
| Clayman et al.[38] | Ad-p53 | II | R HNSCC | Ad-p53 +/– surgery | 34 | RR 11.8% (Patients not treated surgically)<br>Median OS 8.9 mos |
| Nemunaitis et al.[39] | ONYX-015 | II | R HNSCC | ONYX-015 (daily/BID) | 40 | RR 14/10% |

LRA, locoregionally advanced; LRC, locoregional control; RT, radiation therapy; HR, hazard ratio; mos, months; R/M, recurrent/metastatic; CDDP, cisplatin; 5FU, 5-fluorouracil; RR, response rate.

## Monoclonal Antibodies to the Epidermal Growth Factor Receptor

Cetuximab, the first and only FDA-approved targeted therapeutic in HNSCC, is a chimeric monoclonal antibody against the extracellular domain of EGFR. In HNSCC, cetuximab is thought to act through more than one mechanism. By interfering with ligand binding to the extracellular domains of the EGF receptor, cetuximab interferes with receptor dimerization and activation and subsequently reduces downstream mitogenic signaling.[46] In addition, binding of cetuximab induces antibody-dependent cell-mediated cytotoxicity in HNSCC.[47–49]

Early phase II and III studies evaluating cetuximab in HNSCC demonstrated promising clinical activity and improved clinical responses in recurrent and metastatic HNSCC when combined with cisplatin.[21] In 2006, Bonner et al. evaluated the addition of cetuximab to radiation for head and neck cancer.[19] Patients with locoregionally advanced HNSCC were randomized to radiation with or without cetuximab at an initial dose of 400 mg/m2 of body surface area, followed by 250 mg/m2 weekly during radiation. Locoregional control was significantly improved in the cohort receiving combination therapy (24.4 vs. 14.9 months, HR for locoregional progression or death, 0.68, $p = 0.005$). The median overall survival was likewise significantly improved, with a median survival of 49 months in patients treated with cetuximab and radiation versus 29.3 months for those treated with radiation alone (HR for death, 0.70, $p = 0.006$). With the exception of the characteristic acneiform rash, a significant difference in the toxicity of the two treatment arms was not demonstrated.

In recurrent/metastatic HNSCC, cetuximab has been demonstrated to have an objective clinical response rate in the range of 10–20% in cisplatin-refractory disease.[50–52] Based upon these findings, Vermorken et al. performed a randomized clinical trial to test the efficacy of cetuximab in combination with cisplatin and 5-fluorouracil (5-FU) as the initial therapy in metastatic/recurrent HNSCC. In this so-called EXTREME trial, 220 patients were randomized to cisplatin + 5-FU and 222 to cisplatin, 5-FU, and cetuximab. The overall response rate increased from 20% to 36% with the addition of cetuximab. Compared to the doublet of cisplatin and 5-FU, the addition of cetuximab resulted in an improvement in both median overall survival (7.4 months versus 10.1, HR for death 0.8, $p = 0.04$) and progression-free survival (3.3 months versus 5.6, HR for progression 0.54, $p < 0.001$). In contrast to this study, ECOG1395 compared cisplatin to cisplatin and cetuximab in 117 patients with recurrent/metastatic HNSCC (Burtness, JCO). While an improved response rate was noted, no significant difference was found in either PFS or OS, although the magnitude of the differences in survival and hazard ratios were comparable between trials, suggesting the contrasting outcomes may simply reflect differences in statistical power.

In addition to cetuximab, other monoclonal antibodies targeting the EGFR are under clinical investigation in HNSCC. Panitumumab, a fully human monoclonal antibody to EGFR, has been evaluated in the recurrent/metastatic setting with mixed results.[22] In a randomized trial comparing cisplatin and 5-FU alone to the combination with panitumumab (SPECTRUM trial),[22] no significant difference in overall survival could be demonstrated (median overall survival 11.1 months vs. 9.0, HR 0.873, $p = 0.1403$). The median progression-free survival was marginally improved with the addition of panitumumab (4.6 months vs. 5.8, HR 0.78, $p = 0.0036$). In a subset analysis of patients with available p16 data, the addition of panitumumab demonstrated an improvement in overall survival in p16-negative but not p16-positive patients, suggesting an interaction between HPV status and the efficacy of anti-EGFR therapy. Zalutumumab, a human IgG1κ monoclonal antibody targeting the EGFR, has also been shown to prolong progression-free but not overall survival in patients with cisplatin-refractory recurrent/metastatic HNSCC.[23]

## Small-Molecule Inhibitors of the Epidermal Growth Factor Receptor

To date, the efficacy of small-molecule inhibitors of the EGFR has been disappointing. Gefitinib and erlotinib, two tyrosine kinase inhibitors of the EGFR, have been evaluated in both the recurrent/metastatic setting and in combination with cisplatin and radiation in locoregionally advanced HNSCC (Table 22.2). While clinical responses have been consistently noted, they occur in a small percentage of patients,[53] are short-lived and have not been proven to provide significant improvement over traditional second-line chemotherapeutics.[24] In contrast to lung and colorectal cancer, there are currently no biomarkers of response to therapy to allow pre-selection of patients most likely to respond. While these agents remain the subject of ongoing investigation, to date they are not a part of routine treatment of patients with HNSCC outside of the clinical trial setting.

## Targeting the Vascular Endothelial Growth Factor Receptor

Increased expression of one or more isoforms of the vascular endothelial growth factor (VEGF) receptor is a common finding in HNSCC.[54] VEGF receptor expression has been demonstrated to increase with disease progression, with higher expression noted in advanced HNSCCs compared to dysplasia and carcinoma *in situ*[55] and in tumors with lymph node metastases.[56,57] Furthermore, increased VEGF receptor expression has been linked to shortened disease-free survival[56,58] and overall survival[58,59] in case series of patients with HNSCC. Despite strong preclinical evidence supporting the importance of the VEGF pathway in HNSCC, clinical studies to date have failed to demonstrate significant survival improvements with agents targeting the VEGF pathway.

### Monoclonal Antibodies to the Vascular Endothelial Growth Factor Receptor

Bevacizumab, a humanized monoclonal antibody targeting the VEGF-A receptor, is the most studied VEGF-targeting agent in HNSCC. Limited single-agent activity has been noted, although multiple phase II studies examining the role of bevacizumab in combination with radiation,[29] chemotherapy[28] or cetuximab[30] have suggested potential activity. Argiris et al. examined bevacizumab in combination with the pemetrexed as a first-line treatment of recurrent/metastatic HNSCC and noted an overall response rate of 30% with a median overall survival of 11.3 months.[28] In previously treated patients with recurrent/metastatic HNSCC, the combination of cetuximab and bevacizumab resulted in a response rate of 16% and an overall survival rate of 7.5 months.[30] An ongoing phase III trial (ECOG 1305) of a platinum-containing chemotherapy regimen plus or minus bevacizumab should provide a more definitive answer regarding the benefit of bevacizumab in combination with a standard first-line therapy in recurrent/metastatic HNSCC.

### Small-Molecule Inhibitors of the Vascular Endothelial Growth Factor Receptor and Multikinase Inhibition

Despite encouraging preclinical evidence, small-molecule inhibitors with activity against the VEGF receptor have demonstrated limited efficacy in HNSCC. Multiple phase II studies have now been performed with a variety of tyrosine kinase inhibitors targeting the VEGF receptor, among others, with no significant clinical benefit yet demonstrated. Two trials examining the effect of sunitinib, a kinase inhibitor with activity against the VEGF as well as platelet-derived growth factor (PDGF) receptor, were terminated prematurely for a lack of efficacy,[60,61] while a third demonstrated modest effect but was associated with unacceptable toxicity.[32] A separate phase II study in platinum-refractory recurrent/metastatic

HNSCC examined docetaxel plus or minus vandetanib, an inhibitor of the VEGFR, EGFR and RET tyrosine kinases. This trial was stopped early due to a lack of efficacy.[62] Semaxanib, a potent VEGFR kinase inhibitor, and sorafenib, a multikinase inhibitor with activity against BRAF, KIT, FLT-3, RET and PDGFR in addition to the VEGFR, have demonstrated minimal activity in phase II trials in recurrent/metastatic HNSCC.[33,63] While these studies were conducted in heavily pretreated patient populations, the lack of efficacy suggests that the way forward for these targeted therapies in HNSCC is likely to be in a preselected population or in combination therapy if at all.

## Targeting the Proteasome

Bortezomib, a synthetic inhibitor of the 20S proteolytic core of the 26S proteasome, has been shown to inhibit NF-kappa B anti-apoptotic signaling in preclinical studies of HNSCC.[64] This pathway is suggested to play a role in HNSCC survival and treatment resistance,[34,65–67] suggesting a rationale for proteasome inhibition either as monotherapy or in combination with traditional cytotoxic therapy in HNSCC. Unfortunately, overall response rates in early phase I and II studies have been disappointing[34,36,68] and in several cases, the response and treatment efficacy have been worse than expected.[34,35] A phase I trial combining radiation with cetuximab and bortezomib was stopped prematurely due to an unexpectedly high rate of early tumor progression.[35] In tumor biopsy specimens, antagonism of radiation and cetuximab cytotoxicity and EGFR degradation along with an enhancement in prosurvival signaling were noted. Based upon these results, future evaluation of proteasome inhibitors in HNSCC should be considered carefully.

## Targeting TP53a

Mutations in the tumor suppressor TP53 is the single most common genetic alteration to be demonstrated in multiple series of HNSCC patients.[8–10] As a central regulator of genome integrity and cell survival, loss of TP53 function has been demonstrated to be critically important in carcinogenesis and disease progression in HNSCC, as with many other malignancies. Mutations in TP53 have also been demonstrated to have prognostic significance in HNSCC. Patients bearing TP53 mutations that are predicted to significantly affect protein function have been demonstrated to have a worse prognosis.[69,70]

With a complex quaternary structure and numerous protein–protein interactions, finding a way to target TP53 has proven challenging. Strategies to target HNSCCs bearing TP53 mutations have included reintroduction of wild-type protein activity as well as targeting vulnerabilities created by altered TP53 activity. Adjuvant perioperative gene therapy with p53 introduction into the surgical bed of patients with HNSCC using the adenoviral vector IGN201 (Ad5CMV-p53) demonstrated encouraging 1-year progression-free survival rates (92%), although limited patient numbers (n = 13) preclude conclusions regarding efficacy.[37] Previous to this, a study evaluating intratumoral injection of an adenoviral vector containing p53 in unresectable HNSCC demonstrated only modest activity.[38]

Rather than try to reintroduce normal p53 activity, others have tried to capitalize on functional differences and vulnerabilities created by a lack of intact p53 function. In one such trial, ONYX-015, an oncolytic adenovirus with replication ability limited to cells with inactive p53, was evaluated in 40 patients with recurrent HNSCC with a response rate ranging from 10–14% depending upon the dosing schedule.[39] Preclinical data suggest that targeting TP53-mutant HNSCC through cell cycle checkpoint inhibition may preferentially sensitize TP53 mutant tumors to DNA-damaging therapies.[71] Wee1 and Chk1 kinase inhibitors targeting the G2M cell cycle checkpoint are now in early phase clinical trials.

## Conclusions

Cetuximab, the monoclonal antibody directed against the EGFR, is currently the only targeted agent approved by the FDA for use in HNSCC. Despite promising preclinical evidence, the results of early phase clinical trials evaluating targeted agents directed against the tyrosine kinase domains of multiple mitogenic signaling receptors including the EGFR and VEGFR have demonstrated modest activity at best. New targeted agents continue to emerge and to be evaluated in HNSCC, mostly in patients with recurrent/metastatic and locoregionally advanced disease. Given the limited responses in most of these trials, it is clear that future trials will need to incorporate prospective evaluation of markers of response to better delineate patients most likely to respond as well as to consider evaluation of agents earlier in the course of treatment. There remains much work to be done.

## References

1 Ferlay J, Soerjomataram I, Ervik M, et al. GLOBOCAN 2012 v1.0, Cancer Incidence and Mortality Worldwide: IARC CancerBase No. 11 [Internet]. International Agency for Research on Cancer, Lyon, France, 2013. http://globocan.iarc.fr. Accessed March 25, 2015.

2 Sturgis EM, Ang KK. The epidemic of HPV-associated oropharyngeal cancer is here: is it time to change our treatment paradigms? *J Natl Compr Cancer Netw.* 2011;9(6):665–673.

3 Gillison ML, Koch WM, Capone RB, et al. Evidence for a causal association between human papillomavirus and a subset of head and neck cancers. *J Nal Cancer Inst.* 2000;92(9):709–720.

4 Hammarstedt L, Lindquist D, Dahlstrand H, et al. Human papillomavirus as a risk factor for the increase in incidence of tonsillar cancer. *Int J Cancer.* 2006;119(11):2620–2623.

5 Chaturvedi AK, Engels EA, Pfeiffer RM, et al. Human papillomavirus and rising oropharyngeal cancer incidence in the United States. *J Clin Oncol.* 2011;29(32):4294–4301.

6 Surveillance, Epidemiology, and End Results (SEER) Program (www.seer.cancer.gov).

7 Ang KK, Harris J, Wheeler R, et al. Human papillomavirus and survival of patients with oropharyngeal cancer. *N Engl J Med.* 2010;363(1):24–35.

8 Agrawal N, Frederick MJ, Pickering CR, et al. Exome sequencing of head and neck squamous cell carcinoma reveals inactivating mutations in NOTCH1. *Science.* 2011;333(6046):1154–1157.

9 Cancer Genome Atlas N. Comprehensive genomic characterization of head and neck squamous cell carcinomas. *Nature.* 2015;517:576–582.

10 Stransky N, Egloff AM, Tward AD, et al. The mutational landscape of head and neck squamous cell carcinoma. *Science.* 2011;333(6046):1157–1160.

11 Zack TI, Schumacher SE, Carter SL, et al. Pan-cancer patterns of somatic copy number alteration. *Nat Genet.* 2013;45(10):1134–1140.

12 Pickering CR, Zhang J, Yoo SY, et al. Integrative genomic characterization of oral squamous cell carcinoma identifies frequent somatic drivers. *Cancer Discov.* 2013;3(7):770–781.

13 Bernier J, Cooper JS, Pajak TF, et al. Defining risk levels in locally advanced head and neck cancers: a comparative analysis of concurrent postoperative radiation plus chemotherapy trials of the EORTC (#22931) and RTOG (# 9501). *Head Neck.* 2005;27(10):843–850.

14 Bernier J, Domenge C, Ozsahin M, et al: Postoperative irradiation with or without concomitant chemotherapy for locally advanced head and neck cancer. *N Eng J Med.* 2004;350(19):1945–1952.

15 Cooper JS, Pajak TF, Forastiere AA, et al. Postoperative concurrent radiotherapy and chemotherapy for high-risk squamous-cell carcinoma of the head and neck. *N Eng J Med.* 2004;350(19):1937–1944.

16 Ma J, Liu Y, Huang XL, et al. Induction chemotherapy decreases the rate of distant metastasis in patients with head and neck squamous cell carcinoma but does not improve survival or locoregional control: a meta-analysis. *Oral Oncol.* 2012;48(11):1076–1084.

17 Haddad R, O'Neill A, Rabinowits G, et al. Induction chemotherapy followed by concurrent chemoradiotherapy (sequential chemoradiotherapy) versus concurrent chemoradiotherapy alone in locally advanced head and neck cancer (PARADIGM): a randomised phase 3 trial. *Lancet Oncol.* 2013;14(3):257–264.

18 Hitt R, Grau JJ, Lopez-Pousa A, et al. A randomized phase III trial comparing induction chemotherapy followed by chemoradiotherapy versus chemoradiotherapy alone as treatment of unresectable head and neck cancer. *Ann Oncol.* 2014;25(1):216–225.

19 Bonner JA, Harari PM, Giralt J, et al. Radiotherapy plus cetuximab for squamous-cell carcinoma of the head and neck. *N Eng J Med.* 2006;354(6):567–578.

20 Vermorken JB, Mesia R, Rivera F, et al. Platinum-based chemotherapy plus cetuximab in head and neck cancer. *N Engl J Med.* 2008;359:1116–1127.

21 Burtness B, Goldwasser MA, Flood W, Mattar B, Forastiere AA; Eastern Cooperative Oncology G. Phase III randomized trial of cisplatin plus placebo compared with cisplatin plus cetuximab in metastatic/recurrent head and neck cancer: an Eastern Cooperative Oncology Group study. *J Clin Oncol.* 2005;23(34):8646–8654.

22 Vermorken JB, Stohlmacher-Williams J, Davidenko I, et al. Cisplatin and fluorouracil with or without panitumumab in patients with recurrent or metastatic squamous-cell carcinoma of the head and neck (SPECTRUM): an open-label phase 3 randomised trial. *Lancet Oncol.* 2013;14(8):697–710.

23 Machiels JP, Subramanian S, Ruzsa A, et al. Zalutumumab plus best supportive care versus best supportive care alone in patients with recurrent or metastatic squamous-cell carcinoma of the head and neck after failure of platinum-based chemotherapy: an open-label, randomised phase 3 trial. *Lancet Oncol.* 2011;12(4):333–343.

24 Stewart JS, Cohen EE, Licitra L, et al. Phase III study of gefitinib compared with intravenous methotrexate for recurrent squamous cell carcinoma of the head and neck [corrected]. *J Clin Oncol.* 2009;27(11):1864–1871.

25 Argiris A, Ghebremichael M, Gilbert J, et al. Phase III randomized, placebo-controlled trial of docetaxel with or without gefitinib in recurrent or metastatic head and neck cancer: an eastern cooperative oncology group trial. *J Clin Oncol.* 2013;31:1405–1414.

26 Martins RG, Parvathaneni U, Bauman JE, et al. Cisplatin and radiotherapy with or without erlotinib in locally advanced squamous cell carcinoma of the head and neck: a randomized phase II trial. *J Clin Oncol.* 2013;31:1415–1421.

27 Lee NY, Zhang Q, Pfister DG, et al. Addition of bevacizumab to standard chemoradiation for locoregionally advanced nasopharyngeal carcinoma (RTOG 0615): a phase 2 multi-institutional trial. *Lancet Oncol.* 2012;13:172–180.

28  Argiris A, Karamouzis MV, Gooding WE, et al. Phase II trial of pemetrexed and bevacizumab in patients with recurrent or metastatic head and neck cancer. *J Clin Oncol.* 2011;29(9):1140–1145.

29  Fury MG, Lee NY, Sherman E, et al. A phase 2 study of bevacizumab with cisplatin plus intensity-modulated radiation therapy for stage III/IVB head and neck squamous cell cancer. *Cancer.* 2012;118(20):5008–5014.

30  Argiris A, Kotsakis AP, Hoang T, et al. Cetuximab and bevacizumab: preclinical data and phase II trial in recurrent or metastatic squamous cell carcinoma of the head and neck. *Ann Oncol.* 2013;24(1):220–225.

31  Cohen EE, Davis DW, Karrison TG, et al. Erlotinib and bevacizumab in patients with recurrent or metastatic squamous-cell carcinoma of the head and neck: a phase I/II study. *Lancet Oncol.* 2009;10:247–257.

32  Machiels JP, Henry S, Zanetta S, et al. Phase II study of sunitinib in recurrent or metastatic squamous cell carcinoma of the head and neck: GORTEC 2006-01. *J Clin Oncol.* 2010;28(1):21–28.

33  Williamson SK, Moon J, Huang CH, et al. Phase II evaluation of sorafenib in advanced and metastatic squamous cell carcinoma of the head and neck: Southwest Oncology Group Study S0420. *J Clin Oncol.* 2010;28(20):3330–3335.

34  Chung CH, Aulino J, Muldowney NJ, et al. Nuclear factor-kappa B pathway and response in a phase II trial of bortezomib and docetaxel in patients with recurrent and/or metastatic head and neck squamous cell carcinoma. *Ann Oncol.* 2010;21(4):864–870.

35  Argiris A, Duffy AG, Kummar S, et al. Early tumor progression associated with enhanced EGFR signaling with bortezomib, cetuximab, and radiotherapy for head and neck cancer. *Clin Cancer Res.* 2011;17(17):5755–5764.

36  Gilbert J, Lee JW, Argiris A, et al. Phase II 2-arm trial of the proteasome inhibitor, PS-341 (bortezomib) in combination with irinotecan or PS-341 alone followed by the addition of irinotecan at time of progression in patients with locally recurrent or metastatic squamous cell carcinoma of the head and neck (E1304): a trial of the Eastern Cooperative Oncology Group. *Head Neck.* 2013;35(7):942–948.

37  Yoo GH, Moon J, Leblanc M, et al. A phase 2 trial of surgery with perioperative INGN 201 (Ad5CMV-p53) gene therapy followed by chemoradiotherapy for advanced, resectable squamous cell carcinoma of the oral cavity, oropharynx, hypopharynx, and larynx: report of the Southwest Oncology Group. *Arch Otolaryngo Head Neck Surg.* 2009;135(9):869–874.

38  Clayman GL, el-Naggar AK, Lippman SM, et al. Adenovirus-mediated p53 gene transfer in patients with advanced recurrent head and neck squamous cell carcinoma. *J Clin Oncol.* 1998;16(6):2221–2232.

39  Nemunaitis J, Khuri F, Ganly I, et al. Phase II trial of intratumoral administration of ONYX-015, a replication-selective adenovirus, in patients with refractory head and neck cancer. *J Clin Oncol.* 2001;19(2):289–298.

40  Markovic A, Chung CH. Current role of EGF receptor monoclonal antibodies and tyrosine kinase inhibitors in the management of head and neck squamous cell carcinoma. *Expert Rev Anticancer Ther.* 2012;12(9):1149–1159.

41  Lee JW, Soung YH, Kim SY, et al. Somatic mutations of EGFR gene in squamous cell carcinoma of the head and neck. *Clin Cancer Res.* 2005;11(8):2879–2882.

42  He Y, Zeng Q, Drenning SD, et al. Inhibition of human squamous cell carcinoma growth in vivo by epidermal growth factor receptor antisense RNA transcribed from the U6 promoter. *J Natl Cancer Inst.* 1998;90(14):1080–1087.

43  Chung CH, Ely K, McGavran L, et al. Increased epidermal growth factor receptor gene copy number is associated with poor prognosis in head and neck squamous cell carcinomas. *J Clin Oncol.* 2006;24(25):4170–4176.

44  Temam S, Kawaguchi H, El-Naggar AK, et al. Epidermal growth factor receptor copy number alterations correlate with poor clinical outcome in patients with head and neck squamous cancer. *J Clin Oncol.* 2007;25(16):2164–2170.

45  Taoudi Benchekroun M, Saintigny P, Thomas SM, et al. Epidermal growth factor receptor expression and gene copy number in the risk of oral cancer. *Cancer Prev Res.* 2010;3(7):800–809.

46  Li S, Schmitz KR, Jeffrey PD, Wiltzius JJ, Kussie P, Ferguson KM. Structural basis for inhibition of the epidermal growth factor receptor by cetuximab. *Cancer Cell.* 2005;7(4):301–311.

47  Ferris RL, Jaffee EM, Ferrone S. Tumor antigen-targeted, monoclonal antibody-based immunotherapy: clinical response, cellular immunity, and immunoescape. *J Clin Oncol.* 2010;28(28):4390–4399.

48  Lopez-Albaitero A, Ferris RL. Immune activation by epidermal growth factor receptor specific monoclonal antibody therapy for head and neck cancer. *Arch Otolaryngol.* 2007;133(12):1277–1281.

49  Srivastava RM, Lee SC, Andrade Filho PA, et al. Cetuximab-activated natural killer and dendritic cells collaborate to trigger tumor antigen-specific T-cell immunity in head and neck cancer patients. *Clin Cancer Res.* 2013;19(7):1858–1872.

50  Baselga J, Trigo JM, Bourhis J, et al. Phase II multicenter study of the antiepidermal growth factor receptor monoclonal antibody cetuximab in combination with platinum-based chemotherapy in patients with platinum-refractory metastatic and/or recurrent squamous cell carcinoma of the head and neck. *J Clin Oncol.* 2005;23(24):5568–5577.

51  Herbst RS, Arquette M, Shin DM, et al. Phase II multicenter study of the epidermal growth factor receptor antibody cetuximab and cisplatin for recurrent and refractory squamous cell carcinoma of the head and neck. *J Clin Oncol.* 2005;23(24):5578–5587.

52  Vermorken JB, Trigo J, Hitt R, et al. Open-label, uncontrolled, multicenter phase II study to evaluate the efficacy and toxicity of cetuximab as a single agent in patients with recurrent and/or metastatic squamous cell carcinoma of the head and neck who failed to respond to platinum-based therapy. *J Clin Oncol.* 2007;25(16):2171–2177.

53  Perez CA, Song H, Raez LE, et al. Phase II study of gefitinib adaptive dose escalation to skin toxicity in recurrent or metastatic squamous cell carcinoma of the head and neck. *Oral Oncol.* 2012;48(9):887–892.

54  Neuchrist C, Erovic BM, Handisurya A, et al. Vascular endothelial growth factor receptor 2 (VEGFR2) expression in squamous cell carcinomas of the head and neck. *Laryngoscope.* 2001;111(10):1834–1841.

55  Sauter ER, Nesbit M, Watson JC, Klein-Szanto A, Litwin S, Herlyn M. Vascular endothelial growth factor is a marker of tumor invasion and metastasis in squamous cell carcinomas of the head and neck. *Clin Cancer Res.* 1999;5(4):775–782.

56  Mineta H, Miura K, Ogino T, et al. Prognostic value of vascular endothelial growth factor (VEGF) in head and neck squamous cell carcinomas. *Br J Cancer.* 2000;83(6):775–781.

57  O-charoenrat P, Rhys-Evans P, Eccles SA. Expression of vascular endothelial growth factor family members in head and neck squamous cell carcinoma correlates with lymph node metastasis. *Cancer.* 2001;92(3):556–568.

58  Smith BD, Smith GL, Carter D, Sasaki CT, Haffty BG. Prognostic significance of vascular endothelial growth factor protein levels in oral and oropharyngeal squamous cell carcinoma. *J Clin Oncol.* 2000;18(10):2046–2052.

59  Kyzas PA, Cunha IW, Ioannidis JP. Prognostic significance of vascular endothelial growth factor immunohistochemical expression in head and neck squamous cell carcinoma: a meta-analysis. *Clin Cancer Res.* 2005;11(4):1434–1440.

60  Choong NW, Kozloff M, Taber D, et al. Phase II study of sunitinib malate in head and neck squamous cell carcinoma. *Invest New Drugs.* 2010;28(5):677–683.

61  Drugs IN, Fountzilas G, Fragkoulidi A, et al. A phase II study of suni-tinib in patients with recurrent and/or metastatic non-nasopharyngeal head and neck cancer. *Cancer Chemother Pharmacol.* 2010;65(4):649–660.

62  Limaye S, Riley S, Zhao S, et al. A randomized phase II study of docetaxel with or without vandetanib in recurrent or metastatic squamous cell car-cinoma of head and neck (SCCHN). *Oral Oncology.* 2013;49(8):835–841.

63  Fury MG, Zahalsky A, Wong R, et al. A Phase II study of SU5416 in patients with advanced or recurrent head and neck cancers. *Invest New Drugs.* 2007;25(2):165–172.

64  Tamatani T, Takamaru N, Hara K, et al. Bortezomib-enhanced radiosen-sitization through the suppression of radiation-induced nuclear factor-kappaB activity in human oral cancer cells. *Int J Oncol.* 2013;42(3):935–944.

65  Duffey DC, Chen Z, Dong G, et al. Expression of a dominant-negative mutant inhibitor-kappaBalpha of nuclear factor-kappaB in human head and neck squamous cell carcinoma inhibits survival, proinflamma-tory cytokine expression, and tumor growth in vivo. *Cancer Res.* 1999;59(14):3468–3474.

66  Didelot C, Barberi-Heyob M, Bianchi A, et al. Constitutive NF-kappaB activity influences basal apoptosis and radiosensitivity of head-and-neck carcinoma cell lines. *Int J Radiat Oncol Biol Phys.* 2001;51(5):1354–1360.

67  Chang AA, Van Waes C. Nuclear factor-KappaB as a common target and activator of oncogenes in head and neck squamous cell carcinoma. *Adv Otorhinolaryngol.* 2005;62:92–102.

68  Kubicek GJ, Axelrod RS, Machtay M, et al. Phase I trial using the protea-some inhibitor bortezomib and concurrent chemoradiotherapy for head-and-neck malignancies. *Int J Radiat Oncol Biol Phys.* 2012;83(4):1192–1197.

69  Poeta ML, Manola J, Goldwasser MA, et al. TP53 mutations and sur-vival in squamous-cell carcinoma of the head and neck. *N Eng J Med.* 2007;357(25):2552–2561.

70  Skinner HD, Sandulache VC, Ow TJ, et al. TP53 disruptive mutations lead to head and neck cancer treatment failure through inhibition of radiation-induced senescence. *Clin Cancer Res.* 2012;18(1):290–300.

71  Gadhikar MA, Sciuto MR, Alves MV, et al. Chk1/2 inhibition overcomes the cisplatin resistance of head and neck cancer cells secondary to the loss of functional p53. *Mol Cancer Ther.* 2013;12(9):1860–1873.

# CHAPTER 23

# Targeted Therapy in Solid Tumors: Lung Cancer

*Saiama N. Waqar[1], Daniel Morgensztern[1], and Roy S. Herbst[2]*

[1]Department of Medicine, Division of Medical Oncology, Washington University School of Medicine, St. Louis, MO, USA
[2]Department of Medicine, Division of Medical Oncology, Yale Comprehensive Cancer Center, New Haven, CT, USA

Lung cancer is the leading cause of cancer-related death in the United States among men and women.[1] Non-small cell lung cancer (NSCLC) accounts for 87% of lung carcinomas, whereas small cell lung cancer (SCLC) comprises the remaining 13%.[2] NSCLC is divided according to histology into several subtypes, with adenocarcinoma being the most common (41%), followed by squamous cell carcinoma (17%) and large cell carcinoma (8%).[3] Approximately half of patients with NSCLC present with stage IV disease due to either malignant pleural effusion or distant metastases.[4,5] With the exception of rare cases of oligometastatic disease cured with resection of both primary and metastatic sites,[6] treatment for stage IV NSCLC is essentially palliative. Although chemotherapy using mostly platinum-based combinations has been shown to improve the survival in patients with metastatic NSCLC compared to supportive care,[7] this modality reached a plateau with no significant differences in outcomes among the multiple regimens tested.[8,9] Therefore, chemotherapy choices have been empirically based on predictive toxicities and personal preferences. The search for more effective and less toxic therapies for metastatic NSCLC led to the development of several targeted therapies, which have been associated with a significant benefit in molecularly selected patients.

## Angiogenesis

Angiogenesis is defined as the growth of new blood vessels from existing vasculature.[10] Due to its critical role in tumor growth and metastases, the inhibition of angiogenesis has been used as a treatment strategy in solid tumors, including NSCLC. The first antiangiogenesis drug to show benefit in NSCLC was bevacizumab (Avastin), a humanized monoclonal antibody against circulating VEGF. In the initial phase II trial comparing carboplatin plus paclitaxel alone or in combination with bevacizumab, the triplet therapy was associated with increased response rates (31.5% vs. 18.8%), median time to progression (7.4 vs. 4.2 months) and median overall survival (OS) (17.7 vs. 14.9 months).[11] The most serious toxicity was fatal hemoptysis, which was more common in patients with squamous cell histology, tumor cavitation and location close to major vessels. Therefore, subsequent trials included only patients with non-squamous histologies. Two randomized clinical trials, the East-

ern Cooperative Oncology Group (ECOG) 4599[12] and Avastin in Lung (AVAiL)[13] showed improved progression-free survival (PFS) with the addition of bevacizumab to chemotherapy, although only ECOG 4599 was associated with improved overall survival (OS). The benefit from bevacizumab in patients with metastatic however, is modest, transient and there are currently no predictors for response. Multiple trials using small molecule tyrosine kinase inhibitors VEGFR-2 in combination with chemotherapy showed disappointing results in both first- and second-line settings.[14–17]

## Epidermal Growth Factor Receptor

Epidermal growth factor receptor (EGFR; ErbB1) is a transmembrane receptor that belongs to a family of four related proteins also including HER2 (ErbB2), HER 3 (ErbB3), and HER4 (ErbB4). Ligand binding to a single-chain EGFR leads to dimerization, receptor dimerization and signaling through tyrosine kinase activity, resulting in the activation of multiple pathways involved in cell proliferation, survival, metastases, and neoangiogenesis.[18] The two main approaches for targeting EGFR are tyrosine kinase inhibitors (TKIs) and monoclonal antibodies.

The initial studies with the EGFR TKIs were conducted in unselected previously treated NSCLC patients. The response rates for gefitinib (Iressa) as second- or third-line therapy ranged between 11% and 18% in the two Iressa Dose Evaluation in Advanced Lung Cancer (IDEAL) trials, which had no control arm and also showed no significant differences between the two doses of gefitinib (250 mg and 500 mg).[19,20] In the subsequent Iressa Survival Evaluation in Lung Cancer (ISEL), there was no survival benefit from geftinib compared to placebo in previously treated patients with advanced NSCLC.[21] In contrast, the BR.21 trial showed a significant improvement in median PFS and OS for erlotinib (Tarceva) compared to placebo.[22] The major clinical predictors for response to EGFR TKIs were adenocarcinoma histology, East Asian ethnicity, female gender and absence of smoking.[23] In 2004, two groups simultaneously demonstrated that *EGFR* kinase domain mutations were highly predictive for response to EGFR TKIs.[24,25] In a study testing 2105 Spanish patients for activating EGFR mutations, including deletion in exon 19 or L858R on exon 21, there were 350 (16.6%) positive

*Targeted Therapy in Translational Cancer Research*, First Edition. Edited by Apostolia-Maria Tsimberidou, Razelle Kurzrock and Kenneth C. Anderson.
© 2016 John Wiley & Sons, Inc. Published 2016 by John Wiley & Sons, Inc.

**Table 23.1** Comparison between EGFR TKIs and chemotherapy in patients with activating *EGFR* mutations.

| Study | N | EGFR TKI | Chemotherapy | Response | Median PFS | p-value |
|-------|---|----------|--------------|----------|------------|---------|
| IPASS[32] | 261 | Gefitinib | Carb Pac | 71 vs. 47% | 9.8 vs. 6.4 m | <0.001 |
| WJTOG 3405[33] | 172 | Gefitinib | Cisp Doc | 62 vs. 32% | 9.2 vs. 6.3 m | <0.001 |
| NEJ002[34] | 228 | Gefitinib | Carb Pac | 73 vs. 30% | 10.8 vs. 5.4 m | <0.001 |
| OPTIMAL[35] | 154 | Erlotinib | Carb Gem | 82 vs. 36% | 13.1 vs. 4.6 m | <0.001 |
| EURTAC[36] | 173 | Erlotinib | Cis or Carb + Doc or Gem | 58 vs. 15% | 9.7 vs. 5.2 m | <0.001 |

Carb, carboplatin; Cisp, cisplatin; Doc, docetaxel; Gem, gemitabine

cases.[26] Although the frequency of mutations correlated with the clinical predictors, including female gender (30.0%), never smokers (37.7%), and adenocarcinomas (17.3%), all patients with nonsquamous histology had a possibility of harboring the mutations, including current smokers (5.8%) and patients with large cell carcinoma (11.5%).

The use of EGFR TKIs in molecularly selected patients has been associated with response rates ranging from 48% to 90%.[27–31] This significant benefit in earlier studies led to the launching of several randomized trials comparing EGFR TKIs to standard chemotherapy in untreated patients (Table 23.1). The first reported trial, the IRESSA Pan Asia Study (IPASS) compared gefitinib to carboplatin plus paclitaxel in patients with adenocarcinoma who were either nonsmokers defined as less than 100 cigarettes in their lifetime or light smokers, defined as 10 pack-years or less and quitting at least 15 years prior to enrollment.[32] Among the patients without *EGFR* mutation, both the response rates (23.5% vs. 1.1%) and PFS (HR 2.85, $p < 0.001$) favored the chemotherapy arm, whereas among those with *EGFR* mutation, gefitinib was associated with a significant improvement in response rates (71.2% vs. 47.3%) and PFS (HR 0.48, $p < 0.001$). Since then, several other studies showed a PFS benefit from gefitinib or erlotinib compared to platinum doublets in patients with pulmonary adenocarcinoma and activating EGFR mutations.[33–36] Despite the improvement in PFS, maturing data from the trials have not shown an increase in OS for EGFR TKIs compared to standard chemotherapy, most likely due to crossover after disease progression.[37]

Although there is a clear indication for the use of EGFR TKIs in patients with activating *EGFR* mutations, their role in wild-type patients remains undefined. Although chemotherapy has been shown to be significantly superior to EGFR TKIs in previously untreated patients with wild-type *EGFR*,[32] response rates to chemotherapy in the second-line setting are very modest and usually below 10%.[38–40] In the SequentiAl Tarceva in UnResectable NSCLC (SATURN) study, 889 patients with advanced NSCLC who achieved at least stable disease (SD) after four cycles of a platinum-based chemotherapy doublet were randomized to maintenance with erlotinib or placebo.[41,42] There was a significant improvement in PFS for the erlotinib maintenance arm for both adenocarcinomas and squamous cell carcinoma, whereas the OS was improved only in the latter. Nevertheless, when evaluating only patients who achieved SD, there was a significant OS improvement in both histologies.[41] The TArceva Italian Lung Optimization tRial (TAILOR) randomized 222 patients with wild-type *EGFR* and previously treated with one line of platinum-based chemotherapy, to erlotinib or docetaxel with the primary endpoint being OS.[43] Docetaxel was associated with improved response rates (15.5 vs. 3%, $p = 0.003$), disease control rate (44.3 vs. 36%, $p = 0.007$), PFS (2.9 vs. 2.2. months, $p = 0.02$), and median OS (8.2 vs. 5.4 months, hazard ratio [HR] 0.73,

$p = 0.05$). In an attempt to identify predictors for benefit from EGFR TKIs in patient with wild type-disease, the PROSE study compared second-line erlotinib to pemetrexed or docetaxel while stratifying patients according to performance status, smoking history and proteomic profile using VeriStrat into good or poor risk groups.[44] Although patients classified as VeriStrat poor-risk had improved outcomes with chemotherapy compared to erlotinib, there were no significant differences in OS for patients with VeriSrat good. Therefore, despite the improved efficacy for chemotherapy compared to EGFR TKIs in EGFR wild-type tumors, the latter may still have a role in the management of advanced stage NSCLC, either in the maintenance setting or in selected populations.

In contrast to the first-generation EGFR TKIs gefitinib and erlotinib, there are several new EGFR inhibitors characterized by irreversible EGFR inhibition and targeting of additional members of the EGFR family, including HER2 and HER4. The LUX-3 study compared the second-generation EGFR TKI afatinib to cisplatin plus pemetrexed in patients with *EGFR* mutant metastatic pulmonary adenocarcinomas.[45] Afatinib was associated with a significant improvement in PFS (11.1 vs. 6.9 months; HR 0.58, $p = 0.001$), with the median PFS reaching 13.6 months for patients with exon 19 deletions or L858R mutations.

Despite the significant benefit from EGFR TKIs in patients with *EGFR* mutant disease, virtually all patients eventually develop disease progression. The most common cause for secondary resistance is the development of a secondary mutation in T790M on exon 20, which occurs in approximately 50% of patients.[46,47] Other described mechanisms include *PIK3CA* mutations, *MET* amplification, *HER2* amplifications, epithelial to mesenchymal transformation (EMT) and transformation to small cell lung cancer (SCLC). Third generation EGFR TKIs including WZ4002 and CO1686 have been designed specifically to inhibit T790M mutations, with earlier studies showing promising results.[48]

Given the significant benefit of TKIs in the metastatic setting, attempts are being made to incorporate these agents in the curative therapy following surgery, or in combination with chemoradiation. In the National Cancer Institute of Canada (NCIC) BR19 study 503 patients were randomized between 2002 and 2005 to receive adjuvant gefitinib or placebo.[49] Since the study started before the establishment of adjuvant chemotherapy as a standard of care, only 87 patients received chemotherapy. There was no benefit for adjuvant gefitinib on disease-free survival (DFS) or OS, neither in the wild-type EGFR population nor in the 15 patients with activated mutations (seven patients in the gefitinib arm and eight patients in the placebo arm). The RADIANT trial is an ongoing phase III trial comparing erlotinib versus placebo in resected NSCLC with EGFR positivity by IHC or FISH.[50] The phase II SELECT trial is a the first study investigating the role of adjuvant erlotinib in EGFR-mutant NSCLC.[51] The RTOG 1306 study is a phase II trial in which patients with stage III EGFR-mutant lung cancer and ALK-positive NSCLC will be randomized to receive 12 weeks of induction erlotinib (EGFR-mutant) or crizotinib (ALK-positive) followed by chemoradiation, or chemoradiation alone.[52]

Cetuximab (Erbitux) is a monoclonal antibody directed against EGFR that has been evaluated in two large randomized trials. The BMS099 trial showed no benefit from the addition of cetuximab to chemotherapy with carboplatin plus paclitaxel.[53] In contrast, in the First Line ErbituX (FLEX) trial, a multicenter, international phase III trial in patients with advanced EGFR-expressing NSCLC, who were randomized to combination chemotherapy with cisplatin, vinorelbine and cetuximab or cisplatin and vinorelbine without cetuximab,[54] the primary end-point was OS, and patients who were given chemotherapy with cetuximab survived longer than those in the chemotherapy only group (median 11.3 months vs. 10.1 months, HR 0.871 95% CI 0.772–0.996; $p = 0.044$). More recently, the presence of increased EGFR expression by immunohistochemistry (H-score) evaluated in samples from the FLEX study, was found to predict response to cetuximab-based triplets.[55] The median OS was significantly improved for the cetuximab arm in patients with H-score $\geq 200$ (12 vs. 9 months) but not for those with score $<200$ (9.8 vs. 10.3 months). The SWOG 0819 trial is currently comparing chemotherapy with carboplatin plus paclitaxel (and bevacizumab in eligible patients), alone or in combination with cetuximab.

## ALK

*ALK* fusion genes were initially described in 2007 as resulting from a small inversion within chromosome 2p, leading to the expression of a chimeric tyrosine kinase in which the N-terminal portion of the echinoderm microtubule-associated protein-like 4 (*EML4*) gene is fused to the intracellular kinase domain of anaplastic lymphoma kinase (*ALK*).[56] Since the original report, several variants of *ALK-EML4* fusion have been identified and three other partners for *ALK* fusion have been described, including *TGF, KIF5B,* and *KLC1*.[57] ALK fusion proteins activate multiple signaling pathways including the mitogen-activated protein kinase (MAPK) and phosphoinositide 3-kinase (PI3K).[58] *ALK* fusions are more common in men, younger than the usual NSCLC median age, and they have adenocarcinoma histology and a history of light or never smoking.

In the initial targeted study, 82 patients with *ALK* fusion by FISH, defined as more than 15% of scored tumor cells positive, were treated with the ALK inhibitor crizotinib.[59] The overall response rate was 57% with an estimated 6-month PFS of 72% and a median PFS that was not reached at the time of report. In the updated analysis, the PFS rates at 1 year and 2 years were 74% and 54%, respectively.[60] In a randomized clinical trial comparing crizotinib with docetaxel or pemetrexed in previously treated ALK-positive patients, crizotinib was associated with a significant improvement in median PFS (7.7 vs. 3.0 months; HR 0.49, $p < 0.001$).[61] Nevertheless, despite the significant improvement in PFS for patients treated with crizotinib, there was no survival benefit with median OS of 20.3 months and 22.8 months for the crizotinib and chemotherapy arms, respectively. Crizotinib is currently being compared to chemotherapy with platinum plus pemetrexed in patients with *ALK*-positive tumors.

Resistance to crizotinib is essentially universal and has been characterized as ALK-dominant (resistance mutations or ALK copy number gain) or ALK non-dominant (second oncogene, which may be ALK-dependent or independent).[62] Secondary ALK mutations described in patients with acquired resistance to crizotinib include

L1196M and G1269A.[63] New ALK inhibitors that are in clinical trials include LDK378, AP26113, ASP3026, and CH5424802. LDK378 has been studied in patients with ALK-positive NSCLC and was found to have response rates of 60% in crizotinib-naïve patients and 57% in crizotinib pre-treated patients.[64]

## ROS1

ROS1 is a receptor tyrosine kinase belonging to the insulin receptor family. *ROS1* fusions lead to constitutive kinase activity and have been identified as driver mutations in the HCC78 NSCLC cell line and in a sample of one patient with lung cancer.[65] In a screening of 1073 patients with FISH at 4 institutions, there were 18 patients (2%) with *ROS1* rearrangements.[66] *ROS1*-positive patients were younger than the general NSCLC population screened (median age 49.8 vs. 62.0), never smokers (78%), and had adenocarcinoma (100% of the cases). One patient from the cohort had a near complete response to crizotinib by restaging CT scans at 8 weeks, without evidence of recurrence by 6 months. In the initial trial with crizotinib in 14 patients with *ROS1* rearrangements, the overall response rate was 57%, with 1 complete response (CR) and 7 partial responses (PR).[67]

## RET

The fusion gene between *KIF5B* and the *RET* proto-oncogene in lung adenocarcinoma was first described in 2012, with an estimated frequency of 1%.[68–71] *KIF5B-RET* fusion gene overexpresses the chimeric RET tyrosine kinase, which induces cellular transformation.[68] Clinical characteristics of patients with RET fusions include poorly differentiated tumors, small primary tumor $\leq 3$ cm with N2 nodal disease, younger patients, and never-smokers.[72] In the preliminary report for the first three patients enrolled into a phase II trial evaluating the role of cabozantinib in patients with RET fusion positive tumors, 2 patients had PR and another had an SD approaching 8 months.[73]

## BRAF

BRAF is a serine/threonine kinase that lies downstream of RAS in the MAPK signaling pathway. The frequency of *BRAF* mutations in patients with pulmonary adenocarcinomas in two retrospective studies was between 3 and 4.9%, with 50 to 56% represented by V600E mutations.[74,75] Mutations occurred more commonly in current and former smokers. In the phase II BRF113928 study, previously treated patients with *BRAF* V600E mutation received dabrafenib with the primary objective of objective response rate.[76] In the preliminary analysis of the first 20 patients, the PR and SD rates were 40% and 20%, respectively.

## HER2

Unlike the other member of EGFR family, HER2 has no known ligand, participating mostly in heterodimerization with the other receptors upon their ligand binding. In a retrospective study evaluating the frequency of *HER2* in-frame insertion on exon 20, the mutation was observed in 65 (1.7%) of 3800 patients tested.[77] Mutations were more common in women and never smokers. The evaluation of anti-HER2 therapies in this population showed a disease control rate of 96% in the 15 patients treated with trastuzumab-based therapy and 100% for the 4 patients treated with afatinib.

## KRAS

*KRAS* mutations are the most common somatic gene mutation found in pulmonary adenocarcinoma, with a frequency of approximately 30%.[78] In lung cancer, the *KRAS* mutations occur predominantly at codons 12 and 13, with single amino acid substitutions.

There has been minimal success in the targeted treatment of KRAS mutant tumors. In the Biomarker-Integrated Approaches of Targeted Therapy for Lung Cancer Elimination (BATTLE) trial, 341 patients underwent a repeated biopsy and were assigned to erlotinib, vandetanib, erlotinib plus bexarotene or sorafenib, with the first 97 patients being equally randomized and the subsequent 158 patients undergoing adaptive randomization.[79] The primary endpoint was the disease control rate at 8 weeks. Among the 14 patients with *KRAS* or *BRAF* mutations treated with sorafenib, 11 (79%) had no evidence of progression by 8 weeks. In a phase II trial, patients with *KRAS* mutant tumors were randomized to second-line docetaxel alone or in combination with the MEK inhibitor selumetinib with the primary endpoint of OS improvement.[80] The selumetinib arm was associated with a significant improvement in response rate (16% vs. 0%, $p < 0.001$) and PFS (5.3 vs. 2.1 months), but not OS (9.4 vs. 5.2 months, $p = 0.21$). The selumetinib arm was associated with an increased risk of neutropenic fever.

## Other Mutations in Adenocarcinomas

Several additional mutations have been described in patients with pulmonary adenocarcinoma. The Lung Cancer Mutation Consortium (LCMC) is a large multi-institution effort to characterize the recurrent driver mutations in lung adenocarcinoma and match the abnormalities with a specific trial with the goal of offering personalized therapy (Figure 23.1).[81] Other less common driver mutations described by the LCMC include *PIK3CA*, *NRAS*, *AKT1*, and *MEK1*. *MET* amplification has also been categorized as a driver event.

## Squamous Cell Lung Cancer

Although there have been significant improvements in the treatment of lung cancer over the last few years, this benefit has been restricted mostly to patients with adenocarcinoma, with no targeted agent currently approved for the specific therapy of squa-

mous cell lung cancer.[82] Candidate driver mutations in squamous cell carcinoma include *SOX2*, *PIK3CA*, *FGFR1*, *IGF1R*, *MET*, *DDR2*, and *PTEN*. Although there are several drugs currently being tested in patients with squamous cell carcinoma, the results are still unavailable.

The SWOG 1400 (Master protocol) is an intergroup phase II-III biomarker-driven protocol for second-line chemotherapy in squamous cell lung cancer where patients will be randomized according to their genomic markers to receive standard therapy or investigational targeted therapy. Each arm will have a phase II component with the primary endpoint of PFS and a phase III design with OS as the primary endpoint. The initial arms to be compared to standard chemotherapy are expected to be PI3K inhibitors (*PIK3CA* mutations), CD4/6 inhibitors (CDKN2A deletions or mutations, CDK6 amplifications), FGFR inhibitors (*FGFR* mutation, amplification, or fusion), and MET inhibitors (MET overexpression). Patients without matched abnormalities will be randomized to anti-PDL1 checkpoint inhibition or standard therapy. The protocol was activated in 2014.

## Comprehensive Genomic Studies

The use of next-generation sequencing has allowed a comprehensive characterization of tumor genomes with a better understanding of the lung cancer biology and the discovery of new therapeutic targets. In adenocarcinomas, there was a significant difference in the median number of point mutations between smokers and nonsmokers, which were significantly higher in the former (10.5 vs. 0.6 per Mb).[83] More importantly, each patient had a median of 11 (range 7–17) potentially druggable targets. Furthermore, the transcriptome sequencing data identified a novel *KDELR2-ROS1* fusion, which may predict for sensitivity to crizotinib.

The Cancer Genome Atlas (TCGA) research network profiled 178 patients with squamous cell lung cancer.[84] Somatic alterations of potentially targetable genes were found in 114 (64%) of patients. The most commonly altered pathway was the phosphatidylinositol-3-OH kinase (PI3K)-Receptor tyrosine kinase (RTK)-RAS signaling (69%). The *CDKN2A* tumor suppressor gene was inactivated in 72% of patients.

Two large next generation sequencing studies have been recently reported in patients with small cell lung cancer. Pfeifer et al.

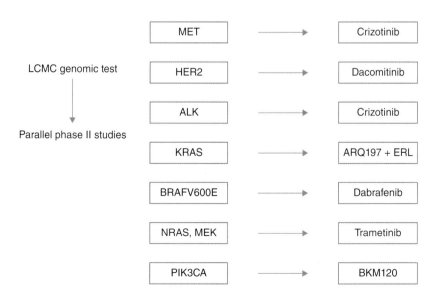

**Figure 23.1** Trial design by Lung Cancer Mutation Consortium. LCMC trials are designed to match a targeted agent to the specific mutation. Crizotinib is an inhibitor of MET, ALK, and ROS1. Dacomitinib is a second-generation EGFR TKI. Both dabrafenib and trametinib are MEK inhibitors. ERL is erlotinib and ARQ197 is a MET inhibitor.

showed mutation and loss of *TP53* and *RB1* in all patients.[85] Other common abnormalities included inactivation of *CREBBP* and *EP300* and *MLL* mutations. Rudin et al. found 22 significantly mutated genes, with the most common being *TP53* (77.4%), *RB1* (30.6%), *COL22A1* (25.8%), and *BCLAF1* (16.1%).[86] There were four recurrent gene fusions, including the fusion between *RLF* and *MYCL1*, which was found in one primary SCLC tumor and four SCLC cell lines. The decreased proliferation of H1097 and CORL47 fusion-positive cell lines with the use of small interfering RNA targeting *MYCL1* supported its role as an oncogene in SCLC.

## Future Perspectives

The use of platinum-based doublets for the treatment of metastatic NSCLC reached a plateau, indicating the need for the development of novel treatment modalities. The initial studies with EGFR and VEGF inhibitors led to a modest benefit in unselected patients. Nevertheless, the subsequent characterization of *EGFR* mutations as predictors for response to EGFR TKIs revolutionized the treatment for NSCLC, with the discovery of additional driver events including the *ALK* and *ROS* fusion genes. Despite this remarkable achievement, however, responses are transient and these targeted agents are not applicable to the majority of patients. The recently reported next generation sequencing studies provide a platform for the discovery of new targets and trials matching the gene abnormalities to the appropriate target drugs, and they may provide the data required for a more rational use of the novel drugs. Once the drugs have an established role and clear predictors for benefit, the next step would be to use them in the earlier stages, where the benefit may be translated into improved cure rates.

## References

1　Siegel R, Ma J, Zou Z, Jemal A. Cancer statistics, 2014. *CA Cancer J Clin*. 2014;64:9–29.

2　Govindan R, Page N, Morgensztern D, et al. Changing epidemiology of small-cell lung cancer in the United States over the last 30 years: analysis of the surveillance, epidemiologic, and end results database. *J Clin Oncol*. 2006;24:4539–4544.

3　Morgensztern D, Waqar S, Subramanian J, Gao F, Govindan R. Improving survival for stage IV non-small cell lung cancer: a surveillance, epidemiology, and end results survey from 1990 to 2005. *J Thorac Oncol*. 2009;4:1524–1529.

4　Morgensztern D, Ng SH, Gao F, Govindan R. Trends in stage distribution for patients with non-small cell lung cancer: a National Cancer Database survey. *J Thorac Oncol*. 2010;5:29–33.

5　Morgensztern D, Waqar S, Subramanian J, et al. Prognostic impact of malignant pleural effusion at presentation in patients with metastatic non-small-cell lung cancer. *J Thorac Oncol*. 2012;7:1485–1489.

6　Ashworth A, Rodrigues G, Boldt G, Palma D. Is there an oligometastatic state in non small cell lung cancer? A systematic review of the literature. *Lung Cancer*. 2013;82:197–203.

7　Group NM-AC. Chemotherapy in addition to supportive care improves survival in advanced non-small-cell lung cancer: a systematic review and meta-analysis of individual patient data from 16 randomized controlled trials. *J Clin Oncol*. 2008;26:4617–4625.

8　Schiller JH, Harrington D, Belani CP, et al. Comparison of four chemotherapy regimens for advanced non-small-cell lung cancer. *N Engl J Med*. 2002;346:92–98.

9　Kelly K, Crowley J, Bunn PA, Jr, et al. Randomized phase III trial of paclitaxel plus carboplatin versus vinorelbine plus cisplatin in the treatment of patients with advanced non–small-cell lung cancer: a Southwest Oncology Group trial. *J Clin Oncol*. 2001;19:3210–3218.

10　Folkman J. Tumor angiogenesis: therapeutic implications. *N Engl J Med*. 1971;285:1182–1186.

11　Johnson DH, Fehrenbacher L, Novotny WF, et al. Randomized phase II trial comparing bevacizumab plus carboplatin and paclitaxel with carboplatin and paclitaxel alone in previously untreated locally advanced or metastatic non-small-cell lung cancer. *J Clin Oncol*. 2004;22:2184–2191.

12　Sandler A, Gray R, Perry MC, et al. Paclitaxel-carboplatin alone or with bevacizumab for non-small-cell lung cancer. *N Engl J Med*. 2006;355:2542–2550.

13　Reck M, von Pawel J, Zatloukal P, et al. Overall survival with cisplatin-gemcitabine and bevacizumab or placebo as first-line therapy for non-squamous non-small-cell lung cancer: results from a randomised phase III trial (AVAiL). *Ann Oncol*. 2010;21:1804–1809.

14　Heymach JV, Paz-Ares L, De Braud F, et al. Randomized phase II study of vandetanib alone or with paclitaxel and carboplatin as first-line treatment for advanced non-small-cell lung cancer. *J Clin Oncol*. 2008;26:5407–5415.

15　Goss GD, Arnold A, Shepherd FA, et al. Randomized, double-blind trial of carboplatin and paclitaxel with either daily oral cediranib or placebo in advanced non-small-cell lung cancer: NCIC clinical trials group BR24 study. *J Clin Oncol*. 2010;28:49–55.

16　Scagliotti GV, Vynnychenko I, Park K, et al. International, randomized, placebo-controlled, double-blind phase III study of motesanib plus carboplatin/paclitaxel in patients with advanced nonsquamous non-small-cell lung cancer: MONET1. *J Clin Oncol*. 2012;30:2829–2836.

17　Herbst RS, Sun Y, Eberhardt WE, et al. Vandetanib plus docetaxel versus docetaxel as second-line treatment for patients with advanced non-small-cell lung cancer (ZODIAC): a double-blind, randomised, phase 3 trial. *Lancet Oncol*. 2010;11:619–626.

18　Ciardiello F, Tortora G. EGFR antagonists in cancer treatment. *N Engl J Med*. 2008;358:1160–1174.

19　Fukuoka M, Yano S, Giaccone G, et al. Multi-institutional randomized phase II trial of gefitinib for previously treated patients with advanced non-small-cell lung cancer (The IDEAL 1 Trial) [corrected]. *J Clin Oncol*. 2003;21:2237–2246.

20　Kris MG, Natale RB, Herbst RS, et al. Efficacy of gefitinib, an inhibitor of the epidermal growth factor receptor tyrosine kinase, in symptomatic patients with non-small cell lung cancer: a randomized trial. *JAMA*. 2003;290:2149–2158.

21　Thatcher N, Chang A, Parikh P, et al. Gefitinib plus best supportive care in previously treated patients with refractory advanced non-small-cell lung cancer: results from a randomised, placebo-controlled, multicentre study (Iressa Survival Evaluation in Lung Cancer). *Lancet*. 2005;366:1527–1537.

22　Shepherd FA, Rodrigues Pereira J, Ciuleanu T, et al. Erlotinib in previously treated non-small-cell lung cancer. *N Engl J Med*. 2005;353:123–132.

23　Sequist LV, Bell DW, Lynch TJ, Haber DA. Molecular predictors of response to epidermal growth factor receptor antagonists in non-small-cell lung cancer. *J Clin Oncol*. 2007;25:587–595.

24　Lynch TJ, Bell DW, Sordella R, et al. Activating mutations in the epidermal growth factor receptor underlying responsiveness of non-small-cell lung cancer to gefitinib. *N Engl J Med*. 2004;350:2129–2139.

25　Paez JG, Janne PA, Lee JC, et al. EGFR mutations in lung cancer: correlation with clinical response to gefitinib therapy. *Science*. 2004;304:1497–1500.

26 Rosell R, Moran T, Queralt C, et al. Screening for epidermal growth factor receptor mutations in lung cancer. *N Engl J Med*. 2009;361:958–967.

27 Fong T, Morgensztern D, Govindan R. EGFR inhibitors as first-line therapy in advanced non-small cell lung cancer. *J Thorac Oncol*. 2008;3:303–310.

28 Sequist LV, Martins RG, Spigel D, et al. First-line gefitinib in patients with advanced non-small-cell lung cancer harboring somatic EGFR mutations. *J Clin Oncol*. 2008;26:2442–2449.

29 Asahina H, Yamazaki K, Kinoshita I, et al. A phase II trial of gefitinib as first-line therapy for advanced non-small cell lung cancer with epidermal growth factor receptor mutations. *Br J Cancer*. 2006;95:998–1004.

30 Cappuzzo F, Ligorio C, Janne PA, et al. Prospective study of gefitinib in epidermal growth factor receptor fluorescence in situ hybridization-positive/phospho-Akt-positive or never smoker patients with advanced non-small-cell lung cancer: the ONCOBELL trial. *J Clin Oncol*. 2007;25:2248–2255.

31 Paz-Ares L, Sanchez JM, Garcia-Velasco A, et al. A prospective phase II trial of erlotinib in advanced non-small cell lung cancer (NSCLC) patients (p) with mutations in the tyrosine kinase (TK) domain of the epidermal growth factor receptor (EGFR). *J Clin Oncol*. 2006;24(suppl.): Abstract 7020.

32 Mok TS, Wu YL, Thongprasert S, et al. Gefitinib or carboplatin-paclitaxel in pulmonary adenocarcinoma. *N Engl J Med*. 2009;361:947–957.

33 Mitsudomi T, Morita S, Yatabe Y, et al. Gefitinib versus cisplatin plus docetaxel in patients with non-small-cell lung cancer harbouring mutations of the epidermal growth factor receptor (WJTOG3405): an open label, randomised phase 3 trial. *Lancet Oncol*. 2010;11:121–128.

34 Maemondo M, Inoue A, Kobayashi K, et al. Gefitinib or chemotherapy for non-small-cell lung cancer with mutated EGFR. *N Engl J Med*. 2010;362:2380–2388.

35 Zhou C, Wu YL, Chen G, et al. Erlotinib versus chemotherapy as first-line treatment for patients with advanced EGFR mutation-positive non-small-cell lung cancer (OPTIMAL, CTONG-0802): a multicentre, open-label, randomised, phase 3 study. *Lancet Oncol*. 2011;12:735–742.

36 Rosell R, Carcereny E, Gervais R, et al. Erlotinib versus standard chemotherapy as first-line treatment for European patients with advanced EGFR mutation-positive non-small-cell lung cancer (EURTAC): a multicentre, open-label, randomised phase 3 trial. *Lancet Oncol*. 2012;13:239–246.

37 Hirsch FR, Janne PA, Eberhardt WE, et al. Epidermal growth factor receptor inhibition in lung cancer: status 2012. *J Thorac Oncol*. 2013;8:373–384.

38 Fossella FV, DeVore R, Kerr RN, et al. Randomized phase III trial of docetaxel versus vinorelbine or ifosfamide in patients with advanced non-small-cell lung cancer previously treated with platinum-containing chemotherapy regimens. The TAX 320 Non-Small Cell Lung Cancer Study Group. *J Clin Oncol*. 2000;18:2354–2362.

39 Shepherd FA, Dancey J, Ramlau R, et al. Prospective randomized trial of docetaxel versus best supportive care in patients with non-small-cell lung cancer previously treated with platinum-based chemotherapy. *J Clin Oncol*. 2000;18:2095–2103.

40 Hanna N, Shepherd FA, Fossella FV, et al. Randomized phase III trial of pemetrexed versus docetaxel in patients with non-small-cell lung cancer previously treated with chemotherapy. *J Clin Oncol*. 2004;22:1589–1597.

41 Cappuzzo F, Ciuleanu T, Stelmakh L, et al. Erlotinib as maintenance treatment in advanced non-small-cell lung cancer: a multicentre, randomised, placebo-controlled phase 3 study. *Lancet Oncol*. 2010;11:521–529.

42 Coudert B, Ciuleanu T, Park K, et al. Survival benefit with erlotinib maintenance therapy in patients with advanced non-small-cell lung cancer (NSCLC) according to response to first-line chemotherapy. *Ann Oncol*. 2012;23:388–394.

43 Garassino MC, Martelli O, Broggini M, et al. Erlotinib versus docetaxel as second-line treatment of patients with advanced non-small-cell lung cancer and wild-type EGFR tumours (TAILOR): a randomised controlled trial. *Lancet Oncol*. 2013;14:981–988.

44 Lazzari C, Novello S, Barni S, et al. Randomized proteomic stratified phase III study of second-line erlotinib (E) versus chemotherapy (CT) in patients with inoperable non-small cell lung cancer (PROSE). *J Clin Oncol*. 2013;31:LBA8005.

45 Sequist LV, Yang JC, Yamamoto N, et al. Phase III study of afatinib or cisplatin plus pemetrexed in patients with metastatic lung adenocarcinoma with EGFR mutations. *J Clin Oncol*. 2013;31:3327–3334.

46 Sequist LV, Waltman BA, Dias-Santagata D, et al. Genotypic and histological evolution of lung cancers acquiring resistance to EGFR inhibitors. *Sci Transl Med*. 2011;3:75ra26.

47 Majem M, Pallares C. An update on molecularly targeted therapies in second- and third-line treatment in non-small cell lung cancer: focus on EGFR inhibitors and anti-angiogenic agents. *Clin Transl Oncol*. 2013;15:343–357.

48 Ohashi K, Maruvka YE, Michor F, Pao W. Epidermal growth factor receptor tyrosine kinase inhibitor-resistant disease. *J Clin Oncol*. 2013;31:1070–1080.

49 Goss GD, O'Callaghan C, Lorimer I, et al. Gefitinib versus placebo in completely resected non-small-cell lung cancer: results of the NCIC CTG BR19 study. *J Clin Oncol*. 2013;31:3320–3326.

50 Richardson F, Richardson K, Sennello G, et al. Biomarker analysis from completely resected NSCLC patients enrolled in an adjuvant erlotinib clinical trial (RADIANT). *J Clin Oncol*. 2009;27(suppl.): Abstract 7520.

51 Neal JW, Pennell NA, Govindan R, et al. The SELECT study: A multicenter phase II trial of adjuvant erlotinib in resected epidermal growth factor receptor (EGFR) mutation-positive non-small cell lung cancer (NSCLC). *J Clin Oncol*. 2012;30(suppl.): Abstract 7010.

52 Devarakonda S, Morgensztern D, Govindan R. Molecularly targeted therapies in locally advanced non-small-cell lung cancer. *Clin Lung Cancer*. 2013;14:467–472.

53 Lynch TJ, Patel T, Dreisbach L, et al. Cetuximab and first-line taxane/carboplatin chemotherapy in advanced non-small-cell lung cancer: results of the randomized multicenter phase III trial BMS099. *J Clin Oncol*. 2010;28:911–917.

54 Pirker R, Pereira JR, Szczesna A, et al. Cetuximab plus chemotherapy in patients with advanced non-small-cell lung cancer (FLEX): an open-label randomised phase III trial. *Lancet*. 2009;373:1525–1531.

55 Pirker R, Pereira JR, von Pawel J, et al. EGFR expression as a predictor of survival for first-line chemotherapy plus cetuximab in patients with advanced non-small-cell lung cancer: analysis of data from the phase 3 FLEX study. *Lancet Oncol*. 2012;13:33–42.

56 Soda M, Choi YL, Enomoto M, et al. Identification of the transforming EML4-ALK fusion gene in non-small-cell lung cancer. *Nature*. 2007;448:561–566.

57 Shaw AT, Engelman JA. ALK in lung cancer: past, present, and future. *J Clin Oncol*. 2013;31:1105–1111.

58 Shaw AT, Solomon B. Targeting anaplastic lymphoma kinase in lung cancer. *Clin Cancer Res*. 2011;17:2081–2086.

59 Kwak EL, Bang YJ, Camidge DR, et al. Anaplastic lymphoma kinase inhibition in non-small-cell lung cancer. *N Engl J Med*. 2010;363:1693–1703.

60 Shaw AT, Yeap BY, Solomon BJ, et al. Effect of crizotinib on overall survival in patients with advanced non-small-cell lung cancer harbouring ALK gene rearrangement: a retrospective analysis. *Lancet Oncol*. 2011;12:1004–1012.

61 Shaw AT, Kim DW, Nakagawa K, et al. Crizotinib versus chemotherapy in advanced ALK-positive lung cancer. *N Engl J Med*. 2013;368:2385–2394.

62 Camidge DR, Doebele RC. Treating ALK-positive lung cancer–early successes and future challenges. *Nat Rev Clin Oncol*. 2012;9:268–277.

63 Kim S, Kim TM, Kim DW, et al. Heterogeneity of genetic changes associated with acquired crizotinib resistance in ALK-rearranged lung cancer. *J Thorac Oncol*. 2013;8:415–422.

64 Shaw AT, Mehra R, Kim D-W, et al. Clinical activity of the ALK inhibitor LDK378 in advanced, ALK-positive NSCLC. *J Clin Oncol*. 2013;31(suppl.): Abstract 8010.

65 Rikova K, Guo A, Zeng Q, et al. Global survey of phosphotyrosine signaling identifies oncogenic kinases in lung cancer. *Cell*. 2007;131:1190–1203.

66 Bergethon K, Shaw AT, Ou SH, et al. ROS1 rearrangements define a unique molecular class of lung cancers. *J Clin Oncol*. 2012;30:863–870.

67 Shaw AT, Camidge DR, Engelman JA, et al. Clinical activity of crizotinib in advanced non-small cell lung cancer (NSCLC) harboring ROS1 gene rearrangement. *J Clin Oncol*. 2012;30(suppl.): Abstract 7508.

68 Ju YS, Lee WC, Shin JY, et al. A transforming KIF5B and RET gene fusion in lung adenocarcinoma revealed from whole-genome and transcriptome sequencing. *Genome Res*. 2012;22:436–445.

69 Lipson D, Capelletti M, Yelensky R, et al. Identification of new ALK and RET gene fusions from colorectal and lung cancer biopsies. *Nat Med*. 2012;18:382–384.

70 Kohno T, Ichikawa H, Totoki Y, et al. KIF5B-RET fusions in lung adenocarcinoma. *Nat Med*. 2012;18:375–377.

71 Takeuchi K, Soda M, Togashi Y, et al. RET, ROS1 and ALK fusions in lung cancer. *Nat Med*. 2012;18:378–381.

72 Wang R, Hu H, Pan Y, et al. RET fusions define a unique molecular and clinicopathologic subtype of non-small-cell lung cancer. *J Clin Oncol*. 2012;30:4352–4359.

73 Drilon A, Wang L, Hasanovic A, et al. Response to Cabozantinib in patients with RET fusion-positive lung adenocarcinomas. *Cancer Discov*. 2013;3:630–635.

74 Paik PK, Arcila ME, Fara M, et al. Clinical characteristics of patients with lung adenocarcinomas harboring BRAF mutations. *J Clin Oncol*. 2011;29:2046–2051.

75 Marchetti A, Felicioni L, Malatesta S, et al. Clinical features and outcome of patients with non-small-cell lung cancer harboring BRAF mutations. *J Clin Oncol*. 2011;29:3574–3579.

76 Planchard D, Mazieres J, Riely GJ, et al. Interim results of phase II study BRF113928 of dabrafenib in BRAF V600E mutation-positive non-small cell lung cancer (NSCLC) patients. *J Clin Oncol*. 2013;31: 8009.

77 Mazieres J, Peters S, Lepage B, et al. Lung cancer that harbors an HER2 mutation: epidemiologic characteristics and therapeutic perspectives. *J Clin Oncol*. 2013;31:1997–2003.

78 Roberts PJ, Stinchcombe TE, Der CJ, Socinski MA. Personalized medicine in non-small-cell lung cancer: is KRAS a useful marker in selecting patients for epidermal growth factor receptor-targeted therapy? *J Clin Oncol*. 2010;28:4769–4777.

79 Kim ES, Herbst RS, Wistuba II, et al. The BATTLE trial: personalizing therapy for lung cancer. *Cancer Discov*. 2011;1:44–53.

80 Janne PA, Shaw AT, Pereira JR, et al. Selumetinib plus docetaxel for KRAS-mutant advanced non-small-cell lung cancer: a randomised, multicentre, placebo-controlled, phase 2 study. *Lancet Oncol*. 2013;14:38–47.

81 Kris MG, Johnson BE, Kwiatkowski DJ, et al. Identification of driver mutations in tumor specimens from 1,000 patients with lung adenocarcinoma: The NCI's Lung Cancer Mutation Consortium (LCMC). *J Clin Oncol*. 2011;29:CRA7506.

82 Rooney M, Devarakonda S, Govindan R. Genomics of squamous cell lung cancer. *Oncologist*. 2013;18:707–716.

83 Govindan R, Ding L, Griffith M, et al. Genomic landscape of non-small cell lung cancer in smokers and never-smokers. *Cell*. 2012;150:1121–1134.

84 Cancer Genome Atlas Research N. Comprehensive genomic characterization of squamous cell lung cancers. *Nature*. 2012;489:519–525.

85 Peifer M, Fernandez-Cuesta L, Sos ML, et al. Integrative genome analyses identify key somatic driver mutations of small-cell lung cancer. *Nat Genet*. 2012;44:1104–1110.

86 Rudin CM, Durinck S, Stawiski EW, et al. Comprehensive genomic analysis identifies SOX2 as a frequently amplified gene in small-cell lung cancer. *Nat Genet*. 2012;44:1111–1116.

# CHAPTER 24

# Targeted Therapy in Melanoma

*Keith T. Flaherty*
Massachusetts General Hospital Cancer Center, Boston, MA, USA

## Introduction

After decades of futility, the pace of advances in systemic therapy for metastatic melanoma has quickened. This is, in part, due to recent advances in the understanding of mechanisms by which tumors escape immune surveillance, but equally because of insights into the genetic changes that give rise to melanoma. In this area, improvements in clinical outcomes have been observed in certain genetically defined patient subsets. Other melanoma subpopulations are still too poorly understood to develop molecular targeted therapeutic strategies. Whereas in years past, prognosis in the setting of metastatic disease was largely determined by measures of disease burden and rate of tumor growth; an increasingly important factor is the presence of a driver oncogene for which targeted therapy is available. In clinical practice, patients are triaged based on the presence or absence of an activating BRAF mutation, a constituent of the MAP kinase pathway, with treatment decisions deferred until this molecular feature has been assessed. Approximately half of the metastatic melanoma population bears a BRAF mutation.[1] Selective, small molecule inhibitors of BRAF and, more recently, regimens inhibiting BRAF and its immediate downstream substrate, MEK, have substantially altered the natural history of metastatic melanoma.[2–4] (Table 24.1).

For an additional 20% of the melanoma population, an activating mutation in the small GTPase, neuroblastoma RAS viral oncogene homolog (NRAS), is the defining oncogenic event.[1] NRAS links receptor tyrosine kinases to the MAP kinase pathway and several other RAS-effector pathways.[9] To date, clinical data with single-agent MEK inhibition and preclinical data demonstrating synergy with other points of intervention points the way toward combination regimens that might accelerate therapeutic progress in that subset as well.[7] (Table 24.1).

An additional small minority of melanomas are characterized by activating tyrosine-protein kinase Kit (CKIT) mutations, some of which are known to be responsive to small molecule CKIT inhibitors, such as those that have been validated in gastrointestinal stromal tumors in which CKIT mutations are present in the majority.[10] Phase II trials of a CKIT inhibitor have demonstrated responses with those agents strictly among patients with activating CKIT mutations.[8,11] (Table 24.1).

For the remaining 30% of melanomas, a driver oncogene and primary therapeutic target have not yet been defined. Recent exploration of the entire melanoma genome has yielded a new list of mutated signaling molecules that can be found in some melanomas that lack a BRAF, NRAS or CKIT mutation.[12,13] Which among them will represent therapeutic targets remains unclear. Thus, the development of targeted therapy in melanoma proceeds at a staggered pace among genetically defined subsets. In the BRAF-mutant population, the first two-drug combination regimen has now been established as effective and the field is now moving to evaluate combination regimens that may include a third point of intervention. This chapter will review the molecular understanding that has been gleaned in preclinical studies and upon application of these targeted therapies, with particular attention to mediators of resistance that may serve as secondary therapeutic targets. This knowledge is nominating additional strategies to assemble rational combination therapy regimens.

## The MAP Kinase Pathway

RAS activation triggers recruitment of RAF kinases and several scaffolding proteins that create the RAF signaling complex.[14] RAF has three known isoforms, ARAF, BRAF, and CRAF, which are expressed to varying degrees in different tissues, but share features such as a RAS-binding domain and a kinase domain. In the absence of mutations, RAF signals as a dimer. RAF kinases directly phosphorylate and activate MEK, which then phosphorylates and activates extracellular signal-regulated kinase (ERK) (Figure 24.1). Both MEK and ERK have multiple isoforms, with MEK1, MEK2, ERK1, and ERK2 being the best characterized.[15] Based on evidence of activation of downstream elements of the MAP kinase pathway, such as phosphorylated ERK, the vast majority of melanomas are characterized by activation of this canonical proliferation pathway. Activated ERK suppresses the expression of p21 and p27, and increases the expression of cyclin D, all of which favor entry into the cell cycle.[16] Two additional functions have been ascribed to CRAF, but not to BRAF or ARAF, other than activation of MEK. At the mitochondrial membrane, CRAF associates with BAD and alters the membrane polarity of the mitochondria in an opposing fashion to proapoptotic BCL-2 family members.[17] Additionally, activated CRAF has been localized to the mitotic spindle where it associates with Aurora A, a regulator of mitosis.[18]

When BRAF mutations were first described and found to constitutively activate MEK and ERK, it was clear that this single mutation accounted for a large proportion of the previously described

*Targeted Therapy in Translational Cancer Research*, First Edition. Edited by Apostolia-Maria Tsimberidou, Razelle Kurzrock and Kenneth C. Anderson.
© 2016 John Wiley & Sons, Inc. Published 2016 by John Wiley & Sons, Inc.

**Table 24.1** Summary of clinical trials demonstrating efficacy with targeted therapies in oncogene-defined melanoma populations.

| Oncogene | Agent | Improved endpoint | Reference |
|---|---|---|---|
| BRAF | Vemurafenib | Response rate, progression-free survival, overall survival | 2,5 |
| | Dabrafenib | Response rate, progression-free survival | 3 |
| | Trametinib | Response rate, progression-free survival, overall survival | 6,37 |
| | Dabrafenib + Trametinib | Response rate, progression-free survival | 4 |
| NRAS | MEK162 | Response rate | 7 |
| CKIT | Imatinib | Response rate | 8,11 |

activated MAP kinase signaling in melanoma.[19] Similarly, activating NRAS mutations result in ERK activation.[20] But even a proportion of BRAF and NRAS wild-type melanomas have activated ERK signaling,[21] suggesting that aberrant signaling in this pathway is nearly ubiquitous in melanoma biology.

However, other recurrent genetic changes resulting in activation of other pathways have been identified in the same melanomas that harbor BRAF or NRAS mutations.[22,23] So, the relative importance of the MAP kinase pathway, particularly in the maintenance of metastatic tumors, was unknown until specific inhibitors of BRAF and MEK became available and demonstrated the dependence on MAP kinase signaling.

## BRAF as a Therapeutic Target

BRAF is a serine threonine kinase. The common mutations in BRAF affect one of two portions of the kinase domain.[19] More than 90% of the BRAF mutations found in human tumors occur in exon 15, at or adjacent to the thymidine residue at position 1796 in the nucleotide sequence. In wild-type BRAF, this codon encodes a valine at the 600 position of the amino acid sequence (referred to as V600). The most commonly identified mutations result in a glutamate (~80%), V600E, or lysine (~15%), V600K.[1,24] Both of these amino acid residues have substantially larger side chains and different charge characteristics which alter the tertiary structure of BRAF, resulting in a kinase that is 800-fold more active than the wild-type structure.[19] These mutated forms of BRAF are thought

to signal as monomers, based on the relatively low RAS-GTP concentrations found in BRAF-mutant melanoma cells.[25] (Figure 24.1). The remaining 5% of BRAF mutations occur in exon 11, a domain that directly interacts with the ATP binding pocket in the three-dimensional structure of BRAF. These also affect the signaling properties of BRAF, but not through direct activation of the kinase domain. Rather, these mutations appear to promote the activation of CRAF,[17] which can then activate MEK or the other described CRAF effector functions. The currently available small molecule, ATP-competitive BRAF inhibitors are designed to inhibit V600E and V600K kinase activity and thus reduce MEK and ERK activation.[3,26] However, these agents do not inhibit BRAF harboring exon 11 mutations and thus they are not considered to be relevant for cancers bearing these types of genetic alterations.[17] Preclinical evidence suggests that MEK inhibitors may be effective at blocking the oncogenic effects of exon 11 BRAF mutations, but this concept has not yet been tested clinically.

Because BRAF appears to exert all of its oncogenic effects on MEK and ERK activation, suppression of ERK phosphorylation has been utilized as the biomarker of BRAF inhibition in preclinical and clinical studies. Supporting that link, our data in BRAF-mutant melanoma cell lines showed that siRNA knockdown of BRAF and MEK produced the same pattern of gene expression.[27] This same profile of altered gene expression is seen with BRAF or MEK small-molecule inhibitors.

*In vitro* and *in vivo*, vemurafenib and dabrafenib, as well as their analogs, profoundly inhibit ERK phosphorylation in melanoma cell

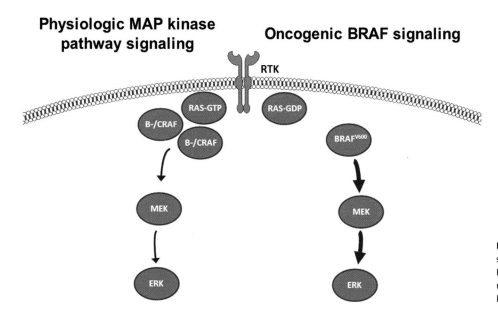

**Figure 24.1** Physiologic MAP kinase signaling and constitutively active BRAF in the setting of a V600 mutation. RTK, receptor tyrosine kinase; B-/CRAF, BRAF or CRAF.

lines harboring V600E mutations.[26, 28] This is associated with cell cycle arrest and induction of apoptosis in a minority of cells. A similar magnitude of ERK inhibition has been observed in serial tumor biopsies taken from patients before and early in the course of therapy with either vemurafenib or dabrafenib treated with maximum tolerated doses.[26]

Among patients with metastatic melanoma harboring activating V600 mutations and treated with standard doses of either vemurafenib or dabrafenib, approximately 90% of patients demonstrate some evidence of disease progression early in the course of therapy.[3, 5] While these data suggest that a 10% subpopulation have primarily refractory disease, functional imaging with fluorodeoxy glucose positron emission tomography suggest that all patients have a metabolic response to BRAF inhibitor therapy even though some go on to have evidence of tumor growth a short time later.[29] This more sensitive measure of antitumor effect seems to indicate that all melanomas that harbor V600 mutations have some degree of dependency on these mutations and activated MAP kinase signaling, though to a highly variable degree. Complete radiographic responses have been documented reproducibly, but in no more than 5% of patients.[3, 5]

Beyond this initial evidence of antitumor effect, vemurafenib and dabrafenib have both been demonstrated to alter the natural history of metastatic melanoma in comparison to conventional cytotoxic chemotherapy. In separate phase III trials, with dacarbazine as the control treatment, vemurafenib or dabrafenib reduce the risk of disease progression by more than 60%.[2] This translated into a median progression-free survival of approximately 6 months for the BRAF inhibitors versus 2 months or less for dacarbazine. Among those cohorts with longer-term follow-up, 10–20% of patients remained progression-free for 18 months or longer demonstrating that single-agent oncogene-targeted therapy can induce durable effects in some patients.[5, 30] But for the majority of patients, resistance manifests within a few to many months. Understanding the molecular mechanisms that mediate resistance to single-agent BRAF inhibitor therapy has been a major focus of translational research efforts. Insights gained from this research and initial attempts to overcome resistance will be discussed later in this chapter. Despite limits in the durability of responses to BRAF inhibitors, survival is clearly prolonged in comparison to conventional melanoma chemotherapy.[2] And for this reason, vemurafenib gained regulatory approval and is currently considered a standard treatment for patients with metastatic melanoma harboring a V600 BRAF mutation.

## Paradoxical MAP Kinase Pathway Activation

Although not anticipated in their early clinical testing, BRAF inhibitors have been consistently observed to cause increased MEK and ERK signaling in cells with either NRAS or KRAS mutation, and some cells with activated receptor tyrosine kinases.[31–33] With increasing concentrations of a BRAF inhibitor, activation of the MAP kinase pathway is observed before inactivation is ultimately achieved with much higher concentrations. It was hypothesized and then experimentally proven that at lower concentrations a RAF dimer will have one of two molecules bound by the BRAF inhibitor, while the other one is not.[31] This hemi-bound state confers increased kinase activity to the unbound RAF molecule. At substantially higher drug concentrations, both binding sites in a dimer are saturated and signaling is inhibited. But, it is not clear that such high concentrations can be achieved *in vivo*. Of note, this problem

of paradoxical activation is only relevant in cells with activated RAS, because RAS is ultimately responsible for facilitating RAF dimerization. In cancer cells that harbor activating BRAF mutations, where RAS is predominantly in the inactive state, mutated BRAF and wild-type RAF are in a monomeric state.

It is likely that this phenomenon of paradoxical activation has both good and bad consequences. The favorable element is that BRAF inhibitors are incapable of inhibiting the MAP kinase pathway in cells that lack BRAF mutation. Therefore, the toxicities observed with BRAF inhibitors are either a consequence of paradoxical activation or relate to inhibition of other kinases once sufficiently high concentrations are achieved. This selective inhibitory signaling effect in tumor cells likely provides the ability to achieve on a drug exposure necessary to profoundly inhibit the MAP kinase pathway and achieve the observed antitumor effects. The negative element is that stimulating the MAP kinase pathway appears to be responsible for the appearance of cutaneous squamous cell carcinomas,[34] raising concerns that other malignancies that were subclinical prior to BRAF inhibitor therapy could have their growth promoted on therapy.

## MEK Inhibitors in BRAF-Mutant Melanoma

Taking advantage of the direct and apparently selective activation of MEK by oncogenic BRAF, it was hypothesized that selective MEK inhibitors would have efficacy in BRAF-mutant melanoma. *In vitro*, this is clearly the case, as potent inhibition of the MAP kinase pathway decreased proliferation and increased cell death.[35] *In vivo*, tumor growth control has been demonstrated in BRAF-mutant melanoma xenografts.[36] And, in clinical trials focused on metastatic melanoma patients harboring V600 BRAF mutations, reproducible efficacy has been documented.

In a cohort of V600 BRAF-mutant melanoma patients treated after completion of dose-finding in a phase I trial, the orally available, selective MEK inhibitor trametinib produced an objective response rate of 20–25% and a median progression-free survival of 4–5 months.[6] These data compared favorably to historical control experience with cytotoxic chemotherapy. Therefore, the phase III trial was undertaken directly comparing trametinib with dacarbazine or paclitaxel in patients with metastatic melanoma that was either previously untreated or refractory to dacarbazine (with paclitaxel as the assigned chemotherapy in such cases).[37] A 55% improvement in progression-free survival was seen for trametinib in comparison with chemotherapy, with associated median progression-free survival of 4.8 months and 1.5 months in the trametinib and chemotherapy arms, respectively. A 46% improvement in survival was also observed despite the fact that patients with progressive disease on chemotherapy could cross over to receive trametinib. The objective response rate in the trametinib arm was 22%.

The clinical evidence clearly supports MEK inhibition as an efficacious approach in V600-mutant BRAF melanoma. It is noteworthy that the objective response rate and median progression-free survival in a patient population that was nearly identical to that observed with selective BRAF inhibitors in a very similar patient population. Unlike BRAF inhibitors, MEK inhibitors inhibit the MAP kinase pathway regardless of the genetic makeup of the cells exposed. And, with trametinib and other MEK inhibitors highly selective for MEK, it is believed that MEK-associated toxicities are due to inhibition of the MAP kinase pathway in normal tissues. With that in mind, it is likely that the maximum safe dose of an MEK inhibitor is defined by the maximum amount of MAP kinase pathway inhibition that can be tolerated in normal tissue. This contrasts with BRAF inhibitors, which cannot inhibit the MAP kinase pathway in normal cells. It seems likely that these differences in effect on the MAP kinase pathway between tumor and normal tissue account for different therapeutic indices for MEK and BRAF inhibitors.

## NRAS

In the formation of melanoma, NRAS mutations appear to be the functional equivalent to BRAF mutations with regard to their oncogenic potential.[38,39] When genetically characterizing advanced melanoma tumors, one rarely, if ever, finds both an NRAS and BRAF mutation.[22,40,41] First identified as a melanoma oncogene in the mid-1980s, a significant amount of insight has been gleaned into the functional consequences of an activating NRAS mutation. It is clear that activated NRAS promotes signaling in the MAP kinase pathway.[20] Again, this helps to explain the mutual exclusivity of BRAF and NRAS mutations in melanoma. It appears that oncogenic NRAS signals predominantly through CRAF, not BRAF.[42] This likely accounts, in part, for the observation *in vitro* that selective BRAF inhibitors have no inhibitory effect on NRAS-mutant melanoma cells. In fact, these drugs may stimulate their growth through paradoxical activation of CRAF.[31] In melanoma cell lines harboring an NRAS mutation, exposure to selective MEK inhibitors blocks ERK phosphorylation and, in some tumor models, significantly blocks cell cycle.[28] However, this effect is visibly observed among NRAS-mutated melanoma cell lines, suggesting that the MAP kinase pathway may not be the most important RAS effector pathway in some cases. Activation of the PI3 kinase pathway and RALGDS has also been ascribed to oncogenic NRAS, but even these do not account for all of the currently known RAS effector pathways.[43,44] The relative importance of each of these forms of activated NRAS has not been established, though some tumors appear to depend largely on the MAP kinase pathway and PI3 kinase pathway simultaneously.

Understanding the signaling inhibitor of NRAS has been a primary focus of therapeutic research because direct RAS antagonists have been elusive. Taking advantage of a required post-translational modification that facilitates RAS localization to the inner surface of the plasma membrane (farnesylation), inhibitors of the enzyme responsible for this modification were developed.[45,46] And while inhibition of mutated RAS signaling could be demonstrated in cancer cell lines *in vitro*, clinical efficacy was nearly nonexistent. In retrospect, it is believed that farnesylation is required for the activation of a large number of signaling molecules. Therefore, farnesyltransferase inhibitors are felt to have widespread effects on numerous unintended targets beyond mutated RAS. This liability likely accounts for the toxicities that limit the dose and drug exposure that could be safely achieved in humans, which then limits the anti-RAS effect of these agents *in vivo*.

The most promising clinical evidence of efficacy with a targeted therapy approach in NRAS-mutant melanoma has been generated with single-agent MEK inhibitor therapy. In a small cohort of metastatic melanoma patients harboring activating NRAS mutations, a selective MEK inhibitor produced objective responses in approximately 20% of patients, with 60% of patients having some degree of tumor regression.[7] The observed median progression-free survival of four months in this cohort summarizes the fact that the efficacy of this therapy is neither widespread nor long-lasting. Nonetheless, these data support evidence from laboratory-based investigations regarding the MAP kinase pathway dependence of a subset of these tumors. What fraction of the NRAS-mutated melanoma population might benefit from MEK inhibition as a component of a targeted therapy approach remains to be determined. Attention has recently turned to identifying additional points of intervention outside of the MAP kinase pathway that might have a greater ability to intercept the critical components of signal transduction downstream of NRAS. As noted previously, one strategy that has been justified based on *in vitro* studies is concomitant targeting of PI3 kinase or mTor, which are thought to be upstream and downstream components of the same RAS effector pathway, respectively.[28] With a large number of PI3 kinase and mTor inhibitors currently in clinical development, investigation of combination regimens containing an MEK inhibitor with an inhibitor of PI3 kinase or mTor is underway at the early stages.

A recent laboratory investigation was undertaken in order to determine which signaling pathway may serve as the critical secondary target in conjunction with MEK inhibition in NRAS-mutant melanoma.[39] A mouse-transgenic model was generated with an activating NRAS mutation, along with inactivation of the CDKN2A tumor suppressor gene, which encodes both p16 and p14, in a reversible fashion in melanocytes. These mice develop advanced melanomas which can be partially controlled with administration of a MEK inhibitor. Analyzing which genes were differentially expressed under MEK treatment or control conditions, as well as activation state of many signaling pathways, a signature of the residual RAS signaling program unaffected by MEK inhibition was described. An analysis of signal transduction networks that might regulate this MEK independent RAS effector function identified cyclin-independent kinase 4 (CDK4) as the most critical node of signaling. Attempts to attenuate CDK4 expression with siRNA or inhibit signaling activity with a small-molecule CDK4/6 inhibitor synergize with MEK inhibition, thereby causing tumor regression in the same mouse-transgenic model. In a human melanoma cell line harboring an activating NRAS mutation in addition to the full complement of somatic genetic alterations, the same combination approach had synergistic activity *in vitro* and *in vivo* in an immunocompromised mouse. One orally available, selective CDK4/6 inhibitor has completed phase I testing,[47] and two others are currently in early clinical development. So, a combination of MEK and CDK4 inhibition is actively being pursued.

Additional laboratory-based investigation is needed to understand if there are other subsets within the NRAS-mutant melanoma population for which different targeted therapy strategies might be explored.

## CKIT

The identification of activating mutations in the CKIT receptor tyrosine kinase in melanoma gave rise to enthusiasm that an additional oncogene-defined subpopulation might have a readily available targeted therapy options. However, initial estimates regarding the prevalence of CKIT mutations in melanoma proved to overstate the actual rate.[10,11] In melanoma, CKIT mutations are restricted to relatively low prevalence clinical subtypes, such as mucosal and acral lentiginous melanomas (arising in the nail beds, palms, and soles). Within these subsets, it is currently estimated that approximately 10% of patients with these types of melanomas have CKIT mutations. Taking into account the proportion of overall melanoma cases with tumors arising at these sites, approximately 1% of all melanomas are currently estimated to have CKIT mutations.

Mutations have been identified in exons 11, 13, 17, and 18.[48] In gastrointestinal stromal tumor, where CKIT mutations were first identified and validated as a therapeutic target, exon 11 and 13 mutations are, by far, the most common.[49] Within these regions, the L576P and K642E mutations have been characterized as sensitive to several small molecule CKIT inhibitors that are currently FDA-approved for patients with advanced gastrointestinal stromal tumors.

In phase II trials with imatinib monotherapy targeting patients with CKIT mutation or amplification, partial and complete responses have been documented in patients with L576P and K642E CKIT mutations.[8,11] However, a significant proportion of patients enrolled had mutations at other sites within exons 11 and 13 or mutations in exons 17 and 18, which are either known to be nonresponsive to imatinib or with uncharacterized sensitivity to imatinib in the gastrointestinal stromal tumor setting. These data indicate that single-agent imatinib therapy can produce objective responses, which are durable in some cases. But, due to the rarity of imatinib sensitive CKIT mutations in advanced melanoma, follow-on clinical trials are proceeding slowly. In gastrointestinal stromal tumor, sunitinib, dasatinib, and nilotinib have all demonstrated efficacy in patients whose tumors harbor imatinib-sensitive mutations, and in some cases with imatinib-insensitive mutations. The efficacy of each of these agents is currently being explored in phase II trials in melanoma.

## Acquired Resistance to BRAF-Targeted Therapy

Following the initial observation of responses to single-agent BRAF inhibitor therapy and subsequent emergence of resistance, identifying the molecular underpinnings of acquired resistance has been the focus of intensive investigation. Ultimately, the goal of this research is to identify points of therapeutic intervention that could render clinical benefit in patients whose tumors were progressing on a BRAF inhibitor. Insight in this area might also provide a basis for developing a combination regimen with the goal of preventing or suppressing tumor escape mechanisms.

Initial characterization of patients' tumors biopsied at the time of disease progression focused on ascertaining the state of MAP kinase pathway signaling. In a cohort of 12 patients who underwent tumor biopsy before treatment, following two weeks of treatment, and again at the time of disease progression, it was observed that nine patients had evidence of reactivation of ERK.[50] While the greatest attention has been paid to defining molecular mediators of ERK reactivation, it is noteworthy that even in this small cohort, biochemical evidence supported the possibility of MAP kinase pathway-independent mechanisms of resistance. Resequencing of all BRAF exons in these tumors failed to identify that mutations might confer resistance to an ATP-competitive BRAF inhibitor.[51] In all cases, the same V600 mutation was present at baseline and identified at disease progression. Based on this evidence, it appears that BRAF inhibitor resistance does not follow the precedent established in chronic myeloid leukemia,[52] gastrointestinal stromal tumor,[53] and 50% of epidermal growth factor receptor-mutated non-small cell lung cancer.[54] In each of these cases, mutations in the kinase domain of the target oncogene have been identified and characterized as blocking the binding of the relevant small molecule inhibitor.

In parallel to these early investigations of melanoma tumors procured from patients with relapsing disease following initial response to a BRAF inhibitor, preclinical studies were undertaken to generate V600E BRAF melanoma cell lines with acquired resistance. These experiments provided a ready source of tumor cells in which genetic alterations and altered signal transduction could be interrogated without concerns of stromal cell contamination or limitations in the amount of material available for analysis. Two mechanisms that might account for reactivation of the MAP kinase pathway were identified using *in vitro* derived resistant cell lines include the emergence of a concomitant activating NRAS mutation and expression of a truncated form of V600E BRAF.[25,51] (Figure 24.2).

As noted previously, in the untreated state, BRAF and NRAS mutations are generally never coexistent. It is thought that a tumor cell clone that harbors both BRAF and NRAS mutation likely has a significant growth disadvantage compared to a BRAF-mutant/NRAS wild-type cell. Experimentally, the simultaneous introduction of oncogenic BRAF and NRAS induces senescence.[55] But, in the presence of a BRAF inhibitor which effectively neutralizes the signaling of mutated BRAF, such a dual mutant clone might gain a growth advantage through the unopposed effect of oncogenic NRAS, signaling the MAP kinase pathway through CRAF.[42] It is currently estimated that approximately 20% of patients whose tumors

## Mechanisms of resistance to BRAF inhibitors

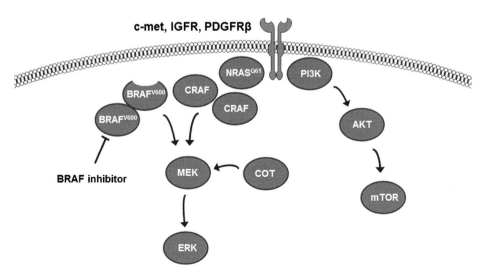

**Figure 24.2** Mechanisms of resistance to BRAF inhibitor therapy.

progress following initial response to a BRAF inhibitor have concomitant NRAS mutation as the putative explanation (Figure 24.2). This phenomenon raises all of the same challenges discussed previously regarding therapeutic approaches in the subpopulation of melanoma tumors for which NRAS is the primary driver oncogene. It is not clear if the dependence on certain RAS effector pathways is different or similar in these tumors with concomitant BRAF and NRAS mutation compared to those with NRAS mutations alone.

The truncated form of V600E BRAF identified in cell lines with acquired resistance *in vitro* provided the first evidence that an alteration in BRAF itself might confer resistance to BRAF inhibitor therapy.[25] (Figure 24.2). It has been speculated that this form of BRAF, referred to as p61 BRAF, represents alternative splicing of oncogenic BRAF mRNA. This hypothesis has been put forward, in part, due to the fact that a similar experience has been described in some normal tissues.[56] Biochemically, p61 BRAF is able to dimerize in the presence of a BRAF inhibitor.[25] This would explain how a cell in which full-length V600E BRAF, which exists in a monomeric state, can be persistently inhibited, while p61 is able to overcome the inhibitory effect of a BRAF inhibitor through paradoxical activation. Structurally, p61 BRAF is lacking the RAS binding domain and regulatory elements of the RAF dimerization domain. To overcome the 61 BRAF signaling directly will likely require the development of an inhibitor of RAF dimerization, which does not currently exist.

In an experiment in which the entire repertoire of kinase domain containing signaling molecules were introduced one by one into a V600E BRAF-mutant melanoma cell line exposed to a BRAF inhibitor, several kinases appeared capable of conferring resistance.[57] Not surprisingly, CRAF is the foremost among them. The kinase next most capable of conferring resistance to a BRAF inhibitor was COT/TPL2. This is a member of the MAP kinase family, and is known to activate MEK and ERK in a RAF-independent fashion (Figure 24.2). Thus, it is plausible that COT activation could bypass the effect of a BRAF inhibitor and allow restoration of MAP kinase pathway signaling. Melanoma tumor samples procured from patients receiving a BRAF inhibitor demonstrated up-regulation of COT early after the initiation of a BRAF inhibitor or at the time of disease progression. But, mutation or amplification of COT have not been described, leaving unanswered the question of how it might be upregulated following BRAF inhibition.

Mutations in MEK1 have also been described in BRAF inhibitor-resistant melanoma cell lines derived *in vitro*, as well as in patient tumor samples.[58,59] One such mutation has been characterized as being able to activate ERK in a RAF-independent fashion and was identified in a single patient's tumor biopsies at the time of progression whereas it was not present at baseline. However, the significance of these mutations in terms of conferring resistance in patients remains unclear, as the same mutations have been identified in the majority of melanoma cells in some patients' tumors prior to the initiation of BRAF inhibitor therapy.

In clinical trials, single-agent MEK inhibition has failed to demonstrate significant efficacy in patients who are refractory to a BRAF inhibitor.[6] However, when combined with a BRAF inhibitor in the BRAF inhibitor naïve setting, this combination approach substantially delays the emergence of resistance compared to BRAF inhibitor monotherapy.[4] Interestingly, several of the BRAF inhibitor and MEK inhibitor associated toxicities are decreased when both agents are given concomitantly.[4] This likely relates to differences in effect on the MAP kinase pathway in normal tissues, with BRAF inhibitor potentially causing paradoxical activation while the MEK inhibitor inhibits ERK activation. These opposing effects may par-

tially cancel out the effect of the other drug, thereby moderating the severe toxicity profile compared to single-agent therapy.

As noted previously, ERK reactivation has not been identified in all BRAF inhibitor refractory tumors.[50] Two mechanisms have been proposed by which receptor tyrosine kinase activation might restore signaling and the MAP kinase pathway through CRAF and/or mediate resistance through activation of the PI3 kinase pathway (Figure 24.2). In one analysis of patient tumor samples biopsied at the time of disease progression and compared to baseline tumor samples from the same patient, PDGF receptor beta was found to be overexpressed in the resistant tumor samples compared to baseline, whereas no other receptor tyrosine kinase overexpression was identified.[51] Curiously, evidence of phosphorylation of the kinase domain was not identified, which is generally considered a marker of an activated PDGF receptor. Subsequent functional studies could not demonstrate the *in vitro* efficacy with a selective PDGF receptor kinase inhibitor, whereas blockade of the PI3 kinase pathway did show antiproliferative effect.[60] In another set of experiments, activation of the insulin-like growth factor receptor was noted when V600E BRAF-mutant melanoma cell lines were cultured in the presence of a BRAF inhibitor.[61] Inhibition of the IGF receptor reversed resistance. Moreover, in one of five patient tumors biopsied at the time of resistance, increased IGFR expression and activation of AKT could be demonstrated.

## Mechanisms of *de novo* BRAF Inhibitor Resistance

Years before BRAF mutations were first identified in melanoma and other cancers, it was known that melanomas commonly harbor activating mutations with deletions in well-described tumor suppressor genes—CDKN2A and PTEN.[62] CDKN2A encodes two proteins with tumor suppressor functions, p16 and p14. Mutation or deletion of this allele is found in the majority of melanoma tumors and the vast majority of melanoma cell lines. p16 is the negative regulator of CDK4 activity, an essential element in cell cycle control. Loss of p16 expression, or an inactivating mutation, allows CDK4 to act in an unopposed fashion, favoring entry into the cell cycle. Supporting the importance of this pathway in melanoma, a smaller subset of tumors harbor amplification of cyclin D,[63] the cofactor necessary for CDK4 activation, and an additional small subset have amplification or activating mutation of CDK4 itself.[64] As noted earlier, CDK4 may mediate a critical element of oncogenic RAS activity,[39] independent of the MAP kinase pathway. It is thought that this may also be the case for BRAF-mutant melanoma and may be a source of *de novo* resistance. Interestingly, the predominant effect of a selective CDK4 inhibitor *in vitro* is induction of senescence.[65] This is consistent with evidence suggesting that introduction of oncogenic BRAF into a melanocyte induces senescence can be reversed by inactivation of p16.[66,67] In advanced melanoma, in which genetic alterations in CDKN2A, BRAF, and numerous other genes, it is unclear what effect a CDK4 inhibitor would have when given in conjunction with a BRAF inhibitor. In patients treated with BRAF inhibitor, loss of p16 is associated with shorter progression-free survival.[68] In aggregate, the available evidence suggests that concomitant targeting of BRAF and CDK4 should be further evaluated.

Approximately 20% of all BRAF-mutant melanoma population has complete loss of PTEN expression.[69] The potential pertinence of this observation is highlighted by the propensity for a transgenic mouse with inducible BRAF mutation and PTEN deletion in melanocytes to develop locally advanced and metastatic melanoma.[38] In melanoma cell lines with concomitant BRAF mutation and PTEN deletion, relatively little cell death is induced with a BRAF inhibitor compared to cells with PTEN intact.[70,71] This relative resistance can be overcome with the addition of a PI3K pathway inhibitor which acts synergistically to induce apoptosis. Considering the limited efficacy observed to date with small molecule inhibitors of all PI3K pathway isoforms, or combined PI3K pathway/mTor inhibitors in patients with PTEN-deleted tumors, it appears that a more selective approach within the PI3K pathway may be needed. siRNA knockdown of p110beta, one of four isoforms of the catalytic domain of PI3K, is selectively toxic to PTEN-deleted tumor cells.[72] And, the same cells are relatively unaffected by knockdown of other p110 isoforms. In patients treated with a BRAF inhibitor as monotherapy, PTEN deletion appears to predict for shorter duration of treatment response.[68] Recently, selective inhibitors of p110beta have entered clinical development and are plausible combination partners with BRAF inhibitors in the subpopulation of BRAF-mutant melanoma patients who have coexisting PTEN deletion.

An intriguing possible mechanism of receptor tyrosine kinase activation was explored using a large screening platform for possible constituents of the tumor microenvironment that might confer resistance to BRAF inhibitors *in vitro*.[73] Simultaneous culturing of V600E BRAF melanoma cell lines in the presence of a BRAF inhibitor with individual cell lines representing cell types known to populate the tumor microenvironment demonstrated that fibroblasts could inhibit BRAF inhibitor-induced cell death. A screen among hundreds of secreted cytokines and growth factors revealed that hepatocyte growth factor had a selective ability to confer resistance in a similar fashion (Figure 24.2). Inhibition of the hepatocyte growth factor receptor (c-met) with a small molecule inhibitor had synergistic antitumor effect with a BRAF inhibitor *in vitro* and *in vivo*. Among patients who had received a BRAF inhibitor, the presence of HGF in the metastatic tumor mass was associated with lesser degrees of tumor regression early in the course of BRAF inhibitor therapy compared to those patients with no evidence of HGF in the tumor microenvironment. This association supported the preclinical observations suggesting that antagonizing HGF directly with a monoclonal antibody or c-met with a small molecule inhibitor might overcome this mechanism of resistance.

## Intersection Between Targeted Therapy and Immune Therapy

In the same timeframe in which BRAF inhibitor therapy has emerged as a new treatment standard, the CTLA-4-blocking antibody ipilimumab has demonstrated survival improvement in patients with metastatic melanoma compared to chemotherapy or vaccine control arms.[74,75] This agent has been FDA approved and represents an additional treatment option for BRAF-mutant melanoma patients and the sole therapeutic advance for patients whose tumors lack a BRAF mutation. Approximately 70% of patients treated with ipilimumab derive no benefit from this therapy and even among the subpopulation of patients who do, responses can require several months to become established. Given the relatively aggressive nature of metastatic melanoma, it would be advantageous to have a cytotoxic therapy that could prevent tumor progression in the short term while an antitumor immune response is being mounted. On these clinical grounds alone, there has been interest in exploring the combination of a BRAF inhibitor and immunotherapy. However, recent evidence suggests that there may

be a mechanistic basis by which BRAF inhibitor therapy might enhance antitumor immunity and synergize with treatments for which the primary mechanism is activation of components of the immune system.

It has previously been described that suppression of oncogenic BRAF expression downregulates transcription factor microphthalmia-associated transcription factor (MITF).[76,77] MITF is the master regulator of melanocyte lineage differentiation pathway which promotes expression of melanocyte lineage antigens including gp100, MART-1, and TYRP-1 and -2.[78] Exposure of V600E BRAF-mutant melanoma cell lines to a BRAF inhibitor relieves the suppression of MITF expression, thereby increasing expression of these melanocyte surface proteins.[79] Furthermore, as will be predicted from the biochemical observations described previously, a BRAF inhibitor is incapable of blocking the MAP kinase pathway in immune cells, an important point when considering that antitumor effector T cells proliferate via the MAP kinase pathway.

In tumor biopsy specimens taken within a few weeks of initiating BRAF inhibitor therapy, there is consistent evidence of a CD8 positive T-cell infiltrate into the tumor.[80] The ability of these T cells to contribute to the antitumor responses observed with BRAF inhibitors is unknown, but their presence suggests that one element of escape from immune surveillance is being blocked by BRAF inhibitor therapy. It is not yet known whether remaining inhibitory factors might prevent an effective antitumor immune response, but understanding these mediators will provide a rational basis for developing targeted therapy/immunotherapy combinations. Absent this insight, clinical trials are being conducted combining BRAF inhibitors with CTLA-4 blockade, high-dose IL-2, and PD-L1 blockade.

## Summary

Targeted therapy has taken hold in melanoma for patients whose tumors harbor activating BRAF mutations. Recent evidence suggests that the combination of a BRAF inhibitor and MEK inhibitor substantially improved outcomes compared to BRAF inhibitor monotherapy, and will likely become the new treatment standard for these patients. In NRAS-mutant melanoma, preliminary data suggest that single-agent MEK inhibition has sufficient antitumor activity to warrant exploration of MEK inhibitor-based combination regimens. For the small subpopulation of patients with activating CKIT mutations, available CKIT inhibitors produce responses in those with particular sensitivity to these agents based on experience in gastrointestinal stromal tumors. However, a full 30% of the melanoma population does not yet have defined driver oncogenes to serve as a primary point of therapeutic intervention. Whether combination targeted therapy regimens will ultimately provide the greatest clinical benefit to patients or the best use of targeted therapies is as a component of a targeted therapy/immunotherapy regimen will require substantially more clinical investigation.

## References

1 Jakob JA, Bassett RL Jr., Ng CS, et al. NRAS mutation status is an independent prognostic factor in metastatic melanoma. *Cancer*. 2012;118(16):4014–4023.

2 Chapman PB, Hauschild A, Robert C, et al. Improved survival with vemurafenib in melanoma with BRAF V600E mutation. *N Eng J Med*. 2011;364(26):2507–2516.

3 Hauschild A, Grob JJ, Demidov LV, et al. Dabrafenib in BRAF-mutated metastatic melanoma: a multicentre, open-label, phase 3 randomised controlled trial. *Lancet*. 2012;380(9839):358–365.

4 Flaherty KT, Infante JR, Daud A, et al. Combined BRAF and MEK Inhibition in Melanoma with BRAF V600 Mutations. *N Eng J Med*. 2012;367(18):1694–1703.

5 Sosman JA, Kim KB, Schuchter L, et al. Survival in BRAF V600-mutant advanced melanoma treated with vemurafenib. *N Eng J Med*. 2012;366(8):707–714.

6 Falchook GS, Lewis KD, Infante JR, et al. Activity of the oral MEK inhibitor trametinib in patients with advanced melanoma: a phase 1 dose-escalation trial. *Lancet Oncol*. 2012;13(8):782–789.

7 Ascierto P, Antonio CB, Agawala SS, et al. Efficacy and safety of oral MEK162 in patients with locally advanced and unresectable or metastatic cutaneous melanoma harboring BRAFV600 or NRAS mutations. *J Clin Oncol*. 2012(suppl.): Abstract 8511.

8 Guo J, Si L, Kong Y, et al. Phase II, open-label, single-arm trial of imatinib mesylate in patients with metastatic melanoma harboring c-Kit mutation or amplification. *J Clin Oncol*. 2011;29(21):2904–2909.

9 Smalley KS. Understanding melanoma signaling networks as the basis for molecular targeted therapy. *J Invest Dermatol*. 2010;130(1):28–37.

10 Curtin JA, Busam K, Pinkel D, Bastian BC. Somatic activation of KIT in distinct subtypes of melanoma. *J Clin Oncol*. 2006;24(26):4340–4346.

11 Carvajal RD, Antonescu CR, Wolchok JD, et al. KIT as a therapeutic target in metastatic melanoma. *JAMA*. 2011;305(22):2327–2334.

12 Berger MF, Hodis E, Heffernan TP, et al. Melanoma genome sequencing reveals frequent PREX2 mutations. *Nature*. 2012;485(7399):502–506.

13 Krauthammer M, Kong Y, Ha BH, et al. Exome sequencing identifies recurrent somatic RAC1 mutations in melanoma. *Nat Genet*. 2012;44(9):1006–1014.

14 Rebocho AP, Marais R. ARAF acts as a scaffold to stabilize BRAF:CRAF heterodimers. *Oncogene*. 2012;32(26):3207–3212.

15 Nikolaev SI, Rimoldi D, Iseli C, et al. Exome sequencing identifies recurrent somatic MAP2K1 and MAP2K2 mutations in melanoma. *Nat Genet*. 2012;44(2):133–139.

16 Dry JR, Pavey S, Pratilas CA, et al. Transcriptional pathway signatures predict MEK addiction and response to selumetinib (AZD6244). *Cancer Res*. 2010;70(6):2264–2273.

17 Smalley KS, Xiao M, Villanueva J, et al. CRAF inhibition induces apoptosis in melanoma cells with non-V600E BRAF mutations. *Oncogene*. 2009;28(1):85–94.

18 Mielgo A, Seguin L, Huang M, et al. A MEK-independent role for CRAF in mitosis and tumor progression. *Nat Med*. 2011;17(12):1641–1645.

19 Davies H, Bignell GR, Cox C, et al. Mutations of the BRAF gene in human cancer. *Nature*. 2002;417(6892):949–954.

20 Eskandarpour M, Kiaii S, Zhu C, Castro J, Sakko AJ, Hansson J. Suppression of oncogenic NRAS by RNA interference induces apoptosis of human melanoma cells. *Int J Cancer*. 2005;115(1):65–73.

21 Satyamoorthy K, Li G, Gerrero MR, et al. Constitutive mitogen-activated protein kinase activation in melanoma is mediated by both BRAF mutations and autocrine growth factor stimulation. *Cancer Res*. 2003;63(4):756–759.

22 Tsao H, Goel V, Wu H, Yang G, Haluska FG. Genetic interaction between NRAS and BRAF mutations and PTEN/MMAC1 inactivation in melanoma. *J Invest Dermatol*. 2004;122(2):337–341.

23 Zhao Y, Zhang Y, Yang Z, Li A, Dong J. Simultaneous knockdown of BRAF and expression of INK4A in melanoma cells leads to potent growth inhibition and apoptosis. *Biochem Biophys Res Commun*. 2008;370(3):509–513.

24 Long GV, Menzies AM, Nagrial AM, et al. Prognostic and clinicopathologic associations of oncogenic BRAF in metastatic melanoma. *J Clin Oncol*. 2011;29(10):1239–1246.

25 Poulikakos PI, Persaud Y, Janakiraman M, et al. RAF inhibitor resistance is mediated by dimerization of aberrantly spliced BRAF(V600E). *Nature*. 2011;480(7377):387–390.

26 Bollag G, Hirth P, Tsai J, et al. Clinical efficacy of a RAF inhibitor needs broad target blockade in BRAF-mutant melanoma. *Nature*. 2010;467(7315):596–599.

27 Joseph EW, Pratilas CA, Poulikakos PI, et al. The RAF inhibitor PLX4032 inhibits ERK signaling and tumor cell proliferation in a V600E BRAF-selective manner. *Proc Natl Acad Sci U S A*. 2010;107(33):14903–14908.

28 Greger JG, Eastman SD, Zhang V, et al. Combinations of BRAF, MEK, and PI3K/mTOR inhibitors overcome acquired resistance to the BRAF inhibitor GSK2118436 dabrafenib, mediated by NRAS or MEK mutations. *Mol Cancer Therap*. 2012;11(4):909–920.

29 McArthur GA, Puzanov I, Amaravadi R, et al. Marked, homogeneous, and early [18F]fluorodeoxyglucose-positron emission tomography responses to vemurafenib in BRAF-mutant advanced melanoma. *J Clin Oncol*. 2012;30(14):1628–1634.

30 Kim K, Flaherty KT, Chapman PB, et al. Pattern and outcome of disease progression in phase I study of vemurafenib in patients with metastatic melanoma (MM). *J Clin Oncol*. 2011;29(suppl.): Abstract 8519.

31 Poulikakos PI, Zhang C, Bollag G, Shokat KM, Rosen N. RAF inhibitors transactivate RAF dimers and ERK signalling in cells with wild-type BRAF. *Nature*. 2010;464(7287):427–430.

32 Hatzivassiliou G, Song K, Yen I, et al. RAF inhibitors prime wild-type RAF to activate the MAPK pathway and enhance growth. *Nature*. 2010;464(7287):431–435.

33 Heidorn SJ, Milagre C, Whittaker S, et al. Kinase-dead BRAF and oncogenic RAS cooperate to drive tumor progression through CRAF. *Cell*. 2010;140(2):209–221.

34 Su F, Viros A, Milagre C, et al. RAS mutations in cutaneous squamous-cell carcinomas in patients treated with BRAF inhibitors. *N Eng J Med*. 2012;366(3):207–215.

35 Solit DB, Garraway LA, Pratilas CA, et al. BRAF mutation predicts sensitivity to MEK inhibition. *Nature*. 2006;439(7074):358–362.

36 Gilmartin AG, Bleam MR, Groy A, et al. GSK1120212 (JTP-74057) is an inhibitor of MEK activity and activation with favorable pharmacokinetic properties for sustained in vivo pathway inhibition. *Clin Cancer Res*. 2011;17(5):989–1000.

37 Flaherty KT, Robert C, Hersey P, et al. Improved survival with MEK inhibition in BRAF-mutated melanoma. *N Eng J Med*. 2012;367(2):107–114.

38 Dankort D, Curley DP, Cartlidge RA, et al. Braf(V600E) cooperates with Pten loss to induce metastatic melanoma. *Nat Genet*. 2009;41(5):544–552.

39 Kwong LN, Costello JC, Liu H, et al. Oncogenic NRAS signaling differentially regulates survival and proliferation in melanoma. *Nat Med*. 2012;18(10):1503–1510.

40 Omholt K, Platz A, Kanter L, Ringborg U, Hansson J. NRAS and BRAF mutations arise early during melanoma pathogenesis and are preserved throughout tumor progression. *Clin Cancer Res*. 2003;9(17):6483–6488.

41 Goel VK, Lazar AJ, Warneke CL, Redston MS, Haluska FG. Examination of mutations in BRAF, NRAS, and PTEN in primary cutaneous melanoma. *J Invest Dermatol*. 2006;126(1):154–160.

42 Marquette A, Andre J, Bagot M, Bensussan A, Dumaz N. ERK and PDE4 cooperate to induce RAF isoform switching in melanoma. *Nat Struct Mol Biol*. 2011;18(5):584–591.

43 Jaiswal BS, Janakiraman V, Kljavin NM, et al. Combined targeting of BRAF and CRAF or BRAF and PI3K effector pathways is required for efficacy in NRAS mutant tumors. *PloS One*. 2009;4(5):e5717.

44  Gyorffy B, Schafer R. Biomarkers downstream of RAS: a search for robust transcriptional targets. *Curr Cancer Drug Targets*. 2010;10(8):858–868.

45  Smalley KS, Eisen TG. Farnesyl transferase inhibitor SCH66336 is cytostatic, pro-apoptotic and enhances chemosensitivity to cisplatin in melanoma cells. *Int J Cancer*. 2003;105(2):165–175.

46  Fokstuen T, Rabo YB, Zhou JN, et al. The Ras farnesylation inhibitor BZA-5B increases the resistance to cisplatin in a human melanoma cell line. *Anticancer Res*. 1997;17(4A):2347–2352.

47  Flaherty KT, LoRusso PM, DeMichele A, et al. Phase 1, Dose-escalation Trial of the Oral Cyclin-dependent Kinase 4/6 Inhibitor PD 0332991, Administered Using a 21-day Schedule in Patients with Advanced Cancer. *Clin Cancer Res*. 2012;18(2):568–576.

48  Kong Y, Si L, Zhu Y, et al. Large-scale analysis of KIT aberrations in Chinese patients with melanoma. *Clin Cancer Res*. 2011;17(7):1684–1691.

49  Demetri GD, von Mehren M, Blanke CD, et al. Efficacy and safety of imatinib mesylate in advanced gastrointestinal stromal tumors. *N Engl J Med*. 2002;347(7):472–480.

50  McArthur GA, Ribas A, Chapman PB, et al. Molecular analyses from a phase I trial of vemurafenib to study mechanism of action and resistance in repeated biopsies from BRAF mutation–positive metastatic melanoma patients. *J Clin Oncol*. 2011;29(suppl.): Abstract 8502.

51  Nazarian R, Shi H, Wang Q, et al. Melanomas acquire resistance to B-RAF(V600E) inhibition by RTK or N-RAS upregulation. *Nature*. 2010;468(7326):973–977.

52  Branford S, Rudzki Z, Walsh S, et al. High frequency of point mutations clustered within the adenosine triphosphate-binding region of BCR/ABL in patients with chronic myeloid leukemia or Ph-positive acute lymphoblastic leukemia who develop imatinib (STI571) resistance. *Blood*. 2002;99(9):3472–3475.

53  Heinrich MC, Corless CL, Blanke CD, et al. Molecular correlates of imatinib resistance in gastrointestinal stromal tumors. *J Clin Oncol*. 2006;24(29):4764–4774.

54  Pao W, Miller VA, Politi KA, et al. Acquired resistance of lung adenocarcinomas to gefitinib or erlotinib is associated with a second mutation in the EGFR kinase domain. *PLoS Med*. 2005;2(3):e73.

55  Petti C, Molla A, Vegetti C, Ferrone S, Anichini A, Sensi M. Coexpression of NRASQ61R and BRAFV600E in human melanoma cells activates senescence and increases susceptibility to cell-mediated cytotoxicity. *Cancer Res*. 2006;66(13):6503–6511.

56  Weisbart RH, Chan G, Heinze E, Mory R, Nishimura RN, Colburn K. BRAF drives synovial fibroblast transformation in rheumatoid arthritis. *J Biol Chem*. 2010;285(45):34299–34303.

57  Johannessen CM, Boehm JS, Kim SY, et al. COT drives resistance to RAF inhibition through MAP kinase pathway reactivation. *Nature*. 2010;468(7326):968–972.

58  Wagle N, Emery C, Berger MF, et al. Dissecting therapeutic resistance to RAF inhibition in melanoma by tumor genomic profiling. *J Clin Oncol*. 2011;29(22):3085–3096.

59  Shi H, Moriceau G, Kong X, et al. Preexisting MEK1 exon 3 mutations in V600E/KBRAF melanomas do not confer resistance to BRAF inhibitors. *Cancer Discov*. 2012;2(5):414–424.

60  Shi H, Kong X, Ribas A, Lo RS. Combinatorial treatments that overcome PDGFRbeta-driven resistance of melanoma cells to V600EB-RAF inhibition. *Cancer Res*. 2011;71(15):5067–5074.

61  Villanueva J, Vultur A, Lee JT, et al. Acquired resistance to BRAF inhibitors mediated by a RAF kinase switch in melanoma can be overcome by cotargeting MEK and IGF-1R/PI3K. *Cancer Cell*. 2010;18(6):683–695.

62  Daniotti M, Oggionni M, Ranzani T, et al. BRAF alterations are associated with complex mutational profiles in malignant melanoma. *Oncogene*. 2004;23(35):5968–5977.

63  Curtin JA, Fridlyand J, Kageshita T, et al. Distinct sets of genetic alterations in melanoma. *N Eng J Med*. 2005;353(20):2135–2147.

64  Smalley KS, Lioni M, Dalla Palma M, et al. Increased cyclin D1 expression can mediate BRAF inhibitor resistance in BRAF V600E-mutated melanomas. *Mol Cancer Therap*. 2008;7(9):2876–2883.

65  Anders L, Ke N, Hydbring P, et al. A systematic screen for CDK4/6 substrates links FOXM1 phosphorylation to senescence suppression in cancer cells. *Cancer Cell*. 2011;20(5):620–634.

66  Michaloglou C, Vredeveld LC, Soengas MS, et al. BRAFE600-associated senescence-like cell cycle arrest of human naevi. *Nature*. 2005;436(7051):720–724.

67  Dhomen N, Reis-Filho JS, da Rocha Dias S, et al. Oncogenic Braf induces melanocyte senescence and melanoma in mice. *Cancer Cell*. 2009;15(4):294–303.

68  Nathanson KL, Martin AM, Letrero R, et al. Tumor genetic analyses of patients with metastatic melanoma treated with the BRAF inhibitor GSK2118436. *J Clin Oncol*. 2011;29(suppl.): Abstract 8501.

69  Davies MA, Stemke-Hale K, Lin E, et al. Integrated Molecular and Clinical Analysis of AKT Activation in Metastatic Melanoma. *Clin Cancer Res*. 2009;15(24):7538–7546.

70  Paraiso KH, Xiang Y, Rebecca VW, et al. PTEN loss confers BRAF inhibitor resistance to melanoma cells through the suppression of BIM expression. *Cancer Res*. 2011;71(7):2750–2760.

71  Xing F, Persaud Y, Pratilas CA, et al. Concurrent loss of the PTEN and RB1 tumor suppressors attenuates RAF dependence in melanomas harboring (V600E)BRAF. *Oncogene*. 2012;31(4):446–457.

72  Jia S, Liu Z, Zhang S, et al. Essential roles of PI(3)K-p110beta in cell growth, metabolism and tumorigenesis. *Nature*. 2008;454(7205):776–779.

73  Straussman R, Morikawa T, Shee K, et al. Tumour micro-environment elicits innate resistance to RAF inhibitors through HGF secretion. *Nature*. 2012;487(7408):500–504.

74  Hodi FS, O'Day SJ, McDermott DF, et al. Improved survival with ipilimumab in patients with metastatic melanoma. *N Eng J Med*. 2010;363(8):711–723.

75  Robert C, Thomas L, Bondarenko I, et al. Ipilimumab plus dacarbazine for previously untreated metastatic melanoma. *N Eng J Med*. 2011;364(26):2517–2526.

76  Garraway LA, Widlund HR, Rubin MA, et al. Integrative genomic analyses identify MITF as a lineage survival oncogene amplified in malignant melanoma. *Nature*. 2005;436(7047):117–122.

77  Wellbrock C, Rana S, Paterson H, Pickersgill H, Brummelkamp T, Marais R. Oncogenic BRAF regulates melanoma proliferation through the lineage specific factor MITF. *PLoS One*. 2008;3(7):e2734.

78  Du J, Miller AJ, Widlund HR, Horstmann MA, Ramaswamy S, Fisher DE. MLANA/MART1 and SILV/PMEL17/GP100 are transcriptionally regulated by MITF in melanocytes and melanoma. *Am J Pathol*. 2003;163(1):333–343.

79  Boni A, Cogdill AP, Dang P, et al. Selective BRAFV600E inhibition enhances T-cell recognition of melanoma without affecting lymphocyte function. *Cancer Res*. 2010;70(13):5213–5219.

80  Wilmott JS, Long GV, Howle JR, et al. Selective BRAF inhibitors induce marked T-cell infiltration into human metastatic melanoma. *Clin Cancer Res*. 2012;18(5):1386–1394.

## CHAPTER 25

# Ovarian Cancer

*Shannon N. Westin[1], Larissa A. Meyer[1], and Robert L. Coleman[1,2]*

[1]Department of Gynecologic Oncology and Reproductive Medicine, The University of Texas MD Anderson Cancer Center, Houston, TX, USA

[2]Center for RNA Interference and Non-Coding RNA, The University of Texas MD Anderson Cancer Center, Houston, TX, USA

## Introduction

Ovarian cancer is the most deadly gynecologic cancer, with approximately 14,720 women predicted to die out of 21,980 diagnosed in 2014. Although there has been a reduction in mortality rates over time, the 5-year survival rates only approach 30%.[1] These dismal survival rates reflect the high proportion of women that are diagnosed at advanced stage (stage III/IV) with epithelial histology, where cure is less likely. The majority of these cancers are chemosensitive in the upfront setting, responding completely to a combination of surgery and chemotherapy 80% of the time.[2–4] However, these tumors are plagued by high recurrence rates with the emergence of drug resistance that makes cure unlikely.[2] In fact, recurrence is frequently characterized by the length of time elapsed from last platinum chemotherapy treatment. Ovarian cancer that recurs 6 months or more after platinum-based therapy is termed platinum-sensitive, while tumors that grow during primary chemotherapy or less than 6 months from chemotherapy completion are classified as platinum-refractory and platinum-resistant, respectively.[5] Nearly all patients with recurrent disease are incurable. However, patients with platinum-resistant and refractory tumors are the most challenging and median overall survival after this diagnosis is under 2 years.[2] Thus, the key unmet needs in ovarian cancer include maximizing the initial success achieved after upfront therapy and lengthening the time to subsequent progression. Further, discovery of new effective agents for the platinum-resistant setting is paramount.

## Ovarian Cancer Histology

Ovarian cancers demonstrate great variation clinically and pathologically. The major histologies of ovarian cancer are derived from the three major components of the developing ovary.[6] Aside from their tissue of origin, the histology types are differentiated based on their pathologic appearance, as well as different molecular and epidemiologic features.[7] The most common histology type is derived from the coelomic epithelium. Approximately 85% of all malignant ovarian tumors are epithelial in nature, including serous, mucinous, endometrioid, clear cell, Brenner, undifferentiated, and carcinosarcomas. Sex cord–stromal tumors arise from the specialized gonadal stroma and include granulosa-theca cell tumors, Sertoli–

Leydig tumors, gynandroblastomas, and lipid cell tumors. The least common histology are tumors originating in the ovarian germ cells, which comprise less than 5% of all ovarian cancers. This cell type includes choriocarcinomas, dysgerminomas, yolk sac, embryonal, and mixed germ cell tumors.

The epidemiology of ovarian cancer varies greatly based on the histology type. In general, germ cell tumors are found in younger women and tend to be highly chemosensitive. These patients present at an early stage and median overall survival is excellent. Sex cord–stromal tumors are found in a middle age population and benefit greatly from surgical therapy. Although they are often sensitive to chemotherapy in the upfront setting, they may recur up to decades after initial diagnosis.

The epithelial histotypes have traditionally been treated with the same therapies and included in the same clinical trials. However, there is growing evidence that these subtypes are quite different molecularly and thus, should be considered separately in clinical decision-making.[8] The most common subtype is high-grade serous (75%). These tumors are found in older women and are associated with estrogen exposure and genetic abnormalities including *BRCA* mutation. High-grade serous tumors tend to present at an advanced stage and often demonstrate an aggressive nature of peritoneal spread. Conversely, low-grade serous tumors are found in younger women (5%) and are sensitive to hormone therapies. Although these tumors have poor sensitivity to chemotherapy, they generally demonstrate an indolent course. Patients with low-grade serous carcinoma have longer median survival compared to those with high-grade histology.[6]

The less common epithelial cell types, including clear cell (5–13%) and carcinosarcoma (1–4%), have similar epidemiologic features to patients with high-grade serous tumors. These tumors are found in older women and are quite aggressive, diagnosed at advanced stages. Both clear cell and carcinosarcoma are typically more likely to be resistant to standard chemotherapies in the upfront setting. Endometrioid histology type (10%) is more common in younger women, and is often found in association with synchronous endometrial cancer. These cancers are diagnosed at early stage and have improved prognosis compared to the other histology types. Mucinous tumors are rare (2–3%) and have been associated with extremely poor prognosis when diagnosed at an advanced stage.

This may be secondary to their historical treatment as a general epithelial ovarian cancer. These tumors appear extremely resistant to standard of care chemotherapy.[6,9] Interestingly, there are growing data to support the use of regimens employed in colorectal carcinoma for this cell type,[9] and results are eagerly anticipated for an ongoing trial comparing standard paclitaxel and carboplatin to XELOX (capcitabine and oxaliplatin) therapy (NCT01081262).

## Molecular Aberrations in Ovarian Cancer

The molecular characterization of ovarian cancer holds the potential to inform future standard of care treatments and clinical trial development. The known molecular aberrations are listed in Table 25.1. By far, the most well-described histology type is high-grade serous ovarian cancer. The Cancer Genome Atlas (TCGA) provided valuable information about the mutations, copy number alterations, and gene expression in this histology type. Although many of the aberrations are not currently actionable, this study helped to frame the direction for agent development.[10] Low-grade serous tumors are characterized by a high fraction of aberrations in the RAS/RAF pathway, providing a promising avenue for targeted treatment of this disease. Mucinous epithelial tumors also harbor a high fraction of KRAS mutations similar to colorectal carcinomas.[11,12] They may also harbor amplification of ErbB2. The phosphatidylinositol 3-kinase (PI3K)/AKT pathway is a promising potential target in clear cell carcinomas, given the number of pathway aberrations found in these tumors.[13–15] Endometrioid histology mimics the aberrations found in endometrioid endometrial cancer, with a high proportion of aberrations in the PI3K/AKT and RAS/RAF pathways.[16,17] Recently, somatic truncating or missense mutations in ARID1A were found in 46% of clear cell and 30% of endometrioid tumors.[18] The downstream loss of nuclear BAF250a expression is being studied as a predictive biomarker for selected therapies. Of the characterized sex cord–stromal tumors, granulosa cell tumors have few known actionable mutations.[19–21] FOXL2 mutations have been recently described in this tumor type; however, a mechanism to target this aberrations is yet to be discovered.[22] Similarly, Sertoli–Leydig tumors have a high proportion of DICER1 mutations, which is not yet actionable in the clinical setting.[23,24] To

date, little data exist describing the molecular landscape of germ cell tumors.

## Targeting Angiogenesis

To date, targets of angiogenesis have been both the most widely studied and the most successful examples of biologic therapies in ovarian cancer. The process of angiogenesis, which is an integral part of normal ovarian physiology, also plays a critical role in the pathogenesis of ovarian cancer via promotion of tumor growth, progression, and metastatic spread.[25,26] Tumors rely on angiogenesis for the supply of nutrients, growth factors, oxygen, and for tumor dissemination. Although the process of angiogenesis in normal tissues leads to the uniform development of new blood vessels, angiogenesis in the tumor microenvironment creates irregular vessels that are dilated, tortuous, leaky, and functionally inferior. This pathologic form of angiogenesis results in unregulated division and growth of normally stable endothelial cells.

Similar to other solid tumors, ovarian tumors express both vascular endothelial growth factor (VEGF) and its receptor, VEGFR.[26,27] VEGF expression has been associated with the development of malignant ascites in ovarian cancer.[26,28] Overexpression of VEGFR is associated with a poor prognosis in ovarian cancer via its association with increased tumor growth, metastases, and mortality.[29] Antiangiogenic therapies capitalize on the overexpression of VEGF/VEGFR.

The most widely studied targeted agent in ovarian cancer is the humanized monoclonal antibody binding to human VEGF, bevacizumab. Bevacizumab has demonstrated single-agent activity in ovarian cancer. Two phase II trials of single-agent bevacizumab were completed in cohorts of women with heavily pretreated, recurrent ovarian cancer demonstrating response rates (RRs) of 16% and 21%, with a median progression-free survival (PFS) of 4.4 and 4.7 months, respectively.[30,31] Enthusiasm over the activity of bevacizumab in these early trials was offset by higher toxicity, with 4 of 44 (11%) patients in the Cannistra study developing gastrointestinal perforation (GIP), which lead to premature termination secondary to concerns regarding toxicity.

**Table 25.1** Molecular characterization of ovarian cancers by histologic subtype.

| Alteration | High-grade serous (%) | Low-grade serous (%) | Endometrioid (%) | Clear cell (%) | Mucinous (%) | Granulosa cell (%) |
|---|---|---|---|---|---|---|
| P53 mutation | 80–96 | 7–10 | 20–30 | 10–50 | 16 | 0 |
| BRCA1/2 mutation | 10–20 | Unknown | Unknown | Unknown | Unknown | Unknown |
| PTEN protein loss | 27 | Unknown | 24 | 40 | Unknown | 0 |
| PTEN mutation | 0.5 | Unknown | 17–33 | 3–5 | Unknown | 0 |
| PIK3CA mutation | 3–12 | 2 | 20 | 20–34 | Unknown | 0 |
| PIK3CA amplification | 68 | 20 | 20 | 20 | Unknown | Unknown |
| PIK3R1 mutation | 1 | Unknown | Unknown | Unknown | Unknown | Unknown |
| AKT mutation | 2 | 2 | Unknown | Unknown | Unknown | 0 |
| AKT amplification | 12–15 | Unknown | Unknown | 14 | Unknown | Unknown |
| KRAS mutation | 0–12 | 19–35 | 4–10 | 5–16 | 40–60 | Unknown |
| BRAF mutation | 1 | 2 | 4 | 1 | 10 | Unknown |
| EGFR amplification | 45 | 17–73 | 10 | 50 | 9 | 74 |
| EGFR mutation | 9 | Unknown | 0 | 15 | 66 | 0 |
| HER2 overexpression | 10–20 | 11 | 0 | 14 | Unknown | Unknown |
| HER2 amplification | 10–20 | 11 | 0 | 14–41 | 45 | Unknown |
| VEGF overexpression | 80 | 40–80 | Unknown | 40–100 | Unknown | Unknown |

**Table 25.2** Comparison of the GOG218 and ICON7 front-line phase III trials in ovarian cancer.

| Study details | GOG 218 | ICON-7 |
|---|---|---|
| Population | Untreated stage III–IV epithelial ovarian, primary peritoneal or fallopian tube cancer | Untreated high risk stage I–IIA and IIB–IV epithelial ovarian, primary peritoneal, or fallopian tube cancer |
| Design | Randomized, placebo-controlled | Randomized |
| Bevacizumab dose | 15 mg/kg IV Q21 days | 7.5 mg/kg IV Q21 days |
| Maintenance | Yes—16 cycles | Yes—12 cycles |
| Sample size | 1873 | 1528 |
| Endpoints | Primary—PFS | Primary—PFS |
| | Secondary—OS, quality of life, correlatives | Secondary—OS, RR, safety, quality of life, cost |

More recent studies, including four pivotal phase III trials, have evaluated the addition of bevacizumab to cytotoxic therapy in the upfront, maintenance, and recurrent setting. Both Gynecologic Oncology Group (GOG) 218 and ICON7 investigated the addition of bevacizumab to the standard carboplatin and paclitaxel combination followed by maintenance bevacizumab for a predetermined period of time for advanced ovarian cancer in the front-line setting. Details of these trials are compared in Table 25.2. In GOG 218, patients who received bevacizumab and cytotoxic chemotherapy followed by maintenance bevacizumab had significantly improved PFS versus those who received chemotherapy alone (median 14.1 vs. 10.3 months; HR, 0.72; 95% CI, 0.63–0.82; $p < 0.001$). Of note, there was no significant difference in PFS between patients who received bevacizumab and chemotherapy without maintenance bevacizumab and those who received chemotherapy alone, suggesting duration of exposure may be important to the treatment strategy.[32]

ICON-7 demonstrated a similar improvement in PFS with an HR of 0.81; $p < 0.004$.[33] Additionally, an overall survival advantage of nearly 8 months (28.8 months vs. 36.6 months; HR, 0.64; 95% CI, 0.48–0.85, $p < 0.002$) was identified in the subgroup of patients designated as high risk given the poor prognostic indicators of FIGO stage IV disease or suboptimally debulked FIGO stage III disease. Overall survival data for both trials have not yet matured; however, preliminary results reveal no OS benefit for bevacizumab plus chemotherapy followed by maintenance bevacizumab versus the control arm. The PFS advantage demonstrated in both trials has led to the acceptance of the addition of bevacizumab to the chemotherapy backbone in first-line therapy for epithelial ovarian cancer.[32,33]

Bevacizumab's role in recurrent ovarian cancer was addressed by the OCEANS study[34] and the AURELIA trial. The OCEANS study,[35] a phase III trial, combined bevacizumab with standard carboplatin and gemcitabine followed by bevacizumab maintenance in platinum-sensitive recurrent ovarian cancer. In this study, a significant improvement in PFS was reported (8.4 vs. 12.4 months).[34] The AURELIA trial, a phase III study comparing bevacizumab in combination with standard second-line chemotherapy agents to the standard agent alone, has reported a statistically significant improvement in PFS (3.4 months vs. 6.7 months) in the challenging platinum-resistant patient population.[35] Although an OS advantage has not been identified, bevacizumab is well accepted as a useful agent in the recurrent setting. GOG 213 is an ongoing bifactorial randomized study to evaluate the role of secondary surgical cytoreduction as well as the impact of the addition of bevacizumab to paclitaxel and carboplatin on OS in patients with recurrent platinum-sensitive ovarian cancer (NCT00565851).

Another useful combination in heavily pretreated patients is bevacizumab and oral metronomic cyclophosphamide.[36] This phase II study demonstrated an RR of 24% at a median follow up of 23.2 months with a PFS at 6 months of 56% with minimal toxicity in patients with multiple prior lines of chemotherapy. Other studies have combined bevacizumab with cyclophosphamide,[37] topotecan,[38] PLD,[39] nab-paclitaxel,[40] and docetaxel.[41]

While bevacizumab's activity in the front-line and recurrent setting is encouraging, the question remains as to whether it is more advantageous to treat with bevacizumab in the front-line setting or in recurrent disease.[42] Additionally, the cost associated with bevacizumab and how to incorporate its use in a cost-effective fashion have been explored and it is suggested that selective treatment of women with suboptimal or stage IV ovarian cancer is more cost-effective in the upfront setting.[42,43] A fraction of patients might be saved the cost and morbidity of bevacizumab if biomarkers with negative predictive value could be identified.

While the majority of data with bevacizumab has focused on epithelial ovarian cancers, bevacizumab has recently been evaluated in a phase II trial (GOG 251) in 36 women with recurrent sex cord–stromal tumors of the ovary with unlimited prior therapies. Brown et al. reported a 16.7% partial response rate with an additional 77.8% with stable disease. The median PFS was 9.3 months, and overall survival was not reached during the reporting period.[44]

Aflibercept is a manufactured protein created via the fusion of the ligand-binding domains of human VEGFR-1 and VEGFR-2 with the constant region of IgG. This agent is unique in its ability to bind all isoforms of VEGF as well as placental growth factor.[45] Two phase II studies of aflibercept as a single agent in platinum-resistant ovarian cancer have demonstrated promising results given a heavily pretreated population.[46,47] A phase II trial of aflibercept in combination with docetaxel in recurrent ovarian cancer demonstrated an overall confirmed RR of 54% (11 CR, 14 PR), with impressive response in platinum-sensitive (RR 77%) and platinum-resistant (RR 45%) patients.[48]

Although VEGF and related receptors have taken center stage thus far, the development of resistance to bevacizumab and like agents, coupled with their failure to achieve complete pathologic response, has led to increasing interest in other targets in the antiangiogenic cascade. For example, the fibroblast growth factor (FGF) pathway has been identified as a key regulator of angiogenesis and ovarian physiology. Further, increased levels of platelet-derived growth factor (PDGF) have been identified in ovarian carcinomas compared to benign tissue and have been associated with poor survival.[49–51] Additionally, both PDGF[52] and FGF signaling[53] have been implicated in resistance to VEGF inhibition, suggesting the possible strategy of the combination of VEGF and PDGF or FGF inhibition may help overcome resistance and block angiogenesis more completely.[52, 54] There are several drugs in development that are capitalizing on this strategy and work by inhibiting multiple angiogenic signaling targets, including pazopanib (VEGFR-1, -2, -3, PDGFR-α/β, FGFR-1 and -3, and c-kit),[55] cediranib (VEGFR-1, -2, -3, c-kit, PDGFR-α/β, and fibroblast growth factor receptor 1 (FGFR-1)),[56] nintedanib (VEGFR-1, -2, and -3, PDGFR-α/β, and FGFR-1, -2, and -3, v-src sarcoma viral oncogene homolog (Src) and fms-like tyrosine kinase 3 (Flt-3),[57] sorafenib (VEGFR-2 and -3, PDGFR-β, c-kit, Flt-3, and Raf),[58] and sunitinib (VEGFR-2, PDGFR-β, c-kit, Flt-3, and the rearranged during transfection (RET) proto-oncogene).[59, 60]

A phase II study of pazopanib in recurrent ovarian cancer achieved a 31% RR by CA125 level and a 56% SD rate. Among 17 patients with measurable disease, 18% reported a PR.[61] Phase II studies in relapsed/resistant ovarian cancer of pazopanib as a single agent (NCT01262014, NCT01227928) and in combination with chemotherapy (NCT01238770 (cyclophosphamide), NCT01600573 (weekly topotecan), NCT01608009 (paclitaxel), NCT01610206 (gemcitabine), and NCT01402271 (carboplatin/paclitaxel) are ongoing. In addition, a phase III study evaluating single-agent pazopanib maintenance to placebo after first-line chemotherapy has recently completed enrollment. While OS data have not yet matured, preliminary results suggest a significant 5.6-month improvement in PFS (HR, 0.77; 95% CI, 0.64–0.91) with pazopanib.[62] The combination of pazopanib and standard carboplatin and paclitaxel chemotherapy for first-line treatment of ovarian cancer was deemed not feasible secondary to excess toxicity.[63] The PACOVAR-trial: a phase I/II study of pazopanib and oral metronomic cyclophosphamide is accruing in the platinum-resistant population (NCT 01238770).[64]

In a phase II study of cediranib in 46 patients with recurrent ovarian cancer, a clinical benefit rate of 30% was reported with eight patients with PR, six patients with SD, and a median PFS of 5.2 months.[65] Hirte et al. reported activity in both platinum sensitive and resistant cohorts with a 41% RR in platinum-sensitive patients and a 29% RR in patients with platinum-resistant ovarian cancer treated with cediranib. The median time to progression and OS in the cohort were 4.1 and 11.9 months, respectively.[66] A phase II/III trial evaluating cediranib in combination with standard platinum doublets and as maintenance therapy in platinum-sensitive recurrent ovarian cancer (NCT00544973 [ICON6]) has finished accrual of 456 patients. Lederman et al. recently reported an improvement in both PFS (median 8.7 vs. 11.1 months, HR, 0.57; 95% CI, 0.45–0.74) as well as a 6-month improvement in OS (median 20.3 vs. 26.3 months, HR, 0.7; 95% CI, 0.51–0.96) in the cediranib plus platinum-based chemotherapy followed by maintenance cediranib.[67]

Phase I and II trials of nintedanib revealed promising single-agent activity and prolonged time to progression in the maintenance setting.[68] Further, nintedanib combined with paclitaxel and carboplatin in patients with advanced or recurrent gynecologic malignancies achieved objective response in five of seven patients with measurable disease.[69] These findings provided the rationale for the randomized placebo-controlled phase III study of nintedanib in combination with paclitaxel and carboplatin in upfront ovarian cancer followed by nintedanib monotherapy as maintenance presented by duBois et al. which revealed significant improvement in PFS in the nintedanib arm.[70] There are several ongoing phase I/II studies investigating the combination of nintedanib and chemotherapy and/or biologic agents in ovarian cancer (NCT01329549; NCT01314105, NCT01485874, NCT01669798, NCT01583322).

Trebananib differs in that it is an antiangiogenic peptibody that fuses an antiangiogenic protein to the Fc region of an antibody, thus inhibiting Ang1/Ang2 binding to the Tie2 receptor and a parallel angiogenic pathway.[71] In a randomized phase II trial evaluating weekly paclitaxel with trebananib versus placebo, a non-significant PFS advantage was seen for the trebananib arm. In the phase III setting, 919 women with recurrent ovarian cancer with three or less prior lines of therapy were randomized to weekly paclitaxel with trebananib or placebo. Overall response rate favored the trebananib arm and there was a statistically significant improvement in PFS. No difference was apparent in median overall survival at interim analysis.[72] Results of a phase III randomized double-blind placebo trial investigating the addition of trebananib to first-line therapy with carboplatin and paclitaxel (NCT01493505) are eagerly anticipated.

Matei et al. reported a phase II trial of sorafenib in recurrent ovarian cancer after 1 or 2 prior therapies. Twenty-two of 59 patients achieved PR or SD and 14 patients with measurable disease were progression-free for 6 months or greater.[73] A phase I study of the combination of sorafenib and bevacizumab had an impressive RR of 46% in heavily pretreated ovarian cancer.[74] A subsequent phase II study of intermittently dosed sorafenib with bevacizumab yielded clinical benefit in 88% of the first 25 response-evaluable patients (including 6 PRs and 16 patients with SD) with recurrent ovarian cancer.[75] Phase II studies combining sorafenib with traditional second-line chemotherapies have not added significant clinical benefit.[76] Sorafenib was not found to be a useful agent for maintenance therapy after complete response to chemotherapy in women with epithelial ovarian cancer.[77]

Single-agent sunitinib has been evaluated in three phase II studies in patients with recurrent or refractory ovarian cancer. RRs among the three trials ranged between 3.3% and 19% and SD rates were between 19% and 53%.[78-80] The utility of this agent in all types of ovarian cancer is unclear; however, due to high levels of VEGF expression in platinum-resistant clear cell carcinoma,[81] sunitinib is under exploration for the treatment of recurrent ovarian cancer of this histology (NCT00979992 [GOG 254]).

## Targeting DNA Repair with Poly-ADP-Ribose Polymerase Inhibition

Increased signaling through DNA damage repair pathways is a known mechanism of chemoresistance. Poly-ADP-Ribose Polymerase 1/2 (PARP1/2) are enzymes that play a critical role in the repair of DNA single-strand breaks through base-excision repair.[82] Loss of PARP activity leads to accumulation of single-strand breaks, subsequent double-stranded breaks, and cellular death. In normal cells, double-stranded breaks are repaired through homologous recombination (HR).[83] Carriers of *breast cancer susceptibility gene 1 (BRCA1)* and *BRCA2* gene mutations, whether germline or somatic, have perturbations in HR repair.[84] The use of PARP inhibitors in these patients presents a rational therapeutic approach, as PARP inhibition in these tumor cells leads to double-stranded DNA accumulation, mitotic catastrophe and cell death. Ordinarily, cells competent in HR will not be dramatically affected by PARP inhibition. However, treatment proves lethal when cells lack HR, through the process of "synthetic lethality." The exact mechanism through which PARP inhibition proves lethal under situations of HR deficiency (HRD) is not completely understood. While one hypothesis stems from accumulation of single-strand breaks leading to double strand breaks and inefficiency of repair via limited HR capacity, another mechanism lies with PARP's normal repressive role of error-prone non-homologous end joining (NHEJ), DNA-PK and Artemis pathways. When PARP is inhibited, under HRD through loss of BRCA1/2, these pathways are released for repair leading to genomic instability and chromosome rearrangement, ultimately promoting cell death.[85] Finally, PARP inhibitors appear to be able to "trap" PARP to DNA complexes disrupting effective repair. This mechanism was discovered when studies of wild-type cells were found to be more sensitive to PARP inhibition when combined with an alkylating agent than cells with intrinsic PARP loss.[86] Regardless of the exact pathway, significant clinical evidence exists to corroborate cellular vulnerability for this class of agents under HRD conditions.

Germline BRCA1 and BRCA2 mutations occur in approximately 10% of patients with ovarian cancer and up to 20% of all patients presenting with high-grade serous ovarian cancer (the most prevalent).[87, 88] In addition, recent findings indicate that somatic mutations in BRCA1 and BRCA2 are also common, suggesting that additional patients may be sensitive to PARP inhibition.[89] Furthermore, hypermethylation of DNA leading to loss of BRCA1 gene function has also been observed in up to 31% of sporadic ovarian cancers.[90] In addition, loss of a number of other genes recruited for successful HR cast a wider potential net for patients in whom inhibitors of PARP would be of value. This "BRCAness" phenotype may account for as many as half of all patients with high-grade serous ovarian cancer.[89, 91]

While several PARP inhibitors are currently being investigated (Table 25.3), the most experience to date in ovarian cancer is with olaparib in patients with BRCA1 and BRCA2 mutations. The first phase I trial of olaparib included all tumors and did not require BRCA mutations. Ten dose levels identified the maximum tolerated dose (MTD) at 400 mg orally twice daily (BID). In the 52-patient expansion cohort (200 mg orally, BID; all confirmed BRCA1/2 mutation carriers; 39 patients with ovarian cancer), objective response or CA125 response was observed in 46%, which was impressive given that 80% of the treatment cohort was considered platinum-resistant or refractory.[92] In the phase II trial, two doses of olaparib were administered to 57 recurrent ovarian cancer patients with confirmed germline BRCA1 and BRCA2 mutations. The overall response rate was 33% in patients receiving olaparib 400 mg twice daily and 13% in patients receiving 100 mg twice daily.[92] However, the median duration of response was 290 days versus 269 days and median PFS was 5.8 months versus 1.9 months. Additional phase II studies of olaparib in recurrent serous ovarian cancer have confirmed favorable response in patients with and without BRCA mutations.[93, 94]

Considering this clinical activity, a small, randomized phase II trial compared two doses of olaparib (200 mg BID, 400 mg BID) to pegylated liposomal doxorubicin (PLD) in patients with BRCA mutations and progression within 12 months of platinum. The trial was limited to just 30 patients per arm and patients receiving PLD were allowed to cross over to olaparib 400 mg BID on progression.

The overall RR was highest in the 400 mg dose versus 200 mg versus PLD (31% vs. 26% vs. 19%) but there was no difference in PFS, the primary endpoint (6.5 and 8.8 months for olaparib 200 and 400 mg, respectively, vs. 7.1 months for PLD).[95]

Three other PARP inhibitors have been evaluated in recurrent ovarian cancer patients, predominately in mixed populations. Veliparib was studied in BRCA1/2 mutation carriers with recurrent platinum-sensitive (40%) and platinum-resistant (60%) ovarian cancer. The overall RECIST confirmed RR was 26%, including 2 CR. The median PFS and OS were 8.1 months and 19.0 months, respectively. Another PARPi, niraparib was recently reported in a phase I/II trial among recurrent platinum-sensitive and -resistant previously treated ovarian cancer patients.[96] Overall RR was 30%, with a higher response rate observed in platinum-sensitive and BRCA1/2 mutation carriers. Finally, a first in human trial of BMN-673, a potent PARPi recently reported in 70 patients with multiple solid tumors (predominately ovarian and breast).[97] BRCA1/2 mutations were characterized in 69% (48/70). Among the 28 patients with ovarian cancer carrying a deleterious germline BRCA1/2 mutation objective response was observed in 44%, including 1 CR. Nearly all of the ovarian cancer responders were platinum-sensitive.

Each of the above trials were designed to treat patients with measurable recurrent and/or assessable disease. However, there has been increasing attention to the potential of these agents to reduce the risk of recurrence following response. The use of olaparib as a maintenance therapy in the platinum-sensitive recurrent setting was recently published with promising findings. Patients, who were not required to carry a germline mutation in BRCA1 or BRCA2, were treated with olaparib or placebo until disease progression after any response to platinum agent. This phase II study found a clear improvement in PFS (HR, 0.35; 95% CI, 0.25–0.49; $p < 0.001$), with a toxicity profile consistent with previous studies.[98] In the interim analysis of overall survival, no difference was observed. However, an update of the trial now accounting for patients with either germline or somatic BRCA1/2 mutation demonstrates an even more dramatic effect on PFS (HR, 0.18; 95% CI, 0.11–0.31), and while not reaching significance for OS, there is a suggestion that a larger sample size may achieve this elusive endpoint. These observations have prompted a robust phase III profile for this class of agent. Indeed, olaparib, neraparib, and rucaparib are each undergoing phase III investigation in the maintenance setting. Table 25.3 demonstrates the agent and setting along with the target patient population.

Given the robust single-agent clinical activity of these agents, there has been a concerted effort to combine them with chemotherapy. The effort has proved difficult due to increased myelosuppression particularly with DNA damaging agents, such as platinum, temozolomide and gemcitabine. One completed randomized phase II trial administered olaparib in ovarian cancer in combination with carboplatin and paclitaxel in the recurrent platinum-sensitive setting.[98] The dose of carboplatin was reduced to AUC of 4 and

**Table 25.3** Phase III trials of PARP inhibitors in ovarian cancer.

| Agent | Setting | Pathology | Patient characteristic | Clinicaltrials.gov ID |
|-------|---------|-----------|------------------------|----------------------|
| Olaparib | Front-line maintenance | HGSOC | BRCAmut only | NCT01844986 |
| Olaparib | Platinum-sensitive maintenance | HGSOC | BRCAmut only | NCT01874353 |
| Niraparib | Platinum-sensitive maintenance | HGSOC | BRCAmut and BRCAwt | NCT01847274 |
| Rucaparib | Platinum-sensitive maintenance | HGSOC and Endometrioid | BRCAmut, genomic "scarring" and BRCAwt | NCT01968213 |

olaparib 200 mg PO BID in order to facilitate multiple cycles of administration. Upon completion of 4 to 6 cycles of chemotherapy (with or without olaparib), those not progressing on therapy were then given maintenance olaparib or placebo. PFS was significantly increased in the olaparib arm compared to placebo producing a 2.6-month improvement in the median PFS (12.2 months vs. 9.6 months. A front-line phase I trial with veliparib in combination with paclitaxel, carboplatin, and bevacizumab is nearly complete (NCT00989651).

Future prospects of PARPi in ovarian cancer are proceeding down several lines of investigation. For instance, regulators of HRD-like states from other tumor suppressor genes, PTEN, have fostered evaluation of PARPi with agents targeting the PI3K pathway.[99] In addition, tumor hypoxia provides a microenvironmental "contextual" synthetically lethal situation, which would support the use of anti-angiogenesis inhibitors in combination.[100] Two phase I studies have been conducted combining olaparib with either bevacizumab or cediranib. In the former, doses of olaparib (100, 200, and 400 PO BID) were administered with bevacizumab 10 mg/kg every 14 days. Twelve patients were enrolled finding the MTD was olaparib 400 mg PO BID with bevacizumab 10 mg/kg every 14 days. In the latter, the recommended phase II dose for olaparib was 200 mg PO BID with cediranib 30 mg daily, after reaching two dose-limiting myelosuppression events at 400 mg PO BID and 30 mg daily for the agents, respectively. Objective responses were observed in this phase I trial (44%) prompting a phase II trial with the same combination, which has completed accrual and awaiting results (NCT01116648). Further, exploration of mechanisms to resistance to PARPi agents will further expand new potential therapeutic options based on specific leveraged pathways.

## Targeting the RAS/RAF Pathway

The RAS-RAF-MEK-ERK signal transduction pathway is a conserved RAS-activated protein kinase cascade that asserts action via the regulation of cell growth, proliferation, and differentiation in response to growth factors, cytokines, and hormones.[101] The pathway is initiated by the binding of a ligand such as a cytokine, growth factor, or mitogen to its cell surface receptor. After RAF activation by RAS-GTP, conformational changes and recruitment to the cell membrane promote changes to RAF phosphorylation that, in combination with its serine/threonine kinase activity, act to trigger sequential phosphorylation and activation of MEK and ERK.[102, 103]

Among all epithelial ovarian cancers, mutations in the RAS/RAF pathway are rare. However, low-grade serous carcinomas differ from their more common high-grade counterpart clinically as well as on the molecular level.[104, 105] Low-grade serous carcinoma have a high frequency of mutations that lead to the constitutive activation of the RAS/RAF pathway.[104, 105] Additionally, up to 50% of mucinous adenocarcinomas of the ovary have been reported to have activating KRAS mutations.[11]

Given the high percentage of women with low-grade serous ovarian cancer with aberrations in the RAS/RAF pathway, a phase II study evaluating selumetinib, an oral MEK-1,2 inhibitor, has been completed in women with recurrent low-grade serous ovarian cancer.[106] Out of 52 eligible patients, 8 (15%) had an objective response with one patient achieving CR. An additional 65% of patients achieved SD.

Based on these positive findings, MEK inhibitors are being fully explored for low-grade serous ovarian cancer. Two randomized phase III trials are currently accruing with patients. One is randomizing women with centrally reviewed recurrent low-grade serous ovarian cancer to either the MEK inhibitor, MEK162, or standard second-line chemotherapy (PLD, paclitaxel or topotecan) (NCT 01849874). The other is randomizing a similar cohort of patients to either trametinib or standard second line chemotherapy or endocrine therapy. Crossover to trametinib is allowed in this second trial (GOG-0281) MEK162 is also being evaluated with weekly paclitaxel in patients with recurrent ovarian cancer (NCT01649336).

Cell line studies combining a dual PI3K with an MEK inhibitor demonstrated synergistic growth inhibition in five of the six cell lines resistant to the PI3K/mammalian target of rapamycin (mTOR) inhibitor as well as two cell lines that were resistant to both single agents.[107] The synergy between the two therapies was supported by xenograft studies. To further assess this approach clinically, a phase Ib clinical trial of the MEK inhibitor trametinib with a PI3K inhibitor is ongoing in women with recurrent ovarian cancer (NCT01155453).

## Targeting the PI3K/AKT Pathway

Targeting the PI3K/AKT pathway has garnered significant attention in patients with ovarian cancer. As in other cancers, this pathway is important in ovarian tumor cell proliferation and survival. The presence of amplification in *PIK3CA* in ovarian cancer has been associated with early cancer-related death.[108] In addition, high expression of downstream targets, such as 4EBP-1, is associated with poor prognosis in ovarian cancer.[109] The importance of the pathway appears to be found across histotypes, as loss of PTEN protein expression has been implicated in the tumorigenesis of endometrioid ovarian cancer.[110] Further, mTORC2 activation is much more common in clear cell compared to high-grade serous ovarian cancer.[111] Thus, exploration of agents against the pathway is ongoing in several histology types.

In ovarian cancer, there may be a "PI3Kness" molecular profile that portends potential response to PI3K-directed agents, the definition of which continues to evolve. PI3Kness may include the presence of mutation in any key pathway member, including *PIK3CA, PTEN, AKT,* or *PIK3R1*. Copy number variations and overexpression of pathway members, including activating receptors such as EGFR, HER2, and IGFR-1, may also play a role.[112] This profile is most common in patients with low-grade, non-serous type tumors, where aberrations in *PIK3CA* and *PTEN* are highly prevalent.[13,16,17] However, high-grade tumors have been found to exhibit copy number variation and/or increased protein expression of PI3KCA and AKT in approximately 46% of cases.[10,112] Further, many ovarian cancers demonstrate increased AKT2 activity with corresponding expression of downstream phosphorylated mTOR and GSK-3β.[113]

In addition to the promising molecular profile, preclinical data support the use of agents that target key pathway members, including mTORC1, mTORC2, and AKT in ovarian cancer. These agents have been found to cause growth inhibition and reduction in expression of angiogenesis-related factors in *in vitro* and *in vivo* models of epithelial and stromal ovarian cancer.[114–116] As in other solid tumors, the use of PI3K/AKT-directed agents to overcome chemotherapy resistance is also of great interest. Several studies have demonstrated that resistance to commonly utilized chemotherapies, such as paclitaxel and cisplatin, may occur through activation of this pathway in ovarian cancer.[117,118] Further, the use of perifostine, an AKT inhibitor, resulted in growth inhibition and increased sensitivity to cisplatin *in vitro*.[119] Additional *in vitro* studies have revealed that cisplatin treatment can induce activation of the PI3K/AKT pathway. Subsequent treatment with LY2904002, a PI3K inhibitor, followed by cisplatin lead to growth inhibition and increased apoptosis.[120]

Thus far, there have been few reported trials of agents targeting the PI3K/AKT pathway in ovarian cancer. A phase II trial of the intravenous mTORC1 inhibitor, temsirolimus, in patients with platinum-resistant recurrent ovarian cancer achieved only a 9% PR rate out of 54 evaluable. An additional 24.1% of patients had clinical benefit as defined by survival progression-free at 6 months.[121] Temsirolimus is currently under exploration in combination with paclitaxel and carboplatin in advanced clear cell carcinoma of the ovary (NCT01196429). A phase II trial is underway to determine the role of temsirolimus and PLD in recurrent ovarian cancer (NCT00982631).

AKT inhibition holds great interest as a target for ovarian cancer. A trial of the highly selective allosteric AKT1/2 inhibitor, MK2206, was started to treat recurrent ovarian cancer with PTEN protein loss. Unfortunately, this trial was closed early secondary to slow accrual. It may be that the use of AKT inhibition holds the most promise in combination with chemotherapy. Perifosine was explored in combination with docetaxel for the treatment of taxane and platinum-resistant ovarian cancer. Only one PR (4.7%) was achieved in a patient with a *PTEN* mutation and three additional patients (14%) had stable disease for greater than 4 months.[122] GSK2110183, an AKT inhibitor, is under investigation in combination with carboplatin and paclitaxel in platinum-resistant ovarian cancer (NCT01653912).

Early success of single agent PI3K-pathway inhibitors may be hampered by the presence of compensatory feedback mechanisms in the pathway. For example, the downstream protein S6K provides negative feedback on mTORC2. mTORC1 inhibition reduces levels of S6K, allowing for activation of AKT by mTORC2. In a preclinical study in high-grade serous and clear cell ovarian cancer cell lines, treatment with everolimus induced AKT activation. AZD8055, an mTORC1/2 inhibitor, inhibited the proliferation of mTORC1-sensitive and -resistant cell lines.[111] Thus, agents that target several nodes along the pathway are of great interest.

NVP-BEZ235 is a novel PI3K and mTORC1/2 inhibitor that demonstrated significant activity in the inhibition of growth of platinum-sensitive and -resistant ovarian cancer cell lines. Of note, the presence of PTEN loss or PI3K-activating mutations was associated with increased sensitivity to this agent. This effect was confirmed in xenograft mouse models, where treatment with NVP-BEZ235 led to reduction in apoptosis, migration, and prolonged survival.[123] Interestingly, Kudoh et al. also found that NVP-BEZ235 was active in mucinous ovarian cancer cell lines and xenograft models.[124]

Resistance to PI3K/AKT agents has also been associated with activation of the RAS/RAF pathway in several solid tumors, including ovarian cancer.[125, 126] Sheppard et al. treated a variety of ovarian cancer cell lines with PF-04691502, a dual PI3K/mTOR inhibitor. Cell lines that were resistant to the PI3K/mTOR inhibitor demonstrated activation of the RAS/RAF pathway. Accordingly, treatment with an MEK inhibitor, PD-0325901, in combination with PF-04691502 achieved growth inhibition in 80% of the resistant cell lines. These findings were confirmed sensitive and resistant xenograft models.[107] Trials of PI3K-directed agents in combination with MEK inhibitors are in development for a variety of solid tumors, including ovarian cancer.

## Targeting the Epidermal Growth Factor Receptor Pathway

The Epidermal Growth Factor Receptor (EGFR) pathway consists of the Type 1 receptors, EGFR (ErbB-1), HER2 (ErbB-2), HER3 (ErbB-3), and HER4 (ErbB-4). Receptor activation requires binding to ligand (epidermal growth factors, neuregulins, amphiregulin, and transforming growth factors) as well as the binding of two identical EGFR family receptors (homodimerization) or two different EGFR family receptors (heterodimerization). Upon activation, these receptors regulate numerous tumorigenic processes through pathways such as RAS/RAF and PI3K/AKT.[127, 128]

It appears that constitutive activation of EGFR family members can contribute to the development and progression of ovarian cancer. This can occur through mutation, overexpression, or amplification of pathway members.[129] EGFR and HER2 overexpression has been found in 30–98% and 20–45% of all ovarian cancers, respectively.[130–133] Further, EGFR ligands may also be overexpressed in this cancer type.[134, 135] In the majority of studies, receptor or ligand expression has been associated with poor prognosis in ovarian cancer.[132, 135, 136] Thus, the exploration of agents that target this pathway was met with great enthusiasm.

Early preclinical data for agents targeting EGFR have not been impressive in ovarian cancer cell lines. Cetuximab, a monoclonal antibody to EGFR, and gefitinib, a tyrosine kinase inhibitor, demonstrated minimal impact on cell proliferation across a variety of ovarian cancer cell lines. Drug effect did not vary based on levels of EGFR expression in each line.[137] The EGFR tyrosine kinase inhibitor, erlotinib, demonstrated higher activity in platinum-resistant compared to platinum-sensitive ovarian cancer cell lines. Interestingly, this did correlate to the level of EGFR and phospho-EGFR expression.[138] Rather than single-agent activity, reversal of resistance to chemotherapy may represent a major opportunity for this class of agents. Benedetti et al. demonstrated that activation of EGFR represented a mechanism of platinum resistance in ovarian cancer cell lines.[139] Treatment with cetuximab and gefitinib has resulted in increased cell death in previously resistant cell lines and xenograft models. However, these same agents may increase resistance to specific chemotherapy agents, indicating that care should be taken in developing combination therapies.[140]

Accordingly, initial studies of single agents targeting EGFR have afforded minimal success in the management of ovarian cancer. In general, trials have been performed in all ovarian cancers regardless of histology. Compounds including gefitinib,[141] erlotinib,[142] and cetuximab[143] achieved few objective responses and only modest clinical benefit through prolonged stable disease. Certainly, this can be explained by the fact that the presence of *EGFR* mutation seems to correlate better with response to EGFR-directed therapy in solid tumors.[144] In fact, the one objective response in the gefitinib study was found in a patient with an EGFR mutation.[141] As the rate of *EGFR* mutation is quite low in ovarian cancer, the potential for success may also be low in an unselected population.[145]

Thus far, combinations of these EGFR-directed agents and chemotherapy has only provided a small amount of improvement over chemotherapy alone,[146–148] Hirte et al. achieved the greatest success in a trial of erlotinib with carboplatin alone in platinum-sensitive and -resistant ovarian cancer. Fifty-seven percent of platinum-sensitive patients achieved response compared to 7% in the platinum-resistant group.[149] Based on the modest success of erlotinib in combination with carboplatin, the European Organization for Research and Treatment of Cancer (EORTC) performed a phase III study of erlotinib versus observation in the maintenance setting after response to first-line platinum-based therapy. Unfortunately, the investigational arm did not provide any benefit for progression-free or overall survival in this setting. Further, activity did not correlate to aberrations in the pathway, including overexpression or mutation.[150]

After significant success in breast cancer, exploration of HER2 as a therapeutic target in ovarian cancer has also been explored given the small fraction of these cancers that express this target.[133,151] Two monoclonal antibodies to HER2, trastuzumab, and pertuzumab have demonstrated activity in ovarian cancer cell lines expressing the target.[152,153] Further, trastuzumab appeared to increase cisplatin sensitivity in the *in vitro* and *in vivo* settings.[151] A phase II trial of trastuzumab in HER2-expressing previously treated ovarian cancer demonstrated a response rate of 7.3% and median progression-free survival of only 2 months.[154] Similarly, pertuzumab was found to have low response rates in the single-agent setting.[155] Studies of pertuzumab in combination with chemotherapy have been the most promising, with improved response rates over chemotherapy alone in platinum-sensitive disease;[156] however, this has not translated into progression-free or overall survival benefit.[157] Low expression of HER3 correlated with response in the combination of pertuzumab and gemcitabine, but this was not confirmed they study of carboplatin-based combination therapy.[156,157]

Alternative strategies to achieve clinical response to EGFR inhibition are being actively explored. The coexpression of both EGFR and HER2 is common in ovarian cancer and dual targeting of the receptors demonstrated synergistic activity *in vitro*.[158] Lapatinib is a dual tyrosine kinase inhibitor of EGFR and HER2 which has been explored in ovarian cancer. Single-agent response has been modest[159] and the combination of this agent and cytotoxic chemotherapy has been limited by poor efficacy and high toxicities.[145,160] Several agents are in development which target all four EGFR family members. Afatinib is a tyrosine kinase inhibitor of EGFR, HER2, and HER4. This agent has had activity in lung cancer and is under development alone and in combination with chemotherapy.[161] Similarly, Neratinib is a pan-Erb inhibitor which is currently under exploration in EGFR-, HER2-, and HER3-mutant or EGFR-amplified advanced solid tumors (NCT01953926).[162]

Prevention of receptor dimerization may be a more successful strategy to achieve successful EGFR inhibition. HER3 expression has been implicated in ovarian cancer cell line resistance to trastuzumab.[163] MM-121 inhibits the dimerization of HER3 and has been found to have significant activity in cancers with ligand-dependent activation of this target.[164] Based on promising early phase data, this agent is under exploration in combination with weekly paclitaxel for platinum-resistant ovarian cancer (NCT01447706). Resistance to chemotherapy and EGFR-directed agents may also occur through activation of alternative pathways such as PI3K/AKT.[165] Thus, the combination of these agents is rational. Glaysher et al. demonstrated promising activity of a PI3K-inhibitor with EGFR inhibitors in ovarian cancer cell lines.[166]

## Targeting Folate

Folate is a lipophobic B-vitamin essential for normal functioning cells, particularly in regard to synthesis of DNA and RNA as well as genomic and proteomic methylation.[167–169] It can be transported into the cell by the reduced folate carrier (RFC), the proton-coupled folate transporter (PCFT), or the folate receptor (FR) of which various isoforms exist. While many normal cells express the RFC and

PCFT, the FR is present only in a small proportion of normal tissues and in these tissues its expression is often low.[170] However, in many types of epithelial cancer, FR expression is prominent, particularly in ovarian cancer, and considering this differential FR is considered a promising anti-tumor target.[171]

There are several proposed mechanisms by which the high-affinity FR promotes the cancer process.[172–174] Since folate is involved in DNA synthesis, the enhanced uptake supports aggressive proliferation. In addition, FR can mediate apoptosis resistance by promoting expression of the anti-apoptotic protein Bcl-2 and inhibiting the proapoptotic protein Bax. Further, FR appears to support anoikis or anchorage-independent growth via downregulation of caveolin-1 expression, which normally inhibits the signaling pathways involved in this process.[175] Finally, FR may increase cancer cell motility through downregulation of E-cadherin. Indeed, FR expression has been found as an adverse prognostic factor for disease-free and overall survival.[176] In light of these observations, therapies targeting or using the FR have entered the clinical domain. Agents in mature clinical development for ovarian cancer include farletuzumab and vintafolide.

Farletuzumab is a monoclonal antibody that induces immune-dependent cell death by binding FRα as a selective marker for tumor cells. Tumor cell death is then mediated by the antibody-dependent cell-mediated cytotoxicity (ADCC) and complement-dependent cytotoxicity (CDC) immune mechanisms.[177,178] In preclinical studies, farletuzumab has shown a high affinity for the FRα isoform and only slight cross-reactivity to non-malignant tissues.[177] In a phase II trial in platinum-sensitive OC patients, farletuzumab treatment (combined with paclitaxel and carboplatin) led to an objective response rate of over 70%, representing an increase in response rate compared to historical outcomes; further, approximately one in five patients (21%) had a longer PFS on recurrence therapy with farletuzumab as compared with their initial PFS with front-line adjuvant chemotherapy.[179]

Based on these phase II trial results, a three-arm phase III trial was initiated in which platinum-sensitive patients were treated with standard chemotherapy combined with two doses of farletuzumab (1.25 mg/kg and 2.5 mg/kg) or placebo (NCT00849667). The results were recently presented showing the primary endpoint, PFS, was not met; the median PFS was 9.0 months versus 9.5 months versus 9.7 months for placebo, farletuzumab 1.25 mg/kg and farletuzumab 2.5 mg/kg, respectively.[180] Another large phase III trial in platinum-resistant patients studying the effects of weekly paclitaxel with or without farletuzumab was discontinued when the trial did not meet pre-specified criteria for continuation (NCT00738699).

Vintafolide is a small-molecule drug conjugate (SMDC) composed of folate linked to the vinca alkaloid desacetylvinblastine monohydrazide (DAVLBH).[181,182] The drug is preferentially taken up by FR-expressing tumor cells and not by FR on non-malignant cells as that expression is often restricted to the luminal membrane. This leads to a targeted delivery of chemotherapy via a stable linker and limited toxicity in non-malignant cells. Preclinical studies showed that vintafolide treatment could lead to regression of FR-expressing human tumor xenografts in the absence of toxicity as measured by weight loss and tissue degeneration.[183] The target-specificity of vintafolide was demonstrated by the fact that no anti-tumor efficacy was observed when folate was co-administered.[183]

These preclinical studies led to a single-arm phase 2 trial in patients with recurrent or persistent epithelial ovarian, fallopian tube, or primary peritoneal carcinoma.[184] This study showed that patient survival seemed to benefit from vintafolide treatment compared to historical controls. A subsequent randomized phase II trial (PRECEDENT), then showed that vintafolide treatment in combination with PLD improved the median PFS of platinum-resistant patients to 5.0 months compared with 2.7 months for patients treated with PLD only (HR = 0.63, $p$ = 0.031).[185] While OS was not demonstrated in this 2:1 randomized trial, stratification by expression of the folate receptor using whole body imaging following administration of a technetium-labeled folate-based small molecule construct (99mTc-etarfolatide) suggested an effect may be seen in those patients whose tumor universally express the FR (median OS 14.6 months vs. 9.6 months; HR, 0.48; 95% CI, 0.17–1.37; $p$ = 0.17). A phase III trial (PROCEED) evaluating the efficacy of vintafolide combined with PLD in FR-expressing platinum-resistant OC patients is currently ongoing (NCT01170650).

Additive or synergistic effects of vintafolide in combination with other cytotoxics have been reported. Vintafolide combined with platinum-based agents, topoisomerase inhibitors or taxanes have led to enhanced anti-tumor effects *in vivo* without significantly increasing toxicity.[186] Another folate-based conjugate with the chemotherapeutic agent tubulysin has been generated as an anti-tumor drug. This FR-targeted drug (EC1456) is currently being tested in a phase 1 dose-escalation trial in patients with advanced solid tumors (NCT01999738).

Alternative strategies to improve the therapeutic window may involve pharmacological manipulation of FR expression.[173] Since estrogen can directly decrease FRα expression and dexamethasone can indirectly increase it, combining FR-targeted drugs with estrogen antagonists and dexamethasone (particularly if combined with histone deacetylase inhibitor) may provide a unique opportunity to further enhance the clinical efficacy of these agents.[173,187,188]

## Targeting Other Pathways of Interest

### SRC Inhibition

Src is a non-receptor protein tyrosine kinase that is involved with the regulation of multiple cellular functions including growth, adhesion, migration.[189] Src activation is associated with a poor prognosis for patients with epithelial ovarian cancer.[190] Advanced mucinous ovarian cancer has a poorer prognosis in comparison with other histologic types of epithelial ovarian cancer.[191] This is hypothesized to be secondary to relative chemoresistance with standard platinum and taxane chemotherapy.[192,193] Efforts are underway to discover more effective treatment strategies for mucinous ovarian cancers. In a mucinous ovarian carcinoma mouse model, targeting Src kinase with dasatinib-inhibited oxaliplatin-induced Src kinase activity and demonstrated synergistic antitumor effects in a mucinous ovarian cancer mouse model.[194] The *in vitro* and *in vivo* effects of KX-01, an agent that blocks the Src pathway and tubulin demonstrated significant inhibition of tumor growth in preclinical mucinous ovarian cancer models.[195]

Dasatinib is an oral Src-family inhibitor. A phase II study of dasatinib was performed by the GOG.[196] In this study of 34 evaluable patients, 21% achieved a PFS interval of at least 6 months, but there were no objective responses to single-agent Dasatinib. A phase I trial evaluated dasatinib with carboplatin and paclitaxel in a mixed cohort of women with recurrent platinum-sensitive and recurrent disease.[197] In this study, there was a 45% response rate (15% CR, 25% PR) with an additional 50% achieving stable disease.

Saracatinib is an oral v-src sarcoma viral oncogene homolog inhibitor. A randomized phase II study of carboplatin and paclitaxel plus or minus saracatinib was performed in a cohort of patients with advanced platinum-sensitive ovarian cancer.[198] The overall response rate in patients with measurable disease was not significantly different and there was no difference in PFS. A trial evaluating the activity of weekly paclitaxel with saracatinib was recently been completed (NCT01196741) and results are pending.

## Leveraging TP53 Mutation

TP53 regulates the G1 cell cycle checkpoint to protect cells from DNA injury and acts as a tumor suppressor gene, relevant to many solid tumors. In the setting of cancer, abrogation of TP53 can lead to chemoresistance. Cells with TP53 dysfunction are dependent on alternative checkpoints to regulate the cell cycle. Aberrations in TP53 are characteristic of high-grade serous carcinoma.[10,199] In addition, lower-grade epithelial histologies may display TP53 alterations in up to 50% of cases.[13,200,201] Inhibition of other regulators of the cell cycle holds the potential to act on p53 aberrations. For example, Wee-1 is a key factor in the repair of DNA damage in p53-deficient tumors. The inhibition of Wee-1 can allow for sensitization of TP53-deficient tumors to cytotoxic chemotherapy.[202] An ongoing randomized phase II study in TP53-deficient platinum-sensitive recurrent ovarian cancer is evaluating the effect of MK-1775, a Wee-1 inhibitor, in combination with standard chemotherapy (NCT01357161). Since one of the mechanisms for abrogation of normal TP53 function is nuclear transport to the cytoplasm, a new class of nuclear exportin inhibitors has been developed.[203] Future clinical work will help to determine their role in tumor control.

## Conclusion

Over the last decade, a growing understanding of the molecular aberrations present in the various histology types of ovarian cancer has yielded significant success for its treatment. Similar to other solid tumors, the use of targeted agents must be considered in the context of mutations, copy number alterations, and RNA/protein expression. Future agent development that is focused on common alterations, specifically TP53 and DNA damage repair, will maximize the impact of targeted therapy for this disease.

## References

1 Siegel R, Ma J, Zou Z, Jemal A. Cancer statistics, 2014. *CA Cancer J Clin*. 2014;64(1):9–29.

2 Guarneri V, Piacentini F, Barbieri E, Conte PF. Achievements and unmet needs in the management of advanced ovarian cancer. *Gynecol Oncol*. 2010;117(2):152–158.

3 Armstrong DK, Bundy B, Wenzel L, et al. Intraperitoneal cisplatin and paclitaxel in ovarian cancer. *N Engl J Med*. 2006;354(1):34–43.

4 Katsumata N, Yasuda M, Takahashi F, et al. Dose-dense paclitaxel once a week in combination with carboplatin every 3 weeks for advanced ovarian cancer: a phase 3, open-label, randomised controlled trial. *Lancet*. 2009;374(9698):1331–1338.

5 Thigpen T. A rational approach to the management of recurrent or persistent ovarian carcinoma. *Clin Obstet Gynecol*. 2012;55(1):114–130.

6 Romero I, Bast RC Jr. Minireview: human ovarian cancer: biology, current management, and paths to personalizing therapy. *Endocrinology*. 2012;153(4):1593–1602.

7 Kurman RJ, Shih Ie M. The origin and pathogenesis of epithelial ovarian cancer: a proposed unifying theory. *Am J Surg Pathol*. 2010;34(3):433–443.

8 Despierre E, Yesilyurt BT, Lambrechts S, et al. Epithelial ovarian cancer: rationale for changing the one-fits-all standard treatment regimen to subtype-specific treatment. *Int J Gynecol Cancer.* 2014;24(3):468–477.

9 Jain A, Seiden MV. Rare epithelial tumors arising in or near the ovary: a review of the risk factors, presentation, and future treatment direction for ovarian clear cell and mucinous carcinoma. *Am Soc Clin Oncol Educ Book.* 2013. doi:10.1200/EdBook_AM.2013.33.e200.

10 Cancer Genome Atlas Research Network. Integrated genomic analyses of ovarian carcinoma. *Nature.* 2011;474(7353):609–615.

11 Gemignani ML, Schlaerth AC, Bogomolniy F, et al. Role of KRAS and BRAF gene mutations in mucinous ovarian carcinoma. *Gynecol Oncol.* 2003;90(2):378–381.

12 Enomoto T, Weghorst CM, Inoue M, Tanizawa O, Rice JM. K-ras activation occurs frequently in mucinous adenocarcinomas and rarely in other common epithelial tumors of the human ovary. *Am J Pathol.* 1991;139(4):777–785.

13 Kuo KT, Mao TL, Jones S, et al. Frequent activating mutations of PIK3CA in ovarian clear cell carcinoma. *Am J Pathol.* 2009;174 (5):1597–1601.

14 Tan DS, Miller RE, Kaye SB. New perspectives on molecular targeted therapy in ovarian clear cell carcinoma. *Br J Cancer.* 2013;108(8):1553–1559.

15 Tan DS, Iravani M, McCluggage WG, et al. Genomic analysis reveals the molecular heterogeneity of ovarian clear cell carcinomas. *Clin Cancer Res.* 2011;17(6):1521–1534.

16 Shih Ie M, Kurman RJ. Ovarian tumorigenesis: a proposed model based on morphological and molecular genetic analysis. *Am J Pathol.* 2004; 164(5):1511–1518.

17 Kolasa IK, Rembiszewska A, Janiec-Jankowska A, et al. PTEN mutation, expression and LOH at its locus in ovarian carcinomas. Relation to TP53, K-RAS and BRCA1 mutations. *Gynecol Oncol.* 2006;103 (2):692–697.

18 Wiegand KC, Shah SP, Al-Agha OM, et al. ARID1A mutations in endometriosis-associated ovarian carcinomas. *N Engl J Med.* 2010;363(16):1532–1543.

19 Bittinger S, Alexiadis M, Fuller PJ. Expression status and mutational analysis of the PTEN and P13K subunit genes in ovarian granulosa cell tumors. *Int J Gynecol Cancer.* 2009;19(3):339–342.

20 Higgins PA, Brady A, Dobbs SP, Salto-Tellez M, Maxwell P, McCluggage WG. Epidermal growth factor receptor (EGFR), HER2 and insulin-like growth factor-1 receptor (IGF-1R) status in ovarian adult granulosa cell tumours. *Histopathology.* 2013;64(5):633–638.

21 Chu S, Alexiadis M, Fuller PJ. Expression, mutational analysis and in vitro response of imatinib mesylate and nilotinib target genes in ovarian granulosa cell tumors. *Gynecol Oncol.* 2008;108(1):182–190.

22 Jamieson S, Butzow R, Andersson N, et al. The FOXL2 C134W mutation is characteristic of adult granulosa cell tumors of the ovary. *Mod Pathol.* 2010;23(11):1477–1485.

23 Witkowski L, Mattina J, Schonberger S, et al. DICER1 hotspot mutations in non-epithelial gonadal tumours. *Br J Cancer.* 2013;109(10):2744–2750.

24 Heravi-Moussavi A, Anglesio MS, Cheng SW, et al. Recurrent somatic DICER1 mutations in nonepithelial ovarian cancers. *N Engl J Med.* 2012;366(3):234–242.

25 Brown LF, Detmar M, Claffey K, et al. Vascular permeability factor/vascular endothelial growth factor: a multifunctional angiogenic cytokine. *EXS.* 1997;79:233–269.

26 Ramakrishnan S, Subramanian IV, Yokoyama Y, Geller M. Angiogenesis in normal and neoplastic ovaries. *Angiogenesis.* 2005;8(2):169–182.

27 Chen H, Ye D, Xie X, Chen B, Lu W. VEGF, VEGFRs expressions and activated STATs in ovarian epithelial carcinoma. *Gynecol Oncol.* 2004;94(3):630–635.

28 Zebrowski BK, Liu W, Ramirez K, Akagi Y, Mills GB, Ellis LM. Markedly elevated levels of vascular endothelial growth factor in malignant ascites. *Ann Surg Oncol.* 1999;6(4):373–378.

29 Kamat AA, Merritt WM, Coffey D, et al. Clinical and biological significance of vascular endothelial growth factor in endometrial cancer. *Clin Cancer Res.* 2007;13(24):7487–7495.

30 Cannistra SA, Matulonis UA, Penson RT, et al. Phase II study of bevacizumab in patients with platinum-resistant ovarian cancer or peritoneal serous cancer. *J Clin Oncol.* 2007;25(33):5180–5186.

31 Burger RA, Sill MW, Monk BJ, Greer BE, Sorosky JI. Phase II trial of bevacizumab in persistent or recurrent epithelial ovarian cancer or primary peritoneal cancer: a Gynecologic Oncology Group Study. *J Clin Oncol.* 2007;25(33):5165–5171.

32 Burger RA, Brady MF, Bookman MA, et al. Incorporation of bevacizumab in the primary treatment of ovarian cancer. *N Engl J Med.* 2011;365(26):2473–2483.

33 Perren TJ, Swart AM, Pfisterer J, et al. A phase 3 trial of bevacizumab in ovarian cancer. *N Engl J Med.* 2011;365(26):2484–2496.

34 Aghajanian C, Blank SV, Goff BA, et al. OCEANS: a randomized, double-blind, placebo-controlled phase III trial of chemotherapy with or without bevacizumab in patients with platinum-sensitive recurrent epithelial ovarian, primary peritoneal, or fallopian tube cancer. *J Clin Oncol.* 2012;30(17):2039–2045.

35 Pujade-Lauraine E, Hilpert F, Weber B, et al. AURELIA: a randomized phase III trial evaluating bevacizumab (BEV) plus chemotherapy (CT) for platinum (PT)-resistant ovarian cancer (OC). *J Clin Oncol.* 2012;30(suppl.): Abstract LBA5002.

36 Garcia AA, Hirte H, Fleming G, et al. Phase II clinical trial of bevacizumab and low-dose metronomic oral cyclophosphamide in recurrent ovarian cancer: a trial of the California, Chicago, and Princess Margaret Hospital phase II consortia. *J Clin Oncol.* 2008;26(1):76–82.

37 Chura JC, Van Iseghem K, Downs LS, Jr., Carson LF, Judson PL. Bevacizumab plus cyclophosphamide in heavily pretreated patients with recurrent ovarian cancer. *Gynecol Oncol.* 2007;107(2):326–330.

38 McGonigle KF, Muntz HG, Vuky J, et al. Combined weekly topotecan and biweekly bevacizumab in women with platinum-resistant ovarian, peritoneal, or fallopian tube cancer: results of a phase 2 study. *Cancer.* 2011;117(16):3731–3740.

39 Kudoh K, Takano M, Kouta H, et al. Effects of bevacizumab and pegylated liposomal doxorubicin for the patients with recurrent or refractory ovarian cancers. *Gynecol Oncol.* 2011;122(2):233–237.

40 Tillmanns TD, Lowe MP, Walker MS, Stepanski EJ, Schwartzberg LS. Phase II clinical trial of bevacizumab with albumin-bound paclitaxel in patients with recurrent, platinum-resistant primary epithelial ovarian or primary peritoneal carcinoma. *Gynecol Oncol.* 2013;128(2):221–228.

41 Wenham RM, Lapolla J, Lin HY, et al. A phase II trial of docetaxel and bevacizumab in recurrent ovarian cancer within 12 months of prior platinum-based chemotherapy. *Gynecol Oncol.* 2013;130(1):19–24.

42 Monk BJ, Pujade-Lauraine E, Burger RA. Integrating bevacizumab into the management of epithelial ovarian cancer: the controversy of frontline versus recurrent disease. *Ann Oncol.* 2013;24(suppl. 10):x53–x58.

43 Mehta DA, Hay JW. Cost-effectiveness of adding bevacizumab to first line therapy for patients with advanced ovarian cancer. *Gynecol Oncol.* 2014;132(3):677–683.

44 Brown J, Brady WE, Schink J, et al. Efficacy and safety of bevacizumab in recurrent sex cord-stromal ovarian tumors: results of a phase 2 trial of the Gynecologic Oncology Group. *Cancer.* 2014;120(3):344–351.

45 Lockhart AC, Rothenberg ML, Dupont J, et al. Phase I study of intravenous vascular endothelial growth factor trap, aflibercept, in patients with advanced solid tumors. *J Clin Oncol.* 2009;28(2):207–214.

46 Gotlieb WH, Amant F, Advani S, et al. Intravenous aflibercept for treatment of recurrent symptomatic malignant ascites in patients with advanced ovarian cancer: a phase 2, randomised, double-blind, placebo-controlled study. *Lancet Oncol.* 2012;13(2):154–162.

47 Tew WP, Colombo N, Ray-Coquard I, et al. VEGF-Trap for patients (pts) with recurrent platinum-resistant epithelial ovarian cancer (EOC): preliminary results of a randomized, multicenter phase II study. *J Clin Oncol.* 2007;25:18(suppl.): Abstract 5508.

48 Coleman RL, Duska LR, Ramirez PT, et al. Phase II multi-institutional study of docetaxel plus afilbercept (AVE0005, NSC# 724770) in patients with recurrent ovarian, primary peritoneal, and fallopian tube cancer. *J Clin Oncol.* 2011;29(suppl.): Abstract 5017.

49 Henriksen R, Funa K, Wilander E, Backstrom T, Ridderheim M, Oberg K. Expression and prognostic significance of platelet-derived growth factor and its receptors in epithelial ovarian neoplasms. *Cancer Res.* 1993;53(19):4550–4554.

50 Apte SM, Bucana CD, Killion JJ, Gershenson DM, Fidler IJ. Expression of platelet-derived growth factor and activated receptor in clinical specimens of epithelial ovarian cancer and ovarian carcinoma cell lines. *Gynecol Oncol.* 2004;93(1):78–86.

51 Matei D, Kelich S, Cao L, et al. PDGF BB induces VEGF secretion in ovarian cancer. *Cancer Biol Ther.* 2007;6(12):1951–1959.

52 Erber R, Thurnher A, Katsen AD, et al. Combined inhibition of VEGF and PDGF signaling enforces tumor vessel regression by interfering with pericyte-mediated endothelial cell survival mechanisms. *FASEB J.* 2004;18(2):338–340.

53 Bergers G, Hanahan D. Modes of resistance to anti-angiogenic therapy. *Nat Rev Cancer.* 2008;8(8):592–603.

54 Lu C, Kamat AA, Lin YG, et al. Dual targeting of endothelial cells and pericytes in antivascular therapy for ovarian carcinoma. *Clin Cancer Res.* 2007;13(14):4209–4217.

55 Sloan B, Scheinfeld NS. Pazopanib, a VEGF receptor tyrosine kinase inhibitor for cancer therapy. *Curr Opin Investig Drugs.* 2008;9(12):1324–1335.

56 Wedge SR, Kendrew J, Hennequin LF, et al. AZD2171: a highly potent, orally bioavailable, vascular endothelial growth factor receptor 2 tyrosine kinase inhibitor for the treatment of cancer. *Cancer Res.* 2005;65(10):4389–4400.

57 Hilberg F, Roth GJ, Krssak M, et al. BIBF 1120: triple angiokinase inhibitor with sustained receptor blockade and good antitumor efficacy. *Cancer Res.* 2008;68(12):4774–4782.

58 Wilhelm SM, Carter C, Tang L, et al. BAY 43–9006 exhibits broad spectrum oral antitumor activity and targets the RAF/MEK/ERK pathway and receptor tyrosine kinases involved in tumor progression and angiogenesis. *Cancer Res.* 2004;64(19):7099–7109.

59 Sun L, Liang C, Shirazian S, et al. Discovery of 5-[5-fluoro-2-oxo-1,2- dihydroindol-(3Z)-ylidenemethyl]-2,4- dimethyl-1H-pyrrole-3-carboxylic acid (2-diethylaminoethyl)amide, a novel tyrosine kinase inhibitor targeting vascular endothelial and platelet-derived growth factor receptor tyrosine kinase. *J Med Chem.* 2003;46(7):1116–1119.

60 O'Farrell AM, Abrams TJ, Yuen HA, et al. SU11248 is a novel FLT3 tyrosine kinase inhibitor with potent activity in vitro and in vivo. *Blood.* 2003;101(9):3597–3605.

61 Friedlander M, Hancock KC, Rischin D, et al. A Phase II, open-label study evaluating pazopanib in patients with recurrent ovarian cancer. *Gynecol Oncol.* 2010;119(1):32–37.

62 du Bois A, Floquet A, Kim JW, et al. Randomized, double-blind, phase III trial of pazopanib versus placebo in women who have not progressed

after first-line chemotherapy for advanced epithelial ovarian cancer (AEOC). Results of an international intergroup trial (AGO-OVAR16). *J Clin Oncol.* 2013;31(suppl.): Abstract LBA5503.

63 du Bois A, Vergote I, Wimberger P, et al. Open-label feasibility study of pazopanib, carboplatin, and paclitaxel in women with newly diagnosed, untreated, gynaecologic tumours: a phase I/II trial of the AGO study group. *Br J Cancer.* 2012;106(4):629–632.

64 Eichbaum M, Mayer C, Eickhoff R, et al. The PACOVAR-trial: a phase I/II study of pazopanib (GW786034) and cyclophosphamide in patients with platinum-resistant recurrent, pre-treated ovarian cancer. *BMC Cancer.* 2011;11:453.

65 Matulonis UA, Berlin S, Ivy P, et al. Cediranib, an oral inhibitor of vascular endothelial growth factor receptor kinases, is an active drug in recurrent epithelial ovarian, fallopian tube, and peritoneal cancer. *J Clin Oncol.* 2009;27(33):5601–5606.

66 Hirte HW, Vidal L, Fleming GF, et al. A phase II study of cediranib (AZD2171) in recurrent or persistent ovarian, peritoneal or fallopian tube cancer: final results of a PMH, Chicago and California consortia trial. *J Clin Oncol.* 2008;26(suppl.): Abstract 5521.

67 Ledermann JA, Raja FA, Embleton A, Rustin GJ, Jayson G, Kaye SB. Randomised double-blind phase III trial of cediranib (AZD 2171) in relapsed platinum sensitive ovarian cancer: results of the ICON6 trial. *Eur J Cancer.* 2013;49(suppl. 3): LBA 10.

68 Ledermann JA, Hackshaw A, Kaye S, et al. Randomized phase II placebo-controlled trial of maintenance therapy using the oral triple angiokinase inhibitor BIBF 1120 after chemotherapy for relapsed ovarian cancer. *J Clin Oncol.* 2011;29(28):3798–3804.

69 du Bois A, Huober J, Stopfer P, et al. A phase I open-label dose-escalation study of oral BIBF 1120 combined with standard paclitaxel and carboplatin in patients with advanced gynecological malignancies. *Ann Oncol.* 2010;21(2):370–375.

70 du Bois A, Kristensen G, Ray-Coquard I, et al. AGO-OVAR 12: a randomized placebo-controlled GCIG/ENGOT-intergroup phase III trial of standard front-line chemotherapy +/− nintedanib for advanced ovarian cancer. *Int J Gynecol Cancer.* 2013;23(suppl. 1): LBA1.

71 Yancopoulos GD, Davis S, Gale NW, Rudge JS, Wiegand SJ, Holash J. Vascular-specific growth factors and blood vessel formation. *Nature.* 2000;407(6801):242–248.

72 Monk BJ, Vergote I, Raspagliesi F, Fujiwara K, Bae DS, Oaknin A. A phase III, randomized, double-blind trial of weekly paclitaxel plus the angiopoietin 1 and 2 inhibitor, trebananib, or placebo in women with recurrent ovarian cancer: TRINOVA-1. *Eur J Cancer.* 2013;49(suppl. 3): LBA 41.

73 Matei D, Sill MW, Lankes HA, et al. Activity of sorafenib in recurrent ovarian cancer and primary peritoneal carcinomatosis: a Gynecologic Oncology Group trial. *J Clin Oncol.* 2011;29:69–75.

74 Azad NS, Posadas EM, Kwitkowski VE, et al. Combination targeted therapy with sorafenib and bevacizumab results in enhanced toxicity and antitumor activity. *J Clin Oncol.* 2008;26(22):3709–3714.

75 Kohn EC, Lee J, Annunziata CM, et al. A phase II study of intermittent sorafenib with bevacizumab in bevacizumab-naïve epithelial ovarian cancer (EOC) patients. *J Clin Oncol.* 2011;29: Abstract 5019.

76 Ramasubbaiah R, Perkins SM, Schilder J, et al. Sorafenib in combination with weekly topotecan in recurrent ovarian cancer, a phase I/II study of the Hoosier Oncology Group. *Gynecol Oncol.* 2011;123(3):499–504.

77 Herzog TJ, Scambia G, Kim BG, et al. A randomized phase II trial of maintenance therapy with Sorafenib in front-line ovarian carcinoma. *Gynecol Oncol.* 2013;130(1):25–30.

78 Baumann KH, du Bois A, Meier W, et al. A phase II trial (AGO 2.11) in platinum-resistant ovarian cancer: a randomized multicenter trial with sunitinib (SU11248) to evaluate dosage, schedule, tolerability, toxicity

and effectiveness of a multitargeted receptor tyrosine kinase inhibitor monotherapy. *Ann Oncol*. 2012;23(9):2265–2271.

79 Biagi JJ, Oza AM, Chalchal HI, et al. A phase II study of sunitinib in patients with recurrent epithelial ovarian and primary peritoneal carcinoma: an NCIC Clinical Trials Group Study. *Ann Oncol*. 2011;22(2):335–340.

80 Campos S, Penson R, Berlin S, Matulonis U, Horowitz N. A phase II trial of sunitinib in recurrent and refractory ovarian, fallopian tube, and peritoneal carcinoma. *Gyn Onc*. 2010;116:S119–S120; Abstract 306.

81 Mabuchi S, Kawase C, Altomare DA, et al. Vascular endothelial growth factor is a promising therapeutic target for the treatment of clear cell carcinoma of the ovary. *Mol Cancer Ther*. 2010;9(8):2411–2422.

82 Schreiber V, Dantzer F, Ame JC, de Murcia G. Poly(ADP-ribose): novel functions for an old molecule. *Nat Rev Mol Cell Biol*. 2006;7(7):517–528.

83 Schultz N, Lopez E, Saleh-Gohari N, Helleday T. Poly(ADP-ribose) polymerase (PARP-1) has a controlling role in homologous recombination. *Nucleic Acids Res*. 2003;31(17):4959–4964.

84 Ashworth A. A synthetic lethal therapeutic approach: poly(ADP) ribose polymerase inhibitors for the treatment of cancers deficient in DNA double-strand break repair. *J Clin Oncol*. 2008;26(22):3785–3790.

85 Patel AG, Sarkaria JN, Kaufmann SH. Nonhomologous end joining drives poly(ADP-ribose) polymerase (PARP) inhibitor lethality in homologous recombination-deficient cells. *Proc Natl Acad Sci U S A*. 2011;108(8):3406–3411.

86 Murai J, Huang SY, Das BB, et al. Trapping of PARP1 and PARP2 by Clinical PARP Inhibitors. *Cancer Res*. 2012;72(21):5588–5599.

87 Ledermann JA, Raja FA. Targeted trials in ovarian cancer. *Gynecol Oncol*. 2010;119(1):151–156.

88 Risch HA, McLaughlin JR, Cole DE, et al. Prevalence and penetrance of germline BRCA1 and BRCA2 mutations in a population series of 649 women with ovarian cancer. *Am J Hum Genet*. 2001;68(3):700–710.

89 Hennessy BT, Timms KM, Carey MS, et al. Somatic mutations in BRCA1 and BRCA2 could expand the number of patients that benefit from poly (ADP ribose) polymerase inhibitors in ovarian cancer. *J Clin Oncol*. 2010;28(22):3570–3576.

90 Baldwin RL, Nemeth E, Tran H, et al. BRCA1 promoter region hypermethylation in ovarian carcinoma: a population-based study. *Cancer Res*. 2000;60(19):5329–5333.

91 Konstantinopoulos PA, Spentzos D, Karlan BY, et al. Gene expression profile of BRCAness that correlates with responsiveness to chemotherapy and with outcome in patients with epithelial ovarian cancer. *J Clin Oncol*. 2010;28(22):3555–3561.

92 Fong PC, Boss DS, Yap TA, et al. Inhibition of poly(ADP-ribose) polymerase in tumors from BRCA mutation carriers. *N Engl J Med*. 2009;361(2):123–134.

93 Ang J, Yap TA, Fong P, et al. Preliminary experience with use of chemotherapy (CT) following treatment with olaparib, a poly(ADP-ribose) polymerase inhibitor (PARPi), in patients with BRCA1/2-deficient ovarian cancer (BDOC). *J Clin Oncol*. 2010;28:15s(suppl.): Abstract 5041.

94 Gelmon KA, Hirte HW, Robidoux A, et al. Can we define tumors that will respond to PARP inhibitors? A phase II correlative study of olaparib in advanced serous ovarian cancer and triple-negative breast cancer. *J Clin Oncol*. 2010;28:15s(suppl.): Abstract 3002.

95 Kaye SB, Lubinski J, Matulonis U, et al. Phase II, open-label, randomized, multicenter study comparing the efficacy and safety of olaparib, a poly (ADP-ribose) polymerase inhibitor, and pegylated liposomal doxorubicin in patients with BRCA1 or BRCA2 mutations and recurrent ovarian cancer. *J Clin Oncol*. 2012;30(4):372–379.

96 Michie CO, Sandhu SK, Schelman WR, et al. Final results of the phase I trial of niraparib (MK-4827), a poly(ADP)ribose polymerase (PARP) inhibitor incorporating proof of concept biomarker studies and expansion cohorts involving BRCA1/2 mutation carriers, sporadic ovarian, and castrate resistant prostate cancer. *J Clin Oncol*. 2013;31(suppl.): Abstract 2513.

97 De Bono JS, Mina LA, Gonzalez M, et al. First-in-human trial of novel oral PARP inhibitor BNM 673 in patients with solid tumors. *J Clin Oncol*. 2013;31(suppl.): Abstract 2580.

98 Ledermann J, Harter P, Gourley C, et al. Olaparib maintenance therapy in platinum-sensitive relapsed ovarian cancer. *N Engl J Med*. 2012;366(15):1382–1392.

99 Mendes-Pereira AM, Martin SA, Brough R, et al. Synthetic lethal targeting of PTEN mutant cells with PARP inhibitors. *EMBO Mol Med*. 2009;1(6–7):315–322.

100 Dean E, Middleton MR, Pwint T, et al. Phase I study to assess the safety and tolerability of olaparib in combination with bevacizumab in patients with advanced solid tumours. *Br J Cancer*. 2012;106(3):468–474.

101 Robinson MJ, Cobb MH. Mitogen-activated protein kinase pathways. *Curr Opin Cell Biol*. 1997;9(2):180–186.

102 Kolch W. Meaningful relationships: the regulation of the Ras/Raf/MEK/ERK pathway by protein interactions. *Biochem J*. 2000;351 Pt 2:289–305.

103 Morrison DK, Cutler RE. The complexity of Raf-1 regulation. *Curr Opin Cell Biol*. 1997;9(2):174–179.

104 Diaz-Padilla I, Malpica AL, Minig L, Chiva LM, Gershenson DM, Gonzalez-Martin A. Ovarian low-grade serous carcinoma: a comprehensive update. *Gynecol Oncol*. 2012;126(2):279–285.

105 Hsu CY, Bristow R, Cha MS, et al. Characterization of active mitogen-activated protein kinase in ovarian serous carcinomas. *Clin Cancer Res*. 2004;10(19):6432–6436.

106 Farley J, Brady WE, Vathipadiekal V, et al. Selumetinib in women with recurrent low-grade serous carcinoma of the ovary or peritoneum: an open-label, single-arm, phase 2 study. *Lancet Oncol*. 2013;14(2):134–140.

107 Sheppard KE, Cullinane C, Hannan KM, et al. Synergistic inhibition of ovarian cancer cell growth by combining selective PI3K/mTOR and RAS/ERK pathway inhibitors. *Eur J Cancer*. 2013;49(18):3936–3944.

108 Woenckhaus J, Steger K, Sturm K, Munstedt K, Franke FE, Fenic I. Prognostic value of PIK3CA and phosphorylated AKT expression in ovarian cancer. *Virchows Arch*. 2007;450(4):387–395.

109 Castellvi J, Garcia A, Rojo F, et al. Phosphorylated 4E binding protein 1: a hallmark of cell signaling that correlates with survival in ovarian cancer. *Cancer*. 2006;107(8):1801–1811.

110 Tanwar PS, Kaneko-Tarui T, Lee HJ, Zhang L, Teixeira JM. PTEN loss and HOXA10 expression are associated with ovarian endometrioid adenocarcinoma differentiation and progression. *Carcinogenesis*. 2013;34(4):893–901.

111 Hisamatsu T, Mabuchi S, Matsumoto Y, et al. Potential role of mTORC2 as a therapeutic target in clear cell carcinoma of the ovary. *Mol Cancer Ther*. 2013;12(7):1367–1377.

112 Bast RC Jr., Mills GB. Dissecting "PI3Kness": the complexity of personalized therapy for ovarian cancer. *Cancer Discov*. 2012;2(1):16–18.

113 Altomare DA, Wang HQ, Skele KL, et al. AKT and mTOR phosphorylation is frequently detected in ovarian cancer and can be targeted to disrupt ovarian tumor cell growth. *Oncogene*. 2004;23(34):5853–5857.

114 Mabuchi S, Altomare DA, Connolly DC, et al. RAD001 (Everolimus) delays tumor onset and progression in a transgenic mouse model of ovarian cancer. *Cancer Res*. 2007;67(6):2408–2413.

115 Gao N, Flynn DC, Zhang Z, et al. G1 cell cycle progression and the expression of G1 cyclins are regulated by PI3K/AKT/mTOR/p70S6K1 signaling in human ovarian cancer cells. *Am J Physiol Cell Physiol.* 2004;287(2):C281–C291.

116 Rico C, Lague MN, Lefevre P, et al. Pharmacological targeting of mammalian target of rapamycin inhibits ovarian granulosa cell tumor growth. *Carcinogenesis.* 2012;33(11):2283–2292.

117 Yang X, Fraser M, Moll UM, Basak A, Tsang BK. Akt-mediated cisplatin resistance in ovarian cancer: modulation of p53 action on caspase-dependent mitochondrial death pathway. *Cancer Res.* 2006;66(6):3126–3136.

118 Fraser M, Bai T, Tsang BK. Akt promotes cisplatin resistance in human ovarian cancer cells through inhibition of p53 phosphorylation and nuclear function. *Int J Cancer.* 2008;122(3):534–546.

119 Al Sawah E, Chen X, Marchion DC, et al. Perifosine, an AKT inhibitor, modulates ovarian cancer cell line sensitivity to cisplatin-induced growth arrest. *Gynecol Oncol.* 2013;131(1):207–212.

120 Peng DJ, Wang J, Zhou JY, Wu GS. Role of the Akt/mTOR survival pathway in cisplatin resistance in ovarian cancer cells. *Biochem Biophys Res Commun.* 2010;394(3):600–605.

121 Behbakht K, Sill MW, Darcy KM, et al. Phase II trial of the mTOR inhibitor, temsirolimus and evaluation of circulating tumor cells and tumor biomarkers in persistent and recurrent epithelial ovarian and primary peritoneal malignancies: a Gynecologic Oncology Group study. *Gynecol Oncol.* 2011;123(1):19–26.

122 Fu S, Hennessy BT, Ng CS, et al. Perifosine plus docetaxel in patients with platinum and taxane resistant or refractory high-grade epithelial ovarian cancer. *Gynecol Oncol.* 2012;126(1):47–53.

123 Santiskulvong C, Konecny GE, Fekete M, et al. Dual targeting of phosphoinositide 3-kinase and mammalian target of rapamycin using NVP-BEZ235 as a novel therapeutic approach in human ovarian carcinoma. *Clin Cancer Res.* 2011;17(8):2373–2384.

124 Kudoh A, Oishi T, Itamochi H, et al. Dual Inhibition of Phosphatidylinositol 3′-Kinase and Mammalian Target of Rapamycin Using NVP-BEZ235 as a Novel Therapeutic Approach for Mucinous Adenocarcinoma of the Ovary. *Int J Gynecol Cancer.* 2014;24(3):444–453.

125 Di Nicolantonio F, Arena S, Tabernero J, et al. Deregulation of the PI3K and KRAS signaling pathways in human cancer cells determines their response to everolimus. *J Clin Invest.* 2010;120(8):2858–2866.

126 Massarelli E, Varella-Garcia M, Tang X, et al. KRAS mutation is an important predictor of resistance to therapy with epidermal growth factor receptor tyrosine kinase inhibitors in non-small-cell lung cancer. *Clin Cancer Res.* 2007;13(10):2890–2896.

127 Mendelsohn J, Baselga J. The EGF receptor family as targets for cancer therapy. *Oncogene.* 2000;19(56):6550–6565.

128 Normanno N, De Luca A, Bianco C, et al. Epidermal growth factor receptor (EGFR) signaling in cancer. *Gene.* 2006;366(1):2–16.

129 Ciardiello F, Tortora G. A novel approach in the treatment of cancer: targeting the epidermal growth factor receptor. *Clin Cancer Res.* 2001;7(10):2958–2970.

130 Moscatello DK, Holgado-Madruga M, Godwin AK, et al. Frequent expression of a mutant epidermal growth factor receptor in multiple human tumors. *Cancer Res.* 1995;55(23):5536–5539.

131 Bartlett JM, Langdon SP, Simpson BJ, et al. The prognostic value of epidermal growth factor receptor mRNA expression in primary ovarian cancer. *Br J Cancer.* 1996;73(3):301–306.

132 Skirnisdottir I, Sorbe B, Seidal T. The growth factor receptors HER-2/neu and EGFR, their relationship, and their effects on the prognosis in early stage (FIGO I-II) epithelial ovarian carcinoma. *Int J Gynecol Cancer.* 2001;11(2):119–129.

133 Slamon DJ, Godolphin W, Jones LA, et al. Studies of the HER-2/neu proto-oncogene in human breast and ovarian cancer. *Science.* 1989;244(4905):707–712.

134 Katso RM, Manek S, O'Byrne K, Playford MP, Le Meuth V, Ganesan TS. Molecular approaches to diagnosis and management of ovarian cancer. *Cancer Metastasis Rev.* 1997;16(1–2):81–107.

135 Scoccia B, Lee YM, Niederberger C, Ilekis JV. Expression of the ErbB family of receptors in ovarian cancer. *J Soc Gynecol Invest.* 1998;5(3):161–165.

136 Nicholson RI, Gee JM, Harper ME. EGFR and cancer prognosis. *Eur J Cancer.* 2001;37(suppl. 4):S9–S15.

137 Bull Phelps SL, Schorge JO, Peyton MJ, et al. Implications of EGFR inhibition in ovarian cancer cell proliferation. *Gynecol Oncol.* 2008;109(3):411–417.

138 Dai Q, Ling YH, Lia M, et al. Enhanced sensitivity to the HER1/epidermal growth factor receptor tyrosine kinase inhibitor erlotinib hydrochloride in chemotherapy-resistant tumor cell lines. *Clin Cancer Res.* 2005;11(4):1572–1578.

139 Benedetti V, Perego P, Luca Beretta G, et al. Modulation of survival pathways in ovarian carcinoma cell lines resistant to platinum compounds. *Mol Cancer Ther.* 2008;7(3):679–687.

140 Knight LA, Di Nicolantonio F, Whitehouse P, et al. The in vitro effect of gefitinib ('Iressa') alone and in combination with cytotoxic chemotherapy on human solid tumours. *BMC Cancer.* 2004;4:83.

141 Schilder RJ, Sill MW, Chen X, et al. Phase II study of gefitinib in patients with relapsed or persistent ovarian or primary peritoneal carcinoma and evaluation of epidermal growth factor receptor mutations and immunohistochemical expression: a Gynecologic Oncology Group Study. *Clin Cancer Res.* 2005;11(15):5539–5548.

142 Gordon AN, Finkler N, Edwards RP, et al. Efficacy and safety of erlotinib HCl, an epidermal growth factor receptor (HER1/EGFR) tyrosine kinase inhibitor, in patients with advanced ovarian carcinoma: results from a phase II multicenter study. *Int J Gynecol Cancer.* 2005;15(5):785–792.

143 Schilder RJ, Pathak HB, Lokshin AE, et al. Phase II trial of single agent cetuximab in patients with persistent or recurrent epithelial ovarian or primary peritoneal carcinoma with the potential for dose escalation to rash. *Gynecol Oncol.* 2009;113(1):21–27.

144 Paez JG, Janne PA, Lee JC, et al. EGFR mutations in lung cancer: correlation with clinical response to gefitinib therapy. *Science.* 2004;304(5676):1497–1500.

145 Kimball KJ, Numnum TM, Kirby TO, et al. A phase I study of lapatinib in combination with carboplatin in women with platinum sensitive recurrent ovarian carcinoma. *Gynecol Oncol.* 2008;111(1):95–101.

146 Pautier P, Joly F, Kerbrat P, et al. Phase II study of gefitinib in combination with paclitaxel (P) and carboplatin (C) as second-line therapy for ovarian, tubal or peritoneal adenocarcinoma (1839IL/0074). *Gynecol Oncol.* 2010;116(2):157–162.

147 Vasey PA, Gore M, Wilson R, et al. A phase Ib trial of docetaxel, carboplatin and erlotinib in ovarian, fallopian tube and primary peritoneal cancers. *Br J Cancer.* 2008;98(11):1774–1780.

148 Secord AA, Blessing JA, Armstrong DK, et al. Phase II trial of cetuximab and carboplatin in relapsed platinum-sensitive ovarian cancer and evaluation of epidermal growth factor receptor expression: a Gynecologic Oncology Group study. *Gynecol Oncol.* 2008;108(3):493–499.

149 Hirte H, Oza A, Swenerton K, et al. A phase II study of erlotinib (OSI-774) given in combination with carboplatin in patients with recurrent epithelial ovarian cancer (NCIC CTG IND.149). *Gynecol Oncol.* 2010;118(3):308–312.

150 Vergote IB, Jimeno A, Joly F, et al. Randomized Phase III Study of Erlotinib Versus Observation in Patients With No Evidence of Disease

Progression After First-Line Platin-Based Chemotherapy for Ovarian Carcinoma: a European Organisation for Research and Treatment of Cancer-Gynaecological Cancer Group, and Gynecologic Cancer Intergroup Study. *J Clin Oncol*. 2014;32(4):320–326.

151 Shepard HM, Lewis GD, Sarup JC, et al. Monoclonal antibody therapy of human cancer: taking the HER2 protooncogene to the clinic. *J Clin Immunol*. 1991;11(3):117–127.

152 Nagumo Y, Faratian D, Mullen P, Harrison DJ, Hasmann M, Langdon SP. Modulation of HER3 is a marker of dynamic cell signaling in ovarian cancer: implications for pertuzumab sensitivity. *Mol Cancer Res*. 2009;7(9):1563–1571.

153 Faratian D, Zweemer AJ, Nagumo Y, Sims AH, Muir M, Dodds M, et al. Trastuzumab and pertuzumab produce changes in morphology and estrogen receptor signaling in ovarian cancer xenografts revealing new treatment strategies. *Clin Cancer Res*. 2011;17(13):4451–4461.

154 Bookman MA, Darcy KM, Clarke-Pearson D, Boothby RA, Horowitz IR. Evaluation of monoclonal humanized anti-HER2 antibody, trastuzumab, in patients with recurrent or refractory ovarian or primary peritoneal carcinoma with overexpression of HER2: a phase II trial of the Gynecologic Oncology Group. *J Clin Oncol*. 2003;21(2):283–290.

155 Gordon MS, Matei D, Aghajanian C, et al. Clinical activity of pertuzumab (rhuMAb 2C4), a HER dimerization inhibitor, in advanced ovarian cancer: potential predictive relationship with tumor HER2 activation status. *J Clin Oncol*. 2006;24(26):4324–4332.

156 Makhija S, Amler LC, Glenn D, et al. Clinical activity of gemcitabine plus pertuzumab in platinum-resistant ovarian cancer, fallopian tube cancer, or primary peritoneal cancer. *J Clin Oncol*. 2010;28(7):1215–1223.

157 Kaye SB, Poole CJ, Danska-Bidzinska A, et al. A randomized phase II study evaluating the combination of carboplatin-based chemotherapy with pertuzumab versus carboplatin-based therapy alone in patients with relapsed, platinum-sensitive ovarian cancer. *Ann Oncol*. 2013;24(1):145–152.

158 Ye D, Mendelsohn J, Fan Z. Augmentation of a humanized anti-HER2 mAb 4D5 induced growth inhibition by a human-mouse chimeric anti-EGF receptor mAb C225. *Oncogene*. 1999;18(3):731–738.

159 Garcia AA, Sill MW, Lankes HA, et al. A phase II evaluation of lapatinib in the treatment of persistent or recurrent epithelial ovarian or primary peritoneal carcinoma: a gynecologic oncology group study. *Gynecol Oncol*. 2012;124(3):569–574.

160 Lheureux S, Krieger S, Weber B, et al. Expected benefits of topotecan combined with lapatinib in recurrent ovarian cancer according to biological profile: a phase 2 trial. *Int J Gynecol Cancer*. 2012;22(9):1483–1488.

161 Dungo RT, Keating GM. Afatinib: first global approval. *Drugs*. 2013;73(13):1503–1515.

162 Lopez-Tarruella S, Jerez Y, Marquez-Rodas I, Martin M. Neratinib (HKI-272) in the treatment of breast cancer. *Future Oncol*. 2012;8(6):671–681.

163 Jia Y, Zhang Y, Qiao C, et al. IGF-1R and ErbB3/HER3 contribute to enhanced proliferation and carcinogenesis in trastuzumab-resistant ovarian cancer model. *Biochem Biophys Res Commun*. 2013;436(4):740–745.

164 Schoeberl B, Faber AC, Li D, et al. An ErbB3 antibody, MM-121, is active in cancers with ligand-dependent activation. *Cancer Res*. 2010;70(6):2485–2494.

165 Qiu L, Wang Q, Di W, et al. Transient activation of EGFR/AKT cell survival pathway and expression of survivin contribute to reduced sensitivity of human melanoma cells to betulinic acid. *Int J Oncol*. 2005;27(3):823–830.

166 Glaysher S, Bolton LM, Johnson P, et al. Targeting EGFR and PI3K pathways in ovarian cancer. *Br J Cancer*. 2013;109(7):1786–1794.

167 Tibbetts AS, Appling DR. Compartmentalization of Mammalian folate-mediated one-carbon metabolism. *Ann Rev Nutr*. 2010;30:57–81.

168 Choi SW, Mason JB. Folate and carcinogenesis: an integrated scheme. *J Nutr*. 2000;130(2):129–132.

169 Stover PJ. Physiology of folate and vitamin B12 in health and disease. *Nutr Rev*. 2004;62(6 Pt 2):S3–S12; discussion S3.

170 Zhao R, Diop-Bove N, Visentin M, Goldman ID. Mechanisms of membrane transport of folates into cells and across epithelia. *Ann Rev Nutr*. 2011;31:177–201.

171 Bagnoli M, Canevari S, Figini M, et al. A step further in understanding the biology of the folate receptor in ovarian carcinoma. *Gynecol Oncol*. 2003;88(1 Pt 2):S140–S144.

172 Siu MK, Kong DS, Chan HY, et al. Paradoxical impact of two folate receptors, FRalpha and RFC, in ovarian cancer: effect on cell proliferation, invasion and clinical outcome. *PLoS One*. 2012;7(11):e47201.

173 Salazar MD, Ratnam M. The folate receptor: what does it promise in tissue-targeted therapeutics? *Cancer Metastasis Rev*. 2007;26(1):141–152.

174 Kelemen LE. The role of folate receptor alpha in cancer development, progression and treatment: cause, consequence or innocent bystander? *Int J Cancer*. 2006;119(2):243–250.

175 Cerezo A, Guadamillas MC, Goetz JG, et al. The absence of caveolin-1 increases proliferation and anchorage- independent growth by a Rac-dependent, Erk-independent mechanism. *Mol Cell Biol*. 2009;29(18):5046–5059.

176 Chen YL, Chang MC, Huang CY, et al. Serous ovarian carcinoma patients with high alpha-folate receptor had reducing survival and cytotoxic chemo-response. *Mol Oncol*. 2012;6(3):360–369.

177 Ebel W, Routhier EL, Foley B, et al. Preclinical evaluation of MORAb-003, a humanized monoclonal antibody antagonizing folate receptor-alpha. *Cancer Immun*. 2007;7:6.

178 Lin J, Spidel JL, Maddage CJ, et al. The antitumor activity of the human FOLR1-specific monoclonal antibody, farletuzumab, in an ovarian cancer mouse model is mediated by antibody-dependent cellular cytotoxicity. *Cancer Biol Ther*. 2013;14(11):1032–1038.

179 Armstrong DK, White AJ, Weil SC, Phillips M, Coleman RL. Farletuzumab (a monoclonal antibody against folate receptor alpha) in relapsed platinum-sensitive ovarian cancer. *Gynecol Oncol*. 2013;129(3):452–458.

180 Vergote I, Armstrong D, Scambia G, et al. Phase 3 double-blind, placebo-controlled study of weekly farletuzumab with carboplatin/taxane in subjects with platinum-sensitive ovarian cancer in first relapse. *Int J Gynecol Cancer*. 2013;2013(23 (8)):supplement 1.

181 Leamon CP, Parker MA, Vlahov IR, et al. Synthesis and biological evaluation of EC20: a new folate-derived, (99m)Tc-based radiopharmaceutical. *Bioconjug Chem*. 2002;13(6):1200–1210.

182 Vlahov IR, Santhapuram HK, Kleindl PJ, Howard SJ, Stanford KM, Leamon CP. Design and regioselective synthesis of a new generation of targeted chemotherapeutics. Part 1: EC145, a folic acid conjugate of desacetylvinblastine monohydrazide. *Bioorg Med Chem Lett*. 2006;16(19):5093–5096.

183 Reddy JA, Dorton R, Westrick E, et al. Preclinical evaluation of EC145, a folate-vinca alkaloid conjugate. *Cancer Res*. 2007;67(9):4434–4442.

184 Morris RT, Joyrich RN, Naumann RW, et al. Phase 2 study of treatment of advanced ovarian cancer with folate-receptor-targeted therapeutic (vintafolide) and companion SPECT-based imaging agent (99mTc-etarfolatide). *Ann Oncol*. 2014; Accepted for publication.

185 Naumann RW, Coleman RL, Burger RA, et al. PRECEDENT: a randomized phase II trial comparing vintafolide (EC145) and pegylated liposomal doxorubicin (PLD) in combination versus PLD alone in patients with platinum-resistant ovarian cancer. *J Clin Oncol*. 2013;31(35):4400–4406.

186 Reddy JA, Dorton R, Dawson A, et al. Rational combination therapy of vintafolide (EC145) with commonly used chemotherapeutic drugs. *Clin Cancer Res*. 2014;20(8):2104–2114.

187 Tran T, Shatnawi A, Zheng X, Kelley KM, Ratnam M. Enhancement of folate receptor alpha expression in tumor cells through the glucocorticoid receptor: a promising means to improved tumor detection and targeting. *Cancer Res*. 2005;65(10):4431–4441.

188 Kelley KM, Rowan BG, Ratnam M. Modulation of the folate receptor alpha gene by the estrogen receptor: mechanism and implications in tumor targeting. *Cancer Res*. 2003;63(11):2820–2828.

189 Summy JM, Gallick GE. Treatment for advanced tumors: SRC reclaims center stage. *Clin Cancer Res*. 2006;12(5):1398–1401.

190 Wiener JR, Windham TC, Estrella VC, et al. Activated SRC protein tyrosine kinase is overexpressed in late-stage human ovarian cancers. *Gynecol Oncol*. 2003;88(1):73–79.

191 Winter WE 3rd, Maxwell GL, Tian C, et al. Prognostic factors for stage III epithelial ovarian cancer: a Gynecologic Oncology Group study. *J Clin Oncol*. 2007;25(24):3621–3627.

192 Shimada M, Kigawa J, Ohishi Y, et al. Clinicopathological characteristics of mucinous adenocarcinoma of the ovary. *Gynecol Oncol*. 2009;113(3):331–334.

193 Pectasides D, Fountzilas G, Aravantinos G, et al. Advanced stage mucinous epithelial ovarian cancer: the Hellenic Cooperative Oncology Group experience. *Gynecol Oncol*. 2005;97(2):436–441.

194 Matsuo K, Nishimura M, Bottsford-Miller JN, et al. Targeting SRC in mucinous ovarian carcinoma. *Clin Cancer Res*. 2011;17(16):5367–5378.

195 Liu T, Hu W, Dalton HJ, et al. Targeting SRC and tubulin in mucinous ovarian carcinoma. *Clin Cancer Res*. 2013;19(23):6532–6543.

196 Schilder RJ, Brady WE, Lankes HA, et al. Phase II evaluation of dasatinib in the treatment of recurrent or persistent epithelial ovarian or primary peritoneal carcinoma: a Gynecologic Oncology Group study. *Gynecol Oncol*. 2012;127(1):70–74.

197 Secord AA, Teoh DK, Barry WT, et al. A phase I trial of dasatinib, an SRC-family kinase inhibitor, in combination with paclitaxel and carboplatin in patients with advanced or recurrent ovarian cancer. *Clin Cancer Res*. 2012;18(19):5489–5498.

198 Poole C, Lisyanskaya A, Rodenhuis S, et al. A randomized phase II clinical trial of the Src inhibitor saracatinib (AZD0530) and carboplatin + paclitaxel (C+P) versus C + P in patients (pts) with advanced platinum-sensitive epithelial ovarian cancer. *Eur Soc Med Oncol*. 2010;21(suppl. 8): Abstract 3715.

199 Matulonis UA, Hirsch M, Palescandolo E, et al. High throughput interrogation of somatic mutations in high grade serous cancer of the ovary. *PLoS One*. 2011;6(9):e24433.

200 Salani R, Kurman RJ, Giuntoli R 2nd, et al. Assessment of TP53 mutation using purified tissue samples of ovarian serous carcinomas reveals a higher mutation rate than previously reported and does not correlate with drug resistance. *Int J Gynecol Cancer*. 2008;18(3):487–491.

201 Schuijer M, Berns EM. TP53 and ovarian cancer. *Hum Mutat*. 2003;21(3):285–291.

202 Leijen S, Beijnen JH, Schellens JH. Abrogation of the G2 checkpoint by inhibition of Wee-1 kinase results in sensitization of p53-deficient tumor cells to DNA-damaging agents. *Curr Clin Pharmacol*. 2010;5(3):186–191.

203 London CA, Bernabe LF, Barnard S, et al. Preclinical evaluation of the novel, orally bioavailable selective inhibitor of nuclear export (SINE) KPT-335 in spontaneous canine cancer: results of a phase I study. *PLoS One*. 2014;9(2):e87585.

## CHAPTER 26

# Molecular Therapeutics: Pancreatic Cancer

*David Fogelman[1], Milind Javle[1], and James Abbruzzese[2]*

[1]Department of Gastrointestinal Medical Oncology, The University of Texas MD Anderson Cancer Center, Houston, TX, USA
[2]Division of Medical Oncology, Duke Cancer Institute, Durham, NC, USA

## Introduction

Pancreatic cancer carries a particularly poor prognosis. Approximately 46,400 new patients were expected to be diagnosed in the year 2012, and of these, 39,600 deaths were anticipated.[1] Most patients present with metastatic disease; chemotherapy prolongs life but does not result in a cure. There have been some recent advances in chemotherapy, notably with the development of the FOLFIRINOX (5-FU, oxaliplatin, irinotecan) regimen, that have improved survival.[2] However, future advances will improve our understanding of the molecular pathways that underlie the growth of cancer, will exploit the mechanisms of DNA repair, and will improve immunotherapy, cancer vaccines, and efforts to address chemotherapy resistance.

Over the past decade, our knowledge of pathways driving pancreatic cancer growth has increased markedly. One recent study has evaluated a group of 24 pancreatic cancers. DNA from these patients' pancreatic cancer was sequenced, after PCR amplification; over 20,000 genes were assessed and over 1300 mutations were identified. From these, a number of core gene pathways common to these tumors were identified, and included KRAS, TGF-ß, Wnt/Notch and Hedgehog, and genes related to integrins, cell adhesion, cell cycling, and GTP-ase-dependent proteins. Hopefully, some of these pathways may lead to therapeutic intervention.[3]

The KRAS pathway is one such example. Early work has demonstrated that activating KRAS mutations are found in the majority of pancreatic intraductal precursor lesions[4] and pancreatic adenocarcinoma specimens,[5] and that these mutations are an early step in carcinogenesis. More recent work has determined that KRAS activates its downstream effectors RAF, MEK, and ERK,[6] and activates the Hedgehog pathway[7,8] through downstream transcription factors.

Multiple other growth pathways contribute to pancreatic cancer formation and propagation. The PI3 kinase/AKT/mTOR pathway may be constitutively active through loss of PTEN, resulting in NF-κB expression and stabilization of c-MYC.[9] The TGF-ß family can act through SMAD dependent and independent pathways to control MYC expression, affect epithelial to mesenchymal transition, and modify the immune response to pancreatic cancer.[10] Likewise, activation of Notch pathway receptors has been shown to regulate cell cycle effectors such as p21, cyclin D1, c-Myc, and NF-κB2.[11]

In addition to signal transduction pathways, DNA repair pathways may be therapeutic targets for pancreatic cancer. Monoallelic mutations in the BRCA2 gene have been found in 27% of patients with pancreatic cancer and cell lines, while biallelic changes in 10%.[12] Mutations in other genes such as PALB2 may also indicate cancers amenable to treatment directed toward DNA repair. For these patients, the emerging class of PARP inhibitors may offer a novel treatment.

In this chapter, we will review agents currently under development targeting each of these pathways. We will focus on "druggable" targets, and will provide a sense of the current state of pathway based pharmaceutical development.

## Therapeutics Currently in Development

### KRAS and Its Effector Pathways

KRAS is one of the most frequently mutated genes in pancreatic cancer. Overall, 70–90% of patients with pancreatic cancer have mutations in the KRAS pathway, most of which are in KRAS itself.[3,13] Mouse models containing an activated KRAS pathway develop premalignant lesions, and when activated in the presence of other pathway mutations (e.g., p53) develop malignancy.[14] Initial efforts to target this pathway have focused on KRAS itself. Attempts to target KRAS directly have included farnesyltransferase inhibitors. Under normal circumstances, the c-terminal of the RAS protein—important for the function of the protein—undergoes post translational modification catalyzed by farnesyltransferase. This protein adds a 15 carbon farnesyl lipid to the c-terminal of a number of proteins, including KRAS. Disappointingly, inhibitors of these proteins were tested by the Southwest Oncology Group (SWOG), and demonstrated a 6-month survival of 19% and a median survival of 2.6 months.[15] It also proved ineffective when combined with gemcitabine,[16] leading investigators to seek other targets in the KRAS pathway.

An alternative strategy is to target the proteins downstream of RAS. With increased understanding of these pathways, we have identified new potential targets, though we have also identified crosstalk between pathways, suggesting that simultaneous inhibition of multiple targets may be required. One such pathway is the RAS→RAF→MEK→ERK pathway. KRAS ordinarily activates

BRAF, which in turn activates MEK, followed by activation of ERK. Mutational activation of BRAF elicits premalignant lesions (PanIN) in a mouse pancreas.[6] Accordingly, RAF and MEK are potential therapeutic targets. KRAS also activates the PIK3CA protein, eliciting subsequent growth of cells, making this phosphatidylinositol-3 kinase (PI3K) and its downstream effector, AKT, which are therefore potential therapeutic targets. In addition, KRAS may activate a chain of proteins including AP-1, IKK2/ß, and NF-κB, which may promote pro-inflammatory and anti-apoptotic responses.[17]

In one mouse model, pharmacologic inhibition of MEK with PD325901 reduces activation of ERK, though individual cell lines exhibit different sensitivities to treatment with this drug as a single agent.[6] In this mouse model, this MEK inhibitor resulted in prolonged survival of the animals. In humans, one study of a MEK inhibitor as a single agent failed to produce a response in a variety of tumor types, suggesting that a multidrug regimen will be required.[18] Such studies are now underway; two examples are gemcitabine in combination with GSK112012 and with BAY86-9766 in patients with pancreatic cancer. MEK inhibitors in development are listed in Table 26.1.

Though MEK inhibitor GSK112012 by itself reduces downstream ERK activation, it may result in increased activation of AKT. One study found that xenografts developing resistance to the drug led to increases in AKT, p38, GSK-3b, FGFR1, and VEGFR1/3,[19] suggesting that combining therapies to inhibit both MEK and AKT may be effective. *In vivo*, such a combination results in synergistic cell death,[6] though AKT inhibition alone seems to be of little potency. This has inspired multidrug combinations, now in testing (Table 26.1).

BRAF is also a possible therapeutic target. Although in pancreatic cancer, BRAF is infrequently mutated, mutational activation of BRAF results in a phenotype similar to that of a KRAS mutation. Targeting BRAF has been challenging. One BRAF inhibitor, GDC-0879, augmented *in vitro* RAF → MEK → ERK expression. Likewise, inhibition of BRAF in KRAS mutant cell lines with GSK2118436A increased phosphorylation of CRAF, MEK, ERK, and p90RSK. Combining BRAF inhibition with MEK inhibition using GSK1120212B resulted in synergistic effects in MIAPACA pancreatic and other (non-pancreatic) cell lines, though the combination was antagonistic in other cell lines. It is not surprising then that little work has been done with single agent BRAF inhibition of pancreatic cancer, though combination therapy may be considered for future testing.

## IGF and PI3K/AKT/pTEN Pathways

The insulin-like growth factor receptor, IGF-IR, is a tyrosine kinase represents a critical component of another pathway frequently activated in pancreatic cancer. IGF-1, IGF-2, and insulin are each capable of binding this receptor, while an antagonist, IGFBP-1, is capable of suppressing its activation.[20] Binding of ligand to this protein results in autophosphorylation of tyrosine, initiating a downstream cascade of both the PI3K and the mitogen-activated protein kinase (MAPK) pathways.

The IGF-I receptor is upregulated in human pancreatic cancer. Its ligand, IGF-I, is a polypeptide that exhibits structural homology to proinsulin. It is also activated with lower affinity by insulin and IGF-II. Application of IGF-1 enhances the growth of pancreatic cancer cell lines in culture, and antibodies to IGF-1R, as well as antisense oligonucleotides, inhibit the growth of these cells.[21] Elevated levels of IGF have been noted in a variety of tumors, including pancreatic cancer, and expression of IGF-IR is required for malignant transformation.[22] Bergmann et al. demonstrated an increase in IGF-I in six of eight cancers. Six of these eight demonstrated an increase in IGF-IR as well. Other authors have also noted that IGF is higher in serum and tissue of pancreatic cancer patients than controls.[23] Elevated levels of IGF-1 receptor promote invasion and metastases in mice models.[24] IGF-I may therefore play autocrine as well as paracrine roles in the stimulation of growth of pancreatic cancer cells.

*In vitro* blockade of IGF-IR by dominant negative blockade results in suppressed tumorigenicity and increased basal apoptosis in cancer cells. It reduced downstream activation of the pathway.[25] The major approach toward targeting this pathway has been the use of monoclonal antibodies directed against IGF-IR. A phase I/II study of one such antibody, MK-0646, has so far demonstrated an increase in median progression-free survival (PFS) from 8 to 17 weeks with the addition of this agent to gemcitabine.[26] Toxicities have so far been mild. A second study, evaluating

**Table 26.1** Drugs currently in development for pancreatic cancer

| Target | Generic Name | Trade Name |
| --- | --- | --- |
| MEK | MEK162/ARRY-438162 | |
| MEK | GDC-0973 | |
| MEK | AZD6244 (ARRY-142886) | |
| MEK | BAY86-9766 | |
| MEK | GSK1120212 | |
| MEK | CI-1040 | |
| MEK | MSC1936369B | Pimasertib |
| MEK | XL518 | |
| | | |
| PI3K | GDC-0941 | |
| PI3K | SAR245409 | |
| PI3K | BEZ235 | |
| PI3K | XL147 | |
| | | |
| AKT | GSK2141795 | |
| AKT | MK2206 | |
| | | |
| RAF | R05126766 | |
| | | |
| ALK1 (TGF-β) | PF-03446962 | |
| | | |
| PARP | ABT-888 | Veliparib |
| PARP | | Olaparib |
| PARP | CEP-9722 | |
| | | |
| Hedgehog | IPI-926 | Saridegib |
| Hedgehog | XL139 | |
| | | |
| IGF (mAB) | AMG479 | |
| IGF (mAB) | MK0646 | Dalotuzumab |
| IGF (mAB) | R1507 | |
| IGF (mAB) | IMC-A12 | Cixutumumab |
| IGF (mAB) | CP-751,871 | Figitumumab |
| | | |
| IGF (TKI) | OSI-906 | |
| IGF (TKI) | XL228 | |
| IGF (TKI) | BMS-754807 | |
| | | |
| MET | XL184 | |
| MET | XL880 | |

gemcitabine and erlotinib with or without cixutumumab (a monoclonal antibody targeting IGF-1 receptor) demonstrated no improvement in PFS or overall survival.[27] In both of these studies, patients were treated without selection based on IGF-R expression or tumor molecular analysis. Future studies may benefit from more refined patient selection, since correlative data suggest that IGF-1R tissue levels may predict response to anti-IGFR antibody therapy.[28] Additional correlative data suggest that IGFBP5 expression, as well as the ratio of IGFBP5/IGFBP4, may predict the efficacy of anti-IGF therapy.[29] Additional anti-IGF-1R monoclonal antibodies are now being tested (Table 26.1). Another potential inhibitor of the IGFR pathway is a molecule called Klotho, a transmembrane protein that may suppress IGFR activity in malignant cells. Animal models have shown a favorable safety profile; human studies have yet to begin.[30]

Activated IGF-RI initiates a cascade of proteins that ultimately result in cell growth and proliferation. It activates KRAS as well as PI3K. It is noteworthy that KRAS itself is also capable of activating PI3K.[9] PI3K, in turn, phosphorylates the 3′ position of the inositol ring of lipids in the plasma membrane, resulting in the generation of two forms of phosphatidylinositol (PIP2 and PIP3). These interact with the pleckstrin homology (PH) domain of intracellular proteins, bringing them to the surface. AKT has such a domain.[31] When recruited to the cell membrane, AKT is phosphorylated at serine and threonine residues, activating this protein. AKT then phosphorylates a wide variety of substrates, notably mTOR. Under normal circumstances, PTEN suppresses PI3K activity. PTEN dephosphorylates PIP2 and PIP3. However, in pancreatic cancer cells, PTEN expression is often lost or reduced (possibly by promoter methylation), resulting in activation of this pathway. As noted above, PI3K may be activated by IGF-R1 activation, which is prevalent in pancreatic cancer. In addition, PI3K is overexpressed in pancreatic cancer,[32] and mediates activation of AKT and its downstream effectors.

Given its role in pancreatic cancer growth, targeting PI3K has been an important therapeutic approach. Agents targeting PI3K are now undergoing phase I testing (Table 26.1). One such agent is NVP-BEZ235, a dual PI3K and mTOR inhibitor, which has been tested in combination with gemcitabine in pancreatic cancer cell lines.[33] This agent reduced phospho-AKT and phospho-mTOR expression in the lines tested, suggesting a potential for decreasing tumor cell growth. Combining this agent with gemcitabine resulted in a synergistic effect on cell viability.[34]

PI3K inhibitors combined with RAS pathway inhibitors are being investigated in clinical trials. In a clinical trial of GDC-0973 (MEK inhibitor), with GDC-0491 (PI3K inhibitor),[35,36] patients with various tumor types were treated. Twenty-six of 46 evaluable patients had decreased tumor activity as noted on PET scans. While the response rate was low (7%), patients were treated with a variety of doses and the study remains in progress. Similar studies are proceeding with other combinations as well (MSC1936369B/SAR245409). However, it is unclear whether the combination of these agents will be sufficient to enhance current chemotherapy regimens. One mouse model demonstrated efficacy roughly equivalent to that of the gemcitabine/erlotinib combination.

## DNA Repair

An intriguing target in pancreatic cancer is DNA repair. The BRCA2 gene has been associated with an increased risk of pancreatic cancer. Families with BRCA2 genes have a 3.5–fold increase in relative risk of pancreatic cancer as compared to families without the mutation.[37] The risk may be higher in Ashkenazi Jewish patients, of whom 5.5% may have such mutations,[38] compared to only 1% of the general population.

BRCA1 and BRCA2 are involved in the repair of double-strand DNA breaks. Patients carrying a heterozygous deficiency of either of these proteins are prone to further loss of the second allele during the development of a malignancy. Loss of expression of either of these two proteins results in impaired homologous recombination. In this instance, DNA repair must be conducted either by single-strand annealing or non-homologous end joining. Both of these techniques are error prone. BRCA2 apparently operates in conjunction with RAD51, while BRCA1 operates independently of this complex.[39]

Poly(ADP-ribose) polymerase (PARP) is a protein involved in single-strand break repair. PARP inhibition is functionally silent in cells capable of homologous recombination, though such cells may be sensitive to alkylating agents. In the absence of homologous recombination (e.g., BRCA-deficient cells), however, inhibition of PARP significantly damages the ability of cells to repair DNA—even with the more error prone SSA or NHEJ mechanisms.

The concept of synthetic lethality is that two non-lethal mutations have no effect when they occur individually, but lead to death of the cancer cell when found in the combination. This may be the case for PARP inhibition and BRCA deficiency. Inhibition of PARP, in the setting of BRCA deficiency, results in the accumulation of unrepaired single-strand breaks. These events result in stalling and collapse of replication forks, which later become double-strand breaks. These accumulate in BRCA-deficient cells, and result in increasing levels of genetic instability and ultimately cell death.[40]

PARP inhibitors are therefore of great interest in patients with innate deficiencies of homologous repair, such as carriers of BRCA1, BRCA2, and PALB mutations. In addition, mutations in NRS1 and ATM, loss of function of PTEN, and overexpression of Aurora Kinase A mutations might predispose cells to death upon inhibition of PARP. A phase I trial of AZD2281, a PARP inhibitor, demonstrated responses in 12 of 19 (63%) patients with BRCA-associated ovarian, breast, or prostate cancers. Two other patients with BRCA mutation in their tumors responded to this treatment. Tumors without BRCA mutation did not respond to this agent.[41] Therefore, it has become of great interest to identify those patients with pancreatic cancer who may have BRCA mutant cancers.

Limited numbers of BRCA-associated pancreatic adenocarcinoma patients have been treated with PARP inhibitors. One retrospective report identified three such patients who received combination chemotherapy with PARP inhibitors; two of these patients responded while the third demonstrated disease stability.[42] In a case report, response to a PARP inhibitor lasted only 8 weeks.[43] It is imperative, therefore, to test for BRCA mutations in pancreatic cancer patients with an appropriate personal or family history. In addition, screening tests for deficiencies of homologous repair may identify additional candidates for PARP inhibitor treatment. Indeed, one such study incorporating gemcitabine, cisplatin, and veliparib is now underway. In this study, patients are treated with standard doses of gemcitabine, accompanied by veliparib administered orally twice daily in increasing dose cohorts. An early report notes that six of nine BRCA patients treated with this regimen demonstrated a response, while the other three had stable disease.[44] In addition, a study of another PARP inhibitor, rucaparib, is currently underway. In this phase II study, patients with BRCA mutations receive a fixed dose of the study drug.

Of note, in addition to BRCA, the Partner and Localizer of BRCA2 (PALB2, also known as FANCN) gene has also been identified as a protein involved in DNA repair that might be sensitive to PARP inhibition. PALB2 binds to BRCA1 and BRCA2 during DNA repair, forming a complex which then binds RAD51, and initiating DNA repair through homologous recombination.[45] While rare in the general population with a prevalence of <1%, patients with familial pancreatic cancers may have a 3–4% chance of carrying such a mutation.[46,47] Such patients also tend to have a family history of breast cancer, further supporting their link with the BRCA pathway. When combined with the prevalence of BRCA mutations, homologous recombination deficits become an important target in pancreatic cancer.

One approach to screening for such mutations may be with the use of pancreatic cancer xenografts. In one study,[48] a patient whose tumor contained a PALB2 mutation was implanted into a mouse and found to be sensitive to mitomycin-C, was then successfully treated with this agent. Such studies allow for screening patients' tumors for sensitivity to such agents, as well as for subsequent DNA analysis. In this case, a sporadically acquired PALB2 mutation was found in addition to a germline frameshift mutation, which successfully predicted the efficacy of mitomycin. Currently, these xenografts remain largely experimental.

### Notch Pathway Inhibition

Under normal circumstances, the Notch pathway prevents cellular differentiation, maintaining a population of undifferentiated precursor cells. Binding of ligand to the Notch receptor leads to cleavage of its intramembranous portion. This cleaved segment of Notch then translocates to the cell nucleus, where it activates a complex of transcription activating proteins. Activation of the Notch pathway has been increasingly recognized in the pathogenesis of pancreatic cancer; specifically, this pathway contributes toward transition of the epithelium from a predominant acinar population to ductal histology. Experimental evidence includes the observation that induction of notch expression results in a shift from acinar to ductal morphology, loss of acinar-specific gene expression, and expression of ductal markers. These steps are critical in the progression toward ductal metaplasia, pancreatic intraepithelial metaplasia, and ultimately to invasive cancer. Similar changes were seen in prior studies upon exposure of pancreatic cells to TGF-α,[49] suggesting that TGF-α may trigger activation of this pathway. In fact, transgenic mice expressing TGF-α demonstrate upregulated expression of Notch pathway ligands, receptors, and target genes as compared to normal mice. HES1, a downstream protein in this pathway, was particularly observed to be present in metaplastic cells and absent in normal in adjacent healthy acinar tissue.

The Notch pathway may be overexpressed in pancreatic cancer. Notch activation precedes the onset of pancreatic intraepithelial neoplasia and represses acinar cell differentiation while mediating the acinar-to-ductal metaplasia.[50] One study comparing pancreatic tumor with healthy tissue found nine Notch-related proteins to be overexpressed in the tumor tissue;[51] These include Notch2, Notch3, Notch4, dkl1, and jag1; conversely, the Notch pathway inhibitor, sel-1L, was downregulated in human cancers. These changes may explain the increase in Notch target gene expression, including Hes1, Hes4, Hey1, and HeyL. Hes1, for example, was expressed in 6 of 10 cancers. Likewise, elevated levels of these proteins were seen in 21 (62%) of 34 specimens using immunohistochemical staining. A separate study of 20 pancreatic cancer cell lines[52] found that while only 40% of pancreatic cancer lines had enhanced expression of

Notch1, and 90% demonstrated overexpression of JAGGED2. The majority of these had >50-fold elevation of this protein, suggesting activation of this pathway. DLL4 was elevated in half the specimens. Likewise, the target genes of the pathway, HES1 and HEY2, were activated in 80% and 65% of the tumors, respectively.

Gamma secretase is an intra-membrane protease required for activation of the Notch pathway. Its normal function is to cleave Notch receptors following ligand binding, in turn activating them, which leads to activation of the downstream pathway. Inhibitors of γ-secretase can prevent TGF-α-induced acinar to ductal metaplasia, while the use of a constitutively activated Notch 1 protein circumvents the effect of γ-secretase.[51] In the previously noted cell line study, treatment with siRNA against Notch1 was able to suppress colony formation in two cell lines tested, while the use of a pharmacologic γ-secretase inhibitor, GSI-18, caused a modest reduction in growth but a more significant reduction in colony formation. The use of a truncated, constitutively activated Notch circumvented this pharmacologic suppression.

A preclinical study of the gamma secretase inhibitor MRK-003[53] evaluated its efficacy against passaged tumor lines. Three of five lines were sensitive; these had reduction in growth, anchorage, engraftment, and stem cell count. Two lines were resistant and did not have these outcomes. Nine additional patient explants were evaluated for growth inhibition based on elevated Notch-1 levels. The combination of MRK-003 and gemcitabine showed enhanced antitumor effects compared to gemcitabine alone in four of nine (44%) pancreatic ductal adenocarcinoma xenografts. Clinical studies of gamma secretase inhibitors are now underway.

### Hedgehog Pathway and JAK/STAT

The Hedgehog pathway also plays a role in human pancreatic adenocarcinoma development. In a normal cell, the Patched (PTCH) protein resides on the cell surface and binds to the Smoothened receptor (SMO), inhibiting the function of the latter. Meanwhile, a downstream protein, Suppressor of Fused (SUFU) binds two proteins, GLI2 and GLI3, subjecting them to proteasomal cleavage from their activated to repressor forms. The Hedgehog ligand (Sonic Hedgehog (SHH)) may then bind to PTCH, which releases the SMO. Once activated, SMO then inhibits the conversion of GLI2 and GLI3 from their active to repressor forms, which enter the nucleus of the cell and facilitate signal transduction.[54]

There is now ample evidence that the Hedgehog pathway plays a role in pancreatic cancer. A thorough evaluation of mutations among 24 pancreatic demonstrated mutations in at least one of the Hedgehog genes in each of the specimens.[55] Xenograft models suggest that activation of the Hedgehog pathway may contribute to pancreatic cancer stem cell development, while inhibition of the pathway reduces the number of cells with the stem cell phenotype.[56] Finally, mouse models have demonstrated an increase in intratumoral vascular density and intratumoral concentration of gemcitabine when given in combination with the Hedgehog inhibitor IPI-926.[57]

IPI-926 is a small molecule that targets the Hedgehog pathway by inhibiting SMO. A phase I trial has demonstrated safety of this compound as a single agent, with an expansion cohort in patients with basal cell carcinomas (BCC). A response rate of 27% was observed in patients with previously untreated BCC.[58] In a phase IB clinical trial, IPI-926 was combined with gemcitabine.[59] Sixteen patients were treated and the median PFS was 7 months. Unfortunately, however, Infinity Pharmaceuticals halted the study of gemcitabine with IPI-926 after an interim analysis of a randomized phase II study demonstrated a survival advantage in the placebo arm. However, it is unclear whether there was *a priori* difference between the study arms. It is possible that the drug was ineffective simply because it is not reaching the target, or because the drug is ineffective in the clinical setting.

A related strategy, now in clinical trials, is to degrade the extracellular matrix that surrounds pancreatic tumors. Hyaluronic acid is found abundantly in the stroma of these cells, though its precise role has remained elusive.[60] Recently, Provenzano et al.[61] have demonstrated that enzymatic targeting of hyaluronic acid using an enzyme (PEGPH20) decreases interstitial fluid pressure, increasing vessel patency and allowing a fluorescent marker to pass. In doing so, treatment with gemcitabine plus PEGPH20 resulted in noticeably smaller tumors than those treated with gemcitabine alone even after a single cycle of therapy. In addition, mice treated with the combination lived longer than mice treated with gemcitabine alone. This has generated considerable enthusiasm, and clinical trials in humans testing this strategy are now in progress. A phase IB study of PEGPH20 with gemcitabine has demonstrated a response rate of 31% (7 of 21) in an early report.[62] Additional studies of this agent combined with gemcitabine and nab-paclitaxel or FOLFIRINOX are ongoing.

The Hedgehog pathway remains important for its downstream activation of the STAT3 pathway. Activated KRAS acts through the SHH ligand and the transcription factor GLI1 to cause malignant *transformation in vitro*.[7] Overexpression of KRAS results in SHH expression. In turn, GLI1 is expressed in both pancreatic cancer and stromal cells, and appears to have a role in oncogenesis as loss of this protein impairs the progression of PanIN into pancreatic cancer.[63] Expression of GLI1 results in an increase in IL-6 mRNA levels in pancreas stromal fibroblasts, with a measurable and robust increase in IL-6 secretion. This is consistent with the identification of GLI1 binding sites in the IL-6 promoter region. In turn, IL-6 is capable of inducing phosphorylation of STAT3; the addition of IL-6 to pancreatic cancer cell lines may stimulate p-STAT3 expression.[64]

JAK/STAT activation in pancreatic cancer begins with cytokine (e.g., IL-6) binding of JAK2 molecules.[65] Once activated, JAK2 phosphorylates a number of effectors including PI3K, RAS, STAT3, and STAT5. STAT3 translocates to the nucleus and binds DNA sequences for genes involved in proliferation and apoptosis such as histone H3 (H3Y41). One known result of this is the increase in expression of oncogene *Imo2*, though other downstream effects are under investigation.

Scholz et al. have demonstrated that p-STAT3 is overexpressed in a variety of pancreatic adenocarcinoma cell lines, but was notably absent from a pancreatic neuroendocrine tumor cell line.[66] Inactivation of pSTAT3 via both dominant negative STAT3 constructs, as well as through inhibition of the upstream Janus kinase 2 (JAK2) results in growth arrest of these cells in G1/S phase, as well as reduced anchorage-independent and -dependent growth. Furthermore, in the setting of constitutive KRAS activation, caerulein-induced STAT3 expression is prolonged, suggesting that insults to cells with such mutations may elicit greater damage from the effects of pSTAT3.[67]

Knockout of STAT3 can reduce some of the changes associated with carcinogenesis. In particular, STAT3-deficient cells demonstrate fewer ductal structures and more acinar structures after exposure to caerulein than STAT3 proficient cells. STAT3-deficient cells demonstrate less fibrotic replacement, fewer KI-67+ cells, and smaller tumor volume in mouse xenograft models. Taken together, this damage may ultimately contribute to carcinogenesis. Consistent with these observations, JAK/STAT inhibitors such as AG490 can decrease markers of cell proliferation such as cyclin D1 and BCL-xL, and can decrease proliferation in cell lines that exhibit significant STAT3 activation.[68]

The observation that JAK inhibition by AG490 produces effects similar to dominant negative STAT3 inhibition *in vitro* provides a rationale for testing JAK/STAT inhibitors in clinical practice. Indeed, one such study[69] of ruxolitinib (Incyte) has demonstrated that, when added to capecitabine in the second-line treatment of metastatic pancreatic cancer, those patients demonstrating systemic inflammation (as noted by an elevated c-reactive protein $\geq 13$) had longer survival compared to others (hazard ratio 0.47 for OS, $p = 0.01$). A larger phase III study has been launched to confirm these results.

## The FGFR Pathway

Fibroblast growth factor receptors (FGFRs) may activate the RAS/MAPK and PI3K/AKT/mTOR pathways. There are multiple, fairly well-conserved FGF ligands that may bind to any of four different receptors (FGFR1–4) that result in complexes containing two receptors and two ligands.[70] These four receptors may themselves take multiple isoforms through alternative splicing.[71] Upon binding their ligands, they activate an adaptor protein, FRS2.[72] Phosphorylated FRS2 in turn activates RAS and PI3K, each of which triggers activation of the downstream pathways. Overexpression of the FGF ligands, notably FGF1, 2, 7, and 10, are commonly noted in pancreatic cancer.[73] In particular, FGF2 and FGF7 expression has been linked to pancreatic cancer via increased cancer cell proliferation, motility, invasion, and stromal hyperplasia.[74,75] Elevated FGFR2 expression, amplification, and phosphorylation have been reported in pancreatic cancer and are associated with an aggressive tumor phenotype.[76–78]

Pancreatic cancer is characterized by desmoplasia that is mediated by activated pancreatic stellate cells (PSCs).[79] FGFR1 and FGFR2 localize to the nucleus in activated PSCs, and promote pancreatic cancer cell invasion into the underlying extra-cellular matrix.[80] Inhibition of these proteins using interfering RNA results in reduced PSC proliferation and also reduced cancer cell invasion. These findings suggest that inhibition of nuclear FGF/FGFR-mediated proliferation and invasion in PSCs may prevent pancreatic cancer cell invasion.

Both pharmacologic and siRNA inhibition of the FGFR pathway results in a significant anti-tumor effect.[81] The effect is pronounced in FGFR2 IIIb overexpressing pancreatic cancer that may be dependent on aberrant stimulation by stromal derived FGF ligands. Therefore, anti-FGF treatment may actually result in antiproliferative but also an "anti-desmoplastic" effect, confirming the validity of FGF/FGFR axis as a potential therapeutic target in pancreatic cancer.

In addition to their role in stimulating growth, FGF may have an effect on angiogenesis.[82] Evidence for this role first came from demonstration of the importance of FGF in wound healing.[83,84] This may be a paracrine effect through the release of FGF by tumor and stromal cells or from the extracellular matrix.[85] Injection of antisense FGF-2 or FGFR-1 cDNA into human melanoma reduced tumor growth, and blocked intratumoral angiogenesis.[86] An earlier clinical trial of bevacizumab, an anti-VEGF agent, demonstrated no significant improvement in survival, PFS, or response rate compared to placebo in patients with pancreatic cancer.[87] It is possible that targeting both VEGF and FGF may offer a superior therapeutic effect than targeting VEGF alone. Indeed, simultaneous expression of FGF-2 and VEGF may be synergistic; such tumors are fast growing with high blood vessel density and permeability.[88] Early work with one such inhibitor, lenvatinib, which targets VEGFR1-3, FGFR1-4, and PDGFRa, demonstrated that 7 of 19 xenografts tested had a reduction in tumor size upon exposure to this agent.[89] Those mice that did respond had a reduction in vessel density in these tumors. Currently, a number of FGF targeting agents are in development, including dovitinib, brivanib, BGJ398, and others. Brivanib in particular has been reported to reduce tumor growth and extend the overall survival in pancreatic neuroendocrine tumors.[90] However, no large clinical trials employing an anti-FGF strategy have been reported to date.

## CDK4/6 Inhibitors

A frequent aberration found in pancreatic cancer is the loss of CDKN2A gene.[91,92] Yachida and others have noted that this mutation may occur soon after the KRAS mutates, and (with KRAS) is sufficient to induce pancreatic intraepithelial neoplasia. CDKN2A encodes the p16 (ink4a) gene, an inhibitor of the cyclin-dependent kinase (CDK) 4 and CDK6 proteins.[93] These in turn regulate the retinoblastoma (RB) tumor suppressor gene. Franco et al.[94] have demonstrated that the use of such an inhibitor suppresses RB and reduces proliferation in sensitive cell lines. Resistance to this pathway appears to be mediated by upregulation of cyclin E1. While there are not yet specific trials of these agents for pancreatic cancer, LEE011 (Novartis) is being tested in a study that does include pancreatic cancer in patients with known aberrations in P16.

## Conclusions

Pancreatic cancer may be unique among malignancies in that much is known about the biology of the illness, and yet the disease has—so far—remained intractable to the slings and arrows of targeted therapy so far directed toward it. However, we are on the verge of clinical progress. The recent development of the FOLFIRINOX and gemcitabine/nab-paclitaxel regimens provides a more effective backbone on which to build trials than we have previously had available. The increasing use of molecular diagnostics is giving us greater insight into the biology of these tumors. There is a growing body of literature to suggest a more rational targeting of these tumors. The most encouraging direction is the increasing use of correlative science that, allows further understanding of which patients may benefit from a given treatment. The hope then is that with progressive iterations of trials, we will continue to learn, refine our future study design, and ultimately improve the outcome of patients with this disease.

## References

1 Siegel R, Ma J, Zou Z, Jemal A. Cancer statistics, 2014. *CA Cancer J Clin.* 2014;64(1):9–29.

2 Conroy T, Desseigne F, Ychou M, et al.; Groupe Tumeurs Digestives of Unicancer; PRODIGE Intergroup. FOLFIRINOX versus gemcitabine for metastatic pancreatic cancer. *N Engl J Med.* 2011;364(19):1817–1825.

3 Jones S, Zhang X, Parsons DW, et al. Core signaling pathways in human pancreatic cancers revealed by global genomic analyses. *Science.* 2008;321(5897):1801–1806.

4 Moskaluk CA, Hruban RH, Kern SE. p16 and K-ras gene mutations in the intraductal precursors of human pancreatic adenocarcinoma. *Cancer Res.* 1997;57(11):2140–2143.

5 Almoguera C, Shibata D, Forrester K, Martin J, Arnheim N, Perucho M. Most human carcinomas of the exocrine pancreas contain mutant c-K-ras genes. *Cell.* 1988;53(4):549–554.

6 Collisson EA, Trejo CL, Silva JM, et al. A central role for RAF->MEK->ERK signaling in the genesis of pancreatic ductal adenocarcinoma. *Cancer Discov.* 2012;2(8):685–693.

7 Ji Z, Mei FC, Xie J, Cheng X. Oncogenic KRAS activates hedgehog signaling pathway in pancreatic cancer cells. *J Biol Chem.* 2007;282(19):14048–14055.

8 Rajurkar M, De Jesus-Monge WE, Driscoll DR, et al. The activity of Gli transcription factors is essential for Kras-induced pancreatic tumorigenesis. *Proc Natl Acad Sci U S A.* 2012;109(17):E1038–E1047.

9 Asano T, Yao Y, Zhu J, Li D, Abbruzzese JL, Reddy SA. The PI 3-kinase/Akt signaling pathway is activated due to aberrant Pten expression and targets transcription factors NF-kappaB and c-Myc in pancreatic cancer cells. *Oncogene.* 2004;23(53):8571–8580.

10 Vaccaro V, Melisi D, Bria E, et al. Emerging pathways and future targets for the molecular therapy of pancreatic cancer. *Expert Opin Ther Targets.* 2011;15(10):1183–1196.

11 Ristorcelli E, Lombardo D. Targeting Notch signaling in pancreatic cancer. *Expert Opin Ther Targets.* 2010;14(5):541–552.

12 Goggins M, Schutte M, Lu J, et al. Germline BRCA2 gene mutations in patients with apparently sporadic pancreatic carcinomas. *Cancer Res.* 1996;56(23):5360–5364.

13 Oliveira-Cunha M, Hadfield KD, Siriwardena AK, Newman W. EGFR and KRAS mutational analysis and their correlation to survival in pancreatic and periampullary cancer. *Pancreas.* 2012;41(3):428–434.

14 Hingorani SR, Wang L, Multani AS, et al. Trp53R172H and KrasG12D cooperate to promote chromosomal instability and widely metastatic pancreatic ductal adenocarcinoma in mice. *Cancer Cell.* 2005;7(5):469–483.

15 Macdonald JS, McCoy S, Whitehead RP, et al. A phase II study of farnesyl transferase inhibitor R115777 in pancreatic cancer: a Southwest oncology group (SWOG 9924) study. *Invest New Drugs.* 2005;23(5):485–487.

16 Van Cutsem E, van de Velde H, Karasek P, et al. Phase III trial of gemcitabine plus tipifarnib compared with gemcitabine plus placebo in advanced pancreatic cancer. *J Clin Oncol.* 2004;22(8):1430–1438.

17 Ling J, Kang Y, Zhao R, et al. KrasG12D-induced IKK2/beta/NF-kappaB activation by IL-1alpha and p62 feedforward loops is required for development of pancreatic ductal adenocarcinoma. *Cancer Cell.* 2012;21(1):105–120.

18 Rinehart J, Adjei AA, Lorusso PM, et al. Multicenter phase II study of the oral MEK inhibitor, CI-1040, in patients with advanced non-small-cell lung, breast, colon, and pancreatic cancer. *J Clin Oncol.* 2004;22(22):4456–4462.

19 Walters DM, Lindberg JM, Adair SJ, et al. Inhibition of the growth of patient-derived pancreatic cancer xenografts with the MEK inhibitor trametinib is augmented by combined treatment with the epidermal growth factor receptor/HER2 inhibitor lapatinib. *Neoplasia.* 2013;15(2):143–155.

20 Rieder S, Michalski CW, Friess H, Kleeff J. Insulin-like growth factor signaling as a therapeutic target in pancreatic cancer. *Anticancer Agents Med Chem.* 2011;11(5):427–433.

21 Bergmann U, Funatomi H, Yokoyama M, Beger HG, Korc M. Insulin-like growth factor I overexpression in human pancreatic cancer: evidence for autocrine and paracrine roles. *Cancer Res.* 1995;55(10):2007–2011.

22 Chu E. The IGF-1R pathway as a therapeutic target. *Oncology (Williston Park).* 2011;25(6):538–539, 543.

23 Karna E, Surazynski A, Orłowski K, et al. Serum and tissue level of insulin-like growth factor-I (IGF-I) and IGF-I binding proteins

as an index of pancreatitis and pancreatic cancer. *Int J Exp Pathol.* 2002;83(5):239–245.

24 Lopez T, Hanahan D. Elevated levels of IGF-1 receptor convey invasive and metastatic capability in a mouse model of pancreatic islet tumorigenesis. *Cancer Cell.* 2002;1(4):339–353.

25 Adachi, Y., Li R, Yamamoto H, et al. Insulin-like growth factor-I receptor blockade reduces the invasiveness of gastrointestinal cancers via blocking production of matrilysin. *Carcinogenesis.* 2009;30(8):1305–1313.

26 Fogelman DR, Holmes H, Mohammed K, et al. Does IGFR1 inhibition result in increased muscle mass loss in patients undergoing treatment for pancreatic cancer? *J Cachexia Sarcopenia Muscle.* 2014;5(4):307–313.

27 Philip PA, Goldman B, Ramanathan RK, et al. Dual blockade of epidermal growth factor receptor and insulin-like growth factor receptor-1 signaling in metastatic pancreatic cancer: phase Ib and randomized phase II trial of gemcitabine, erlotinib, and cixutumumab versus gemcitabine plus erlotinib (SWOG S0727). *Cancer.* 2014;120(19):2980–2985.

28 Javle MM, Varadhachary GR, Fogelman DR, et al. Randomized phase II study of gemcitabine (G) plus anti-IGF-1R antibody MK-0646, G plus erlotinib (E) plus MK-0646 and G plus E for advanced pancreatic cancer. *J Clin Oncol.* 2011. 29:

29 Becker MA, Hou X, Harrington SC, et al. IGFBP ratio confers resistance to IGF targeting and correlates with increased invasion and poor outcome in breast tumors. *Clin Cancer Res.* 2012;18(6):1808–1817.

30 Abramovitz L, Rubinek T, Ligumsky H, et al. KL1 internal repeat mediates klotho tumor suppressor activities and inhibits bFGF and IGF-I signaling in pancreatic cancer. *Clin Cancer Res.* 2011;17(13):4254–4266.

31 Davies MA. The role of the PI3K-AKT pathway in melanoma. *Cancer J.* 2012;18(2):142–147.

32 Edling CE, Selvaggi F, Buus R, et al. Key role of phosphoinositide 3-kinase class IB in pancreatic cancer. *Clin Cancer Res.* 2010;16(20):4928–4937.

33 Ostapoff KT. Effect of NVP-BEZ235, a dual PI3K/mTOR inhibitor, on chemotherapy and antiangiogenic response in pancreatic cancer. *J Clin Oncol.* 2012;suppl. 4:243.

34 Haussmann E, Glienke W, Bergmann L. Combination strategy of gemcitabine with the dual PI3K/mTOR inhibitor NVP-BEZ235 in pancreatic cancer cells. *J Clin Oncol.* 2011;29(suppl.):e14562.

35 Junttila MR, Devasthali V, Cheng JH, et al. Modeling targeted inhibition of MEK and PI3 kinase in human pancreatic cancer. *Mol Cancer Ther.* 2014;14(1):40–47.

36 Lorusso PM. A first-in-human phase Ib study to evaluate the MEK inhibitor GDC-0973, combined with the pan-PI3K inhibitor GDC-0941, in patients with advanced solid tumors. *J Clin Oncol* 2012;30(suppl.): Abstract 2566.

37 Breast Cancer LinkageConsortium. Cancer risks in BRCA2 mutation carriers. *J Natl Cancer Inst.* 1999;91(15):1310–1316.

38 Ferrone CR, Levine DA, Tang LH, et al. BRCA germline mutations in Jewish patients with pancreatic adenocarcinoma. *J Clin Oncol.* 2009;27(3):433–438.

39 Venkitaraman AR. Cancer susceptibility and the functions of BRCA1 and BRCA2. *Cell.* 2002;108(2):171–182.

40 Dedes KJ, Wilkerson PM, Wetterskog D, Weigelt B, Ashworth A, Reis-Filho JS. Synthetic lethality of PARP inhibition in cancers lacking BRCA1 and BRCA2 mutations. *Cell Cycle.* 2011;10(8): 1192–1199.

41 Fong PC, Boss DS, Yap TA, et al. Inhibition of poly(ADP-ribose) polymerase in tumors from BRCA mutation carriers. *N Engl J Med.* 2009;361(2):123–134.

42 Lowery MA, Kelsen DP, Stadler ZK, et al. An emerging entity: pancreatic adenocarcinoma associated with a known BRCA mutation: clinical descriptors, treatment implications, and future directions. *Oncologist.* 2011;16(10):1397–1402.

43 Vyas O, Leung K, Ledbetter L, et al. Clinical outcomes in pancreatic adenocarcinoma associated with BRCA-2 mutation. *Anticancer Drugs.* 2015;26(2):224–226.

44 O'Reilly EM. Phase IB trial of cisplatin (C), gemcitabine (G), and veliparib (V) in patients with known or potential BRCA or PALB2-mutated pancreas adenocarcinoma (PC). *J Clin Oncol.* 2014;32(5S):4023.

45 Hofstatter EW, Domchek SM, Miron A, et al. PALB2 mutations in familial breast and pancreatic cancer. *Fam Cancer.* 2011;10(2):225–231.

46 Tischkowitz MD, Sabbaghian N, Hamel N, et al. Analysis of the gene coding for the BRCA2-interacting protein PALB2 in familial and sporadic pancreatic cancer. *Gastroenterology.* 2009;137(3):1183–1186.

47 Slater EP, Langer P, Niemczyk E, et al. PALB2 mutations in European familial pancreatic cancer families. *Clin Genet.* 2010;78(5):490–494.

48 Villarroel MC, Rajeshkumar NV, Garrido-Laguna I, et al. Personalizing cancer treatment in the age of global genomic analyses: PALB2 gene mutations and the response to DNA damaging agents in pancreatic cancer. *Mol Cancer Ther.* 2011;10(1):3–8.

49 Song SY, Gannon M, Washington MK, et al. Expansion of Pdx1-expressing pancreatic epithelium and islet neogenesis in transgenic mice overexpressing transforming growth factor alpha. *Gastroenterology.* 1999;117(6):1416–1126.

50 Habbe N, Shi G, Meguid RA, et al. Spontaneous induction of murine pancreatic intraepithelial neoplasia (mPanIN) by acinar cell targeting of oncogenic Kras in adult mice. *Proc Natl Acad Sci U S A.* 2008;105(48):18913–18918.

51 Miyamoto Y, Maitra A, Ghosh B, et al. Notch mediates TGF alpha-induced changes in epithelial differentiation during pancreatic tumorigenesis. *Cancer Cell.* 2003;3(6):565–576.

52 Mullendore, ME, Koorstra JB, Li YM, et al. Ligand-dependent Notch signaling is involved in tumor initiation and tumor maintenance in pancreatic cancer. *Clin Cancer Res.* 2009;15(7):2291–2301.

53 Mizuma M, Rasheed ZA, Yabuuchi S, et al. The gamma secretase inhibitor MRK-003 attenuates pancreatic cancer growth in preclinical models. *Mol Cancer Ther.* 2012;11(9):1999–2009.

54 Hidalgo M, Maitra A. The hedgehog pathway and pancreatic cancer. *N Engl J Med.* 2009;361(21):2094–2096.

55 Jones S, Zhang X, Parsons DW, et al. Core signaling pathways in human pancreatic cancers revealed by global genomic analyses. *Science.* 2008;321(5897):1801–1806.

56 Jimeno A, Feldmann G, Suárez-Gauthier A, et al. A direct pancreatic cancer xenograft model as a platform for cancer stem cell therapeutic development. *Mol Cancer Ther.* 2009;8(2):310–314.

57 Olive, KP, Jacobetz MA, Davidson CJ, et al. Inhibition of Hedgehog signaling enhances delivery of chemotherapy in a mouse model of pancreatic cancer. *Science.* 2009.324(5933):1457–1461.

58 Jimeno A, Jacobetz MA, Davidson CJ, et al. Phase I study of the Hedgehog pathway inhibitor IPI-926 in adult patients with solid tumors. *Clin Cancer Res.* 2013;19(10):2766–2774.

59 Richards DA. A phase Ib trial of IPI-926, a hedgehog pathway inhibitor, plus gemcitabine in patients with metastatic pancreatic cancer. *J Clin Oncol.* 2012;suppl. 4:213.

60 Toole BP, Slomiany MG. Hyaluronan: a constitutive regulator of chemoresistance and malignancy in cancer cells. *Semin Cancer Biol.* 2008;18(4):244–250.

61 Provenzano PP, Cuevas C, Chang AE, Goel VK, Von Hoff DD, Hingorani SR. Enzymatic targeting of the stroma ablates physical barriers to treatment of pancreatic ductal adenocarcinoma. *Cancer Cell.* 2012;21(3):418–429.

62 Hingorani SR, Harris WP, Beck JT, et al. A phase Ib study of gemcitabine plus PEGPH20 (pegylated recombinant human hyaluronidase)

in patients with stage IV previously untreated pancreatic cancer. *J Clin Oncol.* 2013;31(suppl.):4010.

63 Mills LD, Zhang Y, Marler RJ, et al. Loss of the transcription factor GLI1 identifies a signaling network in the tumor microenvironment mediating KRAS oncogene-induced transformation. *J Biol Chem.* 2013;288(17):11786–11794.

64 Huang C, Yang G, Jiang T, Huang K, Cao J, Qiu Z. Effects of IL-6 and AG490 on regulation of Stat3 signaling pathway and invasion of human pancreatic cancer cells in vitro. *J Exp Clin Cancer Res.* 2010;29:51.

65 Quintas-Cardama A, Verstovsek S. Molecular pathways: Jak/STAT pathway: mutations, inhibitors, and resistance. *Clin Cancer Res.* 2013;19(8):1933–1940.

66 Scholz A, Heinze S, Detjen KM, et al. Activated signal transducer and activator of transcription 3 (STAT3) supports the malignant phenotype of human pancreatic cancer. *Gastroenterology.* 2003;125(3):891–905.

67 Fukuda A, Wang SC, Morris JP 4th, et al. Stat3 and MMP7 contribute to pancreatic ductal adenocarcinoma initiation and progression. *Cancer Cell.* 2011;19(4):441–455.

68 Toyonaga T, Nakano K, Nagano M, et al. Blockade of constitutively activated Janus kinase/signal transducer and activator of transcription-3 pathway inhibits growth of human pancreatic cancer. *Cancer Lett.* 2003;201(1):107–116.

69 Hurwitz H. A randomized double-blind phase 2 study of ruxolitinib (RUX) or placebo (PBO) with capecitabine (CAPE) as second-line therapy in patients (pts) with metastatic pancreatic cancer (mPC). *J Clin Oncol.* 2014;32(5s):4000.

70 Naski MC, Ornitz DM. FGF signaling in skeletal development. *Front Biosci.* 1998;3:d781–d794.

71 Miki T, Bottaro DP, Fleming TP, et al. Determination of ligand-binding specificity by alternative splicing: two distinct growth factor receptors encoded by a single gene. *Proc Natl Acad Sci U S A.* 1992;89(1):246–250.

72 Wesche J, Haglund K, Haugsten EM. Fibroblast growth factors and their receptors in cancer. *Biochem J.* 2011;437(2):199–213.

73 Kornmann M, Beger HG, Korc M. Role of fibroblast growth factors and their receptors in pancreatic cancer and chronic pancreatitis. *Pancreas.* 1998;17(2):169–175.

74 Escaffit, F., Estival A, Bertrand C, Vaysse N, Hollande E, Clemente F. FGF 2 isoforms of 18 and 22.5 kDa differentially modulate t-PA and PAI-1 expressions on the pancreatic carcinoma cells AR4-2J: consequences on cell spreading and invasion. *Int J Cancer.* 2000;85(4):555–562.

75 Nomura S, Yoshitomi H, Takano S, et al. FGF10/FGFR2 signal induces cell migration and invasion in pancreatic cancer. *Br J Cancer.* 2008;99(2):305–313.

76 Cho K, Ishiwata T, Uchida E, et al. Enhanced expression of keratinocyte growth factor and its receptor correlates with venous invasion in pancreatic cancer. *Am J Pathol.* 2007;170(6):1964–1974.

77 Katoh Y, Katoh M. FGFR2-related pathogenesis and FGFR2-targeted therapeutics (Review). *Int J Mol Med.* 2009;23(3):307–311.

78 Ishiwata T, Matsuda Y, Yamamoto T, et al. Enhanced expression of fibroblast growth factor receptor 2 IIIc promotes human pancreatic cancer cell proliferation. *Am J Pathol.* 2012;180(5):1928–1941.

79 Whatcott CJ, Richard GP, Daniel D. Hoff V, Han H. Desmoplasia and chemoresistance in pancreatic cancer. In Grippo PJ, Munshi HG, eds. *Pancreatic Cancer and Tumor Microenvironment.* Trivandrum, India: Transworld Research Network; 2012.

80 Coleman SJ, Chioni AM, Ghallab M, et al. Nuclear translocation of FGFR1 and FGF2 in pancreatic stellate cells facilitates pancreatic cancer cell invasion. *EMBO Mol Med.* 2014;6(4):467–481.

81 Zhang H, Hylander BL, LeVea C, et al. Enhanced FGFR signalling predisposes pancreatic cancer to the effect of a potent FGFR inhibitor in preclinical models. *Br J Cancer.* 2014;110(2):320–329.

82 Lieu C, Heymach J, Overman M, Tran H, Kopetz S. Beyond VEGF: inhibition of the fibroblast growth factor pathway and antiangiogenesis. *Clin Cancer Res.* 2011;17(19):6130–6139.

83 Broadley KN, Aquino AM, Woodward SC, et al. Monospecific antibodies implicate basic fibroblast growth factor in normal wound repair. *Lab Invest.* 1989;61(5):571–575.

84 Greenhalgh DG, Sprugel KH, Murray MJ, Ross R. PDGF and FGF stimulate wound healing in the genetically diabetic mouse. *Am J Pathol.* 1990;136(6):1235–1246.

85 Presta M, Dell'Era P, Mitola S, Moroni E, Ronca R, Rusnati M. Fibroblast growth factor/fibroblast growth factor receptor system in angiogenesis. *Cytokine Growth Factor Rev.* 2005;16(2):159–178.

86 Wang Y, Becker D. Antisense targeting of basic fibroblast growth factor and fibroblast growth factor receptor-1 in human melanomas blocks intratumoral angiogenesis and tumor growth. *Nat Med.* 1997;3(8):887–893.

87 Kindler HL, Niedzwiecki D, Hollis D, et al. Gemcitabine plus bevacizumab compared with gemcitabine plus placebo in patients with advanced pancreatic cancer: phase III trial of the Cancer and Leukemia Group B (CALGB 80303). *J Clin Oncol.* 2010;28(22):3617–3622.

88 Giavazzi R, Sennino B, Coltrini D, et al. Distinct role of fibroblast growth factor-2 and vascular endothelial growth factor on tumor growth and angiogenesis. *Am J Pathol.* 2003;162(6):1913–1926.

89 Yamamoto Y, Matsui J, Matsushima T, et al. Lenvatinib, an angiogenesis inhibitor targeting VEGFR/FGFR, shows broad antitumor activity in human tumor xenograft models associated with microvessel density and pericyte coverage. *Vasc Cell.* 2014;6:18.

90 Allen E, Walters IB, Hanahan D. Brivanib, a dual FGF/VEGF inhibitor, is active both first and second line against mouse pancreatic neuroendocrine tumors developing adaptive/evasive resistance to VEGF inhibition. *Clin Cancer Res.* 2011;17(16):5299–5310.

91 Cowan RW, Maitra A. Genetic progression of pancreatic cancer. *Cancer J.* 2014;20(1):80–84.

92 Yachida S, Iacobuzio-Donahue CA. Evolution and dynamics of pancreatic cancer progression. *Oncogene.* 2013;32(45):5253–5260.

93 Witkiewicz AK, Knudsen KE, Dicker AP, et al. The meaning of p16(ink4a) expression in tumors: functional significance, clinical associations and future developments. *Cell Cycle.* 2011;10(15):2497–2503.

94 Franco J, Witkiewicz AK, Knudsen ES. CDK4/6 inhibitors have potent activity in combination with pathway selective therapeutic agents in models of pancreatic cancer. *Oncotarget.* 2014;5(15):6512–6525.

# CHAPTER 27

# Targeted Therapies for Pediatric Solid Tumors

*Jasmine Quynh Dao and Patrick A. Zweidler-McKay*

Children's Cancer Hospital, The University of Texas MD Anderson Cancer Center, Houston, TX, USA

## Introduction

Although targeted cancer therapies hold much promise, much of it has been kept "out of reach of children" with cancer. This chapter will focus on some of the successes and challenges in evaluating and incorporating targeted therapies into pediatric oncology. Thankfully childhood cancers are relatively rare, with only 1 in 300 people being diagnosed with cancer during childhood and ~10,000 new cases each year in the United States. However, cancer is the leading cause of death by disease in children.

Just as in adults, there are many types of cancer; however, the spectrum of cancers affecting children differ from those seen in adults with several tumors that occur almost exclusively in childhood, while others are biologically and/or clinically distinct from their adult counterparts. Many of the common cancers in adults, such as carcinomas of the lung, breast, prostate, and colon, occur only rarely in children. More commonly, children are diagnosed with "developmental" cancers, which arise from immature precursor cells during development. For example, neuroblastoma, hepatoblastoma, retinoblastoma, medulloblastoma, and Wilms' tumors occur almost exclusively in children, while Ewing's sarcoma, osteosarcoma, rhabdomyosarcoma, glioma/glioblastoma, and ependymoma each have pathologically related but biologically and/or clinically distinct diseases in children and adults.

Given the diversity and rarity of most childhood cancers, the translational research efforts are, in comparison, relatively limited, and the available pipeline for childhood cancers is just starting to flow. In a few cases, the biology of a childhood cancer has contributed significantly to the development of a therapy, and definitive trials have shown benefit to targeted therapies. However, much more commonly clinical activity has been seen in a small number of patients, providing hope for success but requiring validation in larger trials.

This chapter will present some of the successes and the anecdotal responses seen with targeted therapies for solid tumors in children. Please refer to Table 27.1 which provides a summary of clinical and preclinical successes for targeting specific pathways in particular tumor types. We regret that we could not be comprehensive in reporting every study which is relevant and regret any omissions of important work.

## Neuroblastoma

Neuroblastoma is the most common extra-cranial solid tumor in children and accounts for 15% of childhood cancer-related deaths. Neuroblastoma is a developmental cancer which occurs in early childhood, with 37% of patients being diagnosed in the first year of life, and 90% being diagnosed by 5 years of age. Risk stratification is based on age, MYCN amplification, pathologic features and treatment response. Interestingly, neuroblastoma which occurs in children <18 months of age appears to be biologically and clinically distinct from neuroblastoma in children >18 months old, with spontaneous remissions even from metastatic disease and ~90% survival with little or moderate-intensity chemotherapy. In contrast, the outcomes for children >18 months with neuroblastoma typically have high risk features and outcomes below 60%. Treatment for high-risk neuroblastoma may include five or greater cycles of intense chemotherapy, radiation therapy, surgical resection, myeloablative autologous stem-cell rescue and maintenance with isotretinoin, and immunotherapy. These young children suffer both significant acute and long-term toxicity, and represent an ideal group of patients whose conventional therapies have been maximally intensified and would receive significant benefit from targeted therapies to enhance outcomes and decrease late effects.

Neuroblastoma is a tumor arising from neural crest precursors which carry a number of molecular alterations, including amplification of MYCN, overexpression of TRKB, and recurrent deletions of 11q and 1p36. Familial cases of neuroblastoma have identified mutations in ALK and PHOX2B and the association with specific congenital syndromes has revealed additional potential therapeutic targets, that is, congenital central hypoventilation syndrome (PHOX2B mutations) and Hirschsprung's disease (RET/EDNRB mutations). Recent next generation sequencing of 240 cases of neuroblastoma has identified mutations in ALK (9.2%), PTPN11 (2.9%), ATRX (2.5%, +7.1% focal deletions), MYCN (1.7%), and NRAS (0.8%).[1] In the context of all of these potential targets, currently the most promising targeted therapies for neuroblastoma include anti-GD2 antibodies, I[131]-MIBG, ALK inhibitors, IGF1R inhibitors, mammalian target of rapamycin (mTOR) inhibitors, as well as PI3K/AKT, heat shock protein-90 (HSP90), TEM1, etc.[2]

*Targeted Therapy in Translational Cancer Research*, First Edition. Edited by Apostolia-Maria Tsimberidou, Razelle Kurzrock and Kenneth C. Anderson.
© 2016 John Wiley & Sons, Inc. Published 2016 by John Wiley & Sons, Inc.

**Table 27.1** Targeted therapies in pediatric solid tumors.

| Clinical activity (best responses) | Ependymoma | Ewing's sarcoma | Glioma | Hepatoblastoma | Medulloblastoma | Neuroblastoma | Osteosarcoma | Retinoblastoma | Rhabdomyosarcoma | Wilms' | Targeted agents |
|---|---|---|---|---|---|---|---|---|---|---|---|
| ALK | | | | | | CR | | | | | **Crizotinib** |
| Aurora kinase | | * | | | | * | * | | | | Alisertib |
| BRAF | | | * | | | | | | | | **Vemurafenib** |
| EGFR/ERBB | SD | | SD | | | | | | SD | | **Cetuximab, Lapatinib** |
| FLT3 | | * | | | | | | | * | | **Sunitinib** |
| GD2 | | | | | | CR | CR | | | | ch 14.18, 3F8 |
| HDAC | PR | * | SD | | | CR | SD | * | SD | | **Vorinostat, Depsipeptide** |
| HSP90 | | | * | SD | | * | * | | | | Tanespimycin (17 AAG) |
| IGF1R | | CR | | | | PR | * | | * | | Cixutumumab, Ganitumab |
| Integrins | | | CR | | | | | | | | Cilengitide |
| KIT | | * | | | * | * | * | | * | | **Imatinib, Dasatinib** |
| MDM2 | | | | | | | | * | | | Nutlin-3 |
| MET | | * | | | | * | | | * | | Tivantinib |
| mTOR | | CR | PR | | * | CR | PR | | PR | | **Everolimus, Sirolimus, Temsirolimus** |
| NET | | | | | | CR | | | | | I$^{131}$ MIBG |
| NFKB | | * | | | | | | | | | BAY 11-7082 |
| NOTCH | * | * | | | * | | * | | | | RO4929097, MK-0752 |
| PARP | | * | | | | * | | | | | Olaparib |
| PDGFR | | * | | | * | | PR | | * | | **Sorafenib, Sunitinib**, Tandutinib |
| PI3K/AKT | | | | | * | * | * | | | | MK-2206, PI 103 |
| PLK1 | | | | | | | * | * | | | BI 2536 |
| RAS/RAF/MAPK | SD | | PR | | SD | | * | | * | | **Sorafenib**, Lonafarnib, Selumetinib |
| SHH | | * | | | PR | | * | | | | **Vismodegib**, Erismodegib |
| SRC | | * | | | | | * | | | | **Dasatinib** |
| SYK | | | | | | | | * | | | R406 |
| TNF | | | | | | | | | | CR | rTNF |
| TRAIL | | * | | SD | | | SD | | | | Lexatumumab |
| VEGFR | * | CR | CR | PR | * | PR | PR | | PR | * | **Sorafenib, Pazopanib, Sunitinib** |
| WNT | | | | | | | * | | | * | NC043, ICG001 |

CR, complete response; PR, partial response; SD, stable disease

Bold denotes FDA approved agents

*preclinical activity

## Ganglioside GD2

GD2 is a cell-surface disialoganglioside that is highly expressed on 98% of neuroblastoma cells, while being expressed on few normal tissues. This has made GD2 an attractive targetable tumor antigen. Recent trials demonstrated a profound survival benefit from the addition of the anti-GD2 antibody ch14.18 combined with granulocyte–macrophage colony-stimulating factor (GM-CSF) and interleukin-2 (IL-2) to standard maintenance therapy with isotretinoin in high-risk patients. In a randomized phase III trial enrolling 226 children with high-risk neuroblastoma, event-free survival (EFS) was 66 +/− 5% in the immunotherapy arm, compared to 46 +/− 5% in the control arm.[3] Promising results were also seen with the anti-GD2 antibody 3F8 when combined with GM-CSF and isotretinoin in maintenance therapy, resulting in a progression-free survival (PFS) of 62% in 85 children with stage 4 neuroblastoma in a non-randomized front-line trial.[4] These findings represent a significant improvement in outcome for these patients and this approach

is becoming standard of care. With multiple anti-GD2 antibodies and persistent toxicities, further trials are needed to determine the optimal way to target GD2. Reduction of toxicity was the goal of hu14.18K322A, a humanized anti-GD2 mAb with a mutation that causes less complement-dependent lysis. A recent phase I trial was completed with typical toxicities of the parent antibody ch14.18, except there were no cases of capillary leak syndrome in 38 patients.[5]

An alternate method of targeting GD2 involves adoptive immunotherapy with anti-GD2 chimeric antigen receptor (CAR) T cells which have also shown promise with 3 of 11 children with active high-risk disease attaining a CR.[6] Anti-GD2 CAR NK cells and combination of NK cells with anti-GD2 ch14.18 antibody also show anti-neuroblastoma efficacy in preclinical studies. Further efforts to target GD2 include anti-idiotype antibody vaccination which was tested in high risk neuroblastoma patients and 16 of 21 children remain in remission at >6 years, suggesting clinical activity compared to historical controls. The point mutation reduces complement-dependent lysis. Given the major clinical success seen with anti-GD2 approaches, targeting GD2 in neuroblastoma remains a very active area of interest.

## Meta-iodobenzylguanidine

A successful alternate strategy to target neuroblastoma is through its physiologic uptake of neurotransmitters. Meta-iodobenzylguanidine (MIBG) is a norepinephrine analog that binds to human norepinephrine transporter (NET), which is expressed in 90% of neuroblastoma tumors, reflecting its neural crest origins. Radioactive [123]I-MIBG is used as an imaging tracer to stage neuroblastoma due to their high uptake of MIBG. Subsequently [131]I-MIBG was developed to deliver radiation directly to the neuroblastoma cells. Phase II trials showed 37% of 164 children with relapsed or refractory neuroblastoma had partial or complete responses (CR) to infusions of [131]I-MIBG,[7] and in front-line therapy [131]I-MIBG given before induction had a response rate of 66%.[8] However, significant toxicity is common, with 30% of the phase II patients receiving autologous stem-cell rescue due to severe myelosuppression. Despite this, the remarkable clinical success has led to its incorporation into front-line therapy in centers capable of giving this radiolabeled therapeutic. Phase I combination of [131]I-MIBG with vincristine and irinotecan led to two CR and four partial responses (PR) for an overall response rate (ORR) of 25% in relapsed/refractory neuroblastomas.[9] Preclinical testing shows that exposure to the histone deacetylase (HDAC) inhibitor vorinostat (SAHA) increased expression of NET in neuroblastoma cells, which led to increased MIBG uptake, resulting in additive growth inhibition in mice. With such broad clinical responses, targeting the norepinephrine transporter appears to be a highly successful approach for neuroblastoma and will likely lead to further refinements of MIBG-based therapy and novel molecules in the future.

## Anaplastic Lymphoma Kinase

Recently, targetable kinase mutations have been found in neuroblastoma. Activating anaplastic lymphoma kinase (ALK) mutations were first discovered in cases of familial neuroblastomas, and now are reported in ~10% of sporadic neuroblastomas. ALK mutations are enriched in MYCN-amplified neuroblastomas, and ALK appears to be able to induce MYCN transcription suggesting that these oncogenes cooperate in transformation of neural crest progenitors. Crizotinib (PF-02341066), an ALK/MET inhibitor, has been effective in adult ALK positive tumors such as non-small-cell lung carcinoma (NSCLC) and a single-agent phase I trial of crizotinib in children revealed one CR and three stable disease (SD) responses in 11 patients with ALK-mutated neuroblastoma, hinting at activity in a subset of neuroblastoma patients.[10] Preclinical data shows that ALK amplified neuroblastoma xenografts are sensitive to crizotinib, though neuroblastomas with a subset of ALK mutations, for example, F1174L, are often resistant. The alternative approach of using ALK-inhibiting antibodies, with or without an ALK kinase inhibitor has been validated preclinically, and may overcome crizotinib resistance.[11] Interestingly the mTOR inhibitor Torin2 can sensitize cells carrying ALK mutations to crizotinib, another approach to overcome resistance. With ALK mutations found in the majority of familial cases, and mutations in ~10% of sporadic cases, targeting ALK and its downstream pathways is a very promising approach to a subset of neuroblastomas.

## Insulin-like Growth Factor-1 Receptor

The presence of an IGF1 autocrine loop has been correlated with more aggressive neuroblastomas, and increased insulin-like growth factor-1 receptor (IGF1R) expression was found to correspond with higher rates of bone metastases in murine models. In preclinical studies, neuroblastoma cell lines responded to the IGF1R inhibitors, and adding temozolomide showed an increase in both *in vitro* and *in vivo* efficacy. In a phase II study the anti-IGF1R antibody cixutumumab (IMC-A12) demonstrated a PR in 20% (4 of 20) of neuroblastoma patients.[12] Preclinical studies of the IGF1R kinase inhibitor BMS-754807 demonstrated PRs in neuroblastoma xenografts suggesting that multiple IGF1R approaches hold promise for neuroblastoma.

## Mammalian Target of Rapamycin

Activation of mTOR signaling has been found in a majority of neuroblastoma tumors. In preclinical trials, the mTOR inhibitor sirolimus interrupted G1 to S cell cycle progression in 90% of tested samples, revealing unanticipated preclinical activity. A phase I trial of temsirolimus revealed a CR in one of two refractory neuroblastoma patients[13]; temsirolimus combined with irinotecan showed objective response >15 cycles in one patient and SD for nine cycles in three patients in a COG phase I trial.[14] In the subsequent phase II trial of temsirolimus, one PR and 6 of 19 (32%) SD were seen in neuroblastoma patients, suggesting some single-agent activity, though combinations may be more effective.[15] A COG phase II trial of temsirolimus with irinotecan is underway. A phase I combination of sirolimus with vinblastine led to one patient achieving PR and three patients maintaining SD.[16] Given the significant preclinical activity but modest clinical efficacy, additional approaches for targeting mTOR and novel combinations are under development.

## Topoisomerase I Inhibitors

This family of drugs works by blocking the synthesis of DNA and RNA via disruption of topoisomerase I. Topotecan is one agent that has been used in many CNS tumors. It demonstrates synergistic effects when paired with alkylating agent temozolomide in preclinical studies. The TOTEM phase II study combining temozolomide with topotecan for recurrent neuroblastoma saw PR in 7/38 patients just after two cycles, and overall 68% of patients had either CR, PR, or SD.[17]

## Gliomas

Approximately half of pediatric CNS tumors are gliomas and are associated with two syndromes, for example, neurofibromatosis I (NF1 mutations) and tuberous sclerosis syndrome (TSC mutations). Gliomas occur both in children and adults; however, the majority of pediatric gliomas are low-grade gliomas (LGG) with indolent pilocytic astrocytomas being the most common subtype and the most common pediatric high-grade gliomas (HGG) are diffuse intrinsic pontine glioma (DIPG), not glioblastoma multiforme (GBM). Surgical resection, if feasible, is the most effective therapeutic option, with complete resection of a LGG leading to a >90% survival, while subtotal resection leads to ~60% survival. Meanwhile, unresectable DIPG has a devastating <10% 2-year survival. Radiation therapy with or without chemotherapy may be used for HGG, though radiation provides only transient benefit in DIPG.

The distinct biology of pediatric versus adult gliomas is also becoming clearer. Association with NF1 and TSC1/2 mutations, relative lack of TP53 mutations as well as enhanced RAS/MAPK and mTOR signaling point to targetable biology in pediatric cases. The many pathways of interest are PI3K/AKT, vascular endothelial growth factor (VEGF), mTOR, integrins, HDAC, Ras/Raf/MAPK, epidermal growth factor receptor (EGFR) as well as NOTCH, PDGFR, FGFR1, PTPN11, and NTRK2.[18]

PI3K/AKT: The PI3K/AKT pathway is upregulated in many CNS tumors, including glioma. A phase I trial of the AKT inhibitor MK-2206 was evaluated and found to be tolerated well in patients with malignant glioma, including GBM, and several other CNS tumors.[19] There were no clear responses to the treatment, and no glioma patients had SD. However, combination with other drugs may be more promising.

### Vascular Endothelial Growth Factor

Overexpression of VEGF is commonly seen in gliomas with variable preclinical activity seen in glioma models. In clinical trials, the anti-VEGF antibody bevacizumab induced tumor responses in recurrent pediatric LGGs when used in conjunction with irinotecan, with 70% measurable responses (one CR, three PR, and three minor responses) in 10 patients.[20] Unfortunately, this combination had minimal activity in pediatric HGGs. In another trial, bevacizumab with temsirolimus resulted in 2/5 patients (who had GBM, DIPG) with 4 months of SD/PR suggesting some combined activity.[21]

### Mammalian Target of Rapamycin

Activation of the mTOR pathway has been found in both LGGs and HGGs. In particular, mTOR may be important in gliomas associated with NF1 and tuberous sclerosis. Everolimus demonstrated significant activity against subependymal giant cell astrocytoma in patients with tuberous sclerosis complex, reducing tumor size by at least 50% in 27 patients, compared to the placebo group who had zero objective responses.[22] Incidentally, inhibition of mTOR in glioma was noted to lead to an upregulation of IGF1R signaling, one mechanism of chemoresistance. In preclinical studies, targeting both pathways resulted in a larger decrease in tumor growth.

### Integrins

The avb3/5 inhibitor cilengitide demonstrated promising preclinical activity in pediatric gliomas via anoikis, and a pediatric phase I trial found one GBM CR and two SD.[23] Unfortunately, a phase II trial showed SD for >20 months in only 1 of 24 pediatric HGGs[24] limiting enthusiasm for this approach.

### Histone Deacetylase

The HDACi, SAHA, was tested in patients with recurrent CNS tumors and one patient with HGG and one with ganglioglioma had SD,[25] suggesting limited single-agent activity.

### RAF/RAS/MAPK

Gliomas in patients with neurofibromatosis (NF1 mutation) demonstrate hyperactive RAS/MAPK signaling. In addition, hypermethylation of the RASSF1A gene, activating KRAS mutations, and BRAF activation have all been found in pediatric gliomas. Importantly, translocations of BRAF occur in 70% of pilocytic astrocytomas[26] and the BRAF V600E activating mutation occurs in 10% of pediatric malignant astrocytomas.[27] BRAF mutations in gliomas correlate with high sensitivity to MAPK inhibitors, for example, AZD6244 and BRAF inhibitors synergize preclinically with radiation therapy. Multi-kinase inhibitors which target BRAF, such as sorafenib and sunitinib, have also been promising in preclinical studies. Some clinical activity was seen with lonafarnib, a farne-

syltransferase inhibitor that exerts its effect by post-translational modification of Ras, with one PR and two SD in HGG and two SD in LGG.[28] Unfortunately, there were no responses in two phase II studies of tipifarnib, another farnesyltransferase inhibitor, for recurrent CNS tumors, and no response either when it was given with radiotherapy for intrinsic DIPGs. Although the RAF/RAS/MAPK pathway is a highly compelling target in gliomas, further trials are needed.

### Epidermal Growth Factor Receptor

Overexpression of EGFR is seen in 80% of supratentorial HGGs in children, though the gene amplification is seen in less than 1%. This is in contrast to adult tumors, where over 50% have the EGFR gene amplification. In a clinical trial, the EGFR kinase inhibitor gefitinib (ZD1839, Iressa), led to two SD in children with brainstem gliomas,[29] and when combined with radiation, showed overall survival rates of 56% at 12 months and 20% at 24 months, with three patients with remained progression free for >36 months in children with newly diagnosed brainstem gliomas.[30] An ERBB family inhibitor lapatinib led to SD in two of five children with HGG.[31] Also, the anti-EGFR antibody nimotuzumab showed a 54% 2-year survival in children with HGG[32] and the combination with radiation showed benefit in patients with DIPG.[33]

## Osteosarcoma

Osteosarcoma is the most common malignant bone tumor of childhood. Osteosarcoma typically affects pubertal adolescents, with a peak incidence in childhood of 12 years, and is associated with Li Fraumeni (TP53), hereditary retinoblastoma (RB1) and Rothmund–Thomson (RECQL4) syndromes, and prior radiation therapy to bone. Risk stratification can be made using tumor stage, location, and response to therapy. Survival is highly dependent on the presence of metastatic disease at diagnosis, ranging from 65% for adolescents with localized disease to only 25% for those with metastatic disease. Therapy consists of chemotherapy and surgical resection/amputation.

Osteosarcoma appears to be derived from osteoblasts and frequently produces bone-like material, for example, osteoid. Osteosarcoma is associated with TP53 mutation or loss (Li–Fraumeni syndrome), and mutations in the retinoblastoma gene (RB1). Alterations in TP53 regulators murine double minute 2 (MDM2), cyclin-dependent kinase 4 (CDK4), p14[INK4A] as well as PI3K and WNT pathway genes have been reported in osteosarcomas.[34] Targets that show promise include vascular endothelial growth factor receptor (VEGFR), PI3K/mTOR, GD2, tumor necrosis factor-alpha (TNF-α)-related apoptosis-inducing ligand receptor-2 (TRAIL-R2) activation, as well as NOTCH, RANKL, WNT, WEE1, and ERBB2. Unfortunately, clinical responses remain elusive.

### Vascular Endothelial Growth Factor Receptor

In osteosarcoma, VEGFR3 is highly expressed. In preclinical trials, VEGFR kinase inhibitor cediranib inhibited four of five osteosarcoma xenografts. In a phase I pediatric trial, one of four patients with osteosarcoma demonstrated reduction in pulmonary nodules.[35] Several multi-kinase inhibitors have activity against VEGFR. One example is sorafenib, a VEGFR/PDGFR/FLT3/RET/cKIT inhibitor, which demonstrated preclinical activity in five of six osteosarcoma xenografts, and in a phase II clinical trial 5 of 35 patients (14%) had measurable responses and 12 (34%) had

SD.[36] Thus both VEGFR-specific and multi-kinase inhibition hold promise in osteosarcoma.

## Mammalian Target of Rapamycin

The mTOR pathway appears to be relevant in osteosarcoma murine models, where rapamycin and temsirolimus significantly improved survival, decreased lung metastases, and may effect tumor angiogenesis through interactions between mTOR and VEGF signaling. In a phase II study of the mTOR inhibitor ridaforolimus which enrolled 54 patients with bone tumors, one confirmed PR and one unconfirmed PR in patients with osteosarcoma.[37] With significant preclinical effects but modest clinical activity, work continues to find clinically active combinations.

## Ganglioside GD2

Although perhaps unexpected, GD2 expression is seen in over 90% of osteosarcomas and thus anti-GD2 therapies may be of benefit. In a phase I trial of the anti-GD2 antibody 14.G2a, one of two osteosarcoma patients achieved a CR.[38] Addition efforts are needed to determine whether anti-GD2 therapy will be successful in osteosarcoma; however, as new GD2 targeting approaches are developed for neuroblastoma and melanoma, osteosarcoma appears to present a reasonable secondary disease of interest.

## TRAIL-R2

Another approach to antibody-directed therapy is the use of agonistic/activating antibodies for death receptors. Lexatumumab, an activator of TNF-α-related apoptosis-inducing ligand receptor-2 (TRAIL-R2, DR5), has shown promising preclinical activity in several solid tumors, including osteosarcoma. In a phase I trial, one osteosarcoma patient had resolution of clinical symptoms and PET activity, though this did not meet the criteria for PR.[39] Further studies are needed to validate this novel targeted approach.

## Ewing's Sarcoma

Ewing's sarcoma is the second most common malignant bone tumor in children with most cases being diagnosed between the ages of 5 and 30 years. The most important prognostic factors for Ewing's sarcoma are the presence of metastatic disease and initial response to therapy. With localized disease, survival is 70%. However, patients with metastatic disease at diagnosis have only a <30% survival rate. Treatment includes chemotherapy, surgery with or without radiation therapy.

Ewing's sarcoma is believed to be derived from bone-marrow-derived mesenchymal stem cells, but was often referred to as a primitive neuroectodermal tumor (PNET). Ewing's sarcoma is frequently associated with bone, though soft-tissue primary tumors occur. The t(11;22) translocation which produces the EWS/FLI1 fusion protein is found in over 85% of cases of Ewing's sarcoma, with t(11;21) EWS-ERG in another 10%. These chimeric proteins function as transcription factors altering other pathways such as IGFR via suppression of IGFBP3, sonic hedgehog (SHH) via upregulation of NKX2.2, WNT, NOTCH, TGFb, etc.[40] The most promising targets for Ewing's sarcoma therapy are IGF1R, VEGFR, as well as mTOR, aurora kinases, cKIT, and FAK.

## Insulin-like Growth Factor Receptor

Preclinical studies of anti-IGF1R antibodies have shown promise in Ewing's tumors, alone and in combination with vincristine, doxorubicin, and the mTOR inhibitor sirolimus. In a phase II clinical trial of the anti-IGF1R antibody R1507 in children and adults with Ewing's family tumors, an ORR of 10% with 10 PRs and one CR in 115 patients was observed with most responses seen in patients with bony primary lesions.[41] Similarly, in a phase I/II trial of another anti-IGF1R antibody cixutumumab (IMC-A12) in pediatric Ewing's patients, 10% (3 of 30) of patients had a PR.[42] And in a trial of the anti-IGF1R antibody ganitumab, one PR and eight SD occurred out of 19 young adults with Ewing's tumors again showing consistent though modest activity of IGF1R agents in Ewing's sarcoma.[43] Importantly, in combining cixutumumab with the mTOR inhibitor temsirolimus tumor responses were seen in 29% of 17 young adults with relapsed metastatic Ewing's sarcoma.[44] With multiple clinical responses across several trials, targeting IGF1R appears promising for Ewing's sarcoma.

## Vascular Endothelial Growth Factor

VEGF has been shown to mediate tumor angiogenesis in Ewing's sarcoma and is upregulated by the EWS-FLI1 gene. The anti-VEGF antibody, bevacizumab, combined with chemotherapy induced a partial remission in one out of the two refractory Ewing's patients. In a chemotherapy combination trial, five of the seven had CR or SD after four courses of bevacizumab with vincristine, topotecan, and cyclophosphamide though it is not clear what portion was due to bevacizumab.[45] Combination of bevacizumab with vincristine, oral irinotecan, and temozolomide also led to two responses in Ewing's patients.[46] Once again anti-VEGF therapy appears active, particularly in therapeutic combinations.

## Mammalian Target of Rapamycin

mTOR is a critical pathway in Ewing's sarcoma, and several agents such as everolimus, ridaforolimus, and sirolimus have been investigated. Single-agent mTOR inhibitors have not shown to be effective alone, and thus treatment has involved the use of other chemotherapy agents. Temsirolimus combined with irinotecan and temozolomide evoked a response in one patient for >14 cycles a phase I trial. Such combinations may provide patients more options of treatment as further studies continue.[14]

## Rhabdomyosarcoma

Rhabdomyosarcoma is the third most common non-CNS solid tumor of childhood, following neuroblastoma and Wilms' tumor. Similar to those tumors, two-thirds of rhabdomyosarcomas in children are made before 6 years of age. Although the vast majority of rhabdomyosarcomas are sporadic, a number of syndromes are associated with rhabdomyosarcoma including the Li–Fraumeni syndrome (TP53 mutations), pleuropulmonary blastoma (DICER1 mutations), neurofibromatosis type I, Costello syndrome (HRAS mutations), Beckwith–Wiedemann syndrome (11p15 alterations), and Noonan syndrome (RAS/RAF pathway). Risk stratification relies on age at diagnosis, stage of disease, and histologic subtype (alveolar vs. embryonal). Infants <1 year of age do not tolerate equivalent chemotherapy and radiation therapy, and thus have survival of 57%, while 1–9-year old children with localized disease have survival rates over 80%, and older patients have EFS of 68%. Treatment consists of chemotherapy, surgery, and/or radiation therapy.

Rhabdomyosarcoma arises from skeletal muscle progenitors and carry distinct molecular alterations based on the pathologic subtype. Alveolar subtypes carry translocations of t(2;13) PAX3 or t(1;13) PAX7 to FOXO1 (previously FKHR) in 78% of patients. Embryonal tumors contain losses of 11p15 and 1p11–1q11 but no critical genes have been identified. The most promising pathways for rhabdomyosarcoma include mTOR and VEGF as well as HDACi.

## Mammalian Target of Rapamycin

In preclinical studies, both rapamycin and CCI-779 inhibited tumor growth in mouse models of rhabdomyosarcoma. In a phase II clinical trial, 1 of 16 (6%) patients with rhabdomyosarcoma experienced a PR.[15] In a phase 1 study, a patient with alveolar rhabdomyosarcoma was treated with ridaforolimus and had a PR.[47] Anecdotally temsirolimus combined with irinotecan and temozolomide led to one patient with rhabdomyosarcoma having SD for nine cycles a phase I trial,[14] though the role of mTOR inhibition in this cannot be determined.

## Vascular Endothelial Growth Factor

In a study of bevacizumab for compassionate use, there was radiographic evidence of PR in one patient with rhabdomyosarcoma.[48] Preclinical information on multi-kinase inhibitors such as pazopanib and sunitinib, which target VEGFR1/2 and PDGFR among others, were shown to have intermediate-to-high activity in rhabdomyosarcoma xenografts.

## Wilms' Tumor

Wilms' tumor is the most common kidney tumor in children, representing 90% of childhood renal tumors. The peak incidence is at 3–4 years of age, and the familial type is seen in 1–2% of cases. Up to 10% of children with Wilms' tumor have congenital anomalies with or without associated syndromes, including WAGR (11 loss), Beckwith–Wiedemann (hemihypertrophy, 11p15), Denys–Drash (WT1 mutations), Li–Fraumeni (TP53 mutation), and others. Both WAGR and Beckwith–Wiedemann syndromes involve a defect in chromosome 11, which is the location of the WT1 and IGF2 genes, both thought to be important in the development of Wilms' tumor. Outcomes depend on age and histology, where patients under 10 years of age have a 90% survival, and adolescents and young adults have a 68% survival. Treatment consists of chemotherapy with surgical research with or without radiation therapy.

Wilms' tumor is derived from nephroblasts and can present with synchronous tumors, or with premalignant nephrogeneic rests. However, familial cases are rare. Mutation of the Wilms' tumor 1 gene (WT1, 11p13) or LOH/imprinting of the WT2 locus (11p15, containing IGF2) or mutations in WTX are seen in over 80% of expression of Wilms' tumor and appear to play central roles in Wilms' tumor biology. WT1 interacts with beta-catenin of the WNT pathway, and modulates members of the BCL-2 family. Targets of interest for Wilms' tumor include TNF, EGFR as well as IGF1R, VEGF, WNT/B-catenin, MET, though clinical trial success for targeted agents has been limited.

## Tumor Necrosis Factor

Immune modulation with TNF and chemotherapy has been found to be promising preclinically. In a phase II study, recombinant TNF plus dactinomycin led to CR in 16% (3 of 19) children with relapsed Wilms' tumor, suggesting activity beyond chemotherapy.

## Epidermal Growth Factor Receptor

EGF is expressed at varying levels of Wilms' tumor cells. Anti-EGFR monoclonal antibodies, such as gefitinib, were found to be effective in some xenograft models. In a phase I trial of gefitinib, two patients

with Wilms' tumor demonstrated SD for 8 to >60 weeks,[29] suggesting potential activity in this disease.

## Vascular Growth Factor Receptor

While bevacizumab is not widely effective on its own, a study involving bevacizumab with irinotecan, temozolomide, vincristine led to CR in three patients who received 12 cycles of treatment, and PR in one patient who received eight cycles.[49] Side effects where tolerated well in this patient group.

## Hepatoblastoma

Hepatoblastoma accounts for 80% of liver tumors in children and has a peak incidence at <1 year of age, with the majority of cases occur before age 3 years. Hepatoblastoma has been linked to very-low birth weight, parental exposure to metals, and is associated with multiple syndromes including overgrowth syndromes (Beckwith–Wiedemann, Prader–Willi, Simpson–Golabi–Behmel) as well as familial adenomatosis polypi (APC mutations), glycogen storage diseases I–IV, trisomy 18, tetralogy of Fallot, Goldenhar syndrome. Aggressive surgical resection (including liver transplantation), platinum-based chemotherapy, and radiation therapy are the treatments of choice. Poor outcome is predicted by the presence of non-fetal histology, metastases, residual tumor, and lack of AFP expression. Fortunately, stage I/II fetal histology patients have near 100% survival with complete resection alone; however, those with metastatic disease have 20–50% survival depending on degree of resection of primary and metastatic lesions.

Hepatoblastoma is another developmental tumor and has its origins in multiple hepatic precursors. The two major histologic subtypes are fetal and small-cell undifferentiated type. Fetal histology contains predominantly epithelial precursors, expresses AFP, and confers favorable prognosis. In contrast, small-cell undifferentiated may be of neuroblast origin, often lacks AFP expression, carries 22q11 deletions (containing SMARCB1/INI1), is associated with poor prognosis, and shares features with malignant rhabdoid tumors. Beta-catenin mutations have been found in up to 67% of hepatoblastoma cases, and evidence for WNT pathway activation can be seen in up to 87% of hepatoblastomas, revealing WNT signaling as a major driver of this tumor type.[50] Although VEGF, TRAIL, and HSP90 as well as WNT, MET, and EGFR are therapeutic targets, limited therapeutic success has been seen.

## Vascular Endothelial Growth Factor Receptor

Anti-angiogenic approaches have shown some preclinical in hepatoblastoma. Clinically the decoy VEGFR fusion protein, aflibercept (VEGF trap) resulted with SD in one patient with hepatoblastoma for >13 weeks.[51] Also, in a phase I trial with multikinase inhibitor pazopanib, one patient was able to achieve PR.[52] Also PRs were seen in two patients after 12 cycles of a vincristine, irinotecan, and bevacizumab combination.[49] Though limited, VEGFR-targeted therapy remains promising.

## TRAIL-R2

Lexatumumab is an antibody which activates TRAIL-R2, DR5 and shows promising preclinical activity in several solid tumors. In a phase I trial, one hepatoblastoma patient had a dramatic biomarker response with SD.[39]

## Heat Shock Protein-90

Targeting of this chaperone protein leads to disruption of signaling pathways and induction of apoptosis. In a phase I study of tanespimycin (17-AAG), an antibiotic that interferes with HSP90 function, one patient with hepatoblastoma showed reduction in AFP and SD for three cycles.[53]

## Ependymomas

Ependymomas account for 10% of all pediatric CNS tumors with a peak age of 5 years. In contrast to adults where ependymomas frequently occur in the spine, in children they are typically intracranial, often near the fourth ventricle. Ependymomas are rarely familial and are associated with neurofibromatosis type II (NF2 mutations). Effective treatment relies on surgical resection and radiation therapy, though even with complete resection 5-year PFS remains poor, 25–45%. Prognostic factors include age, tumor location, and resection.

Studies have demonstrated biologic differences between ependymomas in adults and children.[54] In pediatric ependymomas there are numerous chromosomal aberrations and related molecular genetic changes. Gain of 1q25, overexpression of EGFR, hTERT expression, high levels of nucleolin, activation of the Notch pathway or tenascin C, and others have been related to poorer prognosis. In contrast, gains of 9, 15q, and 18, and loss of chromosome 6 were associated with improved prognosis. Promising pathways include ERBB, VEGF, HDAC as well as the Notch, WNT, and SHH pathways.

### ERBB

ERBB2 is expressed on greater than 75% of ependymomas and overexpression correlates with increased proliferation and poorer outcome. In a phase I trial of lapatinib 29% (4 of 14) ependymoma patients had SD.[31] Though modest, this clinical activity is the most promising targeted therapy for pediatric ependymoma.

### Vascular Endothelial Growth Factor

The combination of anti-VEGF antibody bevacizumab with irinotecan in recurrent pediatric ependymoma yielded two SDs for 10–12 months out of 13 evaluable patients.[55]

### Histone Deacetylase

Abnormal deacetylation has been found in ependymomas. In a phase I trial of the HDAC inhibitor SAHA, one patient had a PR and one patient had SD.[25]

## Medulloblastoma

Medulloblastoma is the most common pediatric malignant CNS tumor with a peak age of incidence of 5 years and 80% of medulloblastomas occur before age 15. Medulloblastomas are rarely associated with Gorlin (PTCH mutation, SHH receptor) and Turcot (mismatch repair genes) syndromes. Age <3 years at diagnosis, residual tumor after resection, anaplastic histology, MYC amplification, 17p loss, and disseminated disease may predict poor outcome. Children with localized disease have >80% EFS and disseminated disease have <40% EFS. Treatment typically includes surgical resection, chemotherapy, and radiation in children >3 years old.

Recent genomic studies have identified four subtypes of medulloblastoma with distinct cellular origins, namely WNT, SHH, Group 3, and Group 4, with the WNT subtype having excellent prognosis in both children and adults. Recurrent mutations in CTNNB1, PTCH1, MLL2, SMARCA4, DDX3X, CTDNEP1, KDM6A, and TBR1 have been identified.[56] The pathways of current clinical interest for medulloblastoma include VEGF, SHH as well as WNT, Notch, and ERBB.

### Vascular Endothelial Growth Factor

Anecdotally one child with relapsed medulloblastoma had a near CR with bevacizumab plus irinotecan and another had >30 months of SD.[57] When bevacizumab was combined with irinotecan and temozolomide in children with relapsed medulloblastoma, six of nine (67%) patients had PRs and the other three had SD.[58] Bevacizumab combined with temsirolimus led to 4 months of SD in one patient.[21]

### Sonic Hedgehog

Overexpression of PTCH1, SMO, and suppression of fused homolog mutations are seen in a subtype of medulloblastoma cells. In a preclinical trial, SMO1 inhibitor cyclopamine caused cell cycle arrest *in vitro* and tumor regression *in vivo*. In a phase I trial of vismodegib, an SMO inhibitor, one of three patients with the SHH subtype of medulloblastoma showed anti-tumor activity.[59]

## Retinoblastoma

Retinoblastoma is an embryonal tumor of the eye which has a peak incidence before 2 years of age and 95% are diagnosed by 5 years of age, though rarely cases can occur at any age. Retinoblastoma is one of the most heritable cancers with 30–40% being familial and associated with multi-focal and bilateral tumors and onset <1 year of age. Treatment may include enucleation, external beam radiation, brachytherapy, thermo/cryotherapy, and increasingly effective chemotherapy. Localized tumors amenable to local therapy have a >90% survival, while patients with extracranial metastases have only anecdotal cures despite high-intensity multimodal therapies. Unfortunately, patients with hereditary RB1 mutations have high rates of secondary neoplasms including leiomyosarcoma, osteosarcoma, and melanoma, but not AML. These typically occur >30 years after therapy and have an incidence of 10–25% if non-irradiated and 30–60% if radiation therapy was used to treat the retinoblastoma.

RB1 mutations or deletions occur in >80% of hereditary retinoblastoma tumors, and appears to interact with MDM2/4 alterations, BCOR mutation, and SYK upregulation. The SYK inhibitors R406 and BAY 61-3606 induced caspase-mediated apoptosis in retinoblastoma lines *in vitro*.[60] The most promising preclinical pathways are SYK, AHR, and PLK1[61] though few targeted agents have been tried in retinoblastoma patients, and unfortunately no clinical successes have been reported.

## Conclusions

Although progress in bringing new targeted agents to clinical trial in pediatric cancers has lagged far behind adults, there have been an increasing number of successes in the past few years as can be seen in Table 27.1. As more and more targeted agents are available, access to novel agents will continue to improve for children, and continued efforts to define biologically relevant pathways in pediatric cancers will allow more efficient testing of the agents. With the success of targeting GD2 in neuroblastoma, multiple modest successes in several tumors (e.g., MIBG in neuroblastoma, mTOR in glioma and neuroblastoma, IGF1R in Ewing's sarcoma and neuroblastoma, VEGFR in glioma, sorafenib in osteosarcoma), and numerous anecdotal successes targeting a variety of pathways in a several tumors, targeted therapy appears to hold promise in pediatric solid tumors. Indeed some tumors are associated with multiple compelling targets (e.g., BRAF activation in pilocytic astrocytoma, ALK mutations in neuroblastoma), though clinical success remains elusive, and a few tumors remain a mystery from a targeted therapy perspective, requiring further exploration of their biology and perseverance in clinical trials.

Challenges in pediatric cancer therapies remain as age-related differences in tumor biology, drug metabolism, toxicities, puberty/fertility, and late effects will need to be considered in most cases. As genomic, epigenomic, and proteomic technologies and testing increase, further discovery into rational targeted therapies will continue to emerge. In pediatric solid tumors, predictive-biomarker-based trials are rare and such efforts to enrich potentially responding patient populations may lead to more successes. In a few cases age-related differences in drug metabolism and toxicities have been seen, leading to differences in dose-limiting toxicities and recommended phase II dosing. Adolescence brings challenges to targeted therapy as pubertal changes in drug metabolism, toxicities and issues of fertility preservation become apparent. Finally, with increasing successes, late effects become a critical topic, as these children may survive for >70 years post successful cancer therapy, where neurocognitive impairment, endocrine disruption, subclinical cardiovascular damage, and second malignancies are important considerations. However, despite these challenges and the promise of improved outcomes and decreased toxicities, targeted therapies remain the hope for our children's future.

# References

1 Pugh TJ, Morozova O, Attiyeh EF, et al. The genetic landscape of high-risk neuroblastoma. *Nat Genet*. 2013;45(3):279–284.

2 Matthay KK, George RF, Yu AL. Promising therapeutic targets in neuroblastoma. *Clin Cancer Res*. 2012;18(10):2740–2753.

3 Yu AL, Gilman AL, Ozkaynak MF, et al. Anti-GD2 antibody with GM-CSF, interleukin-2, and isotretinoin for neuroblastoma. *N Engl J Med*. 2010;363(14):1324–1334.

4 Cheung NK, Cheung IY, Kushner BH, et al. Murine anti-GD2 monoclonal antibody 3F8 combined with granulocyte-macrophage colony-stimulating factor and 13-cis-retinoic acid in high-risk patients with stage 4 neuroblastoma in first remission. *J Clin Oncol*. 2012;30(26):3264–3270.

5 Navid F, Sondel PM, Barfield R, et al. Phase I trial of a novel anti-GD2 monoclonal antibody, Hu14.18K322A, designed to decrease toxicity in children with refractory or recurrent neuroblastoma. *J Clin Oncol*. 2014;32(14):1445–1452.

6 Louis CU, Savoldo B, Dotti G, et al. Antitumor activity and long-term fate of chimeric antigen receptor-positive T cells in patients with neuroblastoma. *Blood*. 2011;118(23):6050–6056.

7 Matthay KK, Yanik G, Messina J, et al. Phase II study on the effect of disease sites, age, and prior therapy on response to iodine-131-metaiodobenzylguanidine therapy in refractory neuroblastoma. *J Clin Oncol*. 2007;25(9):1054–1060.

8 de Kraker J, Hoefnagel KA, Verschuur AC, van Eck B, van Santen HM, Caron HN. Iodine-131-metaiodobenzylguanidine as initial induction therapy in stage 4 neuroblastoma patients over 1 year of age. *Eur J Cancer*. 2008;44(4):551–556.

9 DuBois SG, Chesler L, Groshen S, et al. Phase I study of vincristine, irinotecan, and (1)(3)(1)I-metaiodobenzylguanidine for patients with relapsed or refractory neuroblastoma: a new approaches to neuroblastoma therapy trial. *Clin Cancer Res*. 2012;18(9):2679–2686.

10 Mosse YP, Lim MS, Voss SD, et al. Safety and activity of crizotinib for paediatric patients with refractory solid tumours or anaplastic large-cell lymphoma: a Children's Oncology Group phase 1 consortium study. *Lancet Oncol*. 2013;14(6):472–480.

11 Carpenter EL, Haglund EA, Mace EM, et al. Antibody targeting of anaplastic lymphoma kinase induces cytotoxicity of human neuroblastoma. *Oncogene*. 2012;31(46):4859–4867.

12 Weigel B, Malempati S, Reid JM, et al. Phase 2 trial of cixutumumab in children, adolescents, and young adults with refractory solid tumors: a report from the Children's Oncology Group. *Pediatr Blood Cancer*. 2014;61(3):452–456.

13 Spunt SL, Grupp SA, Vik TA, et al. Phase I study of temsirolimus in pediatric patients with recurrent/refractory solid tumors. *J Clin Oncol*. 2011;29(21):2933–2940.

14 Bagatell R, Norris R, Ingle AM, et al. Phase 1 trial of temsirolimus in combination with irinotecan and temozolomide in children, adolescents and young adults with relapsed or refractory solid tumors: a Children's Oncology Group Study. *Pediatr Blood Cancer*. 2014;61(5):833–839.

15 Geoerger B, Kieran MW, Grupp S, et al. Phase II trial of temsirolimus in children with high-grade glioma, neuroblastoma and rhabdomyosarcoma. *Eur J Cancer*. 2012;48(2):253–262.

16 Morgenstern DA, Marzouki M, Bartels U, et al. Phase I study of vinblastine and sirolimus in pediatric patients with recurrent or refractory solid tumors. *Pediatr Blood Cancer*. 2013;61(1):128–133.

17 Di Giannatale A, Dias-Gastellier N, Devos A, et al. Phase II study of temozolomide in combination with topotecan (TOTEM) in relapsed or refractory neuroblastoma: a European Innovative Therapies for Children with Cancer-SIOP-European Neuroblastoma study. *Eur J Cancer*. 2014;50(1):170–177.

18 Jones DT, Hutter B, Jäger N, et al. Recurrent somatic alterations of FGFR1 and NTRK2 in pilocytic astrocytoma. *Nat Genet*. 2013;45(8):927–932.

19 Fouladi M, Perentesis JP, Phillips CL, et al. A phase I trial of MK-2206 in children with refractory malignancies: a Children's Oncology Group study. *Pediatr Blood Cancer*. 2014;61(7):1246–1251.

20 Packer RJ, Jakacki R, Horn M, et al. Objective response of multiply recurrent low-grade gliomas to bevacizumab and irinotecan. *Pediatr Blood Cancer*. 2009;52(7):791–795.

21 Piha-Paul SA, Shin SJ, Vats T, et al. Pediatric patients with refractory central nervous system tumors: experiences of a clinical trial combining bevacizumab and temsirolimus. *Anticancer Res*. 2014;34(4):1939–1945.

22 Krueger DA, Care MM, Agricola K, Tudor C, Mays M, Franz DN. Everolimus long-term safety and efficacy in subependymal giant cell astrocytoma. *Neurology*. 2013;80(6):574–580.

23 MacDonald TJ, Stewart CF, Kocak M, et al. Phase I clinical trial of cilengitide in children with refractory brain tumors: Pediatric Brain Tumor Consortium Study PBTC-012. *J Clin Oncol*. 2008;26(6):919–924.

24 Macdonald TJ, Vezina G, Stewart CF, et al. Phase II study of cilengitide in the treatment of refractory or relapsed high-grade gliomas in children: A report from the Children's Oncology Group. *Neuro Oncol*. 2013;15(10):1438–1444.

25 Hummel TR, Wagner L, Ahern C, et al. A pediatric phase 1 trial of vorinostat and temozolomide in relapsed or refractory primary brain or

spinal cord tumors: a Children's Oncology Group phase 1 consortium study. *Pediatr Blood Cancer*. 2013;60(9):1452–1457.

26 Korshunov A, Meyer J, Capper D, et al. Combined molecular analysis of BRAF and IDH1 distinguishes pilocytic astrocytoma from diffuse astrocytoma. *Acta Neuropathol*. 2009;118(3):401–405.

27 Nicolaides TP, Li H, Solomon DA, et al. Targeted therapy for BRAFV600E malignant astrocytoma. *Clin Cancer Res*. 2011;17(24):7595–7604.

28 Kieran MW, Packer RJ, Onar A, et al. Phase I and pharmacokinetic study of the oral farnesyltransferase inhibitor lonafarnib administered twice daily to pediatric patients with advanced central nervous system tumors using a modified continuous reassessment method: a Pediatric Brain Tumor Consortium Study. *J Clin Oncol*. 2007;25(21):3137–3143.

29 Daw NC, Furman WL, Stewart CF, et al. Phase I and pharmacokinetic study of gefitinib in children with refractory solid tumors: a Children's Oncology Group Study. *J Clin Oncol*. 2005;23(25):6172–6180.

30 Pollack IF, Stewart CF, Kocak M, et al. A phase II study of gefitinib and irradiation in children with newly diagnosed brainstem gliomas: a report from the Pediatric Brain Tumor Consortium. *Neuro Oncol*. 2011;13(3):290–297.

31 Fouladi M, Stewart CF, Blaney SM, et al. Phase I trial of lapatinib in children with refractory CNS malignancies: a Pediatric Brain Tumor Consortium study. *J Clin Oncol*. 2010;28(27):4221–4227.

32 Cabanas R, Saurez G, Rios M, et al. Treatment of children with high grade glioma with nimotuzumab: a 5-year institutional experience. *MAbs*. 2013;5(2):202–207.

33 Massimino M, Bode U, Biassoni V, Fleischhack G. Nimotuzumab for pediatric diffuse intrinsic pontine gliomas. *Expert Opin Biol Ther*. 2011;11(2):247–256.

34 Choy E, Hornicek F, MacConaill L, et al. High-throughput genotyping in osteosarcoma identifies multiple mutations in phosphoinositide-3-kinase and other oncogenes. *Cancer*. 2012;118(11):2905–2914.

35 Fox E, Aplenc R, Bagatell R, et al. A phase 1 trial and pharmacokinetic study of cediranib, an orally bioavailable pan-vascular endothelial growth factor receptor inhibitor, in children and adolescents with refractory solid tumors. *J Clin Oncol*. 2010;28(35):5174–5181.

36 Grignani G, Palmerini E, Dileo P, et al. A phase II trial of sorafenib in relapsed and unresectable high-grade osteosarcoma after failure of standard multimodal therapy: an Italian Sarcoma Group study. *Ann Oncol*. 2012;23(2):508–516.

37 Chawla SP, Staddon AP, Baker LH, et al. Phase II study of the mammalian target of rapamycin inhibitor ridaforolimus in patients with advanced bone and soft tissue sarcomas. *J Clin Oncol*. 2012;30(1):78–84.

38 Frost JD, Hank JA, Reaman GH, et al. A phase I/IB trial of murine monoclonal anti-GD2 antibody 14.G2a plus interleukin-2 in children with refractory neuroblastoma: a report of the Children's Cancer Group. *Cancer*. 1997;80(2):317–333.

39 Merchant MS, Geller JI, Baird K, et al. Phase I trial and pharmacokinetic study of lexatumumab in pediatric patients with solid tumors. *J Clin Oncol*. 2012;30(33):4141–4147.

40 Lessnick SL, Ladanyi M. Molecular pathogenesis of Ewing sarcoma: new therapeutic and transcriptional targets. *Annu Rev Pathol*. 2012;7:145–159.

41 Pappo AS, Patel SR, Crowley J, et al. R1507, a monoclonal antibody to the insulin-like growth factor 1 receptor, in patients with recurrent or refractory Ewing sarcoma family of tumors: results of a phase II Sarcoma Alliance for Research through Collaboration study. *J Clin Oncol*. 2011;29(34):4541–4547.

42 Malempati S, Weigel B, Ingle AM, et al. Phase I/II trial and pharmacokinetic study of cixutumumab in pediatric patients with refractory solid tumors and Ewing sarcoma: a report from the Children's Oncology Group. *J Clin Oncol*. 2012;30(3):256–262.

43 Tap WD, Demetri G, Barnette P, et al. Phase II study of ganitumab, a fully human anti-type-1 insulin-like growth factor receptor antibody, in patients with metastatic Ewing family tumors or desmoplastic small round cell tumors. *J Clin Oncol*. 2012;30(15):1849–1856.

44 Naing A, LoRusso P, Fu S, et al. Insulin growth factor-receptor (IGF-1R) antibody cixutumumab combined with the mTOR inhibitor temsirolimus in patients with refractory Ewing's sarcoma family tumors. *Clin Cancer Res*. 2012;18(9):2625–2631.

45 Leavey P, Glade Bender JL, Mascarenhas L, et al. Feasibility of bevacizumab (NSC 704865, BB-IND# 7921) combined with vincristine, topotecan, and cyclophosphamide in patients with first recurrent Ewing sarcoma (EWS): A Children's Oncology Group (COG) study. *J Clin Oncol*. 2010; 28(15).

46 Wagner L, Turpin B, Nagarajan R, Weiss B, Cripe T, Geller J. Pilot study of vincristine, oral irinotecan, and temozolomide (VOIT regimen) combined with bevacizumab in pediatric patients with recurrent solid tumors or brain tumors. *Pediatr Blood Cancer*. 2013;60(9):1447–1451.

47 Gore L, Trippett TM, Katzenstein HM, et al. A multicenter, first-in-pediatrics, phase 1, pharmacokinetic and pharmacodynamic study of ridaforolimus in patients with refractory solid tumors. *Clin Cancer Res*. 2013;19(13):3649–3658.

48 Benesch M, Windelberg M, Sauseng W, et al. Compassionate use of bevacizumab (Avastin) in children and young adults with refractory or recurrent solid tumors. *Ann Oncol*. 2008;19(4):807–813.

49 Venkatramani R, Malogolowkin M, Davidson TB, May W, Sposto R, Mascarenhas L. A phase I study of vincristine, irinotecan, temozolomide and bevacizumab (vitb) in pediatric patients with relapsed solid tumors. *PLoS One*. 2013;8(7):e68416.

50 Lopez-Terrada D, Gunaratne PH, Adesina AM, et al. Histologic subtypes of hepatoblastoma are characterized by differential canonical Wnt and Notch pathway activation in DLK+ precursors. *Hum Pathol*. 2009;40(6):783–794.

51 Glade Bender J, Blaney SM, Borinstein S, et al. A phase I trial and pharmacokinetic study of aflibercept (VEGF Trap) in children with refractory solid tumors: a children's oncology group phase I consortium report. *Clin Cancer Res*. 2012;18(18):5081–5089.

52 Glade Bender JL, Lee A, Reid JM, et al. Phase I pharmacokinetic and pharmacodynamic study of pazopanib in children with soft tissue sarcoma and other refractory solid tumors: a children's oncology group phase I consortium report. *J Clin Oncol*. 2013;31(24):3034–3043.

53 Weigel BJ, Blaney SM, Reid JM, et al. A phase I study of 17-allylaminogeldanamycin in relapsed/refractory pediatric patients with solid tumors: a Children's Oncology Group study. *Clin Cancer Res*. 2007;13(6):1789–1793.

54 Kilday JP, Rahman R, Dyer S, et al. Pediatric ependymoma: biological perspectives. *Mol Cancer Res*. 2009;7(6):765–786.

55 Gururangan S, Fangusaro J, Young Poussaint T, et al. Lack of efficacy of bevacizumab + irinotecan in cases of pediatric recurrent ependymoma–a Pediatric Brain Tumor Consortium study. *Neuro Oncol*. 2012;14(11):1404–1412.

56 Jones DT, Jäger N, Kool M, et al. Dissecting the genomic complexity underlying medulloblastoma. *Nature*. 2012;488(7409):100–105.

57 Aguilera DG, Goldman S, Fangusaro J. Bevacizumab and irinotecan in the treatment of children with recurrent/refractory medulloblastoma. *Pediatr Blood Cancer*. 2011;56(3):491–494.

58 Aguilera D, Mazewski C, Fangusaro J, et al. Response to bevacizumab, irinotecan, and temozolomide in children with relapsed

medulloblastoma: a multi-institutional experience. *Childs Nerv Syst.* 2013;29(4):589–596.

59 Gajjar A, Stewart CF, Ellison DW, et al. Phase-I study of vismodegib in children with recurrent or refractory medulloblastoma: a Pediatric Brain Tumor Consortium (PBTC) study. *Clin Cancer Res.* 2013;19(22):6305–6312.

60 Zhang J, Benavente CA, McEvoy J, et al. A novel retinoblastoma therapy from genomic and epigenetic analyses. *Nature.* 2012;481(7381):329–334.

61 Ganguly A, Shields CL. Differential gene expression profile of retinoblastoma compared to normal retina. *Mol Vis.* 2010;16:1292–1303.

## CHAPTER 28

# Prostate Cancer

*William G. Nelson, Michael C. Haffner, and Srinivasan Yegnasubramanian*
The Sidney Kimmel Comprehensive Cancer Center and Brady Urological Institute, The Johns Hopkins University School of Medicine, Baltimore, MD, USA

## Introduction

Some 233,000 prostate cancers will be diagnosed in the United States in 2014.[1] The availability of clinical assays for serum prostate-specific antigen (PSA), first used as a tumor biomarker and then later as a screening tool, has increased the fraction of men diagnosed with limited-stage prostate cancer to >90%, leading to more than 75,000 radical prostatectomies each year and even more frequent use of radiation therapy.[2] The increasingly widespread adoption of PSA screening has prompted recent concerns that the disease might be "over-diagnosed" and "over-treated," even though there are now 30% fewer prostate cancer deaths each year since before the test was introduced.[3] However, in spite of this evolution in prostate cancer care, at least 29,480 men will still die of prostate cancer in 2014 in the United States, accounting for 10% of all cancer deaths in men.[1]

Only 5% of men with prostate cancer present now with overt metastatic disease. Instead, most men who ultimately suffer with life-threatening prostate cancer are first diagnosed with localized disease, prompting initial treatment with surgery and/or radiation therapy. For these men, prostate cancer relapses are recognized by detecting increases in serum PSA levels, usually in the absence of clinical or radiological evidence of local or distant recurrence. In one study, by 8 years of follow-up only 29% of men with a rising serum PSA after radical prostatectomy had developed distant metastasis; metastatic progression tended to be heralded by more rapid rates of PSA increases over time.[4] In all, men with recurrent prostate cancer despite local treatment show a median survival >80 months.[5] For men who do develop metastatic disease, prostate cancer progression can threaten symptoms, including bone pain, fatigue, and generally poor performance status. Men with metastatic prostate cancer can expect a median survival in the order of 49 months.[6]

Several systemic treatment options have emerged for prostate cancer, with nine agents earning approval by the Food and Drug Administration (FDA) since 2002 (Table 28.1). Molecular pathways encompassed by current treatments include androgen signaling, microtubule dynamics, bone remodeling, and immune activation. New drugs under development additionally target growth factor/kinase signaling, epigenetics, and immune regulation/checkpoints. To improve prostate cancer outcomes, these new treatments will need to be integrated into existing algorithms and delivered to men most likely to enjoy benefit. Accumulating insights into the molecular pathogenesis of prostate cancer, including into

the heterogeneity of genome alterations between different prostate cancer cases, will likely guide new treatment development by providing molecular diagnostic tools for treatment stratification—hopefully delivering the right treatment to the right man at the right time. This chapter will present a review of the growing portfolio of agents for the systemic treatment of prostate cancer.

## Molecular Pathogenesis of Prostate Cancer

The prostate is a male sex accessory gland that contributes secretions to ejaculate during sexual intercourse. The gland sits in the pelvis between the bladder and the rectum, surrounding the urethra. The prostate is composed of three anatomic zones: (i) the central zone, enveloping the ejaculatory ducts, (ii) the transition zone, near the urethra and the site of benign prostatic hyperplasia/hypertrophy (BPH), and (iii) the peripheral zone, where prostate cancers arise.[7] The prostatic epithelium itself is composed of basal cells, which express the π-class glutathione S-transferase GSTP1, cytokeratins K5/K14, and p63, and of columnar secretory cells, which express the androgen receptor (AR), PSA, cytokeratins K8/K18, prostate-specific membrane antigen (PSMA), and prostate-specific acid phosphatase (PAP).[8] Neuroendocrine cells, which secrete chromogranin A, neuron-specific enolase, and synaptophysin, tend to be scattered about.

Androgenic hormones and an intact AR are both required for normal prostate growth and development, and for maintenance of secretory function. Testosterone (T), the major androgen in the circulation, is mostly produced by testicular Leydig cells upon stimulation by luteinizing hormone (LH). T, in turn, can be converted by 5α-reductase (nicotinamide-adenine dinucleotide-phosphate-dependent $\Delta^4$-3-ketosteroid 5α-oxidoreductase) to 5α-dihydrotestosterone (DHT), a more potent androgen.[9] Both T and DHT act via binding to AR in target cells, triggering a change in receptor shape permitting it to travel to distinct gene regulatory sites in the cell nucleus, to engage co-activators, and to activate selected gene transcription.[10] To turn on genes like *KLK3* (encoding PSA) in prostate cells, AR interacts with genomic DNA at defined androgen-response element (ARE) sequences located within transcriptional promoter and enhancer regions, acting to catalyze marked changes in chromatin organization.[11–13]

Prostate cancer cells arise from the prostatic epithelium and recapitulate many features of the differentiated secretory cell phenotype,

*Targeted Therapy in Translational Cancer Research*, First Edition. Edited by Apostolia-Maria Tsimberidou, Razelle Kurzrock and Kenneth C. Anderson.

**Table 28.1** Drugs approved by the FDA for prostate cancer since 2002.

| Agent | Year of Approval | Class | Indication |
|---|---|---|---|
| Zoledronic acid | 2002 | Bisphosphonate | Reduction in skeletal-disease complications |
| Docetaxel | 2004 | Taxane | Improve survival in CRPC |
| Degarelix | 2008 | Gonadotropin-releasing hormone antagonist | No androgen-mediated "flare" upon initiation |
| Sipuleucel-T | 2010 | Immunotherapy | Improve survival in CRPC |
| Cabazitaxel | 2010 | Taxane | Improve survival in CRPC |
| Abiraterone | 2011 | CYP17 inhibitor | Improve survival in CRPC |
| Enzalutamide | 2012 | Anti-androgen | Improve survival in CRPC |
| Denosumab | 2013 | RANKL antagonist | Reduction in skeletal disease complications |
| $^{223}$Ra | 2013 | Bone-targeted radionuclide | Improve survival in CRPC |

including the expression of AR, PSA, cytokeratins K8/K18, PSMA, PAP.[14] Cancers with basal cell, squamous cell, or neuroendocrine phenotypes are very rare.[15–17] However, unlike normal columnar secretory cells, which use AR signaling to drive terminal differentiation, prostate cancer cells become addicted to AR signaling for growth and survival. One mechanism for this addiction appears to involve somatic translocations between the androgen-regulated gene *TMPRSS2* and various genes, such as *ERG1* and *ETV1*, encoding ETS transcription factors, leading to fusion transcripts in which the oncogenic ETS transcription factor is now regulated by AR.[18,19] The ETS factors promote invasion, undermine terminal differentiation, and redirect the AR transcription program, especially in the setting of additional genome defects like *PTEN* loss.[20] Prostate cancer cell addiction to AR signaling presents an attractive pathway for therapeutic intervention in the vast majority of men with metastatic prostate cancer; reducing circulating androgen levels and/or inhibiting the binding of androgens to AR has been the mainstay systemic treatment for prostate cancer for more than seven decades.[21] The prostate cancer cell addiction to AR signaling can be so strong that progression despite initial androgen deprivation can often be treated with additional hormonal maneuvers.[21] However, for many men with life-threatening disease, prostate cancer ultimately becomes less and less dependent on androgenic hormones, able to grow and survive despite treatment targeting androgen action.

Diet and other lifestyle habits likely drive the epidemic of prostate cancer in the United States. Both incidence and mortality from prostate cancer vary greatly among different regions of the world, with high rates in the United States, particularly among African-Americans, and lower rates in Asia.[22,23] Migrants from Asia to the United States tend to suffer increased risks for prostate cancer, even without inter-marriage, underscoring the dominant effects of the environment on disease development.[24–26] However, inherited susceptibility to prostate cancer also plays a significant role in disease risk; studies comparing concordance for prostate cancer in monozygotic versus dizygotic twins suggest that as many as 40–50% of cases can be attributed to heredity.[27–29] The syndrome of familial prostate cancer, in which the disease shows linkage to rare autosomal or X-linked genes and often presents at an earlier age, likely accounts for only 9% or so of cases.[30,31] Thus far, the combination of genome-wide association (GWAS) and gene mapping studies have hinted that genetic susceptibility to prostate cancer may be complex, with contributions detected from genes involved in cell and genome damage responses (*BRCA2*), host inflammatory responses (*RNASEL*, *MSR1*, and others), prostate development (*HOXB13*), and regulation of *c-MYC* expression.[32–38] When considered together, the environmental and genetic influences on

prostate cancer hint that damage to the prostate, inflicted by dietary carcinogens or infections, may be what initiates disease pathogenesis. This model is supported by the identification of proliferative inflammatory atrophy (PIA) lesions, which arise in response to epithelial damage, as prostate cancer precursors.[7,39]

The prostate is likely barraged by dietary carcinogens, infections, and inflammatory cells for several decades. In autopsy studies, PIA lesions and small prostate cancers have been detected in as many as 30% of men aged 30–40 years, while even with serum PSA screening, most prostate cancers are not diagnosed until men reach 60–70 years of age.[40] Not surprisingly, after years of genome damage, prostate cancer cells accumulate large numbers of somatic genetic and epigenetic defects. In one early report, prostate cancers exhibited a mean of 3866 base mutations (range 3192–5865), 20 non-silent coding sequence mutations (range 13–43), and 108 rearrangements (range 43–213).[41] A case report, in which mutations were surveyed at the time of localized prostate cancer diagnosis, at a time of metastatic progression, and at the time of death, suggested that a single prostate cancer clone was likely to be responsible for malignant lethal progression, acquiring additional somatic genetic defects driving clonal evolution despite many attempts at treatment.[42] Epigenetic defects appear at least as common: somatic DNA hypermethylation has been found in as many as 5408 sites in the genome, with 73% of the regions near genes (5′, 3′, or intron–exon junctions), and 27% of the regions at conserved intergenic loci.[43] As is the case for many other human cancers, the acquired genetic defects catalogued thus far for prostate cancer exhibit significant cell-to-cell, lesion-to-lesion, and case-to-case heterogeneity. Furthermore, which of the genetic changes reflect critical "drivers" of the malignant phenotype, versus "passengers," has been difficult to discriminate. If only ~20 of ~3866 base mutations are non-silent, the fraction of somatic genetic alterations likely to be "drivers" is <1%.[41] Epigenetic alterations may be fundamentally different. Though there are significant case-to-case differences in patterns of DNA hypermethylation, there appears to be markedly less cell-to-cell or lesion-to-lesion heterogeneity.[44] Also, the majority of genes manifesting DNA hypermethylation in prostate cancer may constitute "drivers." Despite the possibility that DNA methylation marks can be actively or passively "erased," hypermethylation patterns in prostate cancer show remarkable stability throughout lethal disease progression.[44]

As described above, the most characteristic somatic genome defect in prostate cancer involves a translocation leading to expression of a fusion transcript between *TMPRSS2* and ETS family of transcription factors, including *ERG1*, *ETV1*, and *ETV4*.[18,45,46] By generating this gene rearrangement, prostate cancer cells co-opt androgen signaling to create an AR-regulated oncogenic "driver." Of

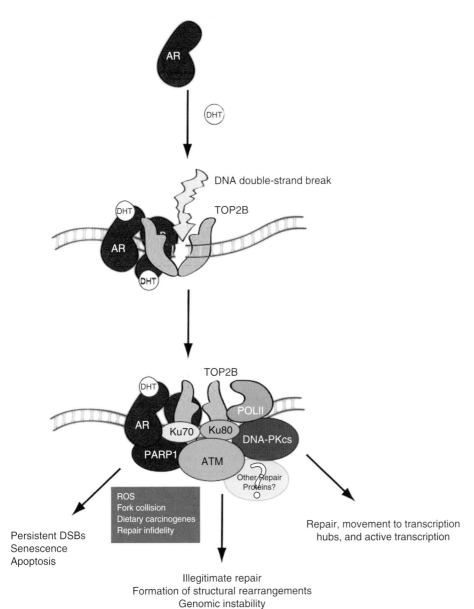

**Figure 28.1** A model for DNA double strand breaks (DSBs) generated by androgen receptor (AR) recruitment of TOP2B during initiation of transcription at target genes. DHT, dihydrotestosterone; DNA-PK, DNA-dependent protein kinase; PARP1, poly(ADP-ribose) polymerase 1; ATM, ataxia-telangiectasia mutated; ROS, reactive oxygen species. *Source:* Reproduced from Haffner et al., 2011, Reference[13] with permission of American Association for Cancer Research (AACR).

interest, the translocations may also be a result of androgen action (Figure 28.1). Androgen-stimulated *trans*-activation of *TMPRSS2* transcription requires AR engagement of TOP2B, an enzyme that uses DNA double-strand breaks to resolve tangling that occurs during assembly of chromatin complexes competent to load RNA polymerase.[47] Inconveniently, TOP2B-mediated DNA double-strand breaks in *TMPRSS2* (and at other sites) appear able to recombine with ETS family partner genes (and others) via non-homologous end-joining, leading to gene fusions preferentially involving AR-regulated genes.[13,47] Among the rearrangements, *TMPRSS2-ERG1* fusions are the most common productive translocations, reported in ~60% of prostate cancers.[48] Nonetheless, neither *TMPRSS2-ERG1* fusions nor *ERG1* expression has great prognostic significance.[48–51] With that in mind, many of the rare genetic changes, such as *SPOP* mutations (6–15%), are found only in prostate cancer cases without *TMPRSS2*-ETS family rearrangements.[52,53]

Most prostate cancer cells express high levels of c-MYC, though the mechanism(s) for *c-MYC* dysregulation during prostatic car-

cinogenesis is not well understood.[54,55] c-MYC in turn promotes activation of ribosomal biogenesis through its target gene *FBL*, encoding the nucleolar protein fibrillarin, leading to a prominently enlarged nucleolus, a hallmark histopathologic feature of prostate cancer.[56] Mice engineered to express c-MYC in prostate cells display a neoplastic phenotype highly reminiscent of human prostate cancer.[57] Another gene subject to dysfunction and somatic alteration in prostate cancer worth mentioning is *PTEN*, the protein and lipid phosphatase which acts to inhibit the phosphatidylinositol 3-kinase/protein kinase B (PI3K/Akt) signaling pathway essential for cell growth and survival.[58–65] PTEN, which is abundantly expressed in normal prostate epithelial cells, tends to disappear in prostate cancer cells as they progress to metastasis.[66] Lethal prostate cancers commonly show somatic *PTEN* alterations, and mice with *Pten* defects display accelerated prostate tumorigenesis.[65,67–69] Loss of *PTEN* in primary prostate cancers may be a harbinger of poor prognosis.[70,71] Of interest, in the absence of PTEN, high-level expression of ERG1 or ETV1 preserved expression of AR-regulated genes, an interaction perhaps capable of sustaining androgen addiction throughout metastatic dissemination.[20]

The most intensively studied, though not the only one, gene target of hypermethylation in prostate cancer is *GSTP1*, encoding the π-class glutathione *S*-transferase.[72,73] Like most genes subjected to epigenetic silencing in human cancers, the protein it encodes, an enzyme capable of catalyzing the detoxification of reactive chemical species via conjugation glutathione, acts as a tumor suppressor. Targeted disruption of π-class GST genes in mice leads to accelerated tumorigenesis in skin treated with the carcinogen 7,12 dimethylbenz(a)anthracene (DMBA) and in intestines of mice with germline *Apc* mutations.[74,75] In nearly all prostate cancer cases, DNA hypermethylation changes encompassing the *GSTP1* transcriptional regulatory region extinguishes GSTP1 expression.[76] Among the many other targets of epigenetic silencing accompanying somatic DNA hypermethylation include genes encoding participants in genome damage and repair, in growth factor signaling, and in cell growth and survival.[77]

## Systemic Prostate Cancer Treatments Targeting Androgen Signaling

The vast majority of prostate cancers show some level of addiction to androgenic hormones. For this reason, treatment approaches intended to antagonize androgen signaling have historically shown great benefit and have gained wide use, both for metastatic prostate cancer and as adjuvant therapy, for high-risk localized or locally advanced prostate cancer. The two general strategies involve androgen deprivation (also referred to as androgen suppression) and administration of AR antagonists. Almost all men with prostate cancer respond, at least initially, to lowering circulating T levels to <50 ng/mL. This response to androgen deprivation is characterized by a rapid fall in serum PSA, a pharmacodynamic biomarker of androgen signaling in prostate cancer cells, and by a reduction in disease-associated symptoms such as bone pain, if present. In rare cases, androgen deprivation fails to trigger such a response. For these men, the prostate cancers appear not to be endowed with "driver" mutations, like *TMRPSS2*-ETS family gene fusions, that co-opt androgen signaling.

Androgen deprivation was historically accomplished via removal of the testis, eliminating the Leydig cells supplying the majority of circulating T. Bilateral orchiectomy, though effective, has largely been supplanted by non-surgical approaches. The first non-surgical strategy for androgen suppression was the use of high doses of estrogens, such as diethylstilbestrol (DES), which lowered T effectively but tended to create cardiovascular complications.[78] Nowadays, surgery and estrogen therapy have been largely replaced by administration of long-acting inhibitors of pituitary gonadotropic hormone production, luteinizing-hormone-releasing hormone (LHRH) analogs (leuprolide, goserelin, and others) and antagonists (abarelix, degarelix, and others). The propensity for LHRH analogs to briefly elevate LH levels before suppressing them has been reported to rarely trigger symptomatic prostate cancer "flares" in men with painful bone metastasis, a property not shared by LHRH antagonists.[79] Despite these minor nuances, data from numerous randomized clinical trials suggests that the various approaches to androgen deprivation tend to be equally effective for prostate cancer treatment. As such, most men in need of systemic treatment for prostate cancer initially receive LHRH agonists or antagonists for androgen suppression.

Unfortunately, for advanced prostate cancer, responses to androgen deprivation to be short-lived (16 months or so) and *castration-resistant prostate cancer (CRPC)* inevitably emerges. In this setting, the serum PSA begins to rise, heralding symptomatic progression if the disease cannot be controlled. *KLK3*, encoding PSA, requires AR for transcription.[12] The rising serum PSA in CRPC thus provides a significant mechanistic clue that addiction to AR has persisted even in the face of low serum T (and DHT) levels.[80] This persistent AR addiction in CRPC was not well recognized until relatively recently, when such a phenotype was encountered in human prostate cancer xenograft models progressing after castration. In these tumors, AR levels were markedly increased, preserving the AR transcriptional output despite low T levels.[81] Both *AR* amplification and *AR* mutation have been detected in progressive CRPC.[80] Increased AR expression appears to lead to CRPC progression by augmenting AR ligand sensitivity and to increasing AR ligand promiscuity.[81] *AR* mutations, particularly those arising in the setting of AR antagonist treatment, often confer an "antagonist-to-agonist switch," in which the mutant AR promotes transcriptional *trans*-activation signal upon antagonist binding.[21] Clinically, this phenomenon appears responsible for an "anti-androgen withdrawal" syndrome, where men with CRPC improve upon discontinuation of anti-androgen treatment.[82] CPRC may also be driven by intratumoral androgen synthesis, by expression of altered AR forms encoded by mRNA splice variants, or by growth factor signaling-associated post-translational modifications of AR.[10,80,83,84]

Production of androgens by the adrenal glands or in the cancer microenvironment, biosynthesis pathways that elude suppression by LHRH analogs and antagonists, can fuel CRPC progression.[10,85] The key molecular participant in both gonadal and extragonadal steroidogenic pathways is CYP17, the enzyme target of ketoconazole, abiraterone, and several new drugs under development.[10,85,86] CYP17 catalyzes the production of androgenic hormones via initial 17-α-hydroxylation of pregnenolone and progesterone followed by C17,20 lyase action to create the T precursors dehydroepiandrosterone and androstenedione. Abiraterone, a potent CYP17 inhibitor, gained FDA approval for CRPC in 2011 (Figure 28.2). Its use has been accompanied by stigmata of mineralocorticoid excess, including fluid retention (30.5%), hypokalemia (17.1%), and hypertension (1.3%), that have been attributed to CYP17 17-α-hydroxylase inhibition.[86,87] Newer CYP17 inhibitors, including galeterone, orteronel, and VT-464, exhibit greater selectivity for the enzyme's C17,20 lyase activity, and may trigger less mineralocorticoid side effects.[88]

In contrast to agents that suppress androgen biosynthesis and indirectly attenuate AR *trans*-activation of target gene transcription, anti-androgens *directly* antagonize AR. The first-generation AR antagonists, bicalutamide, flutamide, and nilutamide, were rarely given as single agents, because feedback production of estrogens was too often complicated by gynecomastia and cardiovascular complications. Instead, the agents were most commonly administered concurrently with LHRH analogs in an attempt to achieve "complete androgen blockade" by both reducing androgen levels and antagonizing binding of non-gonadal androgens to AR.[89] The "complete androgen blockade" effected using first-generation AR antagonists is not likely superior in controlling prostate cancer progression to androgen deprivation alone; a meta-analysis of all published clinical trials testing this hypothesis conducted by the Agency for Health Care Policy and Research (AHCPR; see report number 99-E012 at http://www.ahcpr.gov/clinic/index.html) reported no meaningful differences in survival rates favoring combined

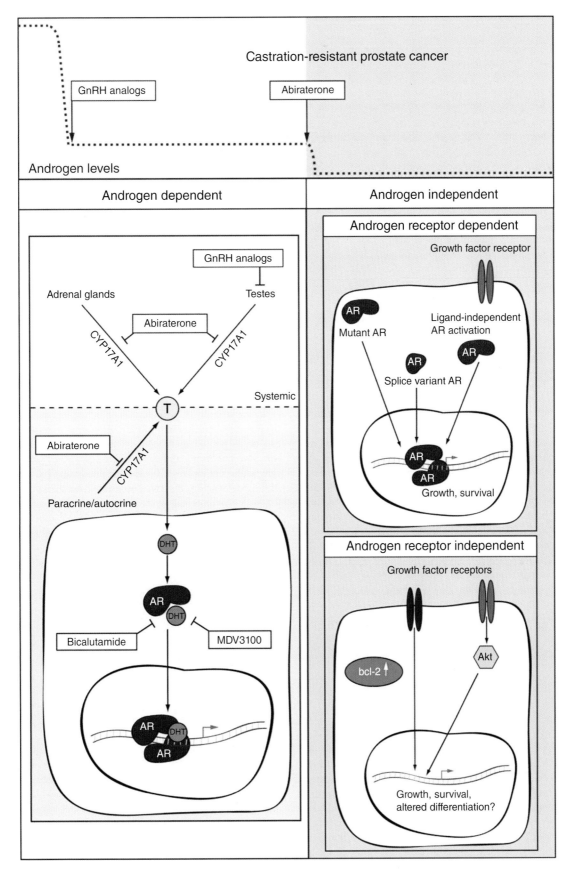

**Figure 28.2** Abiraterone, a CYP17 inhibitor, further reduces androgen levels when used to treat CRPC. Prostate cancers can progress despite abiraterone therapy, becoming androgen independent, either via maintained addiction to AR signaling (androgen-receptor dependent) or by abandoning AR signaling (androgen-receptor independent). *Source:* Reproduced from Nelson et al., 2011, Reference[166] with permission from Elsevier.

treatment.[90] The appearance of newer-generation anti-androgens, with less partial AR agonist properties, may prompt a reassessment of "complete androgen blockade." The first such drug, enzalutamide, was approved by the FDA approval treatment of CRPC in 2012.[91] A second agent, ARN-509, is under active development.[92]

For both first and second-generation anti-androgens, acquired *AR* mutations altering ligand specificity have been described.[93-96] The role of AR mutations responsible for the anti-androgen "withdrawal" phenomenon that accompanies discontinuation of first-generation anti-androgens has already been discussed. However, more recently, a new AR mutation, resulting in an F876L change in the AR ligand-binding region, has been described that may potentially bedevil second-generation anti-androgen treatment of CRPC.[93-95] Both enzalutamide and ARN-509 appear to bind this mutant receptor with increased affinity to trigger agonist receptor function. Alarmingly, mutant *AR* sequences (a C-to-A change at nt 2628 encoding the F876L mutation) appeared in plasma DNA from three men in a phase I clinical trial of ARN-509 for metastatic CRPC who had initially responded to treatment but then ultimately progressed.[93] Of interest, in xenograft tumor models, prostate cancer cells acquiring F876L *AR* mutations grew poorly, raising the possibility that this mutant AR might not persist if enzalutamide or ARN-509 were discontinued.[94] The clinical manifestation of this phenomenon would be a second-generation anti-androgen "withdrawal" syndrome.

For anti-cancer drugs, like anti-microbials, the emergence of treatment resistance despite initial treatment benefit continues to pose a difficult challenge (Figure 28.3). Goldie and Coldman employed fluctuation analysis, first described by Luria and Delbrück decades earlier, to assess the mechanism(s) by which drug-treated cancers acquire resistance to the drugs used.[97,98] For cancer, drug resistance could be ascribed to intrinsic capabilities of cancer cells to adapt to drug exposure, modulating phenotypic properties to elude drug cytotoxicity without altering genome structure or organization, or to spontaneous mutation from ongoing genome instability in cancers before, during, and after initial drug treatment, generating variant cancer cell clones capable of escaping drug killing. The mutant or amplified *AR* genes appearing in the setting of treatments targeting androgen signaling are likely examples of spontaneous mutation followed by selection. However, both mutation/selection and adaptation likely contribute in some way to clinically significant resistance to hormonal treatments for advanced prostate cancer.

Adaptive resistance displayed by prostate cancer cells may resemble physiological mechanisms exhibited by normal prostate epithelial cells upon androgen deprivation and/or anti-androgen administration. In response to castration, mammalian prostates typically undergo involution, characterized by a disappearance of differentiated columnar epithelial cells and a reduction in the number of basal-like epithelial cells.[99,100] The columnar cells undergo a nearly synchronous wave of apoptosis, with the majority of apoptotic cells phagocytosed by adjacent epithelial cells, preventing compromise of epithelial barrier function, and limiting presentation of fragments of tissue-restricted proteins to immune antigen-presenting cells (APCs), attenuating anti-cancer immunity. The remaining basal-like cells possess "stem-cell" properties, capable of renewing an epithelium containing basal, columnar, and neuroendocrine epithelial cells.[8] Among other attributes, the basal-like stem cells express high levels of the anti-apoptotic protein Bcl-2.[101]

Could a prostate cancer "stem-cell" be responsible for resistance to treatments targeting the androgen signaling pathway? Such a stem cell would likely express little or no AR, and not be addicted to AR for survival. Presumably, the administration of T to a man who responded to androgen deprivation would unmask the restorative potential of resistant prostate cancer "stem cells," promoting a rise in serum PSA. In addition, intermittent androgen deprivation should result in recurrent beneficial treatment responses, as more mature prostate cancer cells, expressing high levels of AR, are reproducibly eliminated. Although the "stem-cell" theory for adaptive resistance to androgen deprivation and/or anti-androgen administration has some compelling attributes, controversy remains over whether prostate cancer "stem cells" can be specifically identified or targeted for elimination, and whether the neoplastic prostate "stem cells" exhibit more plasticity than normal prostate cells, able to be recruited from mature prostate cancer cells.[102,103]

Another source of adaptive resistance to abrogation of androgen signaling may be augmented collaborative or compensatory signaling through other cell growth and survival pathways. AR transactivation of target genes can be augmented by co-administration of many polypeptide cytokines and growth factors.[80] Perhaps the most compelling pathway that may be subverted to undermine androgen deprivation and anti-androgen treatment may be PI3K/Akt signaling. As mentioned above, PTEN, typically present in normal prostate cells and in indolent prostate cancers, frequently vanishes as the cancers progress to threaten life.[65-69] Of course, absence of PTEN lipid phosphatase activity can augment PI3K/Akt signals, and mice engineered to express activated Akt in prostate cells manifest prostatic intraepithelial neoplasia, and in the setting of disrupted genes encoding p27, prostate cancer.[104-106] Unfortunately, despite the potential contributions of PI3K/Akt signaling to lethal prostate cancer progression, therapeutic agents targeting the PI3K/Akt pathway have not been very active against CRPC thus far.[107,108] While this may be a reflection of the specific drug or drug target explored, PI3K/Akt signaling may just be difficult to disrupt successfully for the purpose of killing prostate cancer cells. Though the prostatic intraepithelial neoplasia in mice attributable to activated Akt could be ameliorated with an mTOR inhibitor, when these mice were crossed to strains also expressing high levels of c-MYC, small molecule antagonists of the Akt signaling pathway were only weakly effective, and became even less effective as the animals aged, suggesting that dysregulation of c-MYC and other genes might compromise undermine PI3K/Akt inhibitor effects.[109] Perhaps, adaptive resistance to antagonism of androgen action mediated by PI3K/Akt signaling pathways might better be addressed in the setting of *intrinsic* resistance to androgen deprivation or anti-androgen treatment; that is, PI3K/Akt inhibitors might be more effective if administered in conjunction with the initiation of hormonal therapy for prostate cancer.[110] For breast cancer responsive to hormonal therapy, co-administration of the mTOR inhibitor everolimus along with the aromatase inhibitor exemestane has dramatically improved outcomes in a randomized clinical trial.[111]

The generation of variant AR forms in CRPC cells via disruption of physiologic mRNA splicing may present another adaptive resistance mechanism. Several AR splice variants have been identified in CPRC cells that lack a ligand-binding domain (LBD) but can mediate transcriptional *trans*-activation of AR target genes.[112,113] These AR variants arise from mRNAs containing insertions or deletions of exons that encode receptors endowed with DNA-binding domains but not LBDs. In preclinical studies, forced expression of variant ARs promotes growth of CRPC cells, whether or not antagonists such as enzalutamide are present, suggesting that variant ARs can compensate for wild-type AR in maintaining addiction to

## Mechanisms of resistance to AR-directed therapies

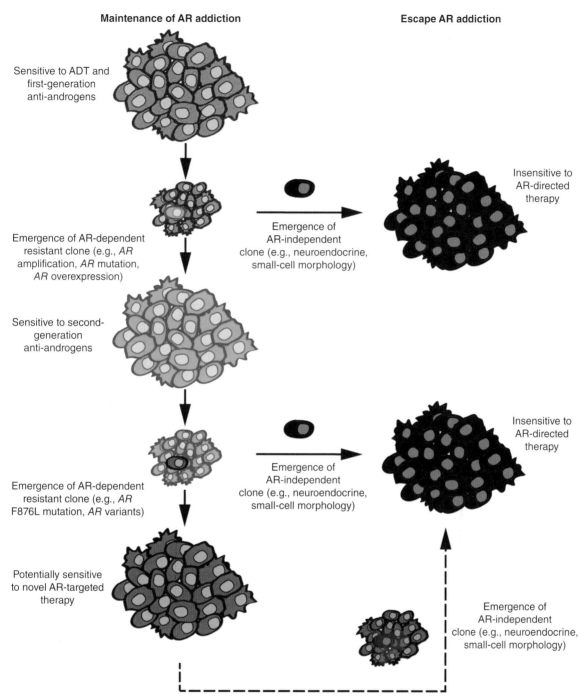

**Maintenance of AR addiction**

**Escape AR addiction**

Sensitive to ADT and first-generation anti-androgens

Emergence of AR-dependent resistant clone (e.g., *AR* amplification, *AR* mutation, *AR* overexpression)

Sensitive to second-generation anti-androgens

Emergence of AR-dependent resistant clone (e.g., *AR* F876L mutation, *AR* variants)

Potentially sensitive to novel AR-targeted therapy

Emergence of AR-independent clone (e.g., neuroendocrine, small-cell morphology)

Insensitive to AR-directed therapy

Emergence of AR-independent clone (e.g., neuroendocrine, small-cell morphology)

Insensitive to AR-directed therapy

Emergence of AR-independent clone (e.g., neuroendocrine, small-cell morphology)

**Figure 28.3** Mechanisms of resistance to AR-directed therapies. Progression to CRPC after initial treatments targeting androgen action often reflects persistent addiction to AR signaling, permitting the successful use of second-generation anti-androgens. Ultimately, both AR-dependent and -independent clones can emerge. *Source:* Reproduced from Reference[21].

AR signaling.[83,114] These splice variant AR forms are likely to be clinically significant. A recent meeting report revealed that the splice variant AR-V7 could be detected in circulating tumor cells (CTCs) from 39% of men with CRPC, including from 55% of men who had also been treated with abiraterone.[115] Astonishingly, when men with detectable AR-V7 were treated with enzalutamide, none responded, while many of the men without AR-V7 showed a benefit to enzalutamide administration, with a decline in PSA or diminution in measurable lesions. The likely contribution of AR-V7 and other splice variants to resistance to androgen deprivation and anti-androgens has motivated an effort to discover and develop agents that target regions of AR other than the LBD.[116]

Finally, some men with CRPC exhibit striking treatment responses to androgen administration.[117] One potential mechanism may be the stabilization of AR by its ligand, particularly in the setting of increased AR levels in CRPC cells, allowing binding to replication complexes in cancer cell nuclei in such a way as to prevent re-licensing of replication initiation sites needed for ongoing cell proliferation.[118] Another mechanism could involve AR stimulation of genome damage mediated by TOP2B.[13] Upon agonist ligand binding, AR recruits TOP2B to its genome-binding sites to resolve DNA tangling generated by creation of looped gene promoter/enhancer structures and by movement of activated target genes to transcriptional hubs.[47] The resultant "trapping" of TOP2B-DNA complexes, recapitulating the action of several notable anti-cancer drugs (including anthracyclines, anthracenes, and epipodophyllotoxins), leads to potentially lethal genome damage (Figure 28.1). The possibility that androgens might benefit men with CRPC has prompted a series of clinical trials aimed at cyclical androgen administration and withdrawal or anti-androgen treatment.

## Non-androgen Signaling-Targeted Systemic Treatments

The most effective cytotoxic chemotherapy drugs for prostate cancer are the taxanes paclitaxel, docetaxel, and cabazitaxel, which interfere with microtubule dynamics to cause cell death.[119] Prostate cancer cells may be exquisitely sensitive to disruptors of microtubule function. Nearly all FDA-approved drugs capable of interfering with microtubule assembly and disassembly, including colchicine and vinca alkaloids in addition to taxanes, exhibit activity against human prostate cancer cells *in vitro*.[120] Historically, microtubule-targeted drugs have been thought to kill cancer cells via interruption of mitotic chromosome segregation needed for cell division. However, the propensity for microtubule-targeted drugs to control prostate cancers, which often have low proliferative rates, has promulgated the notion that the drugs might instead act to attenuate nuclear-cytoplasmic trafficking of critical proteins like AR.[121] The possibility that taxanes, and other microtubule-targeted agents, might treat CRPC by functioning, in part, to interfere with AR signaling, is enticing given the activity of drugs like abiraterone and enzalutamide in this setting.

The survival benefit of docetaxel for CRPC was established in two randomized clinical trials, TAX-327, which tested two different docetaxel single-agent infusion schedules against mitoxantrone and prednisone, and SWOG-9916, which tested docetaxel and estramustine against mitoxantrone and prednisone.[122, 123] In both studies, docetaxel-containing treatment arms outperformed mitoxantrone therapy in terms of serum PSA declines, disease-associated symptom control, and overall survival.[122, 123] Nevertheless, when docetaxel was combined with estramustine, an unacceptably high rate of venous thromboembolism (VTE) was seen that appeared insensitive to prophylactic low-dose warfarin and aspirin. As a result of this and other toxicities, docetaxel is not commonly administered with estramustine; instead, docetaxel is usually given as a single agent for 5–8 treatment cycles to promote disease stabilization. If after a docetaxel "holiday" CRPC again progresses, a significant fraction of men benefit from retreatment with the drug.[124, 125] CPRC felt resistant to docetaxel can be treated with cabazitaxel, a second-generation taxane that was thought to be less susceptible to drug resistance via efflux pumping.[126] The drug gained FDA approval for docetaxel-resistant CRPC by exhibiting improved survival in a randomized comparison with mitoxantrone.[127] Direct comparisons between docetaxel and cabazitaxel in CRPC are currently underway in large randomized trials.

Taxane chemotherapy appears poised for use in androgen-sensitive metastatic prostate cancer in combination with androgen deprivation. Early reports from a randomized trial pitting androgen deprivation therapy alone or with single-agent docetaxel for men with metastatic prostate cancer revealed an increase in median survival from 44 months to 57.6 months as a consequence of adding taxane chemotherapy.[128] Even more astonishingly, among men with high volume metastatic cancer, the improvement in median survival attributable to docetaxel was from 32.2 months to 49.2 months.[128] With this finding almost certain to drive adoption of androgen deprivation plus docetaxel for young men with metastatic prostate cancer, what will comprise the phenotype of CPRC that emerges later? The appearance of a rising serum PSA as evidence of disease progression despite androgen deprivation/docetaxel hints that CPRC emerging in this setting will likely have maintained some addiction to AR.

## Bone-Targeted Systemic Treatments

The skeleton is disproportionately threatened by progressive prostate cancer. Bone metastases are recognized in at least 75% of men with life-threatening CRPC, and treatments targeting androgen signaling used in men with CRPC promote osteopenia and osteoporosis. This combination can and does frequently lead to pain, fractures, and complications like spinal cord compression. Bisphosphonates can be administered to improve skeletal integrity by antagonizing osteoclast action. In the absence of bone metastases, several of the available bisphosphonates can attenuate treatment-associated osteoporosis. However, for men with overt bone metastases, only zoledronic acid has been found to reduce skeletal complications in randomized trials, leading to FDA approval of the drug for men with CRPC and bone metastases.[129, 130] Like other bisphosphonates, zoledronic acid must be used with caution in men with renal impairment. Osteoclasts can be activated to resorb bone by the receptor activator of nuclear factor-$\kappa$B ligand (RANKL), which binds to a cell-surface receptor. Denosumab, an antibody inhibitor of RANKL able to reduce bone resorption by osteoclasts, has been found to lower skeletal complications in men with prostate cancer in a randomized trial.[131–133] Both zoledronic acid and denosumab have been associated with osteonecrosis of the jaw.[134]

Bone-seeking radiopharmaceuticals, which accumulate at sites of bone formation, have also proven useful in the care of men with CRPC complicated by symptomatic bone metastases. Three such agents have gained FDA-approval: $^{89}$Sr, $^{153}$Sm, and $^{223}$Ra. $^{89}$Sr, and $^{153}$Sm, which both emit $\beta$-particles that can travel as far as a few millimeters, relieve pain accompanying widespread prostate cancer bone metastases, but do so at a risk of bone marrow toxicity.[135] As such, these radionuclides, which do not improve survival for men with CRPC as single agents, make poor partners for cytotoxic drugs that also threaten blood-forming cells. $^{223}$Ra is an $\alpha$-particle emitter that can deliver denser ionizing radiation over a substantially narrower range (a few cell diameters).[136] When used to treat prostate cancer, nearly 40–60% of the administered $^{223}$Ra dose ends up at the sites of bone metastases.[137] In a pivotal randomized trial, $^{223}$Ra was compared to placebo for men with CRPC who had been previously treated with docetaxel or were considered unfit for chemotherapy treatment.[138, 139] Among the men who received $^{223}$Ra, an improvement in overall survival was demonstrated, forming the basis for

FDA approval in 2013.[138,139] [223]Ra also appeared very safe, with few adverse events accompanying treatment. If [223]Ra can effectively treat men with CPRC and painful bone metastases, and can do so without interference with hematopoiesis, combination treatment with taxanes (or other cytotoxic agents), may be possible.

## Immunotherapy

There have been many attempts to overcome immune tolerance induced by prostate cancer cells in order to activate effective anti-tumor immune responses that can control prostate cancer progression.[140,141] Prostate cancers likely contain a number of antigens that can be selectively recognized by T cells, including peptides derived from lineage-restricted proteins like PSA and prostatic acid phosphatase (PAP), neopeptides derived from proteins only in present cancer cells containing missense mutations, and peptides derived from proteins otherwise epigenetically silenced in normal adult cells but expressed in cancer cells with reduced DNA methylation levels.[142] Unfortunately, T cells capable of responding to these peptide antigens are stereotypically difficult to activate for the purpose of immune destruction of prostate cancer cells. Mouse models of autochthonous prostate tumorigenesis in the setting of an intact immune system have defined some of the immune tolerance barriers and opportunities.[143] In these models, T-cell tolerance to prostate antigens appears early during tumor development, with reduced CD4+ T-cell responsiveness and emergence of regulatory CD4+ T cells evident even before overt tumors can be detected.[143] However, androgen deprivation seems to create a "window" of reduced T-cell tolerance. Treatment of mouse prostate tumors by castration reduced T-cell tolerance, and maintained the responsiveness of adoptively transferred T cells to antigen-specific vaccination.[143] A similar phenomenon has been detected in human prostates after androgen deprivation, with an influx and expansion of selected T-cell clones hinting at antigen-specific responses.[144-147]

The only immunotherapy currently approved by the FDA is sipuleucel-T, a product generated by loading expanded patient-specific APCs *ex vivo* with a fusion protein formed from PAP linked to granulocyte-macrophage-colony-stimulating factor (GM-CSF). The treatment strategy is to use these APC vaccines to create PAP-directed T-cell responses capable of destroying prostate cancer cells.[148] Unfortunately, though T-cell responses can be elicited in men with CRPC, the benefits of sipuleucel-T treatment are minimal, with few PSA declines (<3%), fewer radiographic responses, and no improvement in time-to-disease progression.[149] A randomized trial sipuleucel-T versus a placebo delivered a survival difference, with 61% of the sipuleucel-T-treated men versus 70.8% of placebo-treated men alive at the time of the trial report.[150] The interpretation of benefit was criticized because men treated with placebo were able to undergo treatment with sipuleucel-T at the time of disease; that is, the trial was more a test of early versus late sipuleucel-T followed by subsequent early versus late docetaxel, than of sipuleucel-T versus placebo *per se*.[151] Provocatively, there has been a report of an impressive response to sipuleucel-T given along with enzalutamide, hinting that antigen-specific T-cell tolerance may be more readily overcome in the setting of antagonism of androgen action.[152] Another lineage antigen-specific vaccine, Prostvac-VF, composed of poxvirus vectors driving expression of PSA and immune co-stimulatory molecules B7.1 (CD80), leukocyte function-associated antigen-3 (CD58), and intercellular adhesion molecule-1 (CD54), has reached phase III trials for prostate cancer.[153]

The immune checkpoint inhibitor ipilimumab, which acts to undermine T-cell tolerance associated with cancer, earned FDA approval for treatment of metastatic melanoma in 2011. Ipilimumab has demonstrated provocative preclinical activity in mouse models of prostate cancer, particularly if administered in conjunction with tumor antigen vaccines or along with radiation therapy.[154-157] However, the behavior of ipilimumab in men with CRPC in a randomized clinical trial was less impressive.[158] The rationale for the trial was to provide prostate cancer antigens via radiotherapy of limited bone metastases, and to allow these antigens to prime anti-cancer immune responses in the presence of ipilimumab. Men were treated with a single 8 Gy fraction of radiotherapy to a bone lesion followed by infusions of ipilimumab or placebo. Unfortunately, there was no survival advantage that could be attributed to ipilimumab, and serious immune-related side effects were seen in 26% of men treated with death in 1%.[158] Despite this disappointing result, further development of immune checkpoint inhibitors, including those targeting PD-1/PD-L1 interactions and others, are ongoing.

## Future Perspectives

The past decade and a half has seen unprecedented systemic treatment development for prostate cancer, and dramatic reductions in United States prostate cancer deaths. The rationale underlying one of the first molecularly targeted approaches to any human cancer, that of lowering androgen levels to treat advanced prostate cancer, continues to dominate the systemic therapy for the disease. New drugs that more dramatically interfere with androgen synthesis and better antagonize AR function have emerged with demonstrated benefit in prolonging survival from life-threatening prostate cancer. Molecular mechanisms for resistance to these new agents are increasingly better understood, with avenues for improving treatment benefits becoming realized. Taxane chemotherapy has become well established. Combinations of androgen signaling antagonists with taxane chemotherapy, and with various other growth factor signaling inhibitors, appear poised to improve outcomes. In addition, various agents that can be used to reduce the morbidity and mortality associated with bone metastases have been introduced and adopted. Finally, immunotherapy for prostate cancer can be readily anticipated, with vaccines and immune checkpoint inhibitors under intense scrutiny for disease control.

On the horizon, epigenetic agents, nanomedicines, selective prodrugs, and other treatment maneuvers can be visualized. Each of these approaches will require meticulous translational research development for success in prostate cancer treatment. For example, as discussed above, hypermethylation of transcriptional regulatory sequences constitutes a pervasive somatic alteration in prostate cancer cells that drives selective expansion of lethal metastatic cancer clones. Yet, available inhibitors of DNA methyltransferases (DNMTs), such as azacitidine and decitabine, only reduce $^{5-m}$CpG density modestly in dividing cancer cells.[159-162] When used in a clinical trial for men with CRPC, decitabine, given at a dose and schedule that may not optimally reduce $^{5-m}$CpG levels in prostate cancer cells, was only able to stabilize disease progression in 2 of the 12 men treated.[163] Clearly, for DNMT inhibitor therapy to be effective against CRPC, a new and different drug, drug administration, or drug combination treatment strategy will be needed that better reduces DNA methylation and reactivates silenced genes. Provocatively, in a clinical trial for non-small cell lung cancer, while treatment with epigenetic drugs really only achieved a modicum of disease stabilization, subsequent administration of chemotherapy drugs or immune checkpoint inhibitors triggered dramatic tumor responses.[164,165] Epigenetic "priming" of responses to immunotherapies or other modes of treatment may offer an exciting direction for CPRC therapy of the future.

# References

1 Siegel R, Ma J, Zou Z, Jemal A. Cancer statistics, 2014. *CA Cancer J Clin.* 2014;64(1):9–29.

2 Sammon JD, Karakiewicz PI, Sun M, et al. Robot-assisted versus open radical prostatectomy: the differential effect of regionalization, procedure volume and operative approach. *J Urol.* 2013;189(4):1289–1294.

3 Etzioni R, Tsodikov A, Mariotto A, et al. Quantifying the role of PSA screening in the US prostate cancer mortality decline. *Cancer Causes Control.* 2008;19(2):175–181.

4 Antonarakis ES, Trock BJ, Feng Z, et al. The natural history of metastatic progression in men with PSA-recurrent prostate cancer after radical prostatectomy: 25-year follow-up. *J Clin Oncol.* 2009;27(15).

5 Makarov DV, Humphreys EB, Mangold LA, et al. The natural history of men treated with deferred androgen deprivation therapy in whom metastatic prostate cancer developed following radical prostatectomy. *J Urol.* 2008;179(1):156–161; discussion 161–162.

6 Hussain M, Tangen CM, Higano C, et al. Absolute prostate-specific antigen value after androgen deprivation is a strong independent predictor of survival in new metastatic prostate cancer: Data from Southwest Oncology Group trial 9346 (INT-0162). *J Clin Oncol.* 2006;24(24):3984–3990.

7 De Marzo AM, Platz EA, Sutcliffe S, et al. Inflammation in prostate carcinogenesis. *Nat Rev Cancer.* 2007;7(4):256–269.

8 De Marzo AM, Nelson WG, Meeker AK, Coffey DS. Stem cell features of benign and malignant prostate epithelial cells. *J Urol.* 1998;160(6 Pt 2):2381–2392.

9 Steers WD. 5alpha-reductase activity in the prostate. *Urology.* 2001;58(6 suppl. 1):17–24; discussion

10 Green SM, Mostaghel EA, Nelson PS. Androgen action and metabolism in prostate cancer. *Mol Cell Endocrinol.* 2012;360(1–2):3–13.

11 Roche PJ, Hoare SA, Parker MG. A consensus DNA-binding site for the androgen receptor. *Mol Endocrinol.* 1992;6(12):2229–2235.

12 Schuur ER, Henderson GA, Kmetec LA, Miller JD, Lamparski HG, Henderson DR. Prostate-specific antigen expression is regulated by an upstream enhancer. *J Biol Chem.* 1996;271(12):7043–7051.

13 Haffner MC, De Marzo AM, Meeker AK, Nelson WG, Yegnasubramanian S. Transcription-induced DNA double strand breaks: both oncogenic force and potential therapeutic target? *Clin Cancer Res.* 2011;17(12):3858–3864.

14 De Marzo AM, Meeker AK, Zha S, et al. Human prostate cancer precursors and pathobiology. *Urology.* 2003;62(5 suppl. 1):55–62.

15 Ali TZ, Epstein JI. Basal cell carcinoma of the prostate: a clinicopathologic study of 29 cases. *Am J Surg Pathol.* 2007;31(5):697–705.

16 Parwani AV, Kronz JD, Genega EM, Gaudin P, Chang S, Epstein JI. Prostate carcinoma with squamous differentiation: an analysis of 33 cases. *Am J Surg Pathol.* 2004;28(5):651–657.

17 Epstein JI, Amin MB, Beltran H, et al. Proposed morphologic classification of prostate cancer with neuroendocrine differentiation. *Am J Surg Pathol.* 2014;38(6):756–767.

18 Tomlins SA, Rhodes DR, Perner S, et al. Recurrent fusion of TMPRSS2 and ETS transcription factor genes in prostate cancer. *Science.* 2005;310(5748):644–648.

19 Rubin MA, Maher CA, Chinnaiyan AM. Common gene rearrangements in prostate cancer. *J Clin Oncol.* 2011;29(27):3659–3668.

20 Chen Y, Chi P, Rockowitz S, et al. ETS factors reprogram the androgen receptor cistrome and prime prostate tumorigenesis in response to PTEN loss. *Nat Med.* 2013;19(8):1023–1029.

21 Nelson WG, Yegnasubramanian S. Resistance emerges to second-generation antiandrogens in prostate cancer. *Cancer Discov.* 2013;3(9):971–974.

22 Hsing AW, Tsao L, Devesa SS. International trends and patterns of prostate cancer incidence and mortality. *Int J Cancer.* 2000;85(1):60–67.

23 Reddy S, Shapiro M, Morton R Jr., Brawley OW. Prostate cancer in black and white Americans. *Cancer Metastasis Rev.* 2003;22(1):83–86.

24 Whittemore AS, Kolonel LN, Wu AH, et al. Prostate cancer in relation to diet, physical activity, and body size in blacks, whites, and Asians in the United States and Canada. *J Natl Cancer Inst.* 1995;87(9):652–661.

25 Haenszel W, Kurihara M. Studies of Japanese migrants. I. Mortality from cancer and other diseases among Japanese in the United States. *J Natl Cancer Inst.* 1968;40(1):43–68.

26 Shimizu H, Ross RK, Bernstein L, Yatani R, Henderson BE, Mack TM. Cancers of the prostate and breast among Japanese and white immigrants in Los Angeles County. *Br J Cancer.* 1991;63(6):963–966.

27 Gronberg H, Damber L, Damber JE. Studies of genetic factors in prostate cancer in a twin population. *J Urol.* 1994;152(5 Pt 1):1484–1487; discussion 7–9.

28 Page WF, Braun MM, Partin AW, Caporaso N, Walsh P. Heredity and prostate cancer: a study of World War II veteran twins. *Prostate.* 1997;33(4):240–245.

29 Lichtenstein P, Holm NV, Verkasalo PK, et al. Environmental and heritable factors in the causation of cancer—analyses of cohorts of twins from Sweden, Denmark, and Finland. *N Engl J Med.* 2000;343(2):78–85.

30 Carter BS, Beaty TH, Steinberg GD, Childs B, Walsh PC. Mendelian inheritance of familial prostate cancer. *Proc Natl Acad Sci U S A.* 1992;89(8):3367–3371.

31 Xu J, Meyers D, Freije D, et al. Evidence for a prostate cancer susceptibility locus on the X chromosome. *Nat Genet.* 1998;20(2):175–179.

32 Ewing CM, Ray AM, Lange EM, et al. Germline mutations in HOXB13 and prostate-cancer risk. *N Engl J Med.* 2012;366(2):141–149.

33 Bambury RM, Gallagher DJ. Prostate cancer: germline prediction for a commonly variable malignancy. *BJU Int.* 2012;110(11 Pt C):E809–E818.

34 Sun J, Wiklund F, Zheng SL, et al. Sequence variants in Toll-like receptor gene cluster (TLR6-TLR1-TLR10) and prostate cancer risk. *J Natl Cancer Inst.* 2005;97(7):525–532.

35 Lindmark F, Zheng SL, Wiklund F, et al. H6D polymorphism in macrophage-inhibitory cytokine-1 gene associated with prostate cancer. *J Natl Cancer Inst.* 2004;96(16):1248–1254.

36 Lindmark F, Zheng SL, Wiklund F, et al. Interleukin-1 receptor antagonist haplotype associated with prostate cancer risk. *Br J Cancer.* 2005;93(4):493–497.

37 Xu J, Lowey J, Wiklund F, et al. The interaction of four genes in the inflammation pathway significantly predicts prostate cancer risk. *Cancer Epidemiol Biomarkers Prev.* 2005;14(11 Pt 1):2563–2568.

38 Zheng SL, Augustsson-Balter K, Chang B, et al. Sequence variants of toll-like receptor 4 are associated with prostate cancer risk: results from the CAncer Prostate in Sweden Study. *Cancer Res.* 2004;64(8):2918–2922.

39 De Marzo AM, Marchi VL, Epstein JI, Nelson WG. Proliferative inflammatory atrophy of the prostate: implications for prostatic carcinogenesis. *Am J Pathol.* 1999;155(6):1985–1992.

40 Sakr WA, Grignon DJ, Crissman JD, et al. High grade prostatic intraepithelial neoplasia (HGPIN) and prostatic adenocarcinoma between the

ages of 20–69: an autopsy study of 249 cases. *In Vivo*. 1994;8(3):439–443.

41 Berger MF, Lawrence MS, Demichelis F, et al. The genomic complexity of primary human prostate cancer. *Nature*. 2011;470(7333):214–220.

42 Haffner MC, Mosbruger T, Esopi DM, et al. Tracking the clonal origin of lethal prostate cancer. *J Clin Invest*. 2013;123(11):4918–4922.

43 Yegnasubramanian S, Wu Z, Haffner MC, et al. Chromosome-wide mapping of DNA methylation patterns in normal and malignant prostate cells reveals pervasive methylation of gene-associated and conserved intergenic sequences. *BMC Genomics*. 2011;12:313.

44 Aryee MJ, Liu W, Engelmann JC, et al. DNA methylation alterations exhibit intraindividual stability and interindividual heterogeneity in prostate cancer metastases. *Sci Transl Med*. 2013;5(169):169ra10.

45 Perner S, Demichelis F, Beroukhim R, et al. TMPRSS2:ERG fusion-associated deletions provide insight into the heterogeneity of prostate cancer. *Cancer Res*. 2006;66(17):8337–8341.

46 Tomlins SA, Mehra R, Rhodes DR, et al. TMPRSS2:ETV4 gene fusions define a third molecular subtype of prostate cancer. *Cancer Res*. 2006;66(7):3396–3400.

47 Haffner MC, Aryee MJ, Toubaji A, et al. Androgen-induced TOP2B-mediated double-strand breaks and prostate cancer gene rearrangements. *Nat Genet*. 2010;42(8):668–675.

48 Cerveira N, Ribeiro FR, Peixoto A, et al. TMPRSS2-ERG gene fusion causing ERG overexpression precedes chromosome copy number changes in prostate carcinomas and paired HGPIN lesions. *Neoplasia*. 2006;8(10):826–832.

49 Hermans KG, van Marion R, van Dekken H, Jenster G, van Weerden WM, Trapman J. TMPRSS2:ERG fusion by translocation or interstitial deletion is highly relevant in androgen-dependent prostate cancer, but is bypassed in late-stage androgen receptor-negative prostate cancer. *Cancer Res*. 2006;66(22):10658–10663.

50 Nam RK, Sugar L, Wang Z, et al. Expression of TMPRSS2 ERG gene fusion in prostate cancer cells is an important prognostic factor for cancer progression. *Cancer Biol Ther*. 2007;6(1):40–45.

51 Petrovics G, Liu A, Shaheduzzaman S, et al. Frequent overexpression of ETS-related gene-1 (ERG1) in prostate cancer transcriptome. *Oncogene*. 2005;24(23):3847–3852.

52 Tomlins SA, Rhodes DR, Yu J, et al. The role of SPINK1 in ETS rearrangement-negative prostate cancers. *Cancer Cell*. 2008;13(6):519–528.

53 Barbieri CE, Baca SC, Lawrence MS, et al. Exome sequencing identifies recurrent SPOP, FOXA1 and MED12 mutations in prostate cancer. *Nat Genet*. 2012;44(6):685–689.

54 Koh CM, Bieberich CJ, Dang CV, Nelson WG, Yegnasubramanian S, De Marzo AM. MYC and prostate cancer. *Gen Cancer*. 2010;1(6):617–628.

55 Nelson WG, De Marzo AM, Yegnasubramanian S. USP2a activation of MYC in prostate cancer. *Cancer Discov*. 2012;2(3):206–207.

56 Koh CM, Gurel B, Sutcliffe S, et al. Alterations in nucleolar structure and gene expression programs in prostatic neoplasia are driven by the MYC oncogene. *Am J Pathol*. 2011;178(4):1824–1834.

57 Iwata T, Schultz D, Hicks J, et al. MYC overexpression induces prostatic intraepithelial neoplasia and loss of Nkx3.1 in mouse luminal epithelial cells. *PloS One*. 2010;5(2):e9427.

58 Li J, Yen C, Liaw D, et al. PTEN, a putative protein tyrosine phosphatase gene mutated in human brain, breast, and prostate cancer. *Science*. 1997;275(5308):1943–1947.

59 Steck PA, Pershouse MA, Jasser SA, et al. Identification of a candidate tumour suppressor gene, MMAC1, at chromosome 10q23.3 that is mutated in multiple advanced cancers. *Nat Genet*. 1997;15(4):356–362.

60 Teng DH, Hu R, Lin H, et al. MMAC1/PTEN mutations in primary tumor specimens and tumor cell lines. *Cancer Res*. 1997;57(23):5221–5225.

61 Myers MP, Pass I, Batty IH, et al. The lipid phosphatase activity of PTEN is critical for its tumor supressor function. *Proc Natl Acad Sci U S A*. 1998;95(23):13513–13518.

62 Myers MP, Stolarov JP, Eng C, et al. P-TEN, the tumor suppressor from human chromosome 10q23, is a dual-specificity phosphatase. *Proc Natl Acad Sci U S A*. 1997;94(17):9052–9057.

63 Maehama T, Dixon JE. The tumor suppressor, PTEN/MMAC1, dephosphorylates the lipid second messenger, phosphatidylinositol 3,4,5-trisphosphate. *J Biol Chem*. 1998;273(22):13375–13378.

64 Cairns P, Okami K, Halachmi S, et al. Frequent inactivation of PTEN/MMAC1 in primary prostate cancer. *Cancer Res*. 1997;57(22):4997–5000.

65 Suzuki H, Freije D, Nusskern DR, et al. Interfocal heterogeneity of PTEN/MMAC1 gene alterations in multiple metastatic prostate cancer tissues. *Cancer Res*. 1998;58(2):204–209.

66 McMenamin ME, Soung P, Perera S, Kaplan I, Loda M, Sellers WR. Loss of PTEN expression in paraffin-embedded primary prostate cancer correlates with high Gleason score and advanced stage. *Cancer Res*. 1999;59(17):4291–4296.

67 Podsypanina K, Ellenson LH, Nemes A, et al. Mutation of Pten/Mmac1 in mice causes neoplasia in multiple organ systems. *Proc Natl Acad Sci U S A*. 1999;96(4):1563–1568.

68 Di Cristofano A, Pesce B, Cordon-Cardo C, Pandolfi PP. Pten is essential for embryonic development and tumour suppression. *Nat Genet*. 1998;19(4):348–355.

69 Kim MJ, Cardiff RD, Desai N, et al. Cooperativity of Nkx3.1 and Pten loss of function in a mouse model of prostate carcinogenesis. *Proc Natl Acad Sci U S A*. 2002;99(5):2884–2889.

70 Chaux A, Peskoe SB, Gonzalez-Roibon N, et al. Loss of PTEN expression is associated with increased risk of recurrence after prostatectomy for clinically localized prostate cancer. *Mod Pathol*. 2012;25(11):1543–1549.

71 Antonarakis ES, Keizman D, Zhang Z, et al. An immunohistochemical signature comprising PTEN, MYC, and Ki67 predicts progression in prostate cancer patients receiving adjuvant docetaxel after prostatectomy. *Cancer*. 2012;118(24):6063–6071.

72 Lee WH, Morton RA, Epstein JI, et al. Cytidine methylation of regulatory sequences near the pi-class glutathione S-transferase gene accompanies human prostatic carcinogenesis. *Proc Natl Acad Sci U S A*. 1994;91(24):11733–11737.

73 Nakayama M, Gonzalgo ML, Yegnasubramanian S, Lin X, De Marzo AM, Nelson WG. GSTP1 CpG island hypermethylation as a molecular biomarker for prostate cancer. *J Cell Biochem*. 2004;91(3):540–552.

74 Henderson CJ, Smith AG, Ure J, Brown K, Bacon EJ, Wolf CR. Increased skin tumorigenesis in mice lacking pi class glutathione S-transferases. *Proc Natl Acad Sci U S A*. 1998;95(9):5275–5280.

75 Ritchie KJ, Walsh S, Sansom OJ, Henderson CJ, Wolf CR. Markedly enhanced colon tumorigenesis in Apc(Min) mice lacking glutathione S-transferase Pi. *Proc Natl Acad Sci U S A*. 2009;106(49):20859–20864.

76 Lin X, Tascilar M, Lee WH, et al. GSTP1 CpG island hypermethylation is responsible for the absence of GSTP1 expression in human prostate cancer cells. *Am J Pathol*. 2001;159(5):1815–1826.

77 Nelson WG, De Marzo AM, Yegnasubramanian S. Epigenetic alterations in human prostate cancers. *Endocrinology*. 2009;150(9):3991–4002.

78 Cox RL, Crawford ED. Estrogens in the treatment of prostate cancer. *J Urol*. 1995;154(6):1991–1998.

79 Thompson IM, Zeidman EJ, Rodriguez FR. Sudden death due to disease flare with luteinizing hormone-releasing hormone agonist therapy for carcinoma of the prostate. *J Urol.* 1990;144(6):1479–1480.

80 Scher HI, Sawyers CL. Biology of progressive, castration-resistant prostate cancer: directed therapies targeting the androgen-receptor signaling axis. *J Clin Oncol.* 2005;23(32):8253–8261.

81 Chen CD, Welsbie DS, Tran C, et al. Molecular determinants of resistance to antiandrogen therapy. *Nat Med.* 2004;10(1):33–39.

82 Kelly WK, Scher HI. Prostate specific antigen decline after antiandrogen withdrawal: the flutamide withdrawal syndrome. *J Urol.* 1993;149(3):607–609.

83 Hu R, Lu C, Mostaghel EA, et al. Distinct transcriptional programs mediated by the ligand-dependent full-length androgen receptor and its splice variants in castration-resistant prostate cancer. *Cancer Res.* 2012;72(14):3457–3462.

84 Montgomery RB, Mostaghel EA, Vessella R, et al. Maintenance of intratumoral androgens in metastatic prostate cancer: a mechanism for castration-resistant tumor growth. *Cancer Res.* 2008;68(11):4447–4454.

85 Mostaghel EA, Page ST, Lin DW, et al. Intraprostatic androgens and androgen-regulated gene expression persist after testosterone suppression: therapeutic implications for castration-resistant prostate cancer. *Cancer Res.* 2007;67(10):5033–5041.

86 de Bono JS, Logothetis CJ, Molina A, et al. Abiraterone and increased survival in metastatic prostate cancer. *N Engl J Med.* 2011;364(21):1995–2005.

87 Ryan CJ, Smith MR, de Bono JS, et al. Abiraterone in metastatic prostate cancer without previous chemotherapy. *N Engl J Med.* 2013;368(2):138–148.

88 Yin L, Hu Q. CYP17 inhibitors–abiraterone, C17,20-lyase inhibitors and multi-targeting agents. *Nat Rev Urology.* 2014;11(1):32–42.

89 Labrie F, Dupont A, Giguere M, et al. Advantages of the combination therapy in previously untreated and treated patients with advanced prostate cancer. *J Steroid Biochem.* 1986;25(5B):877–883.

90 Maximum androgen blockade in advanced prostate cancer: an overview of 22 randomised trials with 3283 deaths in 5710 patients. Prostate Cancer Trialists' Collaborative Group. *Lancet.* 1995;346(8970):265–269.

91 Scher HI, Beer TM, Higano CS, et al. Antitumour activity of MDV3100 in castration-resistant prostate cancer: a phase 1–2 study. *Lancet.* 2010;375(9724):1437–1446.

92 Rathkopf DE, Danila DC, Slovin SF, et al. A first-in-human, open-label, phase I/II safety, pharmacokinetic, and proof-of-concept study of ARN-509 in patients with progressive advanced castration-resistant prostate cancer (CRPC). *J Clin Oncol.* 2011;29:suppl. Abstract TPS190.

93 Joseph JD, Lu N, Qian J, et al. A clinically relevant androgen receptor mutation confers resistance to 2nd generation anti-androgens enzalutamide and ARN-509. *Cancer Discov.* 2013;3(9):1020–1029.

94 Korpala M, Korna JM, Gaob X, et al. A novel mutation in androgen receptor confers genetic and phenotypic resistance to MDV3100 (enzalutamide). *Cancer Discov.* 2013;3(9):1030–1043.

95 Balbas MD, Evans MJ, Hosfield DJ, et al. Overcoming mutation-based resistance to antiandrogens with rational drug design. *eLife.* 2013;2:e00499.

96 Gelmann EP. Molecular biology of the androgen receptor. *J Clin Oncol.* 2002;20(13):3001–3015.

97 Goldie JH, Coldman AJ. A mathematic model for relating the drug sensitivity of tumors to their spontaneous mutation rate. *Cancer Treat Rep.* 1979;63(11–12):1727–1733.

98 Luria SE, Delbruck M. Mutations of bacteria from virus sensitivity to virus resistance. *Genetics.* 1943;28(6):491–511.

99 Kyprianou N, Isaacs JT. Activation of programmed cell death in the rat ventral prostate after castration. *Endocrinology.* 1988;122(2):552–562.

100 Kyprianou N, English HF, Isaacs JT. Activation of a Ca2+-Mg2+-dependent endonuclease as an early event in castration-induced prostatic cell death. *Prostate.* 1988;13(2):103–117.

101 McDonnell TJ, Troncoso P, Brisbay SM, et al. Expression of the protooncogene bcl-2 in the prostate and its association with emergence of androgen-independent prostate cancer. *Cancer Res.* 1992;52:6940–6944.

102 Chen S, Principessa L, Isaacs JT. Human prostate cancer initiating cells isolated directly from localized cancer do not form prostaspheres in primary culture. *Prostate.* 2012;72(13):1478–1489.

103 Frame FM, Maitland NJ. Cancer stem cells, models of study and implications of therapy resistance mechanisms. *Adv Exp Med Biol.* 2011;720:105–118.

104 Majumder PK, Yeh JJ, George DJ, et al. Prostate intraepithelial neoplasia induced by prostate restricted Akt activation: the MPAKT model. *Proc Natl Acad Sci U S A.* 2003;100(13):7841–7846.

105 Majumder PK, Febbo PG, Bikoff R, et al. mTOR inhibition reverses Akt-dependent prostate intraepithelial neoplasia through regulation of apoptotic and HIF-1-dependent pathways. *Nat Med.* 2004;10(6):594–601.

106 Majumder PK, Grisanzio C, O'Connell F, et al. A prostatic intraepithelial neoplasia-dependent p27 Kip1 checkpoint induces senescence and inhibits cell proliferation and cancer progression. *Cancer Cell.* 2008;14(2):146–155.

107 Templeton AJ, Dutoit V, Cathomas R, et al. Phase 2 trial of single-agent everolimus in chemotherapy-naive patients with castration-resistant prostate cancer (SAKK 08/08). *Eur Urol.* 2013;64(1):150–158.

108 Armstrong AJ, Shen T, Halabi S, et al. A phase II trial of temsirolimus in men with castration-resistant metastatic prostate cancer. *Clin Genitourin Cancer.* 2013;11(4):397–406.

109 Clegg NJ, Couto SS, Wongvipat J, et al. MYC cooperates with AKT in prostate tumorigenesis and alters sensitivity to mTOR inhibitors. *PloS One.* 2011;6(3):e17449.

110 Carver BS, Chapinski C, Wongvipat J, et al. Reciprocal feedback regulation of PI3K and androgen receptor signaling in PTEN-deficient prostate cancer. *Cancer Cell.* 2011;19(5):575–586.

111 Baselga J, Campone M, Piccart M, et al. Everolimus in postmenopausal hormone-receptor-positive advanced breast cancer. *N Engl J Med.* 2012;366(6):520–529.

112 Hu R, Dunn TA, Wei S, et al. Ligand-independent androgen receptor variants derived from splicing of cryptic exons signify hormone-refractory prostate cancer. *Cancer Res.* 2009;69(1):16–22.

113 Hu R, Isaacs WB, Luo J. A snapshot of the expression signature of androgen receptor splicing variants and their distinctive transcriptional activities. *Prostate.* 2011;71(15):1656–1667.

114 Cao B, Qi Y, Zhang G, et al. Androgen receptor splice variants activating the full-length receptor in mediating resistance to androgen-directed therapy. *Oncotarget.* 2014;5(6):1646–1656.

115 Antonarakis E, Lu C, Wang H, et al. Androgen receptor splice variant, AR-V7, and resistance to enzalutamide and abiraterone in men with metastatic castration-resistant prostate cancer (mCRPC). *J Clin Oncol.* 2014;325s:5001.

116 Myung JK, Banuelos CA, Fernandez JG, et al. An androgen receptor N-terminal domain antagonist for treating prostate cancer. *J Clin Invest.* 2013;123(7):2948–2960.

117 Denmeade SR, Isaacs JT. Bipolar androgen therapy: the rationale for rapid cycling of supraphysiologic androgen/ablation in

men with castration resistant prostate cancer. *Prostate.* 2010;70(14): 1600–1607.

118 Isaacs JT, D'Antonio JM, Chen S, et al. Adaptive auto-regulation of androgen receptor provides a paradigm shifting rationale for bipolar androgen therapy (BAT) for castrate resistant human prostate cancer. *Prostate.* 2012;72(14):1491–1505.

119 Jordan MA, Wilson L. Microtubules as a target for anticancer drugs. *Nat Rev Cancer.* 2004;4(4):253–265.

120 Platz EA, Yegnasubramanian S, Liu JO, et al. A novel two-stage, trans-disciplinary study identifies digoxin as a possible drug for prostate cancer treatment. *Cancer Discov.* 2011;1(1):68–77.

121 Darshan MS, Loftus MS, Thadani-Mulero M, et al. Taxane-induced blockade to nuclear accumulation of the androgen receptor predicts clinical responses in metastatic prostate cancer. *Cancer Res.* 2011;71(18):6019–6029.

122 Tannock IF, de Wit R, Berry WR, et al. Docetaxel plus prednisone or mitoxantrone plus prednisone for advanced prostate cancer. *N Engl J Med.* 2004;351(15):1502–1512.

123 Petrylak DP, Tangen CM, Hussain MH, et al. Docetaxel and estramustine compared with mitoxantrone and prednisone for advanced refractory prostate cancer. *N Engl J Med.* 2004;351(15):1513–1520.

124 Beer TM, Garzotto M, Henner WD, Eilers KM, Wersinger EM. Intermittent chemotherapy in metastatic androgen-independent prostate cancer. *Br J Cancer.* 2003;89(6):968–970.

125 Meulenbeld HJ, Hamberg P, de Wit R. Chemotherapy in patients with castration-resistant prostate cancer. *Eur J Cancer.* 2009;45(suppl. 1):161–171.

126 Paller CJ, Antonarakis ES. Cabazitaxel: a novel second-line treatment for metastatic castration-resistant prostate cancer. *Drug Des Devel Ther.* 2011;5:117–124.

127 de Bono JS, Oudard S, Ozguroglu M, et al. Prednisone plus cabazitaxel or mitoxantrone for metastatic castration-resistant prostate cancer progressing after docetaxel treatment: a randomised open-label trial. *Lancet.* 2010;376(9747):1147–1154.

128 Sweeney C, Chen YH, Carducci MA, et al. Impact on overall survival (OS) with chemohormonal therapy versus hormonal therapy for hormone-sensitive newly metastatic prostate cancer (mPrCa): An ECOG-led phase III randomized trial. *J Clin Oncol.* 2014;325s:LBA2.

129 Saad F, Gleason DM, Murray R, et al. A randomized, placebo-controlled trial of zoledronic acid in patients with hormone-refractory metastatic prostate carcinoma. *J Natl Cancer Inst.* 2002;94(19):1458–1468.

130 Saad F, Gleason DM, Murray R, et al. Long-term efficacy of zoledronic acid for the prevention of skeletal complications in patients with metastatic hormone-refractory prostate cancer. *J Natl Cancer Inst.* 2004;96(11):879–882.

131 Fizazi K, Carducci M, Smith M, et al. Denosumab versus zoledronic acid for treatment of bone metastases in men with castration-resistant prostate cancer: a randomised, double-blind study. *Lancet.* 2011;377(9768):813–822.

132 Vallet S, Smith MR, Raje N. Novel bone-targeted strategies in oncology. *Clin Cancer Res.* 2010;16(16):4084–4093.

133 Brown JM, Corey E, Lee ZD, et al. Osteoprotegerin and rank ligand expression in prostate cancer. *Urology.* 2001;57(4):611–616.

134 Henry D, Vadhan-Raj S, Hirsh V, et al. Delaying skeletal-related events in a randomized phase 3 study of denosumab versus zoledronic acid in patients with advanced cancer: an analysis of data from patients with solid tumors. *Support Care Cancer.* 2014;22(3):679–687.

135 Goyal J, Antonarakis ES. Bone-targeting radiopharmaceuticals for the treatment of prostate cancer with bone metastases. *Cancer Lett.* 2012;323(2):135–146.

136 Nilsson S, Larsen RH, Fossa SD, et al. First clinical experience with alpha-emitting radium-223 in the treatment of skeletal metastases. *Clin Cancer Res.* 2005;11(12):4451–4459.

137 Bruland OS, Nilsson S, Fisher DR, Larsen RH. High-linear energy transfer irradiation targeted to skeletal metastases by the alpha-emitter 223Ra: adjuvant or alternative to conventional modalities? *Clin Cancer Res.* 2006;12(20 Pt 2):6250s–6257s.

138 Nilsson S, Franzen L, Parker C, et al. Bone-targeted radium-223 in symptomatic, hormone-refractory prostate cancer: a randomised, multicentre, placebo-controlled phase II study. *Lancet Oncol.* 2007;8(7):587–594.

139 Parker P, Nilsson S, Heinrich D, et al. Updated analysis of the phase III, double-blind, randomized, multinational study of radium-223 chloride in castration-resistant prostate cancer (CRPC) patients with bone metastases (ALSYMPCA). *J Clin Oncol.* 2012;30:suppl. Abstract LBA4512.

140 Drake CG. Prostate cancer as a model for tumour immunotherapy. *Nat Rev Immunol.* 2010;10(8):580–593.

141 Antonarakis ES, Drake CG. Current status of immunological therapies for prostate cancer. *Curr Opin Urol.* 2010;20(3):241–246.

142 Yegnasubramanian S, Haffner MC, Zhang Y, et al. DNA hypomethylation arises later in prostate cancer progression than CpG island hypermethylation and contributes to metastatic tumor heterogeneity. *Cancer Res.* 2008;68(21):8954–8967.

143 Drake CG, Doody AD, Mihalyo MA, et al. Androgen ablation mitigates tolerance to a prostate/prostate cancer-restricted antigen. *Cancer Cell.* 2005;7(3):239–249.

144 Mercader M, Bodner BK, Moser MT, et al. T cell infiltration of the prostate induced by androgen withdrawal in patients with prostate cancer. *Proc Natl Acad Sci U S A.* 2001;98(25):14565–14570.

145 Gannon PO, Poisson AO, Delvoye N, Lapointe R, Mes-Masson AM, Saad F. Characterization of the intra-prostatic immune cell infiltration in androgen-deprived prostate cancer patients. *J Immunol Methods.* 2009;348(1–2):9–17.

146 Sfanos KS, Bruno TC, Meeker AK, De Marzo AM, Isaacs WB, Drake CG. Human prostate-infiltrating CD8+ T lymphocytes are oligoclonal and PD-1+. *Prostate.* 2009;69(15):1694–1703.

147 Sfanos KS, Bruno TC, Maris CH, et al. Phenotypic analysis of prostate-infiltrating lymphocytes reveals TH17 and Treg skewing. *Clin Cancer Res.* 2008;14(11):3254–3261.

148 Small EJ, Fratesi P, Reese DM, et al. Immunotherapy of hormone-refractory prostate cancer with antigen-loaded dendritic cells. *J Clin Oncol.* 2000;18(23):3894–3903.

149 Higano CS, Schellhammer PF, Small EJ, et al. Integrated data from 2 randomized, double-blind, placebo-controlled, phase 3 trials of active cellular immunotherapy with sipuleucel-T in advanced prostate cancer. *Cancer.* 2009;115(16):3670–3679.

150 Kantoff PW, Higano CS, Shore ND, et al. Sipuleucel-T immunotherapy for castration-resistant prostate cancer. *N Eng J Med.* 2010;363(5):411–422.

151 Longo DL. New therapies for castration-resistant prostate cancer. *N Engl J Med.* 2010;363(5):479–481.

152 Graff JN, Drake CG, Beer TM. Complete biochemical (prostate-specific antigen) response to sipuleucel-T with enzalutamide in castration-resistant prostate cancer: a case report with implications for future research. *Urology.* 2013;81(2):381–383.

153 Drake CG, Antonarakis ES. Current status of immunological approaches for the treatment of prostate cancer. *Curr Opin Urol.* 2012;22(3):197–202.

154 Kwon ED, Hurwitz AA, Foster BA, et al. Manipulation of T cell costimulatory and inhibitory signals for immunotherapy of prostate cancer. *Proc Natl Acad Sci U S A*. 1997;94(15):8099–8103.

155 Kwon ED, Foster BA, Hurwitz AA, et al. Elimination of residual metastatic prostate cancer after surgery and adjunctive cytotoxic T lymphocyte-associated antigen 4 (CTLA-4) blockade immunotherapy. *Proc Natl Acad Sci U S A*. 1999;96(26):15074–15079.

156 Hurwitz AA, Foster BA, Kwon ED, et al. Combination immunotherapy of primary prostate cancer in a transgenic mouse model using CTLA-4 blockade. *Cancer Res*. 2000;60(9):2444–2448.

157 Grosso JF, Jure-Kunkel MN. CTLA-4 blockade in tumor models: an overview of preclinical and translational research. *Cancer Immun*. 2013;13:5.

158 Kwon ED, Drake CG, Scher HI, et al. Ipilimumab versus placebo after radiotherapy in patients with metastatic castration-resistant prostate cancer that had progressed after docetaxel chemotherapy (CA184–043): a multicentre, randomised, double-blind, phase 3 trial. *Lancet Oncol*. 2014;15(7):700–712.

159 Kaminskas E, Farrell A, Abraham S, et al. Approval summary: azacitidine for treatment of myelodysplastic syndrome subtypes. *Clin Cancer Res*. 2005;11(10):3604–3608.

160 Lin X, Asgari K, Putzi MJ, et al. Reversal of GSTP1 CpG island hypermethylation and reactivation of pi-class glutathione S-transferase (GSTP1) expression in human prostate cancer cells by treatment with procainamide. *Cancer Res*. 2001;61(24):8611–8616.

161 Cheng JC, Matsen CB, Gonzales FA, et al. Inhibition of DNA methylation and reactivation of silenced genes by zebularine. *J Natl Cancer Inst*. 2003;95(5):399–409.

162 Segura-Pacheco B, Trejo-Becerril C, Perez-Cardenas E, et al. Reactivation of tumor suppressor genes by the cardiovascular drugs hydralazine and procainamide and their potential use in cancer therapy. *Clin Cancer Res*. 2003;9(5):1596–1603.

163 Thibault A, Figg WD, Bergan RC, et al. A phase II study of 5-aza-2′deoxycytidine (decitabine) in hormone independent metastatic (D2) prostate cancer. *Tumori*. 1998;84(1):87–89.

164 Wrangle J, Wang W, Koch A, et al. Alterations of immune response of non-small cell lung cancer with azacytidine. *Oncotarget*. 2013;4(11):2067–2079.

165 Juergens RA, Wrangle J, Vendetti FP, et al. Combination epigenetic therapy has efficacy in patients with refractory advanced non-small cell lung cancer. *Cancer Discov*. 2011;1(7):598–607.

166 Nelson WG, Haffner MC, Yegnasubramanian S. Beefing up Prostate Cancer Therapy with Performance-Enhancing (Anti-) Steroids. *Cancer Cell*. 2011;20:7–9.

# CHAPTER 29

# Renal Cell Carcinoma and Targeted Therapy

*Benjamin A. Gartrell[1], Alexander C. Small[2], William K. Oh[2], and Matthew D. Galsky[2]*

[1]Department of Medical Oncology, Montefiore Medical Center, The Albert Einstein College of Medicine, Bronx, NY, USA
[2]Division of Hematology and Medical Oncology, The Tisch Cancer Institute, Mount Sinai School of Medicine, New York, NY, USA

## Introduction

In the United States alone, renal cell carcinoma (RCC) will be diagnosed in approximately 64,770 people and result in 13,570 deaths in 2012.[1] Surgical resection is potentially curative in localized disease, but of these patients, an additional 20% will eventually develop metastatic disease.[2] In addition, approximately 20% of patients will have metastatic disease at the time of presentation.[3] Clear-cell RCC (ccRCC) is the most common histology accounting for 80–90% of tumors. The major non-ccRCC histologies include papillary (10–15%) and chromophobe (~5%) neoplasms.

Renal carcinoma is generally resistant to cytotoxic chemotherapy. Prior to the development of a new generation of systemic therapies in RCC, therapeutic intervention for metastatic disease was limited to immunotherapy with interferon alpha (INF-α) or interleukin (IL-2). However, a greater understanding of the molecular pathogenesis of RCC has led to the introduction of "targeted therapy" into the care of patients with metastatic RCC. This chapter will explore the molecular pathogenesis of RCC, and the targeted therapies that have recently been developed (Figure 29.1).

## Molecular Pathogenesis of RCC

The first insights into the molecular pathogenesis of RCC were derived from observations in von Hippel–Lindau (VHL) disease. VHL disease is inherited in an autosomal dominant fashion and is characterized by the development of hemangioblastomas of the central nervous system and retina, pheochromocytomas, and ccRCC. Clear cell is the most common histologic subtype of RCC and that seen in VHL disease is similar to sporadic ccRCC with the exception that, in patients with VHL disease, ccRCC is often bilateral, multifocal, and occurs at an early age. The frequency of ccRCC in patients with VHL disease led to speculation that the molecular defect was related to that associated with sporadic ccRCC.

The genetics of VHL disease follow the "two hit" model of tumor-suppressor gene function first proposed by Knudson. An affected individual inherits a single defective VHL gene from one parent. Somatic mutation of the remaining wild-type gene leads to complete loss of function of tumor-suppressor gene activity and allows for development of the disease phenotype.

Early studies of families afflicted by a high incidence of ccRCC identified recurring abnormalities on the short arm of chromosome 3 (3p).[4] Subsequently, abnormalities at chromosome 3p were identified in sporadic ccRCC specimens.[5] The VHL gene was later mapped to chromosome 3p25.[6] Thus, the VHL gene was found to be the tumor-suppressor gene responsible for VHL disease and the gene that is most often abnormal in sporadic ccRCC. Mutations in the VHL gene, or epigenetic modifications resulting in gene silencing, have since been shown to be present in the majority of sporadic ccRCC. The protein product of the VHL gene functions as a tumor suppressor primarily through its role in the regulation of hypoxia-inducible factors (HIF). HIF-1 is a heterodimeric transcription factor (HIF-α and HIF-β) that was first found to mediate the hypoxia-induced increased expression of erythropoietin.[7] It was later appreciated that the HIF transcription factors mediate signaling induced by hypoxia in multiple tissue types and serve as a key regulator of the cellular response to hypoxia.[8] Whereas the concentration of HIF-β is generally constant, HIF-α is the target of oxygen-dependent degradation via the ubiquitin-proteasome pathway. HIF prolyl hydroxylase (HPH) enzymes catalyze the hydroxylation of HIF-α using oxygen as a substrate.[9] The protein product of the VHL gene associates with an E3 ubiquitin ligase. The hydroxylated HIF-α is then polyubiquitinated by the protein product of the VHL gene in conjunction with the E3 ubiquitin ligase.[10]

Under normoxic conditions HIF-α is degraded by the proteasome. However, under hypoxic conditions, HIF-α concentrations increase as the prolyl residues remain unhydroxylated and the protein is thus spared from polyubiquitination and proteasome-mediated proteolysis. HIF-α is then free to form a heterodimer with HIF-β and to act as a nuclear transcription factor inducing the increased expression of numerous hypoxia response elements (HREs). In familial RCC, or in sporadic cases of RCC with dysfunction of the VHL gene, HIF levels are elevated, and multiple hypoxia-inducible genes are overexpressed including vascular endothelial growth factor (VEGF), platelet-derived growth factor (PDGF), transforming growth factor-alpha (TGF-α), and TGF-β. Thus, HIF-1 acts a transcription factor that allows untransformed cells to adapt to hypoxic conditions, but is integral to the pathogenesis of RCC when its signal is decoupled from the oxygen-sensing mechanism provided by the VHL gene.

*Targeted Therapy in Translational Cancer Research*, First Edition. Edited by Apostolia-Maria Tsimberidou, Razelle Kurzrock and Kenneth C. Anderson.
© 2016 John Wiley & Sons, Inc. Published 2016 by John Wiley & Sons, Inc.

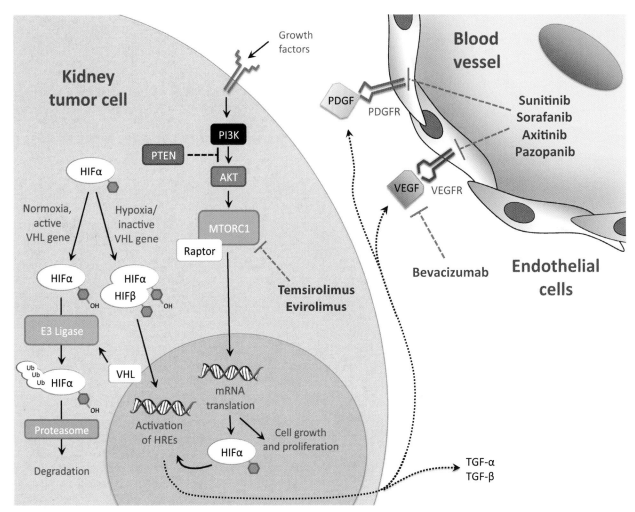

**Figure 29.1** Signaling pathways and targeted agents in the treatment of renal cell carcinoma.

VHL abnormalities are generally limited to ccRCC. Germline mutations in c-MET have been noted in type I papillary RCC. These patients often have a family history of papillary RCC and develop bilateral, multifocal disease at an early age. Somatic mutations in c-MET have also been reported in sporadic papillary RCC.

Next-generation sequencing has been used to evaluate tumor heterogeneity in RCC.[11] Molecular aberrations within primary tumors, and corresponding metastatic lesions, were investigated. Significant intratumoral heterogeneity and a branched evolution pattern were demonstrated. This finding raises concerns that a single tumor biopsy may not adequately represent the mutational profile of a particular malignancy and has potential implications for the development of novel biomarkers and therapeutic approaches. Early genetic events shared by all clones may represent real "drivers" of disease and therefore may be the most attractive therapeutic targets. In addition, stromal elements, not directly impacted by continued clonal evolution of the malignancy, may be targeted to overcome therapeutic resistance.

## Important Signaling Pathways in RCC

### VEGF/VEGFR Signaling

Renal carcinoma is a vascular tumor and VEGF has been detected in high levels in the serum of patients with RCC.[12] The VEGF family of growth factors (VEGF-A, VEGF-B, VEGF-C, VEGF-D, and placental growth factor (PlGF)) transmit an angiogenic signal through interaction with a corresponding family of cell surface receptor tyrosine kinases (RTKs) (VEGFR-1 (Flt-1), VEGFR-2 (KDR/Flk-1), and VEGFR-3 (Flt-4)). VEGF-A is the most significant of the ligands and is often referred to simply as VEGF. VEGF is a 40-kDa disulfide-linked glycoprotein that is a highly selective mitogen for endothelial cells. VEGF/VEGFR signaling is critical to angiogenesis, endothelial cell survival, permeability of the vasculature, and is critical in both physiologic and pathologic processes. VEGF exists is several isoforms as a consequence of alternative splicing of RNA. Each of these splice variants has different biological activity.[13] The VEGF/VEGFR angiogenic signaling pathway has been established as a key target in the treatment of a variety of solid tumors. Both small molecule tyrosine kinase inhibitors (TKIs) (sunitinib, sorafenib, pazopanib, axitinib) and the anti-VEGF monoclonal antibody bevacizumab have been used to interfere with this signaling pathway.

The VEGFR family belongs to the same subclass of cell surface RTKs as fibroblast growth factor receptors (FGFRs) and PDGFRs. VEGFRs interact with the dimerized VEGF ligand and transduce an intracellular signal (reviewed in[14]). The expression of both VEGF-A and VEGFR-1 are directly controlled by HIF. While the gene for VEGFR-2 does not contain a classic HRE promoter sequence, VEGFR-2 levels do increase with hypoxia, and HIF-2α (but not HIF-1α) interacts with the promoter region to increase transcription.[15] Prior to interaction with the VEGF ligand, VEGFR exist as monomers on the cell surface. When bound to a ligand, VEGFR forms homo- or heterodimers allowing for transphosphorylation of the intracellular domains and transduction of intracellular signaling through kinase activity of the VEGFR dimer. The signaling of VEGFRs is dictated by the degree of phosphorylation and this regulated by the opposing activity of phosphatases and kinases. Integrins on the cell surface interact with various components of the extracellular matrix and with phosphatases that inhibit signaling through RTKs including VEGFRs. The signaling of VEGFR-2 is negatively regulated by the tyrosine phosphatases Src-homology phosphatase-1 (SHP1) and SHP2.[16,17] Endorepellin, the C-terminal domain of perlecan (a cell surface heparin sulfate proteoglycan), binds with integrin α2β1 releasing SHP1 to dephosphorylate VEGFR-2 and thereby inhibit its signaling.[16]

The capacity for VEGFR-1 to transduce an intracellular signal is relatively low in comparison to VEGFR-2, whereas VEGFR-1 has a greater affinity for VEGF than does VEGFR-2.[18] This led to speculation that VEGFR-1 may function as a decoy receptor and in this manner may influence VEGF/VEGFR signaling. VEGFR-3 binds VEGF-C but not VEGF-A and appears to be important in the maintenance of lymphatics.

The function of VEGFR-2 is critical for normal angiogenesis and knockout mice die in early embryogenesis.[19] Upon ligand binding and autophosphorylation of several tyrosine residues, VEGFR-2 targets several proteins via their Src homology-2 (SH2) domain for signal transduction including phospholipase-C (PLC), Ras GTPase activating protein (Ras-GAP), and the oncogenic adaptor protein NcK.[20] VEGF has been shown to induce phosphorylation of focal adhesion kinase (FAK) and paxillin both of which contribute to the migration of endothelial cells induced by VEGF.[21] VEGFR-2 induces signaling through the MAPK pathway in a PKC-dependent, but Ras- and phosphatidylinositol 3-kinase (PI3K)-independent, fashion.[22] Ras has since been implicated in the VEGF-mediated activation of the MAPK pathway.[23] A later report implicated PLC-induced activation of protein kinase C (PKC) in the VEGFR-2-mediated upregulation of (MAPK)/extracellular-signal-regulated kinase-1/2 (ERK1/2) cascade.[24] VEGFR-2 signaling has also been shown to activate PI3K and in conjunction with activation of Akt was shown to induce endothelial cell proliferation.[25]

## The Mammalian Target of Rapamycin Pathway in RCC

Rapamycin is a macrolide antifungal antibiotic secreted by the bacteria *Streptomyces hygroscopicus*. Interestingly, this organism was first discovered on Easter Island in the 1970s. Rapamycin was subsequently found to have both anti-proliferative and immunosuppressive properties. Investigation of the mechanism of action led to the discovery of the mammalian target of rapamycin (mTOR) signaling pathway.

mTOR is an evolutionarily conserved intracellular serine/threonine kinase that is structurally related to a group of protein kinases that include ataxia telangiectasia mutated (ATM) gene. mTOR is downstream of multiple signaling pathways, and thus, the function of mTOR is dependent upon multiple upstream regulators. The mTOR pathway incorporates signals from extracellular matrix including nutrients and growth factors and serves as a global regulator of multiple cellular processes that are required to maintain homeostasis. The PI3K/Akt pathway is an important regulator of

mTOR function. mTOR signaling has a multitude of effects on cellular function including regulation of angiogenesis, proliferation, growth, metabolism, and motility.[26]

Rapamycin and its analog tacrolimus (FK506) have two binding surfaces. One binds to FK506-binding protein (FKBP12).[27] This rapamycin/FKBP12 complex then interacts with and inhibits mTOR.[28] mTOR participates in both the mTORC1 and mTORC2 complexes. mTORC1 contains regulatory-associated protein of mTOR (Raptor) and targets of this complex include genes involved in protein translation such as S6K1 and 4EBP1.[29] The mTORC2 complex contains rapamycin-insensitive companion of mTOR (Rictor). This complex does not interact with rapamycin or its analogs and regulates the cytoskeleton.[30] The current armamentarium of approved drugs that target mTOR only inhibit the mTORC1 complex. The PI3K/Akt/mTOR pathway has also been shown to modulate the activation of HIF-1α, which has multiple consequences including augmenting angiogenesis.[31]

The autosomal dominant disorder tuberous sclerosis is associated with increased incidence of RCC. Tuberous sclerosis is a neurocutaneous syndrome associated with the development of benign hamartomas involving multiple organ systems (reviewed in[32]). It is completely penetrant though the degree of expression varies considerably among affected individuals. In this disorder, one of two tumor-suppressor genes (TSC1 and TSC2) is affected. The protein product of these genes (hamartin and tuberin, respectively) interact to form a heterodimer. The hamartin–tuberin heterodimer inhibits signaling through the mTOR pathway.[33] Akt binds to and phosphorylates tuberin, which leads to inhibition of the suppressive capacity of the hamartin–tuberin complex by targeting the complex for proteasome-mediated proteolysis.[34] Signaling through the PI3K/Akt/mTOR pathway is regulated by the tumor repressor gene phosphatase and tensin homologue (pTEN) and, abnormalities in pTEN increase signaling through mTOR.

Thus, the mTOR pathway is critical for responding to cellular stress, nutrient availability, growth factor signaling to control cellular growth, proliferation, and angiogenesis. This pathway is critical in both homeostasis and in malignancy, suggesting that successful targeting may represent an attractive approach to cancer treatment.

## Targeted Therapies in RCC

The results from major randomized studies that have explored the benefit of "targeted therapies" in RCC are presented in this chapter (Table 29.1). As these studies are reviewed, several points should be taken into consideration. First, risk stratification models have been utilized as eligibility criteria for some trials, resulting in non-overlapping patient populations being studied. Historically, the most common prognostic model employed has been the Memorial Sloan-Kettering Cancer Center (MSKCC) model.[47] In this model, elevated lactate dehydrogenase (>1.5 ULN), decreased hemoglobin, increased corrected calcium (>10 mg/dL), decreased Karnofsky performance status (<80%), and time from diagnosis to systemic therapy (<1 year) are used to stratify patients into good (0 risk factors), intermediate (1–2 risk factors), and poor risk (>2 risk factors) groups. Most clinical trials have under-represented patients from the poor risk group. Second, many trials have also excluded patients with brain metastases and those with non-clear cell histologies. Thus, less is known about the potential benefit from "targeted therapy" in patients with these features. Third, a survival benefit has been difficult to evaluate as patients in control arms have often been allowed to receive the experimental agent at progression

**Table 29.1** Phase III trials of approved targeted agents in metastatic RCC.

| Targeted therapeutic | Control | Patient population | ORR (%) | PFS (months) | OS (months) |
|---|---|---|---|---|---|
| Sunitinib[35, 36] | IFN | Treatment-naïve, metastatic ccRCC | 39–47 vs. 9–12 ($p < 0.001$) | 11 vs. 5 ($p < 0.001$) | 26.4 vs. 21.8 ($p = 0.051$). When censored for cross over, 26.4 vs. 20.0 ($p = 0.036$) |
| Sorafenib[37, 38] | Placebo | Prior systemic therapy, metastatic ccRCC, intermediate and low risk | 10 vs. 2 | 5.5 vs. 2.8 ($p < 0.01$) | 17.8 vs. 15.2 ($p = 0.146$). When censored for cross over, 17.8 vs. 14.3 ($p = 0.029$) |
| Pazopanib[39] | Placebo | Treatment-naïve (54%) and cytokine pretreated (46%), advanced/metastatic ccRCC | 30 vs. 3 ($p < 0.001$) | 9.2 vs. 4.2 ($p < 0.0001$) | Not yet reported |
| Axitinib[40] | Sorafenib | Second-line, metastatic ccRCC | 19 vs. 9 ($p < 0.0001$) | 6.7 vs. 4.7 ($p < 0.0001$) | Not yet reported |
| CALGB 90206[41, 42] Bevacizumab/IFN | IFN | Treatment-naïve, metastatic ccRCC | 25.5 vs 13.1 ($p < 0.0001$) | 8.5 vs. 5.2 ($p$ 0.0001) | 18.3 vs. 17.4 ($p = 0.097$) |
| AVOREN[43, 44] Bevacizumab/IFN | Placebo/IFN | Treatment-naïve, metastatic ccRCC, post nephrectomy | 31 vs. 12 ($p < 0.001$) | 10.4 vs. 5.5 ($p < 0.001$) | 23.3 vs. 21.3 ($p = 0.336$) |
| 1) Temsirolimus[45] (25 mg qwk) | 2) Temsirolimus (15 mg qwk) + IFN 3) IFN | Treatment-naïve, metastatic RCC (20% non-clear cell), intermediate and poor risk only | 8.6 vs. 8.1 vs. 4.8 | 5.5 vs. 4.7 vs. 3.1 | 10.9 vs. 8.4 vs. 7.3 (HR for death of 0.73 in Tem vs. IFN, $p = 0.008$) |
| Everolimus[46] | Placebo | Post sunitinib or sorafenib, metastatic ccRCC | 1.8 vs. 0 | 4.9 vs. 1.9 ($p < 0.001$) | 14.8 vs. 14.4 ($p = 0.162$) |

or have been exposed to approved "targeted" agents off protocol. Progression-free survival (PFS) benefit has generally been utilized as the primary endpoint for these trials, and has been acceptable for establishing regulatory approval.

## Targeting VEGF/VEGFR Signaling

Dysregulated oxygen sensing is the central feature in the development and pathogenesis of ccRCC. Impaired function of the VHL gene product inhibits the ability of the cell to inhibit the complex changes in gene expression caused by unopposed activation of HIF. Therefore, focusing on gene products upregulated by HIF was postulated to be a promising strategy for therapeutic targeting in this disease.

The expressions of VEGF and VEGFR are increased in response to tissue hypoxia and VEGF is the most important growth factor for normal and tumor blood vessels. VEGF is increased in the serum of patients with RCC, likely explaining longstanding clinical observations that RCC is a particularly vascular tumor. Several small molecule kinase inhibitors that target VEGFR have been FDA approved for the treatment of RCC (sunitinib, sorafenib, pazopanib, axitinib). In addition, bevacizumab, a monoclonal antibody against VEGF, has also been FDA approved for the treatment of RCC. A variety of additional compounds targeting VEGF/VEGFR signaling are in development. These compounds have revolutionized the treatment of RCC and are now used in the first line and later settings of metastatic disease.

## Sunitinib

Sunitinib is an orally available inhibitor of several tyrosine kinases including VEGFR-2, PDGFRβ, c-kit, and FLT-3. Sunitinib was initially studied, and approved, based on two single-arm phase II trials evaluating the activity of sunitinib in patients with metastatic

RCC who had progressed following cytokine-based therapy. The trials included 63 and 105 patients. The results of these studies were quite similar and were presented in a pooled analysis.[48] An objective response was observed in 42% of patients. The median PFS was 8.2 months. Response rates such as these were unprecedented in RCC and based on the results of these phase II studies, sunitinib was approved by the US Food and Drug Administration (FDA) for use in RCC in 2006.

A phase III trial was subsequently performed comparing sunitinib (50 mg daily for 4 weeks followed by 2 weeks off of treatment) with interferon (IFN, 9 million units subcutaneously three times weekly) in 750 treatment-naïve patients with metastatic ccRCC.[35, 36] The primary end point of this trial was PFS. This study demonstrated an improvement in all outcomes with sunitinib therapy: the objective response rate was 47% versus 12% ($p < 0.001$), PFS was 11 versus 5 months, ($p < 0.001$) and the median overall survival was 26.4 versus 21.8 months ($p = 0.051$), with sunitinib compared with interferon, respectively. The survival endpoint, based on a predefined analysis (unstratified log-rank test), did not reach statistical significance, largely attributed to cross over from placebo to sunitinib. Of note, only 6% and 7% of patients in the sunitinib and IFN groups, respectively, were in the MSKCC poor risk group. Common grade 3–4 events associated with sunitinib use included hypertension (12%), fatigue (11%), diarrhea (9%), hand–foot syndrome (9%), neutropenia (18%), lymphopenia (18%), thrombocytopenia (9%), and anemia (8%).

Sunitinib has also been evaluated in patients that are generally excluded from randomized trials such as those with ECOG performance status ≥2, brain metastases, the elderly, and in those patients with non-clear cell histology.[49] In this international, expanded-access trial, open-label sunitinib was found to be well tolerated in each of these groups of patients. In addition, there was evidence of activity and clinical benefit in all subsets of patients.

## Sorafenib

Sorafenib is an oral multikinase inhibitor that was originally developed as an Raf inhibitor. Additional targets include VEGFR and PDGFR. Sorafenib has been evaluated in a randomized, placebo-controlled, phase III trial in metastatic ccRCC patients who had been treated with prior systemic therapy.[37] This trial enrolled 903 patients with low or intermediate risk disease by MSKCC criteria. Sorafenib was administered at a dose of 400 mg po bid and the primary endpoint was PFS. Though the objective response rate with sorafenib was relatively low, it was higher with sorafenib than placebo (10% vs. 2%), and sorafenib resulted in a statistically significant improvement in PFS (5.5 vs. 2.8 months, $p < 0.01$). Patients were permitted to cross over from placebo to sorafenib at the time of progression. The prolongation in the median overall survival with sorafenib did not reach statistical significance (17.8 vs. 15.2 months, $p = 0.146$). However, when post-placebo cross-over data was censored, statistical significance favoring sorafenib was reached (17.8 vs. 14.3 months, $p = 0.029$).[38] Common grade 3–4 adverse events with sorafenib included the hand–foot syndrome (6%), fatigue (5%), hypertension (4%), and anemia (3%). Based on this trial, sorafenib received regulatory approval for use in advanced RCC by the US FDA in 2005.

A randomized phase II study compared sorafenib and IFN in 189 treatment-naïve patients with metastatic ccRCC.[50] PFS in this trial was a disappointing 5.7 months with sorafenib and 5.6 months with IFN. Tolerability and quality-of-life measures favored sorafenib over IFN. Based on this result, sunitinib largely overtook sorafenib as the preferred first-line treatment for metastatic ccRCC.

## Pazopanib

Pazopanib is an oral inhibitor of VEGFR, PDGFR, and c-kit. Pazopanib has been evaluated in a randomized, placebo-controlled phase III trial of 435 patients with advanced or metastatic ccRCC.[39] Both treatment-naïve (54%) and cytokine-pretreated (46%) patients were enrolled. Only 3% of patients were poor risk by MSKCC criteria. The primary endpoint for this trial was PFS and, similar to other trials in this clinical disease state, cross over was allowed at the time of progression. In the overall study population, PFS was superior with pazopanib compared with placebo (9.2 vs. 4.2 months; $p < 0.0001$), a difference that was even more pronounced in the treatment-naïve population (11.1 vs. 2.8 months, $p < 0.0001$). The objective response rate was 30% with pazopanib and 3% with placebo ($p < 0.001$). Pazopanib was generally well tolerated and was associated with a low incidence of grade ≥3 adverse events including increased ALT (12%), diarrhea (4%), and hypertension (4%). Grade ≥3 cytopenias included neutropenia (<1%), thrombocytopenia (<1%), and lymphopenia (4%). Quality of life was not significantly different in the pazopanib and placebo arms. Pazopanib received regulatory approval for use in advanced RCC in the United States in 2009. A study comparing sunitinib with pazopanib in treatment-naïve metastatic RCC has completed accrual but has not yet been reported.

## Axitinib

Axitinib is a potent and selective second-generation VEGFR inhibitor. Axitinib has been compared to sorafenib in a phase III trial in metastatic ccRCC patients which had progressed despite prior treatment (sunitinib 54%, cytokine 35%, bevacizumab 8%, temsirolimus 3%).[40] This second-line trial included 723 patients with metastatic ccRCC. The primary endpoint of this trial was PFS.

Notably, 33% of patients met criteria for poor risk group by MSKCC criteria. By independent review committee assessment, the median PFS was 6.7 versus 4.7 months ($p < 0.0001$) favoring axitinib. In patients who had prior cytokine-based therapy the PFS was 12.1 versus 6.5 months ($p < 0.0001$) favoring axitinib. In patients who had progressed on prior sunitinib, the PFS was 4.8 versus 3.4 months ($p = 0.0107$) again favoring axitinib. The objective response rate was 19% with axitinib versus 9% with sorafenib ($p < 0.0001$). Grade ≥3 adverse events seen with axitinib included hypertension (16%), diarrhea (11%), fatigue (11%), and hand–foot syndrome (5%). Grade ≥3 lab abnormalities included neutropenia (1%), anemia (<1%), thrombocytopenia (<1%), lymphopenia (3%), and lipase elevation (5%). This trial provides proof of principal that a more potent VEGFR inhibitor (axitinib) is more active than a less potent agent (sorafenib) and also that sequential use of VEGFR inhibitors can yield modest improvements in outcomes. Based on this study, axitinib received regulatory approval for use in the United States, as second-line therapy for metastatic RCC, in 2011.

Several ongoing trials are attempting to answer clinically relevant questions that have emerged as a result of the studies detailed above, including the best sequence of use of these agents, whether combination therapies are of benefit, and the utility of VEGFR TKIs in the adjuvant setting.

## Bevacizumab

Bevacizumab is a humanized, monoclonal antibody that binds and neutralizes VEGF in the serum. Bevacizumab was among the first agents to provide proof of principal that targeting VEGF/VEGFR signaling could yield clinical benefits in ccRCC. In a phase II study, 116 patients with metastatic ccRCC were randomized to bevacizumab (3 or 10 mg/kg) or placebo.[51] The objective response rate was 10% in the high-dose bevacizumab arm. There were no objective responses in the low-dose or placebo arms. The median PFS was 4.8 months in the high-dose arm compared to 2.5 months in the placebo arm ($p < 0.001$).

Bevacizumab was subsequently evaluated in combination with IFN in two phase III studies in metastatic RCC. CALGB 90206 randomized 732 treatment-naïve patients with metastatic ccRCC to receive bevacizumab + IFN or IFN with overall survival as the primary endpoint.[41,42] The objective response rate with bevacizumab + IFN was 25.5% and 13.1% with IFN alone ($p < 0.0001$). While PFS also favored bevacizumab + IFN (8.5 vs. 5.2 months, $p < 0.0001$), the very modest prolongation in the median overall survival with the combination did not reach statistical significance (18.3 vs. 17.4 months, $p = 0.097$). Notable grade ≥3 adverse events with the combination regimen in this trial included hypertension (11%) and proteinuria (15%).

AVOREN (Avastin and Roferon in RCC) was a similarly designed phase III trial that randomized treatment-naïve patients to receive bevacizumab + IFN or placebo + IFN in metastatic ccRCC.[43,44] This trial enrolled 649 patients, 8% of whom were in the MSKCC poor risk group. The primary outcome was overall survival. While the vast majority of patients had resection of their primary tumor in CALGB 90206 (85%), all patients were required to have undergone resection of their primary tumor in AVOREN. The objective response rate was 31% with bevacizumab + IFN and 12% with placebo + IFN ($p < 0.001$). The median PFS was 10.4 versus 5.5 months ($p < 0.001$) favoring the bevacizumab + IFN arm. Following an interim analysis, the study was unblinded and patients in the placebo arm were allowed to initiate treatment with bevacizumab + IFN prior to disease progression ($n = 13$). The final analysis of the median overall survival by an unstratified, intention to treat analysis demonstrated an increase in overall survival with bevacizumab + IFN (23.3 vs. 21.3 months), but did not reach statistical significance ($p = 0.336$). Patient cross over and the availability of off study "targeted therapy" likely both contributed to the failure of this trial to show a statistically significant benefit in the median overall survival with the bevacizumab-containing regimen. Similar to the CALGB trial, grade ≥3 adverse events in the bevacizumab + IFN group included proteinuria (7%) and hypertension (3%). Based largely on the results of the AVOREN trial, bevacizumab + IFN gained regulatory approval for use in advanced RCC by the US FDA in 2009.

## Targeting the mTOR Pathway

The mTOR pathway has been implicated in the molecular pathogenesis of RCC. For this reason, small molecule inhibitors of mTOR have been evaluated in a series of clinical trials in RCC. Currently, two mTOR inhibitors have gained regulatory approval in the United States for the treatment of advanced RCC.

Temsirolimus is a parenterally administered mTOR inhibitor that demonstrated antitumor activity in RCC in a phase II study.[52] Based on a signal from this phase II trial suggesting that patients with poor risk factors might have benefitted disproportionately from temsirolimus, a three-arm trial of temsirolimus versus temsirolimus + IFN versus IFN was initiated in patients with metastatic RCC and poor risk features.[45] Poor risk disease was defined as meeting at least three of six predictors of short survival. These six predictors included the standard five predictors in the MSKCC risk model plus metastases in multiple organs. This trial enrolled 626 treatment-naïve patients; 80% had clear cell histology and 20% had non-clear cell histology. The median overall survival in the IFN, temsirolimus, and combination arms was 7.3 (95% CI, 6.1–8.8), 10.9 (95% CI, 8.6–12.7), and 8.4 months (95% CI, 6.6–10.3), respectively.[37] The hazard ratio for death was 0.73 in the temsirolimus versus the IFN group ($p = 0.008$). Notably, subgroup analysis indicated that patients with non-clear cell histology had similar benefit as those with clear cell histology upon treatment with temsirolimus. Grade ≥3 adverse events seen with single-agent temsirolimus included anemia (20%), fatigue (11%), hyperglycemia (11%), and dypnea (9%). Pneumonitis has emerged as a potentially serious side effect with mTOR inhibitors. A retrospective review of imaging from patients treated with temsirolimus in this study found that 29% had evidence of pneumonitis versus 6% of patients treated with IFN.[53]

Temsirolimus received US FDA approval for the treatment of metastatic RCC in 2007. As the phase III study enrolled treatment-naïve patients with poor-risk features, temsirolimus is most commonly utilized in this patient population.

## Everolimus

Everolimus is an oral mTOR inhibitor that has been evaluated in a randomized (2:1), placebo-controlled, phase III study of 416 patients with metastatic ccRCC who had received prior sunitinib or sorafenib.[46] The primary outcome of this study was PFS and cross over was allowed at the time of progression. By an independent review, PFS was 4.9 versus 1.9 months ($p < 0.001$) favoring everolimus. The median overall survival was 14.8 versus 14.4 months in the everolimus and placebo groups respectively ($p = 0.162$). However, 80% of the patients in the placebo arm were eventually exposed to everolimus, likely obscuring any potential survival benefit. Common grade ≥3 adverse events more common with everolimus included infections (10%), lymphopenia (16%), anemia

(12%), and hyperglycemia (15%). Grade 3 pneumonitis was seen in 4% of patients treated with everolimus. Everolimus received regulatory approval in the United States for treatment of advanced RCC following progression on VEGFR TKIs in 2009.

## Sequence of Therapies

Little is known about the most appropriate sequence of "targeted therapies" in the treatment of metastatic RCC. "Targeted therapies" that have shown efficacy in the first-line setting in phase III trials include sunitinib, pazopanib, bevacizumab, and temsirolimus. Following cytokine-based therapy, phase III trials have shown a benefit from sorafenib, pazopanib, and axitinib. Everolimus and axitinib showed a benefit in PFS in phase III trials following progression on a VEGFR TKI. Beyond this, we have only phase II trials and retrospective analyses to guide the sequencing of "targeted therapies." A number of clinical trials are currently investigating this issue (Table 29.2).

## Combination Regimens

While sequential exposure to single "targeted therapies" is the current standard of care in metastatic RCC, combinations of "targeted therapies" have been investigated. Possible benefits of combining "targeted therapies" include the potential synergistic effects of targeting multiple pathways simultaneously (or multiple targets in one pathway such as VEGF and VEGFR) and the potential to delay acquired resistance. Unfortunately, thus far, most attempts to combine "targeted therapies" have resulted in an increase in toxicity without a clear signal of increased efficacy relative to sequential treatment.

As an example, sorafenib was combined with bevacizumab in a phase I dose escalation study.[54] Due to toxicity, it was not possible to escalate either drug to full dose. The combination of sunitinib with bevacizumab has also been explored. In a phase I study in advanced solid tumors, toxicities with sunitinib + bevacizumab were quite high. Grade ≥3 toxicities included hypertension (47%), fatigue (24%), thrombocytopenia (18%), and proteinuria (13%).[55] This combination was also reported in a phase I trial in RCC patients.[56] Objective responses were seen in 52% of patients, but toxicity required discontinuation of therapy in 48% of patients. There were two cases of microangiopathic hemolytic anemia and grade ≥3 hypertension was seen in 60% of participants.

Combination regimens with mTOR inhibitors have been investigated. A phase I study evaluated the combination of sunitinib with temsirolimus.[57] This resulted in unacceptable toxicity in the initial cohort at low doses of both drugs. Bevacizumab has also been combined with everolimus in a phase II trial in metastatic ccRCC.[58] In this 80 patient trial, bevacizumab (10 mg/kg IV Q2wk) and everolimus (10 mg po daily) could be administered at their standard doses. Based on the promising activity, this combination is now being evaluated in a phase III trial (CALGB 90802) and a randomized phase II trial (RECORD-2) (Table 29.2). Interestingly, the combination of bevacizumab and temsirolimus, both at full dose, has been evaluated in a randomized phase II trial (TORAVA) in untreated RCC and resulted in unacceptable toxicity with grade ≥3 toxicities occurring in 77% of patients.[59] This combination is also being investigated in the phase III INTORACT trial (Table 29.2).

## Cytoreductive Nephrectomy

Two randomized studies, both published in 2001, demonstrated a survival benefit with cytoreductive nephrectomy (CyNx) in patients with metastatic ccRCC that were then treated with INF.[60,61] With

**Table 29.2** Trials of targeted therapies exploring combinations or sequencing in metastatic RCC.

| Trial/sponsor | Arms | Population | Design | Primary Endpoint | Status |
|---|---|---|---|---|---|
| **First line** | | | | | |
| COMPARZ/GSK | 1) Pazopanib<br>2) Sunitinib | Advanced/metastatic ccRCC. First Line | Phase III | PFS | Fully accrued |
| **Second line** | | | | | |
| Torisel 404/Pfizer | 1) Temsirolimus<br>2) Sorafenib | Metastic RCC. Progressed on sunitinib | Phase III | PFS | Fully accrued |
| **Sequence** | | | | | |
| Record-3/Novartis | 1) Everolimus-> Sunitinib<br>2) Sunitinib-> Everolimus | Metastatic RCC. First line | Randomized phase II | PFS | Fully accrued |
| Switch study/GmBH | 1) Sunitinib-> Sorafenib<br>2) Sorafenib-> Sunitinib | Advanced/metastatic RCC. First line | Phase III | PFS | Fully accrued |
| **Combination** | | | | | |
| BeST/ECOG | 1) Bev<br>2) Bev/Tem<br>3) Bev/Sorafenib<br>4) Tem/Sorafenib | Advanced/metastatic ccRCC.<br>No prior targeted therapy.<br>Previous IFN allowed | Randomized phase II | PFS | Fully accrued |
| RECORD-2/Novartis | 1) Bev/Everolimus<br>2) Bev/IFN | Metastatic RCC. First line | Randomized phase II | PFS | Fully accrued |
| CALGB 90802 | 1) Everolimus/Placebo<br>2) Everolimus/Bev | Advanced/metastatic ccRCC.<br>Progressed on one VEGFR TKI.<br>Prior cytokine therapy allowed. | Phase III | OS | Accruing |
| INTORACT/Pfizer | 1) Bev/Tem<br>2) Bev/IFN | Advanced ccRCC. First line. | Phase III | PFS | Fully accrued |

this data, CyNx became the standard of care in patients with metatstatic ccRCC prior to cytokine-based therapy.

In 2005, the first of the "targeted therapies" gained regulatory approval in the United States. There is no randomized clinical trial evidence that addresses the role of CyNx in patients treated with "targeted therapies." However, it should be noted that the vast majority of patients treated in large clinical trials of "targeted therapies" have undergone CyNx and many have required CyNx as an eligibility criteria. Retrospective studies have addressed this issue. One such retrospective study evaluated the role of CyNx in patients treated with VEGF targeted therapy.[62] In a multivariate analysis, CyNx was associated with prolonged survival. The reason for benefit associated with CyNx is unclear, but may be related to a reduction in inflammatory cytokines, reduction in growth factors such as VEGF, or from removal of subclones in the primary tumor that could add to the metastatic burden if left in place.

As the randomized data supporting the survival benefit of CyNx with metastatic ccRCC predated the introduction of "targeted agents," there has been a lack of evidence to support CyNx with these agents. With this uncertainty has come a change in the pattern of use of CyNx. A recent report utilized the Surveillance, Epidemiology, and End Results (SEER) registry to evaluate the use of CyNx before and after the introduction of "targeted agents" into the treatment of RCC.[63] Not surprisingly, a trend toward decreased use of CyNx was noted. Just prior to the approval of the first "targeted agent," 50% of patients with metastatic ccRCC underwent CyNx. This number had decreased to 38% by 2008. There are currently two phase III trials (NCT00930033 and NCT01099423) that are addressing the use of CyNx with "targeted agents." At this time, CyNx is considered in patients with adequate performance status, limited metastatic burden, and good or intermediate risk disease.

## Agents in Development

Several promising TKIs are at various stages of development. Tivozanib is a potent and selective inhibitor of VEGFR that has been recently demonstrated improved outcomes when compared with sorafenib as first-line therapy in a phase III trial (TIVO-1). The publication of the trial results is eagerly anticipated. Dovitinib is a novel TKI that inhibits FGFR in addition to VEGFR and PDGFR. A phase III trial is currently underway comparing dovitinib to sorafenib after progression of metastatic ccRCC following one VEGF-targeted therapy and an mTOR inhibitor. Cabozantinib and foretinib are duel inhibitors of c-Met and VEGFR which are currently being evaluated in RCC.

A number of agents with novel mechanisms of action are currently in development in RCC and include the vascular disrupting agent BNC105P, the angiopoietin inhibitor AMG-386, the VEGF-trap aflibercept, and the anti-carbonic anhydrase IX antibody, girentuximab. Immune checkpoint blockade with monoclonal antibodies against PD-1 (BMS-936558) and CTLA-4 (ipilimumab) have demonstrated very promising initial results.

## Conclusion

Recent years have seen significant advances in the treatment of metastatic ccRCC. With elucidation of key molecular mechanisms of disease, VEGF/VEGFR and mTOR emerged as promising targets which have now been validated in large clinical trials. At this time, seven novel "targeted agents" have gained regulatory approval in the United States since 2005. Outcomes continue to improve in metastatic RCC, but significant challenges remain. The appropriate sequencing of targeted agents and the role for combination regimens remains unclear. New targets are being explored and multiple novel compounds are at various stages of preclinical and clinical development. Biomarkers that add to our ability prognosticate outcomes and to predict benefit from targeted agents are urgently needed. Finally, utilizing these novel therapies earlier in the course of disease has the potential to have a profound impact on the curability of RCC, and trials in this context are ongoing.

# References

1 Siegel R, Naishadham D, Jemal A. Cancer statistics, 2012. *CA Cancer J Clin.* 2012;62:10–29.

2 Umbreit EC, Shimko MS, Childs MA, et al. Metastatic potential of a renal mass according to original tumour size at presentation. *BJU Int.* 2012;109(2):190–194.

3 Kane CJ, Mallin K, Ritchey J, Cooperberg MR, Carroll PR. Renal cell cancer stage migration: analysis of the National Cancer Data Base. *Cancer.* 2008;113:78–83.

4 Cohen AJ, Li FP, Berg S, et al. Hereditary renal-cell carcinoma associated with a chromosomal translocation. *N Engl J Med.* 1979;301:592–595.

5 Zbar B, Brauch H, Talmadge C, Linehan M. Loss of alleles of loci on the short arm of chromosome 3 in renal cell carcinoma. *Nature.* 1987;327:721–724.

6 Seizinger BR, Rouleau GA, Ozelius LJ, et al. Von Hippel-Lindau disease maps to the region of chromosome 3 associated with renal cell carcinoma. *Nature.* 1988;332:268–269.

7 Semenza GL, Wang GL. A nuclear factor induced by hypoxia via de novo protein synthesis binds to the human erythropoietin gene enhancer at a site required for transcriptional activation. *Mol Cell Biol.* 1992;12:5447–5454.

8 Wenger RH. Cellular adaptation to hypoxia: O2-sensing protein hydroxylases, hypoxia-inducible transcription factors, and O2-regulated gene expression. *FASEB J.* 2002;16:1151–1162.

9 Bruick RK, McKnight SL. A conserved family of prolyl-4-hydroxylases that modify HIF. *Science.* 2001;294:1337–1340.

10 Maxwell PH, Wiesener MS, Chang GW, et al. The tumour suppressor protein VHL targets hypoxia-inducible factors for oxygen-dependent proteolysis. *Nature.* 1999;399:271–275.

11 Gerlinger M, Rowan AJ, Horswell S, et al. Intratumor heterogeneity and branched evolution revealed by multiregion sequencing. *N Engl J Med.* 2012;366:883–892.

12 Sato K, Tsuchiya N, Sasaki R, et al. Increased serum levels of vascular endothelial growth factor in patients with renal cell carcinoma. *Jpn J Cancer Res.* 1999;90:874–879.

13 Neufeld G, Cohen T, Gengrinovitch S, Poltorak Z. Vascular endothelial growth factor (VEGF) and its receptors. *FASEB J.* 1999;13:9–22.

14 Olsson AK, Dimberg A, Kreuger J, Claesson-Welsh L. VEGF receptor signalling—in control of vascular function. *Nat Rev Mol Cell Biol.* 2006;7:359–371.

15 Elvert G, Kappel A, Heidenreich R, et al. Cooperative interaction of hypoxia-inducible factor-2alpha (HIF-2alpha) and Ets-1 in the transcriptional activation of vascular endothelial growth factor receptor-2 (Flk-1). *J Biol Chem.* 2003;278:7520–7530.

16 Nystrom A, Shaik ZP, Gullberg D, et al. Role of tyrosine phosphatase SHP-1 in the mechanism of endorepellin angiostatic activity. *Blood.* 2009;114:4897–4906.

17 Mitola S, Brenchio B, Piccinini M, et al. Type I collagen limits VEGFR-2 signaling by a SHP2 protein-tyrosine phosphatase-dependent mechanism 1. *Circ Res.* 2006;98:45–54.

18 Waltenberger J, Claesson-Welsh L, Siegbahn A, Shibuya M, Heldin CH. Different signal transduction properties of KDR and Flt1, two receptors for vascular endothelial growth factor. *J Biol Chem.* 1994;269:26988–26995.

19 Shalaby F, Rossant J, Yamaguchi TP, et al. Failure of blood-island formation and vasculogenesis in Flk-1-deficient mice. *Nature.* 1995;376:62–66.

20 Guo D, Jia Q, Song HY, Warren RS, Donner DB. Vascular endothelial cell growth factor promotes tyrosine phosphorylation of mediators of signal transduction that contain SH2 domains. Association with endothelial cell proliferation. *J Biol Chem.* 1995;270:6729–6733.

21 Abedi H, Zachary I. Vascular endothelial growth factor stimulates tyrosine phosphorylation and recruitment to new focal adhesions of focal adhesion kinase and paxillin in endothelial cells. *J Biol Chem.* 1997;272:15442–15451.

22 Takahashi T, Ueno H, Shibuya M. VEGF activates protein kinase C-dependent, but Ras-independent Raf-MEK-MAP kinase pathway for DNA synthesis in primary endothelial cells. *Oncogene.* 1999;18:2221–2230.

23 Shu X, Wu W, Mosteller RD, Broek D. Sphingosine kinase mediates vascular endothelial growth factor-induced activation of ras and mitogen-activated protein kinases. *Mol Cell Biol.* 2002;22:7758–7768.

24 Takahashi T, Yamaguchi S, Chida K, Shibuya M. A single autophosphorylation site on KDR/Flk-1 is essential for VEGF-A-dependent activation of PLC-gamma and DNA synthesis in vascular endothelial cells. *EMBO J.* 2001;20:2768–2778.

25 Dayanir V, Meyer RD, Lashkari K, Rahimi N. Identification of tyrosine residues in vascular endothelial growth factor receptor-2/FLK-1 involved in activation of phosphatidylinositol 3-kinase and cell proliferation. *J Biol Chem.* 2001;276:17686–17692.

26 Pantuck AJ, Seligson DB, Klatte T, et al. Prognostic relevance of the mTOR pathway in renal cell carcinoma: implications for molecular patient selection for targeted therapy. *Cancer.* 2007;109:2257–2267.

27 Brown EJ, Albers MW, Shin TB, et al. A mammalian protein targeted by G1-arresting rapamycin-receptor complex. *Nature.* 1994;369:756–758.

28 Edinger AL, Linardic CM, Chiang GG, Thompson CB, Abraham RT. Differential effects of rapamycin on mammalian target of rapamycin signaling functions in mammalian cells. *Cancer Res.* 2003;63:8451–8460.

29 Hara K, Maruki Y, Long X, et al. Raptor, a binding partner of target of rapamycin (TOR), mediates TOR action. *Cell.* 2002;110:177–189.

30 Sarbassov DD, Ali SM, Kim DH, et al. Rictor, a novel binding partner of mTOR, defines a rapamycin-insensitive and raptor-independent pathway that regulates the cytoskeleton. *Curr Biol.* 2004;14:1296–1302.

31 Zhong H, Chiles K, Feldser D, et al. Modulation of hypoxia-inducible factor 1alpha expression by the epidermal growth factor/phosphatidylinositol 3-kinase/PTEN/AKT/FRAP pathway in human prostate cancer cells: implications for tumor angiogenesis and therapeutics. *Cancer Res.* 2000;60:1541–1545.

32 Crino PB, Nathanson KL, Henske EP. The tuberous sclerosis complex. *N Engl J Med.* 2006;355:1345–1356.

33 Tee AR, Fingar DC, Manning BD, Kwiatkowski DJ, Cantley LC, Blenis J. Tuberous sclerosis complex-1 and -2 gene products function together to inhibit mammalian target of rapamycin (mTOR)-mediated downstream signaling. *Proc Natl Acad Sci U S A.* 2002;99:13571–13576.

34 Dan HC, Sun M, Yang L, et al. Phosphatidylinositol 3-kinase/Akt pathway regulates tuberous sclerosis tumor suppressor complex by phosphorylation of tuberin. *J Biol Chem.* 2002;277:35364–35370.

35 Motzer RJ, Bacik J, Murphy BA, Russo P, Mazumdar M. Interferon-alfa as a comparative treatment for clinical trials of new therapies against advanced renal cell carcinoma. *J Clin Oncol.* 2002;20:289–296.

36 Motzer RJ, Hutson TE, Tomczak P, et al. Overall survival and updated results for sunitinib compared with interferon alfa in patients with metastatic renal cell carcinoma. *J Clin Oncol.* 2009;27:3584–3590.

37 Motzer RJ, Hutson TE, Tomczak P, et al. Sunitinib versus interferon alfa in metastatic renal-cell carcinoma. *N Engl J Med*. 2007;356:115–124.

38 Escudier B, Eisen T, Stadler WM, et al. Sorafenib in advanced clear-cell renal-cell carcinoma. *N Engl J Med*. 2007;356:125–134.

39 Escudier B, Eisen T, Stadler WM, et al. Sorafenib for treatment of renal cell carcinoma: Final efficacy and safety results of the phase III treatment approaches in renal cancer global evaluation trial. *J Clin Oncol*. 2009;27:3312–3318.

40 Sternberg CN, Davis ID, Mardiak J, et al. Pazopanib in locally advanced or metastatic renal cell carcinoma: results of a randomized phase III trial. *J Clin Oncol*. 2010;28:1061–1068.

41 Rini BI, Escudier B, Tomczak P, et al. Comparative effectiveness of axitinib versus sorafenib in advanced renal cell carcinoma (AXIS): a randomised phase 3 trial. *Lancet*. 2011;378:1931–1939.

42 Rini BI, Halabi S, Rosenberg JE, et al. Bevacizumab plus interferon alfa compared with interferon alfa monotherapy in patients with metastatic renal cell carcinoma: CALGB 90206. *J Clin Oncol*. 2008;26:5422–5428.

43 Rini BI, Halabi S, Rosenberg JE, et al. Phase III trial of bevacizumab plus interferon alfa versus interferon alfa monotherapy in patients with metastatic renal cell carcinoma: final results of CALGB 90206. *J Clin Oncol*. 2010;28:2137–2143.

44 Escudier B, Pluzanska A, Koralewski P, et al. Bevacizumab plus interferon alfa-2 a for treatment of metastatic renal cell carcinoma: a randomised, double-blind phase III trial. *Lancet*. 2007;370:2103–2111.

45 Escudier B, Bellmunt J, Negrier S, et al. Phase III trial of bevacizumab plus interferon alfa-2 a in patients with metastatic renal cell carcinoma (AVOREN): final analysis of overall survival. *J Clin Oncol*. 2010;28:2144–2150.

46 Hudes G, Carducci M, Tomczak P, et al. Temsirolimus, interferon alfa, or both for advanced renal-cell carcinoma. *N Engl J Med*. 2007;356:2271–2281.

47 Motzer RJ, Escudier B, Oudard S, et al. Phase 3 trial of everolimus for metastatic renal cell carcinoma: final results and analysis of prognostic factors. *Cancer*. 2010;116:4256–4265.

48 Motzer RJ, Rini BI, Bukowski RM, et al. Sunitinib in patients with metastatic renal cell carcinoma. *JAMA*. 2006;295:2516–2524.

49 Gore ME, Szczylik C, Porta C, et al. Safety and efficacy of sunitinib for metastatic renal-cell carcinoma: an expanded-access trial. *Lancet Oncol*. 2009;10:757–763.

50 Escudier B, Szczylik C, Hutson TE, et al. Randomized phase II trial of first-line treatment with sorafenib versus interferon Alfa-2 a in patients with metastatic renal cell carcinoma. *J Clin Oncol*. 2009;27:1280–1289.

51 Yang JC, Haworth L, Sherry RM, et al. A randomized trial of bevacizumab, an anti-vascular endothelial growth factor antibody, for metastatic renal cancer. *N Engl J Med*. 2003;349:427–434.

52 Molina AM, Feldman DR, Voss MH, et al. Phase 1 trial of everolimus plus sunitinib in patients with metastatic renal cell carcinoma. *Cancer*. 2012;118:1868–1876.

53 Maroto JP, Hudes G, Dutcher JP, et al. Drug-related pneumonitis in patients with advanced renal cell carcinoma treated with temsirolimus. *J Clin Oncol*. 2011;29:1750–1756.

54 Azad NS, Posadas EM, Kwitkowski VE, et al. Combination targeted therapy with sorafenib and bevacizumab results in enhanced toxicity and antitumor activity. *J Clin Oncol*. 2008;26:3709–3714.

55 Rini BI, Garcia JA, Cooney MM, et al. A phase I study of sunitinib plus bevacizumab in advanced solid tumors. *Clin Cancer Res*. 2009;15:6277–6283.

56 Feldman DR, Baum MS, Ginsberg MS, et al. Phase I trial of bevacizumab plus escalated doses of sunitinib in patients with metastatic renal cell carcinoma. *J Clin Oncol*. 2009;27:1432–1439.

57 Patel PH, Senico PL, Curiel RE, Motzer RJ. Phase I study combining treatment with temsirolimus and sunitinib malate in patients with advanced renal cell carcinoma. *Clin Genitourin Cancer*. 2009;7:24–27.

58 Hainsworth JD, Spigel DR, Burris HA 3rd, Waterhouse D, Clark BL, Whorf R. Phase II trial of bevacizumab and everolimus in patients with advanced renal cell carcinoma. *J Clin Oncol*. 2010;28:2131–2136.

59 Negrier S, Gravis G, Perol D, et al. Temsirolimus and bevacizumab, or sunitinib, or interferon alfa and bevacizumab for patients with advanced renal cell carcinoma (TORAVA): a randomised phase 2 trial. *Lancet Oncol*. 2011;12:673–680.

60 Flanigan RC, Salmon SE, Blumenstein BA, et al. Nephrectomy followed by interferon alfa-2b compared with interferon alfa-2b alone for metastatic renal-cell cancer. *N Engl J Med*. 2001;345:1655–1659.

61 Mickisch GH, Garin A, van Poppel H, de Prijck L, Sylvester R. Radical nephrectomy plus interferon-alfa-based immunotherapy compared with interferon alfa alone in metastatic renal-cell carcinoma: a randomised trial. *Lancet*. 2001;358:966–970.

62 Choueiri TK, Xie W, Kollmannsberger C, et al. The impact of cytoreductive nephrectomy on survival of patients with metastatic renal cell carcinoma receiving vascular endothelial growth factor targeted therapy. *J Urol*. 2011;185:60–66.

63 Tsao CK, Small AC, Kates M, et al. Trends in the use of cytoreductive nephrectomy for metastatic renal cell carcinoma in the VEGFR tyrosine kinase inhibitor era. *J Clin Oncol (Meeting Abstracts)*. 2012; 30:4623.

## CHAPTER 30

# Targeted Therapy in Solid Tumors: Sarcomas

*Anthony P. Conley, Vinod Ravi, and Shreyaskumar Patel*

Department of Sarcoma Medical Oncology, The University of Texas MD Anderson Cancer Center, Houston, TX, USA

## Introduction

Sarcomas comprise less than 1% of all new cancer cases diagnosed each year in the United States and few effective therapies may control, but rarely cure, these neoplasms.[1] These neoplasms are divided into soft-tissue sarcomas and bone sarcomas. Further division involves anatomic location or possible tissue of origin. It is now possible to further classify based on chromosomal aberrations (i.e., translocations or complex cytogenetics) and/or by aberrant signaling pathways (Table 30.1). The exponential development of new agents has led to potential new treatment options for patients with sarcomas in addition to the established therapies. This chapter will focus on signal transduction pathways, including preclinical and clinical data, and the current state of the therapeutic management of patients with sarcoma with targeted therapies. Importantly, compared to carcinomas, sarcomas appear to have a lower incidence of detectable mutational alterations, which may indicate that fewer genomic events are potentially required for sarcomagenesis.[2]

## KIT

Gastrointestinal stromal tumors (GIST) are an example of an oncogene-addicted malignancy. Historically, these tumors have been resistant to doxorubicin-based strategies and prognosis was poor in the pre-imatinib era. Three lines of therapies are now approved by the Food and Drug Administration (FDA) for treatment of advanced, metastatic GIST. Each of these agents (imatinib, sunitinib, and regorafenib) target-mutated c-KIT.

Approximately 85% of sarcomas with c-KIT alterations harbor gain-of-function KIT mutations. In an activated state, c-KIT enables various pathways (AKT, RAS) in order to maintain cellular proliferation and to decrease apoptosis. The most common mutation affects the juxtamembrane domain (exon 11). Mutations may also affect the dimerization motif (exon 9) and the proximal kinase domain (exon 13).[3] Imatinib sensitivity to KIT-mutant GIST is exon-dependent, favoring exon-11 mutations followed by exon-9 mutations.[4] **in contrast, sunitinib** is also KIT exon-dependent and favors exon-9 subset as more responsive, and increases progression-free survival.[5] Rare mutations in the KIT exon 13 have been associated with primary resistance to imatinib, which is often noted in KIT wild-type tumors with mutations in the platelet-derived growth factor receptor alpha (PDGFRA) gene.

Mechanisms of resistance to imatinib in GIST most commonly involve secondary mutations in the KIT gene.[6] The activation loop (exon 17) and the proximal kinase domain (exon 13) represent the most frequent secondary mutations in the KIT gene. Because imatinib competitively inhibits the ATP-binding domain of the c-KIT protein, mutations near or within this region may alter drug binding and, thus, maintain the protein in an activated state.

The so-called "wild type" KIT cohort comprises a small subset (<10%) of patients with GIST, driven by various molecular aberrations. These patients are usually younger individuals with an associated hereditary syndrome such as the Carney's triad (gastric GIST, pulmonary chondromas, paragangliomas), the Carney–Stratakis syndrome (gastric GIST, paraganglioma), hereditary paraganglioma/pheochromocytoma syndromes, and neurofibromatosis type 1.[7] The Carney triad and Carney–Stratakis syndromes are associated with inactivating aberrations involving the succinate dehydrogenase complex, for which no specific targeted therapies are available. Less than 10% of patients with KIT wild-type GIST harbor exon-15 BRAF mutations of unclear significance. Patients with BRAF mutant GIST are currently participating in selective phase I studies with BRAF inhibitors, which will help elucidate the role of BRAF targeted therapy in GIST

### Platelet-Derived Growth Factor and Its Receptors

Platelet-derived growth factor (PDGF), (PDGFRA), and PDGFR beta (PDGFRB) regulate growth and survival in certain cell types during embryologic development.[8] In adult humans, these factors are involved in tissue repair. PDGF are produced by epithelial cells, endothelial cells, smooth muscle cells, activated macrophages, and activated platelets. In both epithelial cells and endothelial cells, PDGF signaling exerts a paracrine effect upon nearby mesenchymal cells such as pericytes or fibroblasts.[9]

PDGFRB is overexpressed in dermatofibrosarcoma protuberans (DFSP), a cutaneous sarcoma with an indolent course in most cases; metastases are rare (<5% of cases).[10] DFSP is associated with a rearrangement involving chromosomes 17 (17q22) and 22 (22q13). This results in a fusion of the COL1A1 gene to the PDGFB gene, which is noted in the normal variant of DFSP and in the fibrosarcomatous transformation of DFSP.[11] This fusion protein stimulates tumor growth in an autocrine manner similar to the effect of PDGF-BB on PDGFRB.[9]

Imatinib can inhibit PDGFR signaling, and it has demonstrated efficacy in several clinical studies. A pooled analysis of two

Table 30.1 Selected sarcomas by histology and genomic aberrations.

| | | Histology | Genomic abnormality |
|---|---|---|---|
| Fusion-positive | Soft tissue | Alveolar rhabdomyosarcoma | PAX3-FOXO1 |
| | | | PAX7-FOXO1 |
| | | Alveolar soft part sarcoma | ASPSCR1-TFE3 (ASPL-TEE3) |
| | | Clear cell sarcoma | EWSR1-ATF1 |
| | | | EWSR1-CREB1 |
| | | Dermatofibrosarcoma protuberans | COL1A1-PDGFB |
| | | Desmoplastic small round cell tumor | EWSR1-WT1 |
| | | Epithelioid hemangioendothelioma | WWTR1-CAMTA1 |
| | | | YAP1-TFE3 |
| | | Inflammatory myofibroblastic tumor | RANBP2-ALK |
| | | Solitary fibrous tumor | NAB2-STAT6 |
| | | Synovial sarcoma | SYT-SSX1 |
| | | | SYT-SSX2 |
| | Bone | Ewing's sarcoma | EWSR1-FLI1 |
| | | | EWSR1-ERG |
| | | Extraskeletal myxoid chondrosarcoma | EWSR1-NR4A3 |
| | | | TAF15-NR4A3 |
| | | Mesenchymal chondrosarcoma | HEY1-NCOA2 |
| Fusion-negative | Soft tissue | Angiosarcoma | KDR, PTPRB, PLCB1 mutations |
| | | Desmoid fibromatosis | CTNNB1 mutations |
| | | Embryonal rhabdomyosarcoma | FGFR4, PIK3CA, RAS, tP53 mutations |
| | | Gastrointestinal stromal tumor | Mutations in KIT, PDGFR, or SDH loss |
| | | PEComa | TSC1/2 loss of function |
| | Bone | Conventional chondrosarcomas | Mutations in IDH1, IDH2, SMO,TP53, & PTCH1 loss |
| | | Osteosarcomas | Chromothripsis; TP53, RB1 |

concurrent phase II trials of imatinib for patients with advanced/metastatic DFSP showed a partial response (PR) rate of 45% by RECIST and a median time to progression of 1.7 years.[12] A neoadjuvant phase II trial of imatinib for patients with DFSP and primary or locally recurrent disease was associated with a complete response (CR) rate of 7.1%, PR of 50%, and stable disease (SD) of 36%[13] Tissue analysis of responders to imatinib showed decreased tumor cellularity and fibrotic formation, while non-responders (7%) exhibited weak PDGFRB activation. Resistance to imatinib is poorly understood. One report demonstrated that the COL1A1-PDGFB fusion persists in the progressive clones without copy number alterations or new point mutations, which suggests that fusion status alone does not account for secondary resistance to imatinib.[14] These imatinib-resistant tumors contained new somatically mutated genes (ACAP2, CARD10, KIAA0556, PAQR7, PPP1R39, SAFB2, STARD9, ZFYVE9) associated with activation in the NF-κB signaling pathway, stress response, and mitotic microtubule formation.[14]

Chordomas express PDGF and PDGFRB without evidence of mutation. In a phase II study of imatinib for advanced chordoma, one of 50 patients had a PR.[15] Rhabdomyosarcomas upregulate PDGFRA, which is associated with a shorter overall survival (OS) compared to patients without PDGFRA overexpression.[16] A subset of patients with GIST and wild-type KIT harbor PDGFRA mutations, generally affecting exons 18 (kinase 2 domain), 12 (juxtamembrane domain), and 14 (kinase 1 domain). The PDGFRA mutations in exon 18 confer decreased sensitivity to imatinib.[3] An analysis of PDGFRA-mutated tumor samples demonstrated that crenolanib, a selective PDGFRA inhibitor, is 135-fold more potent than imatinib.[17] A phase II study of crenolanib for PDGFRA mutant GIST was completed and the final analysis is pending.

## Insulin-Like Growth Factor 1 Receptor

The insulin growth factor (IGF) pathway tightly regulates cellular growth and metabolism. This axis can influence neoplastic development by multiple mechanisms including downstream activation of survival pathways such as the PI3K/AKT pathway and the RAS/MAPK signaling pathway.[18]

IGF1 and IGF2 are produced by multiple tissues of the body, and both bind to IGF1R. IGF1 has a greater binding affinity to insulin-like growth factor 1 receptor (IGF1R) than IGF2. IGF1 secretion is dependent upon growth hormone (GH) binding with its receptor in the liver, while IGF2 is secreted independent of GH secretion or binding. Interestingly, cancer cells may also secrete IGF1 independent of GH signaling.

IGF1R consists of two extracellular alpha chains with ligand-binding capacity and two transmembrane beta chains. IGF1 binds to the alpha subunit of IGF1R, resulting in a conformational change that induces autophosphorylation. Phosphorylation, in turn, recruits adaptor proteins to drive transcription of specific genes via the PI3K/AKT pathway and facilitates recruitment of glucose transporters (GLUT) to the cell surface for entry of glucose from blood for energy consumption.[18] IGF2R does not have kinase activity. IGF-binding proteins (IGFBPs) regulate IGF1/2 levels by sequestering these growth factors in circulation and, thus, removing the ligand which stimulates IGF1R activation.[19]

The IGF1R pathway is important for many sarcomas including alveolar rhabdomyosarcoma, desmoplastic small round cell tumors (DSRCT), Ewing's sarcoma, osteosarcomas, solitary fibrous tumors, and synovial sarcomas.[20] In DSRCT, the EWSR1-WT1 fusion protein can induce promoter activity of IGF1R.[21] The EWSR1-FLI1 fusion protein in Ewing's sarcoma represses IGFBP3, which leads to IGF1R activation.[22]

Inhibitors of IGF1R signaling may directly target IGF ligands, inhibit ligand binding to IGF1R, or inhibit the interactions at the intracellular domain. The monoclonal antibodies targeting the extracellular binding domain of IGF1R are the best studied for this disease. Single-agent activity in Ewing's sarcoma was demonstrated in two phase I trials in heavily pretreated patients. Ganitumab induced a CR in one patient lasting at least 28 months and an unconfirmed PR in another patient, while R1507 induced a PR in two patients that lasted for 11.5 months and 26 months.[23,24]

Unfortunately, these anti-IGF1R antagonists failed to demonstrate substantial activity in the phase II setting. In Ewing's sarcoma or DSRCT, ganitumab had a response rate (RR) of 6% and 49% achieved SD as best response.[25] Only four patients had SD exceeding 24 months. Similarly, a phase II study of R1507 had a RR of 10% and a median duration of response of 29 weeks.[26] Phase II results for other sarcoma histologic subtypes were reported with a RR of 2.5% ($n = 4$ patients; 3 rhabdomyosarcoma, 1 myxoid liposarcoma) and an additional four patients had an unconfirmed response lasting less than 4 weeks.[27]

In these initial studies, no specific marker predicted consistently for response. IGF-1 levels were noted to rise over time in patients treated with anti-IGF1R antibodies. At least one study suggested that increased IGF-1 levels correlated with improvement in PFS.[28] Unfortunately, compensatory mechanisms abrogate the success of initial response. These possibilities include rising levels of ligand, rising insulin levels (which share homology with IGF), and co-activation of other tyrosine kinase receptor pathways. Several studies sought to overcome resistance to IGF1R inhibitors by the addition of mammalian target of rapamycin (mTOR) inhibitors.

In a phase I combination study in Ewing's sarcoma and DSRCT, the addition of temsirolimus to cixutumumab resulted in a SD rate of 35% lasting longer than 5 months of which two patients with Ewing's sarcoma achieved a CR.[29] One had received anti-IGF1R antibody on a prior study. Interestingly, a patient on this study with a prior R1507 exposure, had upregulation of the mTOR pathway in an R1507-progressive lesion noted by morphoproteomic analysis. This same patient responded to the cixutumumab/temsirolimus study suggesting that mTOR upregulation may contribute to resistance to single-agent anti-IGF1R antibodies. A separate phase II study of the same regimen divided patients into three groups: IGF1R-positive soft-tissue sarcomas (by immunohistochemistry), IGF1R-positive bone sarcomas, and IGF1R-negative sarcomas of bone or soft tissue.[30] The study endpoint was PFS at 12 weeks ($PFS_{12\ weeks}$) of at least 40% based on a Simon optimal two-stage design for each treatment arm. The $PFS_{12\ weeks}$ durations for IGF1R-positive soft-tissue sarcomas, IGF1R-positive bone sarcomas, and the IGF1R-negative group were 31%, 35%, and 39%, respectively. Thus, this study failed to achieve its primary endpoint. Furthermore, IGF1R expression failed to correlate with response. The lack of sustained success has halted further development of these agents for Ewing's sarcoma. Better understanding of this signaling pathway and, hopefully, discovery of a biomarker of response may allow us to revisit this treatment strategy for Ewing's sarcoma.

## mTOR Signaling Pathway

As noted earlier, the addition of an mTOR inhibitor to an anti IGF1R antibody appears to improve upon single-agent activity and durability of response to anti-IGF1R antibodies. mTOR is a serine/threonine protein kinase that participates downstream of the phosphatidylinositol 3-kinase (PI3K)-related kinase pathway. Importantly, mTOR represents the catalytic subunit of mTORC1 and mTORC2.[31] Inhibition of mTORC1 alone results in AKT elevation by mTORC2. Thus, inhibition of both mTORC1 and mTORC2 is necessary to decrease resistance by AKT-positive feedback loop.

Multiple sarcoma subtypes exhibit activation of the mTOR/AKT pathway, which led to its study in clinical trials.[32,33] A phase II study of ridaforolimus, an analog of rapamycin, in sarcoma patients with prior systemic therapies resulted in a median PFS of 15.3 weeks and median OS of 40 weeks.[34] The RR was low (1.9%) and the clinical benefit rate (objective responses plus SD), was 28.8%. In terms of safety, grade 3 or 4 adverse events were seen in 38.7% of patients, and anemia was the most common adverse event. Only 11% of patient discontinued the study because of toxicity.

A phase III study of ridaforolimus versus placebo in metastatic sarcoma was performed to determine if mTOR inhibition could be used as a maintenance therapy in individuals with advanced/metastatic sarcoma with response to primary systemic therapy.[35] Overall, 702 of 711 enrolled patients received study drug or placebo. Compared with a median PFS of 14.6 weeks on the placebo arm, ridaforolimus was associated with a modest improvement in survival with a median PFS of 17.7 weeks. The hazard ratio was 0.72 with 95% confidence intervals of 0.61–0.85. After FDA review, an indication for ridaforolimus as maintenance therapy was not granted.

A series of patients with perivascular epithelioid cell tumors (PEComas) treated with sirolimus exhibited radiographic response.[36] Importantly, these tumors exhibited morphoproteomic evidence of mTOR activation (cytoplasmic expression of phosphorylated S6 protein). This was associated with decreased TSC1/TSC2 gene expression and loss of their protein products. Separate case series with other mTOR inhibitors mirrored these results.[37,38]

## Vascular Endothelial Growth Factor/VEGF Receptor Inhibition

Angiogenesis is an extremely complex process utilized by neoplasms, including sarcomas, to aid with growth on a macroscopic level. This system requires factors affecting blood vessel remodeling as well as interactions from the surrounding microenvironment. Several agents targeting the vascular endothelial growth factor (VEGF) pathway have been evaluated for the systemic management of sarcomas, and several of these agents have been impactful.

Pazopanib, a multi-kinase inhibitor with specificity for VEGF receptors (VEGFR1–3), was evaluated in a phase III trial (PALETTE) for soft-tissue sarcoma patients with prior exposure to doxorubicin.[39] Pazopanib resulted in a statistically significant median PFS compared to placebo, (4.6 months versus 1.6 months, respectively) with a hazard ratio of 0.31 (95% CI 0.24–0.40; $p < 0.0001$). There was a trend for improvement in OS with pazopanib compared to placebo, though this was not significant (12.5 months versus 10.7 months; $p = 0.25$). RR was 6% in the pazopanib arm. In a multivariable model evaluating prognostic factors on PFS, good performance status, prior treatment exposure, and histologic grade but histologic subtype was not favorable. Fortunately, the evidence was sufficient for FDA approval of pazopanib for patients with advanced/metastatic soft-tissue sarcoma refractory to at least one prior line of systemic therapy.

Alveolar soft part sarcoma (ASPS), driven by a fusion of ASPL-TFE3, binds the MET promoter resulting in transcriptional upregulation of MET signaling.[40] Primary cultures of ASPS exhibit protein expression of MET, PDGFRB, RET, and VEGFR2.[41] Treatment with sunitinib, an inhibitor of KIT, PDGFR, and VEGFR1–3, results in a decrease in PDGFRB phosphorylation. Five of nine patients

**Table 30.2** Selected studies of anti-vascular agents sarcomas.

| Disease | Agent | Study | Sample size | RECIST RR | Median PFS | Median OS | Ref |
|---------|-------|-------|-------------|-----------|------------|-----------|-----|
| ASPS | Sunitinib | Case series | 9 | 56% | 17 months | 19 months | 41 |
| ASPS | Cediranib | Phase II | 43 | 35% | DCR$_{24\ weeks}$ 84% | NA | 42 |
| SFT | Sunitinib | Case series | 31 | 6.5% | 6 months | 16 months | 43 |
| SFT | Temozolomide Bevacizumab | Case series | 14 | 0% | 10.8 months | 24.3 months | 44 |
| DSRCT | Pazopanib | Case series | 9 | 22% | 9.2 months | 15.4 months | 45 |
| DSRCT | Sunitinib | Case series | 8 | 25% | 2.6 months | NA | 46 |
| EMC | Sunitinib | Case series | 10 | 60% | Not reached | Not reached | 47 |
| AS EHE | Bevacizumab | Phase II | 32 | 17% | 12.4 weeks | 107 weeks | 48 |
| STS | Gemcitabine/Docetaxel Bevacizumab | Phase IB | 38 | 31.4% | 5 months (metastatic) | 11 months (metastatic) | 49 |
| AS | Sorafenib | Phase II | A: 26 B: 15 | 14.6% at 4 months | A: 1.8 months B: 3.8 months | A: 12 months B: 9 months | 50 |
| STS | Sorafenib | Phase II | 122 | 14% (AS) | 3.2 months | 14.3 months | 51 |

ASPS, alveolar soft part sarcoma; AS, angiosarcoma; DCR, disease control rate; DSRCT, desmoplastic small round cell tumor; EMC, extraskeletal myxoid chondrosarcoma; EHE, epithelioid hemangioendothelioma; SFT, solitary fibrous tumor; STS, soft tissue sarcomas; TTP, time to progression.

who received sunitinib experienced a PR by RECIST.[41] A separate ASPS phase II study of cediranib, another inhibitor of VEGFR1–3, resulted in a PR of 35% and a PFS rate of 84%.[42] Activity of VEGF/VEGFR inhibitors have also been observed in other sarcoma subtypes (Table 30.2).[43–51]

## Conclusion

Given the depth of the sarcoma landscape, this chapter focuses on the most relevant areas that have influenced the last decade of clinical development and ongoing work in both the laboratory and clinic. Tyrosine kinase receptor inhibitors clearly play an important role in the management of diseases like GIST or DFSP, but more work is needed to implement these agents into the management of diseases such as Ewing's sarcoma. The IGF1R pathway provided early excitement with the unexpected dramatic responses and the results of several studies clearly demonstrating a need for an improved basic science understanding regarding the mechanisms of resistance to agents targeting the IGF1R pathway. Attempts to implement mTOR inhibitors as maintenance reaffirmed that sarcomas should not be treated as one disease, and that careful selection of patients with specific genomic aberrations (TSC1/2 loss) may enrich the activ-

ity of mTOR inhibitors. Lastly, VEGF/VEGFR1–3 inhibitors have resulted in a new FDA indication for treatment of metastatic soft-tissue sarcoma patients. In selected subtypes, treatment response with delays in progression is also noted.

Future prospects may include a better understanding of cell cycle inhibitors for diseases with intact p53 function and MDM2 amplification as seen with well-differentiated/dedifferentiated liposarcomas.[52] Development of hedgehog inhibitors for chondrosarcomas have yet to yield meaningful results, though enrichment for SMO/PTCH1-mutated tumors may be necessary as seen with mTOR inhibition in sarcoma.[53]

Immunology has become a popular area of interest considering the success of ipilimumab, nivolumab, and pembrolizumab in melanoma. Expression of programmed cell death protein 1 (PD-1) and its ligand, PD-L1, have variable expressions among sarcomas and it is unclear whether response to agents targeting either PD-1 or PD-L1 will result in the same impact as seen with melanomas.[54]

Finally, implementation of next-generation sequencing into the clinic will assist us in the management of sarcomas by identifying actionable targets of therapeutic interest for patients, whose sarcomas are refractory to standard chemotherapy or in rare sarcomas without a standard systemic strategy (Figure 30.1). From a

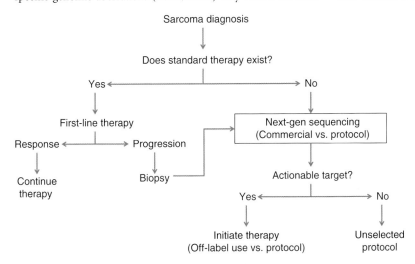

**Figure 30.1** Proposed integration of molecular analysis/next-generation sequencing into clinical practice.

discovery standpoint, these measures have allowed us to uncover mutations in isocitrate dehydrogenase 1 and 2 (IDH1/IDH2) in central chondrosarcomas, and protein tyrosine phosphatase, receptor type B (PTPRB) truncating mutations specific to angiosarcomas.[55,56] Translating these results into the clinic may add to the armamentarium currently used to manage these rare but difficult diseases in the clinic.

# References

1 Amankwah EK, Conley AP, Reed DR. Epidemiology and therapies for metastatic sarcoma. *Clin Epidemiol.* 2013;5:147–162.

2 Sledge GW. The challenge and promise of the genomic era. *J Clin Oncol.* 2012;30:203–209.

3 Gounder MM, Maki RG. Molecular basis for primary and secondary tyrosine kinase inhibitor resistance in gastrointestinal stromal tumor. *Cancer Chemother Pharmacol.* 2011;67:S25–S43.

4 Heinrich MC, Corless CL, Blanke CD, et al. Molecular correlates of imatinib resistance in gastrointestinal stromal tumors. *J Clin Oncol.* 2006;24:4764–4774.

5 Heinrich MC, Maki RG, Corless CL, et al. Primary and secondary kinase genotypes correlate with the biological and clinical activity of sunitinib in imatinib-resistant gastrointestinal stromal tumor. *J Clin Oncol.* 2008;26:5352–5359.

6 Wang WL, Conley A, Reynoso D, et al. Mechanisms of resistance to imatinib and sunitinib in gastrointestinal stromal tumor. *Cancer Chemother Pharmacol.* 2011;67:S15–S24.

7 Nannini M, Biasco G, Astolfi A, Pantaleo MA. An overview on molecular biology of KIT/PDGFRA wild type (WT) gastrointestinal stromal tumours (GIST). *J Med Genet.* 2013;50:653–661.

8 Heldin CH, Westermark B. Mechanism of action and *in vivo* role of platelet-derived growth factor. *Physiol Rev.* 1999;79:1283–1316.

9 Heldin CH. Targeting the PDGF signaling pathway in tumor treatment. *Cell Commun Signal.* 2013;11:97.

10 Baird K, Davis S, Antonescu CR, et al. Gene expression profiling of human sarcomas: insights into sarcoma biology. *Cancer Res.* 2005;65:9226 9235.

11 Rutkowski P, Wozniak A, Switaj T. Advances in molecular characterization and targeted therapy in dermatofibrosarcoma protuberans. *Sarcoma.* 2011;2011:959132.

12 Rutkowski P, van Glabbeke M, Rankin CJ, et al. Imatinib mesylate in advanced dermatofibrosarcoma protuberans: pooled analysis of two phase II clinical trials. *J Clin Oncol.* 2010;28:1772–1779.

13 Ugurel S, Mentzel T, Utikal J, et al. Neo adjuvant imatinib in advanced primary or locally recurrent dermatofibrosarcoma protuberans: a multicenter phase II DeCOG trial with long-term follow-up. *Clin Cancer Res.* 2013;20:499–510.

14 Hong YJ, Liu X, Mao M, et al. Dermatofibrosarcoma protuberans revealed by whole genome sequencing. *PLoS One.* 2013;8:e69752.

15 Stacchiotti S, Longhi A, Ferraresi V, et al. Phase II study of imatinib in advanced chordoma. *J Clin Oncol.* 2012;30:914–920.

16 Armistead PM, Salganick J, Roh JS, et al. Expression of receptor tyrosine kinases and apoptotic molecules in rhabdomyosarcoma: correlation with overall survival in 105 patients. *Cancer.* 2007;110:2293–2303.

17 Heinrich MC, Griffith D, McKinley A, et al. Crenolanib inhibits the drug-resistant PDGFRA D842V mutation associated with imatinib-resistant gastrointestinal stromal tumors. *Clin Cancer Res.* 2012;18;4375–4384.

18 Arnaldez FI, Helman LJ. Targeting the insulin growth factor receptor 1. *Hematol Oncol Clin North Am.* 2012;26:527–542.

19 Tognon CE, Sorensen PH. Targeting the insulin-like growth factor 1 receptor (IGF1R) signaling pathway for cancer therapy. *Expert Opin Ther Targets.* 2012;16:33–48.

20 Maki RG. Small is beautiful: insulin-like growth factors and their role in growth, development, and cancer. *J Clin Oncol.* 2010;28:4985–4995.

21 Karnieli E, Werner H, Rauscher FJ III, et al. The IGF-I receptor gene promoter is a molecular target for the Ewing's sarcoma-Wilm's tumor 1 fusion protein. *J Biol Chem.* 1996;271:19304–19309.

22 Prieur A, Tirode F, Cohen P, et al. EWS/FLI-1 silencing and gene profiling of ewing cells reveal downstream oncogenic pathways and a crucial role for repression of insulin-like growth factor binding protein 3. *Mol Cell Biol.* 2004;24:7275–7283.

23 Tolcher AW, Sarantopoulos J, Patnaik A, et al. Phase I, pharmacokinetic, and pharmacodynamics study of AMG 479, a fully human monoclonal antibody to insulin-like growth factor receptor 1. *J Clin Oncol.* 2009;27:5800–5807.

24 Kurzrock R, Patnaik A, Aisner J, et al. A phase I study of weekly R1507, a human monoclonal antibody insulin-like growth factor-I receptor antagonist, in patients with advanced solid tumors. *Clin Cancer Res.* 2010;16:2458–2465.

25 Tap WD, Demetri G, Barnette P, et al. Phase II study of ganitumab, a fully human anti-type-1 insulin-like growth factor receptor antibody, in patients with metastatic ewing family tumors or desmoplastic small round cell tumors. *J Clin Oncol.* 2012;30:1849–1856.

26 Pappo AS, Patel SR, Crowley J, et al. R1507, a monoclonal antibody to the insulin-like growth factor 1 receptor, in patients with recurrent or refractory ewing sarcoma family of tumors: results of a phase II sarcoma alliance for research through collaboration study. *J Clin Oncol.* 2011;29:4541–4547.

27 Pappo AS, Vassal G, Crowley JJ, et al. A phase II trial of R1507, a monoclonal antibody to the insulin-like growth factor-1 receptor (IGF-1R), in patients with recurrent or refractory rhabdomyosarcoma, osteosarcoma, synovial sarcoma, and other soft tissue sarcomas: results of a sarcoma alliance for research through collaboration study. *Cancer.* 2014;120:2448–2456.

28 Juergens H, Daw NC, Geoerger B, et al. Preliminary efficacy of the anti-insulin-like growth factor type 1 receptor antibody figitumumab in patients with refractory ewing sarcoma. *J Clin Oncol.* 2011;29:4534–4540.

29 Naing A, LoRusso P, Fu S, et al. Insulin growth factor-receptor (IGF-1R) antibody cixutumumab combined with the mTOR inhibitor temsirolimus in patients with refractory ewing's sarcoma family tumors. *Clin Cancer Res.* 2012;18:2625–2631.

30 Schwartz GK, Tap WD, Qin LX, et al. Cixutumumab and temsirolimus for patients with bone and soft-tissue sarcoma: a multicentre, open-label, phase 2 trial. *Lancet Oncol.* 2013;14:371–382.

31 Wullschleger S, Loewith R, Hall M. TOR signaling in growth and metabolism. *Cell.* 2006;124:471–484.

32 Dobashi Y, Suzuki S, Sato E, et al. EGFR-dependent and independent activation of Akt/mTOR cascade in bone and soft tissue tumors. *Mod Pathol.* 2009;22:1328–1340.

33 Hernando E, Charytonowicz E, Dudas ME, et al. The Akt-mTOR pathway plays a critical role in the development of leiomyosarcomas. *Nat Med.* 2007;13:748–753.

34 Chawla SP, Staddon AP, Baker LH, et al. Phase II study of the mammalian target of rapamycin inhibitor ridaforolimus in patients with advanced bone and soft tissue sarcomas. *J Clin Oncol.* 2011;30: 78–84.

35 Demetri GD, Chawla SP, Ray-Coquard I, et al. Results of an international randomized phase III trial of the mammalian target of rapamycin

inhibitor ridaforolimus versus placebo to control metastatic sarcomas in patients after benefit from prior chemotherapy. *J Clin Oncol.* 2013;31:2485–2492.

36 Wagner AJ, Malinowska-Kolodziej I, Morgan JA, et al. Clinical activity of mTOR inhibition with sirolimus in malignant perivascular epithelioid cell tumors: targeting the pathogenic activation of mTORC1 in tumors. *J Clin Oncol.* 2010;28:835–840.

37 Italiano A, Delcambre C, Hostein I, et al. Treatment with the mTOR inhibitor temsirolimus in patients with malignant PEComa. *Ann Oncol.* 2010;21:1135–1137.

38 Benson C, Vitfell-Rasmussen J, Maruzzo M, et al. A retrospective study of patients with malignant PEComa receiving treatment with sirolimus or temsirolimus: thee Royal Marsden Hospital experience. *Anticancer Res.* 2014;34:3663–3668.

39 Van der Graaf WT, Blay JY, Chawla SP, et al. Pazopanib for metastatic soft-tissue sarcoma (PALETTE): a randomized, double-blind, placebo-controlled phase 3 trial. *Lancet.* 2012;379:1879–1886.

40 Landanyi M, Lui MY, Antonescu CR, et al. The der(17)t(X;17)(p11;q25) of human alveolar soft part sarcoma fuses the TFE3 transcription factor gene to ASPL, a novel gene at 17q25. *Oncogene.* 2001;20: 48–57.

41 Stacchiotti S, Negri T, Zaffaroni N, et al. Sunitinib in advanced alveolar soft part sarcoma: evidence of a direct antitumor effect. *Ann Oncol.* 2011;22:1682–1690.

42 Kummar S, Allen D, Monks A, et al. Cediranib for metastatic alveolar soft part sarcoma. *J Clin Oncol.* 2013;31:2296–2302.

43 Stacchiotti S, Negri T, Libertini M, et al. Sunitinib malate in solitary fibrous tumor (SFT). *Ann Oncol.* 2012;23:3171–3179.

44 Park MS, Patel SR, Ludwig JA, et al. Activity of temozolomide and bevacizumab in the treatment of locally advanced, recurrent, and metastatic hemangiopericytoma and malignant solitary fibrous tumor. *Cancer.* 2011;117:4939–4947.

45 Frezza AM, Benson C, Judson IR, et al. Pazopanib in advanced desmoplastic small round cell tumours: a multi-institutional experience. *Clin Sarcoma Res.* 2014;4:7.

46 Italiano A, Kind M, Cioffi A, et al. Clinical activity of sunitinib in patients with advanced desmoplastic round cell tumor: a case series. *Targ Oncol.* 2013;8:211–213.

47 Stacchiotti S, Pantaleo MA, Astolfi A, et al. Activity of sunitinib in extraskeletal myxoid chondrosarcoma. *Eur J Cancer.* 2014;50:1657–1664.

48 Agulnik M, Yarber JL, Okuno SH, et al. An open-label, multicenter, phase II study of bevacizumab for the treatment of angiosarcoma and epithelioid hemangioendotheliomas. *Ann Oncol.* 2013;24:257–263.

49 Verschraegen CF, Arias-Pulido H, Lee SJ, et al. Phase IB study of the combination of docetaxel, gemcitabine, and bevacizumab in patients with advanced or recurrent soft tissue sarcoma: the Axtell regimen. *Ann Oncol.* 2012;23:785–790.

50 Ray-Coquard I, Italiano A, Bompas E, et al. Sorafenib for patients with advanced angiosarcoma: a phase II trial from the French Sarcoma Group (GSF/GETO). *Oncologist.* 2012;17:260–266.

51 Maki RG, D'Adamo DR, Keohan ML, et al. Phase II study of sorafenib in patients with metastatic or recurrent sarcomas. *J Clin Oncol.* 2009;27:3133–3140.

52 Tseng WW, Somaiah N, Lazar AJ, et al. Novel systemic therapies in advanced liposarcoma: a review of recent clinical trial results. *Cancers.* 2013;5:529–549.

53 Italiano A, Le Cesne A, Bellera C, et al. GDC-0449 in patients with advanced chondrosarcomas: a French Sarcoma Group/US and French National Cancer Institute single-arm phase II collaborative study. *Ann Oncol.* 2013;24:2922–2926.

54 Kim JR, Moon YJ, Kwon KS, et al. Tumor infiltrating PD-1 positive lymphocytes and the expression of PD-L1 predict poor prognosis of soft tissue sarcomas. *PLoS One.* 2013;8:e82870.

55 Amary MF, Basci K, Maggiani F, et al. IDH1 and IDH2 mutations are frequent events in central chondrosarcoma and central and periosteal chondromas but not in other mesenchymal tumours. *J Pathol.* 2011;224:334–343.

56 Behjati S, Tarpey PS, Sheldon H, et al. Recurrent PTPRB and PLCG1 mutations in angiosarcoma. *Nat Genet.* 2014;46:376–379.

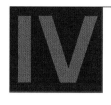

**PART IV**

# Targeted Therapy for Specific Molecular Aberrations

## CHAPTER 31

# RAS-RAF-MEK Pathway: Aberrations and Therapeutic Possibilities

*Javier Munoz[1] and Filip Janku[2]*

[1]Division of Hematology/Oncology, Banner MD Anderson Cancer Center, Gilbert, AZ, USA
[2]Department of Investigational Cancer Therapeutics (Phase I Clinical Trials Program), Division of Cancer Medicine, The University of Texas MD Anderson Cancer Center, Houston, TX, USA

## Introduction

The mitogen-activated protein kinases (MAPK) are part of a family of serine and threonine protein kinases, well preserved among eukaryotes, that form a cascade of molecular signals, eventually leading to proliferation, survival, differentiation, and cell fate determination.[1] The MAPK network is organized hierarchically (Figure 31.1) beginning with cell membrane receptors subject to external stimuli (as hormones, cytokines, and growth factors). These successively initiate proliferation from the cell membrane to the nucleus as MAPKs are phosphorylated by MAPK-kinases (MAPKKs), which in turn are phosphorylated by MAPKK-kinases (MAPKKKs) activated by other protein kinases near the cell membrane.[1] The primary MAPK network is the RAS-RAF-MEK-ERK[2] pathway, composed of rat sarcoma (RAS), rapidly accelerated fibrosarcoma (RAF), MAPK/ERK kinases (MEK), and extracellular signal-regulated kinases (ERK). Once these kinases are up-regulated, carcinogenesis is initiated. An inherited deregulated MAPK pathway, usually due to heterozygous mutations,[3] causes several phenotypic conditions marked by cognitive defects, facial dysmorphism, cardiac defects, and an increased risk of malignancies, known as the neuro-cardio-facial-cutaneous syndrome family.[3] Another component of this intricate network (Figure 31.1) is BRAF (v-raf murine sarcoma viral oncogene homolog B1),[4] whose designation stems from the original identification of RAF during an exploration of retroviral oncogenes. Initially RAF-1 was discovered (now called CRAF) in 1985, then ARAF in 1986, and subsequently BRAF in 1988.[5] Hierarchically, the apex of the cascade is composed of HRAS, KRAS, and NRAS.[5] The next layer is formed by the MAPKKK, including ARAF, BRAF, and CRAF; these can homodimerize or heterodimerize.[5] MEK1 and MEK2 compose MAPKK, which completes the network with ERK1 and ERK2, and MAPK.[5] Although the MAPK network is generally shown as a linear path in cartoons (Figure 31.1), in reality it branches out and interacts with molecular members of other pathways including mTOR (mammalian target of rapamycin).[6]

Germline mutations in the MAPK pathway are associated with developmental abnormalities.[7] Somatic mutations and acquired aberrations in the MAPK pathway, particularly *RAS* and *BRAF* mutations, are associated with malignancies.[8] For example, the MAPK pathway is activated in most melanomas.[9] Furthermore, targeted therapy selectively or nonselectively inhibiting those aberrations with small molecules has shown benefit.[8] Here, the currently known MAPK pathway mutations and therapeutic possibilities suggested by these biomarkers are explicated.

## The RAS Family: HRAS, KRAS, and NRAS

The RAS (rat sarcoma) genes were named because of the similarity of their sequences to the Harvey (HRAS) and Kirsten (KRAS) rat sarcoma viruses.[10] Bos et al.[11] in 1989 reported *RAS* mutations in pancreatic adenocarcinoma (90%), colon cancer (50%), lung cancer (30%), and thyroid tumors (50%). *KRAS* mutations occur most frequently (approximately 85%), then *NRAS* (approximately 15%), and *HRAS* (less than 1%). KRAS, NRAS, and HRAS have a high degree of homology and are expressed in many tissues. On average, somatic *RAS* mutations occur in as many as 30% of human malignancies,[11] although deregulated RAS activation can occur without *RAS* mutation in the setting of upregulated upstream stimuli signal transducers or downregulated downstream negative feedback. These pivotal RAS molecules are small G proteins, or guanosine triphosphate (GTP)/GTP-ases, frontline master regulators activating an intracellular network of signals that ultimately lead to gene expression and proliferation. Small G proteins also include R-RAS, TC21, M-RAS, Rap IA, Rap IB, Rap2A, Rap 2B, RaIA, and RaIB.[12] Guanine nucleotide-exchange factors (GEF) remove guanosine diphosphate (GDP) from inactive GDP-bound RAS. Consequently, RAS has a greater proclivity to bind to the more prevalent GTP that then converts into its active form, GTP-bound RAS. In summary, RAS proteins are governed by binding to GTP or GDP, which subsequently generates active or inactive proteins, respectively.[13] Son-of-sevenless (SOS1), RAS guanine release factor (RASGRF), and RAS guanyl-releasing protein (RASGRP) are examples of GEF. RAS proteins are tightly regulated, due to a fined tuned balance between GDP/GTP switching, activators such as GEF and natural inhibitors such as GTPase activating proteins (GAP).

Members of the RAS family (HRAS, KRAS, and NRAS) can have aberrations that impair the switch between the GTP-active

*Targeted Therapy in Translational Cancer Research*, First Edition. Edited by Apostolia-Maria Tsimberidou, Razelle Kurzrock and Kenneth C. Anderson.
© 2016 John Wiley & Sons, Inc. Published 2016 by John Wiley & Sons, Inc.

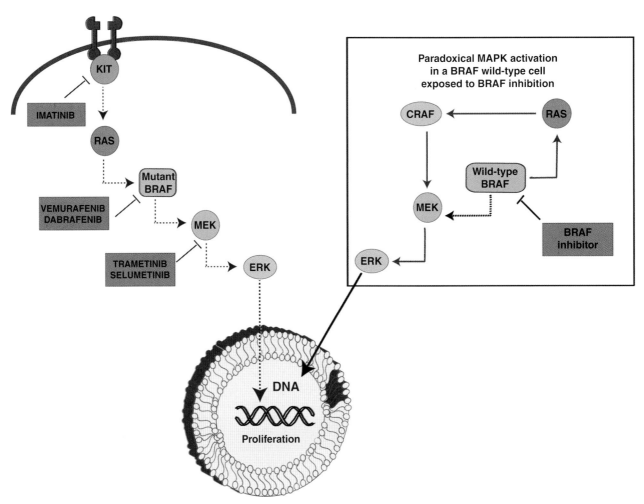

**Figure 31.1** Simplified diagram of the MAPK signaling pathway. Following stimulation of a cell-surface receptor (e.g., KIT), intracellular proteins become activated while recruiting SOS1 which exchanges GTP-GDP in RAS (GDP is the inactive form). RAS activation subsequently stimulates RAF (BRAF, RAF1), MEK (MEK1A1, MEK1A2), and, ERK (ERK1, ERK2). The GDP-GTP balance is regulated by guanine nucleotide exchange factors (GEF) and GTPase activating proteins (GAPs).

and GDP-inactive form of RAS. Missense mutations of residues Gly12 and Gly13 in *HRAS*, for example, are hot spots for oncogenic somatic mutations when RAS becomes perpetually GTP-bound active HRAS from resistance to GAP-induced hydrolysis of GTP. From those mutations, Gly12Val is the most common somatic *HRAS* aberration in human malignancies, accounting for approximately 45% of total somatic *HRAS* gene mutations. The frequency of particular mutations depends on whether aberrations of a particular gene are germline or acquired mutations. Interestingly, germline *KRAS* mutations are rare in human malignancies, where acquired somatic *KRAS* mutations occur far more frequently.

## The Congenital RAS-opathies: Germline Mutations of *RAS*

A phenotypic spectrum is linked to a disturbed MAPK pathway causing genotype–phenotype associations such as *RAS* aberrations[14] and neuro-cardio-facial-cutaneous syndromes. These are known as RAS-opathies and include Noonan syndrome[15] (predisposed to juvenile myelomonocytic leukemia), LEOPARD[16] (lentigines, electrocardiogram conduction abnormalities, ocular hyper-

telorism, pulmonic stenosis, abnormal genitalia, retardation of growth, and sensorineural deafness) syndrome, neurofibromatosis type 1[17] (predisposing individuals to myeloid malignancies such as juvenile myelomonocytic leukemia), Costello syndrome[18] (which can result in solid tumors such as rhabdomyosarcoma), cardiofaciocutaneous syndrome[19,20] (associated with acute lymphoblastic leukemia), and other Noonan-like syndromes.

Each gene in the MAPK pathway, located on different chromosomes, encodes a different protein so it is not surprising that different mutations manifest clinically as different diseases.[14] The clinical presentation of these diseases is not, however, exclusively associated with a particular mutation in these RAS-opathies. An example is the relatively common Noonan syndrome, which has been reported in association with aberrations in seven genes including *PTPN11*, *SOS1*, *KRAS*, *NRAS*, *RAF1*, *BRAF*, and *MEK1*. The *PTPN11* gene encodes SHP2, which is a cytoplasmic protein tyrosine phosphatase that positively regulates the RAS pathway, whereas the SOS1 gene is a type of GEF, which as explained above, alters the GDP/GTP balance involving RAS. Clinical overlap among these hyperactive RAS syndromes[21] is likely due to an interplay among multiple components of the MAPK pathway. Cardiofaciocutaneous syndrome has been linked to a varied array of mutations in *KRAS*, *BRAF*, *MEK1*, and *MEK2* genes in as many as 90% of patients. One exception is a germline missense mutated *HRAS* proto-oncogene causing confirmed Costello syndrome in almost a 100% of affected patients. By the same token, neurofibromatosis type 1 (NF1) is secondary to heterozygous loss-of-function of *NF1* gene, which regulates the expression of neurofibromin, a RAS GTPase, a large ubiquitous protein highly expressed in neurons, Schwann cells, and leukocytes accounting for the clinical stigmata of neurofibromas. *NF1* is a tumor suppressor gene and patients are thus prone to second-hit malignancies as neurofibromin is a protein with GAP activity which works as a negative regulator for MAPK. Patients with type-1 neurofibromatosis have an increased risk of developing benign tumors known as neurofibromas and malignancies such as peripheral nerve sheath tumors,[22] sarcoma, rhabdomyosarcoma, neuroblastoma, gastrointestinal stromal tumors, pheochromocytoma, breast cancer,[23] and juvenile myelomonocytic leukemia.[17] Patients with Costello syndrome can develop embryonic rhabdomyosarcoma, neuroblastoma, and bladder carcinoma.[18]

Even though the genotype–phenotype relationship is not completely clear,[7] mutations in *KRAS* affect the skin with redundant folds, keratinization defects, hair abnormalities, and a small risk of leukemia. Mutations in *HRAS* (such as Costello syndrome) manifest via skin hyperpigmentation, skin growths, and a small risk of soft-tissue tumors. For example, patients with Noonan syndrome have a small increased likelihood of developing rhabdomyosarcoma, neuroblastoma, giant cell tumors, and testicular tumors.[24] LEOPARD syndrome has been associated with acute myeloid leukemia, acute lymphoblastic leukemia, myeloproliferative disorders, neuroblastoma, and melanoma.[24, 25]

## The Acquired RAS-opathies: Melanoma and NRAS

Once a receptor is stimulated by cytokines or growth factors, the receptor binds the Src homology 2 (SH2) domains of SHC, SHP2, and GRB2, which recruit cytoplasmic SOS, subsequently disrupting the homeostatic GDP/GTP balance. Cell receptor stimulation causes RAS to dissociate from GDP and RAS binding to GTP, activating MAPK pathway downstream components including RAF and MEK.[26] RAS activation is restricted by GTP-ase activity or GAPs in a balancing act of active GTP-bound RAS and inactive GDP-bound RAS. Mutations in *RAS* proteins change the amino acids (G12, G13, and Q61), modifying hydrolysis from the binding of RAS to GTP, thus activating the MAPK pathway. *BRAF* mutations are found in 50–70% of melanomas,[27, 28] whereas somatic *NRAS* mutations are found in 15–30% of cases, producing a constitutively active NRAS protein, which stimulates the MAPK pathway. It has been suggested that an interaction exists between NRAS and c-Met, epidermal growth factor receptor (EGFR), and KIT. Most patients with melanoma have a hyperactive MAPK pathway; thus, it is not surprising that an MEK inhibitor such as MEK162 is associated with responses in a subgroup of patients with melanoma and *NRAS* mutations.

## The RAF Family: ARAF, BRAF, and CRAF

The ARAF, BRAF, and CRAF proteins are members of the serine–threonine kinase family downstream from RAS, and upstream from MEK1/2. Even though ARAF, BRAF, and CRAF are members of the same family, they have distinct characteristics; BRAF is a more pow-

erful activator of MEK compared to ARAF and CRAF. For example, BRAF and CRAF have essential differences in binding to RAS[29] and are governed by distinct autoregulatory mechanisms.[30] Of the three RAF isoforms, BRAF is most frequently involved in cancer (approximately 7% in general and up to 70% of melanoma cases).[31] Most *BRAF* mutations are present within the kinase domain, leading to a V600E substitution that activates the MAPK pathway.[32] Somatic *BRAF* mutations have been commonly documented in multiple malignancies; nevertheless aberrations in ARAF and CRAF are rarely seen. Despite the fact that more than 40 germline *BRAF* mutations have been documented, germline *BRAF* mutations rarely promote tumorigenesis as they do not have the malignant potential of the Val600Glu *BRAF* mutation. Interestingly, germline and somatic amino acid shifts may upregulate or downregulate the mutant kinase.

## BRAF Inhibitors

In regard to the importance of RAF in cancer development, even though BRAF is the main RAF isoform, RAF-driven malignancies are likely a minority. Most cancers involving increased MAPK activation do not carry RAF mutations (i.e., KRAS mutant colorectal cancer). Thus it is relevant to document the relative contribution of the different RAF isoforms during carcinogenesis. In the lab, many experiments obviated isoform specificity from RAF. In the clinic, some therapeutic RAF inhibitors do not differentiate between the RAF isoforms. To further complicate the picture, CRAF and BRAF can act in concert through heterodimerization (Figure 31.1). Sorafenib, an RAF inhibitor that also blocks other tyrosine kinases along with vascular endothelial growth factor, was not effective treating patients with melanoma and *BRAF* V600E mutations, and randomized phase III trials did not confirm any benefit from combining sorafenib with chemotherapy[33, 34] despite initial promising results.[35] It may well be that other activated pathways such as PI3K will need to be abrogated to produce a more beneficial response.[36] Vemurafenib spearheads the list of approved BRAF inhibitors and prolonged both progression-free (median 5.3 versus 1.6 months) and overall survival (6-month survival rates of 84% versus 64%) compared to dacarbazine (1000 mg/m$^2$ intravenously every 3 weeks) in patients with *BRAF* V600-mutant metastatic melanoma enrolled in the phase III BRIM-3 trial,[37] results subsequently confirmed by an extended follow-up.[38] Another BRAF inhibitor, dabrafenib, was approved by the US Food and Drug Administration on May 29, 2013, for the treatment of patients with unresectable or metastatic melanoma with a *BRAF* V600E mutation.[39] The approval of dabrafenib (150 mg orally twice daily) was based on improved progression-free survival (median 5.1 vs. 2.7 months) compared to dacarbazine (1000 mg/m$^2$ intravenously every 3 weeks) in an international, open-label phase III trial in 250 patients with unresectable and untreated stage III–IV *BRAF* V600E mutant melanoma.[40]

## Management of Metastatic Melanoma in the Era of BRAF Inhibitors

The management of early-stage cutaneous melanoma is relatively simple. Most cases are cured with local resection plus adjuvant interferon-alfa in the high-risk group.[41] Managing metastatic melanoma is however more complicated. Despite the high toxicity and low cure rate of high-dose interleukin-2, only recently have newer agents revolutionized the management of metastatic melanoma, such as the immunotherapy ipilimumab (a monoclonal antibody directed against CTLA-4) and the targeted therapy vemurafenib. Vemurafenib was approved by the US Food and Drug Administration for the management of patients with melanoma and the V600 driver mutation in the *BRAF* gene, which is found in approximately 50% of patients.[42, 43] This approval was based on clinical trials demonstrating prolongation of overall survival in this population. The substitution of glutamic acid for valine at amino acid 600 (V600E mutation) was found in approximately 80% of cases[43]; whereas the substitution of lysine for valine (V600K mutation) was shown in 20% of cases.

To date, no randomized comparison has been undertaken between immunotherapy with ipilimumab, high-dose interleukin-2, and BRAF inhibitors or the appropriate sequencing of such agents. Nevertheless, it is indicated that all patients be assessed, minimally for *BRAF* mutation, or to test for a more comprehensive panel of mutations. If a comprehensive mutational evaluation is not available, in the absence of *BRAF* V600E mutation, screening for non-V600E *BRAF* mutations, other MAPK aberrations (e.g., *NRAS*), and KIT should be done. Just as distinct malignancies based on their organ of origin have different frequencies of a particular aberration (Figure 31.2)[32], there are particular phenotypic characteristics that correlate with the genotype of patients with melanoma.[44] As an example, an acral melanoma may carry a *KIT* mutation (approximately 15–20%) instead of a *BRAF* mutation. Initial phase II studies of imatinib for unselected patients with advanced melanoma showed limited activity[45–47]; nevertheless a subsequent phase II study with a selected population of patients harboring a *KIT* mutation or amplification showed an overall response rate of 23.3%[48] In general, the MAPK pathway and microphthalmia-associated transcription factor (MITF) have been implicated in the development of melanoma and melanocyte differentiation/survival.[49, 50] MITF is phosphorylated by the MAPK pathway[51] and MITF mutation has been associated with familial and sporadic melanoma.[52] In addition to MITF, specific aberrations have been correlated with particular subtypes of melanoma such as BRAF/NRAS in conjunctival melanomas (*BRAF* mutations in 29% and *NRAS* mutations in 18%),[53] *KIT* mutations or amplifications in acral (36%) and mucosal (39%) melanomas,[54] and *GNAQ/GNA11* in uveal melanomas (*GNAQ* in 45% and GNA11 in 32%)[55] (Figure 31.2). Furthermore, *BRAF* mutations are common in vertical growth phase melanoma and metastatic melanoma

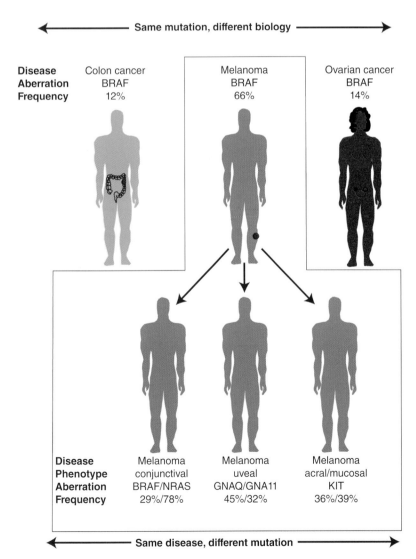

**Figure 31.2** Genotypes and phenotypes in malignant melanomas.

(62–72%),[56] whereas *BRAF* mutations are rare in radial growth phase melanomas (10%)[56] or in *in situ* melanoma (5.6%).[57] Finally, a high frequency of *BRAF* mutations in nonmalignant lesions (82% in nevi)[4,57] suggests that *BRAF* mutations are involved in collaboration with other molecular aberrations in carcinogenesis rather than being solo founder mutations. As an example, *BRAF* mutations were found in 29% of invasive melanomas and in 5.6% of *in situ* melanomas, whereas *NRAS* mutations were found in 5.2% of primary melanomas and in no *in situ* melanomas.[57] These *NRAS* and *BRAF* mutations seem to occur early during melanoma carcinogenesis and remain preserved throughout the progression of disease.[9]

Comorbidities, performance status, drug toxicities, pace of disease progression, and presence of brain metastases are factors to be considered in choosing the appropriate course of therapy. For example, unfit patients with fast-paced bulky disease and central nervous disease involvement are unlikely to benefit from high-dose interleukin-2, although BRAF inhibition can salvage patients in that scenario. Ipilimumab, an antibody-based immunotherapy directed against the CTLA-4 checkpoint, may need a prolonged period of time to show activity and would not be appropriate in the setting of aggressive disease progression. In contrast, BRAF inhibitors are a very attractive targeted therapy in melanoma. Both vemurafenib[58,59] and dabrafenib[60,61] have reported activity in patients with melanoma that has metastasized to the central nervous system.

## The CRAF Story

Downstream of RAS, the next line of activated molecules includes BRAF and CRAF. No reports of activating mutations of CRAF have been documented so far, whereas BRAF kinase domain mutations are as common as 50% in melanoma. As a result, it has been suggested that there is single-step activation between RAS and BRAF, but that multiple-steps might be involved between RAS and CRAF.[62] BRAF inhibitors abrogate the MAPK pathway in *BRAF*-mutant cells, whereas BRAF inhibitors may paradoxically stimulate the MAPK pathway within wild-type BRAF cells.[63–65] Despite being relatively safe, dermatologic side effects[66] have been reported with the use of these inhibitors. These include cutaneous squamous cell carcinoma in 12%,[67] sometimes developing within weeks of starting a BRAF inhibitor suggesting preexisting *RAS* mutations in other skin areas due to paradoxical activation of the MAPK pathway (*HRAS* mutations in 41% of 29 samples with cutaneous squamous cell carcinoma or keratoacanthomas).[68] It has been suggested that combining an MEK inhibitor and a BRAF inhibitor may decrease toxicity caused by paradoxical activation of the MAPK pathway. As a more ominous complication, a patient exposed to vemurafenib developed progression of chronic myelomonocytic leukemia found to have a *RAS* mutation.[69]

## Primary and Secondary Resistance to BRAF Inhibitors

Despite initial responses as high as 48%,[37] primary and secondary resistance to vemurafenib has been reported and most patients with melanoma exposed to vemurafenib eventually develop resistance (Figure 31.3). Thus, combinatorial trials using BRAF inhibitors as a backbone or small molecules targeting other areas of the MAPK pathway are suggested to overcome resistance. Tissue samples obtained during the phase II BRIM-2 trial of vemurafenib showed an association between decreased ERK phosphorylation and objective responses, whereas increased ERK phosphorylation and the development of secondary *NRAS* (Q61) or *MEK1* (Q56P)

or *MEK1* (E203K) mutations were associated with acquired resistance[70] Thus, re-activation of the MAPK pathway seems to be involved in the development of resistance to BRAF inhibitors. Interestingly, resistance has not been associated with developing a second mutation that impairs drug binding to BRAF, a mechanism observed in other malignancies. Other possible mechanisms that can cause resistance include MAPK pathway reactivation via alternative means such as insulin growth factor receptor 1 (IGF-1R)/PI3K pathway activation,[71,72] PD-L1 expression,[73] increased cyclin D1 expression,[74] elevated CRAF protein levels,[75] production of shortened forms of BRAF proteins due to aberrant RNA splicing,[76] *NRAS* (Q61) mutations,[70] *MEK1* (Q56P, E203K, C121S, or F129L) mutations,[70,77,78] and ERK activation through bypassing mechanisms including COT (one of the MAPKKKs that regulates the ERK1/ERK2 pathway) activation and receptor tyrosine kinase as PDGFRβ upregulation.[79,80] Conversely, clinical response associated with BRAF inhibition leads to decreased phosphorylated ERK levels.[81]

## MEK Inhibitors—The MEK Family: MEK1 and MEK2

RAS activation is followed by activation of RAF (ARAF, BRAF, and CRAF), subsequently MEK (MEK1A1, MEK1A2), and finally ERK (ERK1, ERK2). ERK is the last step of the pathway and governs a myriad of proteins. MEK1 and MEK2 genes encode dual specificity kinases that phosphorylate ERK proteins, their only known substrate, at tyrosine and serine-threonine residues. MEK kinase activity has been documented as inducing proliferation, although no *MEK* mutations have been associated with triggering development of cancer or primary resistance to vemurafenib. Interestingly, a *MEK1* C121S mutation was recently seen in a patient with melanoma and acquired resistance to vemurafenib. The mutation was not present before vemurafenib therapy, supporting the role of molecular evolution in therapeutic resistance. MEK aberrations have however been associated with some neuro-cardio-facial-cutaneous syndromes. In melanoma, the *BRAF* V600E mutation correlates with response to MEK inhibitors in preclinical models and clinical studies. Trametinib is a potent specific inhibitor of MEK1/MEK2, initially approved for patients with advanced melanoma, containing a V600E or V600K BRAF mutation, that underwent prior BRAF inhibition.[82] The approval of trametinib (2 mg/day orally) was based on improved progression-free survival (median 4.8 vs. 1.5 months) and overall survival (6-month survival rate of 81% vs. 67%) compared to chemotherapy (dacarbazine or paclitaxel) in the phase III METRIC trial in 322 patients with *BRAF* V600E–positive advanced melanoma.[83] Patients who had received prior chemotherapy or immunotherapy were included, whereas prior BRAF inhibitors were not allowed, because in a previous phase II study, minimal clinical activity was observed with trametinib in patients previously treated with a BRAF inhibitor.[84]

Furthermore, trametinib was approved by the US Food and Drug Administration[82] for use combined with dabrafenib as initial targeted therapy for patients with melanoma carrying a *BRAF* V600E or V600K mutation. The rate of partial and/or complete response with combined dabrafenib (150 mg) plus trametinib (1 or 2 mg) was 76% compared to 54% with dabrafenib monotherapy ($p = 0.03$).[85] Cutaneous squamous cell carcinoma developed less frequently in the combination group compared to monotherapy (7% vs. 19%), whereas pyrexia developed more frequently in the combination group compared to monotherapy (71% vs. 26%).[85]

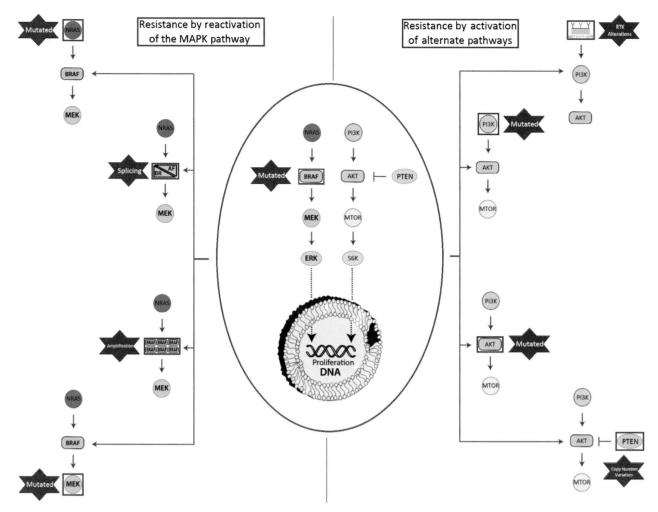

**Figure 31.3**  Primary and secondary resistance to BRAF inhibitors.

Other MEK inhibitors under development are selumetinib, MEK162 and others.[86] The combination of selumetinib plus dacarbazine was compared to single-agent dacarbazine in a randomized phase II study that included 91 *BRAF* mutant patients, showing improved progression-free survival (5.6 vs. 3.0 months) but no improvement in overall survival.[87] Furthermore, a phase II trial assessed MEK162 in 71 patients with advanced melanoma carrying either a V600 *BRAF* mutation (41 cases) or an *NRAS* mutation (30 cases) with partial responses of 20% in both groups (8 of 41 cases with *BRAF* mutations and 6 of 30 patients with *NRAS* mutations).[88]

## Implications of Aberrations in the MAPK Pathway in the Management of Lung Cancer

The personalization of genotype-driven treatments for metastatic nonsmall cell lung cancer is promising, and multiple driver mutations have been identified such as *EGFR*, *ALK*, *ROS1*, *BRAF*, *NRAS*, and *KRAS*. *BRAF* mutations were seen in 1–3% of patients with nonsmall cell lung cancer.[89–91] A study of the selective BRAF inhibitor dabrafenib in *BRAF* V600E-mutant metastatic nonsmall cell lung cancer is ongoing (NCT01336634). *NRAS* mutations were seen in less than 1% (1 of 195) of patients with nonsmall cell lung cancer.[92] *KRAS* mutations seem to be more com-

mon in smokers.[93] Transversion *KRAS* mutations were seen in 22% of smoker patients with lung adenocarcinomas, whereas transition *KRAS* mutations were seen in 15% of nonsmoker patients with lung adenocarcinoma.[94] Mutated *KRAS* on 300 of 1543 patients with early stage nonsmall cell lung carcinoma receiving adjuvant chemotherapy following resection was not associated with a statistically significant difference in overall survival compared to wild-type *KRAS* in a pooled analysis of four clinical trials.[95] In the metastatic setting, mutated *KRAS* conferred a worse prognosis compared to mutated *EGFR*,[96] whereas *KRAS* mutation was prognostic for reduced progression-free survival in patients receiving maintenance erlotinib but showed no statistically significant difference in overall survival compared to wild-type *KRAS*.[97] KRAS mutations herald colon cancer that is resistant to cetuximab. Nevertheless, responses to cetuximab were maintained in phase III trials of patients with nonsmall cell lung cancer.[63,98] In the absence of current KRAS-targeted drugs, the therapeutic emphasis for *KRAS*-mutant lung cancer is to target molecules downstream from activated KRAS, which is supported in preclinical models.[99] Objective partial responses were documented in 16 of 43 patients (37%) treated with docetaxel plus selumetinib compared with none of 40 patients with KRAS-mutant advanced nonsmall cell lung cancer receiving docetaxel plus placebo.[100] Clinical trials evaluating MEK inhibitors combined with chemotherapy in *KRAS*-mutant nonsmall cell lung cancer are underway (NCT01192165, NCT01362296).

## Acquired Mutations in the MAPK Pathway in Other Malignancies

Overall, *RAS* mutations are present in as many as 30% of all malignancies,[5] whereas *BRAF* mutations are found in as many as 60% of melanomas, 50% of thyroid cancers, and 20% of colon cancers.[5] Activating *RAS* oncogenic mutations (*NRAS*, *HRAS*, and *KRAS* in decreasing frequency) are more common in follicular thyroid cancers (80%) than papillary thyroid cancer (20%).[101] *RAS* mutations carry a worse prognosis in thyroid malignancies.[102] On the other hand, 43.8% of 500 patients with papillary thyroid cancers were found to have *BRAF* mutations, which were associated with more invasive disease.[103] The *BRAF* V600E mutation has been linked with high-risk clinicopathological factors[104] and increased cancer-related mortality in patients with papillary thyroid cancer.[105] BRAF inhibition in preclinical mice models of thyroid carcinoma decreased the levels of phosphorylated MEK and ERK.[106] Erdheim-Chester disease is a non-Langerhans cell histiocytosis. Because it may co-exist with Langerhans histiocytosis,[107,108] it is believed that these conditions may overlap pathologically and therapeutically.[109] *BRAF* mutations were found in 54% (13/24) of patients with Erdheim-Chester disease and[110] in 38% (11/29) to 57% (35/61) of patients with Langerhans cell histiocytosis.[111,112] Subsequently, three patients with refractory *BRAF* V600E-mutant Erdheim-Chester disease responded to the BRAF inhibitor vemurafenib.[113] Patients with the classic form of hairy cell leukemia almost always carry the V600E BRAF mutation,[114] whereas approximately 50% of patients with the variant form of hairy cell leukemia carry *MAP2K1* gene (encoding *MEK1*) mutations[115] instead of *BRAF* mutations.[116] It has been suggested that patients with exon 15 *BRAF* V600E-negative hairy cell leukemia should be screened for exon 11 (F468C and D449E) mutations.[63] Case reports of clinical improvement after exposure to the BRAF inhibitor vemurafenib have been described,[63,117] and clinical trials are underway to determine the role of BRAF inhibition in hairy cell leukemia (NCT01711632). Activating mutations of *BRAF* kinase were found in 4% of patients with multiple myeloma.[118] A case report described a patient with *BRAF* V600E-mutant multiple myeloma who responded to low-dose BRAF inhibition with vemurafenib.[119]

## Future Directions: Big Results for Small Molecules

Although aberrations in the MAPK pathway have been known to contribute to deregulated growth, both in inherited developmental disorders and acquired mutations, rendering patients prone to malignancies, only until recently have inhibitors been developed that match their respective targets. Initial investigations on the MAPK pathway were based on preclinical models of acute growth factor exposure in the laboratory, which do not correlate with a normal physiological state *in vivo*, hence, the utility of MAPK pathway inhibitors will have to be tested in the clinic. Three agents have been approved by the Food and Drug Administration for use in patients with *BRAF*-mutated advanced melanoma, the BRAF inhibitors vemurafenib and dabrafenib, and the MEK inhibitor trametinib. Further exploration of MAPK inhibition in other malignancies is eagerly awaited. Molecular stratification and targeted therapy of the MAPK network pose us for success while offering the opportunity to launch a decisive attack against cancer.

## References

1 L'Allemain G. Deciphering the MAP kinase pathway. *Prog Growth Factor Res*. 1994;5(3):291–334.

2 Spirli C, Morell CM, Locatelli L, et al. Cyclic AMP/PKA-dependent paradoxical activation of Raf/MEK/ERK signaling in polycystin-2 defective mice treated with sorafenib. *Hepatology*. 2012;56(6):2363–2374.

3 Tartaglia M, Gelb BD. Disorders of dysregulated signal traffic through the RAS-MAPK pathway: phenotypic spectrum and molecular mechanisms. *Ann NY Acad Sci*. 2010;1214:99–121.

4 Pollock PM, Harper UL, Hansen KS, et al. High frequency of BRAF mutations in nevi. *Nat Genet*. 2003;33(1):19–20.

5 Roskoski R Jr. RAF protein-serine/threonine kinases: structure and regulation. *Biochem Biophys Res Commun*. 2010;399(3):313–317.

6 Faustino A, Couto JP, Pópulo H, et al. mTOR pathway overactivation in BRAF mutated papillary thyroid carcinoma. *J Clin Endocrinol Metab*. 2012;97(7):E1139–E1149.

7 Hernandez-Martin A, Torrelo A. [Rasopathies: developmental disorders that predispose to cancer and skin manifestations]. *Actas Dermosifiliogr*. 2011;102(6):402–416.

8 Dienstmann R, Tabernero J. BRAF as a target for cancer therapy. *Anticancer Agents Med Chem*. 2011;11(3):285–295.

9 Omholt K, Platz A, Kanter L, Ringborg U, Hansson J. NRAS and BRAF mutations arise early during melanoma pathogenesis and are preserved throughout tumor progression. *Clin Cancer Res*. 2003;9(17):6483–6488.

10 Der CJ, Krontiris TG, Cooper GM. Transforming genes of human bladder and lung carcinoma cell lines are homologous to the ras genes of Harvey and Kirsten sarcoma viruses. *Proc Natl Acad Sci U S A*. 1982;79(11):3637–3640.

11 Bos JL, ras oncogenes in human cancer: a review. *Cancer Res*. 1989;49(17):4682–4689.

12 Takai Y, Sasaki T, Matozaki T. Small GTP-binding proteins. *Physiol Rev*. 2001;81(1):153–208.

13 Donovan S, Shannon KM, Bollag G. GTPase activating proteins: critical regulators of intracellular signaling. *Biochim Biophys Acta*. 2002;1602(1):23–45.

14 Tidyman WE, Rauen KA. The RASopathies: developmental syndromes of Ras/MAPK pathway dysregulation. *Curr Opin Genet Dev*. 2009;19(3):230–236.

15 Tartaglia M, Mehler EL, Goldberg R, et al. Mutations in PTPN11, encoding the protein tyrosine phosphatase SHP-2, cause Noonan syndrome. *Nat Genet*. 2001;29(4):465–468.

16 Pandit B, Sarkozy A, Pennacchio LA, et al. Gain-of-function RAF1 mutations cause Noonan and LEOPARD syndromes with hypertrophic cardiomyopathy. *Nat Genet*. 2007;39(8):1007–1012.

17 Burgdorf WH, Zelger B. JXG, NF1, and JMML: alphabet soup or a clinical issue? *Pediatr Dermatol*. 2004;21(2):174–176.

18 Gripp KW. Tumor predisposition in Costello syndrome. *Am J Med Genet C Semin Med Genet*. 2005;137C(1):72–77.

19 van Den Berg H, Hennekam RC. Acute lymphoblastic leukaemia in a patient with cardiofaciocutaneous syndrome. *J Med Genet*. 1999;36(10):799–800.

20 Makita Y, Narumi Y, Yoshida M, et al. Leukemia in Cardio-facio-cutaneous (CFC) syndrome: a patient with a germline mutation in BRAF proto-oncogene. *J Pediatr Hematol Oncol*. 2007;29(5):287–290.

21 Schubbert S, Shannon K, Bollag G. Hyperactive Ras in developmental disorders and cancer. *Nat Rev Cancer*. 2007;7(4):295–308.

22 Evans DG, Baser ME, McGaughran J, Sharif S, Howard E, Moran A. Malignant peripheral nerve sheath tumours in neurofibromatosis 1. *J Med Genet*. 2002;39(5):311–314.

23 Brems H, Beert E, de Ravel T, Legius E. Mechanisms in the pathogenesis of malignant tumours in neurofibromatosis type 1. *Lancet Oncol*. 2009;10(5):508–515.

24 Hasle H. Malignant diseases in Noonan syndrome and related disorders. *Horm Res*. 2009;72(suppl 2):8–14.

25 Seishima M, Mizutani Y, Shibuya Y, Arakawa C, Yoshida R, Ogata T. Malignant melanoma in a woman with LEOPARD syndrome: identification of a germline PTPN11 mutation and a somatic BRAF mutation. *Br J Dermatol*. 2007;157(6):1297–1299.

26 Malumbres M, Barbacid M. RAS oncogenes: the first 30 years. *Nat Rev Cancer*. 2003;3(6):459–465.

27 Dhomen N, Marais R. BRAF signaling and targeted therapies in melanoma. *Hematol Oncol Clin North Am*. 2009;23(3):529–545, ix.

28 Maldonado JL, Fridlyand J, Patel H, et al. Determinants of BRAF mutations in primary melanomas. *J Natl Cancer Inst*. 2003;95(24):1878–1890.

29 Fischer A, Hekman M, Kuhlmann J, Rubio I, Wiese S, Rapp UR. B- and C-RAF display essential differences in their binding to Ras: the isotype-specific N terminus of B-RAF facilitates Ras binding. *J Biol Chem*. 2007;282(36):26503–26516.

30 Tran NH, Wu X, Frost JA. B-Raf and Raf-1 are regulated by distinct autoregulatory mechanisms. *J Biol Chem*. 2005;280(16):16244–16253.

31 Garnett MJ, Marais R. Guilty as charged: B-RAF is a human oncogene. *Cancer Cell*. 2004;6(4):313–319.

32 Davies H, Bignell GR, Cox C, et al. Mutations of the BRAF gene in human cancer. *Nature*. 2002;417(6892):949–954.

33 Hauschild A, Agarwala SS, Trefzer U, et al. Results of a phase III, randomized, placebo-controlled study of sorafenib in combination with carboplatin and paclitaxel as second-line treatment in patients with unresectable stage III or stage IV melanoma. *J Clin Oncol*. 2009;27(17):2823–2830.

34 Flaherty KT, Lee SJ, Zhao F, et al. Phase III trial of carboplatin and paclitaxel with or without sorafenib in metastatic melanoma. *J Clin Oncol*. 2013;31(3):373–379.

35 Eisen T, Ahmad T, Flaherty KT, et al. Sorafenib in advanced melanoma: a phase II randomised discontinuation trial analysis. *Br J Cancer*. 2006;95(5):581–586.

36 Inamdar GS, Madhunapantula SV, Robertson SV. Targeting the MAPK pathway in melanoma: why some approaches succeed and other fail. *Biochem Pharmacol*. 2010;80(5):624–637.

37 Chapman PB, Hauschild A, Robert C, et al. Improved survival with vemurafenib in melanoma with BRAF V600E mutation. *N Engl J Med*. 2011;364(26):2507–2516.

38 McArthur GA, Chapman PB, Robert C, et al. Safety and efficacy of vemurafenib in BRAF(V600E) and BRAF(V600K) mutation-positive melanoma (BRIM-3): extended follow-up of a phase 3, randomised, open-label study. *Lancet Oncol*. 2014;15(3):323–332.

39 Ballantyne AD, Garnock-Jones KP. Dabrafenib: first global approval. *Drugs*. 2013;73(12):1367–1376.

40 Hauschild A, Grob JJ, Demidov LV, et al. Dabrafenib in BRAF-mutated metastatic melanoma: a multicentre, open-label, phase 3 randomised controlled trial. *Lancet*. 2012;380(9839):358–365.

41 Cole BF, Gelber RD, Kirkwood JM, Goldhirsch A, Barylak E, Borden E. Quality-of-life-adjusted survival analysis of interferon alfa-2b adjuvant treatment of high-risk resected cutaneous melanoma: an Eastern Cooperative Oncology Group study. *J Clin Oncol*. 1996;14(10):2666–2673.

42 Smalley KS, Sondak VK. Melanoma—an unlikely poster child for personalized cancer therapy. *N Engl J Med*. 2010;363(9):876–878.

43 Long GV, Menzies AM, Nagrial AM, et al. Prognostic and clinicopathologic associations of oncogenic BRAF in metastatic melanoma. *J Clin Oncol*. 2011;29(10):1239–1246.

44 Curtin JA, Fridlyand J, Kageshita T, et al. Distinct sets of genetic alterations in melanoma. *N Engl J Med*. 2005;353(20):2135–2147.

45 Wyman K, Atkins MB, Prieto V, et al. Multicenter Phase II trial of high-dose imatinib mesylate in metastatic melanoma: significant toxicity with no clinical efficacy. *Cancer*. 2006;106(9):2005–2011.

46 Penel N, Delcambre C, Durando X, et al. O-Mel-Inib: a Cancero-pole Nord-Ouest multicenter phase II trial of high-dose imatinib mesylate in metastatic uveal melanoma. *Invest New Drugs*. 2008;26(6):561–565.

47 Ugurel S, Hildenbrand R, Zimpfer A, et al. Lack of clinical efficacy of imatinib in metastatic melanoma. *Br J Cancer*. 2005;92(8):1398–1405.

48 Guo J, Si L, Kong Y, et al. Phase II, open-label, single-arm trial of imatinib mesylate in patients with metastatic melanoma harboring c-Kit mutation or amplification. *J Clin Oncol*. 2011;29(21):2904–2909.

49 Haq R, Fisher DE. Biology and clinical relevance of the micropthalmia family of transcription factors in human cancer. *J Clin Oncol*. 2011;29(25):3474–3482.

50 Ugurel S, Houben R, Schrama D, et al. Microphthalmia-associated transcription factor gene amplification in metastatic melanoma is a prognostic marker for patient survival, but not a predictive marker for chemosensitivity and chemotherapy response. *Clin Cancer Res*. 2007;13(21):6344–6350.

51 Hemesath TJ, Price ER, Takemoto C, Badalian T, Fisher DE. MAP kinase links the transcription factor Microphthalmia to c-Kit signalling in melanocytes. *Nature*. 1998;391(6664):298–301.

52 Yokoyama S, Woods SL, Boyle GM, et al. A novel recurrent mutation in MITF predisposes to familial and sporadic melanoma. *Nature*. 2011;480(7375):99–103.

53 Griewank KG, Westekemper H, Murali R, et al. Conjunctival melanomas harbor BRAF and NRAS mutations and copy number changes similar to cutaneous and mucosal melanomas. *Clin Cancer Res*. 2013;19(12).3143–3152.

54 Curtin JA, Busam K, Pinkel D, Bastian BC. Somatic activation of KIT in distinct subtypes of melanoma. *J Clin Oncol*. 2006;24(26):4340–4346.

55 Van Raamsdonk CD, Griewank KG, Crosby MB, et al. Mutations in GNA11 in uveal melanoma. *N Engl J Med*. 2010;363(23):2191–2199.

56 Dong J, Phelps RG, Qiao R, et al. BRAF oncogenic mutations correlate with progression rather than initiation of human melanoma. *Cancer Res*. 2003;63(14):3883–3885.

57 Poynter JN, Elder JT, Fullen DR, et al. BRAF and NRAS mutations in melanoma and melanocytic nevi. *Melanoma Res*. 2006;16(4):267–273.

58 Rochet NM, Kottschade LA, Markovic SN. Vemurafenib for melanoma metastases to the brain. *N Engl J Med*. 2011;365(25):2439–2441.

59 Dummer R, Goldinger SM, Turtschi CP, et al. Vemurafenib in patients with BRAF(V600) mutation-positive melanoma with symptomatic brain metastases: final results of an open-label pilot study. *Eur J Cancer*. 2014;50(3):611–621.

60 Falchook GS, Long GV, Kurzrock R, et al. Dabrafenib in patients with melanoma, untreated brain metastases, and other solid tumours: a phase 1 dose-escalation trial. *Lancet*. 2012;379(9829):1893–1901.

61 Long GV, Trefzer U, Davies MA, et al. Dabrafenib in patients with Val600Glu or Val600Lys BRAF-mutant melanoma metastatic to the brain (BREAK-MB): a multicentre, open-label, phase 2 trial. *Lancet Oncol*. 2012;13(11):1087–1095.

62 Garnett MJ, Rana S, Paterson H, Barford D, Marais R. Wild-type and mutant B-RAF activate C-RAF through distinct mechanisms involving heterodimerization. *Mol Cell*. 2005;20(6):963–969.

63 Carnahan J, Beltran PJ, Babij C, et al. Selective and potent Raf inhibitors paradoxically stimulate normal cell proliferation and tumor growth. *Mol Cancer Ther*. 2010;9(8):2399–2410.

64 Poulikakos PI, Zhang C, Bollag G, Shokat KM, Rosen N. RAF inhibitors transactivate RAF dimers and ERK signalling in cells with wild-type BRAF. *Nature*. 2010;464(7287):427–430.

65 Heidorn SJ, Milagre C, Whittaker S, et al. Kinase-dead BRAF and oncogenic RAS cooperate to drive tumor progression through CRAF. *Cell*. 2010;140(2):209–221.

66 Anforth R, Fernandez-Penas P, Long GV. Cutaneous toxicities of RAF inhibitors. *Lancet Oncol*. 2013;14(1):e11–e18.

67 Larkin J, Del Vecchio M, Ascierto PA, et al. Vemurafenib in patients with BRAF mutated metastatic melanoma: an open-label, multicentre, safety study. *Lancet Oncol*. 2014;15(4):436–444.

68 Lacouture ME, Duvic M, Hauschild A, et al. Analysis of dermatologic events in vemurafenib-treated patients with melanoma. *Oncologist*. 2013;18(3):314–322.

69 Callahan MK, Rampal R, Harding JJ, et al. Progression of RAS-mutant leukemia during RAF inhibitor treatment. *N Engl J Med*. 2012;367(24):2316–2321.

70 Trunzer K, Pavlick AC, Schuchter L, et al. Pharmacodynamic effects and mechanisms of resistance to vemurafenib in patients with metastatic melanoma. *J Clin Oncol*. 2013;31(14):1767–1774.

71 Villanueva J, Vultur A, Lee JT, et al. Acquired resistance to BRAF inhibitors mediated by a RAF kinase switch in melanoma can be overcome by cotargeting MEK and IGF-1R/PI3K. *Cancer Cell*. 2010;18(6):683–695.

72 Sanchez-Hernandez I, Baquero P, Calleros L, Chiloeches A. Dual inhibition of (V600E) BRAF and the PI3K/AKT/mTOR pathway cooperates to induce apoptosis in melanoma cells through a MEK-independent mechanism. *Cancer Lett*. 2012;314(2):244–255.

73 Jiang X, Zhou J, Giobbie-Harder A, Wargo J, Hodi FS. The activation of MAPK in melanoma cells resistant to BRAF inhibition promotes PD-L1 expression that is reversible by MEK and PI3K inhibition. *Clin Cancer Res*. 2013;19(3):598–609.

74 Smalley KS, Lioni M, Dalla Palma M, et al. Increased cyclin D1 expression can mediate BRAF inhibitor resistance in BRAF V600E-mutated melanomas. *Mol Cancer Ther*. 2008;7(9):2876–2883.

75 Montagut C, Sharma SV, Shioda T, et al. Elevated CRAF as a potential mechanism of acquired resistance to BRAF inhibition in melanoma. *Cancer Res*. 2008;68(12):4853–4861.

76 Poulikakos PI, Persaud Y, Janakiraman M, et al. RAF inhibitor resistance is mediated by dimerization of aberrantly spliced BRAF(V600E). *Nature*. 2011;480(7377):387–390.

77 Wang H, Daouti S, Li WH, et al. Identification of the MEK1(F129L) activating mutation as a potential mechanism of acquired resistance to MEK inhibition in human cancers carrying the B-RafV600E mutation. *Cancer Res*. 2011;71(16):5535–5545.

78 Wagle N, Emery C, Berger MF, et al. Dissecting therapeutic resistance to RAF inhibition in melanoma by tumor genomic profiling. *J Clin Oncol*. 2011;29(22):3085–3096.

79 Johannessen CM, Boehm JS, Kim SY, et al. COT drives resistance to RAF inhibition through MAP kinase pathway reactivation. *Nature*. 2010;468(7326):968–972.

80 Nazarian R, Shi H, Wang Q, et al. Melanomas acquire resistance to B-RAF(V600E) inhibition by RTK or N-RAS upregulation. *Nature*. 2010;468(7326):973–977.

81 Bollag G, Hirth P, Tsai J, et al. Clinical efficacy of a RAF inhibitor needs broad target blockade in BRAF-mutant melanoma. *Nature*. 2010;467(7315):596–599.

82 Wright CJ, McCormack PL. Trametinib: first global approval. *Drugs*. 2013;73(11):1245–1254.

83 Flaherty KT, Robert C, Hersey P, et al. Improved survival with MEK inhibition in BRAF-mutated melanoma. *N Engl J Med*. 2012;367(2):107–114.

84 Kim KB, Kefford R, Pavlick AC, et al. Phase II study of the MEK1/MEK2 inhibitor Trametinib in patients with metastatic BRAF-mutant cutaneous melanoma previously treated with or without a BRAF inhibitor. *J Clin Oncol*. 2013;31(4):482–489.

85 Flaherty KT, Infante JR, Daud A, et al. Combined BRAF and MEK inhibition in melanoma with BRAF V600 mutations. *N Engl J Med*. 2012;367(18):1694–1703.

86 Kirkwood JM, Bastholt L, Robert C, et al. Phase II, open-label, randomized trial of the MEK1/2 inhibitor selumetinib as monotherapy versus temozolomide in patients with advanced melanoma. *Clin Cancer Res*. 2012;18(2):555–567.

87 Robert C, Dummer R, Gutzmer R, et al. Selumetinib plus dacarbazine versus placebo plus dacarbazine as first-line treatment for BRAF-mutant metastatic melanoma: a phase 2 double-blind randomised study. *Lancet Oncol*. 2013;14(8):733–740.

88 Ascierto PA, Schadendorf D, Berking C, et al. MEK162 for patients with advanced melanoma harbouring NRAS or Val600 BRAF mutations: a non-randomised, open-label phase 2 study. *Lancet Oncol*. 2013;14(3):249–256.

89 Paik PK, Arcila ME, Fara M, et al. Clinical characteristics of patients with lung adenocarcinomas harboring BRAF mutations. *J Clin Oncol*. 2011;29(15):2046–2051.

90 Kinno T, Tsuta K, Shiraishi K, et al. Clinicopathological features of nonsmall cell lung carcinomas with BRAF mutations. *Ann Oncol*. 2014;25(1):138–142.

91 Ohashi K, Sequist LV, Arcila ME, et al. Lung cancers with acquired resistance to EGFR inhibitors occasionally harbor BRAF gene mutations but lack mutations in KRAS, NRAS, or MEK1. *Proc Natl Acad Sci U S A*. 2012;109(31):E2127–e2133.

92 Sasaki H, Okuda K, Kawano O, et al. Nras and Kras mutation in Japanese lung cancer patients: genotyping analysis using LightCycler. *Oncol Rep*. 2007;18(3):623–628.

93 Ahrendt SA, Decker PA, Alawi EA, et al. Cigarette smoking is strongly associated with mutation of the K-ras gene in patients with primary adenocarcinoma of the lung. *Cancer*. 2001;92(6):1525–1530.

94 Riely GJ, Kris MG, Rosenbaum D, et al. Frequency and distinctive spectrum of KRAS mutations in never smokers with lung adenocarcinoma. *Clin Cancer Res*. 2008;14(18):5731–5734.

95 Shepherd FA, Domerg C, Hainaut P, et al. Pooled analysis of the prognostic and predictive effects of KRAS mutation status and KRAS mutation subtype in early-stage resected non-small-cell lung cancer in four trials of adjuvant chemotherapy. *J Clin Oncol*. 2013;31(17):2173–2181.

96 Johnson ML, Sima CS, Chaft J, et al. Association of KRAS and EGFR mutations with survival in patients with advanced lung adenocarcinomas. *Cancer*. 2013;119(2):356–362.

97 Brugger W, Triller N, Blasinska-Morawiec M, et al. Prospective molecular marker analyses of EGFR and KRAS from a randomized, placebo-controlled study of erlotinib maintenance therapy in advanced non-small-cell lung cancer. *J Clin Oncol*. 2011;29(31):4113–4120.

98 Khambata-Ford S, Harbison CT, Hart LL, et al. Analysis of potential predictive markers of cetuximab benefit in BMS099, a phase III study

of cetuximab and first-line taxane/carboplatin in advanced non-small-cell lung cancer. *J Clin Oncol.* 2010;28(6):918–927.

99 Engelman JA, Chen L, Tan X, et al. Effective use of PI3K and MEK inhibitors to treat mutant Kras G12D and PIK3CA H1047R murine lung cancers. *Nat Med.* 2008;14(12):1351–1356.

100 Janne PA, Shaw AT, Pereira JR, et al. Selumetinib plus docetaxel for KRAS-mutant advanced non-small-cell lung cancer: a randomised, multicentre, placebo-controlled, phase 2 study. *Lancet Oncol.* 2013;14(1):38–47.

101 Lemoine NR, Mayall ES, Wyllie FS, et al. Activated ras oncogenes in human thyroid cancers. *Cancer Res.* 1988; 48(16):4459–4463.

102 Garcia-Rostan G, Zhao H, Camp RL, et al. ras mutations are associated with aggressive tumor phenotypes and poor prognosis in thyroid cancer. *J Clin Oncol.* 2003;21(17):3226–3235.

103 Lupi C, Giannini R, Ugolini C, et al. Association of BRAF V600E mutation with poor clinicopathological outcomes in 500 consecutive cases of papillary thyroid carcinoma. *J Clin Endocrinol Metab.* 2007;92(11):4085–4090.

104 Kim TH, Park YJ, Lim JA, et al. The association of the BRAF(V600E) mutation with prognostic factors and poor clinical outcome in papillary thyroid cancer: a meta-analysis. *Cancer.* 2012;118(7):1764–1773.

105 Xing M, Alzahrani AS, Carson KA, et al. Association between BRAF V600E mutation and mortality in patients with papillary thyroid cancer. *JAMA.* 2013;309(14):1493–1501.

106 Salerno P, De Falco V, Tamburrino A, et al. Cytostatic activity of adenosine triphosphate-competitive kinase inhibitors in BRAF mutant thyroid carcinoma cells. *J Clin Endocrinol Metab.* 2010;95(1):450–455.

107 Marchal A, Cuny JF, Montagne K, Haroche J, Barbaud A, Schmutz JL. [Associated Langerhans cell histiocytosis and Erdheim-Chester disease] *Ann Dermatol Venereol.* 2011;138(11):743–747.

108 Haroche J, Arnaud L, Amoura Z. Erdheim-Chester disease. *Curr Opin Rheumatol.* 2012;24(1):53–59.

109 Janku F, Munoz J, Subbiah V, Kurzrock R. A tale of two histiocytic disorders. *Oncologist.* 2013;18(1):2–4.

110 Haroche J, Vibat CR, Kosco K, et al. High prevalence of BRAF V600E mutations in Erdheim-Chester disease but not in other non-Langerhans cell histiocytoses. *Blood.* 2012;120(13):2700–2703.

111 Sahm F, Capper D, Preusser M, et al. BRAFV600E mutant protein is expressed in cells of variable maturation in Langerhans cell histiocytosis. *Blood.* 2012;120(12):e28–e34.

112 Badalian-Very G, Vergilio JA, Degar BA, et al. Recurrent BRAF mutations in Langerhans cell histiocytosis. *Blood.* 2010;116(11):1919–1923.

113 Haroche J, Cohen-Aubart F, Emile JF, et al. Dramatic efficacy of vemurafenib in both multisystemic and refractory Erdheim-Chester disease and Langerhans cell histiocytosis harboring the BRAF V600E mutation. *Blood.* 2013;121(9):1495–1500.

114 Tiacci E, Trifonov V, Schiavoni G, et al. BRAF mutations in hairy-cell leukemia. *N Engl J Med.* 2011;364(24):2305–2315.

115 Waterfall JJ, Arons E, Walker RL, et al. High prevalence of MAP2K1 mutations in variant and IGHV4–34-expressing hairy-cell leukemias. *Nat Genet.* 2014;46(1):8–10.

116 Xi L, Arons E, Navarro W, et al. Both variant and IGHV4–34-expressing hairy cell leukemia lack the BRAF V600E mutation. *Blood.* 2012;119(14):3330–3332.

117 Dietrich S, Glimm H, Andrulis M, von Kalle C, Ho AD, Zenz T. BRAF inhibition in refractory hairy-cell leukemia. *N Engl J Med.* 2012;366(21):2038–2040.

118 Chapman MA, Lawrence MS, Keats JJ, et al. Initial genome sequencing and analysis of multiple myeloma. *Nature.* 2011;471(7339):467–472.

119 Andrulis M, Lehners N, Capper D, et al. Targeting the BRAF V600E mutation in multiple myeloma. *Cancer Discov.* 2013;3(8):862–869.

## CHAPTER 32

# The Phosphatidylinositol 3-Kinase Pathway in Human Malignancies

*Samuel J. Klempner[1], Thanh-Trang Vo[2], Andrea P. Myers[3], and Lewis C. Cantley[4]*

[1] Division of Hematology/Oncology, University of California Irvine Health, Orange, CA, USA
[2] Department of Molecular Biology and Biochemistry, University of California Irvine, Irvine, CA, USA
[3] Novartis Pharmaceuticals, Cambridge, MA, USA
[4] Meyer Cancer Center at Weill Cornell Medical College, New York, NY, USA

## Introduction

Over the last 25 years, the molecular understanding of many of the processes involved in tumorigenesis and cancer progression has been elucidated. Sustained proliferative signaling is one of the hallmarks of cancer and often occurs through transmembrane receptor tyrosine kinases (RTK) and their downstream effectors.[1] The prototypic RTK signaling cascade involves rat sarcoma (RAS) mitogenic signaling and is conserved from flies through humans. It was years after the appreciation of the importance of RAS signaling when one of the important effectors of RTK signaling, phosphatidylinositol 3-kinase (PI3K), was discovered and implicated in cancer through identification of physical PI3K association with the Rous sarcoma (SRC) oncogene encoded protein-tyrosine kinase, pp60[v-src], and with the polyomavirus middle T protein.[2,3] It became rapidly apparent that the PI3K pathway was central to multiple malignant hallmarks including survival, growth, metabolism, motility, and progression.

Over the ensuing years, the fundamentals of PI3K signaling emerged with the characterization of the PI3K heterodimer composed of the regulatory p85 and catalytic p110 subunits discussed in detail below. Since the initial characterization and discovery of the PI3K pathway, there have been numerous insights into both the nuances of the signaling cascade and its potential as a therapeutic target in multiple tumor types. In fact, the PI3K pathway is one of the most frequently mutated pathways in cancer[4] (Figure 32.1). In order to better understand recent PI3K developments, potential pitfalls of inhibition, and future directions, it is important to review the major components of the PI3K signaling cascade, including PI3K, AKT (also known as protein kinase B, PKB), and mammalian target of rapamycin (mTOR). The following chapter will review PI3K signaling in cancer, with particular attention to areas where PI3K inhibitors are actively being developed or already in early phase clinical trials. Finally, we will discuss future challenges and potential limitations of targeting the PI3K/AKT/mTOR pathway in cancer.

## Phosphatidylinositol 3-Kinases

The PI3K family of proteins all catalyzes the phosphorylation of inositol-containing lipids known as phosphatidylinositols (PtdIns) at their 3′ position.[5] It is now known that the PI3K family is composed of three general classes (Class I, II, III) containing multiple subunits and isoforms. Only the class I PI3Ks are known to be involved in malignancy.[6] We will briefly review the class II and III PI3Ks, but further discussion is limited to class I PI3Ks. Briefly, class II PI3K signaling members consist of three isoforms containing a catalytic subunit encoded by the PIK3C2 gene (α, β, γ) and phosphorylate PtdIns and phosphatidylinositol-4-phosphate at the 3′ position of the inositol ring (PI-4-P).[7] The class II PI3Ks are likely involved in membrane trafficking, including receptor internalization. They can also be activated by RTKs, although their downstream effects are not well characterized to date. The class III PI3Ks consist of only a single member, vacuolar protein sorting defective 34 (Vps34), that is conserved from yeast to humans and plays a major role in vesicle trafficking and autophagy.[7] Vps34 phosphorylates PtdIns at the 3′ position of the inositol ring, but does not phosphorylate PI-4-P or phosphatidylinositol-4,5-bisphosphate (PI-4,5-$P_2$).

The class I PI3Ks can phosphorylate the 3′ position of all three phosphoinositides, PtdIns, PI-4-P, and PI-4,5-$P_2$, though the preferred substrate of these enzymes *in vivo* is PI-4,5-$P_2$. Thus, only class I PI3Ks generate the important second messenger phosphatidylinositol (3,4,5) triphosphate (PIP$_3$). The class I PI3Ks can be further subdivided into class IA and class IB, and to date only class IA signaling aberrations have been implicated in human cancers. The class IA PI3Ks are composed of heterodimers of regulatory subunits (p85α, p85β, p50α, p55α, and p55γ) and catalytic subunits (p110α, p110β, p110δ). Three genes encode the regulatory subunits with PIK3R1 coding for p85α (and its alternative transcripts, p55α and p50α),[6] and PIK3R2 and PIK3R3 encode the p85β and p55γ isoforms of the p85 regulatory subunit, respectively.

*Targeted Therapy in Translational Cancer Research*, First Edition. Edited by Apostolia-Maria Tsimberidou, Razelle Kurzrock and Kenneth C. Anderson.
© 2016 John Wiley & Sons, Inc. Published 2016 by John Wiley & Sons, Inc.

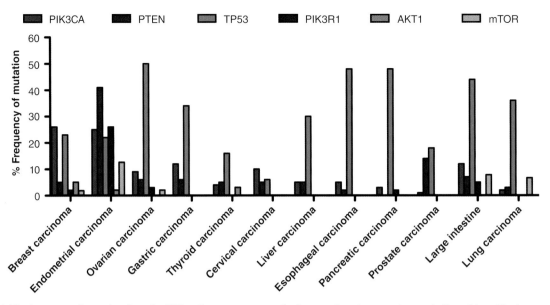

**Figure 32.1** The frequency of mutations in major PI3K pathway components across common cancers. Data from the COSMIC database (http://www.sanger.ac.uk/genetics/CGP/cosmic/) and the Memorial Sloan Kettering cbio database (http://cbio.mskcc.org/gdac-portal/index.do).

Carcinoma categories are not separated by subtype. The tumor suppressor TP53 (p53), the most mutated gene in cancer, is shown for comparison. Deletions and chromosomal rearrangements in PTEN are not included.

Collectively p85α (and its splice variants p55α and p50α), p85β, and p55γ are referred to as p85, and this designation will be used henceforth unless noted specifically. Three genes, PIK3CA, PIK3CB, and PIK3CD, encode the highly homologous p110 catalytic subunit isoforms p110α, p110β, and p110δ and all share a similar 5-domain structure.[5] At the amino (N) terminus, there is an adaptor-binding domain (ABD) that interacts with the p85 regulatory subunit, followed by a Ras-binding domain (RBD) that mediates interaction with the small GTPase Ras. The remaining domains are the C2 domain, thought to be involved in membrane anchoring, a phosphatidylinositol kinase homology (PIK) domain, and finally the

C-terminal catalytic domain. The RBD, C2, PIK, and catalytic domains are highly homologous between the p110 isoforms.[7]

The association of the regulatory p85 subunit with various RTKs occurs via physical interaction between phosphotyrosines in the consensus RTK YxxM sequence, which becomes autophosphorylated by RTK homodimerization, and SRC-homology 2 (SH2) domains on the PI3K p85 regulatory subunit (Figure 32.2). It later emerged that the p85–RTK interaction can also occur indirectly through adaptor proteins such as IRS1 and IRS2 (Figure 32.2).[5] The net effect of p85–RTK binding to RTKs or adaptors is the recruitment of PI3K to the plasma membrane where the substrate,

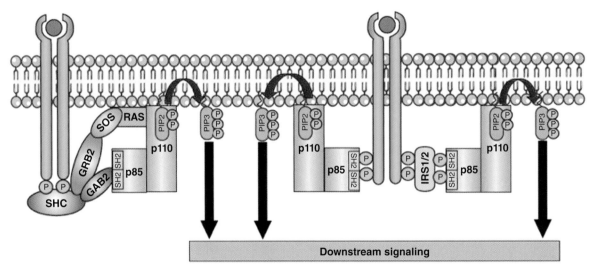

**Figure 32.2** Canonical Class I PI3K activation. RTK ligand binding leads to RTK autophosphorylation and recruitment of class IA PI3K heterodimers via interaction between RTK phosphotyrosine residues and SH2 domains on p85. Binding releases the basal p85 inhibition of the catalytic p110 PI3K subunit, thereby freeing p110 to catalyze the conversion of PIP2 to

PIP3. Also shown is an alternate activation mechanism through adaptor proteins whereby PI3K is bound to activated RAS which stabilizes PI3K plasma membrane localization and activation of the p110 catalytic domain.

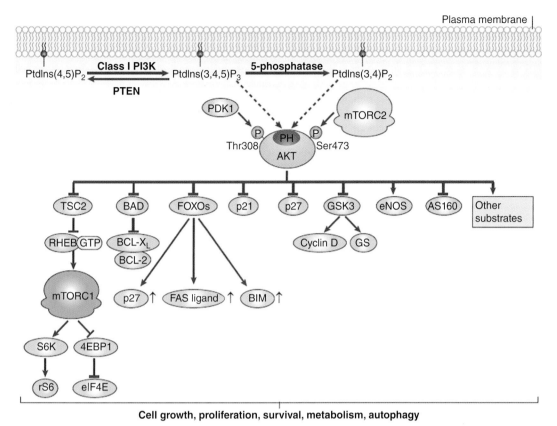

**Figure 32.3** AKT as a primary class I PI3K effector. Following PI3K-mediated conversion of PI-4,5-P2 to PIP3 AKT becomes localized to the plasma membrane via binding of the PH domain of AKT to PIP3. AKT is then fully activated by T308 and S473 phosphorylation by PDK1 and mTORC2, respectively. Numerous AKT substrates are outlined. Source: Vanhaesebroeck et al., 2012.[8] Reproduced with permission from Nature Publishing Group.

PI-4,5-P2 resides, and the induction of a conformational change that relieves the basal inhibition of the catalytic activity of p110 inhibition (Figure 32.2). Upon release of inhibition, the catalytic p110 subunit is free to phosphorylate its major substrate PI-4,5-$P_2$ to produce the second messenger $PIP_3$.[7] A subset of cytosolic proteins contain pleckstrin homology (PH) domains that specifically bind to $PIP_3$ and thereby localize to the plasma membrane in response to PI3K activation. Most notable of these are the AKT family of protein-Serine/Threonine kinases.[9] In the absence of stimulated growth conditions, baseline levels of $PIP_3$ are nearly undetectable in mammalian cells, highlighting how tightly this second messenger is regulated.

The extent and duration of $PIP_3$ elevation at the plasma membrane is primarily regulated by the tumor suppressor phosphatase and tensin homolog (PTEN), whose lipid phosphatase activity converts PIP3 back to PI-4,5-$P_2$ (Figure 32.3). While there are other $PIP_3$ phosphatases such as SHIP1 and SHIP2, it is PTEN activity that is most clearly involved in human cancers. Loss of PTEN function through inactivating mutations, deletion, chromosomal translocation, and epigenetic silencing, is the second most common event in cancer after p53 mutations.[10]

## PI3K Effectors: AKT/mTOR

The serine-threonine protein kinase AKT is the main effector of PI3K activation and exists as three isoforms, AKT1, AKT2, AKT3 encoded by three distinct genes, AKT1, AKT2, and AKT3. The PH domain of AKT directly interacts with $PIP_3$, which induces conformational changes exposing the important residues, threonine 308 (T308) and serine 473 (S473).[11] Upon exposure T308, located in the AKT activation loop, is phosphorylated by phosphoinositide-dependent kinase 1 (PDK1), and S473 (in the hydrophobic AKT motif) is phosphorylated by mTOR complex 2 (mTORC2), leading to full AKT activation and downstream signaling (Figure 32.3).[9] Like AKT, PDK1 directly binds $PIP_3$, thereby localizing to the plasma membrane to facilitate AKT phosphorylation. It is apparent from above that PI3K, mTORC2, and PDK1 inhibition are all potential therapeutic targets to disrupt AKT signaling.

Following full activation AKT phosphorylates multiple targets, recognizing the consensus RxRxxS/TΨ sequence (where Ψ is a hydrophobic residue). There are numerous known and putative AKT substrates, and only the most relevant to cancer will be discussed below.[12] Further, while the AKT isoforms are similar in sequence and *in vitro* substrate specificity, there is evidence that distinct *in vivo* substrate specificity exists for the three isoforms, allowing for fine tuning and/or tissue-specific AKT signaling. AKT signaling has been reviewed in multiple publications, and downstream AKT effects are generally separated into four categories based on their role in controlling cell hypertrophy, cell survival, cell hyperplasia, and cell metabolism. We will briefly review major components in each arena of downstream AKT signaling, as a comprehensive review of all AKT substrates is beyond the scope of this chapter.

In their seminal 2000 review and 2011 update, Hanahan and Weinberg addressed the central importance of cell growth in the development and maintenance of human tumors.[1,13] An increase in cell size, mainly through increased activity of protein and lipid synthesis, is common to many tumors, and the role of AKT in this area must be appreciated. Fully active AKT turns on the protein kinase activity of mTOR complex 1 (mTORC1) via phosphorylating, and thereby turning off the inhibitory protein Tuberin (the protein product of the tuberous sclerosis complex 2 (TSC2) gene, and by phosphorylating PRAS40 (Proline Rich AKT Substrate of 40 kDa).[14,15] The details of this mechanism are discussed below.

Following activation, mTORC1 plays a major role in stimulating protein translation through its substrates, ribosomal protein S6 kinase (S6K) and eukaryotic translation initiation factor 4E-binding protein 1 (4EBP1).[5,14] Phosphorylated 4EBP1 is no longer capable of inhibiting the translation-initiation factor eIF4E, thereby allowing the translation of capped messages.[16] Both the selective advantage and critical importance of cell growth to the maintenance of malignant phenotype have been exploited therapeutically by the mTORC1 inhibitor rapamycin and its analogs.

The highly regulated balance of cell survival and programmed cell death or apoptosis is universally disrupted in cancer. It was readily apparent from early knockdown and rescue experiments that AKT played a role in promoting cell survival and suppressing apoptosis. AKT inhibits the apoptotic pathway via negative regulation of proapoptotic Bcl-2 family proteins, such as Bcl-2-associated death promoter (BAD).[17,18] AKT-mediated BAD phosphorylation causes release of BAD from its antiapoptotic[19] partner BCL-X$_L$, thereby shifting the BAD:BCL-X$_L$ ratio in favor of the antiapoptotic BCL-X$_L$.[19] AKT also phosphorylates the Forkhead box (FOXO) family of transcription factors, which influence the expression of multiple proapoptotic proteins.[20-22] The tumor suppressor p53 is a major regulator of cell survival, and AKT can influence p53 degradation via phosphorylation of MDM2, an E3 ligase that mediates degradation of p53.[23] A review of all known antiapoptotic targets of AKT is beyond the scope of this chapter.

Unconstrained growth is the quintessential property of cancer and ultimately accounts for many of the clinical symptoms produced by tumors. Beyond its antiapoptotic effects, activated AKT can drive cell proliferation via promoting the G1 to S-phase transition of the cell cycle. The most direct mechanism for AKT-driven proliferation is probably the phosphorylation and inactivation of glycogen synthase kinase 3 (GSK3). This kinase processively phosphorylates a host of proteins involved in cell cycle control (including c-Myc, c-Jun, and Cyclin D1), thereby marking them for proteolytic degradation. (Figure 32.3)[21,22] Inactivation of GSK3 via AKT phosphorylation allows stabilization of these proteins and can promote cell cycle progression.

In recent years, it has become increasingly appreciated that in order to sustain high proliferative rates, cancer cells frequently acquire metabolic advantages.[7] The preference of cancer cells for glycolysis and lactate production over aerobic glycolysis potentially provides malignant cells with increased production of ribose-5 phosphate, acetyl-CoA, and NADPH.[24] Isoform-specific AKT signaling is known to be involved in GLUT4 distribution, and catalytic domain mutations in AKT2 cause severe insulin resistance and clinical diabetes in humans.[25] Within cancer cells AKT activation leads to increased plasma membrane GLUT1, as well as increased association of hexose-6-kinase with the mitochondria, thereby promoting glucose entry and increasing glucose-6-phosphate production. These events partially explain the high glycolytic rate characteristic of cancer cells, and the successful use of [18]F-flurodeoxyglucose positron emission tomography (FDG-PET)

for visualization of many cancers.[26-28] The metabolic reprogramming of malignant cells is an active area of therapeutic investigation, and glucose withdrawal via PI3K inhibitors in PIK3CA mutant cells, or starvation causes cell death and tumor regression.[29,30]

The intimate relationship between AKT and mTOR is well established and previously reviewed.[31-33] Briefly, mTOR is the catalytic subunit of two separate complexes known as mTOR complex 1 (mTORC1) and mTOR complex 2 (mTORC2), which are distinguished by their accessory proteins, regulatory-associated protein of mTOR (RAPTOR) and rapamycin-insensitive companion of mTOR (RICTOR).[31,34] The subunit composition of mTORC1 and mTORC2 dictate substrate specificity. There are multiple inputs and regulators of mTOR, and we will restrict the remainder of this chapter to discussion of the PI3K/AKT-relevant inputs.

mTORC1 is a major signal integrator at the intersection of growth, starvation, and cellular stress. Fully active AKT phosphorylates and inactivates Tuberin, a protein that normally stimulates hydrolysis of GTP that is bound to RHEB (Ras homolog enriched in brain). This allows RHEB to accumulate in its GTP-bound state and thereby activate mTORC1[35,36] (Figure 32.3). Activated mTORC1 phosphorylates its major substrates S6 kinase (S6K) and eIF4E-binding protein (4E-BP1) (Figure 32.3), with the net result of increased translation of messenger RNA (mRNA) and ultimately to an increase in global protein synthesis.[37] The related complex mTORC2 does not participate directly in regulation of protein synthesis, but, as discussed above, phosphorylates AKT, thereby contributing to mTORC1 activation. Other major mTORC2 substrates include serum and glucocorticoid-regulated kinase (SGK) family members and protein kinase C (PKC) family members. While mTORC2 substrates are well identified, less is known about upstream regulation of mTORC2. However, insulin stimulation results in increased mTORC2-mediated S473 AKT phosphorylation, suggesting a role for growth factor regulation of mTORC2.[38]

The importance of mTOR as a therapeutic target in cancer has been exploited through the use of rapamycin and its analogies (rapalogs), which preferentially inhibit mTORC1 (Figure 32.4).

## PI3K/AKT/mTOR Mutations

The ability of the PI3K/AKT/mTOR pathway to control numerous processes involved in malignant transformation and progression positions the PI3K/AKT/mTOR axis as a therapeutic target in cancer. Similarly, one can begin to see the potential mechanisms for resistance after inhibition of PI3K pathway components. Researchers have attempted to exploit each component of the signaling cascade with approaches ranging from pan-PI3K inhibition, isoform-specific PI3K inhibitors, mTOR inhibitors, AKT inhibitors, and combination PI3K–mTOR inhibitors. Many other signaling pathways communicate with the PI3K/AKT/mTOR axis and compounds such as PI3K-MEK inhibitors are also being developed. In the following sections we will review common PI3K pathway aberrations in cancer and the results of attempts at targeting the PI3K pathway. A review of all known PI3K/AKT/mTOR mutations and all compounds in development is beyond the scope of this chapter, and we have restricted discussion to the most novel mechanisms of inhibition and the most clinically advanced compounds. Newer databases such as the Genomics of Drug Sensitivity in Cancer (http://www.cancerRxgene.org), the Cancer Cell Line Encyclopedia (http://www.broadinstitute.org/ccle), and http://clinicaltrials.gov will aid in the identification of potential PI3K pathway-modulating compounds.[39,40]

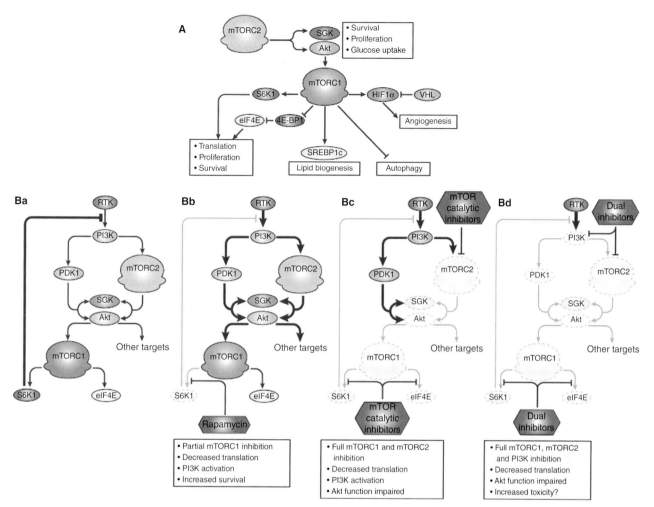

**Figure 32.4** The importance of mTOR in cancer. Panel A shows the major cellular processes regulated by mTORC1 and mTORC2 demonstrating their role in tumorigenesis and progression. Panel Ba depicts the PI3K/AKT/mTOR pathway in the absence of mTOR inhibitors and panel Bb, Bc, and Bd demonstrate effects of rapamycin, mTOR catalytic inhibitors, and dual PI3K/mTOR inhibitors. Source: Zoncu et al., 2011.[31] Reproduced with permission from Nature Publishing Group.

The most common mechanisms of activating the PI3K/AKT/mTOR signaling pathway in cancer are via upstream RTK activation (overexpression of growth factor or receptor, or mutation or amplification of the gene for the RTK) and somatic mutations in components of the signaling network. The frequency of mutations within the PI3K signaling cascade in common cancers is shown in Figure 32.1, although new mutations are likely to be identified in the future. In the cases of increased PI3K signaling resulting from RTK overactivation, the importance of PI3K signaling is highlighted by the fact that for an RTK inhibitor to be effective it typically must turn off PI3K.[41,42] Somatic mutations in PIK3CA, the gene encoding PI3K p110α, occur primarily in the kinase and helical domains and enhance PI3K signaling when RTK signaling is low. Helical domain p110 mutations, most commonly E545 K and E542 K, relieve the inhibitory function of the p85 subunit (Figure 32.2).[43] Kinase domain mutations such as the H1074R mutation appear to enhance PI3K binding to the membrane where its substrate resides. In addition, the genes encoding the p85 regulatory subunit of PI3K, PIK3R1, and PIK3R2, are frequently mutated in a subset of cancers, especially endometrial cancers (Figure 32.1). Some of these mutations appear to relieve the inhibition of p110, thereby

increasing PI3K signaling. Interestingly, in addition to their abilities to bind to p110, p85 subunits can also bind to and stabilize PTEN, indicating a dual role for p85 in modulating PI3K signaling. Some of the p85 mutations observed in endometrial cancers increase PI3K signaling by disrupting p85 binding to PTEN, resulting in the degradation of PTEN.[42] Large genomic and proteomic databases generated from patient samples will likely lead to the identification of further novel PI3K mutations.

Mutations in AKT and mTOR complexes are less commonly observed in cancers (Figure 32.1). However, Carpten and colleagues have shown that the E17 K mutation in the PH domain of AKT1 enhances AKT1 binding to the plasma membrane, independent of PIP3 production, and thereby increases AKT phosphorylation.[44] AKT2 and AKT3 mutations have also been observed in colorectal cancers (CRC) and malignant melanomas. Mutations in the mTOR component of mTORC1 and mTORC2 are even more rare, although they have been detected at >5% in endometrial, colorectal, and lung cancers from TCGA data (Figure 32.1). A recent publication also suggests that mTOR mutations are likely present in renal cell cancers (RCC).[45] Beyond mutations in canonical class IA PI3K components themselves there are numerous mutations that increase input and signaling into the PI3K pathway, for example, Ras-family oncogenes, EGFR mutations, and HER2 gene amplification are all shown to increase PI3K pathway flux.[46, 47]

## PI3K/AKT/mTOR as a Therapeutic Target

Successful drug development and implementation includes target inhibition at bioavailable concentrations, identification of off-target effects and toxicities, understanding of resistance, biomarker development, and ultimately clinical efficacy. PI3K pathway inhibitors have evolved significantly since 1994 when Vlahos et Al. first identified LY294002, a reversible pan-PI3K inhibitor.[48] LY294002 and the irreversible pan-PI3K inhibitor Wortmannin highlighted the early therapeutic potential of PI3K pathway inhibition and have continued use in preclinical studies as toolbox compounds. There are currently numerous PI3K/AKT/mTOR pathway inhibitors in clinical development that have shown *in vitro* and *in vivo* activity in cancer (Table 32.1). As more data emerges regarding mechanisms of resistance to PI3K pathway inhibitors, there has also been an increase in developing drug combinations intended to combat or delay resistance or enhance efficacy.[49, 50] In the following section, we provide examples of PI3K pathway inhibitors in late preclinical or early clinical development and discuss potential limitations.

Both pan-PI3K and isoform-specific PI3K inhibitors are in development (Table 32.1). Pan-PI3K inhibitors such as BKM120 (from Novartis) have shown favorable pharmacokinetic studies at doses of up to 100 mg/day. In a recent phase I study of BKM120, adverse effects include rash, hyperglycemia, nausea, pruritus, and mood alteration.[51] The hyperglycemia is an expected on-target toxicity, since PI3Ks (especially p110α) are required for insulin-dependent glucose uptake into muscle and fat cells and insulin-dependent suppression of gluconeogenesis in the liver. The rash may also be on-target since it is observed with other unrelated PI3K inhibitors. BEZ235, also from Novartis, inhibits both class I PI3Ks and mTOR (both in the context of TORC1 and TORC2). Rational combination studies of BKM120 and BEZ235 with traditional cytotoxic chemotherapies are ongoing at the phase I and II level (see NCT01550380 and NCT01248494 for examples). Importantly, the role of the PI3K pathway in glucose homeostasis, and predictable hyperglycemia from inhibition, may make the readily available and noninvasive serum glucose or C-peptide (a reporter of insulin elevation) potential biomarkers of target inhibition in clinical studies.

**Table 32.1** PI3K/AKT/mTOR inhibitors in advanced clinical development.

| Compound | Target | IC50 (nM) | Phase of clinical development |
|---|---|---|---|
| **p110 inhibitors** | | **IC50 (α, β, δ, γ)** | |
| GDC-0941 | p110 (α, β, δ, γ) | 3, 33, 3, 75 | Phase I–II clinical trials |
| XL147 | p110 (α, β, δ, γ) | 39, 383, 36, 33 | Phase I–II clinical trials |
| ZSTK474 | p110 (α, β, δ, γ) | X, 17, 6, 53 | Phase I clinical trials |
| CAL-101/Idelalisib | p110δ | 2.5 | Phase I–III clinical trials (FDA pending) |
| NVP-BYL719 | p110α >>> β, δ, γ | 5 | Phase I–II clinical trials |
| TGX-221 | p110β | 5 | None |
| PIK-75 | p110α | 5.8 | None |
| NVP-BKM120/Buparlisib | p110 (α, β, δ, γ) | 52-99, 166, 116, 262 | Phase I–III clinical trials |
| **p110/mTOR inhibitors** | | | |
| NVP-BEZ235/Dactolisib | p110 and mTOR | 4-7 (p110α, γ, δ), 16 (mTOR) | Phase I–II clinical trials |
| GSK1059615 | p110 and mTOR | 0.4-5 (p110), 12 (mTOR) | Phase I (terminated) |
| PF-04691502 | p110 and mTOR | 1.6-2.1 (p110), 16 (mTOR) | Phase I clinical trials |
| GDC0980 | p110 and mTOR | 5-27 (p110), 17 (mTOR) | Phase I–II clinical trials |
| XL765 | p110 and mTOR | 9-113 (p110), 157 (mTOR) | Phase I clinical trials |
| GSK2126458 | p110 and mTOR | 0.01-0.06 (p110), 0.2 (mTOR) | Phase I clinical trials |
| **mTOR inhibitors** | | | |
| AZD8055 | mTORC1, mTORC2 (mTOR catalytic site) | 0.8nM (mTOR) | Phase I–II clinical trials |
| AZD2014 | mTORC1, mTORC2 (mTOR catalytic site) | 2.8 (mTOR) | Phase I clinical trials |
| OSI-027 | mTORC1, mTORC2 | 22 (mTORC1), 65nM (mTORC2) | Phase I clinical trials |
| Ridaforolimus | mTORC1>mTORC2 | 0.2 (mTOR) | Phase III clinical trials (rejected by FDA) |
| Everolimus/Temsirolimus | mTORC1 >> mTORC2 | | Phase III, FDA-approved |
| Rapamycin | mTORC1 >> mTORC2 | | Phase III, FDA-approved |
| **AKT inhibitors** | | | |
| MK2206 | AKT | 8 (Akt1), 12 (Akt2), 65 (Akt3) | Phase I–II clinical trials |
| Perifosine | AKT | | Phase I–II clinical trials |
| AT7867 | AKT and p70 S6 Kinase | 32 (Akt1), 17 (Akt2), 47 (Akt3) | Planned phase I |
| PHT-427 | AKT | 2.7 | Planned phase I |
| GSK690693 | AKT | 2 (Akt1), 13 (Akt2), 9 (Akt3) | Phase I clinical trials |

*Source:* Clinical trial data is from published literature and www.clintrials.gov
Compounds are grouped by mechanism of action. Compounds were chosen based on phase of clinical development and mechanism of action. The list shown in the table is not intended to be comprehensive and there are numerous other PI3K pathway inhibitors in preclinical and early clinical development.

As a potential method to minimize toxicities without compromising efficacy, several isoform-specific PI3K inhibitors have been developed. PIK3CA is often mutated in many tumor types, thus development of p110α isoform-specific inhibitors including NVP-BLY719, INK1117, and GDC-0032 are being tested in patients with solid tumors. In early clinical experience, the selective p110α inhibitor NVP-BLY719 causes less hyperglycemia than the pan-PI3K inhibitor NVP-BKM120.[52] Moreover, NVP-BLY719 causes tumor shrinkage in 33% of metastatic breast cancer patients with ER+ PIK3CA mutation in a phase 1 trial.[53] Preclinical data shows that PIK3CA mutation or amplification is the best biomarker for predicting sensitivity to NVP-BLY719.[52] However, the same study showed that p110α inhibitors are not effective in PIK3CA mutated cells that also have a PTEN deletion. This is likely because PTEN deletion tumors are more dependent on p110β than p110α for their growth and survival.[54] Thus, although p110β is not often mutated in cancer cells, inhibitors of p110β like KIN-193 and GSK2636771 are currently being evaluated in PTEN deleted solid tumors. Therefore, patients with PIK3CA gene alterations would benefit from a p110β inhibitor, while patients with PTEN deletion may benefit from p110β inhibition.

As a general rule, p110δ expression is confined to hematopoietic cell types and is more critical than p110α or p110β for the growth of B cells and for the survival of B-cell lineage leukemias and lymphomas, such as chronic lymphocytic leukemia (CLL), an incurable hematologic malignancy.[55] Upon B-cell receptor activation, downstream effectors including p110δ and Bruton's tyrosine kinase (BTK) are activated to promote survival and proliferation of B-cell malignancies. The special dependence of B-cell leukemia on p110δ suggests p110δ-selective inhibition may offer therapeutic benefit, while minimizing off-target effects and potential toxicities. The p110δ isoform-specific PI3K inhibitor CAL-101/idelalisib promotes apoptosis in CLL cells and abrogates the antiapoptotic stimuli from B-cell activating factors such as CD40 ligand and tumor necrosis factor alpha (TNF-α).[56] A phase 3 clinical trial of idelalisib, in combination with monoclonal anti-CD20 (ritiximab) showed that idelalisib increased the overall response rate from 13% to 81% in relapse CLL patients.[57] The progression free survival (PFS) for the rituximab-only arm was 5.5 months, while the PFS for patients also receiving idelalisib was not yet reached by the end of the trial. There was no significant increase in toxicity with the addition of idelalisib.[57] Furthermore, CLL patients with adverse risk characteristics like loss/mutated P53 or mutated IGHV were also responsive to idelalisab, even though they are traditionally poorly responsive to standard chemotherapy. This inhibitor is not only promising in CLL but also in indolent B-cell non-Hodgkin lymphoma (iNHL) and mantle cell lymphoma (MCL).[58,59] As a single agent, up to 90% of patients who had previously failed to respond to standard chemotherapy have experienced a decrease in tumor burden.[58] It seems that targeting survival factors downstream of B-cell receptor activation is a key strategy for targeting B-cell malignancies since idelalisab and the BTK inhibitor ibrutinib have both been successful in clinical trials.[60] Thus the effectiveness of idelalisab as a single agent and in combination is largely due to the significant role of p110δ in B-cell survival upon B-cell receptor activation.

Despite a relative paucity of mutations, the central role of AKT in effecting PI3K signaling has made AKT a potentially attractive therapeutic target. The orally bioavailable allosteric AKT inhibitor MK-2206 has demonstrated AKT inhibition at tolerable doses, with predictable side effects including rash, hyperglycemia, and nausea, and is moving forward in several phase I–II clinical trials (Table 32.1)[61] A recent paper by Rosen et al. suggests that monotherapy with AKT inhibitors may not achieve maximal benefit, as AKT inhibition led to induction of the known PI3K-stimulating RTK HER3 in breast cancer cell lines.[47] In addition to HER3 induction, AKT inhibition led to an increase in IGF-1R and the insulin receptor, possibly mediated by increased FOXO family transcription factors, and this is a suggested escape pathway and resistance mechanism.[62] This observation of increased upstream signaling upon inhibiting a node of the PI3K/AKT/mTOR signaling network or of the MAPK signaling network is more the rule than the exception, and provides a strong argument for the use of combination therapies that anticipate and block the feedback response. Consistent with this point, there is some evidence that this feedback can be overcome with dual inhibition of AKT and the expected RTKs.[47]

Simultaneous proximal (i.e., PI3K) and more distal (mTOR) inhibition has theoretic advantages and is being exploited clinically. It was recently demonstrated that epithelial ovarian cancer cells exposed to the PI3K/mTOR inhibitor BEZ235 showed response, but ultimately developed resistance via drug-induced upregulation of prosurvival cellular programs mediated by FOXO transcription factors.[63] Further, resistance could be eliminated via inhibition of several upregulated proteins such as Bcl-2 and the Epidermal Growth Factor Receptor (EGFR).[63] Examples such as this may also be predicted through large-scale high-throughput synthetic lethal screens.

Prostate cancers commonly carry genomic aberrations in the PI3K pathway, mainly via PTEN loss, and PTEN loss may be associated with resistance to castration.[64,65] Carver et al have shown that BEZ235 causes growth arrest in PTEN negative prostate cancers, but that inhibition of the PI3K pathway leads to activation of androgen receptor (AR) signaling. The converse also appears to be true, with inhibition of AR resulting in promotion of PI3K activity.[65] These examples and others highlight the potential for combination therapies based on targeting known compensatory survival pathways activated in the presence of PI3K pathway inhibition. In CRC, the frequency of KRAS-activating mutations approaches 40%, and KRAS not only activates the RAF/MEK/ERK pathway, but can directly bind PI3K and contribute to activation in some contexts. However, inhibition of the RAF/MEK/ERK pathway typically leads to relief of a negative feedback loop on the IGF1 signaling pathway and causes hyperactivation of PI3K.[66] Because of this, in the presence of KRAS mutations the combined inhibition of MEK and PI3K is superior to either alone.[30] Early results from phase I studies with the isoform-specific class I PI3K-inhibitor GDC-0941 alone in solid tumors demonstrated safety and tolerability with a potential single-agent therapeutic signal in sarcoma, ovarian, and endometrial cancers. Based on the preclinical increase in tumor inhibition with combination MEK/PI3K inhibition and the safety/tolerability of each drug individually, there are ongoing early phase trials combining GDC-0941 with the oral MEK inhibitor GDC-0973 (NCT00996892), as well as combining BKM120 with GSK212, a MEK inhibitor.

A cautionary tale for targeted PI3K/AKT/mTOR monotherapy exists for the naturally occurring mTORC1 inhibitor rapamycin. Following its discovery, rapamycin showed broad anticancer activity in numerous cancer cell lines. However, cell line and xenograft activity has not translated to broad clinical efficacy, and rapamycin is not used as a primary therapy in cancer. What emerged from further rapamycin study was that in many cancers inhibition of mTOR results in increased PI3K activation, again via suppression of negative feedback loops (Figure 32.4).[31,67] Selective mTORC1 inhibition with rapamycin also leads to activation of other prosurvival signals including the MEK-ERK and platelet-derived growth factor receptor (PDGFR), providing a clear cellular escape to mTORC1 inhibition.[62,68,69] Yet, rapamycin analogs (often termed rapalogs) have been shown to have clinical effectiveness in a subset of cancers, typically in combinations with standard of care drugs in renal cell carcinoma and pancreatic neuroendocrine cancers where TSC2 mutations are frequent. The efficacy of rapalogs in combination with standard endocrine therapy for advanced breast cancer was highlighted by the recent landmark BOLERO-2 trial, which showed a median PFS of 6.9 months for everolimus and exemestane versus 2.8 months for exemestane alone.[70] It is likely that further mutational testing will segregate patients and inform the heterogeneity of patient responses to rapalogs and other targeted therapies.

Attempts to overcome the escape of selective mTORC1 inhibition are ongoing with combination mTOR/PI3K inhibitors and mTOR catalytic site inhibitors that target both TORC1 and TORC2 (Figure 32.4, Table 32.1). The catalytic site mTOR inhibitor AZD8055 effectively blocks mTORC1-dependent phosphorylation of 4E-BP1 and TORC2-dependent phosphorylation of the S473 site of AKT.[71] AZD8055 has been shown to induce autophagy and tumor growth inhibition in multiple cell lines including NSCLC, glioblastoma, prostate, and colon cancer xenografts, and is currently being tested in recurrent glioblastoma (NCT01316809).[71] Concomitant with demonstrations of antitumor efficacy, a potential resistance mechanism via enhanced AKT phosphorylation by PDK1 at Thr308 (downstream of PDGFR) and some residual mTORC2 phosphorylation of AKT at Ser473 (from suboptimal dosing) has been shown.[72,73] A logical extension was combined inhibition of PI3K and mTOR.

As in renal cell carcinomas (RCC), mTOR signaling is constitutively activated in several non-Hodgkin lymphomas (NHL) including mantle cell lymphoma (MCL) and diffuse large B-cell lymphoma (DLBCL). However, response to rapalogs is only 30% in DLBCL, which is well below standard therapies.[74] The AKT inhibitor MK-2206 is able to overcome mTOR inhibitor resistance in DLBCL cell lines and is currently in several phase I and II studies in relapsed lymphomas.[75]

As outlined above, there are several promising PI3K pathway inhibitors that have both helped to elucidate existing feedback pathways in the PI3K cascade and to develop rational drug combinations. Ongoing preclinical studies are geared toward identification of tumor mutations that may predict responses or resistance to PI3K pathway inhibitors, and whether or not combination therapy is feasible. Early phase clinical trials with entry criteria linked to tumor mutational status will undoubtedly facilitate further identification of potential resistance pathways.

## From Rational Drug Design to Clinical Efficacy: Lessons and Challenges

Improved diagnostic techniques, the generation of clinically annotated tumor databases, and ongoing high-throughput sequencing and proteomic assays will continue to drive increases in the understanding of cancer biology. The frequency of PI3K/AKT/mTOR aberrations across multiple cancer types solidifies the central importance of this signaling pathway in tumorigenesis and progression. As there are multiple inputs and outputs in the PI3K pathway, there are several compensatory escapes to PI3K/AKT/mTOR inhibition.[62] Single-agent PI3K therapy is unlikely to achieve cures in heterogenous solid tumors although data is mounting for cytostatic effects. Larger phase III trials are required to determine both whether cytostatic therapies will translate into survival benefits and whether combination and/or sequential PI3K pathway inhibition is an effective clinical strategy. It is likely that, as with other targeted agents (trastuzumab, aromatase inhibitors), PI3K pathway inhibitors will have their greatest impact when used in the adjuvant setting to prevent recurrence following initial definitive therapy (i.e., surgery or radiation).

Further research on response biomarkers and mutation–drug sensitivity relationships is likely to more accurately identify patients most likely to achieve maximal benefit from PI3K pathway inhibitors and is a major translational focus.[50] Gene, protein, and phosphoprotein expression data with signatures of sensitivity/resistance are also likely to be informative and some signatures are already emerging.[76]

In the preceding pages, we have attempted to review the PI3K pathway in human cancer and highlight the importance of translational efforts in bringing drug compounds from the bench to the bedside.

## References

1 Hanahan D, Weinberg RA. Hallmarks of cancer: the next generation. *Cell.* 2011;144(5):646–674.

2 Whitman M, Downes CP, Keeler M, Keller T, Cantley L. Type I phosphatidylinositol kinase makes a novel inositol phospholipid, phosphatidylinositol-3-phosphate. *Nature.* 1988;332(6165):644–646.

3 Whitman M, Kaplan DR, Schaffhausen B, Cantley L, Roberts TM. Association of phosphatidylinositol kinase activity with polyoma middle-T competent for transformation. *Nature.* 1985;315(6016):239–242.

4 Yuan TL, Cantley LC. PI3K pathway alterations in cancer: variations on a theme. *Oncogene.* 2008;27(41):5497–5510.

5 Vivanco I, Sawyers CL. The phosphatidylinositol 3-Kinase AKT pathway in human cancer. *Nat Rev Cancer.* 2002;2(7):489–501.

6 Zhao L, Vogt PK. Class I PI3K in oncogenic cellular transformation. *Oncogene.* 2008;27(41):5486–5496.

7 Engelman JA, Luo J. Cantley LC. The evolution of phosphatidylinositol 3-kinases as regulators of growth and metabolism. *Nat Rev Genet.* 2006;7(8):606–619.

8 Vanhaesebroeck B, Stephens L, Hawkins P. PI3K signalling: the path to discovery and understanding. *Nat Rev Mol Cell Biol.* 2012;13(3):195–203.

9 Stephens L, Anderson K, Stokoe D, et al. Protein kinase B kinases that mediate phosphatidylinositol 3,4,5-trisphosphate-dependent activation of protein kinase B. *Science.* 1998;279(5351):710–714.

10 Carracedo A, Alimonti A, Pandolfi PP. PTEN level in tumor suppression: how much is too little? *Cancer Res.* 2011;71(3):629–633.

11 Gonzalez E, McGraw TE. The Akt kinases: isoform specificity in metabolism and cancer. *Cell Cycle.* 2009;8(16):2502–2508.

12 Pearce LR, Komander D, Alessi DR. The nuts and bolts of AGC protein kinases. *Nat Rev Mol Cell Biol.* 2010;11(1):9–22.

13 Hanahan D, Weinberg RA. The hallmarks of cancer. *Cell.* 2000;100(1):57–70.

14 Nave BT, Ouwens M, Withers DJ, Alessi DR, Shepherd PR. Mammalian target of rapamycin is a direct target for protein kinase B: identification of a convergence point for opposing effects of insulin and amino-acid deficiency on protein translation. *Biochem J.* 1999; 344(Pt 2):427–431.

15 Vander Haar E, Lee SI, Bandhakavi S, Griffin TJ, Kim DH. Insulin signalling to mTOR mediated by the Akt/PKB substrate PRAS40. *Nat Cell Biol.* 2007;9(3):316–323.

16 Laplante M, Sabatini DM. mTOR signaling in growth control and disease. *Cell.* 2012;149(2):274–293.

17 Datta SR, Dudek H, Tao X, et al. Akt phosphorylation of BAD couples survival signals to the cell-intrinsic death machinery. *Cell.* 1997;91(2):231–241.

18 Datta SR, Katsov A, Hu L, et al. 14-3-3 proteins and survival kinases cooperate to inactivate BAD by BH3 domain phosphorylation. *Mol Cell.* 2000;6(1):41–51.

19 del Peso L, González-García M, Page C, Herrera R, Nuñez G. Interleukin-3-induced phosphorylation of BAD through the protein kinase Akt. *Science.* 1997;278(5338):687–689.

20 Brunet A, Bonni A, Zigmond MJ, et al. Akt promotes cell survival by phosphorylating and inhibiting a Forkhead transcription factor. *Cell.* 1999;96(6):857–868.

21 Shultz JC, Goehe RW, Wijesinghe DS, et al. Alternative splicing of caspase 9 is modulated by the phosphoinositide 3-kinase/Akt pathway via phosphorylation of SRp30 a. *Cancer Res.* 2010;70(22):9185–9196.

22 Cardone MH, Roy N, Stennicke HR, et al. Regulation of cell death protease caspase-9 by phosphorylation. *Science.* 1998;282(5392):1318–1321.

23 Mayo LD, Donner DB. A phosphatidylinositol 3-kinase/Akt pathway promotes translocation of Mdm2 from the cytoplasm to the nucleus. *Proc Natl Acad Sci U S A.* 2001;98(20):11598–11603.

24 Vander Heiden MG, Cantley LC, Thompson CB. Understanding the Warburg effect: the metabolic requirements of cell proliferation. *Science.* 2009;324(5930):1029–1033.

25 George S, Rochford JJ, Wolfrum C, et al. A family with severe insulin resistance and diabetes due to a mutation in AKT2. *Science.* 2004;304(5675):1325–1328.

26 Majewski N, Nogueira V, Bhaskar P, et al. Hexokinase-mitochondria interaction mediated by Akt is required to inhibit apoptosis in the presence or absence of Bax and Bak. *Mol Cell.* 2004;16(5):819–830.

27 Majewski N, Nogueira V, Robey RB, Hay N. Akt inhibits apoptosis downstream of BID cleavage via a glucose-dependent mechanism involving mitochondrial hexokinases. *Mol Cell Biol.* 2004;24(2):730–740.

28 Wieman HL, Wofford JA, Rathmell JC. Cytokine stimulation promotes glucose uptake via phosphatidylinositol-3 kinase/Akt regulation of Glut1 activity and trafficking. *Mol Biol Cell.* 2007;18(4):1437–1446.

29 Vander Heiden MG. Plas DR, Rathmell JC, Fox CJ, Harris MH, Thompson CB. Growth factors can influence cell growth and survival through effects on glucose metabolism. *Mol Cell Biol.* 2001;21(17):5899–5912.

30 Engelman JA, Chen L, Tan X, et al. Effective use of PI3K and MEK inhibitors to treat mutant Kras G12D and PIK3CA H1047R murine lung cancers. *Nat Med.* 2008;14(12):1351–1356.

31 Zoncu R, Efeyan A, Sabatini DM. mTOR: from growth signal integration to cancer, diabetes and ageing. *Nat Rev Mol Cell Biol.* 2011;12(1):21–35.

32 Shaw RJ, Cantley LC. Ras, PI(3)K and mTOR signalling controls tumour cell growth. *Nature.* 2006;441(7092):424–430.

33 Engelman JA. Targeting PI3K signalling in cancer: opportunities, challenges and limitations. *Nat Rev Cancer.* 2009;9(8):550–562.

34 Hara K, Maruki Y, Long X, et al. Raptor, a binding partner of target of rapamycin (TOR), mediates TOR action. *Cell.* 2002;110(2):177–189.

35 Tee AR, Manning BD, Roux PP, Cantley LC, Blenis J. Tuberous sclerosis complex gene products, Tuberin and Hamartin, control mTOR signaling by acting as a GTPase-activating protein complex toward Rheb. *Curr Biol.* 2003;13(15):1259–1268.

36 Zhang Y, Gao X, Saucedo LJ, Ru B, Edgar BA, Pan D. Rheb is a direct target of the tuberous sclerosis tumour suppressor proteins. *Nat Cell Biol.* 2003;5(6):578–581.

37 Ma XM, Blenis J. Molecular mechanisms of mTOR-mediated translational control. *Nat Rev Mol Cell Biol.* 2009;10(5):307–318.

38 Sarbassov DD, Guertin DA, Ali SM, Sabatini DM. Phosphorylation and regulation of Akt/PKB by the rictor-mTOR complex. *Science.* 2005;307(5712):1098–1101.

39 Barretina J, Caponigro G, Stransky N, et al. The Cancer Cell Line Encyclopedia enables predictive modelling of anticancer drug sensitivity. *Nature.* 2012;483(7391):603–607.

40 Garnett MJ, Edelman EJ, Heidorn SJ, et al. Systematic identification of genomic markers of drug sensitivity in cancer cells. *Nature.* 2012;483(7391):570–575.

41 Yakes FM, Chinratanalab W, Ritter CA, King W, Seelig S, Arteaga CL. Herceptin-induced inhibition of phosphatidylinositol-3 kinase and Akt Is required for antibody-mediated effects on p27, cyclin D1, and antitumor action. *Cancer Res.* 2002;62(14):4132–4141.

42 Mellinghoff IK, Wang MY, Vivanco I, et al. Molecular determinants of the response of glioblastomas to EGFR kinase inhibitors. *N Engl J Med.* 2005;353(19):2012–2024.

43 Huang CH, Mandelker D, Schmidt-Kittler O, et al. The structure of a human p110alpha/p85alpha complex elucidates the effects of oncogenic PI3Kalpha mutations. *Science.* 2007;318(5857):1744–1748.

44 Carpten JD, Faber AL, Horn C, et al. A transforming mutation in the pleckstrin homology domain of AKT1 in cancer. *Nature.* 2007;448(7152):439–444.

45 Gerlinger M, Rowan AJ, Horswell S, et al. Intratumor heterogeneity and branched evolution revealed by multiregion sequencing. *N Engl J Med.* 2012;366(10):883–892.

46 Ramjaun AR, Downward J. Ras and phosphoinositide 3-kinase: partners in development and tumorigenesis. *Cell Cycle.* 2007;6(23):2902–2905.

47 Chandarlapaty S, Sawai A, Scaltriti M, et al. AKT inhibition relieves feedback suppression of receptor tyrosine kinase expression and activity. *Cancer Cell.* 2011;19(1):58–71.

48 Vlahos CJ, Matter WF, Hui KY, Brown RF. A specific inhibitor of phosphatidylinositol 3-kinase, 2-(4-morpholinyl)-8-phenyl-4 H-1-benzopyran-4-one (LY294002). *J Biol Chem.* 1994;269(7):5241–5248.

49 Fruman DA, Rommel C. PI3K and cancer: lessons, challenges and opportunities. *Nat Rev Drug Discov.* 2014;13(2):140–156.

50 Dienstmann R, Rodon J, Serra V, Tabernero J. Picking the point of inhibition: a comparative review of PI3K/AKT/mTOR pathway inhibitors. *Mol Cancer Ther.* 2014;13(5):1021–1031.

51 Bendell JC, Rodon J, Burris HA, et al. Phase I, dose-escalation study of BKM120, an oral pan-Class I PI3K inhibitor, in patients with advanced solid tumors. *J Clin Oncol.* 2012;30(3):282–290.

52 Fritsch C, Huang A, Chatenay-Rivauday C, et al. Characterization of the novel and specific PI3Kα inhibitor NVP-BYL719 and development of the patient stratification strategy for clinical trials. *Mol Cancer Ther.* 2014;13(5):1117–1129.

53 Juric D, Argiles G, Burris HA, et al. Phase I study of BYL719, an alpaspecific PI3K inhibitor, in patients with PIK3CA mutant advanced solid tumors: preliminary efficacy and safety in patients with PIK3CA mutant ER-positive (ER+) metastatic breast cancer (MBC). *Cancer Res.* 2012. 72(24 suppl):P6–10–07.

54 Jia S, Liu Z, Zhang S, et al. Essential roles of PI(3)K-p110beta in cell growth, metabolism and tumorigenesis. *Nature.* 2008;454(7205):776–779.

55 Niedermeier M, Hennessy BT, Knight ZA, et al. Isoform-selective phosphoinositide 3′-kinase inhibitors inhibit CXCR4 signaling and overcome stromal cell-mediated drug resistance in chronic lymphocytic leukemia: a novel therapeutic approach. *Blood.* 2009;113(22):5549–5557.

56 Herman SE, Gordon AL, Wagner AJ, et al. Phosphatidylinositol 3-kinase-delta inhibitor CAL-101 shows promising preclinical activity in chronic lymphocytic leukemia by antagonizing intrinsic and extrinsic cellular survival signals. *Blood.* 2010;116(12):2078–2088.

57 Furman RR, Sharman JP, Coutre SE, et al. Idelalisib and rituximab in relapsed chronic lymphocytic leukemia. *N Engl J Med.* 2014;370(11):997–1007.

58 Brown JR, Byrd JC, Coutre SE, et al. Idelalisib, an inhibitor of phosphatidylinositol 3-kinase p110delta, for relapsed/refractory chronic lymphocytic leukemia. *Blood.* 2014;123(22):3390–3397.

59 Kahl BS, Spurgeon SE, Furman RR, et al. A phase 1 study of the PI3Kdelta inhibitor idelalisib in patients with relapsed/refractory mantle cell lymphoma (MCL). *Blood.* 2014;123(22):3398–3405.

60 Advani RH, Buggy JJ, Sharman JP, et al. Bruton tyrosine kinase inhibitor ibrutinib (PCI-32765) has significant activity in patients with relapsed/refractory B-cell malignancies. *J Clin Oncol.* 2013;31(1):88–94.

61 Yap TA, Patnaik A, Fearen I, et al. First-in-man clinical trial of the oral pan-AKT inhibitor MK-2206 in patients with advanced solid tumors. *J Clin Oncol.* 2011;29(35):4688–4695.

62 Klempner SJ, Myers AP, Cantley LC. What a tangled web we weave: emerging resistance mechanisms to inhibition of the phosphoinositide 3-kinase pathway. *Cancer Discov.* 2013;3(12):1345–1354.

63 Muranen T, Selfors LM, Worster DT, et al. Inhibition of PI3K/mTOR leads to adaptive resistance in matrix-attached cancer cells. *Cancer Cell.* 2012;21(2):227–239.

64 Carver BS, Chapinski C, Wongvipat J, et al. Reciprocal feedback regulation of PI3K and androgen receptor signaling in PTEN-deficient prostate cancer. *Cancer Cell.* 2011;19(5):575–586.

65 Reid AH, Attard G, Ambroisine L, et al. Transatlantic Prostate Group. Molecular characterisation of ERG, ETV1 and PTEN gene loci identifies patients at low and high risk of death from prostate cancer. *Br J Cancer.* 2010;102(4):678–684.

66 Ebi H, Corcoran RB, Singh A, et al. Receptor tyrosine kinases exert dominant control over PI3K signaling in human KRAS mutant colorectal cancers. *J Clin Invest.* 2011;121(11):4311–4321.

67 O'Reilly KE, Rojo F, She QB, et al. mTOR inhibition induces upstream receptor tyrosine kinase signaling and activates Akt. *Cancer Res.* 2006;66(3):1500–1508.

68 Carracedo A, Ma L, Teruya-Feldstein J, et al. Inhibition of mTORC1 leads to MAPK pathway activation through a PI3K-dependent feedback loop in human cancer. *J Clin Invest.* 2008;118(9):3065–3074.

69 Carracedo A, Pandolfi PP. The PTEN-PI3K pathway: of feedbacks and cross-talks. *Oncogene.* 2008;27(41):5527–5541.

70 Baselga J, Campone M, Piccart M, et al. Everolimus in postmenopausal hormone-receptor-positive advanced breast cancer. *N Engl J Med.* 2012;366(6):520–529.

71 Chresta CM, Davies BR, Hickson I, et al. AZD8055 is a potent, selective, and orally bioavailable ATP-competitive mammalian target of rapamycin kinase inhibitor with in vitro and in vivo antitumor activity. *Cancer Res.* 2010;70(1):288–298.

72 Peterson TR, Laplante M, Thoreen CC, et al. DEPTOR is an mTOR inhibitor frequently overexpressed in multiple myeloma cells and required for their survival. *Cell.* 2009;137(5):873–886.

73 Garcia-Martinez JM, Moran J, Clarke RG, et al. Ku-0063794 is a specific inhibitor of the mammalian target of rapamycin (mTOR). *Biochem J.* 2009;421(1):29–42.

74 Smith SM, van Besien K, Karrison T, et al. Temsirolimus has activity in non-mantle cell non-Hodgkin's lymphoma subtypes: The University of Chicago phase II consortium. *J Clin Oncol.* 2010;28(31):4740–4746.

75 Petrich AM, Leshchenko V, Kuo PY, et al. Akt Inhibitors MK-2206 and Nelfinavir overcome mTOR inhibitor resistance in DLBCL. *Clin Cancer Res.* 2012;18(9):2534–2544.

76 O'Brien C, Wallin JJ, Sampath D, et al. Predictive biomarkers of sensitivity to the phosphatidylinositol 3' kinase inhibitor GDC-0941 in breast cancer preclinical models. *Clin Cancer Res.* 2010;16(14):3670–3683.

## CHAPTER 33

# Current Status and Future Direction of PARP Inhibition in Cancer Therapy

*Saeed Rafii[1], Stan Kaye[2], and Susana Banerjee[3]*

[1]Clinical Senior Lecturer and Consultant Medical Oncologist, Institute of Cancer Sciences, The University of Manchester and The Christie Hospital Manchester, UK, Wilmslow Road, Manchester, M20 4BXUK

[2]Professor of Medical Oncology, Drug Development Unit, The Royal Marsden Hospital and The Institute for of Cancer Research, Downs Road, London, UK, SM2 5PT

[3]Consultant Medical Oncologist, Research Lead Gynecological Cancers, The Royal Marsden Hospital, Downs Road, London, UK, SM2 5PT

## Introduction

The identification of *BRCA1* and *BRCA2* genes has not only led to a better understanding of inherited predisposition to breast and ovarian cancer but also has greatly improved our knowledge of DNA repair pathways. This in turn has led to the development of new therapeutic "synthetic lethal" approaches using poly (ADP-ribose) polymerase (PARP) inhibitors (PARPi). In this chapter we review the current understanding of the molecular biology of the key DNA repair pathways, the mechanism of action of PARP inhibition, recent clinical trials of PARPi with a focus on epithelial ovarian cancer (EOC), and how these trials may affect the future treatment of cancer. We also review the mechanisms of resistance to PARPi, the ongoing efforts to identify biomarkers of response, and potential future clinical directions.

## *BRCA1, BRCA2*, and Breast and Ovarian Cancer

Up to 10% of breast and EOC cases are considered to have a strong hereditary component. Patients with hereditary breast and ovarian cancer often have distinct characteristics compared to sporadic cases including younger age at diagnosis, a higher incidence of other cancers and different pattern of response to treatment.[1,2] Studies to find the genetic basis of hereditary breast and ovarian cancer resulted in isolation of the first susceptibility gene *BRCA1* in 1994[3] followed by identification of *BRCA2* in 1995.[4] Up to 90% of hereditary cases of ovarian cancer are associated with mutations in *BRCA1* or *BRCA2*. These genes are tumor suppressor genes as the wild-type *BRCA* allele is lost in cancers. Germline mutations in both *BRCA1* and *BRCA2* genes confer an increased risk of breast and ovarian cancer; female *BRCA1* mutation carriers have up to a 60–80% lifetime risk of developing breast cancer[5,6] and up to a 20–40% lifetime risk of developing ovarian cancer.[6,7] The median age of diagnosis in *BRCA1* mutation carriers is 42 years which is lower than the median age for unselected western European and US women (≥65).[8] The lifetime breast cancer risk for carriers of *BRCA2* muta-

tion is 60–85%[9] and lifetime ovarian cancer risk is 10–20%.[9,10] However, only 15% of breast and/or ovarian cancers are due to mutations in *BRCA2*.[10] Men with germline mutations in *BRCA2* have 6% lifetime risk of developing breast cancer which is 100-fold greater than the risk within the general male population. Carriers of *BRCA2* mutations are also at increased risk for several other cancers, particularly prostate and pancreatic cancers.

The prevalence of carriers of *BRCA1* and *BRCA2* (*BRCA1/2*) mutations varies based on ethnicity. The prevalence of founder mutations in *BRCA1* (185delAG and 5382insC) and *BRCA2* (617delT) is particularly high among people of Ashkenazi Jewish decent and is reported to be around 2.5%.[11,12]

## DNA Damage and Repair

The human genome is constantly exposed to a variety of agents that can cause DNA damage. DNA damage also occurs as a result of normal DNA replication.[13] It is estimated that between $10^4$–$10^5$ episodes of DNA damage occur per cell every day as a result of oxidative endogenous stress.[14,15] These lesions range from a single base alteration to the most deleterious lesions such as double-strand breaks (DSB), which could seriously harm DNA fidelity and cause genomic instability if left unrepaired. Deficiencies in DNA damage signaling and repair pathways are fundamental to the etiology of many human cancers. Genomic instability, caused by a wide range of molecular and/or chromosomal alterations in neoplastic cells, is observed in most human cancers and is suggestive of sustained genetic damage in all cancer cells.[16]

There are different cellular pathways to repair various types of DNA damage and maintain the genomic stability including base excision repair (BER), nucleotide excision repair (NER), mismatch repair (MMR), homologous recombination repair (HRR), and non-homologous end-joining repair (NHEJ). Although each repair pathway is specialized to repair one particular form of DNA damage, repair of DNA lesions is often carried out through multiple and partly overlapping mechanisms dictated by the severity of DNA damage.[13]

*Targeted Therapy in Translational Cancer Research*, First Edition. Edited by Apostolia-Maria Tsimberidou, Razelle Kurzrock and Kenneth C. Anderson.
© 2016 John Wiley & Sons, Inc. Published 2016 by John Wiley & Sons, Inc.

## Role of PARP in DNA Repair

Many nuclear proteins are involved in different repair pathways. Poly (ADP-ribose) polymerase (PARP) is a nuclear protein that belongs to a family of 18 enzymes of which PARP-1 and PARP-2 are the most studied proteins.[17] Its function is essential in BER. When an inappropriate base pair is recognized by damage-specific glycolysis, it is immediately removed, often causing a nick (single-strand break, SSB) in the DNA. PARP-1 then binds to the site of DNA damage and modifies the conformation of chromatin structure to facilitate access of BER proteins to carry out the repair of this SSB.[17,18] Through its enzymatic activity, PARP-1 cleaves nicotinamide adenine dinucleotide (NAD+) to nicotinamide and ADP-ribose. It then transfers and forms a long branch of poly (ADP-ribose) or PAR on itself. This structure attracts BER proteins such as XRCC1, PCNA, and DNA polymerase β in order to repair the SSB.[17–21] Inhibition of PARP-1, however, causes conversion of SSB into deleterious DSBs during the replication process resulting in cell death if left unrepaired.[22] Although PARP-1 binds to DSBs sites, it is not essential for the repair of DSBs as these breaks are repaired by an HRR mechanism which is independent of PARP-1. However, cells lacking PARP-1 show increased rate of sister chromatid exchange and HRR[18,23,24] indicating that inhibition of PARP increases dependency of cells on HRR.

## Molecular Mechanism of HRR

DSBs produced by the conversion of SSBs at the replication fork are normally repaired by HRR as shown in Figure 33.1. Because of chromosomal fragmentation, translocations, and deletions resulting from DSBs, repair of these lesions is of high importance for cell survival and a complex process is employed for high fidelity repair of such lesions.[25] It has been suggested that even a single DSB is sufficient to trigger apoptosis.[26]

During HRR, the damaged ends of DNA are first resected by the RAD50/MRE11/NBS1 complex.[27] Then several proteins including RAD51, RAD52, RAD54, RPA, BRCA1, BRCA2, XRCC2, and XRCC3 localize at the site of the damage and facilitate the identification of homologous sister chromatid sequence. Subsequently the 3′ single-stranded tails invade the intact DNA, and DNA polymerases restore the damaged strand (Figure 33.1).[28] DSBs can also be repaired by nonhomologous end joining (NHEJ) repair which after processing the DNA ends simply ligates the two ends of damaged DNA together and is independent of BRCA function. It is, however, an error-prone mechanism resulting in the inevitable generation of mutations and deletions, which contribute to subsequent genomic instability. In contrast, HRR is an error-free and complex system which provides for high fidelity repair of DSBs and promotes genomic integrity (Figure 33.1).[29]

### BRCA1/2 Genes and HRR

BRCA proteins play a major role in mediation of DNA damage response and repair of DSB by HRR.[30,31] Cells deficient in *BRCA1* or *BRCA2* spontaneously are associated with various chromosome aberrations[30,32,33] indicating that *BRCA1/2* genes are essential for maintaining chromosome structure.[34] Both BRCA1 and BRCA2 interact and co-localize with Rad51.[35–37] BRCA1- and BRCA2-deficient cells are also defective in Rad51 foci formation,[22,38] and there is evidence to show that homologous recombination is less efficient in BRCA1- and BRCA2-deficient cell lines.[30]

### Synthetic Lethality

An intact HRR function provides a safety net for repairing DSBs in cells lacking PARP-1 function. However in *BRCA1/2* mutant cells lacking HRR function to repair the DSBs, inhibition of PARP results in accumulation of SSBs, which are converted into DSBs at the replication fork. This in turn results in cell cycle arrest and cell death. Cancer cells arising in women with heterozygous

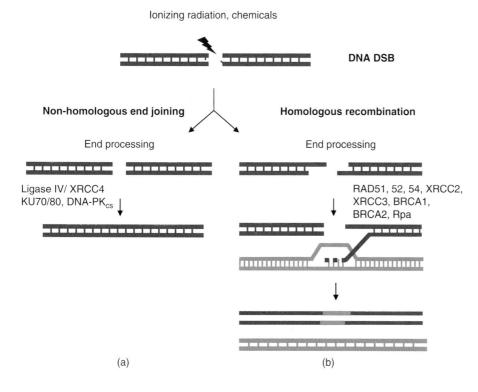

(a)                                   (b)

**Figure 33.1** Repair of double-strand breaks. (a) Double-strand break is rejoined end-to-end. (b) A double-strand break is repaired with the help of a homologous undamaged DNA (shown in orange). Strand invasion allows resynthesis on complementary sequence, followed by a resolution of the strands and rejoining.

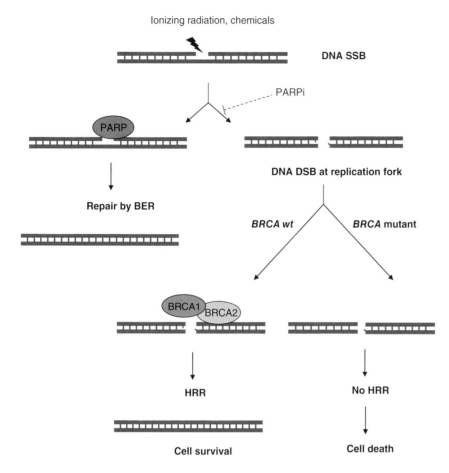

**Figure 33.2** Synthetic lethality. Single-strand DNA breaks can be repaired by BER. PARPi block BER leading to conversion of SSB to DSBs. In *BRCA wt* cells, HR repair DSBs. However, BRCA1/2-mutant cells are deficient in HRR and unable to repair DSBs. Treating cancer cells with mutations in *BRCA1/2* with PARPi causes cell death via synthetic lethality.

germline *BRCA1/2* mutations lose their entire BRCA and HRR function by losing the second wild-type allele, whereas the normal cells with heterozygous BRCA copies retain their HRR function. PARP inhibitors are therefore selectively lethal to cancer cells with homozygous BRCA deficiency, while cells with normal copies of *BRCA1/2* are able to maintain their survival by restoring DSBs through intact HRR (Figure 33.2).[39,40] The exploitation of therapeutic consequences of simultaneous inactivation of two pathways, when inactivation of either one is tolerated in isolation, is also called "synthetic lethality" and has major potential for the treatment of cancer. In theory, the targeting of one of the genes in a synthetic lethal pair, where the other is defective, should be selectively lethal to the cancer cells and minimally toxic to normal cells leading to a significant therapeutic window.[41]

### BRCAness

The concept of synthetic lethality is not restricted to *BRCA*-mutant cells. In fact there is preclinical evidence to show that cells with deficiency in other HRR genes such as *RAD51, XRCC3, ATR, ATM*, and *FANC* genes are also sensitive to PARPi.[39,42,43] Recent research also indicates that mutations in tumor suppressor genes such as *PTEN*, which are not directly involved in HRR, may also cause sensitivity to PARPi through downregulation of RAD51, a key player in HRR.[44,45] It has been shown that a significant proportion of triple negative breast cancer patients with no germline *BRCA1/2* mutations have evidence of HRR deficiency.[46] It has also been reported that as many as 50% of cases of EOC patients, particularly those with the high-grade serous pathological subtype may

have HRR deficiency either from germline or from somatic *BRCA* mutations,[47-49] BRCA methylation,[50-52] epigenetic silencing of fanconi anemia genes[53] or other HRR deficiencies. Taken together, this evidence suggests that a proportion of breast and ovarian cancer patients with wild type copies of *BRCA* genes may in fact have defects in other HRR components that render them HRR deficient. This notion has been described as "*BRCA*ness"[54] and may have great clinical implications. As an example, it has been shown that methylation of *FANCF* promoter region in ovarian cancer cell lines which causes inhibition of FANCF and HRR results in sensitivity to platinum agents while demethylation of this site restores HRR and leads to platinum resistance.[53]

## Clinical Development of PARP Inhibitors

The profound sensitivity of *BRCA*-mutant cells to PARP inhibitors seen in preclinical studies[39,40] led to phase I trials of PARPi which tested the concept of "synthetic lethality." Subsequently, a number of PARP inhibitors have been studied either as a single agent or in combination with chemotherapy or other targeted agents. In this section, we review the clinical development of PARPi in various tumor types with a main focus on PARP inhibition in epithelial ovarian cancer.

## Epithelial Ovarian Cancer

### Olaparib (AZD-2281)

Olaparib is the most extensively studied PARPi and has been studied as a single agent, in combination with other chemotherapeutic agents and also as maintenance therapy.

**Table 33.1** Antitumor efficacy of PARPi in *BRCA*-mutant and sporadic epithelial ovarian cancer in early phase clinical trials.

| Trial | Drug | Pts No. (BRCA) | | Dose of PARPi | Overall | *RECIST and/or CA125 response* Platinum sensitive | Platinum resistant | PFS (months) |
|---|---|---|---|---|---|---|---|---|
| Phase I, Fong et al. 2010[56] | Olaparib | *BRCA* ovary 50 (50) | | 39 pts, 200 mg 11 pts, dose esc | 40% | 61.5% | 41.7% | 6 |
| Phase II, Audeh et al. 2010[57] | Olaparib | *BRCA* ovary 57 (57) | | 33 pts, 400 mg 24 pts, 100 mg | 33% 12.5% | 38% 50% | 30% 0 | 5.8 1.9 |
| Phase II, Kaye et al. 2011[60] | Olaparib vs. PLD | *BRCA* ovary 64 (64) | | 32 pts, 400 mg 32 pts, 200 mg | 59% 38% | Not reported | Not reported | 8.8 6.5 |
| Phase II, Gelmon et al. 2011[58] | Olaparib | Ovary 65 | *BRCA* (17) Sporadic HGSOC | 400 mg | 41% 24% | 60% 50% | 33% 4% | 7.3 |
| Phase I, Sandhu et al. 2013[59] | Niraparib | Ovary 49 | *BRCA* (22) Sporadic HGSOC | Dose escalation (60–400 mg) | 40% 22.7% | 50% 67% | 33% 16% | Not reported |

## Phase I Studies

In a phase I clinical trial which enriched for patients with a *BRCA1* or *BRCA2* mutation, 60 patients with refractory solid tumors enrolled to investigate the safety and tolerability of olaparib.[55] The dose of olaparib increased from 10 mg once a day for 2 weeks in a 3-week cycle and escalated to 600 mg twice daily (BID) continuously. The maximum tolerated dose (MTD) was established at 400 mg BID continuously. The dose-limiting toxicities at this dose were grade 3 mood alteration and fatigue. Grade 4 thrombocytopenia and grade 3 somnolence were noted at 600 mg BID. The investigators demonstrated evidence of over 90% PARP inhibition in patients who received olaparib ≥60 mg BID using peripheral blood mononuclear cells (PBMC), plucked eyebrow-hair follicles and tumor tissue as surrogate samples. PARP inhibition did not significantly increase at doses >100 mg BID.

Patients were not required to have confirmed *BRCA* mutation in this part of the study, however 22 patients had germline *BRCA* mutation and one patient had strong family history of *BRCA*-related cancers but declined genetic testing. 19 *BRCA*-mutant patients with breast, ovarian or prostate cancer were evaluable for response to treatment. Antitumor activity was only observed in patients with *BRCA1/2* mutations. 9/19 patients (47%) derived partial response (RECIST) and 12 patients (63%) showed clinical benefit (either radiological or tumor-marker responses or stable disease for a period of 4 months or more) from olaparib treatment supporting the selective lethality of PARPi in *BRCA*-associated tumors. Notably 8 of 15 advanced ovarian cancer patients showed partial response according to Response Evaluation Criteria in Solid Tumors (RECIST). All of the responses in ovarian cancer were in *BRCA*-mutant patients. This trial showed that olaparib was well tolerated and indicated its activity in *BRCA*-mutant cancers.

A follow up of this trial was reported a year later and investigated the antitumor activity of olaparib in 50 patients (dose-escalation 11 patients; single-stage expansion cohort 39 patients at 200mg BID) with *BRCA*-mutant advanced ovarian cancer.[56] RECIST and CA125 response was observed in 20 patients (40%) and three additional patients had stable disease (SD) of greater than 4 months resulting in a clinical benefit rate of 46%.

In the post hoc analysis, the overall clinical benefit rate decreased significantly with platinum insensitivity (platinum sensitive: 69%, platinum resistant: 46%; platinum refractory 23%) suggesting that

platinum response status may determine response to olaparib (Table 33.1). RECIST and/or GCIG CA125 response rates were 61.5% (8/13) in platinum-sensitive patients, 41.7% (10/24) in platinum-resistant patients, and 15.4% (2/13) in patients with platinum-refractory disease. The association between the platinum-free interval and the response to olaparib was statistically significant (Spearman rank, 0.33; 95% CI, 0.04–0.57; $p = 0.03$). It is noteworthy that although clinical response diminished with shorter platinum-free interval, the antitumor activity of olaparib remained substantial in platinum-resistant and refractory disease.

## Phase II Studies

Phase II clinical trials of olaparib have also shown promising results in the treatment of *BRCA*-mutant epithelial ovarian cancer (Table 33.1). In an international phase II multi-centre single-arm, open-label sequential dosing cohort study (ICEBERG2), 57 heavily pre-treated *BRCA*-mutant (40 *BRCA1* and 17 *BRCA2*) ovarian cancer patients received treatment with olaparib either at 400 mg BID (first cohort, $n = 33$) or 100 mg BID (second cohort, $n = 24$).[57] Allocation to these doses was not randomized and patients in the 100 mg dose cohort had poorer prognostic features compared to patients in the 400 mg group. The objective response rate in the olaparib 400 mg BID cohort was 33% compared to 13% in the 100 mg BID group. Complete response was reported in two patients in the 400 mg cohort and none in the 100 mg group. The investigators reported a clinical benefit rate of 52% in the olaparib 400 mg cohort and 21% in the olaparib 100 mg group. The median progression-free survival was longer in the 400 mg cohort compared to the 100 mg dose (5.8 vs. 1.9 months, respectively). Reported toxicities were mild (grade 1, 2) and were mainly fatigue, nausea, vomiting, and anemia. This trial suggested that olaparib was active even in patients with heavily pretreated disease and that 400 mg BID dose was more active than the 100 mg BID capsule formulation.

Given these promising results, a randomized phase II trial was designed to test the hypothesis that olaparib may be more effective than the current standard of care, pegylated liposomal doxorubicin (PLD), in patients with *BRCA*-mutant advanced ovarian cancer. In this study, 97 women with disease recurrence less than 12 months from their previous platinum-based chemotherapy were randomized to receive olaparib 200 mg BID, olaparib 400 mg BID or PLD

50 mg/m$^2$ every 28 days.[60] The response rates (RECIST/CA125) in the olaparib 200 mg and 400 mg arms were 38% and 59%, respectively. The response rate was significantly higher for olaparib 400 mg BID compared to PLD (59% vs. 39%, odds ratio 2.78, $p = 0.05$) but there were no statistically significant differences in the primary endpoint, PFS (olaparib 200 mg bid 6.5 months; olaparib 400 mg bid 8.8 months; PLD 7.1 months; HR 0.88, $p = 0.66$). The overall response rate for olaparib was, as expected, consistent with previous reports of olaparib response rate in *BRCA*-mutant ovarian cancer.[56,57] However, the PFS in the PLD arm exceeded the predicted efficacy (around 4 months) based on previous studies in unselected patients.[61,62] The lack of clear superiority for olaparib over PLD is supported by recent studies suggesting that patients with BRCA or HR deficiency may have increased sensitivity to anthracycline compared with unselected patients.[63,64] Adams et al. reported a 56.5% response rate to PLD among *BRCA*-mutant ovarian cancer patients, compared to 19.5% response rate in sporadic epithelial ovarian cancer patients,[63] and this improved response was also associated with significantly improved PFS and OS.

The encouraging activity of PARP inhibitors may not be limited to *BRCA*-mutant-associated cancer mutations, and it was postulated that PARP inhibitors may also show meaningful activity in non-*BRCA* germline mutant but HR-deficient cancers ("*BRCA*ness"). Integrated genomic analyses of high-grade serous ovarian cancer (HGSOC) suggest that over 50% of cases of HGSOC may have genomic or epigenomic disruptions that are essential for maintaining HR function.[65] Women with *BRCA1* or *BRCA2* mutations are more likely to develop HGSOC than other histological subtypes. Also 55% of patients with HGSOC were found to have BRCA deficiency as a result of germline or somatic mutations or epigenetic silencing of *BRCA1* or *BRCA2* leading to HR deficiency.[51,65]

Based on these observations a phase II open label nonrandomized trial was designed to investigate the efficacy of olaparib in patients with sporadic HGSOC and triple-negative breast cancer (TNBC). This study stratified 65 patients with advanced HGSOC and/or undifferentiated ovarian carcinoma and 26 patients with TNBC according to *BRCA* status (*BRCA*-mutant vs. *BRCA* wild-type (wt) patients).[58] Patients were enrolled to receive single agent olaparib capsules 400 mg BID continuously. Compatible with previous reports, the objective response was 41% in *BRCA*-mutant ovarian cancer patients. Interestingly 11/47 (24%) germline *BRCA*-negative (*BRCA* wt) patients also achieved radiological response. All responders in the *BRCA* wt cohort had HGSOC confirming the activity of olaparib in women with pre-treated HGSOC without germline *BRCA* mutations. The objective response rate in the *BRCA1/2*-mutant cases was 60% for the platinum-sensitive EOC and 33% for the platinum-resistant group, in line with previous report by Fong et al.[56] In the *BRCA* wt cohort, however, the response to olaparib was significantly higher in the platinum-sensitive group (50%) compared to the platinum-resistant cohort (4%). No difference in progression-free survival (PFS) was observed between the *BRCA*-mutant and *BRCA* wt cohorts. The result of TNBC cohort of this study will be discussed under "Breast cancer" below.

Exploratory analysis of Fong et al. and Gelmon et al. trials suggest that patients with *BRCA1/2* platinum-sensitive ovarian cancer are more likely to respond to subsequent PARP inhibition compared to their platinum-resistant counterparts.[56,58] In contrast to these two trials, response to olaparib 400 mg BID was similar in both platinum-sensitive and platinum-resistant cohorts (38% and 30%, respectively) in the phase II trial by Audeh et al.,[57]

suggesting that the mechanisms of resistance to PARP inhibitors are complex.

## Maintenance Therapy

Considering the favorable toxicity profile of these agents, the long-term use of PARPi for maintaining disease remission has been of particular interest. Recently, a randomized placebo-controlled phase II clinical trial of maintenance therapy with olaparib in women with recurrent platinum-sensitive HGSOC has shown promise in meeting its primary endpoint, PFS.[66] In this 265-patient study, 136 patients were randomized to olaparib 400 mg BID and 129 patients to placebo after having a partial or complete response to their most recent platinum-based chemotherapy. The investigators recruited patients with sporadic disease. Known *BRCA1/2* status was not required for enrollment to the study, however 97 patients (36.6%) had known *BRCA* mutation status. A total of 59 patients (22.3%) had germline *BRCA1/2* mutations and 38 patients (14.3%) were confirmed germline *BRCA* wt. *BRCA* status was not known for the rest of 168 (63.4%) of the cohort. Patients were initially well balanced for *BRCA* mutations between the two arms, 31 patients (22.8%) had *BRCA* mutations in the olaparib arm compared with 28 (21.7%) patients in the placebo arm. PFS by RECIST was significantly longer in the olaparib group than those receiving placebo (median 8.4 vs. 4.8 months; HR, 0.35; 95% CI 0.25–0.49; $p<0.001$). Time to progression by CA125 or RECIST was also significantly longer in the olaparib than the placebo group (median 8.3 vs. 3.7 months; HR, 0.35; 95% CI 0.25–0.47; $p<0.001$). OS was similar between the two arms (29.7 months in the olaparib group and 29.9 months in the placebo group) and statistically not significant (HR, 0.94; 95% CI, 0.63–1.39; $p = 0.75$).

A pre-planned subgroup analysis identified that the improved PFS was even more marked in the *BRCA* mutation carrier subgroup. However, *BRCA* mutation status was only known for 36.6% of patients. Having obtained and stored all the samples prior to randomization, the study investigators then retrospectively analyzed the germline and somatic DNA of all patients for *BRCA* mutations. As a result of this analysis, a total of 136 patients (51.3% of the entire cohort) were found to carry deleterious *BRCA1/2* mutations (96 with germline and 40 with somatic *BRCA* mutations). A total of 118 patients (44.5%) were confirmed *BRCA* wt. The *BRCA* mutation status remained unknown for 11 patients (4.2%).[67] These new data confirmed that the increase in median PFS was most marked in the *BRCA*-mutant patients who had received olaparib 400 mg BID as maintenance treatment compared with the *BRCA*-mutant patients who were on placebo (11.2 vs. 4.3 months, respectively; HR, 0.18; 95% CI, 0.11–0.31; $p<0.00001$). This 6.9-month PFS translates to an 82% reduction in the risk of progression of the disease. The interim OS subgroup data analysis was done at 60% maturity and revealed a trend toward improvement of OS in *BRCA*-mutant compared to *BRCA* wt patients (34.9 vs. 31.9 months, respectively; HR, 0.74; 95% CI, 0.46–1.19; $p = 0.208$). The investigators noted that the improvement in OS may well have been attenuated by cross over from placebo to various PARP inhibitors in 22% of patients at progression.

These studies were performed with the original capsule formulation of olaparib, and at a dose of 400 mg BID, patients were taking 16 capsules per day. A 100-mg tablet formulation has been manufactured, and following bioavailability studies, a dose of 300 mg BID (three tablets twice a day) of the tablet has been chosen to be taken forward for subsequent clinical studies. This will include additional maintenance studies in the first- and second-line settings. Meanwhile consideration is being given to submission of the available data for regulatory approval of olaparib as maintenance therapy in germline *BRCA*-mutant ovarian cancer.

## Other PARPi in Epithelial Ovarian Cancer

### Niraparib (MK4827)

Niraparib is an oral inhibitor of PARP1 and PARP2, and this agent was investigated in a two part multi-institution phase I clinical trial in 100 patients with advanced recurrent solid cancer.[59] In part A, 60 patients with solid cancer were enrolled for the dose escalation; of these, 29 patients were *BRCA1/2* mutations carriers. The MTD of niraparib was established at 300 mg daily, and evidence of PARP inhibition of >50% in PBMC was observed with niraparib >80 mg/day. Significant toxicities comprised of grade 4 thrombocytopenia in 15% of cases and grade 3 pneumonitis in one patient. Other toxicities such as fatigue, anorexia, nausea, and vomiting were mild and manageable. Part B recruited 40 patients with sporadic platinum-resistant HGSOC and sporadic prostate cancer.

In part A, of 49 patients with ovarian and primary peritoneal carcinoma, 22 patients had known germline *BRCA1/2* mutations of which 20 patients were RECIST evaluable. In this subgroup 10 patients were classified as platinum sensitive, 9 patients platinum resistant, and 1 patient as platinum refractory. RECIST or CA125 response was observed in 50% (5 of 10) of platinum-sensitive and 33% (3 of 9) of platinum-resistant *BRCA1/2*-mutant EOC patients (Table 33.1). Median duration of response was reported 431 days for platinum-sensitive and 340 days for platinum-resistant *BRCA1/2*-mutant patients. Additionally the *BRCA1*-mutant patient with platinum-refractory disease had stable disease for 130 days.

Of 22 HGSOC patients eligible for RECIST evaluation in part B, 3 patients had platinum-sensitive and 19 patients had platinum-resistant disease. RECIST/CA125 partial response was seen in 2 of 3 (67%) platinum-sensitive and 3 of 19 patients (16%) platinum-resistant groups. Median duration of time on study was 444 days for the platinum-sensitive and 161 days for the platinum-resistant HGSOC patients. These results are consistent with data from olaparib in platinum-sensitive HGSOC.[58]

Antitumor activity of niraparib is comparable to that of olaparib[55,56,68] and makes it the second PARPi to show activity in *BRCA1/2* tumors.[59] A placebo-controlled randomized clinical trial is currently recruiting patients to investigate maintenance therapy with niraparib in platinum-sensitive EOC (ClinicalTrials.gov identifier: NCT01847274).

### Biomarin BMN-673

BMN-673 is the latest and most potent PARP inhibitor from *in vitro* studies in clinical development. A phase I study of safety and antitumor activity of BMN-673 is currently underway. The investigators studied 39 patients in 9 cohorts which included 23 patients with ovarian or primary peritoneal carcinoma of which 17 women were germline *BRCA1/2* mutation carriers. Preliminary results reported that the DLT was grade 4 thrombocytopenia and MTD was defined at 1000 µg a day. Inhibition of PARP activity in PBMC was observed at a much lower dose, ≥100 µg a day. RECIST and/or CA125 response was reported at dose ≥100 µg a day in 11 of 17 *BRCA1/2*-mutant ovarian and primary peritoneal cancer patients[69] (ClinicalTrials.gov identifier: NCT01286987).

## Breast Cancer

Antitumor activity has been demonstrated for olaparib in *BRCA1/2*-mutant breast cancer patients, although efficacy has been less consistent than in *BRCA*-mutant EOC. In the phase I clinical trial by Fong et al.,[55] a signal of olaparib activity was seen in a *BRCA2*-mutant advanced breast cancer. One patient with *BRCA2* breast cancer had a RECIST complete remission of greater than 60 weeks with resolution of lung and lymph node metastasis. There was also evidence of disease stability in two more patients.

An international phase II proof of concept trial investigated the role of olaparib in recurrent *BRCA1/2*-mutant breast cancer.[68] In this trial, 54 patients with advanced recurrent breast cancer with confirmed deleterious *BRCA1/2* mutations were enrolled into two sequential cohorts to receive olaparib 400 mg BID (cohort 1, n = 27) or olaparib 100 mg BID (cohort 2, n = 27). Confirmed objective response rate was 41% for cohort 1 and 22% for cohort 2. Improvement in PFS (5.7 months for 400 mg BID vs. 3.8 months for 100 mg BID) and clinical benefit rate (52% for 400 mg BID and 26% for 100 mg BID) were observed with the higher olaparib dose. These findings were similar to the companion study in *BRCA*-mutant ovarian cancer which showed reduced antitumor efficacy with the 100 mg BID dose.[57]

Some patients from the 100-mg arm had dose escalation to the 400-mg arm after the interim analysis which reported a difference of 2.5 months in time to treatment withdrawal in favor of the 400-mg arm. Exploratory analysis showed objective response in both *BRCA1/2* carriers, hormone receptor positive and TNBC patients. Also patients with heavily pretreated breast cancer and those who had been treated with platinum agents demonstrated responses to olaparib.

A further phase II study also addressed olaparib in breast cancer. In this study,[58] 26 patients with advanced metastatic or recurrent triple negative or *BRCA*-mutant breast cancer and 65 women with recurrent HGSOC were enrolled. Breast cancer patients were assigned into two groups. Group A consisted of patients with *BRCA wt* TNBC (n = 15), while group B included patients with confirmed germline *BRCA1/2* mutations (n = 11). Two patients in the *BRCA*-mutant group were reclassified as *BRCA wt* after repeated genetic analysis. All patients received olaparib 400 mg BID continuously until disease progression. No RECIST response was observed in breast cancer patients in either cohort. Disease stabilization at 8 weeks was reported in 38% of *BRCA1* carriers, 70% of *BRCA2* carriers, and 19% of *BRCA wt* patients. PFS was 109 days in patients with *BRCA* mutations and 54 days in *BRCA wt* group. The reasons for the reduced efficacy in this trial are not clear, but may relate to the number of lines of prior chemotherapy for breast cancer.

There are currently several trials investigating olaparib mainly in combination with chemotherapy in variety of tumors including breast cancer.

A phase I clinical trial with a potent PARPi, BMN 673, is currently underway. The interim reports from Biomarin indicate RECIST response in 9 of 18 (50%) patients with germline *BRCA1/2*-mutant breast cancer as of July 24, 2013.[70] A phase III clinical trial is being planned to investigate BMN-673 in *BRCA1/2*-mutant breast cancer patients and is expected to start late 2013.

## Prostate Cancer

Emerging data indicates that as well as DNA damage modulation, PARP is also involved in transcription regulation of the androgen receptor (AR) and suppresses AR target-gene expression and tumor proliferation. PARP may also modulate rearranged erythroblast transformation-specific genes, such as *ERG,* and its inhibition has shown activity in preclinical models of *TMPRSS2-ERG* rearranged prostate cancer.[71–73] Early phase clinical trials have confirmed PARPi activities in *BRCA*-deficient castration-resistant prostate cancer (CRPC). In the phase I clinical trial by Fong et al.,[55] a patient with *BRCA2*-associated CRPC who was treated with olaparib demonstrated resolution of his bone metastasis and a reduction of more than 50% in his PSA level and remained on the trial drug for more than 2 years.

In the phase I clinical trial of niraparib as described above[59] (see epithelial ovarian cancer section), of 21 patients with CRPC, 9 patients (43%) showed stable disease for a median duration of 254 days. Although no radiological responses were recorded, a reduction of 30% in the number of circulating tumor cells was observed in several of CRPC patients. Also one patient had reduction of PSA by more than 50%. This study provides preliminary evidence of PARPi activity in CRPC.

## Pancreatic Cancer

About 5–8% of cases of pancreatic cancer have germline mutations in *BRCA1/2* genes. A mutation frequency of up to 17% has been reported in Ashkenazi Jewish families with a history of pancreatic cancer.[74] The lifetime risk of developing pancreatic cancer in *BRCA2* carrier patients is estimated to be 3.5- to 10-fold higher than the general population.

In a single institution study, Lowery et al. identified 15 cases of *BRCA1/2*-associated metastatic pancreatic cancers.[75] Four patients in this cohort were treated with single agent PARPi or combination of PARPi and chemotherapy. Three patients were reported to have RECIST partial response, and one patient had stable disease for six months. Median survival of this cohort was reported as 27.6 months.

The result of a large phase II study in 298 patients with advanced solid cancer with *BRCA1/2* mutations who were treated with single agent olaparib 400 mg BID until disease progression was recently reported.[76] Twenty-three patients in this cohort had pancreatic cancer and had progressed on gemcitabine-based chemotherapy. An objective CR/PR was observed in 21.7% of pancreatic cancer patients. PFS of more than 6 months was observed in 36% of patients. OS at 12 months was 41%. These data indicate that PARP inhibition can be effective in other HR-deficient tumors and highlights the importance of a personalized approach to therapy in pancreatic cancer.

## PARPi Therapy in Other Cancers

Emerging preclinical evidence suggests that PARPi may have activity in cancers other than those usually associated with mutations in *BRCA1/2* genes such as small cell lung cancer (SCLC), gastric cancer, and some sarcomas. Recently, it was shown that PARP1 was highly expressed at the mRNA and protein levels in SCLC.[77] Also a recent observation indicates that ERCC1-deficient cells treated with PARPi show significant delays in repairing DSBs associated with profound and prolonged $G_2/M$ arrest suggesting a possible role for PARPi in the treatment of ERCC1-deficient nonsmall cell lung cancer (NSCLC).[78] Recently the interim results of a phase I clinical trial of the PARPi, BMN 673, reported partial responses in 2 of 11 patients with previously treated SCLC.[79] It has also been shown that Ewing's sarcomas frequently harbor genomic fusions such as EWS-FLI1 or EWS-ERG. Some reports indicate that these

genomic fusions interact with PARP1 and that xenograft models are highly sensitive to PARP inhibition.[80] Clinical evaluation of PARPi in SCLC and Ewing's sarcoma is ongoing.

There are also data from early phase clinical trials suggesting activity of PARPi in gastric cancer. A preclinical study has recently suggested that low levels of ATM expression detected on immunohistochemistry may be associated with response to olaparib.[81] Recently, result of a phase II clinical trial of olaparib plus paclitaxel versus paclitaxel alone as a second-line therapy in patients with recurrent or metastatic gastric cancer was presented at ASCO 2013 (Bang et al., *J Clin Oncol.* 2013;31 suppl; abstract 4013). In this trial, patients were enriched (50% of patients) for low levels of ATM expression detected by IHC (ATM-) and were well balanced between the two arms of the study. A total of 123 patients were randomized to receive olaparib tablet formulation 100 mg BID plus paclitaxel 80 mg/m$^2$ IV on days 1, 8, 15 in a 28-day cycle or placebo plus paclitaxel until progression or investigators' decision. Following combination therapy, patients were treated with maintenance olaparib 200 mg BID or placebo until disease progression. The primary endpoint was PFS and the secondary endpoint was OS. Patients on combination therapy experienced more myelosuppression, treatment delays, and dose reductions. PFS was similar between the olaparib and paclitaxel combination and paclitaxel alone arms (3.9 vs. 3.6 months, respectively, HR = 0.80; 95% CI 0.54, 1.18, $p = 0.261$). However, study investigators reported an intriguing 4.8 months improvement in OS in favor of the olaparib and paclitaxel combination compared to the paclitaxel alone arm (13.1 vs. 8.3 months, respectively, HR = 0.56; 95% CI 0.35, 0.87, $p = 0.010$). The improvement in OS was observed in both the whole cohort and the ATM low subgroup, although the benefit was larger in the ATM low cohort.

There is also a case report of PARPi activity in a patient with metastatic endometrioid endometrial carcinoma, selected by one for treatment with olaparib in an early phase trial, on the basis of prior repeated platinum sensitivity and strong family history of cancer, hypothesized as indicative of deficient DNA repair.[82] The patient had several visceral metastatic diseases including multiple brain metastases which were found during the first 2 weeks of treatment. The patient was continued on olaparib monotherapy 400 mg BID and imaging assessments at 10 weeks showed a significant reduction in the size of her cerebral lesions and RECIST stable disease. This patient had no germline *BRCA1/2* mutations and was reported to have PTEN loss. The clinical observation of response to olaparib in this patient is supported by preclinical data showing that PTEN is involved in maintaining genomic integrity and that cell lines with PTEN loss are unable to repair DNA DSBs induced by ionizing radiation and are sensitive to PARP inhibition.[45,83,84] The response of this patient's brain metastases to olaparib in the absence of any other treatment and also clinical benefit in other metastatic sites suggest that the PARPi may have a role in endometrial cancers which clearly needs further investigations.

## Other PARP Inhibitors in Development

### Veliparib (ABT-888)

Pharmacodynamic data from a phase 0 trial of veliparib has shown more than 48% PARP inhibition in tumor biopsies 24 hours after a single 50 mg dose of veliparib.[85] An open-label, single-arm phase I clinical trial studied the combination of veliparib with metronomic oral cyclophosphamide in patients with advanced solid tumors and lymphoma.[86] This study enrolled 35 patients who had undergone at least four previous lines of anticancer treatment. In total, eight different dose levels with combination therapy were studied. The MTD of the combination was established at veliparib 60 mg with cyclophosphamide 50 mg both once daily in 21-day cycles. In total, 7 of 35 patients in this trial showed PR and another six patients had disease stabilization for six or more cycles including one patient with low-grade lymphoma who had a stable disease for 42 cycles. Of 35 patients in this trial, 13 patients had confirmed germline *BRCA* mutations and the remaining 22 patients had unknown *BRCA* status. In the *BRCA*-mutant cohort, six patients showed PR by RECIST including a *BRCA2*-mutant ovarian cancer patient who showed complete disappearance of her target lesions and reduced, albeit elevated CA125 levels. Further, 3 *BRCA*-mutant patients had prolonged stable disease. Interpolation of the data is difficult because a conventional phase I study has not been performed and the single agent efficacy of ABT-888 has yet not been established. However, based on this phase I trial, a multicenter, randomized phase II study is currently underway investigating metronomic cyclophosphamide alone or in combination with veliparib in patients with *BRCA*-mutant advanced ovarian cancer, HGSOC, TNBC, and low-grade lymphomas (clinicaltrials.gov identifier: NCT01306032).

During the ASCO 2013 annual meeting, design of a phase II clinical trial of cisplatin and gemcitabine with or without veliparib in *BRCA*- or *PALB2*-mutant stage III/IV pancreatic cancer was presented. This study is the first to include a veliparib monotherapy arm. The primary endpoint is RECIST response rate (Abstract TPS4144). The results of phase I trial with a combination of veliparib and carboplatin in 44 patients with triple negative or HER2 negative/hormone receptor positive metastatic breast cancer (with *BRCA*-mutant or fanconi pathway defect) were recently presented. The recommended phase 2 dose of the combination was carboplatin AUC 5 on day 1 and veliparib 250 mg BID on days 1–21 of a 21-day cycle. Thrombocytopenia was a significant toxicity. The investigators reported 18.6% partial response rate in 43 evaluable patients and 25% partial response rate in 16 patients with defective BRCA or fanconi pathway.[87] Other trials are currently investigating veliparib in combination with various chemotherapeutic or targeted agents in advanced ovarian cancer.

### Rucaparib (AG014699, PF0136738)

Rucaparib is another PARP inhibitor with a similar preclinical profile to olaparib. As with veliparib, the initial clinical studies focused on a combination approach. A phase I clinical trial studied the combination of intravenous AG014699 and temozolomide 5 days of 28 days cycles.[88] In the dose escalation part of this study, 17 patients were enrolled. Initially escalating dose of AG014699 was given with temozolomide 100 mg/m². Intravenous AG014699 at 12 mg/m² was reported to inhibit 74–97% of PARP in PBMC. Partial response was observed in patients with melanoma and GIST. In part 2 of this study, dose of AG014699 was kept at 12 mg/m², and temozolomide was escalated to the maximum dose of 200 mg/m². Four patients with melanoma and three patients with prostate cancer, pancreatic cancer, and leiomyosarcoma showed stable disease lasting more than 6 months.

Based on this study a phase II clinical trial evaluated efficacy of intravenous rucaparib 12 mg/m² in combination with oral temozolomide 200 mg/m² on days 1–5 of 28-day cycles in 46 chemotherapy-naïve patients with advanced metastatic melanoma.[89] Confirmed PR was observed in eight patients (17.4%). Additionally eight patients (17.4%) showed disease stability of more than 24 weeks. Median PFS for all patients was 3.5 months and 36%

of patients had PFS of greater than 6 months. Median OS was 9.9 months and 1-year survival rate was 40%. This combination was associated with high rate of bone marrow toxicities. The toxicity profile of this combination has been described under "PARPi combination therapy" section.

As the potential value of PARP inhibition as single agents became clear, a new oral formulation of rucaparib was clearly desirable, and current studies have focused on this. A phase I dose escalation trial of oral rucaparib has identified dose of 600 mg BID as the recommended dose for phase II and III trials. The investigators reported that approximately 50% of patients developed grade 2 and grade 3 myelosuppression including grade 3 anemia (29%), neutropenia (29%), and thrombocytopenia (14%).[90] An encouraging overall disease control rate (CR+PR+SD>24 weeks) of 70% was reported in germline *BRCA*-mutated ovarian cancer patients treated with dose levels above 300 mg daily. Also an interim data for a phase I clinical trial of combination of rucaparib and carboplatin was recently presented.[91] A total of 23 patients were treated with various dose levels of carboplatin AUC 3, 4, and 5 and rucaparib 80, 120, 180, 240, and 360 mg in this dose escalation trial. Despite expected bone marrow suppression, the combination of carboplatin and rucaparib was reported to be well tolerated and active with disease control rate of 50% in ovarian cancer patients across all dose levels.

### Iniparib

Iniparib (4-iodo-3-nitrobenzamide) was initially considered to be a PARPi but subsequent investigations indicated that this was not its primary mode of action. It is a banzamide which is structurally related to nicotinamide and was designated as a PARPi based on this structural similarity.

A phase II trial of iniparib was conducted in patients with metastatic triple-negative breast cancer and showed improvement in median PFS from 3.6 to 5.9 months (HR, 0.59; $p = 0.01$), the OS from 7.7 to 12.3 months (HR, 0.57; $p = 0.01$), and overall response rate (52% vs. 32%, $p = 0.02$).[92] This result was not replicated in a phase III trial and is currently not being pursued for further clinical development.

## Toxicity Profile of PARPi Monotherapy

Single agent therapy with PARPi is usually well tolerated. Hematological toxicities such as anemia and neutropenia have been frequently observed and are mainly grade 1 and 2. Grade 3–4 anemia and neutropenia have been reported between 2% and 10% of cases in different trials.[55–57,59,68] Thrombocytopenia seems to be more frequently seen with niraparib (15% of patients developed grade 3 thrombocytopenia on niraparib).[59] Bone marrow toxicities associated with PARPi seem to be dose related and cumulative.

Nonhematological adverse events have also been reported with various PARP inhibitors in different trials and mainly nausea, fatigue, anorexia, diarrhea or constipation, vomiting, and insomnia. Mood alterations and somnolence have also been reported in a phase I trial of olaparib. A grade 3 pneumonitis has recently been reported in one patient on niraparib. These adverse events are generally mild to moderate and self-limiting or manageable with conservative standard treatments.

## PARPi as Combination Therapy

- **PARPi and cytotoxic drugs.** Preclinical data provide the rationale for combining PARPi and cytotoxic chemotherapy in order to enhance sensitivity of cancer cells to chemotherapy by disrupting their DNA repair machinery.[93–96]

Currently results of only a few combination trials are available and they indicate higher rates of toxicities for the combination therapy compared to PARPi monotherapy. In a phase I clinical trial of AG014699 (rucaparib) and temozolomide, intravenous dose of rucaparib 18 mg/m² resulted in DLT with myelosuppression but the dose of 12 mg/m² was tolerated with no grade 3–4 toxicities.[88] In the phase II of this trial, however, combination of rucaparib 12 mg/m² and temozolomide 200 mg/m² resulted in myelosuppression in 54% of patients necessitating a 25% dose reduction in temozolomide. Grade 3–4 hematologic toxicities included anemia (4%), lymphopenia (30%), thrombocytopenia (57%), and neutropenia (61%). Additionally 54% of patients needed temozolomide dose reduction due to profound or prolong myelosuppression. Two patients died on this study, one due to neutropenic sepsis while pancytopenic and the other due to hepato-renal failure which was felt to be drug related.[89]

Concerns about myelosuppression have also been raised in a phase I clinical trial of olaparib in combination with cisplatin and gemcitabine. The original dose level consisted of olaparib 100 mg BID on days 1–4, Cisplatin 60 mg/m² on day 3, and gemcitabine 500 mg/m² on day 3 and 10 on a 21-day cycle. The dose level had to be amended twice due to persistent thrombocytopenia and neutropenia. The MDT was determined for olaparib at 100 mg BID on day 1 only, cisplatin 60 mg/m² on day 1, and gemcitabine 500 mg/m² on days 1 and 8 on a 21-day cycle. Grade 3–4 neutropenia, lymphopenia, and thrombocytopenia were observed in 61%, 61%, and 57% of patients, respectively. Grade 3–4 anemia and leucopenia were observed in 35% and 30% of patients, respectively. The authors concluded that the combination of olaparib and cisplatin and gemcitabine, even at low dose, is associated with myelosuppression.[97] As well as two patients with pancreatic cancer and one patient with nonsmall cell lung cancer who had RECIST partial response, 13 patients were reported to have stable disease including an ovarian cancer patient with a BRCA1 mutation of unknown significance.

A placebo-controlled randomized phase II trial investigated the efficacy of carboplatin and paclitaxel with or without concurrent and sequential olaparib in 162 women with platinum-sensitive recurrent epithelial ovarian cancer.[98] Patients were stratified by number of prior platinum-based chemotherapy and the platinum-free interval and received six cycles of olaparib 200 mg BID on days 1–10 of a 21-day cycle concurrently with carboplatin (AUC4 IV, day1) and paclitaxel (175 mg/m² IV, day 1) followed by maintenance olaparib monotherapy 400 mg BID (Arm A), or six cycles of carboplatin (AUC6 IV, day1) and paclitaxel (175 mg/m² IV, day 1) with no further therapy (Arm B), until progression. The primary endpoint was PFS by RECIST. A total of 156 patients received treatment (Arm A, $n = 81$; Arm B, $n = 75$) followed by the maintenance or no further therapy in 121 patients (Arm A, $n = 66$; Arm B, $n = 55$). More adverse events such as alopecia, fatigue, and nauseas were observed in Arm A during the combination phase. Also more treatment discontinuation was seen with olaparib arm during the maintenance phase. Preliminary results reported that the overall response rate was similar for Arm A and Arm B (64% vs. 58%). However, the investigators reported an improvement in the median PFS from 9.6 to 12.2 months in favor of maintenance olaparib (median PFS: 12.2 vs. 9.6 months; HR: 0.51, 95% CI 0.34, 0.77; $p$: 0.0012).

Several trials are currently investigating combination of various PARPi and chemotherapeutic agents. Although the results of these trials are yet to be published, synergistic toxicities between PARPi and chemotherapy, in particular myeleosuppression is a common feature, leading to dose reductions and may hinder further development of combination therapies, particularly with alkylating agents.

- **PARPi and PI3K inhibitors**. Phosphoinositide 3-kinase (PI3K) pathway is dysregulated in many cancers as a result of loss of negative regulation by PTEN, mutations in *PIK3CA* gene, or overexpression of EGFR.[99,100] It has been shown that PI3K maintains the steady states of HR and is required for the repair of DSBs.[101] Preclinical studies have investigated the effect of PI3K inhibition on HR pathway and the possibility of combining PI3Ki and PARPi. In a study by Ibrahim et al.,[102] the investigators showed that PI3K inhibition in a BRCA proficient, PTEN null TNBC cell line leads to increased levels of γH2AX, a marker of DNA damage. Additionally they demonstrated that Pan PI3K inhibition with BKM120 results in decreased BRCA1/2 expression, increased PAR formation, and sensitization to PARP inhibition. Furthermore dual PI3K and PARP inhibition with BKM120 and olaparib resulted in reduced tumor growth in two of three patient-derived TNBC xenografts. ERK activation of transcription factor, ETS1, has been proposed as a likely mechanism for reduced BRCA expression.[102]

In another study, a mouse model of BRCA1-deficient breast cancer was utilized. After treatment with PI3K inhibitor BKM120, a median reduction of 46.7% in FDG uptake on the PET scan[103] was reported. Reduction in phosphorylated AKT and the tumor vascularity was observed after BKM120 treatment. Consistent with observation by Ibrahim et al., treatment of mice with *BRCA1*-deleted breast tumors with BKM120 resulted in an increase in phosphorylated H2AX, a marker of DSBs. Combination therapy with olaparib and BKM120 resulted in a synergistic activity, while treatment with olaparib or BKM120 alone showed inferior antitumor efficacy. PI3K inhibition results in impairment of an effective HR repair. With PI3K inhibition, HR deficiency appears to become more prominent in BRCA-deficient tumors that already have a level of background HR deficiency. These cells are more dependent on PARP-mediated repair, and inhibition of PARP in these cells may lead to cell death.

No overt toxicity was observed in the mice treated with the combination of olaparib and BKM120 indicating that this combination, unlike combinations of PARPi and cytotoxic agents, may be tolerated sufficiently to allow adequate dose delivery. The result of a phase I clinical trial of BKM120 and olaparib for TNBC or HGSOC was presented at ASCO 2014.[104] Of 46 patients who received the treatment, 34 patients had HGSOC (24 patients BRCA mutated) and 12 patients had TNBC (11 patients BRCA mutated). The doses in the ongoing expansion phase are BKM120, 50 mg once daily and olaparib tablet 300 mg twice daily. DLTs included grade 3 hyperglycemia and transaminitis. Also one patient developed grade 3 depression. Most observed toxicities were grades 1 and 2 and included nausea, fatigue, depression, hyperglycemia, diarrhea, and anemia. The investigators reported complete response in one TNBC patient (10%) and partial response in two patients (20%) with TNBC and seven (22%) patients with HGSOC. Also 2 (20%) TNBC patients and 15 (47%) HGSOC patients had stable disease with treatment.

- **PARP and anti-vascular therapy**. In ovarian cancer, antivascular therapy has proved to be an effective strategy. Recent preclinical data suggest interaction between the antiangiogenic agents and PARPi. Tentori et al. demonstrated reduction of blood vessel formation in response to angiogenic stimuli in PARP1 knockout mice or in endothelial cells treated with a PARPi, GPI 15427.[105] Also PARP inhibition has been shown to reduce angiogenesis in both *in vitro* and *ex vivo* models.[106]

A recent phase I clinical trial has investigated the combination of olaparib and bevacizumab in patients with advanced solid malignancies.[107] This study enrolled 12 patients to the combination of olaparib (100, 200, and 400 BID capsule) and bevacizumab 10 mg/kg every 2 weeks. The investigators concluded that the combination of olaparib 400 mg BID and bevacizumab 10 mg/kg every 2 weeks was well tolerated with no dose-limiting toxicities. One patient developed bowel perforation due to bevacizumab.

Also recently the result of a phase I/II study of combination of olaparib and the vascular growth factor receptor tyrosine kinase inhibitor cediranib was published.[108] In this study 28 patients with recurrent epithelial ovarian, fallopian tube or primary peritoneal cancer ($n = 20$) or metastatic TNBC ($n = 8$) were enrolled. *BRCA1/2* mutations were noted in both the ovarian cancer and TNBC cohort (60% and 38%, respectively). In the dose escalation the MTD of the combination was determined at cediranib 30 mg daily and olaparib 200 mg BID. Grade 3 or 4 adverse events were reported in 21% of patients and included hypertension in 25%, diarrhea in 18%, and neutropenia in 11% of patients consistent with toxicities expected of antiangiogenesis and PARPi with no evidence of enhanced toxicity for the combination. In the evaluable ovarian cancer cohort ($n = 18$), the overall response rate and clinical benefit rates were 41% and 61%, respectively, with a median PFS of 8.7 months. This is comparable with the response to single agent olaparib. The interim results of a randomized phase 2 trial comparing efficacy of the combination of olaparib and cediranib versus olaparib alone in recurrent platinum-sensitive ovarian cancer were presented at ASCO 2014.[109] Ninety patients with recurrent platinum-sensitive ovarian cancer were randomized to either receive olaparib 400 mg capsules BID or combination of olaparib (200 mg capsules BID) and cedirinib (30 mg daily). The study comprised of a mixture of *BRCA* mutant ($n = 47$) and *BRCA* wt/unknown ($n = 43$) patients. Patients were stratified by their *BRCA* status and prior antiangiogenic treatment. No prior antiangiogeneic treatment in recurrent setting or prior PARPi was allowed. There was a significant improvement in the median PFS with the combination arm compared to the single agent olaparib arm (17.7 months vs. 9.0 months, respectively; HR 0.42; 95% CI 0.23—0.76; $p = 0.005$). Overall response rates were 47.8% in the olaparib arm and 79.6% for the combination arm ($p = 0.002$). In a post hoc analysis, the investigators also investigated the activity of olaparib and cediranib combination in the patients with *BRCA* mutation or *wt*/unknown *BRCA* status. There was a trend toward improved PFS with the combination therapy compared to single agent olaparib in *BRCA*-mutated patients (PFS 19.4 months vs. 16.5 months, respectively; HR 0.55; 95% CI 0.24—1.25; $p = 0.16$). However, the intriguing feature was the striking 10.8 months improvement in PFS with the combination of olaparib and cediranib in *BRCA* wt/unknown patients (median PFS of 16.5 months vs. 5.7 months for combination arm vs. single agent olaparib arm, respectively; HR 0.32; 95% CI 0.14—0.74; $p = 0.008$). These findings indicate that the major benefit in *BRCA* wt/unknown patient is derived from cediranib, while in *BRCA*-mutant patient olaparib is probably the major driver of clinical benefit. Increased grade 3 and grade 4 toxicities associ-

ated with the combination arm compared with olaparib only arm (70% vs. 7%, respectively) including fatigue, diarrhea, and hypertension were seen. Further investigation is needed to investigate if the addition of antivascular therapy might add to the benefit of PARP inhibition particularly in the context of maintenance therapy, where both strategies have yielded positive results in randomized trials.

## Predictive Biomarkers of Response to PARPi

Data from proof of concept trials have confirmed the preclinical evidence that patients with germline deleterious *BRCA1/2* mutations respond to PARP inhibition. In other words germline *BRCA1/2* mutations are predictive markers of response to PARPi. Response to PARPi, however, has been observed in patients with no germline *BRCA* mutations. The identification of markers to predict response to PARPi in *BRCA wt* patients has great clinical implications for instance in patients stratification in prospective clinical trials of PARP inhibitors. However, given the complexity of DNA repair machinery and the number of proteins involved in various DNA repair pathways and their interaction, identification of such biomarkers in patients with wt *BRCA* who have features of *BRCA*ness remains a major challenges in PARPi therapy.[110] There is an ongoing effort for identification of such biomarkers to predict response to PARPi. Examples of different strategies to identify such predictive biomarkers are summarized below.

**1) Functional classifiers of HR deficiency.** Cells with reduced HR capacity show sensitivity to PARPi. Therefore, HR deficiency, in broader terms, may be used as a predictive marker of response to PARPi. Pharmacodynamic assays such as phosphorylated H2AX ($\gamma$H2AX) foci, a marker of DSBs, and Rad51 foci, a marker of proficient HR pathway, have been used in laboratory to quantify the DSBs and also to measure the ability of the cells to repair such DNA damage by HR.[111,112] Rad51 foci consist of DNA repair proteins and its low cellular levels following DNA damage indicates reduced or absent HR proficiency. Preclinical studies have shown that cells with deficiency in HR, including those with *XRCC3* and *BRCA1* mutations or epigenetically silenced *BRCA1*, have significant reduction in RAD51 foci and are sensitive to the PARPi, AG014699.[111–113]

In a preclinical study in cell lines grown from ascitic fluid of women with EOC, Rad51 foci formation has been used as a classifier of HR status and has been shown to correlate with *in vivo* response to PARPi AG014699.[111] Investigators of this study applied this HR classifier to 50 chemotherapy-naïve patients and correlated this with *in vitro* sensitivity to AG014699. Patients were then followed up for the median of 14 months after their primary debulking surgery and adjuvant platinum-based chemotherapy. Response to platinum-based chemotherapy, PFS, and OS in relation to the HR classifier was assessed. Patients who had HR deficiency were found to have more platinum sensitivity compared to the HR-proficient cohort (53.8% vs. 16.7%; $p < 0.063$). The median platinum-free interval was also longer for the HR-deficient patients compared to the HR-proficient group (6 vs. 4 months). HR proficiency was associated with platinum resistance as expected. Sensitivity to PARPi, AG014699 was seen in 98% of HR-deficient and none of the HR-proficient ascitic cell cultures ($p < 0.001$). Patients with HR proficiency characteristics had more progressive disease or relapses at 6 months compared to their HR-deficient counterparts (33.3% vs. 7.7%, respectively, $p < 0.024$). Women with HR-deficient tumors had longer median PFS and OS. The authors concluded that this classifier was able to identify a HR-deficient group. Women with functional characteristics of HR deficiency were more likely to have serous carcinoma, show more platinum sensitivity, and had improved survival.[114]

In a similar study, nuclear foci of RAD51 were quantified in pre- and post-chemotherapy biopsies to predict the response to neoadjuvant chemotherapy in breast cancer. HR deficiency, measured by low RAD51 foci formation score, was identified as one of the possible predictors of response to anthracycline-based chemotherapy.[46]

Prospective clinical studies may be needed to clarify if reduced nuclear RAD51 foci can be used as a predictor of sensitivity to PARP inhibitors. The problem with this form of functional assay is that it is time consuming and difficult to use in routine clinical laboratory settings. It also requires invasive procedures to obtain tissue following treatment with the DNA damaging agents for assessing the HR status of patients.

**2) Gene expression profiling.** Gene expression profiling has also been studied in order to identify markers of PARPi sensitivity. As an example Konstantinopoulos et al.[115] used microarray data to develop a 60 gene signature of *BRCA*ness. They validated this signature in set of *BRCA*-mutant and sporadic ovarian cancer patients and demonstrated that disease-free and overall survival rates were significantly improved in patients with the *BRCA*ness gene signature. Additionally the *BRCA*ness profile was able to predict sensitivity to PARPi in Capan-1 clones.[115] Potential limitation to using the gene expression profiling in clinic is the lack of reproducibility of such gene signatures. Complex methodology and the lack of clear standardization of the techniques and their validation are also other current obstacles in the way of their routine use in clinic at present.

**3) Immunohistochemistry assays.** More recently detection of BRCA1 on immunohistochemistry (IHC) was reported to be a simple method of identifying BRCA dysfunction. In this study, investigators identified 43 patients with *BRCA1/2*-mutant HGSOC from the cancer genome atlas project. They noted that abnormal BRCA1 staining (BRCA1 loss or equivocal) had 100% correlation with *BRCA* germline mutations. The authors then applied this IHC profiling to two validation sets including 70 additional patients, and concluded that abnormal IHC staining was able to predict germline *BRCA1* mutations in 100% of cases and that the BRCA1 IHC staining could be used to stratify patients for germline genetic testing and to detect other mechanisms of BRCA1 dysfunction in high-grade serous ovarian carcinomas.[116] A potential problem with this approach is the lack of consistency and reproducibility due to the subjectivity of the technique and difficulty in interpreting the IHC staining. Also it is not clear if IHC techniques are able to predict gemline *BRCA2* mutations in patients.

## Resistance to PARPi

Although patients with germline BRCA mutations are exquisitely sensitive to PARPi, not all carriers of *BRCA1* or *BRCA2* mutations show response to PARPi[57] and responders eventually acquire resistance after a period of initial response. Since the development of PARP inhibitors is at an early stage, the mechanisms of resistance to PARPi are not completely understood. Those proposed so far can be broadly categorized into those increasing cellular HR capacity or those reducing the effect of PARPi on its target.

- **Increased HR capacity.** Cellular events that can restore HR deficiency may be important in resistance to PARPi. For example, reversal of *BRCA* mutations such as intragenic deletion of *BRCA2* c.6174delT mutation results in restoration of the open reading frame and has been shown to associate with PARPi resistance.[117] In this case, "gain of function" mutation results in lack

of one of the synthetically lethal components and subsequently increases the HR capacity. This has been shown in two cases, one of which is high-grade serous ovarian carcinoma, and indicates that this mechanism may be clinically relevant.[118] However, revertant *BRCA* mutations were not seen in tumor samples from six cases in a further series of *BRCA*-mutated ovarian cancer patients who developed olaprib resistance,[119] suggesting that PARPi resistance is likely to be multifactorial. There is also evidence that tumors carrying certain hypomorphic *BRCA* mutations such as *BRCA1* (C61G) mutation show poor response to PARPi and may confer resistance to treatment.[120]

An alternative mechanism of resistance involves the nuclear protein 53BP1. The 53BP1 and BRCA1 collectively control the balance of DNA repair between the NHEJ or HR pathways. It has been shown that suppression of 53BP1 in *BRCA*-mutant cells with HR deficiency promotes resistance to PARPi through ATM-dependent HR repair.[121,122] Loss of 53BP1 has been demonstrated to cause PARPi resistance in *BRCA1*-mutated mouse mammary tumors.[123]

Also downregulation of microRNA miR-182 can cause resistance to PARPi through its negative regulation of BRCA1 expression.[124] PARP1 regulates BRCA2 function in a negative regulatory manner. Therefore suppression of PARP1 by PARPi may result in overexpression of BRCA2 which could in turn lead to increasing HR capacity and resistance to PARPi.[125]

- **Decreased availability of PARPi or reduced level of its target.** In the context of anticancer therapy PARP1 is the primary target of PARPi and is needed for its effect. Therefore reduced levels of PARP1 or its activity can cause resistance to PARPi. There are reports that cells with normal levels of PARP1, but reduced catalytic activity of PARP1 enzyme (low levels of endogenous PARylation), are resistant to PARPi.[126]

The multidrug resistance protein p-glycoproteins (P-gp) is involved in efflux of PARPi. It has been reported that inhibition of P-gp protein by tariquidar reverses the resistance and re-sensitizes cells to PARPi.[127]

Finally, it has been shown that 6-Thioguanine (6TG) efficiently kills BRCA1-defective tumors that have developed resistance to PARPi due to overexpression of P-gp.[128] The investigators showed that 6TG is lethal to cells which have developed resistance to PARP inhibitors or cisplatin through genetic reversion of the *BRCA2* gene. They suggested that "6TG may be effective in the treatment of advanced tumors that have developed resistance to PARP inhibitors or platinum-based chemotherapy."[128] A phase II clinical trial of 6-mercaptopurine and low dose methotrexate in patients with known *BRCA*-mutated cancer is currently underway in the United Kingdom (ClinicalTrial.gov identifier: NCT01432145).

## Platinum Sensitivity Following PARPi Resistance

With the eventual development of resistance to PARPi in patients with EOC, it is unclear as to what degree PARPi therapy might impact subsequent treatment with platinum agents. This issue is particularly important in the context of maintenance therapy with olaparib since more cases are more likely to go on to receive further platinum chemotherapy at progression. In a retrospective study, Ang et al. have investigated response to chemotherapy following resistance to PARPi.[119] The authors studied 89 PARPi-resistant *BRCA1/2*-mutant EOC patients with a median of three lines of chemotherapy prior to PARPi treatment. Patients were defined as platinum resistant (40%), partial platinum sensitive (43%), and platinum sensitive (17%) based on CGIC criteria. Seventy eight patients were evaluable for response based on CA125 and RECIST. Of these 78 patients, following resistance to PARPi, 53 patients went on to receive platinum-based chemotherapy and the rest received PLD, taxane, or other cytotoxic agents. Overall response rate to platinum-based chemotherapy was 40% and 49% according to RECIST or RECIST/CA125, respectively. The interval between platinum treatment pre- and post-PARPi therapy was a significant factor determining response to platinum-based chemotherapy following resistance to olaparib. There was also a trend for association between the best response to olaparib and post-PARPi platinum response. These data indicate that efficacy of chemotherapy is retained following resistance to PARPi.

Taken together observations from response to PARPi following resistance to platinum agents and the inverse indicate incomplete cross resistance mechanisms between PARPi and platinum agents. Clearly secondary *BRCA* mutations can confer resistance to PARPi but other mechanisms are likely to occur.

## Conclusion and Future Directions

PARP inhibitors have brought the concept of synthetic lethality from the laboratory to the clinical practice. Early phase trials have demonstrated safety and efficacy of PARP inhibitors. In particular, encouraging results have been produced regarding antitumor activity of single agent PARPi therapy in advanced recurrent EOC patients with *BRCA1/2* mutations, even in those with heavily pre-treated disease.

Although higher response rates to PARPi have been reported in platinum-sensitive cases, responses have also been observed in platinum resistant and occasionally in platinum-refractory patients in the form of long-term disease stabilization, suggesting that there may be different as well as overlapping mechanisms of resistance to PARPi and platinum agents. Activity of PARPi in EOC may not be restricted to patients with germline *BRCA* mutations. Clinical trials of PARPi in HGSOC patients with *wt BRCA* have generated data in support of activity of PARPi in this histological subtype, confirming data from TCGA that up to 50% of HGSOC subtype can have genomic and epigenomic abnormalities leading to HR dysfunction.

The PFS advantage is more pronounced in patients with germline or somatic *BRCA1/2* mutations. This has not translated into a significant overall survival benefit but of note, 23% of patients in the placebo arm switched to a PARP inhibitor. Potential toxicities associated with long-term use of PARPi needs to be established but so far, data in this context are reassuring. Also the impact of maintenance PARPi on subsequent sensitivity to platinum agents should be studied more extensively and may indeed differ according to *BRCA* mutation status.

Combination of PARPi and cytotoxic chemotherapy has been effective in preclinical studies; however high rate of myelotoxicity has been a common observation in various clinical trials of combination therapy resulting in frequent dose reductions and delays. Patients' selection, determination of the optimal chemotherapy regimen to combine with PARPi, and identification of an appropriate sequence and schedule of treatment remain major challenges in combination therapy trials. Myelosuppression, particularly at higher doses, is a common feature between different PARP inhibitors. Intermittent scheduling of PARPi monotherapy may be one way of overcoming bone marrow toxicities which could be investigated in future trials.

Preclinical and early phase trials data for combination of PARPi and other targeted agents such as antiangiogenic agents and PI3K inhibitors have been particularly encouraging and may broaden the application of these agents mainly in EOC and warrant further investigations.

Although PARPi activity has been observed in *BRCA1/2*-mutant breast cancer patients, result of single agents PARPi therapy in TNBC does not parallel the HGSOC patients. Current clinical trials only support the use of PARPi in *BRCA1/2*-mutant breast cancer. As well as *BRCA*-mutant cancers, PARPi activity has been observed in cases of prostate and pancreatic cancers in *wt BRCA* patients and further supports the need for identification of predictive biomarkers of response to PARPi in the absence of germline *BRCA* mutations. Efforts for identification of such biomarkers are currently underway. Prospective clinical trials might then validate these biomarkers and also address the relationship of HR status with platinum sensitivity. However, the fastest route to registration for PARP inhibitors seems to be in *BRCA1/2*-mutant ovarian cancer patients at present.

The initial enthusiasm generated by response to PARPi has been borne out by the positive results, particularly of maintenance therapy; however understanding the mechanisms of inherent or acquired resistance to PARPi remains a major challenge. Acquisition of tissue from patients on PARPi to study tumor heterogeneity both in time and space may shed light on possible resistance mechanisms.

## References

1 Alsop K, Fereday S, Meldrum C, et al. BRCA mutation frequency and patterns of treatment response in BRCA mutation-positive women with ovarian cancer: a report from the Australian Ovarian Cancer Study Group. *J Clin Oncol.* 2012;30(21):2654–2663.

2 Byrski T, Gronwald J, Huzarski T, et al. Pathologic complete response rates in young women with BRCA1-positive breast cancers after neoadjuvant chemotherapy. *J Clin Oncol.* 2010;28(3):375–379.

3 Miki Y, Swensen J, Shattuck-Eidens D, et al. A strong candidate for the breast and ovarian cancer susceptibility gene BRCA1. *Science.* 1994;266(5182):66–71.

4 Wooster R, Bignell G, Lancaster J, et al. Identification of the breast cancer susceptibility gene BRCA2. *Nature.* 1995;378(6559):789–792.

5 Easton D, Ford D, Peto J. Inherited susceptibility to breast cancer. *Cancer Surv.* 1993;18:95–113.

6 Struewing JP, Tarone RE, Brody LC, Li FP, Boice JD Jr. BRCA1 mutations in young women with breast cancer. *Lancet.* 1996;347(9013):1493.

7 Easton DF, Ford D, Bishop DT. Breast and ovarian cancer incidence in BRCA1-mutation carriers. Breast Cancer Linkage Consortium. *Am J Hum Genet.* 1995;56(1):265–271.

8 Easton DF, Narod SA, Ford D, Steel M. The genetic epidemiology of BRCA1. Breast Cancer Linkage Consortium. *Lancet.* 1994;344(8924):761.

9 Easton D. Breast cancer genes–what are the real risks? *Nat Genet.* 1997;16(3):210–211.

10 Ford D, Easton DF, Stratton M, et al. Genetic heterogeneity and penetrance analysis of the BRCA1 and BRCA2 genes in breast cancer families. The Breast Cancer Linkage Consortium. *Am J Hum Genet.* 1998;62(3):676–689.

11 King MC, Marks JH, Mandell JB, et al.New York Breast Cancer Study Group. Breast and ovarian cancer risks due to inherited mutations in BRCA1 and BRCA2. *Science.* 2003;302(5645):643–646.

12 Warner E, Foulkes W, Goodwin P, et al. Prevalence and penetrance of BRCA1 and BRCA2 gene mutations in unselected Ashkenazi Jewish women with breast cancer. *J Natl Cancer Inst.* 1999;91(14):1241–1247.

13 Hoeijmakers JH, Genome maintenance mechanisms for preventing cancer. *Nature.* 2001;411(6835):366–374.

14 Hoeijmakers JH, DNA damage, aging, and cancer. *N Engl J Med.* 2009;361(15):1475–1485.

15 Ames BN, Shigenaga MK, Hagen TM. Oxidants, antioxidants, and the degenerative diseases of aging. *Proc Natl Acad Sci U S A.* 1993;90(17):7915–7922.

16 Coleman WB, Tsongalis GJ. The role of genomic instability in human carcinogenesis. *Anticancer Res.* 1999;19(6A):4645–4664.

17 Helleday T, Bryant HE, Schultz N. Poly(ADP-ribose) polymerase (PARP-1) in homologous recombination and as a target for cancer therapy. *Cell Cycle.* 2005;4(9):1176–1178.

18 Lindahl T. Recognition and processing of damaged DNA. *J Cell Sci Suppl.* 1995;19:73–77.

19 Ame JC, Spenlehauer C, de Murcia G. The PARP superfamily. *Bioessays.* 2004;26(8):882–893.

20 El-Khamisy SF, Masutani M, Suzuki H, et al. A requirement for PARP-1 for the assembly or stability of XRCC1 nuclear foci at sites of oxidative DNA damage. *Nucleic Acids Res.* 2003;31(19):5526–5533.

21 Fortini P, Dogliotti E. Base damage and single-strand break repair: mechanisms and functional significance of short- and long-patch repair subpathways. *DNA Repair (Amst).* 2007;6(4):398–409.

22 Haber JE DNA repair. Gatekeepers of recombination. *Nature.* 1999;398(6729):665, 667.

23 Noel G, Giocanti N, Fernet M, Mégnin-Chanet F, Favaudon V. Poly(ADP-ribose) polymerase (PARP-1) is not involved in DNA double-strand break recovery. *BMC Cell Biol.* 2003;4:7.

24 Yang YG, Cortes U, Patnaik S, Jasin M, Wang ZQ, et al. Ablation of PARP-1 does not interfere with the repair of DNA double-strand breaks, but compromises the reactivation of stalled replication forks. *Oncogene.* 2004;23(21):3872–3882.

25 Kanaar R, Hoeijmakers JH, van Gent DC. Molecular mechanisms of DNA double strand break repair. *Trends Cell Biol.* 1998;8(12):483–489.

26 Rich T, Allen RL, Wyllie AH. Defying death after DNA damage. *Nature.* 2000;407(6805):777–783.

27 Paull TT, Gellert M. The 3′ to 5′ exonuclease activity of Mre 11 facilitates repair of DNA double-strand breaks. *Mol Cell.* 1998;1(7):969–979.

28 Khanna KK, Jackson SP. DNA double-strand breaks: signaling, repair and the cancer connection. *Nat Genet.* 2001;27(3):247–254.

29 Helleday T, Lo J, van Gent DC, Engelward BP. DNA double-strand break repair: from mechanistic understanding to cancer treatment. *DNA Repair (Amst).* 2007;6(7):923–935.

30 Moynahan ME, Chiu JW, Koller BH, Jasin M. Brca1 controls homology-directed DNA repair. *Mol Cell.* 1999;4(4):511–518.

31 Moynahan ME, Pierce AJ, Jasin M. BRCA2 is required for homology-directed repair of chromosomal breaks. *Mol Cell.* 2001;7(2):263–272.

32 Moynahan ME, Cui TY, Jasin M. Homology-directed dna repair, mitomycin-c resistance, and chromosome stability is restored with correction of a Brca1 mutation. *Cancer Res.* 2001;61(12):4842–4850.

33 Patel KJ, Yu VP, Lee H, et al. Involvement of Brca2 in DNA repair. *Mol Cell.* 1998;1(3):347–357.

34 Venkitaraman AR. Cancer susceptibility and the functions of BRCA1 and BRCA2. *Cell.* 2002;108(2):171–182.

35 Scully R Role of BRCA gene dysfunction in breast and ovarian cancer predisposition. *Breast Cancer Res.* 2000;2(5):324–330.

36 Scully R, Chen J, Ochs RL, et al. Dynamic changes of BRCA1 subnuclear location and phosphorylation state are initiated by DNA damage. *Cell.* 1997;90(3):425–435.

37 Sharan SK, Morimatsu M, Albrecht U, et al. Embryonic lethality and radiation hypersensitivity mediated by Rad51 in mice lacking Brca2. *Nature.* 1997;386(6627):804–810.

38 Bhattacharyya A, Ear US, Koller BH, Weichselbaum RR, Bishop DK. The breast cancer susceptibility gene BRCA1 is required for subnuclear assembly of Rad51 and survival following treatment with the DNA cross-linking agent cisplatin. *J Biol Chem.* 2000;275(31):23899–23903.

39 Bryant HE, Schultz N, Thomas HD, et al. Specific killing of BRCA2-deficient tumours with inhibitors of poly(ADP-ribose) polymerase. *Nature.* 2005;434(7035):913–917.

40 Farmer H, McCabe N, Lord CJ, et al. Targeting the DNA repair defect in BRCA mutant cells as a therapeutic strategy. *Nature.* 2005;434(7035):917–921.

41 Ashworth A. A synthetic lethal therapeutic approach: poly(ADP) ribose polymerase inhibitors for the treatment of cancers deficient in DNA double-strand break repair. *J Clin Oncol.* 2008;26(22):3785–3790.

42 McCabe N, Turner NC, Lord CJ, et al. Deficiency in the repair of DNA damage by homologous recombination and sensitivity to poly(ADP-ribose) polymerase inhibition. *Cancer Res.* 2006;66(16):8109–8115.

43 Peasland A, Wang LZ, Rowling E, et al. Identification and evaluation of a potent novel ATR inhibitor, NU6027, in breast and ovarian cancer cell lines. *Br J Cancer.* 2011;105(3):372–381.

44 Mendes-Pereira AM, Martin SA, Brough R, et al. Synthetic lethal targeting of PTEN mutant cells with PARP inhibitors. *EMBO Mol Med.* 2009;1(6–7):315–322.

45 Shen WH, Balajee AS, Wang J, et al. Essential role for nuclear PTEN in maintaining chromosomal integrity. *Cell.* 2007;128(1):157–170.

46 Graeser M, McCarthy A, Lord CJ, et al. A marker of homologous recombination predicts pathologic complete response to neoadjuvant chemotherapy in primary breast cancer. *Clin Cancer Res.* 2010;16(24):6159–6168.

47 Baldwin RL, Nemeth E, Tran H, et al. BRCA1 promoter region hypermethylation in ovarian carcinoma: a population-based study. *Cancer Res.* 2000;60(19):5329–5333.

48 Esteller M, Silva JM, Dominguez G, et al. Promoter hypermethylation and BRCA1 inactivation in sporadic breast and ovarian tumors. *J Natl Cancer Inst.* 2000;92(7):564–569.

49 Teodoridis JM, Hall J, Marsh S, et al. CpG island methylation of DNA damage response genes in advanced ovarian cancer. *Cancer Res.* 2005;65(19):8961–8967.

50 Geisler JP, Hatterman-Zogg MA, Rathe JA, et al. Frequency of BRCA1 dysfunction in ovarian cancer. *J Natl Cancer Inst.* 2002;94(1):61–67.

51 Hennessy BT, Coleman RL, Markman M. Ovarian cancer. *Lancet.* 2009;374(9698):1371–1382.

52 Hilton JL, Geisler JP, Rathe JA, Hattermann-Zogg MA, DeYoung B, Buller RE. Inactivation of BRCA1 and BRCA2 in ovarian cancer. *J Natl Cancer Inst.* 2002;94(18):1396–1406.

53 Taniguchi T, Tischkowitz M, Ameziane N, et al. Disruption of the Fanconi anemia-BRCA pathway in cisplatin-sensitive ovarian tumors. *Nat Med.* 2003;9(5):568–574.

54 Turner N, Tutt A, Ashworth A. Hallmarks of "BRCAness" in sporadic cancers. *Nat Rev Cancer*. 2004;4(10):814–819.

55 Fong PC, Boss DS, Yap TA, et al. Inhibition of poly(ADP-ribose) polymerase in tumors from BRCA mutation carriers. *N Engl J Med*. 2009;361(2):123–134.

56 Fong PC, Yap TA, Boss DS, et al. Poly(ADP)-ribose polymerase inhibition: frequent durable responses in BRCA carrier ovarian cancer correlating with platinum-free interval. *J Clin Oncol*. 2010;28(15):2512–2519.

57 Audeh MW, Carmichael J, Penson RT, et al. Oral poly(ADP-ribose) polymerase inhibitor olaparib in patients with BRCA1 or BRCA2 mutations and recurrent ovarian cancer: a proof-of-concept trial. *Lancet*. 2010;376(9737):245–251.

58 Gelmon KA, Tischkowitz M, Mackay H, et al. Olaparib in patients with recurrent high-grade serous or poorly differentiated ovarian carcinoma or triple-negative breast cancer: a phase 2, multicentre, open-label, non-randomised study. *Lancet Oncol*. 2011;12(9):852–861.

59 Sandhu SK, Schelman WR, Wilding G, et al. The poly(ADP-ribose) polymerase inhibitor niraparib (MK4827) in BRCA mutation carriers and patients with sporadic cancer: a phase 1 dose-escalation trial. *Lancet Oncol*. 2013;14(9):882–892.

60 Kaye SB, Lubinski J, Matulonis U, et al. Phase II, open-label, randomized, multicenter study comparing the efficacy and safety of olaparib, a poly (ADP-ribose) polymerase inhibitor, and pegylated liposomal doxorubicin in patients with BRCA1 or BRCA2 mutations and recurrent ovarian cancer. *J Clin Oncol*. 2012;30(4):372–379.

61 Gordon AN, Fleagle JT, Guthrie D, Parkin DE, Gore ME, Lacave AJ. Recurrent epithelial ovarian carcinoma: a randomized phase III study of pegylated liposomal doxorubicin versus topotecan. *J Clin Oncol*. 2001;19(14):3312–3322.

62 Mutch DG, Orlando M, Goss T, et al. Randomized phase III trial of gemcitabine compared with pegylated liposomal doxorubicin in patients with platinum-resistant ovarian cancer. *J Clin Oncol*. 2007;25(19):2811–2818.

63 Adams SF, Marsh EB, Elmasri W, et al. A high response rate to liposomal doxorubicin is seen among women with BRCA mutations treated for recurrent epithelial ovarian cancer. *Gynecol Oncol*. 2011;123(3):486–491.

64 Safra T, Borgato L, Nicoletto MO, et al. BRCA mutation status and determinant of outcome in women with recurrent epithelial ovarian cancer treated with pegylated liposomal doxorubicin. *Mol Cancer Ther*. 2011;10(10):2000–2007.

65 Cancer Genome Atlas Research Network. Integrated genomic analyses of ovarian carcinoma. *Nature*. 2011;474(7353):609–615.

66 Ledermann J, Harter P, Gourley C, et al. Olaparib maintenance therapy in platinum-sensitive relapsed ovarian cancer. *N Engl J Med*. 2012;366(15):1382–1392.

67 Ledermann J, Harter P, Gourley C, et al., Olaparib maintenance therapy in patients with platinum-sensitive relapsed serous ovarian cancer: a preplanned retrospective analysis of outcomes by BRCA status in a randomised phase 2 trial. *Lancet Oncol*. 2014;15(8):852–861.

68 Tutt A, Robson M, Garber JE, et al. Oral poly(ADP-ribose) polymerase inhibitor olaparib in patients with BRCA1 or BRCA2 mutations and advanced breast cancer: a proof-of-concept trial. *Lancet*. 2010;376(9737):235–244.

69 De Bono JS M L, Gonzalez M, et al. First-in-human trial of novel oral PARP inhibitor BMN 673 in patients with solid tumors. *J Clin Oncol*. 2013;(31):abstr 2580.

70 http://investors.bmrn.com/releasedetail.cfm?ReleaseID=780454. Accessed on June 20, 2014

71 Brenner JC, Ateeq B, LiY, et al. Mechanistic rationale for inhibition of poly(ADP-ribose) polymerase in ETS gene fusion-positive prostate cancer. *Cancer Cell*. 2011;19(5):664–678.

72 Schiewer MJ, Goodwin JF, Han S, et al. Dual roles of PARP-1 promote cancer growth and progression. *Cancer Discov*. 2012;2(12):1134–1149.

73 Sebastian de Bono J, Sandhu S, Attard G, Beyond hormone therapy for prostate cancer with PARP inhibitors. *Cancer Cell*. 2011;19(5):573–574.

74 Murphy KM, Brune KA, Griffin C, et al. Evaluation of candidate genes MAP2K4, MADH4, ACVR1B, and BRCA2 in familial pancreatic cancer: deleterious BRCA2 mutations in 17%. *Cancer Res*. 2002;62(13):3789–3793.

75 Lowery MA, Kelsen DP, Stadler ZK, et al. An emerging entity: pancreatic adenocarcinoma associated with a known BRCA mutation: clinical descriptors, treatment implications, and future directions. *Oncologist*. 2011;16(10):1397–1402.

76 Kaufman BS-FR, Schmutzler RK. Olaparib monotherapy in patients with advanced cancer and a germ-line BRCA1/2 mutation: an open-label phase II study. *J Clin Oncol* 2013;(31):abstr 11024.

77 Byers LA, Wang J, Nilsson MB, et al. Proteomic profiling identifies dysregulated pathways in small cell lung cancer and novel therapeutic targets including PARP1. *Cancer Discov*. 2012;2(9):798–811.

78 Postel-Vinay S, Bajrami I, Friboulet L, et al. A high-throughput screen identifies PARP1/2 inhibitors as a potential therapy for ERCC1-deficient non-small cell lung cancer. *Oncogene*. 2013;32(47):5377–5387.

79 Wainberg ZA, Rafii S, Ramanathan RK, et al. Safety and antitumor activity of the PARP inhibitor BMN673 in a phase 1 trial recruiting metastatic small-cell lung cancer (SCLC) and germline BRCA-mutation carrier cancer patients. *J Clin Oncol*. 2014;32(5s): suppl; abstr 7522.

80 Brenner JC, Feng FY, Han S, et al. PARP-1 inhibition as a targeted strategy to treat Ewing's sarcoma. *Cancer Res*. 2012;72(7):1608–1613.

81 Kim HS, Kim MA, Hodgson D, et al. Concordance of ATM (ataxia telangiectasia mutated) immunohistochemistry between biopsy or metastatic tumor samples and primary tumors in gastric cancer patients. *Pathobiology*. 2013;80(3):127–137.

82 Forster MD, Dedes KJ, Sandhu S, et al. Treatment with olaparib in a patient with PTEN-deficient endometrioid endometrial cancer. *Nat Rev Clin Oncol*. 2011;8(5):302–306.

83 Dedes KJ, Wetterskog D, Mendes-Pereira AM, et al. PTEN deficiency in endometrioid endometrial adenocarcinomas predicts sensitivity to PARP inhibitors. *Sci Transl Med*. 2010;2(53):53ra75.

84 Gupta A, Yang Q, Pandita RK, et al. Cell cycle checkpoint defects contribute to genomic instability in PTEN deficient cells independent of DNA DSB repair. *Cell Cycle*. 2009;8(14):2198–2210.

85 Kummar S, Kinders R, Gutierrez ME, et al. Phase 0 clinical trial of the poly (ADP-ribose) polymerase inhibitor ABT-888 in patients with advanced malignancies. *J Clin Oncol*. 2009;27(16):2705–2711.

86 Kummar S, Ji J, Morgan R, et al. A phase I study of veliparib in combination with metronomic cyclophosphamide in adults with refractory solid tumors and lymphomas. *Clin Cancer Res*. 2012;18(6):1726–1734.

87 Wesolowski R, Zhao M, Geyer SM, et al. Phase I trial of the PARP inhibitor veliparib (V) in combination with carboplatin (C) in metastatic breast cancer (MBC). *J Clin Oncol*. 2014;32(5s):suppl; abstr 1074.

88  Plummer R, Jones C, Middleton M, et al. Phase I study of the poly(ADP-ribose) polymerase inhibitor, AG014699, in combination with temozolomide in patients with advanced solid tumors. *Clin Cancer Res.* 2008;14(23):7917–7923.

89  Plummer R, Lorigan P, Steven N, et al. A phase II study of the potent PARP inhibitor, Rucaparib (PF-01367338, AG014699), with temozolomide in patients with metastatic melanoma demonstrating evidence of chemopotentiation. *Cancer Chemother Pharmacol.* 2013;71(5):1191–1199.

90  Kristeleit R, Burris H, LoRusso P, et al. Phase 1/2 study of oral rucaparib: final phase 1 results. *J Clin Oncol.* 2014;32 (5s):suppl; abstr 2573.

91  Molife LR, Roxburgh P, Wilson PH, et al., A phase I study of oral rucaparib in combination with carboplatin. *J Clin Oncol.* 2013;31:abstract 2586.

92  O'Shaughnessy J, Osborne C, Pippen JE, et al. Iniparib plus chemotherapy in metastatic triple-negative breast cancer. *N Engl J Med.* 2011;364(3):205–214.

93  Curtin NJ, Wang LZ, Yiakouvaki A, et al. Novel poly(ADP-ribose) polymerase-1 inhibitor, AG14361, restores sensitivity to temozolomide in mismatch repair-deficient cells. *Clin Cancer Res.* 2004;10(3):881–889.

94  Donawho CK, Luo Y, Luo Y, et al. ABT-888, an orally active poly(ADP-ribose) polymerase inhibitor that potentiates DNA-damaging agents in preclinical tumor models. *Clin Cancer Res.* 2007;13(9):2728–2737.

95  Tentori L, Graziani G. Chemopotentiation by PARP inhibitors in cancer therapy. *Pharmacol Res.* 2005;52(1):25–33.

96  Tentori L, Leonetti C, Scarsella M, et al. Poly(ADP-ribose) glycohydrolase inhibitor as chemosensitiser of malignant melanoma for temozolomide. *Eur J Cancer.* 2005;41(18):2948–2957.

97  Rajan A, Carter CA, Kelly RJ, et al., A phase I combination study of olaparib with cisplatin and gemcitabine in adults with solid tumors. *Clin Cancer Res.* 2012;18(8):2344–2351.

98  Oza AM, Cibula D, Oaknin A, et al. Olaparib plus paclitaxel plus carboplatin (P/C) followed by olaparib maintenance treatment in patients (pts) with platinum-sensitive recurrent serous ovarian cancer (PSR SOC): A randomized, open-label phase II study. *J Clin Oncol* 2012;(30):Abstract 5001.

99  Courtney KD, Corcoran RB, Engelman JA. The PI3K pathway as drug target in human cancer. *J Clin Oncol.* 2010;28(6):1075–1083.

100  Gewinner C, Wang ZC, Richardson A, et al. Evidence that inositol polyphosphate 4-phosphatase type II is a tumor suppressor that inhibits PI3K signaling. *Cancer Cell.* 2009;16(2):115–125.

101  Kumar A, Fernandez-Capetillo O, Carrera AC. Nuclear phosphoinositide 3-kinase beta controls double-strand break DNA repair. *Proc Natl Acad Sci U S A.* 2010;107(16):7491–7496.

102  Ibrahim YH, Garcia-Garcia C, Serra V, et al. PI3K inhibition impairs BRCA1/2 expression and sensitizes BRCA-proficient triple-negative breast cancer to PARP inhibition. *Cancer Discov.* 2012;2(11):1036–1047.

103  Juvekar A, Burga LN, Hu H, et al. Combining a PI3K inhibitor with a PARP inhibitor provides an effective therapy for BRCA1-related breast cancer. *Cancer Discov.* 2012;2(11):1048–1063.

104  Matulonis UWG, Birrer MJ, et al. Phase I study of oral BKM120 and oral olaparib for high-grade serous ovarian cancer (HGSC) or triple-negative breast cancer (TNBC). *J Clin Oncol.* 2014. 32(5s):suppl; abstr 2510.

105  Tentori L, Lacal PM, Muzi A, et al. Poly(ADP-ribose) polymerase (PARP) inhibition or PARP-1 gene deletion reduces angiogenesis. *Eur J Cancer.* 2007;43(14):2124–2133.

106  Rajesh M, Mukhopadhyay P, Batkai S, et al. Pharmacological inhibition of poly(ADP-ribose) polymerase inhibits angiogenesis. *Biochem Biophys Res Commun.* 2006;350(2):352–357.

107  Dean E, Middleton MR, Pwint T, et al. Phase I study to assess the safety and tolerability of olaparib in combination with bevacizumab in patients with advanced solid tumours. *Br J Cancer.* 2012;106(3):468–474.

108  Liu JF, Tolaney SM, Birrer M, et al. A phase 1 trial of the poly(ADP-ribose) polymerase inhibitor olaparib (AZD2281) in combination with the anti-angiogenic cediranib (AZD2171) in recurrent epithelial ovarian or triple-negative breast cancer. *Eur J Cancer.* 2013;49(14):2972–2978.

109  Liu J, Barry W, Birrer M, et al. A randomized phase 2 trial comparing efficacy of the combination of the PARP inhibitor olaparib and the antiangiogenic cediranib against olaparib alone in recurrent platinum-sensitive ovarian cancer. *J Clin Oncol.* 2014;32(5s):suppl; abstr LBA5500.

110  Wang X, Weaver DT. The ups and downs of DNA repair biomarkers for PARP inhibitor therapies. *Am J Cancer Res.* 2011;1(3):301–327.

111  Mukhopadhyay A, Elattar A, Cerbinskaite A, et al. Development of a functional assay for homologous recombination status in primary cultures of epithelial ovarian tumor and correlation with sensitivity to poly(ADP-ribose) polymerase inhibitors. *Clin Cancer Res.* 2010;16(8):2344–2351.

112  Redon CE, Nakamura AJ, Zhang YW, et al. Histone gammaH2AX and poly(ADP-ribose) as clinical pharmacodynamic biomarkers. *Clin Cancer Res.* 2010;16(18):4532–4542.

113  Drew Y, Mulligan EA, Vong WT, et al. Therapeutic potential of poly(ADP-ribose) polymerase inhibitor AG014699 in human cancers with mutated or methylated BRCA1 or BRCA2. *J Natl Cancer Inst.* 2011;103(4):334–346.

114  Mukhopadhyay A, Plummer ER, Elattar A, et al. Clinicopathological features of homologous recombination-deficient epithelial ovarian cancers: sensitivity to PARP inhibitors, platinum, and survival. *Cancer Res.* 2012;72(22):5675–5682.

115  Konstantinopoulos PA, Spentzos D, Karlan BY, et al. Gene expression profile of BRCAness that correlates with responsiveness to chemotherapy and with outcome in patients with epithelial ovarian cancer. *J Clin Oncol.* 201028(22):3555–3561.

116  Garg K, Levine DA, Olvera N, et al. BRCA1 immunohistochemistry in a molecularly characterized cohort of ovarian high-grade serous carcinomas. *Am J Surg Pathol.* 2013;37(1):138–146.

117  Edwards SL, Brough R, Lord CJ, et al. Resistance to therapy caused by intragenic deletion in BRCA2. *Nature.* 2008;451(7182):1111–1115.

118  Barber LJ, Sandhu S, Chen L, et al. Secondary mutations in BRCA2 associated with clinical resistance to a PARP inhibitor. *J Pathol.* 2013;229(3):422–429.

119  Ang JE, Gourley C, Powell CB, et al. Efficacy of chemotherapy in BRCA1/2 mutation carrier ovarian cancer in the setting of PARP inhibitor resistance: a multi-institutional study. *Clin Cancer Res.* 2013;19(19):5485–5493.

120  Drost R, Bouwman P, Rottenberg S, et al. BRCA1 RING function is essential for tumor suppression but dispensable for therapy resistance. *Cancer Cell.* 2011;20(6):797–809.

121  Bouwman P, Aly A, Escandell JM, et al. 53BP1 loss rescues BRCA1 deficiency and is associated with triple-negative and BRCA-mutated breast cancers. *Nat Struct Mol Biol.* 2010;17(6):688–695.

122  Bunting SF, Callen E, Wong N, et al. 53BP1 inhibits homologous recombination in Brca1-deficient cells by blocking resection of DNA breaks. *Cell.* 2010;141(2):243–254.

123 Jaspers JE, Kersbergen A, Boon U, et al. Loss of 53BP1 causes PARP inhibitor resistance in Brca1-mutated mouse mammary tumors. *Cancer Discov.* 2013;3(1):68–81.

124 Moskwa P, Buffa FM, Pan Y, et al. miR-182-mediated downregulation of BRCA1 impacts DNA repair and sensitivity to PARP inhibitors. *Mol Cell.* 2011;41(2):210–220.

125 Wang W, Figg WD. Secondary BRCA1 and BRCA2 alterations and acquired chemoresistance. *Cancer Biol Ther.* 2008;7(7):1004–1005.

126 Oplustilova L, Wolanin K, Mistrik M, et al. Evaluation of candidate biomarkers to predict cancer cell sensitivity or resistance to PARP-1 inhibitor treatment. *Cell Cycle.* 2012;11(20):3837–3850.

127 Rottenberg S, Jaspers J E, Kersbergen A, et al. High sensitivity of BRCA1-deficient mammary tumors to the PARP inhibitor AZD2281 alone and in combination with platinum drugs. *Proc Natl Acad Sci U S A.* 2008;105(44):17079–17084.

128 Issaeva N, Thomas HD, Djureinovic T, et al. 6-thioguanine selectively kills BRCA2-defective tumors and overcomes PARP inhibitor resistance. *Cancer Res.* 2010;70(15):6268–6276.

## CHAPTER 34

# Targeting the c-Met Kinase

*Chad Tang[1], M. Angelica Cortez[2], David Hong[3], and James W. Welsh[1]*

[1] Department of Radiation Oncology, The University of Texas MD Anderson Cancer Center, Houston, TX, USA
[2] Department of Experimental Radiation Oncology, The University of Texas MD Anderson Cancer Center, Houston, TX, USA
[3] Department of Investigational Cancer Therapeutics, The University of Texas MD Anderson Cancer Center, Houston, TX, USA

## Role of c-Met in Carcinogenesis and Tumor Progression

The expression of the cell membrane receptor and proto-oncogene c-Met has been linked to numerous aspects of cancer development. Although c-Met has been implicated in the initial stages of carcinogenesis, two of its best characterized functions are in the development of metastasis and the development of resistance toward molecularly targeted therapeutics, as discussed further in this chapter.

A correlation between increased c-Met expression and metastatic behavior has been identified in numerous types of cancer, including melanoma,[1] colon cancer,[2] and lung cancer.[3] The association of increased c-Met expression with liver metastasis underscores this correlation. One proposed mechanism by which c-Met promotes metastasis is through the enhanced production of hepatocyte growth factor (HGF, the cleavage product and ligand of c-Met) by hepatocytes, which enhances paracrine signaling and produces an environment that favors the clonal selection of metastatic cells with higher c-Met expression.[4] This hypothesis has been functionally tested in preclinical models in which mice that had been subjected to hepatectomy, which stimulates liver regeneration, were found to exhibit higher rates of cancer engraftment corresponding with higher c-Met expression.[5] The functional importance of c-Met signaling within the metastatic microenvironment is further emphasized by reports of increased c-Met expression in metastatic sites in the absence of increased expression by the primary tumor.[4,6]

Some of the earliest reports of c-Met function focused on its physiologic role in normal development. Montesano et al. studied the role of c-Met activation in canine kidney cells grown on collagen or Matrigel matrices.[7] The addition of HGF resulted in a loss of cell anchoring and polarity, facilitating increased cellular migration and scattering. The end result was the formation of complex tubular structures reminiscent of the nascent kidney *in vitro*.[7] Bladt et al. further showed that limb muscle formation during mouse embryogenesis was abrogated in homozygous MET mutants, in which skeletal muscle precursors lacking MET do not migrate normally, thereby preventing limb bud invasion.[8] The developmental processes promoted by c-Met have been described as the epithelial–mesenchymal transition (EMT),[9] in which epithelial cells that are normally structurally anchored and physiologically polarized detach from their neighboring cells and take on a migratory mesenchymal phenotype.

A phenomenon akin to physiologic EMT has also been observed in cancer metastasis. In analogous processes, cancerous epithelial cells experience upregulation of molecules involved in migration and downregulation of those involved in attachment, effectively recapitulating the EMT.[9] C-Met was shown to be a major facilitator of this pathologic EMT by Rong et al., who induced ectopic c-Met expression in fibroblast cultures and noted the development of an invasive phenotype characterized by enhanced serine protease activity and migratory behavior. When these transformed cells were implanted into nude mice, they exhibited greater tumorigenicity with a tendency toward metastatic behavior.[10] Moreover, inhibition of c-Met function in cancer cell lines has been shown to induce the opposite phenotype, reducing motility *in vitro* and rates of metastasis *in vivo*.[11,12]

In addition to its role in metastasis, c-Met has also been implicated in the development of resistance toward targeted therapies. As a receptor tyrosine kinase, the intracellular pathways activated by c-Met are often redundant and exhibit cross talk with numerous other oncogenic surface receptors, such as the epidermal growth factor receptor (EGFR), the human epidermal growth factor receptor (HER2, also known as ERBB2), WNT, and the insulin-like growth factor receptor 1 (IGF1R), as discussed further below.[13] Evidence of this cross talk has been demonstrated on several levels. *In vitro* studies have shown that EGFR activation leads to c-Met phosphorylation and activation.[14] Similarly, activation of the WNT-β-catenin pathway leads directly to *MET* transcription.[15] Conversely, c-Met activation can also promote other growth receptor pathways, including ERBB3-PI3K-AKT signaling.[16]

As result of intracellular cross talk, c-Met activation has been linked to the development of resistance to several tyrosine kinase inhibitors (TKIs), including sunitinib,[17] gefitinib,[16] and erlotinib.[18] Engelman et al. identified a gefitinib-sensitive lung cancer cell line that was later shown to develop resistance via *MET* amplification. Subsequent c-Met inhibition restored cellular sensitivity to gefitinib. In subsequent analyses of 18 specimens of lung cancer from patients whose tumors initially responded to gefitinib or erlotinib but later developed resistance, four specimens (22%) were found to have MET amplification, and further analysis of samples available both before and after treatment from two patients showed that MET alterations were present only in the post-treatment samples. These results suggest that MET amplification in these patients (and perhaps in others) represented an acquired event during oncogenesis.[16]

## c-Met Expression in Various Tumor Types

Upregulation of c-Met, HGF expression, or both has been identified in almost every type of solid tumor.[19] On the genomic level, increased c-Met expression has been linked with gene amplification, and c-Met constitutive activation with gene mutation. In addition to direct genomic alterations, several epigenetic processes facilitate c-Met overexpression, including stimulation by tumor-secreted growth factors, hypoxia, and activation of other oncogenes.[19,20] The use of several therapeutic modalities such as radiation therapy and molecularly targeted systemic agents has also been associated with c-Met upregulation.[16,21]

Current evidence indicates that most c-Met mutations are a result of sporadic somatic alterations acquired during cancer development.[4,6,16,18] However, a subset of cancers has been identified as having germ line MET mutations, the best characterized of which is papillary renal cell carcinoma (RCC). Schmidt et al. identified several missense mutations in the tyrosine kinase domain in members of families with hereditary papillary RCC.[22] Additional mutations were also identified in cases of sporadic RCC. To determine the functional consequences of these alterations, Jeffers et al. induced the specific mutations identified by Schmidt et al. into cultured fibroblast cells and noted that mutated c-Met exhibited increased tyrosine phosphorylation and enhanced kinase activity, resulting in greater tumorigenicity *in vivo*.[23] Similar germ line mutations have also been identified in familial gastric and colorectal cancer.[24,25]

Numerous groups have demonstrated the prognostic significance of c-Met and its ligand HGF. Upregulation of both receptor and ligand has been linked with overall and metastasis-free survival in several types of solid tumors.[19] Independent studies have linked c-Met and HGF levels with metastasis and survival in breast cancer[26–28] as well as in gastric,[29] lung,[30] and hepatocellular[31] cancers, among others. The major functions of c-Met in these types of cancer are thought to be promotion of metastatic potential and development of resistance to therapy.

## Cross Talk Among Signaling Pathways

Cross talk between c-Met and other cell surface proteins, including receptor tyrosine kinases, contributes to both tumorigenesis and treatment resistance. For example, interaction of c-Met with the c-Met-related tyrosine kinase macrophage-stimulating 1 receptor (MST1R, also known as the RON receptor) causes phosphorylation of the c-Met receptor in the absence of HGF.[32] Notably, transactivation of RON by c-Met was suggested to be a feature of cancer cells "addicted" to c-Met pathway signaling.[33] Transactivation between c-Met and both platelet-derived growth factor receptor (PDGFR) and Axl was found recently to be involved in bladder cancer.[34] Semaphorin receptors, including the plexins and neuropilins, can also transactivate c-Met in the absence of HGF when stimulated by their semaphorin ligands.[35–37]

Importantly, c-Met has also been shown to interact directly with EGFR, allowing activation of c-Met after cells have been stimulated with the EGFR ligands EGF or transforming growth factor-alpha (TGF-α).[38,39] Indeed, both EGFR and c-Met can cooperate to enhance cellular functions such as proliferation, cell motility, and downstream signal transduction. In one study, treatment of cells expressing both c-Met and EGFR with EGF resulted in activation of c-Met and synergistic effects on proliferation, suggesting mutual activation of these two pathways.[39] Previous studies showed that HGF can transactivate EGFR and phosphorylation of EGFR can

activate c-Met, resulting in synergistic effects on tumor growth.[40] On the other hand, inhibition of both c-Met and EGFR leads to enhanced growth inhibition and apoptosis.[41] c-Met also interacts with ERBB2 and ERBB3, causing transactivation of both receptors.[42,43] These findings are particularly important in lung cancer therapy, because c-Met amplification is present in more than 20% of cases of acquired resistance to EGFR inhibitors in nonsmall cell lung cancer (NSCLC).[18,44] Interestingly, the mTOR and Wnt signaling pathways were recently shown to contribute to acquired EGFR/c-Met TKI resistance; indeed, combination therapy might be able to prevent the development of secondary resistance in many patients with lung cancer.[40] Specifically, inhibition of either mTOR or Wnt signaling in NSCLC sensitized cells to EGFR/c-Met TKIs. Studies such as these indicate that cross talk among pathways such as c-Met and EGFR is important in the efficacy of targeted therapy, and a better understanding of these interactions is needed to improve our current therapeutic approaches and to develop new drug combinations for lung cancer.

## c-Met Pathways as Therapeutic Targets

As is true for other receptor kinases that are overexpressed on tumor cell surfaces, c-Met is an attractive therapeutic target for several types of solid tumors. Given the involvement of c-Met in cancer initiation, progression, and metastasis, coupled with the relative ease of targeting extracellular receptors with both small-molecule inhibitors and monoclonal antibodies, several types of therapeutic agents have been designed to target c-Met signaling. Indeed, some therapeutics designed against either the c-Met receptor or its specific ligand HGF are already in clinical use. Although some such agents seem to be specific to this pathway, others are more promiscuous and block other pathways in addition to c-Met. As described in the previous section, the discovery of cross talk between c-Met and other receptor kinases such as EGFR[45] has emphasized that EGFR signaling can confer resistance to therapeutic approaches that block c-Met and, conversely, that c-Met signaling can mediate resistance to agents that target both EGFR and the vascular endothelial growth factor (VEGF).[17,38,39] Given the ability of cancer cells to rapidly adapt to specific pathway inhibitors, interest has been expressed in developing approaches in which c-Met blocking agents are combined with other targeted therapeutics and with more generally cytotoxic agents such as radiation.

Perhaps the best characterized anti-c-Met therapeutic to date is MetMAb (onartuzumab), a single-armed monoclonal antibody developed by Genentech that specifically binds to the c-Met receptor. A phase II trial of erlotinib given with MetMAb or a placebo for advanced NSCLC in which crossover was allowed at disease progression showed that this combination improved progression-free survival and overall survival among patients with Met-positive tumors but not among patients with Met-negative tumors.[46] Overall the combination of MetMAb plus erlotinib was well tolerated, with little increased toxicity aside from peripheral edema. These encouraging findings led to implementation of a similar randomized phase III trial for patients with Met-positive NSCLC.

Interestingly, two agents currently approved by the US Food and Drug Administration as c-Met-targeting therapeutics have been approved for other indications as well. One of these agents, crizotinib, is a small-molecular inhibitor initially developed to target c-Met (and indeed is highly specific in this targeting) that has also been approved for the treatment of ALK-positive NSCLC. Several clinical trials, including the CREATE trial, are underway to evaluate crizotinib for patients with c-Met-positive tumors. Another c-Met therapeutic, cabozantinib, was developed by Exelixis and approved in 2012 for medullary thyroid cancer; this agent is unique in that it blocks not only c-Met but also VEGFR2.[47] Because c-Met has been implicated in the development of resistance to the VEGF pathway,[17] cabozantinib could have a therapeutic advantage over agents that target only the c-Met receptor.

The c-Met pathway also confers resistance to cytotoxic therapies such as radiation, and blocking c-Met signaling has been shown to reduce double-strand DNA repair capacity and thus increase the therapeutic ratio of radiation *in vitro*.[21,48] Radiation has further been shown to induce the c-Met pathway as a stress response; as such, blocking c-Met could be useful for tumors that express either high or low levels of c-Met when used in combination with radiation therapy.[49] Blockade of other kinase receptors such as EGFR[50] in combination with radiation has been shown to increase the therapeutic ratio, and studies of triple-combination therapy are underway in the BATTLE-XRT trial, in which personalized, tumor-specific anti-c-Met and anti-EGFR targeted therapeutics are used with radiation to treat patients with stage III NSCLC.

## HGF/c-Met-Targeted Therapies Now in Development

Three classes of molecules that target the HGF-c-Met axis are currently in development: antibodies against HGF; antibodies against c-Met; and synthetic small-molecule TKIs that specifically target the tyrosine kinase domain of c-Met. Examples of each of these three classes of therapeutics are given in the following sections.

### HGF Antibodies

Three leading HGF antibodies are currently in development: AMG-102 (rilotumumab), AV-299 (ficlatumzumab), and TAK-701. Rilotumumab is perhaps the most clinically advanced of the current HGF antibodies. A phase I trial showed that the maximum tolerated dose for this antibody was 20 mg/kg, given every 2 weeks. Although to date rilotumumab has shown little activity as single-agent therapy, its use in combination with panitumumab increased the response rate over that obtained with panitumumab alone (31% vs. 21%) in KRAS wild-type colorectal cancer.[51]

### c-Met Antibodies

Most of the anti-c-Met antibodies currently in development (OA5D5 (MetMAb, onartuzumab), LY-2875358, h224G11A, and DN30) primarily target the c-Met extracellular domain. A phase II trial of single-agent erlotinib with or without onartuzumab (MetMAb) for patients with refractory NSCLC and immunohistochemical evidence of c-Met overexpression by the primary tumor showed significant improvement in both progression-free and overall survival; these encouraging findings have led to a phase III trial, now ongoing.[46]

### Synthetic Small-Molecule Tyrosine Kinase Inhibitors

At least 12 c-Met TKIs were under development when this chapter was written, including both unselective and selective agents. The unselective agents (crizotinib, foretinib, cabozatinib, MGCD-265) also inhibit kinases other than c-Met such as VEGFR2, PDGFR, KIT, RON, ALK, RET, and TIE2. As noted previously, both crizotinib and cabozatinib have been approved for other indications as well. Selective c-Met TKIs in early development at this time include tivatinib, JNJ-38877605, AMG337, AMG208, PF-04217903, EMD-1214063, LY-2801653, and INC-280. Tivatinib, given in combination with erlotinib for nonsquamous NSCLC, showed a potential survival benefit in a phase II trial and is now being tested in a phase III clinical trial.[52]

## Mechanisms of Resistance

Therapeutic resistance is the primary factor limiting the effectiveness of current therapies for solid tumors, and thus strategies designed to overcome this resistance should readily translate into improved outcomes. Mechanisms underlying acquired resistance to pathway-targeted drugs are the subject of intense study, with the goal of being able to identify biomarker-defined patient subpopulations who are most likely (or least likely) to benefit from a particular therapy.[53] For instance, mechanisms of acquired resistance to kinase inhibitors in NSCLC and other types of cancer include amplification of the target kinase (*KIT* or *BCR-ABL*), overexpression of other kinases downstream of the target kinase (e.g., *LYN* in chronic myelogenous leukemia),[54,55] or secondary mutations in the kinase itself (*BCR-ABL, KIT, or EGFR*). EGFR inhibitors such as erlotinib and gefitinib can prolong survival in patients with *EGFR*-mutant NSCLC, but acquired resistance limits the long-term clinical efficacy of these drugs. The first mechanism of acquired resistance to EGFR TKIs, the EGFR T790 M mutation, was identified by investigators at Harvard Medical School[56] and at Memorial Sloan-Kettering Cancer Center[57] in 2005. Another mechanism of TKI resistance, amplification of c-Met, was discovered in 2007.[16,18]

HGF/c-Met overexpression has been linked with poor prognosis in NSCLC as well as in treatment resistance; cancer progression; and cell scattering, migration, and invasion.[58] Although amplification of c-Met is less common in untreated NSCLC,[59] both c-Met expression and mutations have been detected in NSCLC.[3] About 20% of patients with mutations in EGFR and acquired resistance to gefitinib or erlotinib also have acquired amplification of c-Met, but most untreated patients do not present with c-Met amplification.[16,18] Mechanistically, c-Met interacts with ERBB3 and activates downstream signals mediated by AKT that bypass the inhibited EGFR.[16] Inhibition of c-Met signaling by RNA interference can restore sensitivity to gefitinib, and dual inhibition of EGFR and c-Met with TKIs can overcome c-Met-amplified resistance to EGFR TKIs.[16] Interestingly, in about half of the patients with c-Met amplification, T790M was identified in biopsy specimens from both the primary tumor and other sites of metastatic disease.[16,18] In addition, patients with EGFR-activating mutations and primary resistance to gefitinib can have concomitant c-Met amplification,[60] suggesting that MET-amplified clones are selected in the presence of gefitinib or erlotinib.

C-Met activation has also been implicated in resistance to DNA-damaging agents.[61–63] Further, we and others have shown that c-Met expression is increased by radiation treatment[64,65] and that c-Met blockade radiosensitizes cancer cells to radiation.[49,66] Specifically, we found that blocking c-Met with the small-molecule inhibitor MP470 mitigated radiation resistance, increased cell death, and suppressed the double-stranded DNA repair enzyme RAD51 *in vitro*. In *in vivo* models, radiation plus c-Met blockade with MP470 led to substantial absolute growth delays, with an enhancement ratio of 2.9.[48] Further, when we irradiated lung cancer cells with low endogenous expression of c-Met (A549), we found a rapid and sustained expression of c-Met protein, which we assume is a stress response to radiation and contributes to further radiation resistance.[49] Even though c-Met antagonists did not radiosensitize cell lines with low endogenous c-Met expression, we nevertheless showed that the c-Met axis could still contribute to radiation resistance in these cell lines.[21,49]

These findings, plus the observation that radiation could influence radioresistance by increasing the expression of EGFR, led us to develop a phase II trial to evaluate the addition of erlotinib to whole-brain RT and found that erlotinib extended median overall survival time to 12 months versus 3.9 months for controls.[50] Findings from another phase II trial suggest that anti-EGFR therapy with erlotinib radiosensitized lung tumors in patients with stage III NSCLC, resulting in extended median overall survival times (Komaki et al., in preparation).

Ongoing clinical studies of c-Met inhibitors such as cabozantinib, foretinib, and tivantinib have shown some promising results,[67] but like many other targeted therapies, use of c-Met inhibitors as monotherapy can lead to treatment resistance.[68] Results of studies in which c-Met inhibitors are used in combination with chemotherapy or radiation are eagerly awaited, as they will increase our understanding of how signaling pathways interact with each other to promote therapy resistance and perhaps bring profound changes to current therapeutic approaches for lung cancer and other solid tumors.

## Future Perspectives

It seems clear that treatments targeting the c-Met pathway are likely to become an integral weapon in the oncologist's arsenal for treating solid tumors. However, what remains to be defined are which patients will derive benefit from c-Met-targeted therapies (e.g., those with mutations in c-Met, or perhaps those with elevated c-Met protein expression) and which combinations of therapy will best overcome the development of resistance. To date c-Met signaling has been shown to contribute to resistance to EGFR- and VEGF-targeted therapeutics, and thus these pathways may be good candidates to combine with c-Met blocking approaches. Other future developments could include new combinations of c-Met antibodies conjugated to drugs, similar to trastuzumab emtansine (T-DM1),[69] or targeting the c-Met pathway via microRNAs that regulate this pathway, such as miR-34a.[70] This powerful microRNA regulates several important oncologic proteins in addition to c-Met and is already in clinical trials for patients with metastatic disease to the liver. Because a single microRNA can regulate multiple pathways and hundreds of different proteins, use of microRNAs may have the potential to overcome resistance resulting from complex processes with multiple redundant feedback loops. Finally, in addition to its role in cancer therapeutics, c-Met may also be useful in molecular imaging and detection. GE recently developed a fluorodeoxyglucose-c-Met tracer for positron emission tomography that can be used to visualize c-Met expression on cellular surfaces in real time, *in vivo*. This technology could one day provide information helpful for disease staging, for defining areas at higher risk of recurrence, for identifying patients who are likely to benefit from c-Met antagonists, and finally for assessing response to treatment.

## References

1 Otsuka T, Takayama H, Sharp R, et al. c-Met autocrine activation induces development of malignant melanoma and acquisition of the metastatic phenotype. *Cancer Res.* 1998;58(22):5157–5167.

2 Takeuchi H, Bilchik A, Saha S, et al. c-MET expression level in primary colon cancer: a predictor of tumor invasion and lymph node metastases. *Clin Cancer Res.* 2003;9(4):1480–1488.

3 Ma PC, Jagadeeswaran R, Jagadeesh S, et al. Functional expression and mutations of c-Met and its therapeutic inhibition with SU11274 and small interfering RNA in non-small cell lung cancer. *Cancer Res.* 2005;65(4):1479–1488.

4 Di Renzo MF, Olivero M, Giacomini A, et al. Overexpression and amplification of the met/HGF receptor gene during the progression of colorectal cancer. *Clin Cancer Res.* 1995;1(2):147–154.

5 Harun N, Costa P, Christophi C. Tumour growth stimulation following partial hepatectomy in mice is associated with increased upregulation of c-Met. *Clin Exp Metastasis.* 2014;31(1):1–14.

6 Di Renzo MF, Olivero M, Martone T, et al. Somatic mutations of the MET oncogene are selected during metastatic spread of human HNSC carcinomas. *Oncogene.* 2000;19(12):1547–1555.

7 Montesano R, Matsumoto K, Nakamura T, Orci L. Identification of a fibroblast-derived epithelial morphogen as hepatocyte growth factor. *Cell.* 1991;67(5):901–908.

8 Bladt F, Riethmacher D, Isenmann S, Aguzzi A, Birchmeier C. Essential role for the c-met receptor in the migration of myogenic precursor cells into the limb bud. *Nature.* 1995;376(6543):768–771.

9 Kalluri R. EMT: when epithelial cells decide to become mesenchymal-like cells. *J Clin Invest.* 2009;119(6):1417–1419.

10 Rong S, Segal S, Anver M, Resau JH, Vande Woude GF. Invasiveness and metastasis of NIH 3T3 cells induced by Met-hepatocyte growth factor/scatter factor autocrine stimulation. *Proc Natl Acad Sci U S A.* 1994;91(11):4731–4735.

11 Christensen JG, Schreck R, Burrows J, et al. A selective small molecule inhibitor of c-Met kinase inhibits c-Met-dependent phenotypes in vitro and exhibits cytoreductive antitumor activity in vivo. *Cancer Res.* 2003;63(21):7345–7355.

12 Previdi S, Abbadessa G, Dalo F, France DS, Broggini M. Breast cancer-derived bone metastasis can be effectively reduced through specific c-MET inhibitor tivantinib (ARQ 197) and shRNA c-MET knockdown. *Mol Cancer Ther.* 2012;11(1):214–223.

13 Gherardi E, Birchmeier W, Birchmeier C, Vande Woude G. Targeting MET in cancer: rationale and progress. *Nat Rev Cancer.* 2012;12(2):89–103.

14 Yamamoto N, Mammadova G, Song RX, Fukami Y, Sato K. Tyrosine phosphorylation of p145met mediated by EGFR and Src is required for serum-independent survival of human bladder carcinoma cells. *J Cell Sci.* 2006;119(Pt 22):4623–4633.

15 Boon EM, van der Neut R, van de Wetering M, Clevers H, Pals ST. Wnt signaling regulates expression of the receptor tyrosine kinase met in colorectal cancer. *Cancer Res.* 2002;62(18):5126–5128.

16 Engelman JA, Zejnullahu K, Mitsudomi T, et al. MET amplification leads to gefitinib resistance in lung cancer by activating ERBB3 signaling. *Science.* 2007;316(5827):1039–1043.

17 Shojaei F, Lee JH, Simmons BH, et al. HGF/c-Met acts as an alternative angiogenic pathway in sunitinib-resistant tumors. *Cancer Res.* 2010;70(24):10090–100100.

18 Bean J, Brennan C, Shih JY, et al. MET amplification occurs with or without T790M mutations in EGFR mutant lung tumors with acquired resistance to gefitinib or erlotinib. *Proc Natl Acad Sci U S A.* 2007;104(52):20932–20937.

19 Christensen JG, Burrows J, Salgia R. c-Met as a target for human cancer and characterization of inhibitors for therapeutic intervention. *Cancer Lett.* 2005;225(1):1–26.

20 Pennacchietti S, Michieli P, Galluzzo M, Mazzone M, Giordano S, Comoglio PM. Hypoxia promotes invasive growth by transcriptional

activation of the met protooncogene. *Cancer Cell.* 2003;3(4):347–361.

21  Bhardwaj V, Cascone T, Cortez MA, et al. Modulation of c-Met signaling and cellular sensitivity to radiation: potential implications for therapy. *Cancer.* 2013;119(10):1768–1775.

22  Schmidt L, Duh FM, Chen F, et al. Germline and somatic mutations in the tyrosine kinase domain of the MET proto-oncogene in papillary renal carcinomas. *Nat Genet.* 1997;16(1):68–73.

23  Jeffers M, Schmidt L, Nakaigawa N, et al. Activating mutations for the met tyrosine kinase receptor in human cancer. *Proc Natl Acad Sci U S A.* 1997;94(21):11445–11450.

24  Lee JH, Han SU, Cho H, et al. A novel germ line juxtamembrane Met mutation in human gastric cancer. *Oncogene.* 2000;19(43):4947–4953.

25  Neklason DW, Done MW, Sargent NR, et al. Activating mutation in MET oncogene in familial colorectal cancer. *BMC Cancer.* 2011;11:424.

26  Kang JY, Dolled-Filhart M, Ocal IT, et al. Tissue microarray analysis of hepatocyte growth factor/Met pathway components reveals a role for Met, matriptase, and hepatocyte growth factor activator inhibitor 1 in the progression of node-negative breast cancer. *Cancer Res.* 2003;63(5):1101–1105.

27  Ghoussoub RA, Dillon DA, D'Aquila T, Rimm EB, Fearon ER, Rimm DL. Expression of c-met is a strong independent prognostic factor in breast carcinoma. *Cancer.* 1998;82(8):1513–1520.

28  Lee WY, Chen HH, Chow NH, Su WC, Lin PW, Guo HR. Prognostic significance of co-expression of RON and MET receptors in node-negative breast cancer patients. *Clin Cancer Res.* 2005;11(6):2222–2228.

29  Nakajima M, Sawada H, Yamada Y, et al. The prognostic significance of amplification and overexpression of c-met and c-erb B-2 in human gastric carcinomas. *Cancer.* 1999;85(9):1894–1902.

30  Masuya D, Huang C, Liu D, et al. The tumour-stromal interaction between intratumoral c-Met and stromal hepatocyte growth factor associated with tumour growth and prognosis in non-small-cell lung cancer patients. *Br J Cancer.* 2004;90(8):1555–1562.

31  Ueki T, Fujimoto J, Suzuki T, Yamamoto H, Okamoto E. Expression of hepatocyte growth factor and its receptor, the c-met proto-oncogene, in hepatocellular carcinoma. *Hepatology.* 1997;25(3):619–623.

32  Follenzi A, Bakovic S, Gual P, Stella MC, Longati P, Comoglio PM. Cross-talk between the proto-oncogenes Met and Ron. *Oncogene.* 2000;19(27):3041–3049.

33  Benvenuti S, Lazzari L, Arnesano A, Li Chiavi G, Gentile A, Comoglio PM. Ron kinase transphosphorylation sustains MET oncogene addiction. *Cancer Res.* 2011;71(5):1945–1955.

34  Yeh CY, Shin SM, Yeh HH, et al. Transcriptional activation of the Axl and PDGFR-alpha by c-Met through a ras- and Src-independent mechanism in human bladder cancer. *BMC Cancer.* 2011;11:139.

35  Conrotto P, Valdembri D, Corso S, et al. Sema4D induces angiogenesis through Met recruitment by plexin B1. *Blood.* 2005;105(11):4321–4329.

36  Hu B, Guo P, Bar-Joseph I, et al. Neuropilin-1 promotes human glioma progression through potentiating the activity of the HGF/SF autocrine pathway. *Oncogene.* 2007;26(38):5577–5586.

37  Sierra JR, Corso S, Caione L, et al. Tumor angiogenesis and progression are enhanced by Sema4D produced by tumor-associated macrophages. *J Exp Med.* 2008;205(7):1673–1685.

38  Jo M, Stolz DB, Esplen JE, Dorko K, Michalopoulos GK, Strom SC. Cross-talk between epidermal growth factor receptor and c-Met signal pathways in transformed cells. *J Biol Chem.* 2000;275(12):8806–8811.

39  Puri N, Salgia R. Synergism of EGFR and c-Met pathways, cross-talk and inhibition, in non-small cell lung cancer. *J Carcinog.* 2008;7:9.

40  Fong JT, Jacobs RJ, Moravec DN, et al. Alternative signaling pathways as potential therapeutic targets for overcoming EGFR and c-Met inhibitor resistance in non-small cell lung cancer. *PLoS One.* 2013;8(11):e78398.

41  Xu H, Stabile LP, Gubish CT, Gooding WE, Grandis JR, Siegfried JM. Dual blockade of EGFR and c-Met abrogates redundant signaling and proliferation in head and neck carcinoma cells. *Clin Cancer Res.* 2011;17(13):4425–4438.

42  Bachleitner-Hofmann T, Sun MY, Chen CT, et al. HER kinase activation confers resistance to MET tyrosine kinase inhibition in MET oncogene-addicted gastric cancer cells. *Mol Cancer Ther.* 2008;7(11):3499–3508.

43  Khoury H, Naujokas MA, Zuo D, et al. HGF converts ErbB2/Neu epithelial morphogenesis to cell invasion. *Mol Biol Cell.* 2005;16(2):550–561.

44  Turke AB, Zejnullahu K, Wu YL, et al. Preexistence and clonal selection of MET amplification in EGFR mutant NSCLC. *Cancer Cell.* 2010;17(1):77–88.

45  Belalcazar A, Azana D, Perez CA, Raez LE, Santos ES. Targeting the Met pathway in lung cancer. *Exp Rev Anticancer Ther.* 2012;12(4):519–528.

46  Spigel DR, Ervin TJ, Ramlau RA, et al. Randomized phase II trial of onartuzumab in combination with erlotinib in patients with advanced non-small-cell lung cancer. *J Clin Oncol.* 2013;31(32):4105–4114.

47  Bentzien F, Zuzow M, Heald N, et al. In vitro and in vivo activity of cabozantinib (XL184), an inhibitor of RET, MET, and VEGFR2, in a model of medullary thyroid cancer. *Thyroid.* 2013;23(12):1569–1577.

48  Welsh JW, Mahadevan D, Ellsworth R, Cooke L, Bearss D, Stea B. The c-Met receptor tyrosine kinase inhibitor MP470 radiosensitizes glioblastoma cells. *Radiat Oncol.* 2009;4:69.

49  Bhardwaj V, Zhan Y, Cortez MA, et al. C-Met inhibitor MK-8003 radiosensitizes c-Met-expressing non-small-cell lung cancer cells with radiation-induced c-Met-expression. *J Thorac Oncol.* 2012;7(8):1211–1217.

50  Welsh JW, Komaki R, Amini A, et al. Phase II trial of erlotinib plus concurrent whole-brain radiation therapy for patients with brain metastases from non-small cell lung cancer. *J Clin Oncol.* 2013;31(7):895–902.

51  Tebbutt NC, Cutsem EV, Eng C, et al. A randomized, phase Ib/II trial of rilotumumab (AMG 102; ril) or ganitumab (AMG 479; gan) with panitumumab (pmab) vs pmab alone in patients with wild-type (WT) KRAS metastatic colorectal cancer (mCRC): primary and biomarker analyses (abstract). *J Clin Oncol.* 2011;29(suppl 15):221s (abstr 3500).

52  Sequist LV, von Pawel J, Garmey EG, et al. Randomized phase II study of erlotinib plus tivantinib versus erlotinib plus placebo in previously treated non-small-cell lung cancer. *J Clin Oncol.* 2011;29(24):3307–3315.

53  Lackner MR, Wilson TR, Settleman J. Mechanisms of acquired resistance to targeted cancer therapies. *Future Oncol.* 2012;8(8):999–1014.

54  Kosaka T, Yatabe Y, Endoh H, et al. Analysis of epidermal growth factor receptor gene mutation in patients with non-small cell lung cancer and acquired resistance to gefitinib. *Clin Cancer Res.* 2006;12(19):5764–5769.

55  Donato NJ, Wu JY, Stapley J, et al. BCR-ABL independence and LYN kinase overexpression in chronic myelogenous leukemia cells selected for resistance to STI571. *Blood.* 2003;101(2):690–698.

56  Kobayashi S, Boggon TJ, Dayaram T, et al. EGFR mutation and resistance of non-small-cell lung cancer to gefitinib. *N Engl J Med.* 2005;352(8):786–792.

57  Pao W, Miller VA, Politi KA, et al. Acquired resistance of lung adenocarcinomas to gefitinib or erlotinib is associated with a second mutation in the EGFR kinase domain. *PLoS Med.* 2005;2(3):e73.

58  Siegfried JM, Weissfeld LA, Singh-Kaw P, Weyant RJ, Testa JR, Landreneau RJ. Association of immunoreactive hepatocyte growth factor with poor survival in resectable non-small cell lung cancer. *Cancer Res.* 1997;57(3):433–439.

59 Beau-Faller M, Ruppert AM, Voegeli AC, et al. MET gene copy number in non-small cell lung cancer: molecular analysis in a targeted tyrosine kinase inhibitor naive cohort. *J Thorac Oncol.* 2008;3(4):331–339.

60 Sequist LV, Lynch TJ. EGFR tyrosine kinase inhibitors in lung cancer: an evolving story. *Annu Rev Med.* 2008;59:429–442.

61 Li Y, Lal B, Kwon S, et al. The scatter factor/hepatocyte growth factor: c-met pathway in human embryonal central nervous system tumor malignancy. *Cancer Res.* 2005;65:9355–9362.

62 Laterra J, Rosen E, Nam M, et al. Scatter factor/hepatocyte growth factor expression enhances human glioblastoma tumorigenicity and growth. *Biochem Biophys Res Commun.* 1997;235:743–747.

63 Koochekpour S, Jeffers M, Rulong S, et al. Met and hepatocyte growth factor/scatter factor expression in human gliomas. *Cancer Res.* 1997;57:5391–5398.

64 Qian LW, Mizumoto K, Inadome N, et al. Radiation stimulates HGF receptor/c-Met expression that leads to amplifying cellular response to HGF stimulation via upregulated receptor tyrosine phosphorylation and MAP kinase activity in pancreatic cancer cells. *Int J Cancer.* 2003;104(5):542–549.

65 De Bacco F, Luraghi P, Medico E, et al. Induction of MET by ionizing radiation and its role in radioresistance and invasive growth of cancer. *J Natl Cancer Inst.* 2011;103(8):645–661.

66 Buchanan IM, Scott T, Tandle AT, et al. Radiosensitization of glioma cells by modulation of Met signalling with the hepatocyte growth factor neutralizing antibody, AMG102. *J Cell Mol Med.* 2011;15(9):1999–2006.

67 Underiner TL, Herbertz T, Miknyoczki SJ. Discovery of small molecule c-Met inhibitors: evolution and profiles of clinical candidates. *Anticancer Agents Med Chem.* 2010;10(1):7–27.

68 Liu X, Newton RC, Scherle PA. Developing c-MET pathway inhibitors for cancer therapy: progress and challenges. *Trends Mol Med.* 2010;16(1):37–45.

69 Krop I, Winer EP. Trastuzumab emtansine: a novel antibody-drug conjugate for HER2-positive breast cancer. *Clin Cancer Res.* 2014;20(1):15–20.

70 Li N, Fu H, Tie Y, et al. miR-34a inhibits migration and invasion by down-regulation of c-Met expression in human hepatocellular carcinoma cells. *Cancer Lett.* 2009;275(1):44–53.

## CHAPTER 35

# KIT Kinase

*Scott E. Woodman*
Departments of Melanoma Medical Oncology and Systems Biology, The University of Texas MD Anderson Cancer Center, Houston, TX, USA

## KIT Biology

The *KIT* (*c*-kit) tyrosine kinase receptor gene was identified in 1987 based on sequence similarity to the oncogenic transforming Hardy–Zuckerman 4 feline sarcoma virus (*v-kit*).[1,2] Human *KIT* is located on chromosome 4q11 and consists of 21 exons that encode for a 976 amino acid protein. Of the fifty-eight receptor tyrosine kinases (RTKs) in the human genome,[3] KIT (a.k.a., CD117) is a member of the class III RTKs along with the platelet-derived growth factor alpha and beta receptors (PDGFR α/β), Fms-like tyrosine kinase 3 receptor (FLT3), and colony stimulating factor 1 receptor (CSF1R). Type III RTKs are characterized by a glycosylated extracellular ligand-binding domain containing five immunoglobulin-like (Ig-like) repeats, a single hydrophobic transmembrane domain, an intracellular juxtamembrane inhibitory domain, and two regions that constitute the tyrosine kinase domain (see Figure 35.1).[4] Alternative splicing of *KIT* can result in the loss of a GNNK amino acid sequence at the 5′ end of the extracellular domain and/or the loss of a serine amino acid residue in the kinase domain.[5,6] Thus four possible isoforms of the *KIT* gene can be expressed in human cells. There is some data to suggest that the isoform without the GNNK amino acid sequence has greater transforming and oncogenic properties.[5] The KIT protein undergoes post-translational N-linked glycosylation at multiple sites in the extracellular juxtamembrane region.

The cognate ligands for the class III RTKs are each dimers. Stem cell factor (SCF, a.k.a., kit ligand, steel factor, or mast cell growth factor) is a glycosylated transmembrane protein identified to be the ligand for KIT. Alternative splicing results in the presence or absence of a proteolytic cleavage site within SCF.[7] If splicing results in the presence of the cleavage site, the cleaved SCF can be released from the cell surface. Both the cleaved and membrane-bound forms of SCF are capable of serving as a ligand for KIT.

Unbound KIT exists mostly as an autoinhibited monomer at the cell surface with very low affinity for other KIT monomers.[8] Autoinhibition in the unbound state is facilitated by two major biophysical mechanisms: (1) repulsive electrostatic interactions of the extracellular juxtamembrane region and (2) structural interference imposed on the activation loop within the kinase domain by the intracellular juxtamembrane domain. The dimeric SCF ligand binds and couples the KIT Ig-like domains 1–3 highly favoring KIT dimerization. In the extracellular portion of KIT, the conformational change is most dramatic in the regions between the 3–4th and the 4–5th

Ig-like domains, bringing the 4th and 5th Ig-like domains of each KIT in proximity.[9] Upon dimerization, each KIT molecule transactivates the adjacent KIT molecule through ATP-driven autophosphorylation at specific tyrosines (Y568 and Y570) within the intracellular juxtamembrane domain relieving the inhibition imposed on the activation loop. Further transphosphorylation ensues on multiple tyrosines (e.g., Y703, Y721, Y730, Y823, Y900, Y936) which serve to directly or indirectly (through adaptor proteins) activate downstream signaling molecules.[8] It has been shown that binding of the soluble form of SCF causes KIT activation, internalization, and degradation, whereas binding of the membrane-bound form of SCF results in prolonged KIT activation, however, the ultimate effect of SCF–KIT interaction can be cell specific.[10] Activated KIT has been shown to initiate multiple downstream signaling pathways (e.g., MAPK/MEK, PI3K/AKT, JAK/STAT, SRC) that can vary depending on the cellular context in which KIT is activated.[11–14]

The necessity of KIT for particular cellular development and function is eloquently revealed through the phenotypic defects that result from its loss or reduced activity in mice, most notably mice harboring the "W" white spotting locus.[15] Following the identification of the *KIT* gene, mutations in *KIT* were shown to be the cause of W mice phenotypes. The complete loss of KIT activity results in in utero or perinatal death. Of those mice which survive, the severity of the phenotype expressed correlates with the degree of KIT activity. The W locus was identified based upon the observation that some pigmented mice develop a hypopigmented white spot on the ventral surface. In addition to pigment alterations, the W mice were infertile, deaf, and developed hematopoietic defects (macrocytic anemia, mast cell loss). These "loss of function" phenotypes were all the result of a failure of particular stem cell populations to migrate and survive and would foreshadow the cancers observed to have somatic "gain-of-function" mutations in particular cell types.

## KIT in Cancer

Gain-of-function *KIT* mutations were first identified in the human mast cell leukemia cell line HMC-1 .[16] The mutations localized to exon 11 (intracellular juxtamembrane domain) and exon 17 (kinase domain), and each was shown to result in constitutive SCF-independent activation of KIT. Decades of assessing the *KIT* gene mutation status in multiple tumor types have demonstrated that *KIT* gain-of-function mutations are present in many cancers at low

*Targeted Therapy in Translational Cancer Research*, First Edition. Edited by Apostolia-Maria Tsimberidou, Razelle Kurzrock and Kenneth C. Anderson.
© 2016 John Wiley & Sons, Inc. Published 2016 by John Wiley & Sons, Inc.

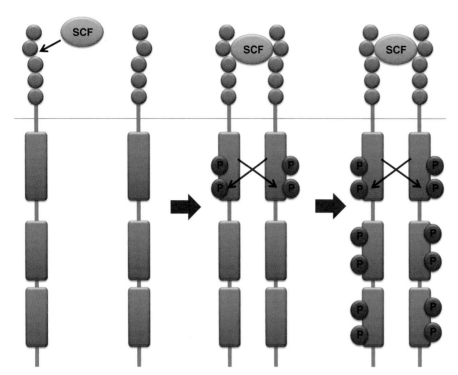

**Figure 35.1** Activation of the KIT tyrosine kinase receptor. The natural ligand for KIT, stem cell factor (SCF, orange oval) binds to the extracellular region of KIT resulting in dimerization and autophosphorylation of intracellular tyrosine residues. The conformational change resulting from autophosphorylation perpetuates the further phosphorylation of other tyrosine residues that serve as sites that initiate downstream signaling. Activating mutations in the KIT gene result in the constitutive activation (not needing SCF initiation) of the KIT protein.

frequency, but have a significantly higher frequency in mastocytosis, gastrointestinal stromal tumor (GIST), and particular subsets of melanoma, acute myeloid leukemia (AML), and germ cell tumors.[11-14] Thus many of the cell types in which *KIT* gain-of-function mutations have been identified are the same as those in which *KIT* loss-of-function mutations result in developmental pathology, suggesting the link between the stem cell and cancer cell states.

Consistent with biological structure and function, activating mutations in the *KIT* gene occur in the exons that encode for regulatory or activating regions in the protein (Figure 35.1). It is of note, however, that the *KIT* mutations in different cancers tend to be enriched in particular exons, be of a particular type (e.g., missense, indel), and in some cases, primarily alter a specific amino acid. Overall, these mutations result in constitutive ligand-independent activation of KIT, however, there may be significant differences in the particular signaling cascades associated with different mutations and the sensitivity of particular mutations to small-molecule inhibition.[15]

### Gastrointestinal Stromal Tumor

Activating mutations in the *KIT* gene are present in up to 80% of GIST tumors.[17] Approximately two-thirds of these mutations localize to exon 11 resulting in dysfunction of the intracellular autoinhibitory juxtamembrane domain.[18] Insertions or deletions (indels) and substitution mutations have all been observed, but the majority of *KIT* exon 11 mutations are indels. Among *KIT* Exon 11 mutations, deletion mutations correlate with a shorter progression-free and overall survival.[19,20] Approximately 10–15% of *KIT* mutations in GIST occur in the extracellular region encoded by exon 9 resulting in a conformational change that is thought to mimic SCF binding.[9] Mutations in exon 9, unlike exon 11 mutations, do not appear to significantly alter the kinase domain. Of note, Exon 9 mutations are rarely observed in gastric GIST, and are primarily seen in intestinal GIST.[21] Primary mutations in exons 13, 17, or 18 of *KIT* are rare

in GIST, but when present serve to stabilize the active state of the kinase.[22]

### Acute Myeloid Leukemia

*KIT* mutations have been identified in approximately 20–40% of adults and 20% of pediatric cases of the core binding factor (CBF) subset of AML.[23,24] CBF–AMLs are correlated with the fusion genes AML-ETO or CBFB-MYHII that result from the chromosomal aberrations t,[8;21] or inv,[16] respectively. The *KIT* mutations in CBF–AMLs are mostly missense mutations (affecting primarily the D816 amino acid) within activation loop encoded by exon 17 or indels within the extracellular domain encoded by exon 8 resulting in the conformational mimicking of KIT being bound by SCF. The co-occurrence of an activating *KIT* mutation in CBF–AMLs has been reported to result in worse clinical outcomes prompting the National Comprehensive Cancer Network's (NCCN) guidelines to list CBF–AMLs with a *KIT* mutation as an intermediate prognosis group compared to the favorable prognostic status of having CBF–AML alone.[23-25] Although the presence of a *KIT* mutation is associated with a higher incidence of relapse, there are competing results regarding overall survival.[26,27]

### Mastocytosis

Mastocytosis is a subset of myeloproliferative disease and is classified as either cutaneous (most frequent and good prognosis) or systemic. Systemic mastocytosis (SM) is further characterized by the clinical course: indolent (ISM) versus advanced (consisting of aggressive (ASM), SM associated with clonal hematologic non-mast cell lineage disease (SM-AHNMD) and mast cell leukemia (MCL)).[28,29] Each of the more advanced forms of mastocytosis is associated with a worse median survival: ASM 41 months, SM-AHNMD 24 months, and MCL 2 months.[30] Approximately 90%+ with advanced SM harbor an activating *KIT* mutation. By far the most frequent somatic *KIT* mutations in SM are missense mutations in exon 17 that affect the D816 amino acid (most commonly

D816V) within the activation loop.[29] The presence of a *KIT* D816V mutation is associated with a higher mast cell burden in the bone marrow and disease aggressiveness, made worse by the number of cell lineages involved.[30,31] As with CBF–AML, the sensitivity of the method used to detect *KIT* mutations is very important.

## Melanoma

Multiple studies have identified *KIT* mutations in subsets of melanoma: acral lentiginous (ALM), mucosal (MM), and chronic sun-damaged (CSD).[14,32–34] ALM and MM are distinct from other subsets of melanoma in that they do not have a predilection for fair skinned, light-eyed individuals, but rather are essentially proportionately distributed across populations of all skin tones and races.[35] ALM and MM do not appear to be UV radiation mediated. In addition, these subtypes of melanoma tend to be associated with a worse prognosis than sun-damaged melanomas, although the factors appear to be multifactorial and not purely biological. Activating *KIT* mutations are identified in approximately 20% of ALM and MM melanomas. CSD melanoma is contrasted with nonchronic sun-damaged melanoma and is associated with a relatively higher degree of solar elastosis upon histological evaluation.[36] The term "lentigo maligna" is used to describe melanomas that arise after long-term sun exposure, typically on fair-skinned older individuals, and many lentigo maligna lesions are determined to be CSD upon histological review. *KIT* mutations are present in up to 10% of CSD cases. CSD melanoma accounts for approximately 10–15% of all melanomas, and although CSD tends to have a better prognosis than non-CSD, it can still be a very lethal form of melanoma. Unlike the other neoplasias, *KIT* mutations in melanoma are dispersed across the hotspot exons with greater frequency: exon 9 (5%), exon 11 (45%), exon 13 (25%), exon 17 (10%), exon 18 (15%). Over 90% of *KIT* mutations in melanoma are missense mutations.[14,32,33,37,38]

## Seminoma

Reports of activating *KIT* mutations in germ cell tumors vary in frequency, with ranges from <5–40%, however, the data clearly show that the majority of *KIT* mutations occur in testicular seminomas (vs. nonseminomas) and unilateral ovarian dysgerminomas.[39–41] These mutations are typically located in exon 17 of the *KIT* gene, primarily at the D816 amino acid position. A COSMIC database review found *KIT* mutations in 20% of seminomas, with nearly twice as many (38%) extragonadal seminomas harboring *KIT* mutations, and no extragonadal nonseminomas having *KIT* mutations.[42] More divergent results have been reported as to whether *KIT* mutations are more prevalent in bilateral testicular seminomas, and therefore, identification of a *KIT* mutation may not serve as a predictor of contralateral tumor risk.[43–45]

## KIT as a Therapeutic Target

With the success of small-molecule kinase inhibition of the constitutively activated ABL kinase in CML, researchers went on to test other gain-of-function mutant kinases. It was observed that imatinib inhibited the growth of activated mutant *KIT*-driven cells, and soon after that imatinib administration had a profound impact on advanced *KIT*-mutant GIST tumors.[17] Imatinib binds directly to the ATP-binding site within KIT, competitively inhibiting ATP binding, stabilizing the kinase in the inactive conformation.[15] As nearly all primary *KIT* mutations in GIST localize to the intracellular juxtamembrane (exon 11) or extracellular juxtamembrane (exon 9) domains, and not the kinase domains (exons 13/14 and 17/18),

inhibition targeted directly at the kinase domain (ATP-binding site) was an effective molecular strategy in GIST. In the pre-imatinib era, advanced GIST was essentially refractory to therapy and the median survival was no more than 1.5 years. The current median survival for advanced GIST patients treated with imatinib is approximately 5 years, with about 35% of patients alive at a 9.4-year median follow-up.[46] In addition, recent data shows that adjuvant treatment decreases the risk of relapse after surgery with curative intent.[47,48] A review of long-term follow-up results from major clinical studies not only revealed the extended efficacy and safety of imatinib treatment, but also showed that imatinib treatment should not be interrupted, as efficacy following reintroduction is inferior.[46]

About 10% of GIST patients exhibit primary resistance to imatinib treatment (progression within the first 6 months). The probability of primary resistance is approximately threefold higher for *KIT* exon 9 mutant tumors than *KIT* exon 11 mutant tumors, although it is possible that treating *KIT* exon 9 mutant tumors with a lower than optimal dose may underlie part of this difference.[49] Primary imatinib resistance is not associated with the presence of another mutation in the *KIT* gene. Secondary imatinib resistance (disease progression after initial benefit), however, is typically associated with the presence of an acquired mutation in the same allele as the original *KIT* mutation. Acquired *KIT* resistance mutations occur in one of two regions of the kinase domain: (1) ATP-binding site (exons 13/14), interfering with imatinib binding or (2) activation loop (exons 17/18), stabilizing the active conformation of KIT.[17,50] Since imatinib can only inhibit KIT when the kinase is in the inactive conformation, long-term response is not typically achieved by increasing the dose of imatinib. Sunitinib, a TKI with a broader range of kinase targets (including the VEGFR family members) showed significant improvement in the median time to progression compared to placebo in imatinib-resistant GIST tumors and gained FDA approval for this setting.[51] Sunitinib is proposed to have efficacy in the setting of secondary resistance caused by exon 14 "gatekeeper" mutations because it is smaller than imatinib and thus avoids the steric hindrance imposed by these specific mutations.[52] Sunitinib does not inhibit activation loop mutants. The other tyrosine kinases targeted by sunitinib may also play a role, as non-*KIT*-mutant GIST tumors also showed response to sunitinib treatment. However, resistance to sunitinib ultimately develops. The most recently FDA-approved agent for TKI-resistant GIST is regorafenib, also a multikinase inhibitor. Treatment of TKI-resistant GIST with regorafenib resulted in a median PFS of 4.8 months compared with 0.9 months for the placebo group.[53] As with sunitinib, the non-KIT kinase targets of regorafenib may account for the activity observed. With the exception of nilotinib, which did not show significant activity in the third-line setting,[54] TKIs that target KIT (e.g., dasatinib, sorafenib) have not been sufficiently tested in third-line clinical trials to draw universal conclusions, but clinical activity has been observed.

Multiple studies examining the efficacy of imatinib in unselected populations of advanced melanoma patients did not reveal a significant response rate.[55–57] However, the identification of activating *KIT* mutations in the ALM, MM, and CSD melanoma subtypes generated interest in testing the effect of KIT inhibition in *KIT*-mutant melanoma. Early case studies showed responses in tumors with *KIT* mutations to TKIs (imatinib, sunitinib, sorafenib, and dasatinib) with known activity against particular activating *KIT* mutations.[58–63] Recently, three prospective phase II studies evaluating the efficacy of imatinib in melanoma tumor subsets enriched with *KIT* mutations were recently reported.[64–66] Taken together, these three studies support the concept that melanoma tumors that display sensitivity to imatinib treatment tend to harbor recurrent activating mutations in exons 11 and 13 of *KIT* (particularly, *KIT* L576P and K462E, respectively). Tumors with amplification of the wild-type *KIT* gene did not show significant sensitivity to imatinib treatment. These observations hold for much smaller studies looking at the effect of sunitinib or nilotinib.[67,68] Clear caveats from these studies (and multiple case reports) are that the presence of a *KIT* exon 11 or 13 mutation in a melanoma tumor does not ensure tumor response to these TKIs. In the two phase II clinical studies that specified which amino acid position was altered by a mutation in *KIT*, 7 of 11 (64%) of *KIT* L576P and 3 of 7 (43%) of *KIT* K642E-mutant tumors responded to imatinib. Despite response rates not being on par with imatinib-treated *KIT*-mutant GIST, the rates of response, even accounting for the varied responses observed in nonrecurrent *KIT*-mutant tumors, are far beyond any chemotherapy ever attempted in these subtypes of melanoma and are a very encouraging starting point. However, the duration of the response and overall survival observed in mutant *KIT* melanoma, with a few exceptions, do not begin to compare to imatinib-treated GIST. In addition, it is clear tumors with other *KIT* mutations, typically in exon 11 (e.g., V559X, V560D), can also show sensitivity to imatinib, and even a *KIT* mutation in exon 17 (D820Y) has been reported to respond to imatinib.[64] A clearer sense of the frequency of response in tumors harboring "nonrecurrent" *KIT* mutations awaits the assessment of larger cohorts. The report by Carvajal et al. suggests that recurrent activating mutations with a greater mutant to wild-type allele ratio may be more sensitive to imatinib therapy, but this observation awaits validation with greater numbers of samples.[65] Finally, it is of note, that although insertion/deletion mutations in *KIT* are rare in melanoma, tumors harboring such mutations (in exon 11, akin to common *KIT* mutations found in GIST) have been reported to show marked response to KIT-inhibiting TKIs (also, unpublished observations).

The vast majority of patients with systemic mastocytosis show the presence of a *KIT* D816V mutation in mastocytosis cells and multiple hematopoietic cell lineages within the bone marrow.[29] This exon 17 mutation confers relative resistance to imatinib. However, imatinib is FDA approved for adult patients with systemic mastocytosis with a non-*KIT* D816V mutation (or with unknown *KIT* mutation status), as less common *KIT* mutations tend to occur in exons 9 or 11. For the far more prevalent *KIT* D816V-mutant systemic mastocytosis cases, other TKIs that may have greater efficacy against this mutation are under evaluation. Early preclinical data showed dasatinib to have marked *in vitro* activity against the *KIT* D816V mutation.[69,70] As part of a phase II clinical trial, patients with mastocytosis harboring a *KIT* D816V mutation have been shown to gain symptomatic benefit.[71] In addition, some mastocytosis tumors without a *KIT* mutation also benefited from dasatinib treatment, revealing that kinases other than *KIT* may be involved in mastocytosis. Midostaurin, another TKI that targets KIT, has been reported to result in high response rates in advanced mastocytosis; with a median duration of response of 29 months and a median survival of 41 months. These results come from an update of the global D2201 Trial (NCT00782067).

## KIT Future Strategies

As this review focuses specifically on the *KIT* oncogene, only future strategies that entail the KIT molecule or its immediate downstream mediators will be considered. A deep interrogation

into the molecular underpinnings that mediate *KIT*-mutant-driven cancers, especially GIST, has revealed the mechanisms by which some of these cancers respond or do not respond to TKIs, as well as, develop resistance to specific TKIs. Knowing the exon location of a *KIT* mutation and the specific amino acid alteration(s) that results has been very predictive of which GIST tumors will respond to imatinib. However, there is considerable heterogeneity within and between tumors. Imatinib-resistant GIST tumors within the same individual can harbor different acquired *KIT* mutations. In addition, an imatinib-resistant GIST tumor can harbor different acquired *KIT* mutations in different regions of the tumor.[72,73] Both inter- and intratumor-resistant clones support the observation that complete eradication of GIST cells is not achieved under the selective pressure of imatinib treatment. Although other TKIs with a broader range of efficacy against some of the acquired *KIT* mutations are employed in acquired imatinib resistance, the heterogeneity of *KIT* mutations within these tumors will require a therapy that inhibits the variety of secondary mutations that emerge.

A strategy to approach the given heterogeneity of tumors is to inhibit the downstream mediators of activated mutant *KIT*, regardless of the specific mutation. The MAPK and PI3K pathways have clearly been shown to be mediators of activated KIT in numerous cell types. Recent *in vivo* preclinical data shows the combination of imatinib with a selective class I PI3K inhibitor to result in a marked antiproliferative and apoptotic effect, not observed with either agent alone.[74] This effect showed durability after drug discontinuation. It is important when testing combinatorial strategies to determine which member(s) of a particular pathway to target. For example, the PI3K pathway can be inhibited at the level of the PI3K or AKT molecules. Each of these molecules has at least multiple distinct isoforms which may be differentially activated. In addition the PI3K pathway is highly regulated by the tumor suppressor PTEN which may be variably expressed across tumors. Another potential strategy to combat the heterogeneity of acquired TKI-resistant tumors is the use of a monoclonal antibody that specifically disables the KIT receptor by inducing receptor internalization and degradation, as well as, potentially initiating an immune response against the cell expressing the KIT receptor.[75] The function of many normal cells requires activation of the MAPK and PI3K pathways, and KIT activity plays important role in normal tissue function. For either the "downstream inhibitor" or "antibody targeting" strategies to be clinically relevant, the "off-target" effects will have to be outweighed by the clinical efficacy.

Although GIST serves as an illuminating model of how to approach KIT mutations in other cancers, the cellular milieu in which activating *KIT* mutations function may significantly alter the efficacy of approaches attempting to be translated from the GIST experience. This is suggested by early data from *KIT*-mutant melanoma, where imatinib treatment of "imatinib-sensitive" *KIT*-mutant tumors does not appear to result in the frequency of durable tumor responses/stability observed in GIST. Thus, it will be important to properly model each KIT-mutant cancer to account for the cancer-specific differences.

## References

1 Besmer P, Murphy JE, George PC, et al. A new acute transforming feline retrovirus and relationship of its oncogene v-kit with the protein kinase gene family. *Nature.* 1986;320(6061):415–421.

2 Yarden Y, Kuang WJ, Yang-Feng T, et al. Human proto-oncogene c-kit: a new cell surface receptor tyrosine kinase for an unidentified ligand. *EMBO J.* 1987;6(11):3341–3351.

3 Choura M, Rebai A. Receptor tyrosine kinases: from biology to pathology. *J Recept Signal Transduct Res.* 2011;31(6):387–394.

4 Ronnstrand L. Signal transduction via the stem cell factor receptor/c-Kit. *Cell Mol Life Sci.* 2004;61(19–20):2535–2548.

5 Crosier PS, Ricciardi ST, Hall LR, Vitas MR, Clark SC, Crosier KE. Expression of isoforms of the human receptor tyrosine kinase c-kit in leukemic cell lines and acute myeloid leukemia. *Blood.* 1993;82(4):1151–1158.

6 Reith AD, Ellis C, Lyman SD, et al. Signal transduction by normal isoforms and W mutant variants of the Kit receptor tyrosine kinase. *EMBO J.* 1991;10(9):2451–2459.

7 Huang EJ, Nocka KH, Buck J, Besmer P. Differential expression and processing of two cell associated forms of the kit-ligand: KL-1 and KL-2. *Mol Biol Cell.* 1992;3(3):349–362.

8 Verstraete K, Savvides SN. Extracellular assembly and activation principles of oncogenic class III receptor tyrosine kinases. *Nat Rev Cancer.* 2012;12(11):753–766.

9 Yuzawa S, Opatowsky Y, Zhang Z, Mandiyan V, Lax I, Schlessinger J. Structural basis for activation of the receptor tyrosine kinase KIT by stem cell factor. *Cell.* 2007;130(2):323–334.

10 Miyazawa K, Williams DA, Gotoh A, Nishimaki J, Broxmeyer HE, Toyama K. Membrane-bound Steel factor induces more persistent tyrosine kinase activation and longer life span of c-kit gene-encoded protein than its soluble form. *Blood.* 1995;85(3):641–649.

11 Lennartsson J, Jelacic T, Linnekin D, Shivakrupa R. Normal and oncogenic forms of the receptor tyrosine kinase kit. *Stem Cells.* 2005;23(1):16–43.

12 Corless CL, Heinrich MC. Molecular pathobiology of gastrointestinal stromal sarcomas. *Annu Rev Pathol.* 2008;3:557–586.

13 Orfao A, Garcia-Montero AC, Sanchez L, Escribano L. Recent advances in the understanding of mastocytosis: the role of KIT mutations. *Br J Haematol.* 2007;138(1):12–30.

14 Woodman SE, Davies MA. Targeting KIT in melanoma: a paradigm of molecular medicine and targeted therapeutics. *Biochem Pharmacol.* 2010;80(5):568–574.

15 Lennartsson J, Ronnstrand L. Stem cell factor receptor/c-Kit: from basic science to clinical implications. *Physiol Rev.* 2012;92(4):1619–1649.

16 Furitsu T, Tsujimura T, Tono T, et al. Identification of mutations in the coding sequence of the proto-oncogene c-kit in a human mast cell leukemia cell line causing ligand-independent activation of c-kit product. *J Clin Invest.* 1993;92(4):1736–1744.

17 Corless CL, Barnett CM, Heinrich MC. Gastrointestinal stromal tumours: origin and molecular oncology. *Nat Rev Cancer.* 2011;11(12):865–878.

18 Mol CD, Dougan DR, Schneider TR, et al. Structural basis for the autoinhibition and STI-571 inhibition of c-Kit tyrosine kinase. *J Biol Chem.* 2004;279(30):31655–31663.

19 Singer S, Rubin BP, Lux ML, et al. Prognostic value of KIT mutation type, mitotic activity, and histologic subtype in gastrointestinal stromal tumors. *J Clin Oncol.* 2002;20(18):3898–3905.

20 Andersson J, Bumming P, Meis-Kindblom JM, et al. Gastrointestinal stromal tumors with KIT exon 11 deletions are associated with poor prognosis. *Gastroenterology.* 2006;130(6):1573–1581.

21 Antonescu CR, Viale A, Sarran L, et al. Gene expression in gastrointestinal stromal tumors is distinguished by KIT genotype and anatomic site. *Clin Cancer Res.* 2004;10(10):3282–3290.

22 Lasota J, Corless CL, Heinrich MC, et al. Clinicopathologic profile of gastrointestinal stromal tumors (GISTs) with primary KIT exon 13

or exon 17 mutations: a multicenter study on 54 cases. *Mod Pathol.* 2008;21(4):476–484.

23 Park SH, Chi HS, Min SK, Park BG, Jang S, Park CJ. Prognostic impact of c-KIT mutations in core binding factor acute myeloid leukemia. *Leuk Res.* 2011;35(10):1376–1383.

24 Pollard JA, Alonzo TA, Gerbing RB, et al. Prevalence and prognostic significance of KIT mutations in pediatric patients with core binding factor AML enrolled on serial pediatric cooperative trials for de novo AML. *Blood.* 2010;115(12):2372–2379.

25 Paschka P, Marcucci G, Ruppert AS, et al. Cancer and Leukemia Group B. Adverse prognostic significance of KIT mutations in adult acute myeloid leukemia with inv(16) and t(8;21): a Cancer and Leukemia Group B Study. *J Clin Oncol.* 2006;24(24):3904–3911.

26 Allen C, Hills RK, Lamb K, et al. The importance of relative mutant level for evaluating impact on outcome of KIT, FLT3 and CBL mutations in core-binding factor acute myeloid leukemia. *Leukemia.* 2013;27(9):1891–1901.

27 Cairoli R, Beghini A, Turrini M, et al. Old and new prognostic factors in acute myeloid leukemia with deranged core-binding factor beta. *Am J Hematol.* 2013;88(7):594–600.

28 Carter MC, Metcalfe DD, Komarow HD. Mastocytosis. *Immunol Allergy Clin North Am.* 2014;34(1):181–196.

29 Verstovsek S. Advanced systemic mastocytosis: the impact of KIT mutations in diagnosis, treatment, and progression. *Eur J Haematol.* 2013;90(2):89–98.

30 Lim KH, Tefferi A, Lasho TL, et al. Systemic mastocytosis in 342 consecutive adults: survival studies and prognostic factors. *Blood.* 2009;113(23):5727–5736.

31 Garcia-Montero AC, Jara-Acevedo M, Teodosio C, et al. KIT mutation in mast cells and other bone marrow hematopoietic cell lineages in systemic mast cell disorders: a prospective study of the Spanish Network on Mastocytosis (REMA) in a series of 113 patients. *Blood.* 2006;108(7):2366–2372.

32 Curtin JA, Busam K, Pinkel D, Bastian BC. Somatic activation of KIT in distinct subtypes of melanoma. *J Clin Oncol.* 2006;24(26):4340–4346.

33 Beadling C, Jacobson-Dunlop E, Hodi FS, et al. KIT gene mutations and copy number in melanoma subtypes. *Clin Cancer Res.* 2008;14(21):6821–6828.

34 Torres-Cabala CA, Wang WL, Trent J, et al. Correlation between KIT expression and KIT mutation in melanoma: a study of 173 cases with emphasis on the acral-lentiginous/mucosal type. *Mod Pathol.* 2009;22(11):1446–1456.

35 Bastian BC. The molecular pathology of melanoma: an integrated taxonomy of melanocytic neoplasia. *Annu Rev Pathol.* 2014;9:239–271.

36 Bastian BC, Esteve-Puig R. Targeting activated KIT signaling for melanoma therapy. *J Clin Oncol.* 2013;31(26):3288–3290.

37 Omholt K, Grafstrom E, Kanter-Lewensohn L, Hansson J, Ragnarsson-Olding BK. KIT pathway alterations in mucosal melanomas of the vulva and other sites. *Clin Cancer Res.* 2011;17(12):3933–3942.

38 Kong Y, Si L, Zhu Y, et al. Large-scale analysis of KIT aberrations in Chinese patients with melanoma. *Clin Cancer Res.* 2011;17(7):1684–1691.

39 Holst VA, Marshall CE, Moskaluk CA, Frierson HF, Jr. KIT protein expression and analysis of c-kit gene mutation in adenoid cystic carcinoma. *Mod Pathol.* 1999;12(10):956–960.

40 Kemmer K, Corless CL, Fletcher JA, et al. KIT mutations are common in testicular seminomas. *Am J Pathol.* 2004;164(1):305–313.

41 Hoei-Hansen CE, Kraggerud SM, Abeler VM, Kaern J, Rajpert-De Meyts E, Lothe RA. Ovarian dysgerminomas are characterised by frequent KIT mutations and abundant expression of pluripotency markers. *Mol Cancer.* 2007;6:12.

42 Forbes S, Clements J, Dawson E, et al. Cosmic 2005. *Br J Cancer.* 2006;94(2):318–322.

43 Coffey J, Linger R, Pugh J, et al. Somatic KIT mutations occur predominantly in seminoma germ cell tumors and are not predictive of bilateral disease: report of 220 tumors and review of literature. *Genes Chromosomes Cancer.* 2008;47(1):34–42.

44 McIntyre A, Summersgill B, Grygalewicz B, et al. Amplification and overexpression of the KIT gene is associated with progression in the seminoma subtype of testicular germ cell tumors of adolescents and adults. *Cancer Res.* 2005;65(18):8085–8089.

45 Looijenga LH, de Leeuw H, van Oorschot M, et al. Stem cell factor receptor (c-KIT) codon 816 mutations predict development of bilateral testicular germ-cell tumors. *Cancer Res.* 2003;63(22):7674–7678.

46 Patel S. Long-term efficacy of imatinib for treatment of metastatic GIST. *Cancer Chemother Pharmacol.* 2013;72(2):277–286.

47 Bednarski BK, Araujo DM, Yi M, et al. Analysis of prognostic factors impacting oncologic outcomes after neoadjuvant tyrosine kinase inhibitor therapy for gastrointestinal stromal tumors. *Ann Surg Oncol.* 2014;21(8):2499–2505.

48 Joensuu H. Adjuvant treatment of GIST: patient selection and treatment strategies. *Nat Rev Clin Oncol.* 2012;9(6):351–358.

49 Heinrich MC, Corless CL, Demetri GD, et al. Kinase mutations and imatinib response in patients with metastatic gastrointestinal stromal tumor. *J Clin Oncol.* 2003;21(23):4342–4349.

50 Chen LL, Trent JC, Wu EF, et al. A missense mutation in KIT kinase domain 1 correlates with imatinib resistance in gastrointestinal stromal tumors. *Cancer Res.* 2004;64(17):5913–5919.

51 Demetri GD, van Oosterom AT, Garrett CR, et al. Efficacy and safety of sunitinib in patients with advanced gastrointestinal stromal tumour after failure of imatinib: a randomised controlled trial. *Lancet.* 2006;368(9544):1329–1338.

52 Gajiwala KS, Wu JC, Christensen J, et al. KIT kinase mutants show unique mechanisms of drug resistance to imatinib and sunitinib in gastrointestinal stromal tumor patients. *Proc Natl Acad Sci U S A.* 2009;106(5):1542–1547.

53 Demetri GD, Reichardt P, Kang YK, et al.GRID study investigators. Efficacy and safety of regorafenib for advanced gastrointestinal stromal tumours after failure of imatinib and sunitinib (GRID): an international, multicentre, randomised, placebo-controlled, phase 3 trial. *Lancet.* 2013;381(9863):295–302.

54 Reichardt P, Blay JY, Gelderblom H, et al. Phase III study of nilotinib versus best supportive care with or without a TKI in patients with gastrointestinal stromal tumors resistant to or intolerant of imatinib and sunitinib. *Ann Oncol.* 2012;23(7):1680–1687.

55 Wyman K, Atkins MB, Prieto V, et al. Multicenter phase II trial of high-dose imatinib mesylate in metastatic melanoma: significant toxicity with no clinical efficacy. *Cancer.* 2006;106(9):2005–2011.

56 Kim KB, Eton O, Davis DW, et al. Phase II trial of imatinib mesylate in patients with metastatic melanoma. *Br J Cancer.* 2008;99(5):734–740.

57 Ugurel S, Hildenbrand R, Zimpfer A, et al. Lack of clinical efficacy of imatinib in metastatic melanoma. *Br J Cancer.* 2005;92(8):1398–1405.

58 Lutzky J, Bauer J, Bastian BC. Dose-dependent, complete response to imatinib of a metastatic mucosal melanoma with a K642E KIT mutation. *Pigment Cell Melanoma Res.* 2008;21(4):492–493.

59 Hodi FS, Friedlander P, Corless CL, et al. Major response to imatinib mesylate in KIT-mutated melanoma. *J Clin Oncol.* 2008;26(12):2046–2051.

60 Woodman SE, Trent JC, Stemke-Hale K, et al. Activity of dasatinib against L576P KIT mutant melanoma: molecular, cellular, and clinical correlates. *Mol Cancer Ther.* 2009;8(8):2079–2085.

61 Kluger HM, Dudek AZ, McCann C, et al. A phase 2 trial of dasatinib in advanced melanoma. *Cancer.* 2011;117(10):2202–2208.

62 Quintas-Cardama A, Lazar AJ, Woodman SE, Kim K, Ross M, Hwu P. Complete response of stage IV anal mucosal melanoma expressing KIT Val560Asp to the multikinase inhibitor sorafenib. *Nat Clin Pract Oncol.* 2008;5(12):737–740.

63 Satzger I, Kuttler U, Volker B, Schenck F, Kapp A, Gutzmer R. Anal mucosal melanoma with KIT-activating mutation and response to imatinib therapy—case report and review of the literature. *Dermatology.* 2010;220(1):77–81.

64 Hodi FS, Corless CL, Giobbie-Hurder A, et al. Imatinib for melanomas harboring mutationally activated or amplified KIT arising on mucosal, acral, and chronically sun-damaged skin. *J Clin Oncol.* 2013;31(26):3182–3190.

65 Carvajal RD, Antonescu CR, Wolchok JD, et al. KIT as a therapeutic target in metastatic melanoma. *JAMA.* 2011;305(22):2327–2334.

66 Guo J, Si L, Kong Y, et al. Phase II, open-label, single-arm trial of imatinib mesylate in patients with metastatic melanoma harboring c-Kit mutation or amplification. *J Clin Oncol.* 2011;29(21):2904–2909.

67 Minor DR, Kashani-Sabet M, Garrido M, O'Day SJ, Hamid O, Bastian BC. Sunitinib therapy for melanoma patients with KIT mutations. *Clin Cancer Res.* 2012;18(5):1457–1463.

68 Cho JH, Kim KM, Kwon M, Kim JH, Lee J. Nilotinib in patients with metastatic melanoma harboring KIT gene aberration. *Invest New Drugs.* 2012;30(5):2008–2014.

69 Shah NP, Lee FY, Luo R, Jiang Y, Donker M, Akin C. Dasatinib (BMS-354825) inhibits KITD816V, an imatinib-resistant activating mutation that triggers neoplastic growth in most patients with systemic mastocytosis. *Blood.* 2006;108(1):286–291.

70 Schittenhelm MM, Shiraga S, Schroeder A, et al. Dasatinib (BMS-354825), a dual SRC/ABL kinase inhibitor, inhibits the kinase activity of wild-type, juxtamembrane, and activation loop mutant KIT isoforms associated with human malignancies. *Cancer Res.* 2006;66(1):473–481.

71 Verstovsek S, Tefferi A, Cortes J, et al. Phase II study of dasatinib in Philadelphia chromosome-negative acute and chronic myeloid diseases, including systemic mastocytosis. *Clin Cancer Res.* 2008;14(12):3906–3915.

72 Wardelmann E, Thomas N, Merkelbach-Bruse S, et al. Acquired resistance to imatinib in gastrointestinal stromal tumours caused by multiple KIT mutations. *Lancet Oncol.* 2005;6(4):249–251.

73 Liegl B, Kepten I, Le C, et al. Heterogeneity of kinase inhibitor resistance mechanisms in GIST. *J Pathol.* 2008;216(1):64–74.

74 Floris G, Wozniak A, Sciot R, et al. A potent combination of the novel PI3K Inhibitor, GDC-0941, with imatinib in gastrointestinal stromal tumor xenografts: long-lasting responses after treatment withdrawal. *Clin Cancer Res.* 2013;19(3):620–630.

75 Edris B, Willingham S, Weiskopf K, et al. Use of a KIT-specific monoclonal antibody to bypass imatinib resistance in gastrointestinal stromal tumors. *Oncoimmunology.* 2013;2(6):e24452.

# CHAPTER 36

# TP53

*Kensuke Kojima and Michael Andreeff*

Section of Molecular Hematology and Therapy, Department of Leukemia, The University of Texas MD Anderson Cancer Center, Houston, TX, USA

## Introduction

p53 was discovered in 1979 when it was initially considered an onco-gene, but subsequently it was established to be a tumor suppres-sor.[1-4] p53 is a transcription factor that controls the cellular response to stress signals through the induction of cell cycle arrest, apoptosis, or senescence. Furthermore, p53 has been found to be involved in diverse biological processes, including metabolism, stem-cell repro-gramming, longevity, fertility, germ-line fidelity, autophagy, necro-sis, angiogenesis, and cancer invasion. p53-induced growth arrest is primarily mediated through upregulation of p21, GADD45, and 14-3-3σ. p53-induced apoptosis is mediated by the mitochondrial pathway through transcription-dependent and -independent mech-anisms and by the death receptor pathway through transcriptional activation of FAS and DR5. p53 induces proapoptotic BH3 pro-teins PUMA, NOXA, and BAX and represses antiapoptotic BCL-2 and MCL-1, leading to mitochondrial outer membrane perme-ability and apoptosis. p53 can also trigger mitochondrial apoptosis in the absence of transcription, through direct activation of Bax or Bak or through binding to Bcl-2 or Bcl-XL. The mechanisms of p53-dependent cellular senescence are still poorly understood, but p21, DCR2, PAI-1, and DEC1 appear to mediate senescence downstream of p53. Since p53 elicits life or death decisions, an exquisite mech-anism has evolved to prevent its erroneous activation and to initi-ate prompt stress responses when necessary. To achieve delicate and precise control of p53, many proteins are involved in the regulation of p53 (Figure 36.1). MDM2 and MDMX are the major and essen-tial negative regulators of p53. ARF stabilizes p53 by antagonizing MDM2. ATM and ATR are sensors of DNA damage and activate p53 through its posttranslational modifications.

p53 prevents cancer development, which is initiated by a multi-tude of oncogenic events. Considerable efforts have been focused on the p53 pathway because nearly all cancers show defects in p53 and/or the p53 pathway.[5-7] *TP53* is the most frequently altered gene in human cancer and *TP53* mutations have been found in approx-imately 50% of human solid tumors. p53 mutations usually lack DNA binding and transcriptional activities. The remaining human cancers possess wild-type p53, but have defects in the p53 pathway that render p53 incapable of exerting its tumor-suppressive func-tions. Therefore, inactivation of p53 functions is an almost univer-sal feature of human cancers. Most of the recently developed agents targeting cancer-related abnormalities, including imatinib, gefitinib,

sorafenib, trastuzumab, and rituximab, represent enormous advan-tages in cancer therapy, but their efficacy is limited to small patient populations. Considering that almost all cancers exhibit defects in the p53 pathway, an alternative strategy targeting universal cancer-related abnormalities like p53, may benefit a large population of can-cer patients.

In this chapter, we discuss p53 pathway abnormalities in can-cer and p53-activating cancer therapies that either have reached the clinic, demonstrated preclinical efficacy, or represent novel approaches.

## p53 Pathway Abnormalities in Malignancies

Considering the potent tumor suppressing activity of p53, it is not surprising that disruption of the p53 pathway is a common denominator in many malignancies. In malignancies, p53 function is impaired by *TP53* alterations or defective p53 pathway regula-tion. While approximately 50% of human solid cancers carry *TP53* mutations, hematological malignancies present a rather low inci-dence of genetic alterations in *TP53*, with the exception of acute myeloid leukemia (AML) with complex karyotype and mantle-cell lymphoma (MCL). Neoplastic cells carrying wild-type p53 fre-quently have abnormalities in p53 regulatory proteins, including MDM2/MDMX overexpression, *CDKN2A* alterations, and ATM inactivation.

### p53 Mutations

Germline mutations of *TP53* cause the Li–Fraumeni syndrome, a genetic disorder that greatly increases the risk of developing several types of cancer in children and young adults. The cancers most often associated with the Li–Fraumeni syndrome include breast cancer, sarcomas, and hematologic malignancies. Genetically engineered mice that lack p53 or express p53 mutants have been found to be prone to early onset of tumor development. The latest International Agency for Research on Cancer (IARC) *TP53* mutation database (R17) contains 28,000 somatic mutations and 750 germline muta-tions as of November 2013[8] The majority of p53 mutations (>95%) are clustered in the central DNA-binding domain and 75% of the mutations are mis-sense mutations. *TP53* mutations are expected to abrogate the tumor suppressor function of the affected *TP53*

*Targeted Therapy in Translational Cancer Research*, First Edition. Edited by Apostolia-Maria Tsimberidou, Razelle Kurzrock and Kenneth C. Anderson.
© 2016 John Wiley & Sons, Inc. Published 2016 by John Wiley & Sons, Inc.

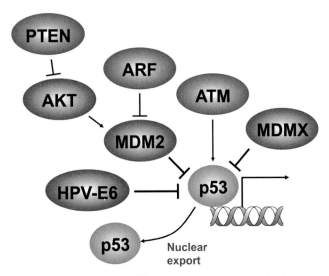

**Figure 36.1** Inactivation of wild-type p53 in cancer. p53 inactivation may be achieved at least by MDM2/MDMX overexpression, reduced ATM/ARF expression, HPV infection, and nuclear exclusion of p53. HPV-E6, human papillomavirus E6 protein.

allele. Furthermore, some mutants may exert dominant negative effects over coexpressed wild-type p53 or even gain new properties that promote tumorigenesis (mutant p53 gain-of-function). Epidemiologic studies have identified some cancers specifically associated with exogenous carcinogens, including sunlight-associated skin cancers, tobacco-associated lung cancers, and aristolochic acid–related urothelial tumors.[9] Carcinogens critically determine *TP53* mutation types. For example, ultraviolet insult induces tandem CC to TT substitutions, which are characteristics of nonmelanoma skin tumors. Tobacco smoke carcinogens are linked to G to T mutations on codons 157, 158, 248, and 273 in lung cancer. In hepatocellular carcinoma, a specific G-to-T transversion on codon 249 is classically described as a fingerprint of aflatoxin exposure. Chinese herb nephropathy is characterized by A-to-T mutations in urothelial tumors. Mutations of p53 have been demonstrated to be associated with poor prognosis in cancers such as breast, colorectal, head and neck, and hematologic malignancies.[10]

### MDM2/MDMX Overexpression

The homologs MDM2 and MDMX are essential negative regulators of p53. MDM2 and MDMX proteins bind the N-terminal transactivation domain of p53 and inhibit its transcriptional activity. In addition, MDM2 has E3 ubiquitin ligase activity and promotes ubiquitin-dependent proteasomal degradation of p53. Since MDM2 is transcriptionally activated by p53, MDM2 and p53 mutually regulate their protein levels through a negative feedback loop. A p53 response element has also been found in the MDMX promoter. MDM2 is more broadly responsive to p53 activation and p53-dependent increases in MDMX expression occur only under certain conditions.[11] In addition to inhibition of p53-mediated transcription and p53 ubiquitination, MDM2 also promotes nuclear export of p53.

Through p53 inactivation, MDM2 and MDMX overexpression contributes to cancer initiation, maintenance, and progression. Some authors have described that high levels of *MDM2* or *MDMX* gene amplification are mutually exclusive, whereas low levels of amplification of both genes can coexist in a tumor cell.[12] In mouse

models, overexpressed MDM2 or MDMX have resulted in hematologic malignancies.[13,14] Gene amplification can lead to increased protein levels of MDM2 or MDMX, which is most typically seen in atypical lipomatous tumors. MDM2 gene is amplified in nearly 100% of well-differentiated and dedifferentiated liposarcoma.[15] On the other hand, MDMX gene amplification has been reported in retinoblastoma, brain tumors, breast cancers, soft-tissue tumors, and diffuse large B-cell lymphoma.[16–18] Secondary MDMX gene amplifications may promote leukemic transformation in myeloproliferative neoplasms.[19] Importantly, many tumors exhibit high MDM2 and MDMX protein expression without increased copy number, including melanoma, Ewing's sarcoma, colon carcinoma, retinoblastoma, and leukemia.[7] An SNP in the MDM2 gene has been associated with MDM2 overexpression.[20] It has been thought that cancer-specific signaling pathways activate MDM2 and MDMX proteins via posttranslational stabilization. In some cancer types, the frequency of MDM2/MDMX protein deregulation has been higher in tumors that retain wild-type p53, suggesting that overexpressed MDM2 or MDMX can sufficiently inhibit p53 and promote cancer development.

### CDKN2A Alterations

The *CDKN2A* tumor suppressor locus on 9p21 encodes two tumor suppressor genes: *p16INK4A* and *p14ARF* (*p19ARF* in the mouse).[21] p16INK4A is an inhibitor of the cyclin D-dependent kinases and regulates cell cycle progression. p14ARF binds MDM2, sequesters it in the nucleolus, and thus inhibits its p53 regulatory function. Germline mutations in *CDKN2A* have been reported in melanoma and pancreatic cancer families (melanoma-pancreatic carcinoma syndrome). Homozygous deletions of *CDKN2A* have been found to be associated with glioblastoma and lymphoid malignancies (acute lymphoblastic leukemia and lymphoid blast crisis of chronic myeloid leukemia (CML) and lymphomas).[22–24] In CML, *CDKN2A* deletion frequently occurs in lymphoid crisis but has not been reported in CML-CP or myeloid blast crisis, underscoring its lineage-specific occurrence.[23]

### ATM Alterations

ATM is a serine/threonine protein kinase that is activated in response to DNA double-strand breaks and synchronizes DNA repair with the induction of p53-dependent apoptosis. ATM directly phosphorylates p53 on Ser15 and induces phosphorylation at Ser9, Ser20, and Ser46 through activation of additional protein kinases, including Chk2. The protein is named for the disorder ataxia telangiectasia caused by *ATM* mutations. ATM inactivation leads to increased radiosensitivity, radioresistant DNA synthesis, loss of cell cycle checkpoints, and p53 dysfunction. Ataxia telangiectasia is characterized by cerebellar degeneration, extreme cellular sensitivity to radiation, and a predisposition to cancer. Approximately 0.5–1% of the general population has been estimated to be heterozygous for a germline mutation in the *ATM* gene, and women heterozygous for mutations in *ATM* are reported to have a fourfold to fivefold increased risk of breast cancer compared with noncarriers of the mutations.[25] Somatic ATM alterations (point mutations or deletions) have been reported in lymphoid malignancies such as chronic lymphocytic leukemia (CLL), T-prolymphocytic leukemia (T-PLL) and MCL.[26,27] In CLL, a deletion of the long arm of chromosome 11 (*ATM* gene located at 11q22.3 to q23.1) is found in 10–20% of patients and identifies a group with poor outcome.[26] Furthermore, *ATM* is mutated in 30–40% of CLL cases with 11q deletion.

## HPV Infection

Various DNA viruses, such as SV40, human papillomaviruses (HPVs) or adenoviruses, encode proteins that target p53 protein.[28] HPVs have been shown clinically to cause cancer in humans. HPVs are a group of more than 150 related viruses and some high-risk HPV types (especially HPV types 16 and 11) are closely associated with cancer development. High-risk HPVs cause virtually all cervical cancers, most anal cancers, and some vaginal, vulvar, penile, and oropharyngeal cancers. High-risk HPV infection is estimated to account for approximately 5% of all cancers worldwide. The Food and Drug Administration (FDA) has approved two HPV vaccines (Gardasil and Cervarix) for the prevention of cervical and some other types of cancers. Both vaccines are highly effective in preventing infections with HPV types 16 and 18. The E6 viral protein expressed by HPV binds to the p53 protein and promotes its degradation through the ubiquitin–proteasome pathway. HPV infection represents an alternative and is functionally comparable with p53 mutations, as HPV infection and p53 mutations are often mutually exclusive. Prospective studies of head and neck squamous cell carcinoma have found a more favorable prognosis for patients with HPV-positive, than HPV-negative tumors.[29] Importantly, inactivation of p53 by E6 protein leads to the loss of functional p53 but not to altered p53 and therefore, p53 protein and transcriptional activity are potentially inducible. p53 inactivation by a viral protein has not been formally demonstrated in other human cancers associated with viral infection, such as HCC (associated with HBV) or Burkitt's lymphoma (associated with EBV).

## Nuclear Exclusion

p53 is shuttled between the nucleus and the cytoplasm. In inflammatory breast cancers or neuroblastomas, molecular and immunohistochemical analyses demonstrate accumulation of wild-type p53 in the cytoplasm of tumor cells, leading to functional inactivation of p53.[30] Exportin-1 (chromosomal region maintenance 1, CRM1) is involved in nuclear export of p53, and CRM1 overexpression has been associated with poor prognosis of solid cancers including osteosarcoma, glioblastoma, ovarian, and cervical cancer. p53-associated parkin-like cytoplasmic protein (PARC) that exists as part of a large complex in the cytoplasm, anchors p53 in the cytoplasm, and prevents the tumor suppressor from entering the nucleus. It has been reported that neuroblastoma cells express high cytoplasmic levels of PARC.[31]

## Targeting p53 for Cancer Therapy

The tumor-suppressive function of p53 is originated from its ability to activate a program that directs cells to undergo cell cycle arrest, apoptosis, or senescence. DNA damage-induced p53 activation has been a major component in cancer treatment by using anticancer drugs and irradiation. Here we discuss several strategies to restore and/or activate p53 functions in cancer cells, including (i) TP53 gene therapy, (ii) p53 vaccines, (iii) rescue of mutant p53 function, and (iv) wild-type p53 stabilization and activation.

### TP53 Gene Therapy

Adenovirus is one of the most commonly used vectors for gene therapy and replication-incompetent, p53-expressing adenovirus (Ad5CMV-p53, Gendicine) has been approved for clinical use in China in 2003[32] for the treatment of head and neck squamous cell carcinoma. Its counterpart Advexin has not been approved in the United States or Europe. More than 2500 patients have received

Gendicine in China, but a definitive report of phase IV safety and efficacy has not yet been published. Conditionally replicating adenoviruses (ONYX-015) that can replicate only in p53 mutant cells have been also been tested in clinical trials. Due to inefficient systemic delivery and limited therapeutic efficacy, however, the development was abandoned in the United States. In 2005, Shanghai Sunway Biotech (Shanghai, China) announced the approval of H101 (Oncorine) by Chinese government regulators, specifically for the treatment of nasopharyngeal carcinoma in combination with cisplatin-based chemotherapy. H101 is an oncolytic adenovirus with an E1B-55kD gene deletion, similar to that present in ONYX-015. The relatively small phase III oncology trial (just over 100 patients) did not result in significant improvements in overall survival. As noted, TP53 gene therapy has not been granted approval yet in the United States, and recent preclinical studies have used mesenchymal and neural stem cells as delivery vehicles for oncolytic viruses or combined siRNAs with oncolytic adenovirus.[33]

### p53 Vaccines

p53 has been a target for cancer vaccination therapy. p53 mutants lose their DNA binding and the ability to transactivate MDM2, the major negative regulator of p53, leading to prolonged half-life and abnormal accumulation of p53 in cancer cells. Because of the tumor specificity and high expression levels, p53 mutants may present a more visible signal to the immune system and hence provide a better target for immunotherapy. p53 autoantibodies and p53-reactive T cells have been found in cancer patients. The mixture of 10 long synthetic p53-dervied peptides (p53-SLP) has been shown to induce p53-specific T-cell responses in patients with solid cancers.[34] It has been suggested that responses to chemotherapy might improve in patients with vaccine-induced immune responses in lung cancer.[35] Vaccination of cancer patients with a p53-modified adenovirus-transduced dendritic cell vaccine (INGN-225) has shown p53 immune responses and chemosensitization in patients with small-cell lung cancer.[36]

### Reactivation of Mutant p53

p53 mutations either change wild-type p53 conformation (conformation mutants) or abolish its DNA contact (contact mutants). Approaches using phenotypic and biochemical screens have been taken to identify molecules that can restore mutant p53 activity, and specific small peptides or small molecules have been reported to restore wild-type function mainly in conformation mutants.[37] PRIMA-1 (p53 reactivation and induction of massive apoptosis-1) and its derivative PRIMA-1MET/APR-246 are believed to react covalently with thiols in mutant p53 and restore wild-type function to p53. APR-246 has been shown to be safe, well tolerated, and induced in vivo biologic and clinical effects in patients with hematologic malignancies and prostate cancer.[38] CP-31398 has been selected from a biochemical screen for molecules promoting the stability of p53's DNA-binding domain. CP-31398 has been proposed to bind to p53, stabilize the structure of p53, and inhibit cell growth both in p53 wild type and mutant cells. Other mutant p53-targeting compounds include MIRA-1 (mutant p53-dependent induction of rapid apoptosis-1)/MIRA-3 and STIMA-1 (SH group targeting and induction of massive apoptosis), whose mechanisms of action have not been well established. An alternative approach would be to activate p53 downstream targets, such as TRAIL or the TRAIL receptor, DR5, in the presence of inactivated p53. One such compound, TIC10 (also known as ONC-201), has recently been identified.[39]

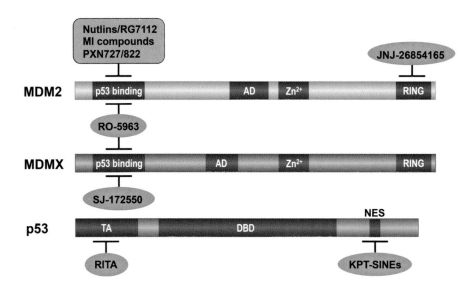

**Figure 36.2** Agents targeting wild-type p53, MDM2, or MDMX. p53 binding, p53-binding domain; AD, acidic domain; Zn2+, zinc finger domain; RING, RING domain; TA, transactivation domain; DBD, DNA-binding domain; NES, nuclear export signal; RITA, reactivation of p53 and induction of tumor cell apoptosis.

## Wild-Type p53 Stabilization and Activation

Several pharmacological strategies have been proposed for the activation of wild-type p53 (Figure 36.2). One promising strategy to reactivate wild-type p53 in cancer cells is blockade of the MDM2–p53 interaction.[38] Disruption of MDM2–p53 interaction has been shown to stabilize p53, activate p53 functions and induce cell cycle arrest, apoptosis, or senescence in cancer cells at least partially in cell type-specific manner.[40–42] Using structure-based design and high-throughput screening, several small-molecule inhibitors of p53–MDM2 interaction have been developed including RG7288 and the structurally unrelated RO5503781, Nutlin-3a/RG7112, MI compounds (MI-43, MI-63, MI-219, and MI-319), and PXN727/822 that bind MDM2 in its p53-binding pocket of MDM2. RG7112 has been tested in phase I trials in patients with hematologic malignancies (NCT00623870) and advanced solid tumors (NCT00559533). MI compounds and PXN727/822 represent different series of MDM2–p53-binding inhibitors, currently at the preclinical stage of investigation.[43,44] Another p53 activator that reportedly blocks MDM2–p53 interaction is the small-molecule RITA (reactivation of p53 and induction of tumor cell apoptosis), which is proposed to disrupt the MDM2–p53 interaction by binding to p53 (not MDM2).[45] Although RITA has been shown to induce p53 activation, the mechanism of action has not been well defined and is still controversial. RITA has been reported to exhibit p53-independent functions.

JNJ-26854165, originally reported as MDM2 antagonist that reactivate p53 by inhibiting MDM2 E3 activity, has been assessed in phase I studies as an oral agent for advanced or refractory solid tumors.[46] Although JNJ-26854165 was well tolerated in these patients, no objective responses were observed. JNJ-26854165 induces S-phase delay and apoptosis preferentially of S-phase cells. JNJ-26854165 exhibits p53-dependent and -independent apoptotic activities, and the mechanism of action is not fully understood.[47]

Although the p53-binding regions of MDM2 and MDMX are similar, MDM2 antagonists do not sufficiently disrupt the MDMX–p53 interaction. The p53-binding pocket of MDMX is relatively shallower and less accessible to MDM2 antagonists such as Nutlin than that of MDM2. This is likely to be clinically relevant, since overexpression of MDM2, MDMX are mutually exclusive events in a significant fraction of human tumors, and the low affinity of MDM2 antagonists for MDMX binding may limit reactivation of

p53 in cancer cells. Indeed, p53 wild-type cancer cells with high MDMX may show relative resistance to Nutlin-3a treatment.[48,49] A dual MDM2/MDMX antagonist, RO-5963, has been recently identified.[50] RO-5963 blocks p53 interaction with both MDM2 and MDMX by inhibitor-driven homo and/or heterodimerization of MDM2 and MDMX. SJ-172550 was identified as a selective antagonist of MDMX–p53 interaction, but subsequent studies have shown that SJ-172550 forms covalent adducts with cysteine residues in the p53-binding domain of both MDM2 and MDMX.[51,52] The thiol reactivity precludes this chemical scaffold from further development and optimization as a selective MDMX inhibitor.

Leptomycin B is a potent inhibitor of CRM1, an exportin required for nuclear export of proteins containing nuclear export signals. p53 contains a functional nuclear export signal within its tetramerization domain and leptomycin B activates p53-dependent transcription in cells through nuclear accumulation of stabilized p53. Despite significant *in vitro* potency against cancer cells, the clinical development was abandoned in phase I due to toxicity and poor pharmacokinetic properties. Recently, less toxic CRM1 inhibitors with improved therapeutic windows have been developed. KPT-330 is a potent and irreversible small-molecule selective inhibitor of CRM1 currently in phase I trials in patients with advanced or metastatic solid cancer (NCT01607905) and hematologic malignancies (NCT01607892) that shows clinical activity in AML and non-Hodgkin's lymphomas.[53]

## Nutlin-3a/RG7112

Nutlin-3a is a cis-imidazoline compound that binds specifically and with high affinity to the p53-binding pocket of MDM2 by mimicking critical residues of p53 essential for MDM2 binding (Phe19, Trp23, Leu26).[40] Nutlin-3 induces cell cycle arrest, apoptosis and/or senescence in cancer cells, and is less toxic to normal cells. This favorable activity profile suggests that induction of the p53 response in transformed cells may offer a novel approach to treat tumors that retain a functional p53 pathway. Although the Nutlin-induced activation of E2F1, p73, and apoptosis have been reported in p53 defective cells, the primary activity of MDM2 inhibitors depends on wild-type p53. Other reported determinants of response to MDM2 inhibition are MDM2 and MDMX expression levels. High levels of MDM2 in tumor cells seem to be associated with increased sensitivity to Nutlin in some malignancies.[41] On the other hand, high MDMX expression has been associated with low susceptibility to Nutlin.[48,49] Alterations of *CDKN2A* or *ATM* have not affected Nutlin sensitivity.[54,55] Nutlin has shown synergism with conventional chemotherapeutic agents, anthracyclines, cytarabine, fludarabine, chlorambucil, and imatinib.

The advanced clinically relevant Nutlin analog RG7112 has been tested in phase I trials in patients with liposarcoma and hematologic malignancies.[56,57] p53 activation by RG7112 was demonstrated by MIC-1 induction in serum and p53 target gene induction including *MDM2*, *CDKN1A (p21)*, and *PUMA*. Common adverse events were gastrointestinal (nausea, vomiting, and diarrhea) and hematological (neutropenia and thrombocytopenia). RG7112 showed clinical activities. In the clinical study of 20 patients with liposarcoma, one patient had a confirmed partial response and 14 had stable disease. In the phase I extension study, 3 out of 28 patients with AML achieved complete remissions, and the overall response rate was 46%.

MDM2 inhibition can also exert a reversible cytostatic effect in normal cells, which leads to the accumulation of cells in G1 and G2, and may shield them from the cytotoxicity and genomic damage caused by clinically used S and M phase-specific poisons.[58] This provides rationale for the potential use of MDM2 inhibitors in patients with p53-null or mutant cancers. In this concept of p53-induced cell cycle arrest using MDM2 inhibitors, pretreatment of p53 defective cancer with MDM2 inhibitors leads to cell cycle arrest in normal tissues but allows tumor cells to continue proliferation. Subsequent exposure to drugs that target proliferating cells would then selectively kill the tumor cells while sparing normal cells. This concept has not yet been well developed and the cytopenias observed in patients with solid tumors treated with MDM2 inhibitors would suggest that timing and exposure are critical for this concept to be clinically beneficial. However, investigators have shown that in elegant murine models the transient disruption of the p53–MDM2 interaction could be exploited as a potential strategy for protecting hematologic stem cells.[59]

Long-term exposure to Nutlin has been reported to induce or select p53 mutant clones in originally p53 wild-type cancer cells.[60,61] This potential disadvantage appears to be due to the high selectivity of Nutlin for MDM2–p53 interaction and reinforces the idea that the antitumor activity is mostly dependent on p53 activation. Treatment with selective small-molecule MDM2 antagonists may require monitoring for possible emergence or selection of p53-mutated clones.

### MI Compounds

The MI compounds (MI-43, MI-63, MI-219, and MI-319) are a class of MDM2 inhibitors, which similar to Nutlins, selectively block the MDM2–p53 interaction.[43] MI compounds can act like Nutlin to produce a nongenotoxic reversible G1 arrest in normal cells, while inducing p53-dependent apoptosis in p53 wild-type tumor cells. Oral administration of MI-219/319 led to tumor regression in mouse tumor models at nontoxic doses.[62] MI compounds have been combined with etoposide, doxorubicin, and cisplatin against solid tumors and with cytarabine against AML; and the combinations have been reported to have potent antineoplastic effect with minimal toxicity in normal cells. In this regard, it is noteworthy that recently developed MDM2 inhibitors show greater affinity to human, rather than murine MDM2, and hence preclinical studies in murine xenograft models would underestimate the effects on normal tissues.

### RO-5963

Overexpressed MDMX has been associated with low susceptibility to MDM2 inhibition, raising the possibility that dual inhibition of MDM2 and MDMX would have an advantage over selective MDM2 inhibition in some cancers. The dual MDM2/MDMX antagonist RO-5963 blocks p53 interaction with both MDM2 and MDMX, by inhibitor-driven homo and/or heterodimerization of MDM2 and MDMX.[50] The novel mode of inhibiting protein–protein interactions effectively activated p53 signaling in cancer cells, leading to cell cycle arrest and apoptosis. Since RO-5963 has exhibited better cell death activity against MCF7 and other solid tumor cell lines with higher MDMX levels than the MDM2-specific inhibitor Nutlin, dual inhibition of MDM2 and MDMX may offer a more effective therapeutic modality for MDMX-overexpressing cancers. Similar to MDM2 inhibitors, RO-5963 activity largely depends on wild-type p53 status. RO-5963 and related dual MDM2 and MDMX inhibitors are still in preclinical development, but this novel class of compounds may be advantageous over pure MDM2 inhibitors in cancers expressing high MDMX, including retinoblastoma, brain tumors, breast cancers, soft-tissue tumors, and lymphoma.[7,16–18]

### KPT Compounds

CRM1 is a nuclear export receptor involved in the active transport of tumor suppressors (e.g., p53), whose function is altered in cancer because of increased expression and overactive transport. CRM1 overexpression has been associated with poor prognosis of solid cancers including osteosarcoma, glioblastoma, ovarian cancer, and cervical cancer.[63,64] The KPT compounds (i.e., KPT-185, KPT-127, KPT-205, KPT-227, KPT-251, and KPT-330, Karyopharm Therapeutics Inc., Inc., Natick, MA, USA) are novel selective and irreversible CRM1 inhibitors with improved therapeutic window.[53] KPT compounds induce apoptosis and block proliferation in malignant cell lines and patient-derived cells, including pancreas, colon, and breast cancer as well as leukemias.[53,65,66] KPT-330 is currently in phase I trials in patients with advanced or metastatic solid cancer (NCT01607905) and hematologic malignancies (NCT01607892). Since CRM1 is involved in nuclear export of more than 200 proteins including p53, p21, p27, p73, nucleophosmin-1, PP2A, FOXO, β-catenin/APC, topoisomerase II, and NFκB/IκB, the extent of contribution of p53 signaling to the total apoptotic potential of CRM1 inhibition needs to be determined.[66] However, synergistic effects of KPT-185 and Nutlin-3a in leukemias have been reported.[67] It is unknown whether p53 cellular localization affects cell sensitivity to CRM1 inhibitors, as inflammatory breast cancer and neuroblastoma cells frequently show accumulation of wild-type p53 in the cytoplasm.

## Concluding Remarks

Recent advances in the understanding of p53 structure and function have clarified almost universal loss of p53 activity in cancers and led to various approaches to p53-based cancer therapy. The next decade holds the prospect of new p53-based therapies that will have wide utility in malignant diseases.

## Acknowledgments

The authors acknowledge Dr. Numsen Hail Jr. for his editorial assistance with the manuscript.

# References

1 Lane D, Levine A. p53 Research: the past thirty years and the next thirty years. *Cold Spring Harb Perspect Biol*. 2010;2(12):a000893. doi:10.1101/cshperspect.a000893.

2 Levine AJ, Oren M. The first 30 years of p53: growing ever more complex. *Nat Rev Cancer*. 2009;9(10):749–758. doi:10.1038/nrc2723.

3 Aylon Y, Oren M. New plays in the p53 theater. *Curr Opin Genet Dev*. 2011;21(1):86–92. doi:10.1016/j.gde.2010.10.002.

4 Beckerman R, Prives C. Transcriptional regulation by p53. *Cold Spring Harb Perspect Biol*. 2010;2(8):a000935. doi:10.1101/cshperspect.a000935.

5 Cheok CF, Verma CS, Baselga J, Lane DP. Translating p53 into the clinic. *Nat Rev Clin Oncol*. 2011;8(1):25–37. doi:10.1038/nrclinonc.2010.174.

6 Li Q, Lozano G. Molecular pathways: targeting Mdm2 and Mdm4 in cancer therapy. *Clin Cancer Res*. 2013;19(1):34–41. doi:10.1158/1078-0432.CCR-12-0053.

7 Wade M, Li YC, Wahl GM. MDM2, MDMX and p53 in oncogenesis and cancer therapy. *Nat Rev Cancer*. 2012;13(2):83–96.

8 Petitjean A, Mathe E, Kato S, et al. Impact of mutant p53 functional properties on TP53 mutation patterns and tumor phenotype: lessons from recent developments in the IARC TP53 database. *Hum Mutat*. 2007;28(6):622–629.

9 Pfeifer GP, Besaratinia A. Mutational spectra of human cancer. *Hum Genet*. 2009;125(5–6):493–506. doi:10.1007/s00439-009-0657-2.

10 Petitjean A, Achatz MI, Borresen-Dale AL, Hainaut P, Olivier M. TP53 mutations in human cancers: functional selection and impact on cancer prognosis and outcomes. *Oncogene*. 2007;26(15):2157–2165.

11 Phillips A, Teunisse A, Lam S, et al. HDMX-L is expressed from a functional p53-responsive promoter in the first intron of the HDMX gene and participates in an autoregulatory feedback loop to control p53 activity. *J Biol Chem*. 2010;285(38):29111–29127. doi:10.1074/jbc.M110.129726.

12 Arjona D, Bello MJ, Alonso ME, et al. Real-time quantitative PCR analysis of regions involved in gene amplification reveals gene overdose in low-grade astrocytic gliomas. *Diagn Mol Pathol*. 2005;14(4):224–229.

13 Jones SN, Hancock AR, Vogel H, Donehower LA, Bradley A. Overexpression of Mdm2 in mice reveals a p53-independent role for Mdm2 in tumorigenesis. *Proc Natl Acad Sci U S A*. 1998;95(26):15608–15612.

14 Xiong S, Pant V, Suh YA, et al. Spontaneous tumorigenesis in mice overexpressing the p53-negative regulator Mdm4. *Cancer Res*. 2010;70(18):7148–7154. doi:10.1158/0008-5472.CAN-10-1457.

15 Coindre JM, Pédeutour F, Aurias A. Well-differentiated and dedifferentiated liposarcomas. *Virchows Arch*. 2010;456(2):167–179. doi:10.1007/s00428-009-0815-x.

16 Laurie NA, Donovan SL, Shih CS, et al. Inactivation of the p53 pathway in retinoblastoma. *Nature*. 2006;444(7115):61–66.

17 Toledo F, Wahl GM. Regulating the p53 pathway: in vitro hypotheses, in vivo veritas. *Nat Rev Cancer*. 2006;6(12):909–923.

18 Monti S, Chapuy B, Takeyama K, et al. Integrative analysis reveals an outcome-associated and targetable pattern of p53 and cell cycle deregulation in diffuse large B cell lymphoma. *Cancer Cell*. 2012;22(3):359–372. doi:10.1016/j.ccr.2012.07.014.

19 Harutyunyan A, Klampfl T, Cazzola M, Kralovics R. p53 lesions in leukemic transformation. *N Engl J Med*. 2011;364(5):488–490. doi:10.1056/NEJMc1012718.

20 Bond GL, Hu W, Levine A. A single nucleotide polymorphism in the MDM2 gene: from a molecular and cellular explanation to clinical effect. *Cancer Res*. 2005;65(13):5481–5484.

21 Matheu A, Maraver A, Serrano M. The Arf/p53 pathway in cancer and aging. *Cancer Res*. 2008;68(15):6031–6034. doi:10.1158/0008-5472.CAN-07-6851.

22 Cancer Genome Atlas Research Network. Comprehensive genomic characterization defines human glioblastoma genes and core pathways. *Nature*. 2008;455(7216):1061–1068. doi:10.1038/nature07385.

23 Williams RT, Sherr CJ. The INK4-ARF (CDKN2A/B) locus in hematopoiesis and BCR-ABL-induced leukemias. *Cold Spring Harb Symp Quant Biol*. 2008;73:461–467. doi:10.1101/sqb.2008.73.039.

24 Jardin F, Jais JP, Molina TJ, et al. Diffuse large B-cell lymphomas with CDKN2A deletion have a distinct gene expression signature and a poor prognosis under R-CHOP treatment: a GELA study. *Blood*. 2010;116(7):1092–1104. doi:10.1182/blood-2009-10-247122.

25 Tamimi RM, Hankinson SE, Spiegelman D, Kraft P, Colditz GA, Hunter DJ. Common ataxia telangiectasia mutated haplotypes and risk of breast cancer: a nested case-control study. *Breast Cancer Res*. 2004;6(4):R416–R422.

26 Austen B, Skowronska A, Baker C, et al. Mutation status of the residual ATM allele is an important determinant of the cellular response to chemotherapy and survival in patients with chronic lymphocytic leukemia containing an 11q deletion. *J Clin Oncol*. 2007;25(34):5448–5457.

27 Jares P, Campo E. Advances in the understanding of mantle cell lymphoma. *Br J Haematol*. 2008;142(2):149–165. doi:10.1111/j.1365-2141.2008.07124.x.

28 Parkin DM. The global health burden of infection-associated cancers in the year 2002. *Int J Cancer*. 2006;118(12):3030–3044.

29 Fakhry C, Westra WH, Li S, et al. Improved survival of patients with human papillomavirus-positive head and neck squamous cell carcinoma in a prospective clinical trial. *J Natl Cancer Inst*. 2008;100(4):261–269. doi:10.1093/jnci/djn011.

30 Zaika A, Marchenko N, Moll UM. Cytoplasmically "sequestered" wild type p53 protein is resistant to Mdm2-mediated degradation. *J Biol Chem*. 1999;274(39):27474–27480.

31 Nikolaev AY, Li M, Puskas N, Qin J, Gu W. Parc: a cytoplasmic anchor for p53. *Cell*. 2003;112(1):29–40.

32 Shi J, Zheng D. An update on gene therapy in China. *Curr Opin Mol Ther*. 2009;11(5):547–553.

33 Tyler MA, Ulasov IV, Sonabend AM, et al. Neural stem cells target intracranial glioma to deliver an oncolytic adenovirus in vivo. *Gene Ther*. 2009;16(2):262–278. doi:10.1038/gt.2008.165.

34 Vermeij R, Leffers N, Hoogeboom BN, et al. Potentiation of a p53-SLP vaccine by cyclophosphamide in ovarian cancer: a single-arm phase II study. *Int J Cancer*. 2012;131(5):E670–E680. doi:10.1002/ijc.27388.

35 Antonia SJ, Mirza N, Fricke I, et al. Combination of p53 cancer vaccine with chemotherapy in patients with extensive stage small cell lung cancer. *Clin Cancer Res*. 2006;12(3 Pt 1):878–887.

36 Chiappori AA, Soliman H, Janssen WE, Antonia SJ, Gabrilovich DI. INGN-225: a dendritic cell-based p53 vaccine (Ad.p53-DC) in small cell lung cancer: observed association between immune response and enhanced chemotherapy effect. *Expert Opin Biol Ther*. 2010;10(6):983–991. doi:10.1517/14712598.2010.484801.

37 Lehmann BD, Pietenpol JA. Targeting mutant p53 in human tumors. *J Clin Oncol*. 2012;30(29):3648–3650. doi:10.1200/JCO.2012.44.0412.

38 Lehmann S, Bykov VJ, Ali D, et al. Targeting p53 in vivo: a first-in-human study with p53-targeting compound APR-246 in refractory hematologic malignancies and prostate cancer. *J Clin Oncol*. 2012;30(29):3633–3639. doi:10.1200/JCO.2011.40.7783.

39 Allen JE, Krigsfeld G, Mayes PA, et al. Dual inactivation of Akt and ERK by TIC10 signals Foxo3a nuclear translocation, TRAIL gene induction, and potent antitumor effects. *Sci Transl Med*. 2013;5(171):171ra17. doi:10.1126/scitranslmed.3004828.

40 Vassilev LT, Vu BT, Graves B, et al. In vivo activation of the p53 pathway by small-molecule antagonists of MDM2. *Science*. 2004;303(5659):844–848.

41 Kojima K, Konopleva M, Samudio IJ, et al. MDM2 antagonists induce p53-dependent apoptosis in AML: implications for leukemia therapy. *Blood*. 2005;106(9):3150–3159.

42 Villalonga-Planells R, Coll-Mulet L, Martínez-Soler F, et al. Activation of p53 by nutlin-3a induces apoptosis and cellular senescence in human glioblastoma multiforme. *PLoS One*. 2011;6(4):e18588. doi:10.1371/journal.pone.0018588.

43 Shangary S, Qin D, McEachern D, et al. Temporal activation of p53 by a specific MDM2 inhibitor is selectively toxic to tumors and leads to complete tumor growth inhibition. *Proc Natl Acad Sci U S A*. 2008;105(10):3933–3938. doi:10.1073/pnas.0708917105.

44 Schilling D, Düwel M, Molls M, Multhoff G. Radiosensitization of wild-type p53 cancer cells by the MDM2-inhibitor PXN727 is associated with altered heat shock protein 70 (Hsp70) levels. *Cell Stress Chaperones*. 2013;18(2):183–191.

45 Issaeva N, Bozko P, Enge M, et al. Small molecule RITA binds to p53, blocks p53-HDM-2 interaction and activates p53 function in tumors. *Nat Med*. 2004;10(12):1321–1328.

46 Tabernero J, Dirix L, Schöffski P, et al. A phase I first-in-human pharmacokinetic and pharmacodynamic study of serdemetan in patients with advanced solid tumors. *Clin Cancer Res*. 2011;17(19):6313–6321. doi:10.1158/1078-0432.CCR-11-1101.

47 Kojima K, Burks JK, Arts J, Andreeff M. The novel tryptamine derivative JNJ-26854165 induces wild-type p53- and E2F1-mediated apoptosis in acute myeloid and lymphoid leukemias. *Mol Cancer Ther*. 2010;9(9):2545–2557. doi:10.1158/1535-7163.MCT-10-0337.

48 Bernal F, Wade M, Godes M, et al. A stapled p53 helix overcomes HDMX-mediated suppression of p53. *Cancer Cell*. 2010;18(5):411–422. doi:10.1016/j.ccr.2010.10.024.

49 Bo MD, Secchiero P, Degan M, et al. MDM4 (MDMX) is overexpressed in chronic lymphocytic leukaemia (CLL) and marks a subset of p53wild-type CLL with a poor cytotoxic response to Nutlin-3. *Br J Haematol*. 2010;150(2):237–239. doi:10.1111/j.1365-2141.2010.08185.x.

50 Graves B, Thompson T, Xia M, et al. Activation of the p53 pathway by small-molecule-induced MDM2 and MDMX dimerization. *Proc Natl Acad Sci U S A*. 2012;109(29):11788–11793. doi:10.1073/pnas.1203789109.

51 Reed D, Shen Y, Shelat AA, et al. Identification and characterization of the first small molecule inhibitor of MDMX. *J Biol Chem*. 2010;285(14):10786–10796. doi:10.1074/jbc.M109.056747.

52 Bista M, Smithson D, Pecak A, et al. On the mechanism of action of SJ-172550 in inhibiting the interaction of MDM4 and p53. *PLoS One*. 2012;7(6):e37518. doi:10.1371/journal.pone.0037518.

53 Lapalombella R, Sun Q, Williams K, et al. Selective inhibitors of nuclear export show that CRM1/XPO1 is a target in chronic lymphocytic leukemia. *Blood*. 2012;120(23):4621–4634. doi:10.1182/blood-2012-05-429506.

54 Kojima K, Konopleva M, McQueen T, O'Brien S, Plunkett W, Andreeff M. Mdm2 inhibitor Nutlin-3a induces p53-mediated apoptosis by transcription-dependent and transcription-independent mechanisms and may overcome Atm-mediated resistance to fludarabine in chronic lymphocytic leukemia. *Blood*. 2006;108(3):993–1000.

55 Sugihara E, Shimizu T, Kojima K, et al. Ink4a and Arf are crucial factors in the determination of the cell of origin and the therapeutic sensitivity of Myc-induced mouse lymphoid tumor. *Oncogene*. 2012;31(23):2849–2861. doi:10.1038/onc.2011.462.

56 Ray-Coquard I, Blay JY, Italiano A, et al. Effect of the MDM2 antagonist RG7112 on the P53 pathway in patients with MDM2-amplified, well-differentiated or dedifferentiated liposarcoma: an exploratory proof-of-mechanism study. *Lancet Oncol*. 2012;13(11):1133–1140. doi:10.1016/S1470-2045(12)70474-6.

57 Andreeff M, Drummond MW, Vyas P, et al. Results of the Phase 1 trial of RG7112, a small-molecule MDM2 antagonist, in acute leukemia. *ASH Annual Meeting Abstracts*. 2012;120:675.

58 van Leeuwen IM, Rao B, Sachweh MC, Laín S. An evaluation of small-molecule p53 activators as chemoprotectants ameliorating adverse effects of anticancer drugs in normal cells. *Cell Cycle*. 2012;11(9):1851–1861. doi:10.4161/cc.20254.

59 Pant V, Xiong S, Jackson JG, et al. The p53-Mdm2 feedback loop protects against DNA damage by inhibiting p53 activity but is dispensable for p53 stability, development, and longevity. *Genes Dev*. 2013;27(17):1857–1867. doi:10.1101/gad.227249.113.

60 Michaelis M, Rothweiler F, Barth S, et al. Adaptation of cancer cells from different entities to the MDM2 inhibitor nutlin-3 results in the emergence of p53-mutated multi-drug-resistant cancer cells. *Cell Death Dis*. 2011;2:e243. doi:10.1038/cddis.2011.129.

61 Aziz MH, Shen H, Maki CG. Acquisition of p53 mutations in response to the non-genotoxic p53 activator Nutlin-3. *Oncogene*. 2011;30(46):4678–4986. doi:10.1038/onc.2011.185.

62 Mohammad RM, Wu J, Azmi AS, et al. An MDM2 antagonist (MI-319) restores p53 functions and increases the life span of orally treated follicular lymphoma bearing animals. *Mol Cancer*. 2009;8:115. doi:10.1186/1476-4598-8-115.

63 Yao Y, Dong Y, Lin F, et al. The expression of CRM1 is associated with prognosis in human osteosarcoma. *Oncol Rep*. 2009;21(1):229–235.

64 Noske A, Weichert W, Niesporek S, et al. Expression of the nuclear export protein chromosomal region maintenance/exportin 1/Xpo1 is a prognostic factor in human ovarian cancer. *Cancer*. 2008;112(8):1733–1743.

65 Etchin J, Sanda T, Mansour MR, et al. KPT-330 inhibitor of CRM1 (XPO1)-mediated nuclear export has selective anti-leukaemic activity in preclinical models of T-cell acute lymphoblastic leukaemia and acute myeloid leukaemia. *Br J Haematol*. 2013;161(1):117–127. doi:10.1111/bjh.12231.

66 Inoue H, Kauffman M, Shacham S, et al. CRM1 blockade by selective inhibitors of nuclear export (SINE) attenuates kidney cancer growth. *J Urol*. 2013;189(6):2317–2326. doi:10.1016/j.juro.2012.10.018.

67 Kojima K, Kornblau SM, Ruvolo V, et al. Prognostic impact and targeting of CRM1 in acute myeloid leukemia. *Blood*. 2013;121(20):4166–4174. doi:10.1182/blood-2012-08-447581.

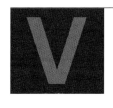

**PART V**

# Future Perspectives

# CHAPTER 37

# Future Perspectives

*Rabih Said[1,2] and Apostolia-Maria Tsimberidou[1]*

[1]Department of Investigational Cancer Therapeutics, The University of Texas MD Anderson Cancer Center, Houston, TX, USA
[2]Department of Internal Medicine, The University of Texas Health Science Center Houston, TX, USA

## Introduction

Precision medicine uses traditional as well as emerging concepts of the genetic and environmental basis of disease to individualize prevention, diagnosis, and treatment.[1–4] It integrates tumor molecular data into medical practice decision making. The conventional model of treating unselected patients is rapidly evolving toward selective targeted interventions in patients whose tumors have specific genotypic and biologic biomarkers. The selective use of targeted therapy, combined with other therapeutic strategies based upon the tumor biology of individual patients, holds the promise of improving clinical outcomes and patient care.[5] The exponential growth of the molecular therapeutic field integrates advances in basic science with translation to clinic.

Targeted therapy—the use of molecules that target specific enzymes, growth factor receptors, and signal transducers and thereby interfere with a variety of cellular processes—has transformed the treatment of cancer. Characterization of genomic, transcriptional, proteomic, and epigenetic changes[6,7] has led to the discovery of targeted therapies which have increased response, progression-free survival (PFS), and/or overall survival in selected patients with cancer.[8–10] The discovery and implementation of imatinib mesylate more than a decade ago in the treatment of chronic myeloid leukemia (CML) and gastrointestinal stromal tumor (GIST) was associated with significant improvement in clinical outcomes in patients.[11–13] Inspired by the discovery that imatinib mesylate targets the Bcr-Abl oncoprotein and dramatically improves the overall survival of patients with CML, translational research efforts have focused on understanding individualized patient tumor biology, and selecting the appropriate therapy for patients with solid tumors.[1] In recent years, several targeted agents have been approved by the Food and Drug Administration (FDA) for the treatment of solid tumors and hematologic malignancies with specific molecular alterations, based on their antitumor activities and safety profiles.[8–10,14]

Given the multiple identifiable tumor alterations that are associated with human cancers and the relatively small number of specific alterations in certain tumor types,[15–19] the development of targeted agents is suboptimal. Resistance to targeted therapy is often noted and it is attributed to acquisition of additional genetic alterations,[20–23] the activation of downstream signaling pathways bypassing the inhibited effect of targeted therapy,[24–26] and the activation of redundant signaling pathways,[27] or other mechanisms. To prevent the development of resistance mechanisms, or to circumvent them, combinations of targeted agents are rapidly evolving (Chapter 1). Ongoing clinical trials investigate combinations of novel agents targeting various signaling pathways,[28–30] immune therapeutic molecules,[31–34] chemotherapeutic agents, or radiotherapy.

Specific markers predicting clinical response to targeted agents (even by targeting more than one signaling pathway) based on an identified genomic alteration is suboptimal and needs further investigation.[35,36] Pharmacogenomics provide crucial information in the development of targeted therapy and resistance to therapy to understand the association of genomic alterations and clinical response to targeted therapies.[37–39] Discoveries of genetic polymorphisms have not yet widely translated into a meaningful, clinically useful tool.[35,36,40,41] In addition, drug–drug interactions and geographic factors (pharmacoethnicity) may affect patients' response to therapy.[42]

Optimization of technology to enable real-time, accurate, inexpensive, and efficient assessment of tumor tissue profiling will lead to better selection of appropriate therapy. Next-generation sequencing, circulating DNA, circulating tumor cells, and other profiling (DNAs, RNAs, proteins, and metabolites)[43] are critical components to permit precise bioinformatics analyses of patients' tumors.

Currently, the regulatory drug approval process can be cumbersome, expensive, and lengthy. In rare diseases, clinical trials are not encouraged because they affect small number of patients. Therefore, the available resources should be efficiently used, and policy and practice should be harmonized. Effective strategies are needed to close the gap between the plethora of preclinical data and the relative paucity of their clinical applications. Overall, a small proportion of patients has access to targeted therapies due to lack of agents that effectively target "driver" alterations of human cancer, the high cost of commercially available drugs, and limited access of patients to clinical trials with promising anticancer agents. Ongoing clinical trials with innovative adaptive study design will improve our understanding of the molecular basis of cancer and ultimately lead to effective treatments.

We envision that breakthroughs in cancer therapy over the next two decades will be associated with widespread use of new technology and bioinformatics analyses to define tumor pathophysiology, leading to the discovery of novel drugs and therapeutic strategies.[44] Dynamic changes in biology and tumor plasticity will require treatment adjustment to obtain optimal results. Importantly, tailoring of treatment is more challenging and complex than simply matching biomarkers and targeted therapy.[45–47] The key limitations of these concepts are related to the lack of complete understanding of tumor biology; our limited ability to generate, analyze, and manage large amounts of data with precision in a timely manner; and the lack of consistently effective targeted therapies. Other factors related to the patient tumor microenvironment and unknown pathophysiologic factors of cancer should be considered.

In this chapter, we will summarize the advances in cancer biology using genomic profiling technologies and computational techniques that collectively improve the selection and development of targeted therapies. We will also discuss proposed mechanisms for providing wide access to targeted personalized medicine. Finally, we will present future scenarios or strategies to improve patient care based upon our understanding of tumor biology, big data, and new drug development.

## Study of Tumor Biology

The pathophysiology of cancer involves interactions between various environmental factors and malignant cells with diverse and complex genetic and epigenetic changes.[48] Accumulating evidence supports the dynamic interaction between the tumor genome and the epigenome,[49,50] and that genes' functions and expressions are directly related to the ongoing stimulus of the surrounding microenvironment.[50,51]

Computational sciences have dramatically improved our knowledge about the complex dynamics of cancer,[52] including the analysis of signaling pathways and genotypic–phenotypic interactions. Signaling pathways represent the major determinants of cancer phenotypes and treatment responsiveness.

The main role of computational sciences in drug development is to establish methods to characterize the cancer genome data and various molecular interactions and processes. This characterization is based on analyzing a large amount of collected data using mathematical and correlation networks.[53–60] The value of systems biology in cancer treatment is to consider various components simultaneously, rather than compartmentalizing individual biological systems.

## Molecular Testing for Clinical Use

Molecular testing is a powerful tool in understanding the driver molecular alterations of patients' tumors.[44] It includes qualitative assays for single target detection, quantitative assays for response monitoring, and multiplexed assays to detect more than one analyte in the same specimen. To ensure accurate and precise molecular analysis results for the therapeutic management of patients, Clinical Laboratory Improvement Amendments (CLIA)-certification of laboratories is required.[61] More importantly, molecular testing should have specific characteristics including analytical and clinical validity, as well as clinical utility.[62,63] As such, many efforts have been made by various professional societies to establish evidence-based molecular tests for specific molecular alterations.[64–66] As molecular analysis evolves and more complex testing such as whole genome sequencing becomes available, we need to establish evidence-based guidelines to assure validity and utility,[67] and to standardize and harmonize results obtained from CLIA-certified laboratories.

With the main focus on accuracy, sensitivity, and validity by fulfilling CLIA-certification requirements, major efforts are still needed to ensure routine use of molecular testing for all patients with cancer. Results of these tests should be available in a timely manner to inform therapeutic decisions. Ongoing clinical trials will assess the effectiveness of molecular profiling to select targeted therapy. Data from these studies will in turn contribute to the development of regulations, which are necessary for the use of molecular testing in clinical practice and coverage by health care insurance policies.

## Tumor Monitoring

Access to tumor specimens from sequential biopsies to study the evolution of tumor biology, and the emergence of significant subclones during treatment is critical for the adjustment of anticancer therapy.[68,69] In certain tumor types, simultaneous biopsies from different metastatic sites to assess tumor heterogeneity are also informative.[68] Insufficient tissue from biopsy represents a major barrier to comprehensive, accurate, and clinically useful molecular testing, especially in advanced-stage cancer.[70] The role of using peripheral blood (circulating DNA, circulating tumor cells) as an easier source of biological components is rapidly evolving,[71–73] and its clinical utility needs to be validated using systematic studies correlating molecular profiling data from individual patients' matched tumor tissue versus peripheral blood. Delays can occur at multiple steps in the tumor-monitoring process including acquisition of tissue, reporting of results of molecular testing, and selection of the appropriate treatment. Standardization of the procedures involved in molecular testing is essential for the successful management of patients with cancer.[63]

## Use of Bioinformatics

Bioinformatics analysis of a patient's tumor involves global biologic components such as DNA, various RNA components, structural and functional proteins; as well as the dynamic interactions of the biological components in space and time. Skilled bioinformaticians with experience in managing complex biological data with precision in a timely manner are required. The goal of deciphering the biological complexity is to create a fundamental knowledge database of the dynamic causes of cancer in order to direct clinical management and ultimately develop preventative and curative therapies.

The rapid accumulation of data of activated pathways, as well as the cross talk and interactions between various components of the cancer intracellular machinery, has an enormous impact on clinical outcomes.[74–79] Different tumor types respond differently to targeted agents against driver molecular alterations.[80] It is therefore critical to accurately use all the available data in a clinical approach. Large-scale genomic and proteomic data should be integrated with the patient's individual clinical characteristics and they should be taken into consideration when making treatment decisions.[74]

To achieve this goal, several initiatives are under way, including MD Anderson's APOLLO[81] (Adaptive Patient-Oriented Longitudinal Learning and Optimization) and ASCO's CancerLinQ.[82,83] CancerLinQ is compiling and analyzing data from millions of electronic health records in real time; assembling the latest research, guidelines, and other expert knowledge; and updating them in real time as new evidence becomes available. CancerLinQ is designed to reduce fragmentation, inconsistency, and unnecessary costs, and to deliver personalized, clinical guidance for every patient based on the best expert evidence coupled with the analysis of many similar patient experiences. These efforts are expected to standardize the treatment of patients and to improve the quality of patient care and patient outcomes.

## Innovative Clinical Trials

The clinical development of anticancer drugs is a complex process that might require a new algorithm for designing and conducting clinical trials.[84] A high rate of failure in the late stages of development is common,[85] as various targeted agents that showed promising results in early phase clinical trials failed to demonstrate clinical improvement in phase III clinical trials.[86–91] This high failure rate is attributed to the design of the study, statistical validity, the definition of success, and lack of interest to develop drugs that would be used by small proportions of patients.[92] These facts emphasize the need for integrating biomarkers in early phase clinical trials for better selection of patients for appropriate treatment.[93] Sequential biomarker-guided molecular targeted therapies also represent an innovative strategy that needs further investigation and validation.[94] A multidisciplinary approach that includes the input of experts in molecular biology and clinical investigators from multiple oncology specialties is needed. Currently, various early phase clinical trials are prospectively integrating biomarkers in the selection of targeted agents.[95]

In addition to advances in technologies and cancer research, biomarker-guided trials require a partnership between regulatory agencies, academic institutions, pharmaceutical companies, scientific groups, and other stakeholder organizations to conduct efficient clinical research for drug development and to expedite approval of new targeted molecules.[96] For example, the European Organization for Research and Treatment of Cancer (EORTC) is evaluating a collaborative molecular screening platforms model in order to facilitate the delivery of optimal targeted therapy to matched patients with specific cancer molecular alterations, involving a partnership between various registered stakeholder institutions across Europe.[97]

## Optimal Access to Drugs

Access to targeted agents varies significantly among geographic areas, institutions, and community practices, and is largely related to health policies and programs to cover the cost of the drugs and availability of clinical trials.[46,98–101] Until 2009, the median times from filing of an investigational new drug (IND) to FDA regular and accelerated approval of the drug were 7.3 and 7.2 years, respectively.[102] Access to investigational or FDA-approved drugs is available via (i) clinical trials, (ii) compassionate use (providers contact the drug company and submit an application to the FDA), and (iii) expanded access studies (offered to patients who do not qualify for the clinical trials). Despite these regulations, access to investigational cancer drugs is limited, and only a small proportion of patients have the privilege to receive new drugs. A more efficient strategy needs to be implemented to shorten the process of drug development without compromising patient safety, and to facilitate access of patients to drugs with documented promising antitumor activity outside the academic setting.

Efforts should be directed toward partnership and collaboration between various stakeholder organizations and clinical settings to facilitate the delivery of matched molecular targeted agents in both community and academic clinical practices. For example, some experts have suggested a national access program and registry that allows off-label use of approved molecular targeted agents in

patients without available treatment options whose tumor genome profiling has been performed and validated in a CLIA-certified laboratory.[63]

## Drug Development Regulations

Drug development includes several steps[103] including preclinical studies filing for an IND, collaborations between clinical investigators with pharmaceutical companies and clinical research organizations, with guidance of the FDA through all steps of drug development.[104] In recent years, pharmaceutical research and development has increased substantially.[105] The existing process is associated with prolonged time to approval and is expensive.[102,106,107] Factors that contribute to the high price[107] include the capacity of the market, presence of various components involved in the development process, and the price of marketing. Other factors not related to drug development *per se* include the inability of Medicare to negotiate lower prices and the strategy of paying to delay the introduction of competing generic drugs.[107] Some investigators have proposed that changes should be implemented to decrease the cost of these drugs,[107] including allowing Medicare to negotiate the price with pharmaceutical companies and revising the guidelines to decrease the cost of research procedures.[107] Furthermore, improving the implementation of existing regulations, such as the accelerated approval process, as well as developing new regulations to expedite drug development and to shorten the timeline from IND filing to NDA registration, will have a great impact on the access to newer drugs.[102] Other regulations might be needed to facilitate access to targeted therapies and decrease the timeline for approval.[63,84,102,107]

Although pharmaceutical companies sponsor programs to help patients get access to cancer drugs, these programs are available to only a small proportion of patients. The economic analysis of cancer treatment will require collaborative efforts to assess and accumulate accurate data about the relative effectiveness of treatments in the community, outside the clinical trial environment. Future efforts should be directed toward development of cancer policy, defining economic determinants such as social and cultural values, participation of cancer advocacy groups, and mobilizing political influence to wisely direct cancer research and expenditures.

## Economic Considerations

The high cost of cancer care can be attributed to direct (e.g., therapeutic interventions) and indirect (e.g., associated with complications and morbidity of both cancer and therapy) expenses. The cancer expenditure in the United States alone is estimated to reach $158 billion by 2020 compared to $124 billion in 2010.[108] The US population changes and the increased number of cancer survivors represent approximately 27% of the cost increase.[108] Innovation of technologies, expensive therapeutic modalities, and increases in other medical services contribute to increased cost.[109]

The fundamentals of health economics are based on two established concepts: cost-minimization and cost-effectiveness.[110] Cost-minimization implies the choice of the therapeutic approach with the lowest cost, when equal clinical effectiveness is shown. Cost-effectiveness implies the choice of a specific intervention among others when clinical effectiveness varies; life gain per cost spent is considered and the goal is to identify the greatest clinical effectiveness with the lowest cost. Safety and efficacy should always be the main focus and drivers for any therapeutic choice; however, cost should be considered in such an expensive health-care system,[111] especially when multiple options are available. The most practical approach to determine the cost/benefit of any therapeutic approach is to include an economic analysis in randomized clinical trials.[112,113]

The financial impact of cancer treatment is critical for patients.[114] In a survey, 15% of patients had a discussion with their oncologist about the cost of their treatment and the out-of-pocket expenses, while 63% of patients wish to discuss these expenses.[115] A wide variety of barriers exist, including discomfort for both physicians and patients, insufficient time, the belief that no viable solution is available, and concerns about the impact of such discussions on quality of care.[116] Clinical research should be directed to identify efficient communication methods to discuss the cost of care with patients. Various models have been proposed based on communication skills, expressing empathy which builds trust and aids disclosure, and understanding and acceptance of the patient's feelings, values, and ideas.[116,117]

## Value of Cancer Care

The outcome of cancer care is better assessed in the clinical trial setting, and the clinically significant outcome is critical and vital for therapeutic guidelines. However, the evaluation of outcome is complicated because it depends on the clinical effectiveness of various therapeutic models, safety versus toxicity, patient preference, and the cost/benefit ratio. The term minimum clinically meaningful outcome (mCMO) was recently introduced to assess the value of any cancer therapeutic model introduced into practice.[118] The mCMO value not only takes into consideration the survival benefit of any therapeutic intervention, but also assesses the survival benefit in light of harm and costs.[118]

In a recent study[118] in which the mCMO value was applied to 43 completed phase III clinical trials using different drugs approved by the FDA, only two studies met the high-benefit criteria of mCMO, and none met the large-benefit criteria in absolute and proportional survival at 2–3 years. In a recent evaluation, an ASCO working group emphasized the role and importance of clinically meaningful outcome for patients, including survival, quality of life, or both.[119] In addition to the importance of biomarker-driven trials to prospectively determine a subpopulation with significant clinical benefit, the working group also emphasized the role of defining and raising the bar of the clinical outcomes in phase III clinical trials.[119]

In summary, large collaborative efforts and changes in existing regulations are needed in order to achieve significant clinical health value (related to goals of patient care), which should be patient-centric in the context of cost-effectiveness.[120]

## Centralized Big Data

The exponential development of innovative technology provides unlimited opportunities to evaluate the effects of global sets of biological molecules including DNAs, RNAs, proteins, and metabolites on the therapeutic management of patients with cancer[121–124]; and sharing these data between basic scientists and clinical investigators will solidify understanding of tumor biology and inform treatment. The wealth of collected data, coupled with the rapid improvement in computational analysis and bioinformatics, has created an enormous amount of data, known as big data,[123] with complex aspects for scientists and policy makers.[124]

Maximizing the use of existing data with minimal cost, and avoiding duplicate efforts while maintaining confidentiality, is vital. Data sharing is emerging with various clinical research projects, including the human genome project[125] and The Cancer Genome Atlas (TCGA).[126] This model increases the statistical power of research questions and consequently accelerates the implementation of discoveries and translational research in medical practice.[127,128]

Given the critical importance of data sharing, international collective efforts have been initiated.[129–131] Some experts argue that a model involving a certified third party can be successful in balancing privacy and the need for data sharing.[124] The power of computational medicine and data sharing is stimulating investigators to develop promising projects that involve the implementation of both bioinformatics and big data. In this scenario, all specific data for a patient with cancer (DNA, RNA, proteins, -omics, clinical, etc.) will be collected and analyzed in real time via computer with a superfast network in the context of previously established big data; this process will expedite the selection of appropriate therapy.

In conclusion, breakthroughs in technology to optimally characterize the biology and pathophysiology of an individual patient's cancer, along with the discovery of effective drugs, have provided an epic opportunity in the war against cancer. The use of these discoveries has led to exponential success in the diagnosis and therapeutic management of patients with specific tumor types. The implementation of exponential advances in technology related to tumor biology and big data analyses is allowing for the selection and development of effective therapeutic strategies, carefully designed clinical trials, and collaborative efforts among key stakeholders in cancer therapy, and ultimately holds the promise of curing cancer.

## References

1 Garraway L, Verweij J, Ballman KV. Precision oncology: an overview. *J Clin Oncol*. 2013;31(15):1803–1805. doi:10.1200/JCO.2013.49.4799.

2 Baselga J. Bringing precision medicine to the clinic: from genomic profiling to the power of clinical observation. *Ann Oncol*. 2013;24(8):1956–1957. doi:10.1093/annonc/mdt273.

3 Tsimberidou AM, Iskander NG, Hong DS, et al. Personalized medicine in a phase I clinical trials program. the MD Anderson Cancer Center initiative. *Clin Cancer Res*. 2012;18(22):6373–6383. doi:10.1158/1078-0432.CCR-12-1627.

4 Von Hoff DD, Stephenson JJ, Jr, Rosen P, et al. Pilot study using molecular profiling of patients' tumors to find potential targets and select treatments for their refractory cancers. *J Clin Oncol*. 2010;28(33):4877–4883. doi:10.1200/JCO.2009.26.5983.

5 Vanneman M, Dranoff G. Combining immunotherapy and targeted therapies in cancer treatment. *Nat Rev Cancer*. 2012;12(4):237–251. doi:10.1038/nrc3237.

6 Lander ES, Linton LM, Birren B, et al. Initial sequencing and analysis of the human genome. *Nature*. 2001;409(6822):860–921. doi:10.1038/35057062.

7 Garraway LA, Lander ES. Lessons from the cancer genome. *Cell*. 2013;153(1):17–37. doi:10.1016/j.cell.2013.03.002.

8 Chapman PB, Hauschild A, Robert C, et al. Improved survival with vemurafenib in melanoma with BRAF V600E mutation. *N Eng J Med*. 2011;364(26):2507–2516. doi:10.1056/NEJMoa1103782.

9 Shaw AT, Kim DW, Nakagawa K, et al. Crizotinib versus chemotherapy in advanced ALK-positive lung cancer. *N Eng J Med*. 2013;368(25):2385–2394. doi:10.1056/NEJMoa1214886.

10 Shepherd FA, Rodrigues Pereira J, Ciuleanu T, et al. Erlotinib in previously treated non-small-cell lung cancer. *N Eng J Med*. 2005;353(2):123–132. doi:10.1056/NEJMoa050753.

11 Druker BJ, Talpaz M, Resta DJ, et al. Efficacy and safety of a specific inhibitor of the BCR-ABL tyrosine kinase in chronic myeloid leukemia. *N Eng J Med*. 2001;344(14):1031–1037. doi:10.1056/NEJM200104053441401.

12 Demetri GD, von Mehren M, Blanke CD, et al. Efficacy and safety of imatinib mesylate in advanced gastrointestinal stromal tumors. *N Eng J Med*. 2002;347(7):472–480. doi:10.1056/NEJMoa020461.

13 Bjorkholm M, Ohm L, Eloranta S, et al. Success story of targeted therapy in chronic myeloid leukemia: a population-based study of patients diagnosed in Sweden from 1973 to 2008. *J Clin Oncol*. 2011;29(18):2514–2520. doi:10.1200/JCO.2011.34.7146.

14 Kantarjian H, Shah NP, Hochhaus A, et al. Dasatinib versus imatinib in newly diagnosed chronic-phase chronic myeloid leukemia. *N Eng J Med*. 2010;362(24):2260–2270. doi:10.1056/NEJMoa1002315.

15 Wang E. Understanding genomic alterations in cancer genomes using an integrative network approach. *Cancer Lett*. 2013;340(2):261–269. doi:10.1016/j.canlet.2012.11.050.

16 Albertson DG, Collins C, McCormick F, Gray JW. Chromosome aberrations in solid tumors. *Nat Genet*. 2003;34(4):369–376. doi:10.1038/ng1215.

17 Biankin AV, Waddell N, Kassahn KS, et al. Pancreatic cancer genomes reveal aberrations in axon guidance pathway genes. *Nature*. 2012;491(7424):399–405. doi:10.1038/nature11547.

18 Wang G, Huang CH, Zhao Y, et al. Genetic aberration in primary hepatocellular carcinoma: correlation between p53 gene mutation and loss-of-heterozygosity on chromosome 16q21-q23 and 9p21-p23. *Cell Res*. 2000;10(4):311–323. doi:10.1038/sj.cr.7290058.

19 Kim TM, Xi R, Luquette LJ, Park RW, Johnson MD, Park PJ. Functional genomic analysis of chromosomal aberrations in a compendium of 8000 cancer genomes. *Genome Res*. 2013;23(2):217–227. doi:10.1101/gr.140301.112.

20 Heinrich MC, Owzar K, Corless CL, et al. Correlation of kinase genotype and clinical outcome in the North American Intergroup Phase III Trial of imatinib mesylate for treatment of advanced gastrointestinal stromal tumor: CALGB 150105 Study by Cancer and Leukemia Group B and Southwest Oncology Group. *J Clin Oncol*. 2008;26(33):5360–5367. doi:10.1200/JCO.2008.17.4284.

21 Poulikakos PI, Persaud Y, Janakiraman M, et al. RAF inhibitor resistance is mediated by dimerization of aberrantly spliced BRAF(V600E). *Nature*. 2011;480(7377):387–390. doi:10.1038/nature10662.

22 Yauch RL, Dijkgraaf GJ, Alicke B, et al. Smoothened mutation confers resistance to a Hedgehog pathway inhibitor in medulloblastoma. *Science*. 2009;326(5952):572–574. doi:10.1126/science.1179386.

23 Pao W, Miller VA, Politi KA, et al. Acquired resistance of lung adenocarcinomas to gefitinib or erlotinib is associated with a second mutation in the EGFR kinase domain. *PLoS Med*. 2005;2(3):e73, doi:10.1371/journal.pmed.0020073.

24 Eichhorn PJ, Gili M, Scaltriti M, et al. Phosphatidylinositol 3-kinase hyperactivation results in lapatinib resistance that is reversed by the mTOR/phosphatidylinositol 3-kinase inhibitor NVP-BEZ235. *Cancer Res*. 2008;68(22):9221–9230. doi:10.1158/0008-5472.CAN-08-1740.

25 Nazarian R, Shi H, Wang Q, et al. Melanomas acquire resistance to B-RAF(V600E) inhibition by RTK or N-RAS upregulation. *Nature*. 2010;468(7326):973–977. doi:10.1038/nature09626.

26 Prahallad A, Sun C, Huang S, et al. Unresponsiveness of colon cancer to BRAF(V600E) inhibition through feedback activation of EGFR. *Nature*. 2012;483(7387):100–103. doi:10.1038/nature10868.

27 Stommel JM, Kimmelman AC, Ying H, et al. Coactivation of receptor tyrosine kinases affects the response of tumor cells to targeted therapies. *Science*. 2007;318(5848):287–290. doi:10.1126/science.1142946.

28 Villanueva J, Vultur A, Lee JT, et al. Acquired resistance to BRAF inhibitors mediated by a RAF kinase switch in melanoma can be overcome by cotargeting MEK and IGF-1R/PI3K. *Cancer Cell*. 2010;18(6):683–695. doi:10.1016/j.ccr.2010.11.023.

29 Wee S, Jaqani Z, Xiang KX, et al. PI3K pathway activation mediates resistance to MEK inhibitors in KRAS mutant cancers. *Cancer Res*. 2009;69(10):4286–4293. doi:10.1158/0008-5472.CAN-08-4765.

30 Yu K, Toral-Barza L, Shi C, Zhang WG, Zask A. Response and determinants of cancer cell susceptibility to PI3K inhibitors: combined targeting of PI3K and Mek1 as an effective anticancer strategy. *Cancer Biol Ther*. 2008;7(2):307–315.

31 Disis ML, Wallace DR, Gooley TA, et al. Concurrent trastuzumab and HER2/neu-specific vaccination in patients with metastatic breast cancer. *J Clin Oncol*. 2009;27(28):4685–4692. doi:10.1200/JCO.2008.20.6789.

32 Boni A, Coqdill AP, Dang P, et al. Selective BRAFV600E inhibition enhances T-cell recognition of melanoma without affecting lymphocyte function. *Cancer Res*. 2010;70(13):5213–5219. doi:10.1158/0008-5472.CAN-10-0118.

33 McNeel DG, Smith HA, Eickhoff JC, et al. Phase I trial of tremelimumab in combination with short-term androgen deprivation in patients with PSA-recurrent prostate cancer. *Cancer Immunol immunother* 2012;61(7):1137–1147. doi:10.1007/s00262-011-1193-1.

34 Jaffee EM, Hruban RH, Biedrzycki B, et al. Novel allogeneic granulocyte-macrophage colony-stimulating factor-secreting tumor vaccine for pancreatic cancer: a phase I trial of safety and immune activation. *J Clin Oncol*. 2001;19(1):145–156.

35 Nebert DW, Jorge-Nebert L, Vesell ES. Pharmacogenomics and "individualized drug therapy": high expectations and disappointing achievements. *Am J pharmacogenomics*. 2003;3(6):361–370.

36 Wang L, McLeod HL, Weinshilboum RM. Genomics and drug response. *N Eng J Med*. 2011;364(12):1144–1153. doi:10.1056/NEJMra1010600.

37 Ganapathi RN, Ganapathi MK. Pharmacogenomics: New paradigms for targeted therapy based on individual response to drugs. *Urol Oncol*. 2014;32(1):1–4. doi:10.1016/j.urolonc.2013.08.027.

38 Longley DB, Allen WL, Johnston PG. Drug resistance, predictive markers and pharmacogenomics in colorectal cancer. *Biochim Biophys Acta*. 2006;1766(2):184–196. doi:10.1016/j.bbcan.2006.08.001.

39 Zheng Y, Zhou J, Tong Y. Gene signatures of drug resistance predict patient survival in colorectal cancer. *Pharmacogenomics J*. 2014. doi:10.1038/tpj.2014.45.

40 Monte AA, Heard KJ, Vasiliou V. Prediction of drug response and safety in clinical practice. *J Med Toxicol*. 2012;8(1):43–51. doi:10.1007/s13181-011-0198-7.

41 Crews KR, Hicks JK, Pui CH, Relling MV, Evans WE. Pharmacogenomics and individualized medicine: translating science into practice. *Clin Pharmacol Therapeut*. 2012;92(4):467–475. doi:10.1038/clpt.2012.120.

42 O'Donnell PH, Dolan ME. Cancer pharmacoethnicity: ethnic differences in susceptibility to the effects of chemotherapy. *Clin Cancer Res*. 2009;15(15):4806–4814. doi:10.1158/1078-0432.CCR-09-0344.

43 Micheel CM, Nass sj, Omenn GS. Evolution of Translational Omics: Lessons Learned and the Path Forward (2012). ISBN: 978-0-309-22418-5.

44 MacConaill LE. Existing and emerging technologies for tumor genomic profiling. *J Clin Oncol*. 2013;31(15):1815–1824 doi:10.1200/JCO.2012.46.5948.

45 Meric-Bernstam F, Farhangfar C, Mendelsohn J, Mills GB. Building a personalized medicine infrastructure at a major cancer

center. *J Clin Oncol.* 2013;31(15):1849–1857. doi:10.1200/JCO.2012.45.3043.

46 Van Allen EM, Wagle N, Levy MA. Clinical analysis and interpretation of cancer genome data. *J Clin Oncol.* 2013;31(15):1825–1833. doi:10.1200/JCO.2013.48.7215.

47 Bast RC Jr, Mills GB. Dissecting "PI3Kness": the complexity of personalized therapy for ovarian cancer. *Cancer Discov.* 2012;2(1):16–18. doi:10.1158/2159-8290.CD-11-0323.

48 Knox SS. From 'omics' to complex disease: a systems biology approach to gene-environment interactions in cancer. *Cancer Cell Int.* 2010;10(11):11. doi:10.1186/1475-2867-10-11.

49 Shen H, Laird PW. Interplay between the cancer genome and epigenome. *Cell.* 2013;153(1):38–55. doi:10.1016/j.cell.2013.03.008.

50 Feil R, Fraga MF. Epigenetics and the environment: emerging patterns and implications. *Nat Rev Genet.* 2012;13(2):97–109. doi:10.1038/nrg3142.

51 Herceg Z. Epigenetics and cancer: towards an evaluation of the impact of environmental and dietary factors. *Mutagenesis.* 2007;22(2):91–103. doi:10.1093/mutage/gel068.

52 Vandin F, Upfal E, Raphael BJ. Finding driver pathways in cancer: models and algorithms. *Algorithms Mol Biol.* 2012;7(1):23. doi:10.1186/1748-7188-7-23.

53 Calvano SE, Xiao W, Richards DR, et al. A network-based analysis of systemic inflammation in humans. *Nature.* 2005;437(7061):1032–1037. doi:10.1038/nature03985.

54 Brown KR, Jurisica I. Unequal evolutionary conservation of human protein interactions in interologous networks. *Gen Biol.* 2007;8(5):R95. doi:10.1186/gb-2007-8-5-r95.

55 Kanehisa M, Goto S, Kawashima S, Nakaya A. The KEGG databases at GenomeNet. *Nucleic Acids Res.* 2002;30(1):42–46.

56 Cerami EG, Bader GD, Gross BE, Sander C. cPath: open source software for collecting, storing, and querying biological pathways. *BMC Bioinformatics.* 2006;7:497. doi:10.1186/1471-2105-7-497.

57 Vastrik I, D'Eustachio P, Schmidt E, et al. Reactome: a knowledge base of biologic pathways and processes. *Gen Biol.* 2007;8(3):R39. doi:10.1186/gb-2007-8-3-r39.

58 Subramanian A, Tamayo P, Mootha VK, et al. Gene set enrichment analysis: a knowledge-based approach for interpreting genome-wide expression profiles. *Proc Natl Acad Sci U S A.* 2005;102(43):15545–15550. doi:10.1073/pnas.0506580102.

59 Solvang HK, Lingjaerde OC, Frigessi A, Borresen-Dale AL, Kristensen VN. Linear and non-linear dependencies between copy number aberrations and mRNA expression reveal distinct molecular pathways in breast cancer. *BMC Bioinformatics.* 2011;12:197. doi:10.1186/1471-2105-12-197.

60 Glaab E, Baudot A, Krasnogor N, Valencia A. Extending pathways and processes using molecular interaction networks to analyse cancer genome data. *BMC Bioinformatics.* 2010;11:597. doi:10.1186/1471-2105-11-597.

61 Burd EM. Validation of laboratory-developed molecular assays for infectious diseases. *Clin Microbiol Rev.* 2010;23(3):550–576. doi:10.1128/CMR.00074-09.

62 Teutsch SM, Bradley LA, Palomaki GE, et al. The Evaluation of Genomic Applications in Practice and Prevention (EGAPP) Initiative: methods of the EGAPP Working Group. *Genet Med.* 2009;11(1):3–14. doi:10.1097/GIM.0b013e318184137c.

63 Schilsky RL. Implementing personalized cancer care. *Nat Rev Clin Oncol.* 2014;11(7):432–438. doi:10.1038/nrclinonc.2014.54.

64 Hammond ME, Hayes DF, Dowsett M, et al. American Society of Clinical Oncology/College Of American Pathologists guideline recommendations for immunohistochemical testing of estrogen and proges-

terone receptors in breast cancer. *J Clin Oncol.* 2010;28(16):2784–2795. doi:10.1200/JCO.2009.25.6529.

65 Wolff AC, Hammond ME, Hicks DG, et al. Recommendations for human epidermal growth factor receptor 2 testing in breast cancer: American Society of Clinical Oncology/College of American Pathologists clinical practice guideline update. *J Clin Oncol.* 2013;31(31):3997–4013. doi:10.1200/JCO.2013.50.9984.

66 Lindeman NI, Cagle PT, Beasley MB, et al. Molecular testing guideline for selection of lung cancer patients for EGFR and ALK tyrosine kinase inhibitors: guideline from the College of American Pathologists, International Association for the Study of Lung Cancer, and Association for Molecular Pathology. *J Thorac Oncol.* 2013;8(7):823–859. doi:10.1097/JTO.0b013e318290868f.

67 McShane LM, Cavenagh MM, Lively TG, et al. Criteria for the use of omics-based predictors in clinical trials. *Nature.* 2013;502(7471):317–320. doi:10.1038/nature12564.

68 Gerlinger M, Rowan AJ, Horswell S, et al. Intratumor heterogeneity and branched evolution revealed by multiregion sequencing. *N Eng J Med.* 2012;366(10):883–892. doi:10.1056/NEJMoa1113205.

69 Almendro V, Marusyk A, Polyak K. Cellular heterogeneity and molecular evolution in cancer. *Ann Rev Pathol.* 2013;8:277–302. doi:10.1146/annurev-pathol-020712-163923.

70 Tam AL, Kim ES, Lee JJ, et al. Feasibility of image-guided transthoracic core-needle biopsy in the BATTLE lung trial. *J Thorac Oncol.* 2013;8(4):436–442. doi:10.1097/JTO.0b013e318287c91e.

71 Plaks V, Koopman CD, Werb Z. Cancer. Circulating tumor cells. *Science.* 2013;341(6151):1186–1188. doi:10.1126/science.1235226.

72 Newman AM, Bratman SV, To J, et al. An ultrasensitive method for quantitating circulating tumor DNA with broad patient coverage. *Nat Med.* 2014;20(5):548–554. doi:10.1038/nm.3519.

73 Bettegowda C, Sausen M, Leary RJ, et al. Detection of circulating tumor DNA in early- and late-stage human malignancies. *Sci Transl Med.* 2014;6(224):224ra24, doi:10.1126/scitranslmed.3007094.

74 Wu D, Rice CM, Wang X. Cancer bioinformatics: a new approach to systems clinical medicine. *BMC Bioinformatics.* 2012;13:71. doi:10.1186/1471-2105-13-71.

75 Wang X, Liotta L. Clinical bioinformatics: a new emerging science. *J Clin Bioinformatics.* 2011;1(1):1. doi:10.1186/2043-9113-1-1.

76 Holford ME, McCusker, JP, Cheung KH, Krauthammer MA. A semantic web framework to integrate cancer omics data with biological knowledge. *BMC bioinformatics.* 2012;13(suppl 1):S10, doi:10.1186/1471-2105-13-S1-S10.

77 Ebbert MT, Bastien RR, Boucher KM, et al. Characterization of uncertainty in the classification of multivariate assays: application to PAM50 centroid-based genomic predictors for breast cancer treatment plans. *J Clin Bioinforma.* 2011;1:37. doi:10.1186/2043-9113-1-37.

78 Haustein V, Schumacher U. A dynamic model for tumour growth and metastasis formation. *J Clin Bioinforma.* 2012;2(1):11. doi:10.1186/2043-9113-2-11.

79 Wang X. Role of clinical bioinformatics in the development of network-based Biomarkers. *J Clin Bioinformatics.* 2011;1(1):28. doi:10.1186/2043-9113-1-28.

80 Lito P, Rosen N, Solit DB. Tumor adaptation and resistance to RAF inhibitors. *Nat Med.* 2013;19(11):1401–1409. doi:10.1038/nm.3392.

81 http://www.mdanderson.org/newsroom/news-releases/2013/ibm-watson-to-power-moon-shots-.html. Accessed on 2013.

82 Kolacevski A, Mann JT, Hauser R, Schilsky RL. Using big data to track trends in medical practice. *J Oncol Pract 2014;.* doi:10.1200/JOP.2014.001541.

83 Schilsky RL, Michels DL, Kearbey AH, Yu, PP, Hudis, CA. Building a rapid learning health care system for oncology: the regulatory

framework of CancerLinQ. *J Clin Oncol.* 2014;32(22):2373–2379. doi:10.1200/JCO.2014.56.2124.

84  Doroshow JH, Sleijfer S, Stupp R, Anderson K. Cancer clinical trials–do we need a new algorithm in the age of stratified medicine? *Oncol.* 2013;18(6):651–652. doi:10.1634/theoncologist.2013-0190.

85  Wehling M. Drug development in the light of translational science: shine or shade? *Drug Discov Today.* 2011;16(23–24):1076–1083. doi:10.1016/j.drudis.2011.07.008.

86  Van Cutsem E, Bajetta E, Valle J, et al. Randomized, placebo-controlled, phase III study of oxaliplatin, fluorouracil, and leucovorin with or without PTK787/ZK 222584 in patients with previously treated metastatic colorectal adenocarcinoma. *J Clin Oncol.* 2011;29(15):2004–2010. doi:10.1200/JCO.2010.29.5436.

87  Hecht JR, Trarbach T, Hainsworth JD, et al. Randomized, placebo-controlled, phase III study of first-line oxaliplatin-based chemotherapy plus PTK787/ZK 222584, an oral vascular endothelial growth factor receptor inhibitor, in patients with metastatic colorectal adenocarcinoma. *J Clin Oncol.* 2011;29(15):1997–2003. doi:10.1200/JCO.2010.29.4496.

88  Thatcher N, Chang A, Parikh P, et al. Gefitinib plus best supportive care in previously treated patients with refractory advanced non-small-cell lung cancer: results from a randomised, placebo-controlled, multicentre study (Iressa Survival Evaluation in Lung Cancer). *Lancet.* 2005;366(9496):1527–1537. doi:10.1016/S0140-6736(05)67625-8.

89  Van Cutsem E, van de Valde H, Karasek P, et al. Phase III trial of gemcitabine plus tipifarnib compared with gemcitabine plus placebo in advanced pancreatic cancer. *J Clin Oncol.* 2004;22(8):1430–1438. doi:10.1200/JCO.2004.10.112.

90  Bergh J, Bondarenko IM, Lichinitser MR, et al. First-line treatment of advanced breast cancer with sunitinib in combination with docetaxel versus docetaxel alone: results of a prospective, randomized phase III study. *J Clin Oncol.* 2012;30(9):921–929. doi:10.1200/JCO.2011.35.7376.

91  Crown JP, Dieras V, Staroslawska E, et al. Phase III trial of sunitinib in combination with capecitabine versus capecitabine monotherapy for the treatment of patients with pretreated metastatic breast cancer. *J Clin Oncol.* 2013;31(23):2870–2878. doi:10.1200/JCO.2012.43.3391.

92  Amiri-Kordestani L, Fojo T. Why do phase III clinical trials in oncology fail so often? *J Natl Cancer Inst.* 2012;104(8):568–569. doi:10.1093/jnci/djs180.

93  Freidlin B, McShane LM, Korn EL. Randomized clinical trials with biomarkers: design issues. *J Natl Cancer Inst.* 2010;102(3):152–160. doi:10.1093/jnci/djp477.

94  Sahin O, Wang Q, Brady SW, et al. Biomarker-guided sequential targeted therapies to overcome therapy resistance in rapidly evolving highly aggressive mammary tumors. *Cell Res.* 2014;24(5):542–559. doi:10.1038/cr.2014.37.

95  www.clinicaltrials.gov. (NCT02152254, NCT01827384, NCT01771458, NCT01248247, NCT01042379, NCT02117167). Last accessed on 2015.

96  Burock S, Meunier F, Lacombe D. How can innovative forms of clinical research contribute to deliver affordable cancer care in an evolving health care environment? *Eur J Cancer.* 2013;49(13):2777–2783. doi:10.1016/j.ejca.2013.05.016.

97  Lacombe D, Teipar S, Salgado R, et al. European perspective for effective cancer drug development. *Nat Rev Clin Oncol.* 2014;11(8):492–498. doi:10.1038/nrclinonc.2014.98.

98  ESMO. Market access for cancer drugs and the role of health economics. *Ann Oncol.* 2007;18 (suppl 3): iii55–iii66.

99  Chafe R, Culyer A, Dobrow M, et al. Access to cancer drugs in Canada: looking beyond coverage decisions. *Healthc Policy.* 2011;6(3):27–36.

100  Bengt Jönsson NW. New cancer drugs in Sweden: Assessment, implementation and access. *J Cancer Policy.* 2014;2.

101  Lopes Gde L Jr, de Souza JA, Barrios C. Access to cancer medications in low- and middle-income countries. *Nat Rev Clin Oncol.* 2013;10(6):314–322. doi:10.1038/nrclinonc.2013.55.

102  Richey EA, Lyons EA, Nebeker JR, et al. Accelerated approval of cancer drugs: improved access to therapeutic breakthroughs or early release of unsafe and ineffective drugs? *J Clin Oncol.* 2009;27(26):4398–4405. doi:10.1200/JCO.2008.21.1961.

103  Lanthier ML, Sridhara R, Johnson JR, et al. Accelerated approval and oncology drug development timelines. *J Clin Oncol.* 2010;28(14):e226–e227. author reply e228, doi:10.1200/JCO.2009.26.2121.

104  Keng MK, Wenzell CM, Sekeres MA. A drug's life: the pathway to drug approval. *Clin Adv Hematol Oncol.* 2013;11(10):646–655.

105  DiMasi JA, Hansen RW, Grabowski HG. The price of innovation: new estimates of drug development costs. *J Health Econ.* 2003;22(2):151–185. doi:10.1016/S0167-6296(02)00126-1.

106  Pfister DG. The just price of cancer drugs and the growing cost of cancer care: oncologists need to be part of the solution. *J Clin Oncol.* 2013;31(28):3487–3489. doi:10.1200/JCO.2013.50.3466.

107  Kantarjian HM, Fojo T, Mathisen M, Zwelling LA. Cancer drugs in the United States: Justum Pretium–the just price. *J Clin Oncol.* 2013;31(28):3600–3604. doi:10.1200/JCO.2013.49.1845.

108  Mariotto AB, Yabroff KR, Shao Y, Feuer EJ, Brown ML. Projections of the cost of cancer care in the United States: 2010–2020. *J Natl Cancer Inst.* 2011;103(2):117–128. doi:10.1093/jnci/djq495.

109  Aggrawal AG, Fojo T. Cancer economics, policy and politics: What informs the debate? Perspectives from the EU, Canada and US. *J Cancer Policy.* 2014;2:1–11.

110  Lyman GH. Understanding economic analyses. *Evid Based Oncol.* 2001;2:2–5.

111  Lyman GH. Economics of cancer care. *J Oncol Pract.* 2007;3:113–114. doi:10.1200/JOP.0731501.

112  Lyman GH. *Methodological issues related to health economic analysis in controlled clinical trials.* In: Crowley J, ed. Handbook of Statistics in Clinical Oncology. Marcel Dekker; 2001;291–320.

113  Lyman GH. Economic analysis of randomized, controlled trials. *Curr Oncol Rep.* 2001;3:396–403.

114  AD M. Price becomes factor in cancer treatment. *Wall Street J.* 2004;97:D1–D7.

115  Alexander GC, Casalino LP, Meltzer DO. Patient-physician communication about out-of-pocket costs. *JAMA.* 2003;290(7):953–958. doi:10.1001/jama.290.7.953.

116  Alexander GC, Casalino LP, Tseng CW, McFadden D, Meltzer, DO. Barriers to patient-physician communication about out-of-pocket costs. *J Gen Intern Med.* 2004;19(8):856–860. doi:10.1111/j.1525-1497.2004.30249.x.

117  Hardee JT, Platt FW, Kasper IK. Discussing health care costs with patients: an opportunity for empathic communication. *J Gen Intern Med.* 2005;20(7):666–669. doi:10.1111/j.1525-1497.2005.0125.x.

118  Sobrero AF, Pastorino A, Sargent DJ. Bruzzi P. Raising the bar for antineoplastic agents: how to choose threshold values for superiority trials in advanced solid tumors. *Clin Cancer Res.*2015;21(5):1036–1043. doi:10.1158/1078-0432.CCR-14-1505.

119  Ellis LM, Bernstein DS, Voest EE, et al. American Society of Clinical Oncology perspective: Raising the bar for clinical trials by defining clinically meaningful outcomes. *J Clin Oncol.* 2014;32(12):1277–1280. doi:10.1200/JCO.2013.53.8009.

120  Porter ME. What is value in health care? *N Eng J Med.* 2010;363(26):2477–2481. doi:10.1056/NEJMp1011024.

121 Costa FF. Social networks, web-based tools and diseases: implications for biomedical research. *Drug Discov Today*. 2013;18(5—6):272–281. doi:10.1016/j.drudis.2012.10.006.

122 Knoppers BM, Zawati MH, Kirby ES. Sampling populations of humans across the world: ELSI issues. *Ann Rev Genom Hum Genet*. 2012;13:395–413, doi:10.1146/annurev-genom-090711–163834.

123 Costa FF. Big data in biomedicine. *Drug Discov Today*. 2014;19(4):433–440. doi:10.1016/j.drudis.2013.10.012.

124 Kosseim P, Dove ES, Bagaley C, et al. Building a data sharing model for global genomic research. *Genome Biol*. 2014;15(8):430. doi:10.1186/s13059-014-0430-2.

125 Mello MM, Francer JK, Wilenzick M, Teden P, Bierer BE, Barnes M. Preparing for responsible sharing of clinical trial data. *N Eng J Med*. 2013;369(17):1651–1658. doi:10.1056/NEJMhle1309073.

126 Ledford H. End of cancer-genome project prompts rethink. *Nature*. 2015;517(7533):128–129, doi:10.1038/517128a.

127 Kaye J, Heeney C, Hawkins N, de Vries J, Boddington P. Data sharing in genomics–re-shaping scientific practice. *Nat Rev Genet*. 2009;10(5):331–335. doi:10.1038/nrg2573.

128 Knoppers BM, Harris JR, Tasse AM, et al. Towards a data sharing Code of Conduct for international genomic research. *Genome Med*. 2011;3(7):46. doi:10.1186/gm262.

129 Dove ES, Knoppers BM, Zawati MH. An ethics safe harbor for international genomics research? *Genome Med*. 2013;5(11):99, doi:10.1186/gm503.

130 Colledge F, Elger B, Howard HC. A review of the barriers to sharing in biobanking. *Biopreserv Biobank*. 2013;11(6):339–346. doi:10.1089/bio.2013.0039.

131 Kaye J. The tension between data sharing and the protection of privacy in genomics research. *Ann Rev Genom Hum Genet*. 2012;13:415–431, doi:10.1146/annurev-genom-082410-101454.

# Index

---